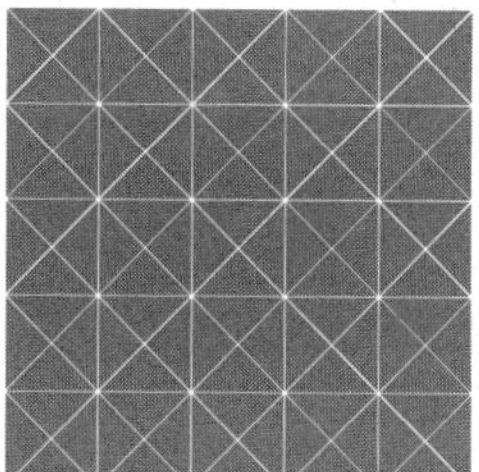

Keane's Essentials of Medical-Surgical Nursing

Keane's Essentials of Medical-Surgical Nursing

Susan C. deWit, MSN, RNCS
Instructor of Nursing
El Centro College
Dallas, Texas

Third Edition

W.B. SAUNDERS COMPANY
A Division of Harcourt Brace & Company

Philadelphia London Toronto Montreal Sydney Tokyo

W. B. Saunders Company
A Division of
Harcourt Brace & Company
The Curtis Center
Independence Square West
Philadelphia, Pennsylvania 19106

Library of Congress Cataloging-in-Publication Data

deWit, Susan C.

Keane's essentials of medical-surgical nursing.—3rd. ed. / Susan C. deWit.
p. cm.
Rev. ed. of: Essentials of medical-surgical nursing / Claire Brackman Keane. 2nd ed. 1986.
Includes bibliographical references and index.

ISBN 0-7216-3451-6

1. Nursing. 2. Surgical nursing. I. Keane, Claire Brackman. Essentials of medical-surgical nursing. II. Title. III. Title: Essentials of medical-surgical nursing.
[DNLM: 1. Nursing. 2. Surgical Nursing. WY 150 D521k]
RT41.D44 1992
610.73--dc20
DNLM/DLC 91-25733

Editor: Ilze Rader
Developmental Editor: Martha Tanner
Designer: Bill Donnelly
Cover Designer: Kevin Curry
Production Manager: Linda R. Garber
Manuscript Editors: Kendall Sterling, David Harvey
Illustration Specialist: Brett MacNaughton
Indexer: Linda Van Pelt

Keane's Essentials of Medical-Surgical Nursing, 3rd edition ISBN 0-7216-3451-6

Printed in the United States of America

Last digit is the print number: 9 8 7 6 5 4 3

To Kristen, who is a very special person
and a wonderful daughter.

Preface

With nursing becoming more complex in theory and practice, the revision of a textbook claiming to present the *essentials* of nursing is a tremendous challenge. Decisions regarding which topics to expand within the text and which new topics to include have been based on suggestions from reviewers, nursing instructors, and students. In this third edition, nursing process has become even more prominent with increased emphasis on nursing assessment, use of nursing diagnosis, creation of outcome criteria, expansion of specific nursing interventions, and guidelines for evaluating the effectiveness of the plan of care. All nursing diagnoses have been updated per the 1990 NANDA list. All nursing care plans have been revised and many new ones have been added. In this edition, each nursing diagnosis is supported with appropriate data. An evaluation section has been included for each nursing diagnosis to show properly the flow of the nursing process. Chapters with parts have now been reworked into individual free-standing chapters.

With the trend toward early discharge from the hospital, health maintenance, home care, patient teaching, and discharge planning have been considerably expanded.

Learning objectives have been revised to reflect changes in content and to better meet criteria for measurability. The vocabulary lists at the beginning of each chapter have been rewritten to introduce key words pertinent to the content of the chapter. Illustrations have been updated as needed to reflect current practice. Other study aids include clinical case problems related to common disorders and a detailed study outline at the end of each chapter. The Glossary has been expanded and separated from the index in this edition.

Diagnostic tests in the major medical-surgical chapters have been placed in a Table format for ease of reference and to help keep the text down to a usable size. A listing of the most common laboratory tests and normal values has been added to the Appendix so that users will be able to refer to them quickly.

This third edition has been written to broaden the focus in order to include more suggestions for psychosocial care, including cultural factors and sexuality.

With the increase in our aging population, the chapter on care of older patients has been reorganized and expanded. A brief section on concerns of the elderly, which points out important assessment factors and physiologic changes that might have a bearing on nursing care, has been added to each of the pertinent medical-surgical nursing chapters.

In Unit I, the basic concepts of human nature, health, and society and their relevance to nursing care are presented. An effort has been made to present the nursing process with greater clarity, giving practical examples wherever possible. Documentation has become crucial to the financial health of hospitals and of increasing importance legally. A look is taken at how nurses across the country are trying to meet the requirements while still having time for patient care. The increasing morbidity of patients and technical tasks of nurses make communication between staff members paramount. A section on communication and "report" has been added to this edition. This unit now includes a section on self-esteem for both nurse and patient and has an expanded content on the psychosocial aspects of nursing. Chapters in this unit could be optional if the content has already been covered in a previous course of study.

Unit II focuses on helping a patient strengthen and maintain his natural resources for defense, repair, and healing. The content on the autoimmune deficiency syndrome (AIDS) has been increased and updated. Unit III provides a more in-depth discussion of the internal environment and the homeostatic mechanisms that are essential to the life and normal functioning of each cell. In each chapter the emphasis is on nursing interventions to prevent or mitigate the effects of various factors in the external and internal environments that can threaten a patient's health. Rationale is correlated to the nursing interventions.

Unit IV is larger in this third edition. Content has been added on assessment, signs and symptoms, specific nursing interventions, new medications, new therapies, additional diagnostic tests, observation for common potential complications, discharge planning, and patient teaching. More common diseases and problems have been added at the request of users of the text. Where there are differences in care of a patient in the home, or pertinent adaptations that should be made in interventions, these have been included. Nursing research is constantly providing scientifically validated knowledge on which interventions are based. The material in this unit is intended to reflect that growth in our knowledge base and to foster professional confidence and competence in the performance of the tasks of nursing.

Although patients and nurses alike include both men and women, for ease of expression and conservation of space, the nurse is referred to as "she" and, unless otherwise identified in scenarios, the patient is spoken of as "he."

The Study Guide written to accompany this text has also been totally revised. It is designed to facilitate study of the text and evaluate students' comprehension and ability to apply what has been learned.

It is hoped that this text will help many individuals to gain the knowledge needed to skillfully and compassionately care for patients so that they may share the joy that I have found in nursing.

SUSAN C. DEWIT

Acknowledgments

Many people have been involved in this third revision of Claire Keane's *Essentials of Medical-Surgical Nursing*. It would be impossible to update a comprehensive text adequately without suggestions and input from a variety of people. I am most grateful to each of the following people for their contributions:

Reviewers

Madelon O'Rawe Amenta, BA, MN, MPH, Dr.PH • School of Nursing, Pennsylvania State University, McKeesport, Pennsylvania

Roslyn Mary Atkin, RN • Director of Neurological ICU, Presbyterian Medical Center, Dallas, Texas

Roxanne Aubol Batterden, BSN, RN, CCRN • Franklin Square Hospital Center, Baltimore, Maryland

Jimmie C. Borum, BS, RN • Staff Nurse and Diabetic Educator, Presbyterian Medical Center, Dallas, Texas

Hardenia J. Childrey, BSN, MS, RN • School of Practical Nursing, Trenholm State Technical College, Montgomery, Alabama

Jody A. Eckler, BSN, RN • Instructor, Sandusky School of Practical Nursing, Sandusky, Ohio

Sandra K. Harting, RN, CEN • Assistant Unit Director Emergency Services, Presbyterian Medical Center, Dallas, Texas

Deitra L. Lowdermilk, PhD, RNC • Department of Women's and Children's Health, School of Nursing, University of North Carolina, Chapel Hill, North Carolina

Karen Moser, MSN, RN, CCRN • Clinical Specialist, Presbyterian Medical Center, Dallas, Texas

Ruth Nicholson, BS, MA, RN • School of Practical Nursing, Elizabeth Seton School of Iona College, Yonkers, New York

Pamela S. Schremp, MSN, RN, CRNO • Clinical Instructor, Bolton School of Nursing, Case Western Reserve University, Clinical Nurse Specialist, University Hospitals of Cleveland, Cleveland, Ohio

Donna J. Shallenberger, RN • Instructor, Practical Nurse Program of Canton City Schools, Canton, Ohio

Diane L. Thomas, MSN, RN • Clinical Specialist, Presbyterian Medical Center, Dallas, Texas

Linda N. Tunks, RN • Unit Director, Telemetry, Presbyterian Medical Center, Dallas, Texas

Kathleen Murphy White, MS, RN • School of Nursing, University of Maryland, Baltimore, Maryland

Judith M. Young, BSN, MSN, RN • Instructor, Practical Nursing Program, Upper Bucks County Area Vocational-Technical School, Perkasie, Pennsylvania

Consultants

Gustavio Dascanio, M.D. • Internist, Solvang, California

Onesimo Hernandez, M.D., F.A.C.S. • General Surgeon, Dallas, Texas

Thanks also to Louise Hucks, Director of the Licensed Practical Nursing Program of El Centro College, Dallas, Texas and to Dr. Barbara Horner, Director of Nursing Programs at Alan Hancock College, Santa Maria, California, for their input and gracious loan of materials.

Heartfelt thanks go to my aunt, Marjorie Wiester, who has put up with my computer in her livingroom, provided a beautiful place to work here in the Santa Ynez Valley, and provided both physical and emotional support during this project. The encouragement and emotional support provided by "The Camaradas" group of Solvang has also been invaluable.

I am very grateful for the fine job that Claire Keane did on the previous editions, which made this revision much easier. Kudos to the outstanding staff at W. B. Saunders Company who all have given personal attention and professional expertise to this project: Ilze Rader, Senior Editor; Marie Thomas, Editorial Assistant; Martha Tanner, Developmental Editor; Kendall Sterling and David Harvey, Manuscript Editors; David Nazaruk, Marketing Manager; and Linda R. Garber, Production Manager.

SUSAN C. DEWIT

Contents in Brief

Contents in Detail

CHAPTER 9

Problems of Immobility 183

UNIT FOUR

MEDICAL-SURGICAL PATIENT CARE PROBLEMS 203

CHAPTER 10

Care of Patients With Pain 205

CHAPTER 11

Care of Surgical Patients 223

CHAPTER 12

Care of Older Patients 250

CHAPTER 13

Care of Patients With Cancer 266

CHAPTER 14

Care of Terminally Ill and Dying Patients 297

CHAPTER 15

Care of Patients With Neurologic Disorders 322

CHAPTER 16

Care of Patients With Disorders of the Nose and Throat 375

CHAPTER 17

Care of Patients With Respiratory Disorders 386

CHAPTER 18

Care of Patients With Disorders of the Blood, Blood-Forming Organs, and Lymphatic System 436

CHAPTER 22

Care of Patients With Urologic Disorders 520

CHAPTER 23

Care of Patients With Disorders of the Digestive Tract 555

CHAPTER 27

Care of Patients with Endocrine Disorders: Thyroid and Parathyroid Glands 680

CHAPTER 28

Care of Patients With Diabetes Mellitus and Hypoglycemia 696

CHAPTER 29

Care of Patients With Disorders of the Adrenal and Pituitary Glands 722

CHAPTER 30

Care of Patients With Disorders of the Female Reproductive System 731

CHAPTER 31

Care of Patients With Disorders of the Male Reproductive System 767

CHAPTER 32

Care of Patients With Sexually Transmitted Diseases 781

CHAPTER 33

Care of Patients With Disorders of the Skin 791

CHAPTER 34

Care of Patients With Disorders of the Eyes 819

CHAPTER 35

Care of Patients With Disorders of the Ears 849

CHAPTER 36

Care of Accident and Emergency Patients 867

Appendix: Table of Most Common Laboratory Test Values 899

Glossary 908

Index 921

Nursing Care Plans

Concerns for the Elderly

UNIT ONE

PERSPECTIVES, THEORIES, AND PROCESS

We spend a large part of our lives dealing with ideas, things (objects), and people. In this beginning section of the text we are going to discuss ideas—that is, abstract notions or concepts that are significant to and influential in the practice of nursing. Throughout the remainder of the text we will continue to present and explore ideas and how they are applied to the delivery of nursing care. Sometimes we also will talk about things—for example, equipment, diagnostic tests, and procedures—useful to the nurse in the care of her patients. And we will certainly talk about people.

Some of the concepts most reflected in the development of definitions of nursing and theories about the practice of nursing are based on the views one holds of *human nature, society, health and illness,* and, of course, *nursing* itself.

Your personal ideas about the meaning of these terms have a definite impact on your judgments about what a nurse does or should be doing when she is engaged in the nursing process. Although it is not necessary that all nurses agree on the meaning and implications of these concepts, it is important that we understand what thoughts other people have had about them and how they have influenced leaders in the field of nursing.

Concepts are vehicles of thought. In fact, thinking about any subject in an abstract way requires having some basic concept or general idea of the nature of that subject: what it is like, its purpose, and how it might influence your life. Concepts are general impressions that evolve from particular experiences and information acquired from the world around us. They are logical descriptive terms that help explain why we feel and act as we do in a particular situation.

As an example of what we are talking about here, Florence Nightingale's concept of environment was central to her definition of nursing and its goals. This is understandable when we consider the environment of the soldiers of the Crimean War who were her patients. Before she put into effect some much-needed changes, the wounded soldiers were being cared for in enormous, drafty barracks hospitals where they lay amidst filth, vermin, and the stench of death. In her writings about nursing, Nightingale stressed ventilation, cleanliness, warmth, and quiet so that the natural powers of healing could work most effectively to restore health to the wounded. Although she wrote *Notes on Nursing* in 1859, much of what she had to say about the relationship between a clean, orderly environment and the promotion of health is as true today as it was then. Her concept of environment and its relationship to health and illness still influences current thought on the subject.

In this unit we will look at some old and new thoughts about human nature, society, health and illness, and how they relate to nursing. It should be pointed out that no theory of nursing is appropriate for every nursing care situation and every nurse-patient relationship. There is far too much variety in nursing for that. The purpose of learning about different views of nursing and nursing theories is to arm oneself with a variety of approaches from which to select the one (or more) that seems best suited for a particular situation and best meets the needs of an individual patient.

In the last chapter of this unit we will consider the characteristics, purposes, major components, and documentation of the nursing process. To engage in the nursing process is to systematically approach the health problems a patient has and to intervene deliberately and thoughtfully on his behalf to help him deal with them. Documenting what she observes about and does for her patient, as well as his response to medical and nursing intervention, is essential to coordination of all the activities concerned with the patient's care.

In this first unit of study you are challenged to start developing your own view of nursing and begin to make some decisions about how you want to practice nursing so that your patients are cared for in a systematic but very personal way. It is in truly caring for and about one another that we find meaning and purpose in our own lives.

CHAPTER 1

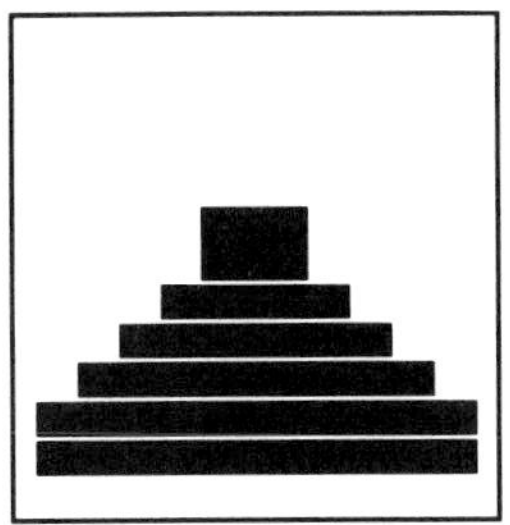

Concepts of Health and Illness

VOCABULARY

acute illness
adaptation
chronic illness
continuum
feedback
health behavior
homeostasis
noncompliance
pathologic
spectrum

Upon completion of this chapter the student should be able to:

1. Compare traditional and current views of the meanings of health and illness.
2. State in his or her own words a definition of health that reflects the current concept of the term.
3. Cite two major goals of the complex living system that is a person.
4. Identify at least three characteristics common to all living systems.
5. State some ways in which positive and negative feedback contribute to individualized and personalized nursing care.
6. Discuss reasons why nurses need to be aware of any cultural, educational, and social differences that might exist between themselves and their patients.
7. List three areas of health care in which differences among races and cultures are most apparent.

The word *health* means many different things to people. For some it is simply the absence of disease; for others it encompasses optimum functioning on every level. It is derived from a word that means "wholeness." A dictionary might define health as a state in which "all functions of the body and mind are active" (Taber's, 1981). Each person must develop his own concept of the term.

It is important that you have a mental picture of what you believe health and illness to mean, because your concept of these terms influences everything you say and do in the service of your patients. When you make judgments about a person's state of health, plan and implement nursing care to improve his health status, and evaluate the effectiveness of planned nursing intervention, you must have some understanding of what the word *health* really means. The results that you expect to achieve through nursing care are based on your vision of what your patient might be able to do and what he might become because of the care you give. If you view health and wellness in a narrow and limited sense, you will be inclined to set health care goals accordingly. If you have a broader perspective of health and see it as something more than merely the absence of disease, you can be far more creative in helping each of your patients reach a higher level of wellness and a more satisfying sense of well-being. When you view health as something more than freedom from disease, you and your patient can feel less defeated when the medical diagnosis is a chronic disease that cannot be cured but can be managed so that the patient can live with his illness and experience life more fully.

If you truly believe that your task is to work with the patient to help him achieve his personal goals for health and wellness, it is essential that you know how he views health and wellness. And you should know what he thinks are important and realistic goals for meeting his health needs. The basic concept of health is a very personal one and can vary from person to person. One's goals for healthful living, for being alive and well, also are highly individualized and based on values and beliefs.

Because of cultural, educational, and social differences, you and your patient could have totally different ideas about health and illness and what constitutes "good" health and effective health practices. Before you can work with your patient to accomplish his health care goals, you should try to find out how he feels about health and illness and what he believes to be true about these concepts. If there are differences of opinion, you owe it to your patient to try to reconcile your differences. If that is not possible, you still must acknowledge that the differences exist and that your goals might not be the same as his.

Comprehension of the full meaning of any idea is improved when one becomes more aware of the truths discovered by others in their search for its meaning. Many theories have been proposed to help explain what it means to be well and healthy, fully alive and satisfied with one's life, or to be deprived of a healthy state of body, mind, or spirit. All of the more recent theories about the meaning of health and illness recognize how complex these concepts are. The human body, mind, and spirit are parts of a living system. The elements of the human system interact with one another in ways we still do not completely understand. We can, however, begin to appreciate how powerfully the thoughts, emotions, and experiences of a person influence his state of physical health. Because every human is a complex living system, the basic rules of general systems theory have been included in this chapter as a foundation for understanding the concepts of health and illness. Thoughtful consideration of these laws and principles should help you appreciate more fully the mysteries of human life, health, and illness and apply what you have learned to the systematic care of your patients.

TRADITIONAL VIEWS OF HEALTH AND ILLNESS

The traditional view of health in Western culture was influenced by Plato, Aristotle, and other philosophers who were concerned only with biologic well-being. For many years an acceptable definition of health was simply the absence of disease. Hence health and illness were dealt with as two separate entities.

In 1946 the World Health Organization redefined health as: "the state of complete physical, mental, and social well-being and not merely the absence of disease or infirmity."

It was not until 1974, however, that a change was made in the Federal Employees Compensation Act to reimburse federal employees for treatment by psychologists and psychiatrists. This change reflected a recognition of treatment of mental illness as a legitimate medical cost. Following the lead of the federal government, other third-party payers (such as insurance companies) made similar changes in the 1970s. This willingness to pay for medical care for illnesses other than clearly defined physical diseases reflected a new and expanded understanding of the nature of health.

Current concepts of health and illness still do not give a clear idea of the nature of health.

They do, however, increase our understanding of and appreciation for the complexity of human life. We look around us and see that people are not always either sick or well, diseased or healthy. Throughout the entire span of life from conception to the final hour of death, the health status of an individual can vary from day to day or even hour to hour. There are people who are partially or completely paralyzed, suffering from a chronic illness, deaf or blind, or living with an anatomic defect who think of themselves as fairly healthy and who are capable of living full and productive lives. None of these people can be labeled as "sick," nor can any one of them be called completely healthy. There also are others who have no identifiable organic disease who nevertheless do not feel well and are not able to live their lives to the fullest.

Current concepts of health and illness still do not provide all the answers to questions about what it means to be healthy, but they can help us realize more fully the wisdom of the ancient definition of health: that is, "hale," "sound," and "whole." Somewhere in history this meaning was lost, and man was compartmentalized into body, mind, and soul. Current thought brings us back to a view of our patients and ourselves as wholly integrated and dynamic beings in a continuous state of change and growth and with potential for becoming something more in every dimension of our lives.

A comparison of the consequences of traditional and current views of health and illness is presented in Table 1–1.

CURRENT VIEWS OF HEALTH AND ILLNESS

Contemporary definitions of health and illness are more abstract and philosophical, and therefore more vague, than the precise definitions based on the measurable criteria of the scientist.

In general, being healthy means being able to function well physically and mentally and to express the full range of one's potentialities within the environment in which one is living.

This concept takes health beyond the level of meeting basic physiologic needs and recognizes man's need to accept himself as worthwhile, to live in harmony with others, and to express his personality fully, thereby becoming more self-actualized and fulfilled. In the words of René Dubos, "health is primarily a measure of each person's ability to do [what he wants to do] and become what he wants to become."

Current views of health and illness are based on the thoughts and ideas of men such as Dubos and Halbert Dunn, who urged their readers to look at these concepts in a new and different way. Realizing that people are dynamic beings whose state of health changes daily and even hourly, they suggest that it is better to think of each person as being located somewhere on a graduated scale or continuous spectrum (continuum) ranging from obvious disease through the absence of discernible disease to a state of optimum functioning in every aspect of their lives.

TABLE 1–1 **COMPARISON OF TRADITIONAL AND CURRENT VIEWS OF HEALTH AND ILLNESS**

Traditional View	Current View
1. Health and illness are absolute, unconditional, and separate entities.	1. Health and illness are relative, ever-changing states of being.
2. Sees a person as either sick or well.	2. Sees a person as being somewhere on a continuum ranging from high-level wellness to death.
3. Focus is on biologic and physiologic aspects of disease.	3. Considers all factors affecting the total person and all levels of human need. Based on a holistic view of man.
4. Tendency to treat the disease rather than the person.	4. Patient seen as a person with unique health care needs.
5. Focus is on crisis management of disease.	5. Emphasizes maintenance of health and prevention of disease and injury.
6. Emphasizes cure of existing illness or injury.	6. Supports the common theme of nursing as a caring profession.
7. Limits options for action in the management of disease.	7. Allows for creativity in developing ways to manage illnesses that cannot be cured and to contribute to the continued growth and development of the total personality.

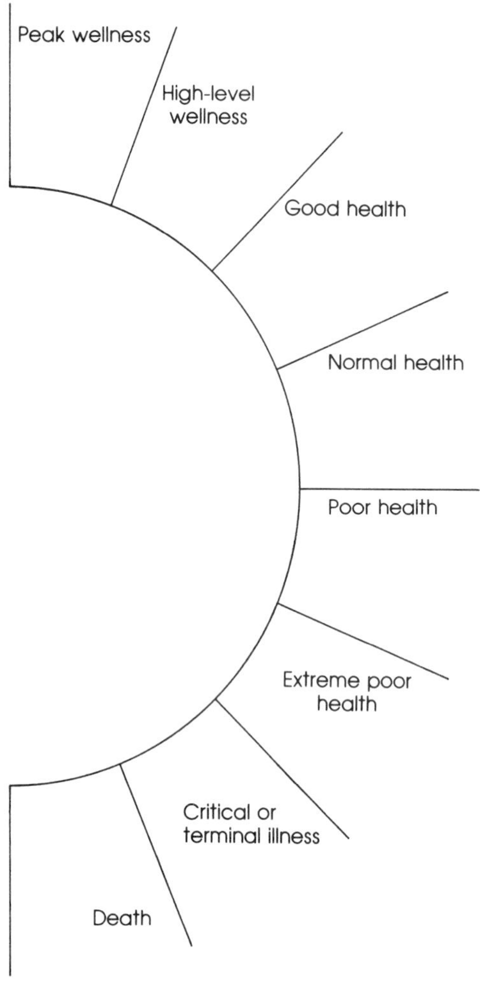

Figure 1–1 Health-illness spectrum.

Figure 1–1 shows a model for the current view of health and illness as dynamic states of being. The phrase *high-level wellness* was first used by Dunn to signify the ideal state of health in every dimension of man's personality. Dunn does not consider high-level wellness to be the same as good health. He thinks of health as being a relatively passive state, one that a person enjoys because of hereditary and environmental factors that are essentially beyond the control of the person. High-level wellness, on the other hand, is described as a dynamic and active movement toward fulfillment of one's potential.

In Dunn's view each person accepts responsibility for and takes an active part in improving and maintaining his own state of wellness. A person who enjoys a high level of wellness does so by virtue of his own efforts. When a person works at achieving high-level wellness, he improves his self-esteem, is able to accept and give love and concern for others, and lives each day of his life to its fullest insofar as he is able to do so. We all know or have heard about people who suffer from a physical illness or impairment and yet are able to enjoy a higher level of wellness than others who are physically sound but are somehow "crippled" socially, emotionally, or spiritually.

In the contemporary view, health and illness are relative, rather than absolute, terms. This means that each person's state of health depends on many different things beyond his biologic fitness. Among the personal, psychosocial, and spiritual factors that influence a person's state of health at any given moment are his values and beliefs about what it means to be healthy and what it means to be sick, his image of himself, his ability to reach out and relate to others, and his ability to search for and find meaning and purpose in his own life. From this point of view, health is never the same for everyone for all time and in all circumstances.

IMPLICATIONS OF CURRENT VIEWS

It readily becomes apparent that these views of the nature of health and illness greatly add to the complexity of health care. They challenge traditional methods of health care delivery and the single-minded goal of curing disease. In the delivery of nursing care, current concepts of health and illness reinforce the value of nursing as primarily a caring profession.

A common theme in all of nursing theory is that nursing is concerned with helping people cope with adverse physiologic, psychosocial, and spiritual responses to illness, rather than with treating the illness itself, which is in the realm of medical practice.

Although the nurse is involved in the curing of those who are ill or injured, this goal is primarily in the domain and under the control of the physician. Nurses have traditionally been concerned with promoting good health habits in their patients and giving them the support they need to cope with illness. Since Florence Nightingale, nurses have encouraged a wholesome environment in the home, hospital or other health care agency, and community.

The assistance and support typically provided by nurses are given with the knowledge that ultimately it is the inner resources of the individual that determine whether he will be able to function at his optimum level.

The essential task of nursing is to enhance and reinforce these healing strengths: to help people use their available resources to adapt at an optimum level of functioning and achieve goals they have set for themselves.

In short, as Dubos has said, the central task is to help people "do and become what they want to become."

A major advantage of the current concepts of health and illness is the hope such views offer and the added meaning they can give to the interaction between a nurse and her patient. The patient with a chronic and incurable illness can be helped to minimize its harmful effects and can be encouraged to continue to set and attain goals in other dimensions of his life. A patient who is permanently disabled because of traumatic injury is not necessarily limited in every other aspect of his life, and it is possible for the terminally ill patient to live his final days more fully and perhaps with greater meaning and purpose than during any other stage of his life.

GENERAL SYSTEMS THEORY AS A BASIS OF CURRENT VIEWS

The current definitions of health and illness just described have evolved from a wide range of theories. One way of looking at a person is to think of him as a living system. All systems, from the simplest to the most complex, must obey certain fundamental laws and principles if they are to survive. By becoming familiar with some of these basic laws we can better understand human anatomy and physiology, psychology, the behavioral sciences and, in fact, all of the life sciences. We also are better able to grasp the meaning and intent of nursing as a systematic process and to engage in that process for the benefit of our patients.

In 1937 Ludwig von Bertalanffy proposed the theory that there could be a single conceptual systems model that would be useful to all who study the life sciences, regardless of their particular area of interest. The main purpose of the systems model is to organize the findings of researchers in the various sciences into one set of laws and principles and to provide a common language for describing research results. Thus scientists in the various disciplines could communicate with one another more easily and benefit from the knowledge and truths each had discovered through research.

Since they were first proposed by von Bertalanffy, the unifying principles of general systems theory have been useful in many different fields, including anthropology, sociology, biology, psychology, and nursing. Some of the underlying principles or laws of general systems theory are presented in the text that follows.

DEFINITION AND PURPOSE

What is a system? Although we have heard the word *system* used in hundreds of different ways, many people do not have a clear idea of what is meant by the word.

The most simple and direct definition of a system is* an organized whole composed of interacting parts or components. *A system has content, purpose, and process.

The various parts that form the structure of a system are called the system's *content*. For example, the content of the circulatory system in the human body includes the heart and blood vessels and the blood that is pumped through them. The content of nursing as a system includes the patient, the nurse, and the knowledge and skills each one contributes to the nursing process.

The purpose of a system gives it meaning and direction; that is, it determines its goals. The purpose of the circulatory system is to distribute blood throughout the body. The purpose of nursing is to assist patients in their response to real or potential health problems. All of nursing's activities and functions should be directed toward accomplishing its goals and thereby fulfilling its purpose.

The goals of a system are accomplished by the process or function of the system. When a nurse and her patient are engaged in the nursing process, each has certain functions to perform. Goals are set by the nurse and the patient, and plans are made for certain activities to be carried out to meet the goals. During the process the plan is implemented and evaluated to determine whether or not the goals were accomplished. The nursing process is discussed in more detail in Chapter 4, in which the relationship between general systems theory and the nursing process should become more clear.

SUBSYSTEMS, SYSTEMS, AND SUPRASYSTEMS

Earlier we spoke of a human as a living system, and so one might ask how the total person can be a system and at the same time only one part of his body—such as the circulatory system—can also be called a system. In general systems theory there are two terms that can be used to indicate whether one is talking about a complex system or a system within a system.

A *suprasystem* usually means a highly complex system; for example, a nation or society. A *subsystem* is a smaller system within a larger one; for example, the health care delivery system of a society. A subsystem has a purpose of its own, but it also contributes to the overall purpose of the system to which it belongs. If it does not do this, the system becomes impaired and less efficient and may eventually die. Evidence that this is so can be found if one considers what happens when the body's circulatory system (or subsystem) fails to distribute blood. If the situation is not corrected, the system (the individual person) becomes ill and may ultimately die. The same can be said of a health care delivery system. If its subsystems such as nursing and medicine do not perform their functions, the health care system is less able to accomplish its goals. Because patients also are part of the health care system, if they fail to accept responsibility for their own welfare and refuse or are unable to do what they should to avoid, recover from, or manage illness, the system cannot accomplish its goals. Figure 1–2 shows the relationships among various systems and subsystems in a society, which would be considered the suprasystem. Included in the health care delivery system are people and agencies concerned with health care.

HUMANS AS COMPLEX LIVING SYSTEMS

> ***In regard to its health and survival, the human system has two major goals: (1) to maintain internal constancy (that is, a dynamic state of equilibrium called*** **homeostasis,** ***which will be discussed later); and (2) to live in harmony with the world.***

In order to accomplish these goals, there are many different processes taking place within the human system and its subsystems. A person who remains healthy does so by continuous adaptation. Being healthy allows the human system to use what it has (structure) to do whatever is necessary (process) to fulfill its purpose. The human system also shares some general characteristics and functions with all other systems.

GENERAL CHARACTERISTICS AND FUNCTIONS OF LIVING SYSTEMS

All living systems exist in space. The space or environment of a system includes all factors that affect the system and also all factors affected by the system. Another way of saying this is, *all living systems continuously interact with their environments.* A living system has an external and an internal environment.

The external environment is, of course, outside the system itself, but the system is in communication with and responds to changes in its environment. The external environment of humans plays an important role in human growth and development and has a direct influence on a person's state of health in every dimension of his life.

The internal environment of the human body is composed of the fluids that surround each cell and are within each cell. There must be continuous exchange in the internal environment to provide life-giving substances and to remove wastes. The internal environment is discussed in more depth in Chapter 8.

Living systems also exist in time. Change in any system must take place over a period of time, and because all living systems continuously interact with and adapt to elements in their external and internal environments so they can

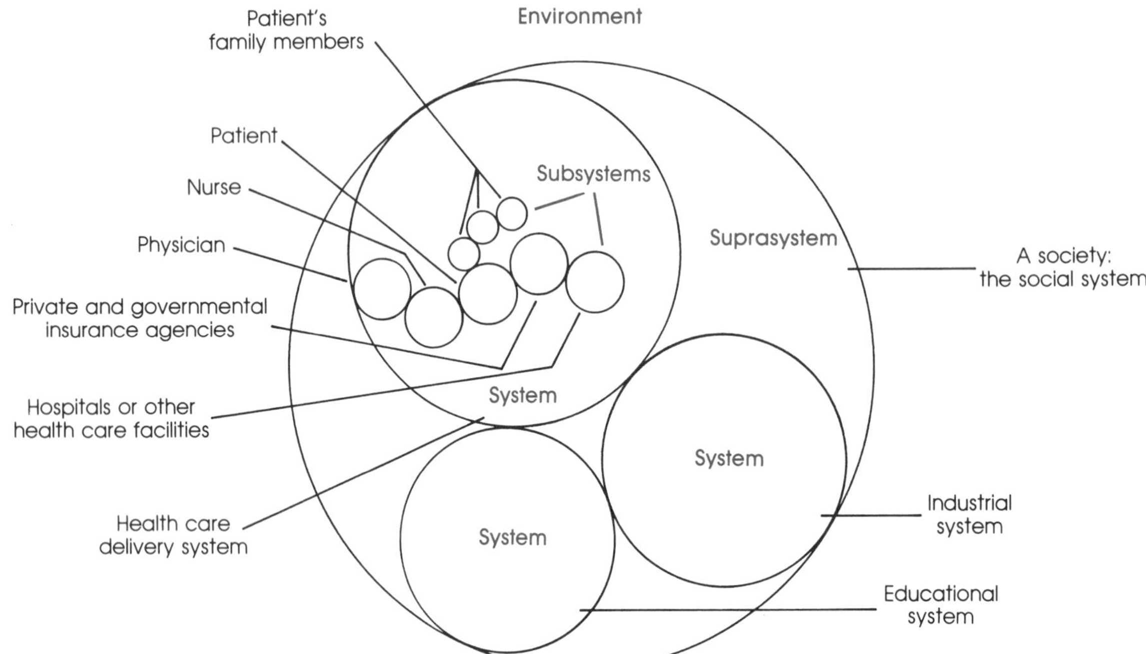

Figure 1–2 Within the environment there are suprasystems (e.g., human society) and systems within the suprasystem such as the educational and industrial systems and the health care delivery system. Within the health care delivery system are subsystems (e.g., the patient, his family members, the nurse, the physician, and allied health care paraprofessionals).

survive, change is inevitable. There can be no standing still, no stagnation in a living system. It must either grow or deteriorate, progress or regress, live or die. Changes can be short-term or long-term, but they must occur if the system is to survive.

Matter and energy are integral parts of a living system and its environment. Matter consists of anything that has mass and occupies space. Energy is the ability to do work or overcome resistance. The exchange of matter and energy between the system and its environment is a life-giving process. The intake of food and air and the performance of physical activity are good examples of this characteristic of the living human system. Without the exchange of nutrients and wastes and some degree of physical motion, the human system deteriorates and dies.

A living system needs to have information. It needs information in order to make the correct adjustments and changes for life, adaptability, and growth. As we have noted, a living system must adapt and make changes, or it will cease to exist. If the changes are not appropriate or are based on false information, the system becomes disorganized and dies.

In general systems theory, *information* is a broad term that denotes any event or agent that activates the system's processes. Let's say, for example, that after a person has eaten a high-carbohydrate meal his blood glucose level is abnormally high. This information about the blood sugar level is sent to the hypothalamus, which notifies the beta cells of the pancreas, which in turn produce insulin. In response to the information that more insulin is needed, the beta cells produce this hormone to return the blood sugar to the normal range.

In the human body there are many such physiologic processes functioning on a continuous basis to maintain health. Communication within the internal environment of the human system is performed by the nervous system, by hormones and enzymes, and by variations in the pressure in the vascular system. Each of these components sends messages to controllers in the system. The function of these controllers is to regulate the system's processes or functions so that its chemical and physiologic components will stay within normal limits.

However, because the human system has psychosocial and spiritual components, it also uses information from its external environment to adjust and make changes to maintain well-being so that its goals and purpose can be accomplished. Nursing is concerned with the total person and all aspects of human life. The complexity of the human system presents some very real challenges to the nurse. She is more likely to meet these challenges successfully if she is familiar with the characteristics and functions of all living systems.

OPEN AND CLOSED SYSTEMS AND FEEDBACK

There are two major types of systems: closed and open. A *closed* system does not exchange matter, energy, and information with its environment; nothing enters the system and nothing leaves it. Many electronic systems, such as closed-circuit television, are closed systems.

All living systems are *open* systems. The matter, energy, and information that enter the system are called *input*; that which leaves the system is called *output*. *Feedback* gives a system information about its output. The system can then evaluate its output and make the necessary adjustments, adaptations, or modifications. Figure 1-3 illustrates the concept of input, output, and feedback in a nurse-patient system. All humans need food for energy (input) and must excrete waste materials of metabolism (output). Data such as weight, number of bowel movements, and character and quantity of urine give us feedback on how the system is operating. There are many examples of physical feedback systems in the body. The angiotensin-renin mechanism is an example of how sensors in the body determine whether more or less of these substances is needed to control blood pressure; when the data are processed, the substances are released or secretion is slowed as necesssary.

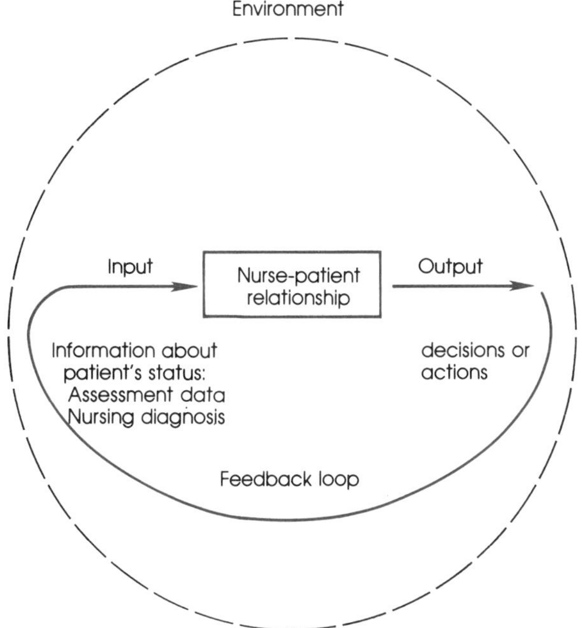

Figure 1-3 Feedback in a patient care system. Input influences interaction and output, which is evaluated and returned as input.

The concept of feedback is very important to an understanding of how a living system regulates and controls its functions to accomplish its purpose. There are two general kinds of feedback: negative and positive.

Negative feedback ***is a corrective action. It informs a controller in the system that things are not as they should be and a change must be made to return a factor within the system to a normal range or acceptable level.***

For example, the serum concentration of oxygen is affected in part by the rate and depth of respirations and is therefore an output of the respiratory system. If the content of oxygen drops below normal, this information is transmitted as input by the nerve cells to the respiratory control center in the brain. The control center is thereby stimulated to increase the respiratory rate so that more oxygen will be inhaled.

Positive feedback ***informs the system that its output is satisfactory.***

This is fine as long as there is no deviation from acceptable norms, but if there is some excess or deficiency outside the normal limits, positive feedback will accelerate and perpetuate the deviation. Because this is true of all living systems, continued positive feedback can be fatal to a system in which there is some abnormality. Fortunately, most of the vital mechanisms of the body are regulated by a continuous-circuit, negative-feedback control system that can overcome a mild degree of positive feedback. If these control systems fail, however, death will ensue. For example, positive feedback can encourage the division and multiplication of malignant cells, resulting in growth and spreading of cancer within the body.

The ability of a living system to regulate itself by controlling its activities is fundamental to accomplishment of its purpose. In the nursing process, feedback can be used to evaluate the effectiveness of planned nursing intervention. If there is negative feedback in the form of subjective and objective information indicating that the intervention is not having the desired effect, decisions can be made about revising the plan of care. The subjective and objective data are the input of the system, and the decisions and actions taken are its output.

HOMEOSTASIS AND HARMONY

Earlier in this chapter it was stated that two major goals of the human system are stability in the internal environment and harmony with elements in the external environment. *Homeostasis* is a term first coined by Cannon to describe a tendency of biologic systems to maintain stability of the internal environment while continuously adjusting to changes necessary for survival. The term is considered by some authorities to be misleading, because the suffix *-stasis* implies a static, or fixed and unmoving, state, whereas the process actually involves continuous adaptation, movement, and change. Cannon did not intend to suggest that homeostasis is a condition of stagnation, but instead that the term implies a "steady state" in which there are variations within preset limits. These variations take place in a predictable manner—for example, variations in body temperature, changes in the acidity and alkalinity of body fluids, hormonal production and release, and other changes that occur during every 24-hour period. In health, continuous adaptation and change must take place in the internal environment in order to maintain its "steady state."

The internal environment of the human body is composed of blood, lymph, and fluid in the spaces surrounding each cell. The substances dissolved in the body fluids are essential to the life of the cell. The cell takes in nutrients and discharges wastes, as well as substances it has synthesized that are essential to normal function of other cells and organs. Thus the internal environment serves to integrate and unify all body cells and their activities. More detailed discussions of homeostatic mechanisms and the internal environment are presented throughout the text, especially in those chapters dealing with fluid and electrolyte balance, hormonal activities, the neurologic system, and the cardiovascular system.

In order to enjoy some degree of health and sense of well-being, a person must adapt to factors in his *external environment*. In other words, he needs to be in harmony with elements outside himself, and he does this by interacting with these elements and integrating them into his life. These elements include the physical, biologic, and psychosocial factors in the world in which he lives and works.

To live in harmony with external environmental factors requires both adaptability and stability.

Wellness is maintained or regained, at least in part, when a person is able to keep a sense of balance while at the same time adapting to factors that can upset that balance. These factors include such life experiences as socialization, education, mental and physical stress, satisfactions, and rewards. Perhaps one of the most crucial of factors in today's world is change. When change is required, additional stress is put on a person's inner resources, and this in turn can increase his susceptibility to illness. Health and illness are dynamic states; hence, adaptability to a changing external environment is essential to stability and health.

THE CONSUMER'S CONCEPT OF HEALTH AND ILLNESS

Up to this point we have taken a shallow dip into a wide and deep pool of theories proposed by philosophers and scientists and have briefly explored their thoughts about what constitutes health and illness. Now we turn our attention to the consumer's point of view. All efforts toward achieving health-related goals should begin with the person for whom these goals are intended. His views and opinions are at least as important, if not more so, as those of the professional health care provider.

> *A major goal of nursing is to foster* voluntary action *on the part of the consumer to take positive steps toward improving his own health status and achieving higher levels of wellness.*

Nursing care, more than any other form of health care, places a high value on working with the consumer to help him become more independent and better able to meet his own health-care needs.

> *If the goals of health promotion, disease prevention, and recovery from the effects of illness and injury are to be achieved, the consumer must be both able and willing to accept responsibility for his health-related behavior.*

HEALTH AND ILLNESS BEHAVIOR

Health and illness behaviors, like all types of human behavior, are the outcome of complex responses to internal and external stimuli. Basic to this behavior is what a person knows and believes about health and illness and how he assesses his own state of health.

Health behavior can be defined as any action undertaken in order to promote health, prevent disease, or detect disease in an early asymptomatic stage.

Illness behavior, in contrast, is any activity a person who believes himself to be ill takes in order to determine his actual state of health and to seek a suitable remedy.

Some examples of health behavior might include watching one's dietary intake to avoid becoming overweight, engaging in a regular program of exercise, taking care to obtain available immunizations against communicable diseases, and monthly self-examination of the breasts. These behaviors are encouraged by health care providers, because they are perceived by them as valuable. When such behaviors are not undertaken by a consumer for whom they have been recommended, the nurse should consider whether there is a conflict of values. Because of cultural and personal differences, not everyone views certain health practices and behaviors in the same way. What one eats or refuses to eat can be influenced by religious and cultural beliefs. Whether one allows himself or his children to be immunized can be dictated by religious convictions and restrictions. Furthermore, early detection of disease can depend on what one knows about normal physiology and psychology, abnormal conditions of the body and mind, and whether one perceives suggested measures and treatments as effective and worthwhile.

Illness behavior is equally complex. Because it involves actions undertaken by a person who believes himself to be ill, the underlying question to be answered by the person is, "What does it mean to be ill?" or, "How do I know I am ill?" Again, the nurse must consider what the person knows about health and deviations from health, and what he believes to be an appropriate remedy for his health problems. Examples of illness behavior include consulting a physician or nurse, visiting a neighborhood health care clinic, and taking prescribed medications.

CULTURAL INFLUENCES ON CONCEPTS OF HEALTH AND ILLNESS

In the United States, perhaps more than in any other developed nation, there is much cultural diversity among its citizens. There are many differences between the values and practices of white, middle-class Americans and those of the minority groups in this country. Effective nursing care, whatever the setting, is dependent on an appreciation of these differences and successful accommodation of and adaptation to these differences.

Some of the areas in which differences among racial and ethnic groups are most apparent are attitudes and practices related to birth, death, and general health care; susceptibility to specific diseases; responses to pain and suffering; personal hygiene and sense of privacy; acceptance of number of children in the family; rate of growth of children; and adjustment to life changes. Additionally, the words and concepts used to communicate feelings and behaviors related to health practices and remedies for sickness are quite different in each cultural subgroup.

The attitudes, beliefs, and practices of a cultural subgroup may or may not conform to the nurse's idea of what constitutes a productive and beneficial action. Typically, health care professionals in the United States and other countries influenced by Western medical science have been taught according to the values and beliefs of a white, middle-class society. At the same time, the minority groups that they deal with in the United States do not necessarily share these values and beliefs. Unless this conflict is resolved in some way, there is certain to be a problem in communication and in meeting the goals of health care. There will be problems for the nurse, because she might have unrealistic expectations of what she will be able to do for and with those she hopes to help, and there will be problems for the patient, because he will probably be denied the quality of care he needs and deserves.

Many cultural health beliefs are based on "folk medicine" passed down through the generations within a culture. Many cultures have their own "healers" in the form of a medicine man, shaman, or curandera. Those within the culture often seek the advice of this person before going to a health professional. Beliefs in the various cures that the cultural "healer" suggests are difficult to overcome. Respect for the person's cultural beliefs in all areas is necessary on the part of the nurse for her advice and teaching to be acted upon.

The most obvious source of information about the patient's perception of his own health status is the patient himself.

Whatever the technique of assessing a patient's health status—interview, history taking, or simply observation of behavior—it must be done without criticism, with an open mind, and with a listening heart. Judgmental terms such as *noncompliant, uncooperative, ignorant, lazy,* or *unmotivated* are not acceptable descriptions of another person's health behavior.

There should be no conditions or "strings attached" to the unspoken contract between a nurse and the person or persons she is trying to help. This is not to say that she must always condone what a patient is doing or not doing to maintain or restore his health or that she will not try to present her own point of view and provide him with information about what she considers to be good health practices. Differences between professional care and folk care that could be sources of conflict are shown in Table 1–2.

TABLE 1–2 COMPARISON OF FOLK HEALTH CARE AND PROFESSIONAL HEALTH CARE AS PERCEIVED BY CLIENTS

Folk Care Emphases	Professional Health Care Emphases
1. Primarily a humanistic approach.	1. Primarily a scientific approach.
2. Emphases on *familiar, practical,* and *concrete facts.*	2. Emphases on *unfamiliar, less practical,* and *abstract facts.*
3. Uses a *holistic* integrated health-illness focus (i.e., culture, religious, kinship, economics, social aspects) with people.	3. Uses a *fragmented and nonintegrated approach* with people, except for nursing's partially holistic approach.
4. Primarily a *caring* attitude.	4. Primarily a *curing* attitude with some caring.
5. Primarily *nontechnical* in services; more *sociocultural* relationships are stressed.	5. Primarily *technical treatments* and *diagnostic services.*
6. *Prevention of illness* and disabilities by cultural taboos.	6. *Diagnosis and treatment* of diseases emphasized.
7. *Modest cost* for care or cure services in home setting.	7. *High costs* for physician and hospital services.
8. *Health assessment* done in relation to cultural, social, political, and economic conditions.	8. *Illness assessment* done mainly on physical and psychological problems.
9. Folk practitioners continue to be the *primary* or *first-line* caregivers.	9. Professional practitioners perform mainly *secondary and tertiary services.*
10. Uses *diverse explanations* to interpret wellness and illness.	10. Uses *focused cause(s)* to explain illness and health problems.

Adapted from Leininger, M. M.: Transcultural nursing: Its progress and its future. Nursing & Health Care, Sept., 1981, p. 370.

TRANSCULTURAL NURSING

The need for consideration of cultural factors as an integral part of providing total and individualized health care services for all patients is recognized throughout the health care industry. This has resulted in specialists who are adding to the knowledge base of a subfield called *transcultural nursing*.

The body of knowledge needed to ensure total, holistic care for all people of all cultures is incredibly large. Much research is under way to validate the proposed theories of appropriate caring behaviors for various cultural groups. Nurses knowledgeable in transcultural nursing are invaluable resource persons for the practitioner of general nursing. The nurse must recognize the need to deal with each patient as a unique individual whose concepts of health and illness and health care might be different from her own.

BIBLIOGRAPHY

Byrne, M. L., and Thompson, L. F.: Key Concepts for the Study and Practice of Nursing, 3rd ed. St. Louis, C. V. Mosby, 1978.

Cannon, W. B.: The Wisdom of the Body. New York, Morton & Co., Inc., 1939.

Dubos, R.: Man Adapting. New Haven, CT, Yale University Press, 1965.

Dunn, H. L.: High Level Wellness. Arlington, VA, R. W. Beatty , Ltd., 1959.

Harron, F., et al.: Health and Human Values. New Haven, CT, Yale University Press, 1983.

Hazzard, M. E.: An overview of systems theory. Nurs. Clin. North Am., Sept., 1971, p. 385.

Leininger, M.: Cultural diversities of health and nursing care. Nurs. Clin. North Am., March, 1977, p. 5.

Taber's Cyclopedic Medical Dictionary, 14th ed. Philadelphia, F. A. Davis Co., 1981.

Yura, H., and Walsh, M. B.: The Nursing Process, 6th ed. New Haven, CT, Appleton-Lange, 1989.

STUDENT STUDY AIDS

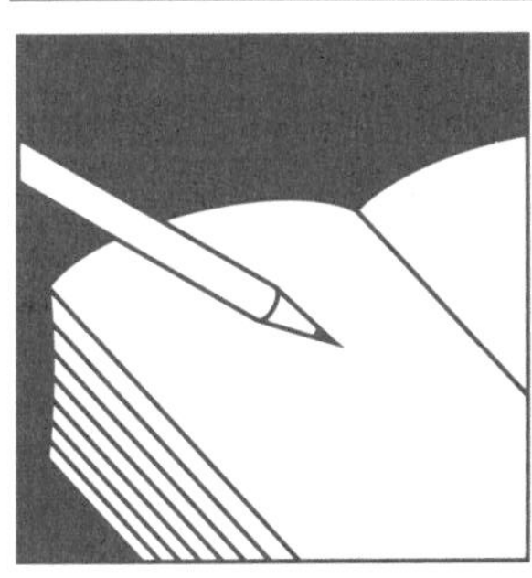

PROBLEMS FOR DISCUSSION

Read each situation and discuss the questions with your classmates.

1. Mr Moses, age 67, is a neighbor of yours who has arthritis and mild congestive heart failure. He has recently retired and spends his days working in his garden. He and his wife occasionally visit the local center for senior citizens and often take day-long trips with other members. Mr. Moses fertilizes his garden and controls insects without using inorganic chemicals. He likes to discuss his methods of gardening and is very enthusiastic about pollution control.

- How would you describe Mr. Moses' position on the health-illness continuum?
- There is no cure for either of Mr. Moses' health problems, nor is there a single cause for either of them. Compare the traditional and current views of Mr. Moses' health status and how each might affect the kind of health care he would receive.

---

2. Consider the educational system of which your school is a subsystem. Write down as briefly and simply as you can (a) the purpose of the system, (b) the content of the system, (c) the process or series of actions that take place within the system. Next, try to identify the characteristics of your educational system that show it is a living system.

---

3. Mrs. Hoy, a Vietnamese refugee, is admitted to the hospital for delivery of her ninth child. She is obviously frightened and intimidated by the physicians and nurses. She has never been in a modern hospital and does not understand the negative attitude of the nursing staff toward her willingness to have so many children. She refuses to eat most of the food brought to her from the diet kitchen, politely saying that she is not hungry.

- Can you imagine what it was like for Mrs. Hoy when she delivered her other eight children in Vietnam?
- Why do you think she is intimidated by the doctors and nurses?
- Why does she refuse to eat?
- What nursing interventions could help with Mrs. Hoy's cultural differences?

STUDY OUTLINE

I. Introduction

A. Each nurse's understanding of the meaning of health and illness influences the quality of care she provides.

B. A narrow view of health and illness can have a limiting effect on all phases of the nursing process.

C. Consideration of the patient's perspectives on health and illness is essential to cooperative assessment of his health needs and successfully setting realistic goals.

D. Cultural and social differences can result in conflict of opinions about the quality of health care provided.

II. Traditional views of health and illness

A. Concepts based on biologic aspects of disease.

B. Health defined as the absence of disease; hence a person is either sick or well.

C. Traditional scientific view does not consider all dimensions of human life and health.

D. Consequences of traditional view (see Table 1–1).

III. Current views of health and illness

A. More philosophical, abstract, and vague than traditional view.

B. Hold that health is a highly subjective and relative term; describe a state of being that is continuously changing and is not the same for everyone for all time in all circumstances.

C. In general, being healthy means being able to function well in one's environment and to do and become what one wants to become.

D. A person's state of health is located on a health-illness continuum extending from obvious disease through the absence of discernible disease to a state of optimum functioning in every aspect of life.

E. Good health is a passive state; high-level wellness requires active participation of the person who strives to achieve fulfillment of his potential.

F. Implications of current views.

1. Greatly add to the complexity of health care.
2. Help explain consumers' dissatisfaction with the traditional health care delivery system.
3. Reinforce the value of nursing as primarily a *caring*, rather than a *curing*, profession.
4. Essential task of nursing is to support and enhance the patient's inner resources and strengths for healing.
5. Expected outcomes of current views (see Table 1–1).

IV. General systems theory as basis of current views

A. Humans can be thought of as living systems.

B. Being familiar with basic laws of general systems theory can improve understanding of the life sciences.

C. General systems theory—proposed by von Bertalanffy as a conceptual model for all the behavioral and life sciences, regardless of the special area of interest.

1. Organizes research data into one set of laws or principles.
2. Common terminology improves communication among the various disciplines.
3. Definition and purpose of systems.
   a. System defined as an organized whole made up of interacting components or parts.
   b. Components or parts from the *content* of a system.

c. *Purpose* of a system gives it direction or meaning and provides its goals.
d. *Process*, or function, is a series of actions that help a system achieve its goals.

D. Suprasystems, systems, and subsystems.
1. Suprasystem: term sometimes used to denote a large and complex system (e.g., a society).
2. A subsystem is a system within a larger system (e.g., medicine system and nursing system within the health care system).

E. Humans as complex living systems.
1. Major health-related goals of human systems are to maintain internal equilibrium and live in harmony with the outside world.
2. Being healthy allows the human system to use its structure (content) and process (functions) to accomplish its goals and fulfill its purpose.

F. General characteristics and functions of living systems.
1. All living systems exist in space, their environment; they affect their environments and are affected by them.
2. Living systems exist in time. There must be continuous exchange between a system and its environment if it is to grow, develop, and survive.
3. Matter and energy are integral parts of a living system.
4. A living system needs *information* in order to make appropriate changes and adjustments for health and survival.

G. Open and closed systems and feedback.
1. A living system uses information obtained by feedback to make needed changes.
2. Closed systems do not exchange matter, energy, and information with their environments; open systems do.
3. Input is the matter, energy, or information received into the system.
4. Output is the matter, energy, or information that passes out of the system.
5. Feedback is essential to the self-regulating and self-correcting functions of a living system.
   a. Negative feedback is a corrective action.
   b. Positive feedback perpetuates or accelerates an existing condition, even if it is harmful to the system (e.g., continued division and growth of malignant cells).
   c. Self-regulation is essential to accomplishment of the living system's purpose, which is to maintain homeostasis in the internal environment and exist in harmony with the world around it.

H. Homeostasis and harmony.
1. Homeostasis is the tendency of biologic systems to maintain stability in the internal environment.
   a. Not a condition of stagnation or equilibrium but a "steady state" in which there are variations within preset limits (e.g., body temperature or acid-base levels in the body fluids).
   b. Variations take place in a predictable manner.
   c. Internal environment composed of body fluids that serve to integrate and unify cells and their activities throughout the whole body.
   d. Harmony with external environment.
      (1) External environment: physical, biologic, and psychosocial factors.

(2) Health requires adaptability and stability to maintain harmony with external environmental factors.

V. The consumer's concept of health and illness

A. Important to fostering voluntary action to meet health-related goals.

B. Health and illness behavior.

1. Health behavior: any action taken by person who thinks of himself as relatively healthy; done for the purpose of promoting health, preventing disease, or detecting disease in its early stages.
2. Illness behavior: undertaken by one who believes himself to be ill.
   a. Action taken to determine his state of health and to seek a suitable remedy.
   b. Person must answer the question, "What does it mean to be ill?" or "How do I know I am ill?"
3. Examples of health behavior: maintaining normal body weight, being immunized against communicable diseases, self-examination of the breast.
4. Examples of illness behavior: consulting physician or nurse practitioner, visiting neighborhood clinic, taking prescribed medications.

C. Cultural influences on health-illness behavior.

1. Effective nursing care depends on appreciation of cultural differences and adaptation to these differences among clients.
2. Cultural differences among racial and ethnic groups are apparent in attitudes and health practices (e.g., those related to birth, death, and general health care, responses to pain and suffering, adjustment to life changes).
3. Cultural attitudes, beliefs, and practices of patient may not be the same as those of a typical white, middle-class health care professional.
4. Patient is most obvious and valid source of information about his perception of health and evaluation of health care practices.
5. Views of consumer must be accepted with an open mind and listening heart.

D. Transcultural nursing.

1. Developed in response to need for meeting the challenge to know about and understand cultural differences.
2. Important that the nurse deal with each person as an individual whose views may not be the same as hers.

CHAPTER 2

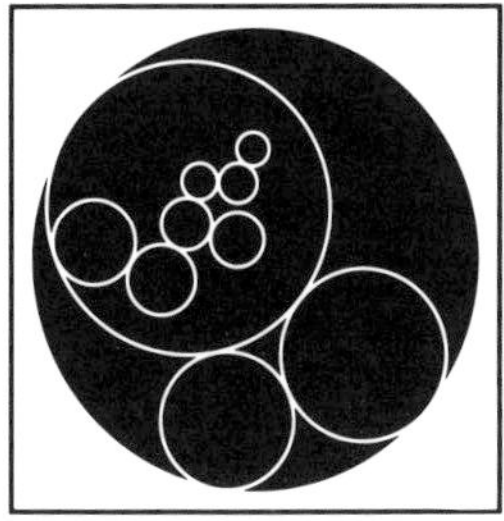

Concepts, Theories, Issues, and Trends Significant to Nursing

VOCABULARY

abstract
concept
hierarchy
holism
integration
intervene
process
proliferation
rationale
theory
validate

Upon completion of this chapter the student should be able to:

1. Describe how the theoretical frameworks of nursing contribute to the practice of the profession.
2. List three basic assumptions on which the philosophy of holistic nursing care is based.
3. Identify the interrelationship of basic human needs and the planning of nursing care.
4. From the American Nurses' Association definition of nursing, identify the components of holistic philosophy, human needs theory, and the concept of self-care.
5. After determining your feelings about the concepts and theories presented in this chapter, formulate your own definition of nursing.

Although nursing activities can be documented as far back as the written word records, the history of nursing really begins with Florence Nightingale (1820–1910), who crusaded to change the public's view of the nurse. Her belief in education, proper hygiene techniques, and preventive health practices and her theories regarding nursing practice still influence the nursing profession.

Throughout the twentieth century, the concepts and theories that make nursing practice what it is today have evolved and changed. Because of its nature, being integral to other health care professions, nursing has borrowed and adapted theories from other sciences and disciplines such as biology, psychology, and sociology.

Concepts are general ideas about the nature of something. They are derived from impressions received from the world around us through our senses and intellect. Your "concept" of family is derived from your own experience, what you have seen of other families around you, and what you have read and heard about families.

The word *theory* evolved from the Greek word *theoria*, which means the act of viewing, contemplating, or considering. Current definitions interpret the word to mean beliefs or underlying principles proposed or followed as the foundation for action. Theories of nursing are sets of beliefs or underlying principles that a particular individual has proposed as the basis of nursing practice.

When a person theorizes about something, he compares, experiments, and finds significant relationships that lead to a conclusion. In this sense, anyone who thinks extensively about a subject, comes to some conclusions, and tries them out in practice could be considered a theorist. However, the development of a theory should lead to the discovery of a truth. Nightingale's theory about the importance of a clean and orderly environment to the recovery of health was validated (shown to be true) when she proved that because of changes she initiated in the environment of her patients, the death rate among them dropped from a staggering 42 per 100 to 22 per 1,000.

Theories help describe and explain the relationship of concepts and make it possible to look at a particular phenomenon in a different, creative way. This is one reason the various scientific disciplines "borrow" theories from one another and apply them to situations in their own field of study. Nursing is no exception. It has taken advantage of theories in the biologic, physical, and behavioral sciences, as well as in the humanities, to develop its own unique theory for practice. When used appropriately, theories from other sciences have provided logical explanations for various approaches to patient care problems, helped to improve nursing practice, and served to predict with some accuracy the effects (outcomes) of specified nursing interventions.

In its broadest sense, the word* nursing *means nurturing.

To nurture is to provide nourishment, protection, and a wholesome environment in order to promote healing, growth, and development. Throughout human history there have always been some people who have chosen the role of nurturer in response to the needs of others. Out of this desire to give aid to those who are suffering, to prevent disease, and to promote health, the profession of nursing has evolved.

Nurturing is woven into the essense of nursing. However, the profession of nursing has taken portions of theories from other disciplines and interwoven them into a framework for practice. Central to the theoretical framework of nursing are the theories of holism, basic human needs, adaptation, and self-care. A brief description of these theories follows.

The modern practice of nursing focuses on the whole person: on helping him meet his physiologic, psychosocial, and spiritual needs. Modern definitions of nursing are derived, in part, from the belief that each person is a unified whole (the *holistic view*) and from acceptance of the theory that all humans share basic needs (*human needs theory*).

THE HOLISTIC VIEW

The fundamental idea of holism, that each person is a unified whole, has been with us for thousands of years. However, only within recent decades has it reemerged as a philosophy on which to base certain health care practices. Perhaps the one person most responsible for renewed interest in holism is Jan Smuts, a noted South African who formulated a philosophic theory of holism. Although he died in 1950, his writings continue to influence current thought about human nature and the maintenance of health.

It is important that we all clarify in our own minds what we believe about human nature and what each person is meant to be.

The value we place on human life, our ability to deal with sickness and death, and our decisions about how to behave toward other people are all profoundly influenced by our basic beliefs about other humans and our relationships with them.

Some basic beliefs about people and health that are typical of the holistic view are:

- Each person is a unique integration of body, mind, and spirit, and the unified whole is more than the sum of the body parts. Hence a change in one aspect of a person's life brings about change in every aspect of his being and alters the quality of the whole.
- Each person has potential for growth in knowledge and skills and in becoming more loving toward himself and others.
- Humans are naturally inclined to be healthy; each of us has responsibility for his own well-being, self-healing, and self-care.
- The "person" of an individual belongs to himself; therefore decisions about what happens to that person rightfully belong to the owner.
- The focal point of healing efforts is the person, not the disease or injury.
- The relationship between health care professionals and their patients should be one of mutual cooperation. Health care providers intervene in behalf of the adult patient only when their help is sought by the patient or when he cannot meet his health needs unaided and is unable to request their help.

From these basic beliefs about human nature have evolved a host of changes in the selection of approaches to health care problems. In holistic health care, traditional methods of surgical intervention and drug prescription are being integrated with or replaced by acupuncture, acupressure, biofeedback, meditation to reduce tension and stress, and various relaxation techniques for the management of pain, to name but a few of the less traditional approaches.

In some instances modern scientific research has found a physiologic explanation for the effectiveness of both ancient and new techniques that are employed in holistic health care. An example is the discovery of pain-killing *endorphins* (morphinelike substances produced within the body), which are released in response to such measures as massage, contrastimulation, and other practices that nurses have used for years to promote relaxation and relieve discomfort. (The management of pain through stimulation of the body's own natural pain relievers is discussed more fully in Chapter 10.)

When we think about the essential meaning of holism, the dignity it imparts to human beings, and the respect it has for human rights, it is easy to see why the concept has served as a foundation for many nursing practices and contributed to the development of virtually all theories of nursing.

HUMAN NEEDS THEORY

Proponents of human needs theory view the individual as an integrated whole who shares with all other humans some basic needs for survival and personal growth. A *need* is a lack, a desire, or a sense of something missing. When a need is perceived by an individual, tension is created within the person. This internal tension motivates the person to do something about his situation so that the felt need is partially or completely satisfied. In other words, the person's behavior is a goal-directed response; the goal is gratification of an unmet need. The manner in which a person behaves to meet his basic human needs is influenced by his cultural background, education, experience, present environment, and the opportunities available to him at any given moment.

MASLOW'S HIERARCHY OF HUMAN NEEDS

Abraham Maslow, a psychologist, philosopher of science, and leading spokesman for humanistic psychology, proposed a hierarchy of human needs as an explanation for the motivational forces that act as stimuli to human behavior. Since publication of his theory of human needs in the 1950s, Maslow's hierarchy has been revised, amplified, and applied to a wide variety of situations in the fields of nursing, the humanities, and management, to name but a few. Figure 2–1*A* illustrates the nature of the hierarchy and the various levels of human needs proposed by Maslow and adapted for nursing.

> ***A* hierarchy *is defined as the arrangement of objects, elements, or values in a graduated series.***

The hierarchy of human needs shown in Figure 2–1 identifies five levels arranged according to priority for the maintenance of human life. Theoretically, the physiologic needs such as food, air, water, and rest must be satisfied before the higher level needs emerge. This is true in general, but the order in which needs are felt and become important to an individual varies considerably from person to person and from situation to situation. For example, we usually do not expect a person who is starving, in pain, or suffering from a high fever to be concerned about his social status at the moment or about the development of his potential for becoming an outstanding concert pianist. Yet we have all known or heard about people who have become so absorbed in their work that they have forgotten to eat and sleep or have failed to notice that they are working in an uncomfortably hot or cold room. Another example of reversed priority of need is the infant who fails to thrive because of a lack of love and attention. Being loved and having human contact are more important needs for the infant than food and water. Lacking love and attention, he refuses to eat.

It also should be pointed out that once a

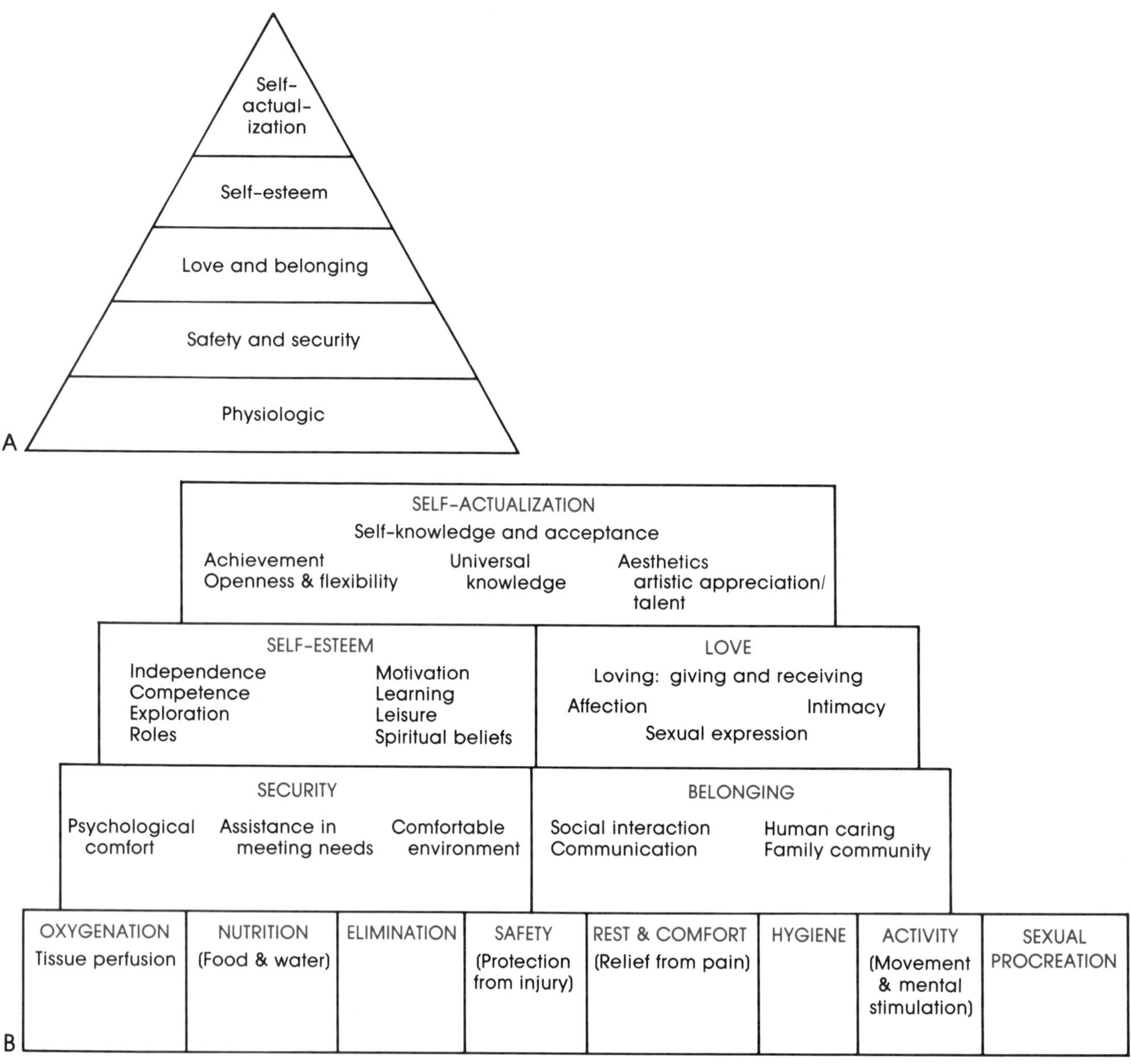

Figure 2-1 *A,* Maslow's original hierarchy of needs. Maslow's hierarchy has been adapted by nursing to help determine priorities of care. *B,* Fluid hierarchy for prioritization of patient care. Which needs take precedence at a particular time greatly depends on the individual patient's perception of his situation. Most of the time the first level of needs (physiologic) takes precedence, but sometimes higher needs are of greater importance to the patient. Priorities should be set according to patient input and perception of his own needs, along with consideration of the physician's orders and the nurse's assessment.

human need is met, it does not remain satisfied forever. This is obviously true in regard to food, water, air, and other first-level physiologic needs. Having one good meal, one drink of water, or one breath of air does not satisfy a person for very long. Requirements for satisfaction of higher level needs might not be obvious. The patient who feels isolated from other caring humans during hospitalization is not satisfied once and for all with a visit from a nurse making her daily rounds. He needs continued assurance that he is important, held in esteem, safe, and secure from harm.

Gratification of higher level needs can be postponed or modified while the more vital lower level needs are being attended to, but it cannot be put off indefinitely.

In essence, the arrangement of basic human needs in a hierarchy is based on the strength of each level, but the individual responds as a unified whole. Therefore the needs cannot be isolated, nor can we act as if the gratification of one need is the only thing happening to a person. A critically ill person whose circulation and respiration are being supported artificially continues to need personal contact with loving and caring people.

Levels of Human Needs

The relationships of the nursing process to each level of human needs will be discussed in greater detail in this and other chapters of this unit. In fact, the theory of human needs is incorporated into most, if not all, of nursing theory and practice. Maslow's hierarchy provides a framework for determining what a patient needs at any given time and how the nurse can help him meet his particular needs.

As a result of the evolvement of nursing theory and years of working with patients, it seems that an adaptation of Maslow's hierarchy in a more fluid form serves as a better basis for determining patient care priorities (see Fig. 2–1*B*). The nurse must remember that each patient views his needs somewhat differently and must be consulted about what he views as his priorities of care. For some patients a sense of security and belonging will be more important than having their physical needs met.

Physiologic Needs

Fundamental physical needs are considered to be the most influential, primarily because the life of the individual or the group of which he is a member cannot be sustained without their being satisfied. Everyone must take in food and liquids, inhale air, eliminate bodily wastes, have a balance of rest and activity, and be relatively free of pain. The first physiologic need is for oxygen and is immediately followed by the need for adequate cardiovascular function to provide for tissue perfusion. The needs for adequate nutrition and for elimination come next.

Basic safety needs are almost as important as physiologic needs. If the patient cannot be protected from the dangers of a high fever or a severe fall, attending to his physiologic needs is useless. Protection from physical harm, from a nursing standpoint, is equivalent in importance to (i.e., at the same level as) physical needs.

The need for rest comes next and includes freedom from pain, which can greatly interfere with rest. Hygiene needs follow the need for rest, as good hygiene is integral in providing comfort and adds a measure of safety and protection against the invasion of bacteria.

Musculoskeletal activity is also a basic physiologic need, for without activity of the muscles and joints, atrophy and deformity will occur, preventing normal function of the human being. Nurses therefore attend to assisting the patient with movement and ambulation or perform passive range-of-motion exercises for patients who are totally immobile.

Sexual expression is a physiologic and psychological need. Survival of a group in society clearly depends on sexual intercourse as a means of gratifying the sexual needs of at least some members of the group, if the group is to exist for more than one generation. Self-gratification of sexual needs fits best in the areas of self-esteem and love.

Security and Belonging

Once basic physiologic needs are satisfied, the needs for security and belonging demand attention. Security for patients mainly depends on the reassurance that their physiologic and safety needs will be met. Security also includes protection from psychological harm; freedom from anxiety and fear; and the need for structure, order, and a peaceful environment. The hospitalized child and the elderly person are particularly susceptible to stress created by an unfamiliar, disorderly, or hazardous environment. People value order, routine, and rhythm in their daily lives and thrive more readily in an environment in which they believe that these things are present, although it should be remembered that orderliness and routine are much more important to some people than to others.

Adults who suddenly become ill might be anxious about finances, loss of control, change in their body image, continuation of employment, and what will happen to them in the future if they must cope with the effects of a permanently disabling lllness or injury. Therefore emotional support from the nurse is very important. Active listening on the part of the nurse is essential in meeting the patient's security needs, because to feel secure, he must feel that his needs are being accurately perceived.

All human beings have a need for contact with others and to feel self-confident and worthwhile. Each person needs to feel that he belongs or is attached to others. People need to feel cared about, and they function best if they feel a sense of community with others. Some social interaction is essential to a sense of well-being and psychological balance.

Communication is the cornerstone by which human interaction takes place and is therefore very important. Providing a means of communication, encouraging sharing of thoughts and feelings, and therapeutically interacting with the patient is the core of good nursing practice. One can perhaps meet the basic physiologic needs of a patient without communication, but it is impossible to meet other needs if good communication is not present. Adequate feedback and clarification and validation of communication are essential.

Self-esteem and Love

Self-esteem and love are interrelated, for it has become apparent that one cannot truly love others until one first loves or accepts oneself. Self-esteem develops from feelings of independence, competence, and self-respect and from recognition, appreciation, and respect from others. One's employment, or work, and his various roles (e.g., as husband, father, brother, child, community leader, etc.) all contribute to his self-esteem. For many, spiritual belief systems are an integral part of the sense of self and of one's relationship to the universe. Gratification of sexual needs contributes to the feeling of wholeness of the individual and to one's identification and behavior as a male or a female.

Freedom from boredom, mental stimulation, motivation to seek knowledge, and learning play a role in self-esteem also. People have a desire and a need to explore the environment and universe around them. Illness often brings about the need for new knowledge in order to provide for adequate self-care. Without this necessary learning, self-esteem will decrease. The nurse must then become the teacher, helping the patient to meet these needs.

Balance in a person's life and self-image is brought about by the ability to enjoy leisure activity, to play, and to seek things that bring a measure of happiness.

Illness and adversity, particularly physical adversity, often damage the patient's self-esteem. The nurse can be very instrumental in helping him rebuild his feelings of competence, independence, and self-respect.

Love consists of both giving and receiving. We know that without love and attention, an infant will withdraw and gradually decline, despite having its physiologic needs met. Adults are not as dependent on receiving love as infants, but perhaps that is because they have the capacity to give love, and therefore feeling confident is not contingent on receiving it. Certainly being loved adds a tremendous dimension to the life and well-being of an individual, and losing love can cause discouragement, depression, and despair. Too often an elderly person who no longer has a mate or family and whose close friends have all died will give up on life, for he feels there is nothing left for which to live. Extreme prolonged deprivation of love and esteem can bring about neurotic behavior and organic illness.

Intimacy, that greater degree of connectedness, of feeling that one understands and is understood by another, is one of the fibers of love. The achievement of intimacy is the developmental task of the teenager and young adult. However, illness can greatly interfere with intimacy for all adults. Nurses need to provide ways for intimacy needs to be fulfilled, especially in patients with long-term or chronic illnesses.

Self-Actualization

Self-actualization is an area to which people do not advance until the physiologic, security and belonging, and self-esteem and love needs have been met. Self-actualization occurs when a person is very comfortable with himself and is certain of his beliefs and values but is flexible; he is self-reliant but open to new ideas and has sought and come to terms with areas of universal knowledge and truth and is functioning at a level akin to his full potential. Creative expression, be it in an area of performance or appreciation, is part of the self-actualization process. Self-actualization is an ongoing process, not something reached at a particular point in time. Maslow says that "self-actualization is a matter of degree, or little accessions accumulated one by one"

TABLE 2–1 MASLOW'S PROFILE OF THE SELF-ACTUALIZED PERSON

1. Healthy; polite; versatile, expressive; lets go when he wishes to; can drop controls, inhibitions, and defenses when deemed desirable; can relate interpersonally on a deeper level.
2. In control of himself and his impulses; can avoid hurting others; can have fun or give up fun.
3. Thinks in the present and the future; has a large array of responses and can move toward full humanness.
4. Efficient and superior in his perception of reality and his relations with reality; can see concealed and confused realities more swiftly and more accurately than others.
5. Superior in his ability to reason, to perceive truth, to make conclusions, and to be logically and cognitively efficient; can discriminate between good and evil, means and ends.
6. Accepts self, others, nature; is natural, simple, and spontaneous in his behavior.
7. Strongly focuses on problems outside himself, is not a problem to himself or generally concerned with himself; has a mission in life, a task to fulfill—some problem outside himself that uses his energies.
8. Displays a quality of detachment, of a desire for privacy, autonomy, independence of the culture and the physical and social environment; has the capacity for fresh appreciation of the basic things of life; has a philosophical, nonhostile sense of humor.
9. Capable of intense peak or even mystic experiences (problem-centering; intense concentration; self-forgetfulness; intense enjoyment of music, art, and sensations).
10. Able to feel an identification, sympathy, and affection for human beings in the world (in spite of occasional anger, disgust, or impatience); has a democratic character and a desire to be of genuine help to the human beings in the world.

Adapted from Maslow, A. H.: Motivation and Personality. New York, Harper & Row, 1954.

(Maslow, 1971). Nursing actions that facilitate self-actualization are pertinent mainly during rehabilitation periods when the nurse assists the patient to strive to achieve his full potential.

We are self-actualizing rather than fully self-actualized at any given point in our lives. Maslow states that self-actualization is not a matter of achieving one great moment when the potential of a person is finally and for all time fully developed. As he writes: "It is not that on Thursday at four o'clock the trumpet blows and one steps into the pantheon forever and altogether. Self-actualization is a matter of degree, or little accessions accumulated one by one." Table 2–1 presents Maslow's profile of the self-actualized person.

Theories of human need are based on the assumption that humans are rational, decision-making beings. A person is believed to want to have control over his life, even when he chooses dependence over independence. Although a person is indeed free to choose, there is no guarantee that every choice will be a wise one. Patients can and do decide not to take doctor-prescribed medications, to continue drinking to excess, or to ignore advice of any kind offered by health care professionals.

The notion that every person has the potential for choosing that which is harmful to him, as well as that which is beneficial, is crucial to our understanding of how good health habits are developed, wholesome lifestyles are adopted, and disease is prevented. It is not enough to inform people of the dangers of obesity, the risks inherent in excessive drinking and smoking, or the folly of any other life-threatening behavior. Nurses must understand that behavior is based on what one perceives to be a need and how highly a person values satisfaction of that need.

NURSING THEORY AND HUMAN NEEDS THEORY

Human needs theory is integrated into much of nursing theory. In 1954, Virginia Henderson wrote: "The unique function of nurse is to assist the individual, sick or well, in the performance of those activities contributing to health or its recovery (or to a peaceful death) that he would perform unaided if he had the necesssary strength, will, or knowledge. And to do this in such a way as to help him gain independence as rapidly as possible." She defined nursing within the framework of 14 components of basic nursing care based on how the nurse could help the patient meet his basic human needs.

Faye Abdellah extended her definition of nursing to include not only individuals, but also family groups and society. She was concerned with basic human needs and applied a holistic approach to nursing care problems, working toward a goal of independence within the limits of the patient's capabilities. She formulated a list of 21 nursing problems that served as the foundation of nursing practice.

With time it has become apparent that it is essential to view nursing in terms of the patient and what the nurse can help him achieve, rather than what the nurse can achieve for him. With this change in thought came the beginnings of *nursing process*. Nursing process is the orderly method by which nursing care is delivered.

A nursing leader in the development of the concept of nursing as process, Helen Yura, combined several of the concepts and theories presented in this chapter. She defines nursing as "an encounter with the client and his family in which the nurse observes, reports, supports, communicates, administers, and teaches; she contributes to the maintenance of optimum health, and provides care during illness until the client is able to assume full responsibility for the fulfillment of his own basic human needs; when necessary she provides compassionate assistance with dying" (Yura, 1988).

Reflected in Yura's definition are the concepts of nursing as process, the specific roles of the nurse who is engaged in the process, the patient as a member of a family or group in society, the recognition of basic human needs, the goal of self-care, and the realization that death is an inevitable and natural aspect of life. Throughout this text we will continue to explore the influence of these concepts in the nursing process.

THE PERSON AS AN ADAPTIVE BEING

Adaptation is a process by which a person changes in response to factors in his environment (internal or external) and yet remains whole. Nursing theorists Myra Levine and Sister Callista Roy have developed theories of nursing that are based on adaptation as the central theme. They basically state that a patient is affected by factors in his environment and, using his own particular strengths and abilities, changes (adapts) to present conditions. Nursing activities are geared to assist the patient to adapt in a positive manner.

THE CONCEPT OF SELF-CARE

Other traditional definitions of nursing have focused on what the nurse does *for* a patient, rather than what she does to work *with* the patient as a partner. The notion of helping a patient reach some level of self-care has always been incorporated into definitions of nursing, but only recently has self-care been a major concern in providing nursing care. No matter what the health status of a person might be, he will need instruction, support, and guidance to help him care for himself.

Self-care is defined here as the process whereby laypersons (individuals who are not health-care professionals) initiate and carry out certain health practices on their own in order to maintain life, health (prevent illness), and personal well-being. The ability to perform these kinds of functions depends on how well informed the layperson is about good health practices and the prevention of disease and illness.

Implementation of the concept of self-care requires that the nurse assume the role of assistant or teacher to the patient. The patient is in control of what is happening to him insofar as this is possible. The patient, or the nurse and patient together, make decisions based on the patient's perception of the kind of help he needs from the professional. He becomes an active participant in his health care and status.

The concept of self-care fosters independence and contributes to personal growth, fuller development of human potential, and maturity of the individual. The outcome is an enhancement of the person's self-image and strengthening of his self-esteem. The professional caregiver brings expert knowledge and skills and provides support, counseling, and instruction as needed.

EXAMPLES OF SELF-CARE ACTIVITIES

Self-care involves activities for disease prevention, health restoration, and health maintenance. Examples of disease prevention include obtaining immunizations against polio, measles, tetanus, or influenza. Maintaining good, balanced nutrition and obtaining sufficient rest and daily exercise would also assist an individual in disease prevention. Health restoration self-care activities include taking prescribed medication on schedule, keeping medical appointments, losing excess weight, treating a wound as instructed, and obtaining extra rest after surgery. Health maintenance activities include self-catheterization, breast self-examination, home glucose monitoring for better control of diabetes, adherence to a diabetic diet, cessasion of smoking, and performing ambulatory peritoneal dialysis for management of chronic renal failure. Additionally, self-help groups, which promote self-care, have been successful in helping many of their members overcome a variety of problems ranging from obesity to drug and alcohol abuse.

OREM'S THEORY OF SELF-CARE

Throughout the evolution of professional nursing, leaders in the field have incorporated some elements of self-care into the development of their theories.

Dorothea Orem's theory of nursing is directly related to the concept of self-care. Orem recognizes that no person is completely self-sufficient; all humans depend on others to help meet some of their needs. According to Orem, there are three categories of self-care that a patient might have: basic needs, developmental needs, and needs that are a result of alteration in health status. Nurses operate within one of three systems to help the patient meet these self-care needs, or *requisites.* In the wholly compensatory system, the patient is unable to do much for himself and must depend on the nurse to act on his behalf. In the partly compensatory system, the patient participates in his self-care to the extent that he is mentally and physically able and seeks the assistance of the nurse to complete actions as necessary. The supportive-educative system is where the patient makes decisions about what knowledge or skills he needs and what support is necessary to carry out self-care activities. The nurse acts as the patient's agent in carrying out the patient's self-care activities (Fig. 2–2).

Orem's theory serves as a framework for developing instructions for a patient who must cope with the lasting effects of an illness or injury. For example, a patient who has suffered a spinal cord injury resulting in paralysis of the lower half of his body (paraplegia) will need assistance in learning new ways to meet such universal self-care needs as control of bowel and bladder function, protection from hazards, and normalcy. It should be pointed out that in this context the word *normal* does not have the same meaning for everyone. Self-catheterization can be normal for a person who accepts responsibility for handling his own routine procedures for elimination of urine from the bladder.

The paraplegic patient used as an example above will also need help in performing other activities related to health-deviation self-care. He will need to learn how to move about in his enviroment by transferring from bed to wheelchair, how to bathe and dress himself with minimum help, and how to revise his other routines of daily living. He also will need to modify his self-image, especially if he had been an active and independent person before the spinal cord injury, and he may or may not need to develop a new lifestyle. Decisions about the learning needs of the patient striving for independence and self-care are made on the basis of each individual's capacity for and willingness to accept responsibility for his own care.

Application of Orem's concept of self-care to the practice of nursing requires that the nurse focus on doing for the patient only those things that he cannot do for himself.

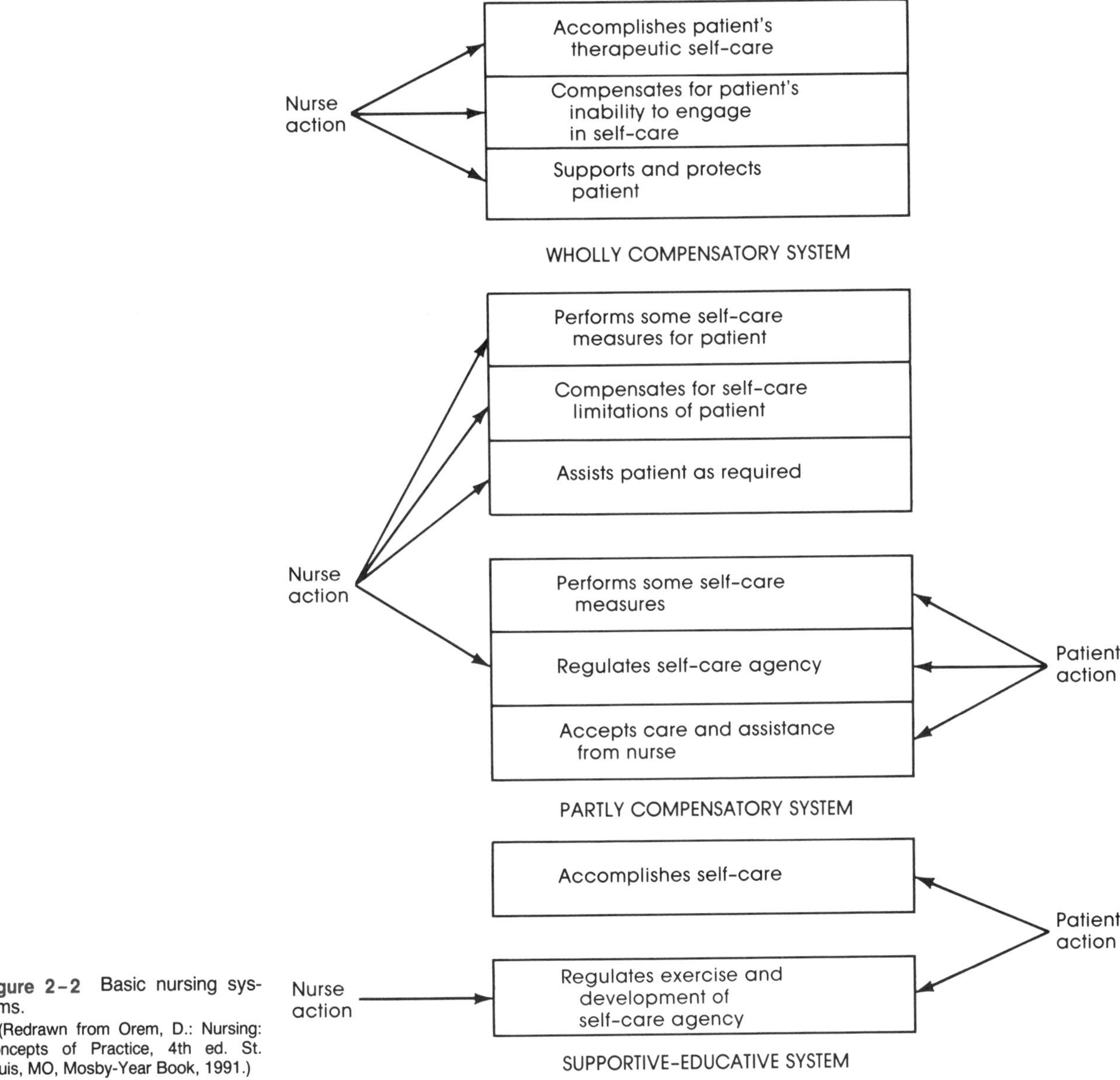

Figure 2-2 Basic nursing systems.
(Redrawn from Orem, D.: Nursing: Concepts of Practice, 4th ed. St. Louis, MO, Mosby-Year Book, 1991.)

Translation of self-care theory into nursing practice in an acute-care facility is essentially a matter of the nurse asking herself two critical questions as she works with patients: why is the activity being done, and how is the activity helping the patient take charge of his own self-care?

By focusing on the purpose of the assistance being given and the goal of maintaining, restoring, or increasing the self-care ability of the individual, the nurse can establish continuity of care that is goal-directed, rather than haphazard or routine.

ECONOMICS OF HEALTH CARE

As the cost of health care has sky-rocketed in the United States and elsewhere, the health care industry has placed more emphasis on self-care, health promotion, and disease prevention. Teaching and assistance for disease prevention and health maintenance should be the primary goals of each nurse from the minute she begins work with a new patient. "What can I do to assist this patient with his self-care both now and in the future?" should be the primary question in the nurse's mind.

CURRENT CONCEPTS OF NURSING PRACTICE

Nursing leaders continue their efforts to define and describe the practice of nursing and clarify the direction in which nursing has evolved. A major goal of these activities is to identify those things unique to the profession of nursing or to focus on what nurses fix.

The Social Policy Statement of the American Nurses' Association's (ANA's) Cabinet on Nursing Practice defines nursing as "the diagnosis and treatment of human responses to actual or potential health problems" (American Nurses' Association, 1983).

This definition focuses the attention of nurses on meeting each patient's needs, rather than those of an institution, another member of the health care team, or even of the nurse herself. Fundamental to acceptance of this definition is the belief that professions are granted rights, responsibilities, and privileges by the society to which they belong and which they purport to serve.

For one to have a clear concept of nursing, it is necessary to first think about the concepts of man, health, and environment, for these three are crucial to a definition of nursing. Various theorists have utilized different views of these components to formulate their particular definition of nursing. Florence Nightingale defined nursing as "the act of utilizing the environment of the patient to assist him in his recovery" (Nightingale, 1859).

The definition supported by the ANA allows for great variation in nursing practice, but the central theme is concern for human response and needs. For example, diagnosing an illness and prescribing medical or surgical treatment is within the domain of the physician. The patient's response to uncomfortable or tedious diagnostic procedures, the fears that arise when he learns of his diagnosis, any self-care limitations, impaired functioning, and the management of pain and other effects of chronic illness are all within the domain of nursing. Once a person learns, for example, that he has diabetes mellitus, the impact of the medical diagnosis can have far-reaching physiologic and psychosocial effects. The patient and his family will need special nursing care to help him adjust to changes in his diet, learn to administer his own insulin or have a family member do this for him, monitor his own urine and blood sugar levels, and undertake a special exercise program.

In the definition proposed by the ANA it is assumed that nurses assess each patient's health status and identify specific problems that are amenable to functions and goals within the realm of nursing practice. Assessment and nursing diagnosis as components of the nursing process are discussed in more detail in Chapter 4.

BIBLIOGRAPHY

Abdellah, F. G., et al.: New Directions in Patient-Centered Nursing. New York, Macmillan, 1973.

American Nurses' Association: A Social Policy Statement. Publ. no. NP-63. Kansas City, American Nurses' Association, 1983.

Chisholm, D.: Patient Classification: Why? Adv Clin Care, July/Aug., 1990, p. 4.

Donnelly, G. F., et al.: The Nursing System: Issues, Ethics and Politics. New York, John Wiley & Sons, 1980.

Dunston, J.: How managed care can work for you. Nursing 90, Oct., 1990, p. 56.

Henderson, V.: The nature of nursing. Am. J. Nurs., Aug., 1954, p. 64.

Joseph, L. S.: Self-care and the nursing process. Nurs. Clin. North Am., March, 1980, p. 131.

Lamonica, E. L.: The Nursing Process: A Humanistic Approach. Menlo Park, CA, Addison-Wesley, 1979.

Maslow, A. H.: Motivation and Personality. New York, Harper & Row, 1954.

Nightingale. F.: Notes on Nursing. London, Harrison & Sons, 1859. Reprinted by Dover Publications, Inc., New York, 1969.

Orem, D.: Nursing Concepts of Practice, 4th ed. St. Louis, Mosby-Year Book, 1991.

Yura, H.: The Nursing Process, 5th ed. East Norwalk, CT, Appleton & Lange, 1988.

STUDENT STUDY AIDS

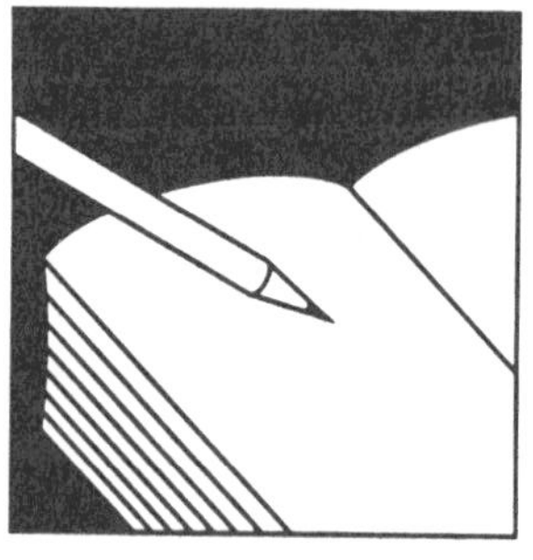

CLINICAL CASE PROBLEMS

Read each clinical situation and discuss the questions with your classmates.

1. Jan Cornell, age 26, suffered a fractured femur and head injuries in an automobile accident. She was transferred from the intensive care unit to an orthopedic unit 1 week after recovery from her head injury. She was in traction and experienced moderate discomfort at the site of the fracture.

Jan expressed concern about her daughter at home and said she was afraid she could never be a "good mother" again. She did not show any interest in her personal hygiene, activities of daily living, feeding herself, or recovering from her injuries. She cried often and behaved in a very childish manner.

- What are some of the basic human needs that Jan cannot meet for herself right now?
- Devise a holistic nursing care plan for Jan.
- What are some interventions that might help Jan become less dependent and better able to care for herself?

---

2. James Neaby, age 48, has cerebral palsy. He is confined to a wheelchair but bathes, dresses, and feeds himself. He sings in a choral group, practices law, and is a volunteer tutor for disadvantaged children. His hobbies include fishing and making up recipes for his sister, who is a gourmet cook. Mr. Neaby is a deeply spiritual person and has a delightful sense of humor.

- Considering Maslow's profile of a self-actualized person, which of these criteria do you think Mr. Neaby seems to meet?
- What could be some reasons why Mr. Neaby is unable to meet those criteria remaining on the profile?

STUDY OUTLINE

I. Introduction

A. A *concept* is a general idea or view of a particular entity.
B. A *theory* is a belief, policy, or principle proposed or followed as the basis of action.
C. Theorizing involves comparing, experimenting, and finding significant relationships.
D. Theories make it possible to develop creative approaches to the resolution of problems.
E. Scientists often apply theories from other disciplines to situations in their own field of study.
F. Theories from other disciplines have (1) provided logical explanations for nursing approaches, (2) helped improve nursing practice, and (3) helped predict nursing outcomes.

II. The holistic view

A. Basic tenets of holistic philosophy:
   1. Each person is a unique and unified whole that is different from and more than the sum of his body parts.
   2. Each person has potential for growth regardless of his state of development and maturity.
   3. Humans are meant to be healthy; each person has responsibility for his own well-being, self-healing, and self-care.
   4. The "person" of an individual belongs to himself or herself.
   5. The focal point of healing is the person, not the illness or injury.
   6. Health care is provided in mutual cooperation with the patient and only when it is sought by an individual who feels he cannot meet his own health needs unaided.

B. Holistic health care incorporates ancient and new, conventional and nontraditional methods.

III. Human needs theory

A. All people share common basic needs, rather than only biologic drives for survival.
B. A need is a lack, or sense that something is missing; this creates internal tension that acts as a powerful motivator and brings about goal-directed behavior. The goal is satisfaction of the unmet need.
C. Behavior in response to a felt need is influenced by culture, education, experience, and available opportunities.

D. The individual responds to felt needs as an integrated whole.
E. Maslow's hierarchy of human needs:
   1. A hierarchy is an arrangement of objects, etc., in a graduated series.
   2. Maslow's hierarchy (see Fig. 2–1).
F. Nursing theory and human needs theory:
   1. Most theories of nursing incorporate human needs theory.
   2. Yura's definition of nursing reflects the concepts of nursing as a process, man as a social being, human needs as the framework for determining how the nurse can assist the patient so that he can live his life more fully, and the belief that death is a natural aspect of life.

IV. The person as an adaptive being

A. Adaptation: process in which a person changes in response to factors in his environment and yet remains whole.
B. Nursing theorists Myra Levine and Sister Callista Roy have used adaptation as the core for their theories of nursing. Nursing activities are directed to assist the patient to adapt in a positive manner.

V. The concept of self-care

A. Self-care is the process whereby laypersons initiate and carry out certain health practices on their own to maintain health.
   1. Ability to carry out the roles of self-care requires a well-informed layperson.
   2. When illness or injury occurs, self-care includes actions the patient takes to restore and maintain as high a level of wellness as possible.
B. The patient remains in control and makes decisions based on his perception of what he needs from the professional.
C. The professional caregiver brings expert knowledge and skills and serves as a resource for the patient, who is an active participant in planning and implementing his health care.
D. Advantages of self-care concept:
   1. Fosters independence; contributes to personal growth, development of human potential, and maturation.
   2. Enhances self-image and improves self-esteem.
E. Examples of nursing intervention to assist the patient with self-care activities:
   1. Disease prevention: obtaining immunizations against disease, maintaining nutrition, getting sufficient rest and exercise.
   2. Health restoration: taking prescribed medication correctly, losing excess weight, treating a wound as instructed.
   3. Health maintenance: self-catheterization, breast self-examination, home glucose monitoring for diabetes control, cessation of smoking, performing ambulatory peritoneal dialysis.
   4. Self-help groups assist in overcoming problems such as obesity or drug or alcohol abuse.
F. Orem's theory of self-care
   1. Throughout nursing history self-care has been incorporated into nursing theory.
   2. Orem's theory recognizes that no person is completely self-sufficient.
   3. Three categories of self-care:
      a. Basic needs
      b. Developmental needs
      c. Needs that result from alteration of health status

4. Nurses operate within one of three systems to help patients meet their self-care requisites.
    a. Wholly compensatory system; patient is unable to do much for himself.
    b. Partly compensatory system; patient participates in self-care to the extent of his mental and physical abilities and seeks nurse's assistance to complete actions.
    c. Supportive-educative system; patient directs his self-care and seeks skills and support he needs for those activities.
5. Translation of philosophy of self-care into nursing practice demands focusing on the patients. The nurse asks: "Why am I doing this nursing activity?" and "How is this activity helping the individual to be his or her own self-care agent?"

VI. Current concepts and definitions of nursing

A. ANA defines nursing as "the diagnosis and treatment of human responses to actual or potential health problems."
1. Focus is on meeting patient's needs, rather than those of other members of the health team, the institution, or the nurse herself.
2. ANA definition allows for great variation in nursing practice.
3. Assumption is that each patient is assessed to identify specific problems amenable to nursing activities.

CHAPTER 3

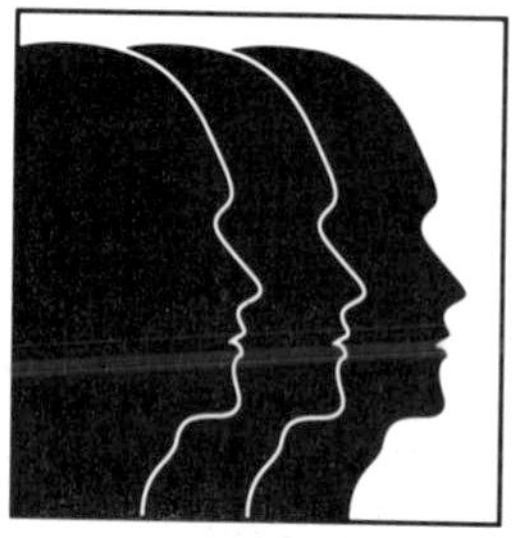

Psychosocial Aspects of Nursing

VOCABULARY

accountability
colleague
compassion
competence
dependency
esteem
humanistic
placebo effect
psychotic
vulnerable

Upon completion of this chapter the student should be able to:

1. Cite two reasons why humans need social interaction with other people.
2. Describe in own words the concept of "self" and the ways in which the nurse uses her "self" in the practice of nursing.
3. Use Carl Rogers' evaluative questions to assess her own ability to use "self" when caring for patients and their significant others.
4. List at least five expectations patients have of their nurses.
5. Discuss the rights and responsibilities of hospitalized patients.
6. Identify relationships among withdrawn, dependent, and hostile behaviors and specific unmet needs.
7. Assess the needs of patients exhibiting extreme inappropriate behaviors.
8. Develop and implement plans for nursing interventions to meet the identified needs of patients exhibiting inappropriate behaviors.

As was pointed out in Chapter 2, human need theory recognizes that people have basic needs that are dependent on social interaction with other humans. Once physical needs are satisfied, a person usually directs his attention and energy toward the world around him and seeks satisfaction of his emerging social needs. These needs are more likely to be met in a peaceful and safe environment (that is, one in which there is harmony among people and safety from physical and psychological violence).

A person must have interaction with other people to help him develop a good self-image and to see himself as worthy of the respect and esteem of others. His love and belonging needs are met when there is satisfaction of his desire for affection, intimacy, togetherness, and face-to-face encounter with others.

A nurse-patient interaction that goes beyond meeting the physical needs of the patient engages the personhood of both the nurse and the patient. Each brings to the situation his or her own unique self, the whole person each one is at the moment and is in the process of becoming.

In this chapter we will discuss the nurse's use of self in nursing; that is, how she uses the person that she is in a helping and healing way, and how she can contribute to fuller development of her own potential, as well as that of the patient.

In personalized nursing care the patient's feelings, values, and expectations for his own care are of primary concern to the nurse. Institutions that provide health care services also are interested in knowing what the consumers of their services perceive as important to their satisfaction with the care they receive. The results of surveys and studies conducted by professional nurses and by health care agencies are discussed and their implications for nursing care explored later in this chapter.

USE OF THE SELF IN NURSING

The word *self* has many meanings. In the context of this discussion it is intended to mean the entire person of an individual, the sum of the physical, psychological, social, and spiritual dimensions of one's personality—and then some. It includes those personal characteristics of which one might be conscious and those that transcend consciousness and enter the realm of mystery.

A nurse-patient interaction is a dynamic encounter between two people. As the word interaction ***implies, there is active participation on the part of both persons involved in the process.***

The patient is not merely a passive body to which things are done to help him survive an illness or injury and recover from its effects. He is, instead, a partner and the center of all activities related to improving or maintaining his well-being.

In an address to a group of nurses in 1955, Lydia Hall, who introduced the concept of total patient care, used four prepositions to describe the quality of nursing care from its least desirable to its most desirable. She spoke of nursing *at* the patient, *to* the patient, *for* the patient, and *with* the patient (Hall, 1955). Implied in Hall's words is the assumption that the patient can make a significant contribution to planning, implementing, and evaluating his nursing care and that he must be allowed the opportunity to do so insofar as he is able. Since Hall's suggestion that the ideal nurse-patient relationship is that of a partnership, research studies have borne out her theory that a collaborative effort between the nurse and patient results in more effective health care. In the process of collaborating with her patient, the nurse brings to the interaction her own unique self.

In general, the nurse uses her self in three broad areas: in the knowledge she has acquired through study and experience; in the hands-on skills she possesses; and in the values and beliefs she holds dear and the attitudes toward herself and others that she expresses in her behavior. Although each of us acts and responds as a whole person, the three areas just mentioned will be considered separately.

USE OF KNOWLEDGE

The nurse uses her knowledge of the physical, biologic, social, and behavioral sciences to promote health, prevent disease, and give the best care of which she is capable to those who are unable to meet their own health needs.

When it is appropriate to do so, she shares her knowledge with patients and their families, with members of the community in which she works and lives, and with her colleagues on the health care team. Preventive health care and preparation of a patient for self-care are but two of the important tasks requiring a giving of one's personal knowledge, insights, wisdom, and understanding. Throughout her professional life the nurse is obligated to continued learning and expanding her store of knowledge and to use it for her own benefit and that of others.

HANDS-ON SKILLS

The nurse uses her psychomotor (hands-on) skills in therapeutic procedures for the purpose of ministering to her patients efficiently, safely, and gently.

The hands of the nurse can themselves be a tool of healing when used with compassion and competence. The nurse who gives this part of herself in the practice of her profession must continually learn how to perform new procedures and develop facility in using new equipment and supplies. Technologic advances within the past few decades have dramatically changed and will continue to change the clinical settings for patient care, particularly in emergencies and for those who are critically ill. Nurses are expected to be adept in their handling of sophisticated monitoring devices and complex instruments that provide information about the physiologic status of a patient and in manipulating machines that give life-sustaining support to those who cannot maintain vital physiologic processes on their own.

CULTURE, VALUES, BELIEFS, AND ATTITUDES

The culture that each person was raised in has a direct influence on the development of that person's attitudes, values, and beliefs. The Oriental woman has a much greater degree of modesty ingrained from childhood than the white American woman. The Hispanic man grows up with a much greater emphasis on the "macho" image than does the white male in America. Cultural beliefs are intertwined in each person's entire being and need to be considered by the nurse when she works with each patient. She needs to review what effect her own culture has on her perspective of the patient and his problems, as well as consider the impact of the patient's cultural background and beliefs on his view of his illness and recommended treatment.

A person's values, beliefs, and attitudes are outwardly expressed in the behavior of that person. Every day of their professional lives nurses deal with situations that require value judgments. There can be no such thing as "value-free" professional behavior for the nurse, because the choices she makes, her responses to requests for help and guidance, and her ability to give emotional and spiritual support are greatly influenced by her personal beliefs and values. The many ways in which a nurse might share her values and personal beliefs are not easily defined and measured. Of all the health care professionals, it is the nurse who spends the most time with the patient, is closest to him, and deals most intimately with him.

It is understandable, then, that it is most often the nurse who is called upon when the patients and their families and loved ones must cope with the sadder aspects of human existence. In order to give strength and support in times of pain and human suffering, the nurse herself must have some inner resources of faith and hope to draw upon. One cannot give to others that which she does not have.

A person's values and personal convictions are developed in a host of ways. For some, many of their values were acquired through religious education and from the examples of moral and ethical behavior set before them by their parents, teachers, and other authority figures and by their peers. Others have rebelled against religious teachings and parental guidance or have not received much help in this area of their personal growth. Many have either developed their own value system without formal training and guidance or remained unclear as to what they really do hold sacred.

The professional nurses' code of ethics and standards for practice recognize a person as a whole being with needs other than the purely physical (Table 3–1). They challenge the nurse to assist the individual in all facets of his life, through joy and sorrow, fear and anxiety, anger, hope and despair, and pain and suffering. In

TABLE 3–1 **CODE FOR NURSES**

1. The nurse provides services with respect for human dignity and the uniqueness of the client, unrestricted by considerations of social or economic status, personal attributes, or the nature of health problems.
2. The nurse safeguards the client's right to privacy by judiciously protecting information of a confidential nature.
3. The nurse acts to safeguard the client and the public when health care and safety are affected by the incompetent, unethical, or illegal practice of any person.
4. The nurse assumes responsibility and accountability for individual nursing judgments and actions.
5. The nurse maintains competence in nursing.
6. The nurse exercises informed judgment and uses individual competence and qualifications as criteria in seeking consultation, accepting responsibilities, and delegating nursing activities to others.
7. The nurse participates in activities that contribute to the ongoing development of the profession's body of knowledge.
8. The nurse participates in the profession's efforts to implement and improve standards of nursing.
9. The nurse participates in the profession's efforts to establish and maintain conditions of employment conducive to high-quality nursing care.
10. The nurse participates in the profession's effort to protect the public from misinformation and misrepresentation and to maintain the integrity of nursing.
11. The nurse collaborates with members of the health professions and other citizens in promoting community and national efforts to meet the health needs of the public.

From Code for Nurses with Interpretive Statements. Kansas City, MO, American Nurses' Association, 1985.

order to accept that challenge, the nurse must know what she believes in, have the strength of her convictions, and be able to express them to others. Otherwise, she has limited personal resources to depend on when either she or those who look to her for help are experiencing mental and physical anguish.

Most people, when confronted with pain and human suffering, ask why such things must happen. The patient with an incurable terminal illness asks, "Why me?" The parents of a seriously ill child ask, "Why us?" And the nurses caring for a vivacious teenager suddenly and permanently disabled and disfigured in an accident caused by a drunk driver ask, "Why her and not the person responsible for this tragedy?" There are no logical answers, no reasonable explanations for such heartbreaking calamities. Each person must deal with the mysteries of life and death and the meaning of pain and suffering in his or her own way. How this is done depends in large part on the person's previous experiences and thoughtful contemplation of these mysteries. Boros suggested an answer when he said, "Life's ultimate questions—and among them are certainly sickness, suffering, and death—must be dealt with in the light of the fundamental insights of our faith; otherwise the answers are not merely too superficial, but simply false" (Boros, 1966).

Whatever her source of strength, when a nurse uses the self therapeutically, she shares her hope in the face of apparent hopelessness; she shares her understanding of the meaning of life, death, illness, and suffering; and she shares her faith and confidence in powers beyond those of human endeavor. This implies a sense of her own worth and an understanding of the purpose of her own life and how she is fulfilling that purpose.

This kind of inner strength and self-understanding is exemplified in an encounter between a nurse and the son of one of her terminally ill patients. One evening the young man, who was about her age, became distraught over his father's imminent death. He approached her in the hall and asked how she could do nothing to save them, and how she could stand to be around people who were dying, how she slept at night knowing she could do nothing to save them, and how she could continue working in a place filled with such hopelessness. The nurse replied that she did indeed spend some miserable nights grieving over the loss of those whom she had come to know and love as her patients. But she knew that her task was to be there with them during their final days and not desert them, to ease their final passage whenever and however she could, and to provide whatever support her presence might give. She was committed to sticking with them to the end. The young man looked at her intensely for a long moment, nodded, and with tears in his eyes hugged her, turned, and walked back to his father's room.

Perhaps this young man, the nurse, and others like her understood the sense of the words of Alfred Delp: "When through one person a little more love and goodness, a little more light and truth come into the world, then that person's life has meaning."

Giving of the self can make one extremely vulnerable and at risk for misunderstanding and rejection. One who is willing to take that risk has a reasonably high level of self-esteem and self-confidence and a wholesome appraisal of his or her own strengths and limitations. Most successful people, whatever their field of endeavor, see themselves as good and their accomplishments in life as worthwhile. They have a positive self-perception that gives them a hopeful outlook and an acceptance of themselves as they are. In short, in the words of Don Hamachek, "They see themselves as fundamentally and basically 'enough.'" They are, therefore, prepared to take the risk of committing themselves to and caring for and about other people. They have learned from experience that it is in taking risks and experiencing failure and success, rejection and acceptance, uncertainty and certainty, that one grows to fuller maturity and greater wisdom.

THE HELPER ROLE

Therapeutic use of self involves entering into a special kind of relationship with another person.

In the nurse-patient relationship the nurse most often, but not always, is in the role of helper (Fig. 3-1). Carl Rogers, a humanistic psychologist, suggested that the type of helping relationship that exists between the psychotherapist and his patient can be therapeutic in all kinds of situations in which one person reaches out to help another, whether it be teacher to student, parent to child, or nurse to patient. He defined a helping relationship as one "in which at least one of the parties has the intent of promoting growth, development, maturity, improved functioning, and improved coping in the life of another" (Rogers, 1961).

In an effort to identify the qualities one needs to be helpful to another, Rogers formulated a set of evaluative questions the helper might ask of herself. These questions, listed below and followed by some explanatory questions, can be used by the nurse to measure her own ability to use the self and to establish some goals for improving her skills as helper.

- "Can I *be* in some way that will be perceived by the other person as dependable or con-

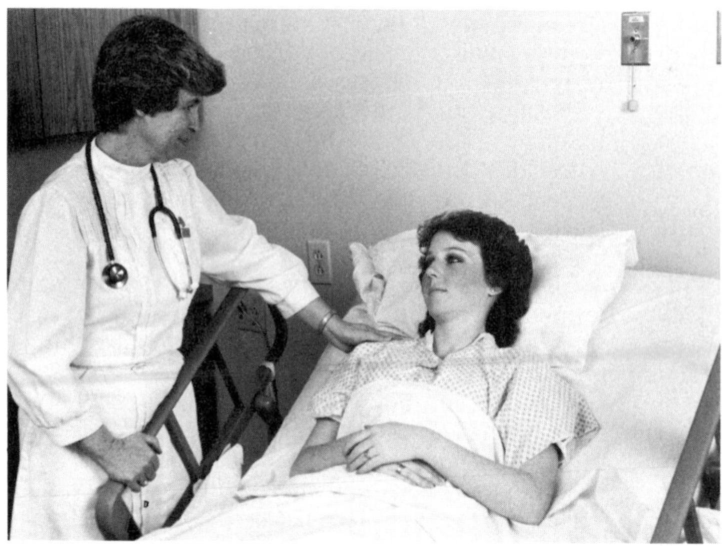

Figure 3-1 The nurse enters into a special kind of therapeutic relationship with her patient by being there when needed and showing care and concern. (Photo by Ken Kasper.)

sistent in some sense?" Am I punctual? Do I do what I say I will do? Do I keep my promises? Am I even-tempered or moody and unpredictable?

- "Can I be expressive enough as a person that what I *am* will be communicated unambiguously?" Am I honest, direct, and true to the attitudes of total acceptance that I claim to be ideal? Or do I send conflicting messages in what I say and do?
- "Can I let myself experience positive attitudes toward this other person—attitudes of warmth, caring, liking, interest, and respect?" Or do I remain professionally aloof and cool toward the other person? Am I afraid of becoming involved or misunderstood? Can I take the risk of loving? Am I afraid to care?
- "Can I be strong enough as a person to be separate from the other?" Can I accept our differences in values, behavior, and attitudes? Do I have the strength of my own convictions and the courage to remain true to them? Do I recognize and accept my own strengths and limitations?
- "Have I sufficiently identified and understood my own emotional and evaluative reactions so that I am not engulfed and overwhelmed by another's depression, anger, or dependency needs?" Can I allow the other person to be angry, sullen, and ungrateful without taking his behavior as a personal insult? Do I realize that I cannot always find the perfect solution to every problem? Am I able to recognize who owns the problem and who is responsible for finding ways to either resolve or cope with it?
- "Can I let myself enter into the world of his feelings and personal meanings and see these as he does?" Even though I cannot always condone what the other person does, can I try to understand how he might think or feel? Can I avoid labeling him or putting him into some category? Can I acknowledge his very personal concerns without making a judgment about them?
- "Can I receive him as he is? Can I communicate this attitude?" Am I frightened, embarrassed, or threatened by his statements about how he feels or what he thinks?
- "Can I meet this other individual as a person who is in the process of *becoming*, or will I be bound by his past and my past?" Am I willing to help him develop his potential more fully and become something more than he is? Can I help him adapt to the periods of adjustment and change that are stages of growth in every person's life?

Each of us is in the process of developing our potential. Few, if any, of us can answer each of the above questions with an honest and resounding "yes." It is possible, however, that with experience in the therapeutic use of self and in knowing our strengths and weaknesses, progress can be made toward a freer, more helpful, and more satisfying relationship with those who come to us for help.

SELF-ESTEEM: THE NURSE AND THE PATIENT

Self-concept, *self-esteem*, or *self-image* is an integral part of each person's personality and greatly influences a person's mental and physical health. People who have a positive self-image are more capable of developing and maintaining warm interpersonal relationships. They can also resist psychological and physical illness better than those who have poor self-esteem. It is the responsibility of the nurse to assess her patient's level of self-esteem and, if it is low, to assist the person to develop a more positive self-image.

The nurse's self-concept is also very important. The nurse who has a positive self-image is better equipped to help patients meet their needs, because she can respond to them in a healthy and positive manner.

Essentially, *self-concept* and *self-image* mean how a person sees himself. *Self-esteem* indicates how a person feels overall about himself. Table 3-2 lists some behaviors that are associated with low self-esteem.

People with low self-esteem tend to be critical of themselves and their ideas and actions. The nurse can assist them to develop more positive thoughts and images about themselves by providing a model for them with positive statements about herself, such as, "I did a really good job redecorating the family room last weekend," or "I finally cooked a pie with a really good crust yesterday" and then asking what the patient has done lately that he feels good about—no matter how small the example. She can also give the patient honest, positive feedback such as "You managed more of your bath by yourself today!" Talking with the patient and getting him to express things he feels good about in his life can help him focus on positive, rather than negative, aspects of himself.

Another technique for helping the person to improve self-esteem is to use thought stopping. This is done by having the person say "stop" or "no" to himself every time he finds himself thinking or saying something negative about himself. One way for the nurse to do this for herself is to put a rubber band on her wrist for a few weeks, and every time she thinks a negative thought, she gives the band a "snap." She can also ask her close friends to snap the band if they hear her saying anything negative about herself. This method simply makes the person more aware of how negative they are being and gives her an opportunity to rephrase the thoughts or words into something more positive. It is a matter of changing a habit. Positive affirmations of even the smallest kind, if used frequently, can set a person on the path to thinking positively about himself. By telling oneself "I'm clever," "I'm bright," "I'm pretty," "I'm a good person," or "I did that well" over and over can begin to change negative trends in thinking into positive ones.

Another tool for improving self-esteem is imagery, or visualization, in which a person visualizes positive images of the desired change in himself, and over time it becomes easier to be that image. For example, the person who finds it difficult to ask her family for help around the house can use this technique to become comfortable asking for help—and getting it! A positive goal is set: the family will help around the house. While quietly sitting, the visual image of asking each family member to help with a specific chore around the house is brought to mind. The words of the request are practiced several times, and with the eyes closed, the vision of the actual requesting is run through the mind. After utilizing this technique several times, the person will be more comfortable asking for the help and can reach the goal of getting it.

TABLE 3-2 BEHAVIORS ASSOCIATED WITH POOR SELF-ESTEEM

Avoids direct eye contact
Poor grooming; appears unkempt
Stooped posture
Makes statements critical of self
Has difficulty accepting compliments
Apologizes frequently
Avoids interacting with others
Fails to complete or follow through with projects
Is indecisive; has difficulty making up mind about things
Overly dependent
Verbalizes inability to cope
Displays lack of energy
Poor problem-solving ability
Verbalizes feelings of guilt

PATIENTS' EXPECTATIONS

The public demands that teachers, nurses, physicians, and other professionals who provide a service to the public be held personally responsible for the quality of service they provide. Nurses have traditionally been interested in providing a high level of care for their patients; however, the source of information about how well they have met their goal has typically been the nurses themselves. It was assumed that if they performed their nursing tasks according to established procedure, the quality of nursing care would be satisfactory to the consumer. However, as people have become more knowledgeable, more articulate in expressing their needs, more aware of the rising costs of health care, and more interested in the accessibility of the kind of care they want, they have become more insistent on having a say in the evaluation of their care.

In response to this trend toward consumerism, nurses and their organizations have set standards and criteria for evaluation of nursing care that focus *less on efficient performance* of specific nursing procedures and tasks, and *more on pa-*

tients' evaluations of the effectiveness of the end results or outcome of nursing activities.

Hospitals and other health care facilities also are concerned about how the people they serve view the quality of care they received in their institutions. Administrators and staff members are genuinely concerned about the quality of care they give and are interested in having satisfied consumers. There are, of course, many reasons for their concern, not the least of which is minimizing or eliminating altogether the possibility of lawsuits against them. People are less likely to take legal action against an individual or institution if they perceive the individual practitioner caring for them or those who work in the institution as friendly, helpful, and striving to do their best. In the days of the family doctor, who often was a friend of the family, knew each patient intimately, and was a respected and well-known member of the community, malpractice suits against physicians were rare. As medical and nursing care have become more depersonalized, legal action against physicians and nurses has increased greatly. Insurers of medical facilities, physicians, and nurses estimate that poor interpersonal relationships among practitioners and their clients and patients are a major contributing factor in more than half the malpractice suits brought against doctors and other staff members in hospitals.

SURVEYS OF HOSPITAL PATIENTS

Because health care facilities are interested in how patients and clients rate their effectiveness in the delivery of care, numerous studies and surveys have been conducted to find out what is important to the patients and their families and how they rate the quality of care and services provided by the facility.

In reporting results of a survey of hospital patients, the writer of one article was surprised to note that not a single respondent commented on the skill and expertise of the nurses. Instead, they repeatedly and spontaneously chose to evaluate the interpersonal skills and personal characteristics of the nurses. Positive comments included such words as "kind," "courteous," "helpful," and "concerned." In their negative comments the respondents used such words as "rude," "hateful," and "slow." These kinds of comments are typical of patients' and relatives' responses to questions routinely asked about hospital care.

Based on documented evidence received from numerous studies throughout the United States, it is safe to say that, above all, consumers of health care want that which we all want when we are being served—courtesy and respect.

NURSING'S STUDIES OF PATIENT EXPECTATIONS

One of the first studies conducted by nurses was done by Faye Abdellah and Myra Levine, who were interested in finding out what patients expect from their nurses. Their findings and the implications for nursing care are briefly summarized below.

First, the patient wants to be treated as an individual; that is, he wants personalized care that is designed to meet his needs.

He does not want care planned to provide the most efficient service to the most people in the shortest period of time. He wants to be called by name, not by room number or diagnosis. He wants to be recognized as a person, not a case study or locality.

Perhaps one answer to the question of dehumanized nursing care is preoccupation with routine tasks, policies, and procedures, which are as much a structural part of every institution as the bricks and stones of which it is made. Many nursing actions are carried out automatically and routinely. In recognition of the contrast between generalized and individualized nursing care, Orlando identified two major kinds of nursing action: automatic and deliberative. As a measure of whether her actions are automatic or deliberative, the nurse asks herself, "Why am I doing this?"

Automatic actions are done for reasons other than meeting the individual needs of the patient. For example, morning baths are insisted upon for every patient in spite of the fact that ambulatory patients may wish to have a shower at night, or a sedative is given because the doctor ordered it and not because the patient needs or wants sedation.

Deliberative actions are planned according to accurately assessed needs of the patient. He is asked whether the action is likely to meet his need, if it has been tried before, and if he thinks it could be helpful. How the patient feels about the action and what he thinks his need might be are clarified before the action is either carried out by the nurse or refused by the patient. Finally, the patient is asked to evaluate the effectiveness of the action once it has been carried out. An example might be a patient who is suffering mild discomfort but does not want to take an analgesic drug. The nature of the pain is explored with the patient, and the nurse suggests repositioning and a back rub to help him relax. The patient asks that he not have any visitors or treatments for the next hour so that he can rest quietly. Together they plan to try to relieve the discomfort using the nurse's suggestion for comfort measures and the patient's request for restriction of visitors. The plan is put into effect.

Later, the nurse talks with the patient about the effectiveness of their plan and learns that the patient did indeed find relief and rest. These measures then become a part of the nursing care plan so that all nurses caring for the patient can utilize these effective actions when the patient experiences discomfort. These deliberative actions illustrate the assessment, planning, implementation, and evaluation phases of the nursing process.

Another factor in the dehumanizing of patient care is the increased use of advanced technologic instruments for diagnostic and therapeutic purposes. Although the use of sophisticated equipment has greatly improved the efficiency of health care, it has at the same time presented the hazards of a machine-oriented society. In many instances the proper functioning of monitoring and support equipment means the difference between recovery and death. A major problem facing nurses today is that of maintaining a happy balance between attention to the machinery surrounding the patient and tending to the personal needs of the patient.

A major consideration of all health care workers should be the human rights of the patient. The first of the 12 patient's rights listed in the American Hospital Association's (AHA's) *Statement on a Patient's Bill of Rights* (Table 3–3) is "The right to considerate and respectful care." In a reference to the kind of dehumanizing effect hospitalization can have on a person, a distinguished physician has written:

> A stay in the hospital exposes an individual to a condition of passivity and impotence unparalleled in adult life, this side of prison. You are dressed in an uncomfortable garment, leaving you exposed and ludicrous; told when you must sleep and when you must rise; informed of what you may eat and when you have to eat it; notified as to when you can have visitors, who they shall be, and how long they can stay. You are discussed in the third person in your presence as though you were some idiot child or inanimate object. If you are unfortunate enough to have an interesting case, you will be presented to a group of strangers who may take the invasion of your privacy as their privilege (Gaylin, 1973).

Hospitals and other health agencies are required to have some rules and regulations that provide a safe and therapeutic environment for their clients. However, the mindless adherence to rules for the sake of legality, rather than for the welfare of the patients, can lead to the violation of the rights of those whom the agency and its health personnel have contracted to care for.

A second wish of the patient is to be given an explanation of his care.

He wants to know what is going to be done to and for him, why it is being done, and how he is expected to cooperate before, during, and after the procedure. He wants to know the expected outcome of treatments and asks that explanations be given to him in language he can understand. The second and third rights listed in the AHA's *Patient's Bill of Rights* refer to this issue (Table 3–3).

Although these statements are primarily concerned with communication between the patient and his physician, the basic principles of the patient's right to be informed about his health care apply to all aspects of that care. From the outset of their training in nursing, students are taught to explain procedures to patients. Perhaps it is the repetition of that or a similar statement at the beginning of every nursing procedure that has caused it to lose its meaning for many nurses. Regardless of the reason for the omission, the patient who is not given an adequate explanation of what is to be done has been denied his rights as a human being.

A third wish of the patient—to be treated as a partner—might well be the most important factor in his recovery and his ability to care for himself.

This is closely related to the will to live and is the essence of what has been described by Lydia Hall as the best kind of nursing care: nursing *with* the patient.

When a patient is treated as a partner, he is being told that he is a worthwhile individual whose thoughts and ideas count for something. The partnership recognizes our human need to have some control over what happens to us and some voice in the decisions that directly affect us. It implies a cooperative effort and a mutual conviction that the therapy being employed can and will have a desirable effect.

We do not yet know why a firm belief in the efficacy of a particular drug or treatment greatly improves its effectiveness, but what is known as the *placebo effect* cannot be ignored. If a patient believes that a treatment or drug will provide relief from his symptoms, the chances of the patient's experiencing that relief are vastly increased. Patients who are informed about the nature of their illness and given opportunities to participate in decisions concerning treatment are strongly motivated to follow the prescribed regimen. However, there is more to the partnership than giving the patient opportunities to set his own goals and plan for their attainment. The body has an innate ability to heal itself. A factor that has been called *the wisdom of the body* implies that the drive for self-preservation permeates every cell of our being. The mind and its powerful influence on the body's healing powers cannot be discounted when we deal with patients. Those who are treated with respect and trusted to know what is best for them are receiv-

TABLE 3-3 **A PATIENT'S BILL OF RIGHTS**

1. The patient has the right to considerate and respectful care.
2. The patient has the right to obtain from his physician complete current information concerning his diagnosis, treatment, and prognosis in terms the patient can be reasonably expected to understand. When it is not medically advisable to give such information to the patient, the information should be made available to an appropriate person in his behalf. He has the right to know, by name, the physician responsible for coordinating his care.
3. The patient has the right to receive from his physician information necessary to give informed consent prior to the start of any procedure and/or treatment. Except in emergencies, such information for informed consent should include but not necessarily be limited to the specific procedure and/or treatment, the medically significant risks involved, and the probable duration of incapacitation. Where medically significant alternatives for care or treatment exist, or when the patient requests information concerning medical alternatives, the patient has the right to such information. The patient also has the right to know the name of the person responsible for the procedures and/or treatment.
4. The patient has the right to refuse treatment to the extent permitted by law and to be informed of the medical consequences of his action.
5. The patient has the right to every consideration of his privacy concerning his own medical care program. Case discussion, consultation, examination, and treatment are confidential and should be conducted discreetly. Those not directly involved in his care must have the permission of the patient to be present.
6. The patient has the right to expect that all communications and records pertaining to his care should be treated as confidential.
7. The patient has the right to expect that within its capacity a hospital must make reasonable response to the request of a patient for services. The hospital must provide evaluation, service, and/or referral as indicated by the urgency of the case. When medically permissible, a patient may be transferred to another facility only after he has received complete information and explanation concerning the needs for and alternatives to such a transfer. The institution to which the patient is to be transferred must first have accepted the patient for transfer.
8. The patient has the right to obtain information as to any relationship of his hospital to other health care and educational institutions insofar as his care is concerned. The patient has the right to obtain information as to the existence of any professional relationships among individuals, by name, who are treating him.
9. The patient has the right to be advised if the hospital proposes to engage in or perform human experimentation affecting his care or treatment. The patient has the right to refuse to participate in such research projects.
10. The patient has the right to expect reasonable continuity of care. He has the right to know in advance what appointment times and physicians are available and when. The patient has the right to expect that the hospital will provide a mechanism whereby he is informed by his physician or a delegate of the physician of the patient's continuing health care requirements following discharge.
11. The patient has the right to examine and receive an explanation of his bill regardless of source of payment.
12. The patient has the right to know what hospital rules and regulations apply to his conduct as a patient.

No catalog of rights can guarantee for the patient the kind of treatment he has a right to expect. A hospital has many functions to perform, including the prevention and treatment of disease, the education of both health professionals and patients, and the conduct of clinical research. All these activities must be conducted with an overriding concern for the patient, and, above all, the recognition of his dignity as a human being. Success in achieving this recognition assures success in the defense of the rights of the patient.

Reprinted with permission of the American Hospital Association, copyright 1972.

ing physical and psychological support of a very special kind. They are being encouraged to will their own health—to use their whole being to repair and restore the body's tissues.

Fourth, but no less important, is the patient's desire to have his behavior accepted as part of his illness and not necessarily typical of the way he might react under more normal conditions.

If we understand that a person's response to a particular situation is the best he is capable of at that particular time, it is easier to accept his behavior, even though we might not condone it. The task of the nurse is to recognize the patient's behavior as resulting from the demands being placed on him at the moment. This requires kindness, understanding, and often firmness on the part of the nurse. People tend to become childlike and fearful when they are ill, and they appreciate having someone with them who can guide them through their ordeal gently and kindly.

The two major facets of nursing are *compassion* and *competence*. Patients want to be cared for by caring individuals who are fully competent in the skills of nursing. *They want a nurse to know what she is doing and to act as if she knows what to do.* They expect her to have the necessary equipment at hand before she begins a procedure, to be skillful and adept in using it, and to perform repeated procedures in the same manner and sequence as much as possible. Performing nursing procedures with consistency can reduce the patient's anxiety and build his confidence in the competence of the nurses. Even patients who appear to be semiconscious and unaware of most of the treatments being administered might know what is happening to them but be unable to communicate their awareness. If a tracheostomy is suctioned the same way each time according to a step-by-step procedure, the process becomes familiar to the patient. It might cause brief discomfort for him, but if it is done consistently he knows what to expect, and he is reassured of the competence of his nurses and the relief their efforts bring to him.

Finally, and perhaps most important to a patient's need for safety and security, is the nurse's ability to assess a situation quickly, make a decision, and act promptly to solve the problem.

There is perhaps nothing as exasperating to a patient as indecisiveness on the part of the nurse when a situation arises that the patient perceives as a crisis calling for immediate action.

In summary, patients expect and have a right to competent, confident, and caring professional help from nurses and other providers of health care.

MAINTAINING A PATIENT'S RIGHTS

One way in which the nurse can help the patient maintain his "rights" is to communicate effectively and to integrate teaching into every facet of her care. To be optimally effective, patient teaching must begin with admission and continue until discharge. It should not be left for a 5- to 15-minute segment of time the day of discharge.

During her initial admission assessment, the nurse should begin thinking about the various topics of health teaching that will be appropriate for this patient. Providing some general information is a start: how the television works, how to call the nurse, what the mealtime schedule is, and so on.

A review of the initial physician's orders will give clues to other topics. Teaching regarding what to expect for scheduled diagnostic tests or upcoming surgery and about each prescribed medication should come next. Before beginning teaching on any given topic, it is necessary to assess what the patient already knows about it. After a diagnosis is finalized, assessment of his perception of what the physician has told him is made and reinforcement teaching done regarding his disorder and its impact on his lifestyle.

An assessment of the patient's educational level, cultural biases, and personality type is necessary in order to determine what methods of teaching will be most effective for him. Some patients will need simple, concrete explanations; others do better with an audiovisual presentation or written materials.

Discharge teaching regarding diet, level of activity, continued medications, signs and symptoms to report, and the importance of follow-up care is begun as soon as the patient is well enough to retain the information.

A major part of patient teaching is taking the time to obtain feedback from the patient about what you have taught. What he has learned must be validated, errors in perception corrected, and reinforcement given in order for him to integrate what you have taught into his daily living. Return demonstration of a motor skill is essential and will make the patient more confident in his ability to carry out the procedure correctly once he is home.

COPING WITH "DIFFICULT" PATIENTS

Being hospitalized for any illness or injury can create emotional problems and unacceptable behaviors in patients who, under less trying circumstances, are mentally sound and emotionally mature. A holistic and personalized approach to nursing care certainly must respect a patient's need for emotional as well as physiologic support and provide planned nursing intervention to meet each patient's emotional needs.

Identifying and meeting a patient's emotional needs does not necessarily require an extensive knowledge of psychiatric nursing.

Patients whose primary illness is a physiologic rather than psychological disorder can sometimes behave in ways that are uncomfotable for the nurse who is not prepared to intervene effectively when a patient's emotional discomfort is expressed by dependent, withdrawn, hostile, or manipulative behavior.

The nurse who is able to provide effective planned intervention to meet a patient's emotional needs has learned to respond in an appropriate and therapeutic manner when a patient's extreme behavior is uncomfortable for her. In short, she is able to respond positively to the evaluative questions proposed by Rogers and listed earlier in this chapter.

There are techniques and interventions that nurses can effectively use to deal with patients who exhibit dependent, withdrawn, hostile, or manipulative behaviors, but first and foremost the nurse must remember that the patient needs to have his behavior accepted. The nurse should look for what is underlying the behavior. If the patient is extremely dependent, often he is extremely frightened. If he is withdrawn and depressed, he frequently needs help in bolstering his coping techniques. Hostility is sometimes an expression of anger toward the illness or oneself. Manipulation just might be a grasping for some control over a part of life when everything else seems out of control.

DEPENDENCY BEHAVIOR

Patients exhibiting extreme dependency behavior are attempting to satisfy an unmet need to depend on someone other than themselves.

In its extreme form the patient may refuse to do anything for himself. He might be unreasonably demanding of the nurse's time and attention, show little or no initiative in performing the simplest of self-care activities, or exhibit flirtatious behavior to attract attention to himself. This is the patient who is constantly ringing for the nurse and can't seem to do anything for himself.

Attempts to force the patient to do things for himself and develop some independence usually have the opposite effect, causing further regression into an even more dependent state and an escalation of unacceptable attention-getting behaviors.

Nursing interventions for dependent behavior are first directed toward meeting the patient's dependency needs and then gradually fostering independence once the dependency needs are met and the patient feels secure. Nursing actions initially include increasing the amount of time spent with the patient, establishing trust, anticipating his needs and wants, utilizing therapeutic touch, and assuring him that his needs will be met. Next, the nurse should encourage him to do one small task of daily care on his own, such as wash his own face or put on his own gown. When this is accomplished, lavish praise should be given. It is also helpful to focus on the patient's abilities and to praise each and every thing he does for himself. If constant ringing for the nurse is a problem, sometimes this can be cured by setting limits. Meet all of the patient's current requests and then tell him that you will check on him in 30 minutes if he will not use the call bell. Be sure that you check on him in exactly 30 minutes. By turning up as promised, you help him feel secure that his needs will be met, and the time period between checks can be lengthened to 45 minutes and then to 1 hour.

WITHDRAWN BEHAVIOR

Withdrawn behavior is a withdrawal from contact with others.

Extreme withdrawn behavior reflects a need to feel safe and secure and can be indicative of feelings of anxiety, fear, or sometimes anger. However, depression can also cause this type of behavior.

Although some degree of caution in establishing close contact with a stranger is natural when a relationship is new, continued withdrawal from the nursing staff can interfere with effective care and prohibit a therapeutic nurse-patient relationship.

Withdrawn behavior is characterized by silence, failure to make eye contact, recoiling from touch, superficial conversation without any self-disclosure or sharing of feelings, and denial of feelings. The patient also may deny a reality such as his own illness and its effects on his life.

Nursing interventions to meet a patient's need to feel safe and secure include providing a consistent routine of care so the patient knows what to expect; reducing environmental stress, confusion, and disorder; and limiting the number of health care providers the patient must interact with. Primary nursing as a mode of care is ideal for this kind of behavior problem.

Because these patients have a need for structure and trust, it is important that their nurses develop a reliable and trusting relationship with them. Whispering and secretive behavior on the part of the nurse can destroy trust. Teasing, joking, and otherwise failing to establish a bond of real friendship with the patient also can damage a trusting relationship and the patient's confidence in the nurse.

THE DEPRESSED PATIENT

Depression can range from occasionally feeling "blue" and sad to unrelenting despair and suicidal tendencies. Although some degree of depression might be expected in hospitalized patients, symptoms of depression should not be ignored.

A person's frame of mind can directly affect his rate of recovery and will to live.

Depression is usually expressed in withdrawn behavior. Signs and symptoms of depression are not always readily recognized. Loss of appetite, fatigue, vague aches and pains, insomnia, poor posture, gazing into space, and difficulty making decisions are all possible signs of depression. Sometimes the patient will make a statement such as, "I don't have anything to live for anymore," "I don't feel like eating or going anywhere," or "I don't care whether I get better or not."

Many times a depressed patient becomes more and more withdrawn and uncommunicative. Physical appearance and personal hygiene begin to deteriorate, and the patient has no interest in what is going on around him.

The truly depressed patient is a psychiatric problem and should be dealt with accordingly. One helpful nursing action is just spending silent time with the patient. This assures him that someone cares and is there for him, yet respects his desire to be withdrawn and silent.

Several other nursing interventions are sometimes helpful in relieving a patient's depression:

- Encourage and help the patient to engage in activities of daily living.
- Work at a slower pace and be patient and gentle.
- Emphasize the patient's good qualities and point out his accomplishments and strengths.
- Do not overdo being bright and cheerful in his presence or admonish him to "cheer up and look at the bright side of things."
- Show that you care by being with the patient and interacting with him.
- Encourage exercise and social interaction with others.
- Be alert for signs of self-destruction and the potential for suicide.

HOSTILE BEHAVIOR

Hostile behavior is an expression of the patient's need to have control over what is happening to him.

It can arise from fear, desperation, anger, and frustration. Illness inevitably represents some degree of loss. For some patients it is a loss of independence, loss of control over some body functions, or loss of the means to care for and financially support themselves or their family members. Others suffer a loss of self-esteem or a disturbance in self-image because of functional changes brought about by illness, disability, or surgical removal of a body part.

Losses of any kind can intensify the need to regain power and control over one's life. Behaviors that indicate a need to gain power or control include shouting, criticism, threats to "report" the nurse, and constant complaints about the care provided. Under a barrage of this kind of behavior it sometimes is extremely difficult for the nurse to be compassionate toward and concerned about the abusive patient. Planned and consistent nursing intervention often can change the patient's behavior to a more acceptable and comfortable level, and make his hostile behavior less uncomfortable for the nurse.

Sometimes it is not the patient who exhibits this kind of behavior, but a family member who is upset over a serious, rapidly progressing, or perhaps fatal illness of a loved one. In either case, no matter who is the aggressor, the natural reaction is to either become defensive or to counterattack and wage a power struggle. Neither of these reactions is an appropriate response to the patient's or family member's need for control.

Nursing interventions for expressions of anger that represent hostile behavior should begin with letting the person know you are aware of his anger and allowing him to express his feelings freely. The person could be asked what is upsetting him and what can be done to help him feel less angry and frustrated. It is important to listen *actively* to the person who is exhibiting hostile behavior. Usually the opportunity to release some of his pent-up anger provides some relief and permits a calmer and more reasoned approach to his problem.

Other interventions include allowing the patient to make suggestions about his care and giving in to his demands when they are not unreasonable and will not jeopardize his recovery. Physical activity can help release the pent-up energy associated with frustration and anger. Providing the patient with opportunities to participate in decisions and make choices in regard to his care can give the patient a sense of power and control.

Patients or family members who have a need for power and control sometimes feel better when they can talk to a supervisor or other person in a position of authority. This is not to say that the nurses caring for the patient are not providing the best of care, but rather that the patient or family member has a need to exercise some power and control and they perceive summoning an authority figure as a way to satisfy that need.

THE MANIPULATIVE PATIENT

Manipulative patients may use charm or flattery, seductiveness, lies, or threats to get what they want from the nurse. Sometimes they play one staff member against another ("splitting"). Examples of these various behaviors include: "Gee Paula, you do such a good job! They ought to promote you. Couldn't I have an extra dessert tonight?" "A hug would make me feel so much better." (Tomorrow he wants a full body clinch.) "The doctor said I only have to walk to the door." "If I don't get more pain medicine I'll kill myself." "I'm so glad you are here! Sally didn't come into my room all night. You are the only one who understands me."

This type of behavior has various causes. It may be a learned behavior that the patient uses as a way of communicating and responding to stress, or it may be a manifestation of a psychiatric disorder. However, many times it is based on fear of losing control. The manipulative person fears losing total control of himself or his environment.

Suggested ways of dealing with the manipulative patient include: (1) help decrease the need for control; (2) help him use alternate ways of coping; and (3) maintain an environment in which he feels safe, regardless of his behavior (Pelletier and Kane, 1989).

Specific interventions include the following:

- Set limits. Respond to the undesirable behavior as calmly as possible. Indicate that you will not tolerate the behavior. Tell him "Don't swear at me" or "Your screaming is inappropriate and disturbing to other patients and is making it impossible for me to help you; please stop and then tell me how I can help you."
- Be consistent and firm. Tell him when someone can help him and how often someone can check on him, and remind him of that when he demands attention between scheduled times.
- Don't take insults personally or become defensive. Take any threat of suicide seriously. Explore the situation by saying something like "That threat sounds like you are experiencing a lot of feelings you are not talking about. Can you tell me about them?" This lets him know you care.
- Be aware of your own feelings. This patient may remind you of a family member or friend who has used such tactics on you before.

If all of the above fail, rather than get into a shouting match or promote further hostility, tell the patient you are leaving the room because of his behavior and that you will be back when he has calmed down. State when you will be back and be sure you arrive on time. Of course, this can only be done if the patient is not in need of some immediate care.

BIBLIOGRAPHY

Antai-Otong, D.: What you should and shouldn't do when your patient is angry. Nursing 88, Feb., 1988, p. 44.

American Hospital Association: Statement on a Patient's Bill of Rights. Chicago, American Hospital Association, 1976.

Boros, L.: Pain and Providence. Translated by Quinn, E. Baltimore, Helicon, 1996.

Fertz, G. G., and Taylor, P. B.: When your patient needs spiritual comfort. Nursing 88, April, 1988, p. 48.

Fish, S., and Shelley, J. A.: Spiritual Care: The Nurse's Role. Downers Grove, IL, Intervarsity Press, 1978.

Gaylin, W.: Editorial: The Patient's Bill of Rights. Sat. Rev. Science, March, 1973, p. 22.

Hall, L. E.: Quality of nursing care. Presented at the meeting of the New Jersey League of Nursing, Feb. 7, 1955. Published in Public Health News, New Jersey State Dept. of Health, June, 1955.

Hirst, S. P., and Metcalf, B. J.: Promoting self-esteem. J. Gerontolog. Nurs., Feb., 1984, p. 72.

Kozier, B., and Erb, G.: Fundamentals of Nursing Concepts and Procedures, 3rd ed. Menlo Park, CA, 1987.

Lewis, S., et al.: Saving the suicidal patient from himself. RN, Dec., 1986, p. 26.

Muhlenkamp, A. F., and Sayles, J. A.: Self-esteem, social support, and positive health practices. Nurs. Res., Nov./Dec., 1986, p. 334.

Murray, R. B., and Zentner, J. P.: Nursing Concepts for Health Promotion, 5th ed. Englewood Cliffs, NJ, Prentice-Hall, 1988.

Norris, J., and Kunes-Connell, M.: Self-esteem disturbance. Nurs. Clin. North Am., Dec., 1985, p. 745.

Pelletier, L. R., and Kane, J. J.: Strategies for handling manipulative patients. Nursing 89, May, 1989, p. 81.

Reale, J.: Life changes: Can they cause disease? Nursing 87, July, 1987, p. 52.

Redman, B. K.: The Process of Patient Teaching, 5th ed. St. Louis, C. V. Mosby, 1985.

Richardson, J. T., and Berline-Nauman, D.: In the face of anger. Nursing 84, Feb., 1984, p. 66.

Roberts, C. S.: Identifying the real patient problems. Nurs. Clin. North Am., Sept., 1982, p. 481.

Rogers, C.: On Becoming a Person. Boston, Houghton Mifflin Co., 1961.

Townsend, M. C.: Nursing Diagnoses in Psychiatric Nursing: A Pocket Guide for Care Plan Construction. Philadelphia, F. A. Davis, 1988.

Valente, S. M., and Saunders, J. M.: Dealing with serious depression in cancer patients. Nursing 89, Feb., 1989, p. 44.

Ward, D. B.: Why patient teaching fails, fails, fails. RN, June, 1986, p. 45.

Yura, H, and Walsh, M.: The Nursing Process, 5th ed. East Norwalk, CT, Appleton-Lange, 1988.

STUDENT STUDY AIDS

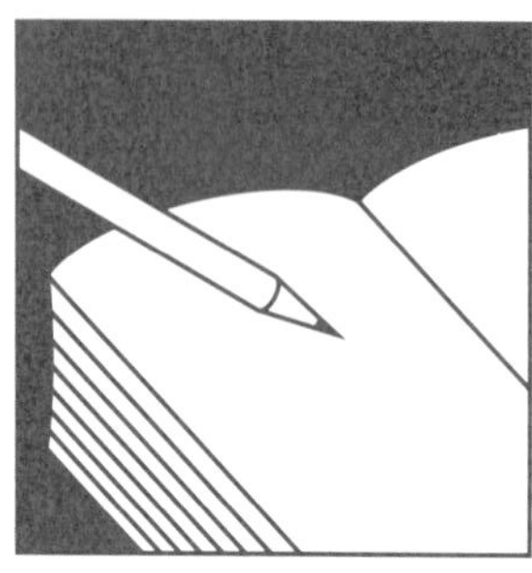

CLINICAL CASE PROBLEMS

Read each clinical case problem and discuss the questions and complete the exercise with your classmates.

1. Mary is a 16-year-old who dove into the shallow end of a swimming pool and sustained a cervical fracture and paralysis. She is almost totally dependent on others for the most basic of self-care activities.

Alfred Delp has written: "When through one person a little more love and goodness, a little more light and truth come into the world, then that person's life has meaning."

- Considering Mary's physical limitations and extremely poor prognosis for recovery, how can her life have meaning?
- Considering what little you can do as a nurse to improve Mary's prognosis, how could what you do for her give meaning to your own life?

2. Mr Porter has been hospitalized many times in the past few years and has earned the label "difficult patient" because of his abrasive and demanding personality.

- What do you think Mr. Porter's expectations of nurses might be?
- Conduct a survey among yourselves in the classroom to determine what each person thinks a patient should reasonably expect of nurses. Ask each person to list five expectations. After the survey, compare these expectations with those you listed for Mr. Porter and those listed in this chapter.

---

3. Sally is a 10-year-old Korean girl who is hospitalized with a fracture of the right tibia that she received in a bicycle accident. She also has a weeping wound of the left knee. She is to be discharged home on Friday.

- How would you assess what teaching will need to be done before discharge?
- Who will need to be included in the teaching sessions?
- How can you determine whether learning about cast care, medications, and wound care has taken place?
- What cultural implications related to the care of this patient might need to be considered in your teaching?

STUDY OUTLINE

I. Introduction

A. All humans have basic needs related to social interaction.
  1. Love and belonging needs are met when there is satisfaction of the desire for affection, togetherness, and face-to-face encounter.
  2. Nurse-patient interaction goes beyond meeting the patient's physical needs.
  3. Nurse and patient each brings his or her unique self to the situation (i.e., the person each *is* and is in the process of *becoming*).
  4. Interaction can bring about growth and self-fulfillment in both parties.

II. Use of the self in nursing

A. Self defined as the entire person of an individual, the sum of the physical, psychosocial, and spiritual dimensions, and then some.
B. Nurse-patient interaction is a dynamic encounter.
C. Active participation of the patient is essential for effective health care. Ideally, the nurse works *with* the patient.
D. Three general ways in which the nurse uses the self:
  1. Her knowledge: information that is important to the patient and can benefit him through the nurse's actions and in what he can be taught to do for himself.
  2. Skills in hands-on nursing activities affect the efficiency, effectiveness, and gentleness with which healing procedures are performed.
  3. Culture, values, beliefs, and attitudes: those things considered important to the nurse as sources of inner strength. They are the basis for ethical and moral action. A major task of nursing is to support others who are struggling with questions of life, death, pain, and suffering.
E. Use of the self gives opportunities for growth and self-actualization by taking risks and learning from failures as well as successes.
  1. Life's ultimate questions must be dealt with in the light of what one believes, trusts, and has faith in.
  2. The "good" nurse sees herself as basically "enough."

III. **The helper role**
   A. The nurse enters into a helping relationship with her patient, not unlike other relationships such as parent and child, teacher and student.
   B. Carl Rogers defines a helping relationship as one in which one person has the intent of helping another grow and develop psychologically and socially and mature so that he or she can function better in the world and cope more effectively.
      1. Evaluative questions formulated by Rogers can serve as criteria by which the nurse can judge her own effectiveness as helper and identify her own strengths and weaknesses.
      2. The questions are related to acceptance of oneself and others, risk taking, caring, and self-fulfillment.

IV. **Self-esteem and its impact on health**
   A. Self-esteem influences mental and physical health.
   B. Certain behaviors may indicate low self-esteem (Table 3–1).
   C. Methods for assisting patient to increase self-esteem:
      1. Modeling with positive statements and behaviors.
      2. Give honest, positive feedback.
      3. Teach him to use thought stopping for negative thoughts.
      4. Teach him to use positive affirmations.
      5. Use imagery and visualization for positive development of positive actions.

V. **Patients' expectations of nurse-patient interaction**
   A. Factors influencing interest in the consumer's evaluation of the care he receives.
      1. A more knowledgeable public.
      2. Rising costs of health care.
      3. Public's desire for accessibility of and contribution to the quality of health care.
   B. American Nurses' Association has developed standards and criteria for measuring quality of care that focus on the outcome of nursing actions and patients' evaluations of the effectiveness of care.
   C. Hospitals and other agencies are concerned about the quality of care they give and the problem of legal actions against them by the consumer.
   D. People are less likely to initiate lawsuits against institutions or individuals if they perceive them to be friendly, helpful, and striving to do their best.
   E. Surveys of hospital patients show that in general, people are more interested in the personal characteristics and interpersonal skills of their nurses than in their clinical expertise.
   F. Surveys conducted by nurses show that the typical patient wants:
      1. To be treated as an individual and his care to be personalized. Orlando identifies two major types of nursing actions: those that are carried out *automatically* for reasons other than meeting the identified personal needs of the patient, and those planned and implemented according to assessed needs of the patient (*deliberative* actions),
      2. To be given an explanation of his care.
      3. To be treated as a partner.
      4. To have his behavior accepted as part of his illness and not necessarily typical of the way he might respond under more normal circumstances.
      5. The nurse to be able to act decisively and accurately in a crisis.

VI. Coping with "difficult" patients

A. Illness and injury amplify unmet emotional needs, which can be identified through nursing assessment and handled by planned nursing interventions.

B. Effective nursing intervention for unacceptable behaviors does not necesssarily require in-depth knowledge of psychiatric nursing.

C. The patient needs to have his behavior accepted by the staff.

D. Help patients maintain their rights by communicating effectively and integrating teaching into all facets of care.

1. Assess teaching-learning needs on initial assessment; use patient interview and chart information to identity needs.
2. Assessment of educational level, cultural biases, and personality type is needed to determine most effective teaching methods.
3. Areas to be covered in discharge teaching include diet, level of activity, medications, treatments, signs and symptoms to report, and follow-up care.
4. Obtaining feedback about material taught is essential; return demonstrations of motor skills aids confidence when at home.

E. Dependency behavior is used to satisfy an unmet need.

1. The patient's needs must be consistently met by the nurse; establishing trust is vital.
2. Behavior modification is then used to alter the dependent behavior.
3. Lavish praise for self-care actions is important.

F. Withdrawn behavior.

1. Withdrawal can be an expression of anxiety, fear, anger, or depression and reflects a need to be safe and secure.
2. Characterized by silence, failure to make eye contact, recoiling from touch, superficial conversation, denial of reality.
3. Nursing interventions include providing structure and developing trust.
   a. Provide consistent routine of care.
   b. Reduce environmental stress, disorder, and confusion.
   c. Assign primary nurse for patient care.
   d. Avoid secretive behavior, teasing, and joking with patient.

G. The depressed patient: symptoms should not be ignored.

1. Depression affects recovery from illness.
2. Suicide assessment should be done if patient is deeply depressed.
3. Symptoms of depression include loss of appetite, fatigue, vague aches and pains, insomnia, poor posture, difficulty making decisions, withdrawal, and poor hygiene.
4. Spending time just in silence with patient can be helpful.
5. Chronic depression requires psychiatric intervention.
6. Nursing interventions can be helpful in alleviating patient's depression.
   a. Encourage engagement in activities of daily living and exercise.
   b. Do not rush patient.
   c. Emphasize his good qualities and point out accomplishments and strengths.
   d. Do not be too cheerful and bright.
   e. Encourage social interaction.
   f. Be alert for signs of self-destruction and suicidal tendencies.

H. Hostile behavior: an expression of a need for control over what is happening.

1. Hostile behavior can arise from fear, desperation, frustration, and

anger. Patient experiences sense of loss as a result of incapacitating illness or injury.

2. Characterized by shouting, criticism, threats, and constant complaints. Family members also can exhibit hostile behavior because of concern for patient.
3. Nursing interventions aimed at allowing person to ventilate pent-up feelings. Constructive help includes giving patient choices and opportunities for exercising control.
   a. Actively and nonjudgmentally listen to person.
   b. Allow person to make decisions and give in to demands that will not jeopardize his welfare.
   c. Encourage physical activity.
   d. Respect person's need to speak with authority figure.
4. Do not take anger or hostility personally.
5. Assist to find source of anger.
6. Set limits on patient's expressions of anger and hostility when necessary.
7. Seek help when unable to deal effectively with another person's anger or hostility.
8. If anger is getting out of control and harm may ensue, get help immediately.

I. The manipulative patient: may use charm, flattery, seductiveness, lies, or threats to get what he wants.

1. Manipulative behavior has various causes; it may be a learned behavior and used as a method of communication.
2. May be a manifestation of a psychiatric disorder.
3. May be based on fear of losing control.
4. Suggestions for dealing with the manipulative patient include:
   a. Help decrease the need for control.
   b. Assist with alternate ways of coping.
   c. Maintain a safe environment regardless of the behavior.
   d. Set limits; respond to undesirable behavior calmly.
   e. Be consistent and firm.
   f. Don't take insults personally or become defensive.
   g. Be aware of own feelings.

CHAPTER 4

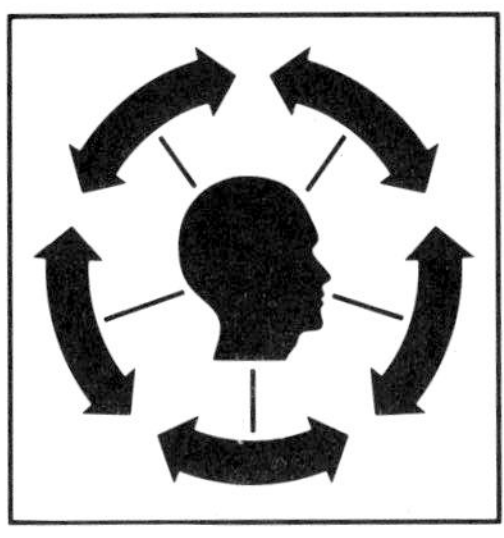

The Nursing Process and Documentation

VOCABULARY

assessment
chronologic
deviation
diagnosis
documentation
dynamic
evaluation
implementation
inference
intervention
nursing diagnosis
objective
outcome criteria
PEMS
planning
POMR
priority
problem oriented
process
regimen
SOAP

Upon completion of this chapter the student should be able to:

1. Define the nursing process and its goals.
2. Identify the role and functions of the nurse as a teacher.
3. State seven assumptions that are fundamental beliefs underlying the nursing process.
4. Give three reasons why nursing is considered a science.
5. List the five major components of the nursing process.
6. Describe the various methods by which a nurse performs an assessment of the patient.
7. Identify ways in which nurses participate in a quality assurance program.
8. List the steps in the teaching-learning process.
9. State four reasons why complete, accurate, and objective documentation by nurses is important.
10. Compare the SOAP method and systems charting of documenting nursing care.
11. Identify the kinds of information that make up a data base in a POMR system.

Nursing is essentially a problem-solving endeavor that should be approached and carried out in a scientific and orderly manner. Thinking of nursing as a problem-solving process provides the nurse with a framework for identifying and dealing with the actual or potential problems presented by her patients. The components of the nursing process give organization and direction to the activities that are in the realm of nursing care. The nurse enters into the process when she accepts responsibility for the care of each patient, recognizes him as a unique individual, and plans the care she will give according to his specific health care needs at any given moment. Additionally, the orderly approach inherent in the nursing process provides the means by which outcomes can be predicted and the results of nursing activities evaluated.

Communication is an essential part of any effective interaction between people. Documentation of the nursing process is the method by which vital information is communicated to all who provide health care to a patient. Written records provide continuity of care. Accurate and complete written records tell others on the health care team what is planned, what has been done, and how the patient has responded to whatever was done.

In the first portion of this chapter we will discuss the characteristics and goals of the nursing process, its basic components, and specific nursing activities for each phase. In the last portion we will discuss the reasons why documentation is necessary, some systems for recording nursing care, and some systematic ways of thinking about and writing information regarding nursing care given and the patient's response to his illness and care.

CHARACTERISTICS AND GOALS OF THE NURSING PROCESS

Process can be defined as a series of actions that move forward from one point to another on the way to accomplishment of a goal. In a process there is continuous progress through stages, each stage being dependent on the other and leading to a specific result, outcome, or product. In every process there is a moving force that controls and systematically directs activities so that the goal is ahieved, the desired result attained. The actions taking place in a process are deliberately and consciously carried out in a logical way. If a process is without a goal or there are no deliberate efforts to achieve it, the process has neither meaning nor substance and will sooner or later break down. The *nursing process* is a goal-directed series of activities whereby the practice of nursing is approached in a systematic and orderly way.

The goal of the nursing process is to alleviate, minimize, or prevent real or potential problems of health.

The problems that are identified in the nursing process are those that the nurse is qualified to treat by virtue of her education, experience, and commitment to the goals of nursing.

The nursing process is deliberate. It is not haphazard, routine, or unmindful of the needs of the patient. It demands careful thought about what is happening to the patient and how he is responding to activities intended to improve his health and well-being. It is, therefore, a rational and logical approach to the task of helping a patient meet his health needs.

The nursing process demands knowledge, skills, and a belief in the worth of every person.

The actions of the nurse are based on her knowledge of nursing theory, her competence in performing the techniques of nursing practice, and her understanding of and commitment to the basic philosophical beliefs and scientific principles derived from theories of nursing and other disciplines.

The sequence of events taking place in each phase of the nursing process promotes orderly progression from assessment for specific nursing care problems and formulation of nursing diagnoses to planning how to deal with them, implementing the plan, and evaluating the outcome.

The American Nurses' Association (ANA) provides measures to judge the competency of its membership and to evaluate the quality of services nurses give. These measures are the Standards of Practice, which were written to provide assurance that service of a high quality will be provided by nurses. These Standards are continually revised to reflect the emerging scope of practice for nurses.

The ANA Standards for Medical-Surgical Nursing Practice in an acute care setting are presented in the discussion of each phase of the nursing process.

DIFFERENCES IN ROLES IN THE NURSING PROCESS

Because of differences in their educational preparation for nursing practice, graduates, of 1-, 2-, 3-, and 4-year programs are expected to perform at different levels when engaged in the nursing process. In actual practice these role differences are not nearly so clearly defined as they might be; there remains some question about who is qualified, and therefore expected, to perform at what level. The National League of Nursing (NLN) is presently working to clarify roles and expectations for the graduates of these programs.

In addition to differences in formal educational preparation for the practice of nursing, there are differences in the amount of experience each nurse has and in the setting in which she practices. In general, graduates of 1- and 2-year programs mostly work in acute health care settings, long-term care facilities, or clinics, where they use the nursing process to achieve goals related to recovery from sickness and injury. Graduates of baccalaureate programs are more likely to practice in community-oriented settings where they deliver primary health care and practice independently and without direct supervision.

The essential tasks of the beginning nurse are: (1) contributing to an assessment data base for the patient by collecting information using a standardized form, performing basic psychosocial assessment, and taking objective measurements of body functions; (2) assisting with development of nursing care plans and then implementing the established plan of care by (3) performing basic therapeutic and preventive nursing measures; and (4) participating in evaluation of the care given by reporting observed outcomes and making necessary changes according to the results of the evaluation.

The information presented in this chapter and the remainder of this text is intended to help prepare the beginning nurse for competent performance of these tasks. They are relatively complex tasks within the nursing process and demand a sound knowledge of nursing principles and a commitment to the basic assumptions and beliefs presented below.

UNDERLYING ASSUMPTIONS OR BELIEFS

The nursing process is based on some fundamental beliefs about human life, the role of nursing, and the delivery of health care. These beliefs are:

- Every person is endowed with worth and dignity.
- Every person has basic needs common to all humans, and these needs must be met to some degree if a person is to survive and enjoy an acceptable level of wellness.
- Meeting one's basic human needs may require assistance from someone else until one is able to resume responsibility for oneself.
- Every person has the right to service of high quality, regardless of his socioeconomic status, cultural background, race or religious beliefs.
- A patient and his family prefer a patient-centered approach that actively seeks their input and respects their thoughts, feelings, and needs.
- The focus of nursing should be on maintaining health, preventing disease, and rendering help to the sick and injured.
- The nurse who engages in the nursing process will continue to work toward her own self-fulfillment through continuing study, learning, and improving competence.

NURSING PROCESS AND THE SCIENTIFIC METHOD

Nursing is a science. It uses scientific methodology as a framework for organizing the many activities performed by the nurse on behalf of her patient.

Typically, the scientific method involves recognizing that a problem, question, or relationship exists or might exist. The problem or question is then stated in such a way that it has meaning for the problem solver and can be understood by others familiar with the problem area. Once the problem is stated, the remaining steps are: determining the nursing diagnosis, deciding on a plan of action to deal with the problem or find the relationship, carrying out the plan, and evaluating the results. The components of the nursing process are similar to these steps in the scientific method (Table 4-1).

Scientists in many different fields use the

TABLE 4-1 **THE RELATIONSHIP OF THE NURSING PROCESS TO SCIENTIFIC METHODOLOGY**

Nursing Process	Scientific Method
ASSESSMENT	PROBLEM FINDING
	Gathering information
Data Base	Examining information
	Interpreting information
	Identifying the problem
NURSING DIAGNOSES	Stating the problem
Priority Setting	
Goals	PROBLEM SOLVING
	Developing alternatives
	Making a decision
	Deciding on a plan of action
PLANNING	
IMPLEMENTATION	Executing the plan
EVALUATION	Evaluating the results
REVISION	Revising as necessary

Adapted from Fredette, S., and O'Connor, K.: Nursing diagnosis in teaching and curriculum planning. Nurs. Clin. North Am., Sept., 1979, p. 544.

time-honored scientific method. Physicians and nurses may use essentially the same sequence of activities, but the kinds of information gathered by each, the activities performed, and the methods of evaluation are different. Most of us are familiar with the medical process that begins when the physician evaluates his patient's physical condition. At the initial visit to the doctor the patient's medical history is taken, and a physical examination is done. Any number of diagnostic tests might be done by the clinical laboratory staff, radiologist, and others involved in diagnostic testing. On the basis of information obtained through these procedures the physician makes a medical diagnosis and decides on a plan of treatment. This might consist of prescriptions for drugs, surgical intervention, therapeutic treatments such as physical therapy, and other procedures carried out by the physician himself or delegated to others.

When she is engaged in the nursing process the nurse is aware of the patient's medical diagnosis, the medical care plan, and the rationale for the prescribed medical regimen. However, her primary concern is for patient care problems and nursing measures to deal with these problems. She develops her nursing care plan so that it is in conjunction with and complementary to the physician's plan of care. Integration of the medical plan and the nursing care plan results in the total patient care plan.

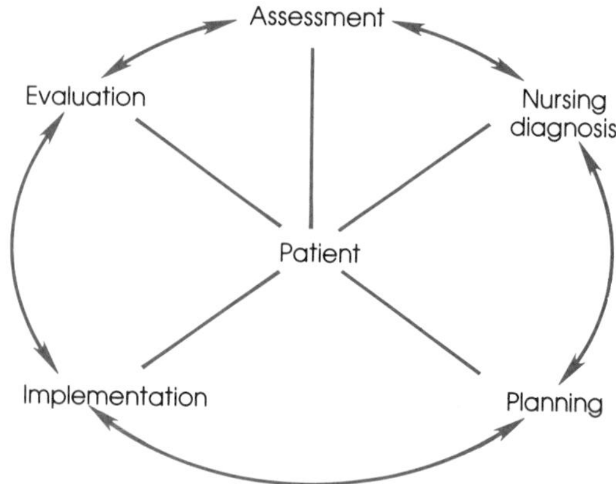

Figure 4–1 The five-step nursing process. The nursing process is set in motion at the time of the initial assessment. There is continuous interaction among the components. The patient is the center and focus of all activities within the process. Arrows point in both directions, indicating that the process is always in motion. Thus each component is subject to revision as new information is obtained through interaction with the patient.

There are currently five components of the nursing process: (1) assessment, (2) nursing diagnosis, (3) planning, (4) implementation or intervention, and (5) evaluation. Some theorists have used a four-step model of the nursing process, in which diagnosis was considered part of the assessment component. In keeping with current usage, however, the five-step model will be discussed here.

COMPONENTS OF THE NURSING PROCESS

The components of a system are its structural parts or elements.

For example, the components of a heating system are the thermostat, the furnace, the fan, radiators, or other structures that bring heat into a room. The components of the nursing process are sometimes called *phases* or *stages* through which the process moves toward achievement of its goal. Although there is a beginning and an end to each phase, none stands alone. Each phase is dependent on the others, and there is continuous interaction among them as information and energy flow through them (Fig. 4–1).

Because the nursing process is dynamic, its components represent points at which action can take place in response to feedback. It is a continuous process in which evaluation and revision of the plan occur constantly. As a patient's status changes and some problems are alleviated, other problems can arise, requiring a change in the plan and in the actions that are taken. The process is cyclical, with each component reacting to input from, and providing output for, each of the other components.

ASSESSMENT (DATA GATHERING)

ANA Standard 1. The collection of data about the health status of the patient is systematic and continuous. These data are communicated to appropriate persons, recorded, and stored in a retrievable and accessible system.

The purpose of a nursing assessment is to collect a complete, relevant data base from which a nursing diagnosis can be made. Information for the data base is gathered in a purposeful way, not accumulated just for the sake of collecting facts. In general, the more relevant information one has about a problem, the more likely one is to identify the problem correctly and arrive at a satisfactory resolution. However, in a life-threatening situation requiring immediate intervention, the nurse quickly assesses the patient's needs and determines the appropriate action to take.

During the nursing process assessment and reassessment are ongoing tasks. An *initial* assessment is made at the time of admission to the hospital or clinic. The information or data gathered at this time are used to establish a *data base* from which nursing diagnoses can be formulated. The data base also can be used later to determine whether the patient is progressing or regressing.

For example, the nurse might learn through her initial assessment that the patient with heart disease is 100 pounds overweight. This information is useful in setting a realistic goal for a return to normal weight and in deciding whether the goal has been reached.

Sources and Techniques for Assessment

There are several sources of assessment data available to the nurse. If nursing care is to be patient-centered, the most obvious source is the patient, his family members, and other persons significant in the life of the patient (significant others). Information-gathering techniques include (1) review of records, (2) the interview, (3) psychosocial assessment, (4) spiritual assessment, (5) observation, (6) physical examination (including objective measurement of vital signs and other bodily functions), (7) review of laboratory data, and (8) consultation with other health team members.

Records

At the time of admission some information about the patient will be available on an admission form. This will tell the admitting nurse such things as the patient's name, age, religious affiliation, and medical diagnosis; the reason for admission; and other pertinent information. If the patient has had previous admissions, medical records and documentation of care received will be available for the nurse making an initial assessment. Numerous previous admissions usually give an idea of the chronic nature of the illness or illnesses suffered by the patient and his long-term needs for nursing intervention. The physician's history and physical examination report will contain valuable information about the overall health of the patient.

Interview

The *interview* is conducted with the patient and, whenever possible, one or more family members. At this time a nursing history is obtained. This is sometimes referred to as an *admissions interview, health appraisal,* or *assessment questionnaire.* The interview is conducted in a systematic and orderly manner, using a printed format so that the nursing data base will be as complete as possible. The printed form might be organized according to body systems, a "head to foot" appraisal, or patterns of health-related behaviors such as nutrition, elimination, activity and exercise, sleep and rest, and so on. A nursing history and assessment form that is organized under nine health-related categories and that facilitates nursing diagnosis is shown in Figure 4–2. Additionally, information regarding health problems in relatives is sought.

Before starting the interview the nurse should gather as much information about the patient as she can from his admission forms, physician's orders accompanying the patient (if any), and previous hospitalization records (if available). This is done to avoid repetition of data gathering. Having to answer the same kinds of questions posed by several different people can be exasperating to the patient and can give the impression that members of the health care team are not in communication with one another.

The nurse begins the interview by introducing herself and explaining why she is going to be asking the questions. The patient should be told that his responses will be recorded and the information used to help his nurses get to know him better and plan his care more effectively. He is assured that he is free to answer or not answer any of the questions asked and that he may add any pertinent information at any time he thinks it would be helpful. The interview should be conducted in a place in which there will be some privacy and freedom from distraction and should take about 20 to 30 minutes to complete.

At the end of the interview the nurse briefly summarizes the data she has gathered and clarifies with the patient any important points or questions she might have. Summarizing the information with the patient shows him that the nurse has been an interested and attentive listener and is concerned about him. It could be at this point that the patient begins to trust the nurse and is able to express his feelings more openly and ask questions more freely. As a final gesture the nurse might ask if there is anything that has been missed during the interview that the patient thinks is important to his care or his problem.

Psychosocial Assessment

In order to holistically care for the patient, the nurse must gather sufficient data regarding the psychological and sociological areas of the patient's life.

Sociological data include the patient's educational level; his employment status; his marital status; the number of children, their ages, and whether they are living at home; whether the patient has health insurance; where he lives and what the household is like; whether he has a pet; what his hobbies or leisure activities are; with whom he has significant relationships; and any significant problems he might presently have other than his state of health. Cultural beliefs and values, especially in relation to illness and health care, need to be assesseed. It is essential to determine whether the patient has a solid support system.

NURSING ASSESSMENT

Chief complaint as stated by patient: ____ Patient's understanding of condition ____
Secondary health problems: ____
PHYSICAL ASSESSMENT TIME ____ T ____ P ____ R ____ BP: L. Arm ____ R. Arm ____ Ht. ____ Wt. ____
Neurological: No known problem ___ Oriented ___ Lethargic ___ Comatose ___ Muscular weakness ___ Paralysis ___
Headaches: ____ Seizures ____ Vertigo ____ Syncope ____
COMMENTS: ____
Sensory Deficit: No known problem ___ Speech ___ Tactile ___ Pain ___ Hearing ___ Vision ____
COMMENTS: ____
Integumentary: No known problem ___ Intact ___ Color ____ Diaphoretic ___ Dry ___ Temperature ____ Drainage ___
COMMENTS: ____
Muscuolskeletal: No known problem ___ COMMENTS: ____
Respiratory: No known problem ___ Dyspnea ___ Productive Cough ___ Non-productive cough ___ Char. of Resp. ____
Breath Sounds ____ COMMENTS: ____
Cardiac: No known problem ___ Angina ___ Irregular Rhythm ___ Palpitations ___ COMMENTS: ____
Circulatory: No known problem ___ Cyanotic ___ Pain ___ Varicosities ___ Bleeding ___ Edema ___ Pulses ___
COMMENTS: ____
Endocrine: No known problem ___ Diabetes ___ Thyroid Dysfunctions ___ COMMENTS: ____
G.I.: No known problem ___ Abd: Soft ___ Tender ___ Firm ___ Distended ___ Nausea ___ Vomiting ___
Present Diet (cultural considerations): ____ Food Allergies ____
Diarrhea ___ Normal Bowel Pattern: ____ Aids: ____
Bowel Sounds: ____ COMMENTS: ____
G.U.: No known problem ___ Freq. ___ Dysuria ___ Hematuria ___ Nocturia ___ COMMENTS: ____
Reproductive/Genital: Do you do monthly: self breast exam? Yes ___ No ___ Testicular exam? Yes ___ No ___ Changes Noted ___
Date of last breast exam by physician: ____ Date of last pap smear ____
Breasts: No change ___ Lumps ___ Discharge ___ COMMENTS: ____
LMP ____ Contraception ____ Grav ___ Living ___ Para ___
No known problem ___ Rash ___ Tenderness ___ Swelling ___ Discharge ___ Itching ___ Sores ___
COMMENTS: ____

CONDITION OF SKIN
Abrasions/Bruises •
Lacerations/Scars —
Decubiti O
Reddened Areas □
Burns ★
Rash △
COMMENTS:

Locomotion: Independent? YES ____ NO ____
Dependent due to: ____
Aids used: ____

CURRENT MEDICATIONS				
NAME	DOSE	FREQ.	HOW LONG?	LAST DOSE

Brought to Hospital? Yes ___ No ___ Sent to Pharmacy Yes ___ No ___
ALLERGIES (what and type of reaction) ____

PREVIOUS MEDICAL/SURGICAL HISTORY AND COMPLICATIONS	
DATE	Chronic illnesses or diseases and surgeries

PREVIOUS MEDICAL/SURGICAL HISTORY AND COMPLICATIONS	
DATE	CONTINUED

Tobacco Use: (#PPD, # Years, Type) ____ Alcohol: (Type, Amt., Freq.) ____
ENVIRONMENTAL EXPOSURE: Toxic Chemicals: ____ Infections: ____
Environmental Allergies ____

FAMILY HEALTH HISTORY: Diabetes: ____ Heart: ____ Hypertension: ____ Epilepsy: ____
Cancer: ____ Respiratory: ____ Kidney: ____ Mental Health Problems: ____ Other: ____

Psychological Data: Are you worried about anything now? ____ Behavior observed: ____
How do you handle stress/worries? ____ What do you do to relax? ____
What can we do to help you feel more comfortable during this hospital stay? ____
Name of Physician Notified: ____ Date/Time ____ Family Physician ____
Nurse's Signature and Title ____ Date/Time ____

ADDRESSOGRAPH

PATIENT'S STRENGTHS

SIGNIFICANT SOCIOCULTURAL DATA
MARITAL STATUS: | SIGNIFICANT OTHER:
OCCUPATION:
INSURANCE:
SPIRITUAL DATA: (Sources of Strength) | LIVING ARRANGEMENTS:

DISCHARGE PLANS
Projected Date: | Discharge To:
Potential Problems | Projected Needs

CARE PLAN REVIEWED/UPDATED
Date and Initial Appropriate Box When Updated

DATE	SIGNIFICANT CLINICAL EVENTS

Referrals/Date
( ) Social Service ____
( ) Clergy ____
( ) Home Health Care ____
( ) ____
( )

ADM. DATE	DIAGNOSIS	HOSPITAL #	SURGERY/DATE	PT. CLASSIFICATION INITIAL	DISCHARGE

ROOM	NAME	AGE	DOCTOR	DRUG ALLERGIES

Figure 4-2 Sample form for recording data from nursing history and initial assessment. (Courtesy St. Mary's Hospital, Athens, GA.)

Psychological data focus on how the patient perceives his state of health, his coping abilities, his past pattern of reacting to stress, his level of self-esteem, his perceived roles, and the dynamics of family relationships. Are there signs of extreme nervousness, anxiety, or depression? Each of these states can interfere with the patient's ability to take in information and to quickly progress to wellness.

Many times home or work problems affect the patient just as much as or more than his current health problem. An effective care plan can be devised only if the entirety of the patient's life is considered.

Educational level can be assessed by determining how well the patient reads, paying attention to the vocabulary he uses, determining his occupation or profession, or asking him about his school years. Level of education plays a key part in determining how the patient can best be taught what he needs to know in order to take care of himself.

When seeking information about past response to stress and usual coping patterns, find out what stresses he has experienced in the past and then ask him how he reacted and made decisions. Does he gather data, withdraw, and carefully consider the facts before making a decision and taking action? Or does he quickly assess the situation and make a snap decision? Does he lose his temper and yell? Or is he cool and calm? Does he adapt to almost any situation and make the best out of it that he can?

Spiritual Assessment

Regardless of whether one agrees that spiritual care is within the realm of nursing care, commitment to meeting the needs of the whole person must take into account the spiritual aspect of human nature.

Assessment of spiritual needs and planning for their gratification are not emphasized in nursing literature. One reason usually given for this reluctance to confront spiritual concerns and distress in a patient is that religion and matters of spirituality are personal and private. It is feared that patients and their families might resent having a nurse enquire into their beliefs and practices. Many nurses assume that they and their patients would be uncomfortable dealing with the subject. However, as has been pointed out by several authors, nurses usually have no difficulty asking the most intimate questions about their patients' bodily functions and sexual feelings and practices.

Another reason frequently given for failure to help a patient spiritually is that nurses are not qualified to handle problems of this kind. However, of all health care personnel, it is nurses who spend the most time with their patients, are most readily available in times of spiritual and emotional crises, and are presumably the most committed to holistic health care. Additionally, it is reasonable to expect a competent nurse to be able to use her "self" as a source of strength and hope when her patient is trying to cope with questions about the meaning of life and death and of sickness and suffering. Such competence is gained only by actively seeking answers for oneself and by sharing one's insights and beliefs with others.

During the assessment phase of the nursing process it is most often the case that spiritual assessment is limited to finding out from the admission sheet whether the patient is affiliated with some religion. This is obviously not enough information to do any more than pay lip service to nursing the whole patient. At the time of the initial interview to obtain a nursing history, the nurse might more thoroughly assess her patient's spiritual needs once she has gained his trust and confidence. Stoll suggests that questions about values and beliefs be asked toward the end of the interview (Stoll, 1979). Furthermore, she stresses the importance of respecting the patient's religious beliefs and his right to remain silent if he does not wish to talk about the spiritual dimension of his life.

Another approach is to question the patient about whether spirituality is important to him. What does he do to nurture his spiritual self? Does he meditate? What sources of spirituality does he feel give him strength? Does he have a spiritual adviser?

Table 4–2 lists four general areas of concern with pertinent questions in each area. The table is a summary of Stoll's suggestion for a spiritual history guide to be used during assessment. The guidelines can be used on admission or at any point during nurse-patient interaction when it seems appropriate to help a patient deal with his spiritual needs.

Once a patient's needs have been identified, the nurse can draw on a number of sources of help for her patient. She can, as previously stated, depend on the use of self and her personal inner strengths and resources. Other sources include praying with the patient, reading

TABLE 4–2 SPIRITUAL ASSESSMENT GUIDE

Area of concern: Concept of God or deity.
Pertinent questions: Is religion or God significant to you? If yes, can you describe how? Is prayer helpful to you? In what way is it helpful? Does a God or deity have influence on your personal life? How would you describe your God or what you worship?

Area of concern: Sources of help and strength.
Pertinent questions: Who is the most important person to you? To whom do you turn when you need help? How do they help? What is your source of strength and hope? What helps you most when you are afraid or need special help?

Area of concern: Religious practices.
Pertinent questions: Do you feel your faith (or religion) is helpful to you? If yes, can you tell me how? Are there any religious practices that are important to you? Has being sick made any difference in your practice of praying? Your religious practices? What religious books or symbols are helpful to you?

Area of concern: Relation between spiritual beliefs and health.
Pertinent questions: What has bothered you most about being sick (or what is happening to you)? What do you think is going to happen to you? Has being sick (or what has happened to you) made any difference in your feelings about God or the practice of your faith? Is there anything that is especially frightening or meaningful to you now?

Data from Stoll, R. I.: Guidelines for spiritual assessment. Am. J. Nurs., Sept., 1979, p. 1574.

religious passages, and referral to and consultation with clergy or another spiritual adviser.

Observation

Observation might be considered the most important of all assessment activities

Florence Nightingale, in describing the role of the nurse, said, "Without the habit of ready and correct observation we [nurses] shall be useless for all our devotion."

Much can be learned simply by observing a patient's general appearance. Many an experienced nurse has sensed that something was wrong with her patient by noticing his facial expression, posture in bed, bodily movements, and ability or inability to cooperate or respond appropriately.

There also are specific signs the nurse looks for when she first encounters her patient and during the time she is caring for him. These signals of deviation from health are called *symptoms*; they can be either subjective or objective. *Subjective symptoms* are those the patient must tell us about. They include itching, fatigue, pain, and nausea, to mention but a few. *Objective symptoms* are those that can be detected through the senses of sight, smell, touch, taste, and hearing or measured through the use of instruments, such as a thermometer, blood pressure apparatus, and clinical laboratory equipment. Pallor, rash, scratching, high blood pressure, and elevated blood sugar are examples of objective symptoms.

The observant nurse uses all her senses to obtain data for assessment of a patient's condition and identification of the problem. By touching the patient, she can distinguish between normal, healthy skin and skin that is coarse, dry, dehydrated, edematous, or cold and clammy. She feels the extremities and other body parts to determine if they are cold because of poor circulation or hot because of a localized inflammation.

She listens for normal breathing and distinguishes between a cough that is dry and hacking and one that is moist and "bubbly." She hears the wheezing of an asthmatic patient or the crowing sound produced by an obstruction of the air passages. These are just a few of the ways in which the nurse uses her hearing to evaluate a patient's condition.

In some instances, specific odors can be helpful in diagnosing certain disorders. For example, the sweetish, fruity odor of acetone can indicate diabetic acidosis; the smell of newly mown clover can accompany hepatic coma. The odor of alcohol is usually detected rather easily in acute alcoholism, unless the person has been drinking vodka, which is relatively odorless. A patient who is suffering from acute alcoholism also might smell of Sterno, lighter fluid, after-shave lotion, or other sources of alcohol.

Mouth odors that are foul or metallic usually indicate poor oral hygiene and periodontal disease (disease of the tissues around the teeth). A nasal odor can be caused by chronic sinusitis with postnasal drip or an obstruction in the nasal passages. In children, one might suspect a foreign object such as a bean or pea in the nose when there is a distinctly foul nasal odor. The patient who wears excessive amounts of perfume or cologne may be hiding a serious body odor problem that is symptomatic of anemia, endocrine dysfunction, or an abnormality of the central nervous system. If the nurse suspects that the patient is trying to hide an embarrassing odor, she should seek to gain the patient's confidence and trust so that he can talk freely about his problem and receive help in coping with it.

Physical Examination

Measurement of body temperature, pulse, respiration, and blood pressure are included in the physical examination. Familiarity with these routine procedures can cause the nurse to overlook their importance to the overall assessment of a patient's condition, but they are truly "vital signs" that are significant indicators of what is happening to a patient at any given moment.

Other procedures used in the physical examination involve auscultation, percussion, and palpation. A stethoscope is used to amplify the sounds heard through auscultation, for example, in assessing bowel sounds and in listening to breath sounds through the chest wall. The extent to which physical examination is performed by a particular nurse depends on the agency in which she works and her experience and expertise in the techniques. Many nurses have become quite proficient in this area. Records of vital signs establish, along with other data, a baseline with which to compare results of assessments performed later on.

Assessment is a very complex task, and the beginning nurse might not be as proficient at some aspects of the physical examination and the interview as the more experienced nurse or one with more advanced clinical skills. She should, however, be aware of the importance of this phase of the nursing process and the valuable contribution she can make toward determining the nursing needs of the patient. Because she is frequently at the patient's bedside and communicates personally with the family, she can use her knowledge and skills in interpersonal relationships, observation, and communication to augment the collection of information about the patient. There are many occasions when the nurse is in an excellent position to clarify a patient's statement and verify data already obtained. In this way, she can make sure that the information being used for the patient care plan is indeed factual and not misunderstood.

Laboratory Data

Information about test results, radiologic studies, and other diagnostic procedures performed by other departments within the hospital or clinic can be helpful to the nurse who is continually assessing the status of her patient. She can use the information so obtained to identify general areas in which a patient might have a health care problem or to validate a nursing diagnosis. For example, she might note activity intolerance, self-care deficit, ineffective breathing pattern, and other nursing diagnoses common to anemia. A review of laboratory findings after blood analysis might verify that the patient does indeed have a pathologic condition causing these kinds of responses.

Consultation

In the process of assessing her patient's needs the nurse uses a variety of sources for information. These include persons on the health team, as well as nursing textbooks, professional journals, and other forms of nursing literature. Members of the health team who might be consulted include pharmacists, social workers, dietitians, occupational therapists, clinical specialists, physical therapists, respiratory therapists, physicians, and pastoral counselors or chaplains.

ANALYSIS AND NURSING DIAGNOSIS

Standard II. The nursing diagnosis is derived from health status data.

In the analysis phase of the nursing process, the nurse looks at the data base, synthesizes and analyzes all the data, and determines where problems exist. Next she determines what the appropriate nursing diagnoses should be.

A nursing diagnosis is a concise statement of "a patient's actual or potential health problem which nurses, by virtue of their education and experience, are capable and licensed to treat (Gordon, 1979)." The concept of nursing diagnosis is relatively new in the field of nursing and still is not totally accepted and used by all health care professionals. The idea of a classification system for problems related to health disorders treatable by nursing intervention was first introduced by Abdellah in 1960. A list of 21 common nursing problems was eventually developed through a National League for Nursing study conducted by Abdellah and others.

The original 21 problems were stated as therapeutic goals for the practice of nursing. Later it was decided that there should be a common diagnostic classification system that focuses on the patient and his problems. In 1972 the First National Conference on Classification of Nursing Diagnoses met to begin the task of identifying problems amenable to nursing intervention. This classification system continues to be developed and refined. The National Group for Classification of Nursing Diagnoses has as its goal the standardization of diagnostic descriptions so that nurses can communicate with one another more easily. Eventually it is hoped that standardized nursing diagnoses will lead to the identification of specific outcome criteria and nursing interventions for each diagnosis. Once this is accomplished, nursing will have a sounder scientific basis for its practice.

The categories of nursing diagnoses shown in Table 4–3 describe the *general area* of a patient's problem. They are *not* statements of an individual patient's problems; that cannot be known without an assessment of the patient's health status. Standard II of the American Nurses' Association Standards of Nursing Practice clearly states that "nursing diagnoses are dervied from health status data." Arriving at a nursing diagnosis requires much skill and a thorough knowledge of nursing theory and practice. Identifying patient care problems and establishing nursing diagnoses are the responsibility of the nurse assigned to admit or care for the patient and are derived from data collected by other nurses as well as herself and other health team members.

The nursing diagnosis focuses on the patient's response to the pathologic condition diagnosed by the physician or to other factors that can adversely affect or have the potential for interfering with the attainment and maintenance of optimal wellness. Nursing diagnoses and interventions are primarily concerned with (1) physical, psychosocial, and spiritual comfort and well-being; (2) prevention of complications; and (3) patient education. Nursing diagnoses do not include health problems that are treatable by surgery, medications, or other forms of therapy that have been legally defined as the practice of medicine.

An example of how the medical and nursing diagnoses complement one another is presented below.

- Medical diagnosis: chronic obstructive pulmonary disease.
- Assessment data: shortness of breath; cough; thick, tenacious, yellow sputum; pursed-lip breathing; respirations at 24 per minute; unable to walk for more than a short distance

TABLE 4-3 APPROVED NURSING DIAGNOSES

Activity intolerance
Activity intolerance, potential
Adjustment, impaired
Airway clearance, ineffective
Anxiety
Aspiration, potential for
Body image disturbance
Body temperature, potential altered
Breast-feeding, effective
Breast-feeding, ineffective
Breathing pattern, ineffective
Cardiac output, decreased
Communication, impaired verbal
Conflict, decisional (specify)
Conflict, parental role
Constipation
Constipation, colonic
Constipation, perceived
Coping, defensive
Coping, family, ineffective: compromised
Coping, family, ineffective: disabled
Coping, family, potential for growth
Coping, ineffective individual
Denial, ineffective
Diarrhea
Disuse syndrome, potential for
Diversional activity deficit
Dysreflexia
Family processes, altered
Fatigue
Fear
Fluid volume deficit
Fluid volume deficit, potential
Fluid volume excess
Gas exchange, impaired
Grieving, anticipatory
Grieving, dysfunctional
Growth and development, altered
Health maintenance, altered
Health-seeking behaviors (specify)
Home maintenance management, impaired
Hopelessness
Hyperthermia
Hypothermia
Incontinence, bowel
Incontinence, functional
Incontinence, reflex
Incontinence, stress
Incontinence, total
Incontinence, urge
Infection, potential for
Injury, potential for
Knowledge deficit (specify)
Mobility, impaired physical
Noncompliance (specify)
Nutrition, altered: less than body requirements
Nutrition, altered: more than body requirements
Nutrition, altered: potential for more than body requirements
Oral mucous membrane, altered
Pain
Pain, chronic
Parenting, altered
Parenting, altered: potential
Personal identity disturbance
Poisioning, potential for
Posttrauma response
Powerlessness
Protection, altered
Rape-trauma response
Rape-trauma syndrome: compound reaction
Rape-trauma syndrome: silent reaction
Role performance, altered
Self-care deficit: bathing/hygiene, dressing/grooming, feeding, toileting
Self-esteem, chronic low
Self-esteem disturbance
Self-esteem, situational low
Sensory/perceptual alterations (specify: visual, auditory, kinesthetic, gustatory, tactile, olfactory)
Sexual dysfunction
Sexuality patterns, altered
Skin integrity, impaired
Skin integrity, potential impaired
Sleep pattern disturbance
Social interaction, impaired
Social isolation
Spiritual distress
Suffocation, potential for
Swallowing, impaired
Thermoregulation, ineffective
Thought processes, altered
Tissue integrity, impaired
Tissue perfusion, altered (specify: cardiopulmonary, cerebral, gastrointestinal, peripheral, renal)
Trauma, potential for
Unilateral neglect
Urinary elimination, altered patterns of
Urinary retention
Violence, potential for: self-directed or directed at others

From the Ninth Conference of the North American Nursing Diagnosis Association, 1990.

without stopping to rest and catch his breath; sleeps with three pillows behind his back.

- Appropriate nursing diagnoses:
  1. Ineffective breathing pattern related to dyspnea and copious sputum.
  2. Potential for infection related to retained secretions.
  3. Activity intolerance related to shortness of breath.
  4. Self-care deficit related to inability to perform ADL without shortness of breath.

Nursing diagnoses provide the basis for planning nursing interventions that will help prevent, minimize, or alleviate specific health problems. In the above example, physical well-being will be the major focus of the interventions.

PLANNING

Standard III. Goals for nursing care are formulated.

Standard IV. The plan for nursing care prescribes nursing actions to achieve the goals.

The planning phase of the nursing process provides a blueprint for nursing interventions to achieve designated goals. If no problems have been identified during assessment (as with a client in a community health care clinic), the nurse and client sit down together and discuss goals for maintenance of wellness. In a hospital setting it is fairly certain that the patient will have some health-deficit problems that are amenable to nursing care. After all, one of the main reasons for hospitalization is to make 24-hour nursing care available to patients who need such care.

The steps included in the planning phase of the nursing process are (1) determining priorities from the list of nursing diagnoses, (2) setting short-term and long-term goals for dealing with problems associated with each diagnosis, (3) developing objectives to reach the goals or outcome criteria by which success of the interventions can be measured, and (4) writing nursing orders.

Priorities are decided according to what is most important for the well-being of the patient and are set according to (1) Maslow's hierarchy of needs and (2) what is perceived as important to the patient. For example, although eradication of infection (physiologic need) might be seen as most important by the nurse, the patient might feel that obtaining a good night's sleep after several sleepless nights is more important.

Goals should be stated in terms of observable outcomes. They are formulated by the patient and the nurse and are in line with the patient's ability to achieve them. Goals are achievable within a specifically stated time frame and relate to one of three aspects of care: (1) restoration to health when there is a deviation from health, (2) maintenance of health when the patient needs to continue using his resources to stay healthy, and (3) promotion of health when the patient's resources can and should be maximized. Goals may be long-term or short-term, meaning that some are achievable in the near future and others will take considerably more time for the patient to reach. For example, a long-term goal for a stroke patient who has right-sided paresis might be: "Patient will feed himself without assistance." A short-term goal might be: "Patient will feed himself finger foods at lunch time before discharge."

Objectives are steps toward accomplishment of major goals and are placed on the care plan in the form of outcome criteria. They should be stated in behavioral terms; that is, they should describe what the patient should be able to do, or how he has improved, as a result of nursing actions. They relate directly to the goal that is derived from the nursing diagnosis. For example, if the nursing diagnosis is "Potential for infection related to surgical incision," the goal is prevention of infection. The outcome criteria might be:

- White blood cell (WBC) count within normal limits at discharge.
- Temperature within normal limits by third postoperative day.
- Incision clean, dry, and without signs of infection such as redness or swelling at discharge.

Outcome criteria are written with a subject, a verb, conditions or modifiers, and the criterion for desired performance. (A criterion is a standard against which judgments are made.) They should include the following elements: (1) patient activity that can be observed by the nurse or patient knowledge that can be assessed (e.g., medication side effects), and (2) a description of how the patient's behavior will be measured—for example, the time when the objective will be met and the accuracy or quality of performance. By writing outcome criteria that are very specific, it is easy to determine whether the planned nursing interventions have worked to achieve the goal. If so, the outcome criteria will have been met.

Nursing orders are the nursing actions and patient activities prescribed by the nurse to help achieve the stated goals and objectives.

INTERVENTION (IMPLEMENTATION)

Standard V. The plan for nursing care is implemented.

During the implementation phase the plan of action is put into effect. The nurse coordinates her activities with other members of the health care team who are directly concerned with the patient. Procedures and activities involving the patient should be carefully timed so that he is allowed sufficient rest and his natural healing and recuperative powers can do their work to restore him to a higher level of wellness.

In some instances implementation will include ordered medical treatments such as medications, irrigations, and oxygen therapy. At times, nursing intervention will involve unplanned and prompt intervention, as when a crisis arises that demands immediate and decisive action on the part of the nurse.

During implementation the nursing care plan is tested for effectiveness and accuracy. Nursing interventions may not have the intended effect, or a change in the patient's condition may present more crucial problems. The implementation phase concludes with the documentation of nursing care. This includes the nursing action performed, the outcome of the activity, and the patient's response. Documentation is discussed in more detail later in this chapter.

EVALUATION

Standard VI. The plan for nursing care is evaluated.

Evaluation is the process of judging or appraising the effectiveness of what has been done. In the nursing process, to evaluate means to identify whether or to what degree the patient's goals and outcome criteria have been met. The nurse continually evaluates as she goes about giving patient care and performing nursing interventions. She should continually ask, "Is this action effective? Is the outcome of the action I performed expected or unexpected? Does the plan of care need to be revised and the nursing orders rewritten?" If the outcome criteria have been met, the nursing diagnoses and nursing orders for that problem can be noted "achieved," and that portion of the care plan can be closed or deleted from the plan of care. Each nursing intervention under a nursing diagnosis should be evaluated to see whether it is effective and is still needed. Once each day the data obtained regarding the patient's response to the nursing interventions are examined, and a decision is made as to whether the various interventions should be continued, stopped, or changed. Consider, for example, a nursing diagnosis of "fluid deficit related to nausea and vomiting," and an outcome criterion of "takes in 3,000 mL of fluid each 24 hrs." Then during evaluation the nurse would note how much fluid the patient took in during the previous 24 hours and also would assess whether the patient was able to keep the fluid down. If the patient could only take in 2,200 mL but managed to keep the fluid down, then the nursing intervention is appropriate and should be continued until the patient is taking 3,000 mL per day for several days without difficulty. If the patient has been drinking 3,000 mL of fluid but is vomiting most of it, then the nursing care plan must be revised to assist the patient with this problem. Perhaps the nurse will need to obtain a different order for an antiemetic or give it more frequently than twice a day.

Another broader aspect of evaluation pertinent to nursing practice is the overall evaluation done to determine whether the hospital unit is performing as well and as efficiently as possible. Quality assurance audits are a form of evaluation in which various nursing and hospital services are scrutinized to see if they are meeting standards. The structure of the unit and its physical facilities, equipment, staffing, and other characteristics that affect the quality of nursing care are evaluated periodically. The Joint Commission on Accreditation of Hospitals is a governing body that reviews care given by hospitals. Within this procedure is a series of retrospective audits. (Retrospective means dealing with the past). An *audit* is an examination of a record or chart. Objective criteria are applied to a patient's chart after he is discharged to see if the care he received met set standards for the type of problem he had. Every hospital must do both medical and nursing audits in order to achieve and maintain accreditation.

Each hospital has a quality assurance board or committee that coordinates audit activities. Generally each nursing unit must do a number of chart audits for data to see whether a particular standard practice of nursing is being met. An example would be an audit to see how often intravenous (IV) tubing is being changed. The procedure manual may state that all IV tubing is to be changed every 48 hours. A review of charts for a specific period of time will identify how often this "standard" or criteria is being met. One nursing unit may be meeting it 98% of the time, while another that has a shortage of nurses as a result of illness for that time period may have met the criteria only 78% of the time.

Process evaluations center on the activities of the nurse and what she has done to assess, plan, implement, and evaluate nursing care. The criteria used in process evaluation are the Standards of Nursing Practice developed by the American Nurses' Association.

An important question that should have a part in evaluating nursing care is, "What can be done to improve the care?" Evaluation is not done so that someone can be blamed for inefficiency, carelessness, or incompetence. It is done for the purpose of improvement, by identifying specific areas that need change for the better. Some weaknesses that might be found include vague or inaccurate statements of the problem because of poor assessment or inability to analyze data correctly, unrealistic goal-setting caused by overestimating what a patient is capable of doing, and well-intentioned but ineffective nursing interventions that simply do not accomplish the desired goal. Whatever the results of an evaluation, they should be seen as a means of improving the quality of nursing care.

Nursing Care Plan 4–1 shows how the components of the nursing process can be used to provide a systematic plan of care for an individual patient. Sample care plans are provided throughout this text to familiarize the reader with the manner in which each phase of the process is recorded in order to document and communicate to others the planned care of patients with specific problems and nursing diagnoses related to their health status.

PATIENT EDUCATION

The model for carrying out the nursing process can also be used, with slight modifications, for teaching patients.

During assessment of any patient the nurse should ask herself what this patient needs to know to perform self care, get well, or maintain health. The nursing diagnosis "knowledge deficit" should always be considered when formulating the nursing care plan.

The overall goals of patient education are concerned with helping him to (1) promote his own and his family's health, (2) maintain his current health status and improve it as much as possible, and (3) learn to care for himself and participate as actively as he can in his health care plan.

The specific objectives of patient education are dictated by each patient's individual needs. The patient who suffers from hypertension (high blood pressure) will need to know about the nature of his illness, the purposes and expected actions of the medications that are prescribed for him, how he can change his living habits to help keep his hypertension under control, and what is expected of him in following the medical regimen designed for him.

Other patients, such as stroke victims, might need instruction in self-help so that rehabilitation is possible. The patient with diabetes has many instructional needs if he is to participate in monitoring and controlling the symptoms of his illness and preventing complications.

COMPONENTS OF THE TEACHING-LEARNING PROCESS

The teaching-learning process is similar to the nursing process in that both are flexible and dynamic—that is, subject to change whenever the patient's needs and problems require attention. The components of the teaching-learning process are (1) assessment, (2) planning, (3) instruction, and (4) evaluation (Fig. 4–3).

Assessment

The nurse must have some idea of what the patient needs to learn before she can begin to teach him. There are three general areas (domains) of learning that she should be concerned with: (1) cognitive (knowing), (2) psychomotor (doing), and (3) affective (feeling). Perhaps you can remember these best as the "three Hs"—head, hands, and heart.

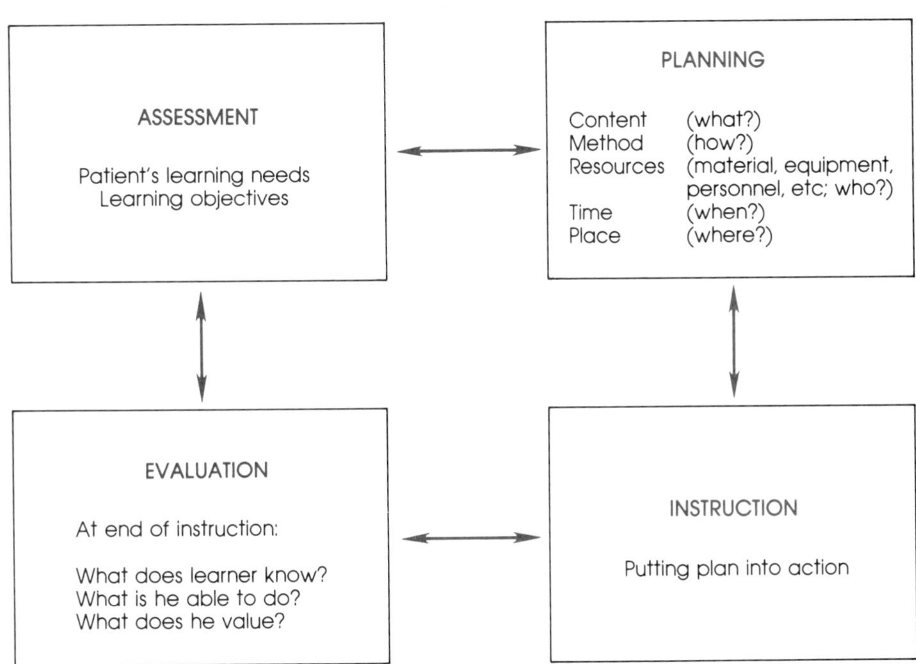

Figure 4–3 The teaching-learning process.

The three learning domains take into account what the patient should know, what he should be able to do, and how he should feel. As an example, consider the diabetic patient who wants to learn to administer his own insulin at home. He should know the action of the various types of insulin, how to calculate the dosage, and when and how it is administered. He should be able to administer the insulin under aseptic conditions without injuring his tissues unnecessarily, and with a minimum of pain. He should realize that the administration of insulin is a valuable part of his total care.

It is necessary to determine whether the pa-

NURSING CARE PLAN 4–1

Selected nursing diagnoses, goals/outcome criteria, nursing interventions, and evaluations for a patient with hypertension

Situation: 53-year-old male with a blood pressure of 170/100 found during routine screening of all employees at a local plant. A visit to the hypertension clinic reveals that he is hypertensive, is 75 pounds overweight, smokes two packs of cigarettes a day, and eats snacks during the day and in the evening while watching television. The physician prescribes a low-sodium diet and a mild antihypertensive. During her interview with the patient the nurse notes that he does not understand the nature of his illness, how his lifestyle is related to hypertension, and the purpose of the low-sodium diet and the expected action of the diuretic.

Nursing Diagnosis	Goals/Outcome Criteria	Nursing Intervention	Evaluation
Altered systemic tissue perfusion related to increased peripheral vascular resistance. SUPPORTING DATA BP, 172/102; P, 96; feet cool and pale; pedal pulses, 1+; capillary refill > 4 s.	Patient will maintain adequate tissue perfusion as evidenced by: 1. BP within normal limits at end of 1 week. 2. Pulse returns to normal range by discharge. 3. Skin of feet warm and dry at discharge. 4. Capillary refill time less than 3 s within 2 weeks. Patient will quit smoking within one month.	Administer antihypertensive as ordered; monitor vital signs q 4 hr. Assess skin and peripheral pulses q shift. Discourage smoking; encourage him to quit smoking. Discourage intake of foods high in caffeine. Maintain sodium restrictions. Weigh daily	BP, 156/96; P, 86; skin on feet pale and cool; smoked only five cigarettes this shift; weight down 2 lbs. Continue plan.
Altered nutrition, exceeding body requirements; related to overeating and lack of exercise. SUPPORTING DATA Weight, 285 lbs; height, 6 ft; consumes lots of junk food between meals; no daily exercise program; watches television a lot.	Patient will lose 2 lbs before discharge. Consultation with dietitian before discharge. Patient will maintain 2-lb/wk weight loss until normal weight of 210 lbs is attained. Patient will have developed daily exercise plan by discharge.	Explain need to lose excess weight; encourage him to participate in weight loss plan. Assist with development of daily exercise plan.	Weight, 283 lbs; is considering options for daily exercise plan.
Knowledge deficit related to self-care aspects of hypertension: how to take blood pressure, medication rationale and side effects, low-sodium diet, need for exercise, need for continued medical follow-up SUPPORTING DATA Does not know how to take blood pressure; has never taken antihypertensive medication; unaware of sodium content of foods and sodium's relationship to hypertension; unaware of the benefits of exercise on the cardiovascular system; complains of cost of going to doctor for a check-up.	Patient will demonstrate correct technique for taking own blood pressure within 1 week of teaching. Patient will explain action of antihypertensive medication and possible side effects 3 days after teaching session. Patient will describe effects of exercise on cardiovascular system after teaching session. Patient will state which foods are high in sodium when given a list from which to choose foods after teaching session. Before discharge patient will give three reasons why continued follow-up is necessary for patients with hypertension.	Develop teaching plan covering the following points: 1. How to take own blood pressure. 2. Action and side effects of antihypertensive medication. 3. Beneficial effects of exercise program on cardiovascular system. 4. How sodium increases water retention and elevates blood pressure. 5. Foods to avoid that contain excess sodium. 6. Potential complications of uncontrolled blood pressure and reason for physician examination to detect beginning complications.	First teaching session completed; verbalizes action and three side effects of antihypertensive medication; can pick foods high in sodium from a list. Continue teaching and plan.

NURSING CARE PLAN 4–1, *Continued*

Nursing Diagnosis	Goals/Outcome Criteria	Nursing Intervention	Evaluation
Potential ineffective individual coping related to lack of desire to quit smoking, even though he is hypertensive. SUPPORTING DATA States that he does not wish to quit smoking and doesn't really see the need to do so. All of his friends smoke.	Patient will verbalize how smoking affects the blood vessels 3 days after teaching session. Patient will verbalize desire to quit smoking before discharge. Patient will institute a "no smoking" program within 1 month of discharge.	Teach how nicotine constricts the blood vessels, elevating blood pressure and decreasing blood flow to the periphery of the body. Encourage patient to quit smoking. Obtain American Heart Association, American Lung Association, and American Cancer Society materials regarding the dangers of smoking. Familiarize the patient with available community "Quit Smoking" programs. Encourage him to join support group for those who are quitting smoking.	Discussed effect of smoking on vessels; gave patient AHA materials to read; encouraged him to quit smoking; scheduled another session tomorrow. Continue plan.

tient learns best from an oral presentation, a demonstration, reading printed material, or watching a video presentation. Usually a combination of media will be best for most patients. If there is a language barrier, an interpreter must be obtained and all printed materials translated for the patient.

Assessment of readiness for learning must also include a search for factors that might interfere with learning. Pain, extreme fear, anxiety, a room that is too warm or too cold, too much noise, and too many interruptions can all interfere with learning and need to be remedied before teaching begins. If the patient usually wears a hearing aid, it should be in place. The patient who wears glasses should have them on during a learning session.

After you have assessed a patient's readiness for learning and determined what his learning needs are, you work with him in setting up learning objectives. These objectives become the basis for the teaching-learning plan.

Planning

In planning, you must consider not only what you will teach but how you will help your patient to learn. The information needed by the patient should be organized in a logical sequence from the simple to the complex. Try to start with what the patient already knows (he might have a lot of misinformation and confusion) and proceed toward acquisition of new information and skills. If he is to learn some skill requiring equipment, be sure the necessary tools are at hand.

The amount of time required for teaching a patient will depend on how much he needs to know and how easily he learns. It might be necessary to reteach the patient if your first attempts are not successful. He should not be exhausted by long periods of instruction. He should set the pace and feel free to express his opinions on how he learns best. His input during the planning phase of instruction can be extremely valuable.

Nurses often hesitate to become involved in patient education, because they think it must be done in a formal setting. Teaching and learning can take place in any setting at any time. For example, a nurse can teach foot care to a diabetic patient while bathing him. She can teach a patient who has had surgery to avoid complications of inactivity while helping him to get out of bed and walk.

Instruction

This phase involves implementing your plan of instruction. If you are well organized, you will know what you expect the patient to learn. You will have the teaching material and equipment readily at hand.

It is important not to be too rigid in following your teaching plan. You might find that the patient is more confused than enlightened by your teaching efforts. If that is so, you might need to review your objectives and ask him to help you determine exactly what it is that is confusing him. At this point, you might need to revise your plan and try a different approach. Perhaps showing a film, having him talk with another patient who has similar health problems, or giving him additional reading material will facilitate his learning. Encourage the patient to ask questions and express his feelings about learning to care for himself.

Evaluation

The means by which you measure the effectiveness of your teaching depends on which area of learning you are evaluating. One often-repeated concept of education is that learning produces a change in behavior. In other words, if someone is able to answer questions, perform a certain task, and show that he appreciates the value of what he has learned by acting in a certain way, he has learned in each of the three learning domains.

If a change in behavior is valid proof that learning has taken place, a measurement of behavior would be a basis for evaluating instruction. For example, to evaluate a patient's ability to walk with crutches, you would ask him to demonstrate that ability by walking with crutches while you observe him. You would not administer a written test, nor would you simply ask questions about how he walks with crutches. Any learning that involves psychomotor skills should be evaluated by observing the learner as he demonstrates those skills.

Evaluation of a person's feelings and attitudes is more difficult, but it is not impossible. One drawback is that we all have a tendency to tell others what we think they want to hear. A patient who knows how important it is to stay on his diet might tell you he feels it is very important to his health, because he knows that is what you want him to feel. If, however, a patient tells you that he has been explaining his diet to his wife and would like some help in teaching her so she will prepare the right kind of meals for him, it is probably safe to assume that he attaches some importance to staying on his diet. If his goal is to control his diabetes by diet and exercise, and he is able to do so over a period of time, he apparently values dietary control. He has demonstrated a knowledge of and a commitment to following the prescribed regimen.

Evaluation of the teaching-learning process provides a means for improvement. It should help the nurse to improve her teaching competence and help the patient either to improve or to maintain his health status.

It must be understood that the teaching-learning process is a complex system that involves several factors. Some of these are beyond the control of the nurse—for example, the physical, mental, and emotional capabilities of the patient. This is not to imply, however, that patient education is better "left to the experts." We cannot speak of humanized, patient-centered care of the total individual without recognizing that he has learning needs that directly affect his health. We must do more than pay lip service to the patient's desire to be treated as a partner in his care and his right to be treated as a person worthy of respect.

DOCUMENTATION

Documentation of the teaching plan is done either under the nursing diagnosis of "knowlege deficit" on the patient's nursing care plan or on a separate flow sheet especially designed to track patient teaching.

It is essential that each nurse record material taught, patient response, and evaluation of the process and the patient's progress after each teaching session. The amount of time the nurse spends teaching the patient should also be specified, as this information is important for insurance company reimbursement.

Documentation of every part of the nursing process and communication among staff members is crucial to quality patient care. With the current emphasis on accountability and insurance company scrutiny of charges for services rendered, the old adage, "If it isn't charted, it wasn't done," holds more clout than ever.

DOCUMENTATION AND INTERSTAFF COMMUNICATION

Communication regarding what has been done for the patient, pertinent observations, data regarding physical parameters such as vital signs and input and output, how the patient is reacting to medication and other treatments, his psychological and emotional state, and his present needs is vital to good patient care. Two to three different sets of staff on a unit are in charge of the care of each patient during a 24-hour period. Rarely does a patient have the same nurse for each shift for several consecutive days. If communication is inadequate, patient care will be very fragmented.

Good, thorough documentation is one way in which continuity of care can be achieved. The other way is through adequate verbal communication between staff members. Usually, each type of communication complements the other, and it is only with attention to thoroughness in each area, written and verbal, that high-quality, holistic care can be given to the patient.

VALUE OF DOCUMENTATION

Throughout every nursing program students are taught to record significant information on the patient's chart. Documentation is important for a number of reasons. The rationale for documentation usually falls within four broad areas of concern: (1) the quality of care given to each patient, (2) continuity of care, (3) legal consequences of failure to document accurately and completely, and (4) verification of services rendered for Medicare and insurance payment.

SOURCE-ORIENTED AND PROBLEM-ORIENTED RECORD KEEPING

Source-oriented records are arranged according to the source of the information written on the patient's chart. The source can be the nurse, attending physician, pathologist, radiologist, social worker, rehabilitation specialist, or any other health team member. Each person or department has a section of the chart in which certain kinds of records are kept. Each set of records is arranged in chronologic order without regard for its meaning to the overall care of the patient and his response to the care.

A person interested in following the progress of the patient is obliged to shuffle back and forth through the chart to locate isolated bits of information. He must then take these scattered notes and try to fit them together to get some idea of what has happened and is happening to the patient. The reader must coordinate the data in his own mind in order to know what has been and is being done, why it has been done, and how the many diagnostic tests and forms of therapy have helped the patient deal with his health problems.

Problem-oriented records are organized according to specific problems presented by the patient at the time he seeks medical help. This system of record keeping was first introduced by Dr. Lawrence Weed in the 1960s. Its purpose is to integrate all the notes kept on a patient in a hospital, clinic, or community health care center. In the traditional, source-oriented system of record keeping, the medical diagnosis—for example, congestive heart failure—serves as the point of reference. However, patients do not present themselves to physicians with a medical diagnosis. They consult the physician because they have one or more specific problems that adversely affect their health and therefore their ability to do what they want to do. The patient with congestive heart failure might be able to function at an acceptable level in his life, or he might be experiencing shortness of breath, swelling of the feet and ankles, and mental confusion. Records of what is done to help him cope with these specific problems are organized around the problems. More information about problem-oriented record keeping is presented later.

Whatever the system for recording data might be, the nurse is obliged to make notes related to activities within the nursing process and the effect of these activities on her patient. Additionally she is responsible for recording any treatments delegated to her by the physician. Documentation in the nurses' notes should therefore include (1) all treatments and care given, including medications not charted elsewhere; (2) diagnostic procedures performed at the bedside, on the unit, or someplace else inside or outside the facility; (3) the patient's reaction to therapeutic and diagnostic procedures; (4) observations of the nurse; (5) subjective and objective symptoms experienced by the patient; (6) evidence of changes in the patient's physical, psychosocial, and spiritual needs and status; and (7) any irregularities or unusual incidents during his stay at the hospital or health care agency.

FORMATS FOR DOCUMENTATION

Nurses document assessments, care given (including teaching), observations, and other pertinent information in the patient's chart on a variety of forms. A note is made, usually each shift, on the "Nurse's Notes" page, and notations are made on several "flow sheets." There is often an "Activity Sheet" with space for notations on meals, bath, safety devices used, and treatments, where the nurse simply puts a check mark or initials to indicate that the item was accomplished.

Methods of nursing documentation are undergoing considerable transformation at the present time. Nursing care and assesment have become so complex that nurses have had to spend an excessive amount of time on documentation, which has taken time away from working directly with the patient. An effort is being made to design systems that adequately and efficiently document the necessary data while fulfilling legal requirements.

SYSTEMS CHARTING

With the systems charting method the nurse charts pertinent data regarding each physical system of the patient and then adds relevant data regarding psychosocial aspects. Included are the neurologic, respiratory, cardiovascular, gastrointestinal, renal, endocrine, musculoskeletal, and integumentary systems. Most of the nurse's notes will focus on the system in which there is a specific patient problem. A system does not need any notation at all if that system is functioning without problems. Usually a note is made regarding neurologic, respiratory, and cardiovascular function, as these systems are vital to life.

PEMS

Another systematic approach to charting is the Physical problems, Emotional needs, Mental status, and Safety needs (PEMS) approach. It is suggested that information in each of these areas be recorded at least once during every shift. The authors of this system also recommend charting additional information about teaching and evidence of learning, doctor's visits, discontinued treatments (e.g., intravenous fluids), removal of sutures, isolation precautions, and other significant events that indicate something special or unusual is being done or is happening to the patient.

FOCUSED CHARTING

Focused charting utilizes a narrative format for documenting data about the "focus" of the patient's problem and then noting other data on activity or other flow sheets. The purpose of this method is to cut down the time the nurse spends on the chart, thereby allowing more time to be spent directly with the patient.

HIERARCHY OF HUMAN NEEDS

Another systematic way of thinking about the data that need to be documented is to consider the hierarchy of basic human needs. The acronym RN'S HOPE provides a guide: Rest and activity, Nutrition, Safety and self-care deficit, Hygiene and skin, Oxygenation, Psychosocial, Elimination. By mentally running through this list, the nurse considers all areas of patient needs and can decide whether there are any data that need to be recorded. It is also useful to consider each area when thinking about whether anything else needs to be added to the patient's nursing care plan. Adequate fluid intake might be difficult for the patient with mild nausea and almost certainly impossible for a patient with prolonged nausea and vomiting. A nursing diagnosis of "potential fluid volume deficit related to nausea or vomiting" should be added to the care plan. A patient with a chronic lung disorder might not be able to meet his need for oxygen because of accumulations of mucus and ineffective coughing, or because he has difficulty breathing without sitting upright in a chair or bed. A nursing diagnosis of "impaired gas exchange related to ineffective coughing" may be needed on the care plan.

On the next level of need are safety and security needs. Is the patient confused, under the influence of a sedative, or otherwise unable to be responsible for his actions? Should he have siderails up on his bed? Does he need a padded headboard to protect him during convulsive seizures? assistance when getting up to the bathroom? restraints to prevent his pulling out a catheter or tube? Perhaps his security needs can be met by assuring him that someone will come as soon as he calls (and then following through on that promise!). Or he might feel more secure if time is spent explaining hospital routine to him, or answering his questions about the series of radiographs he will have in the morning or telling him that arrangements have been made to have someone come in and help take care of him when he returns home.

A clean and orderly environment, having the same nurses care for him day in and day out, and having procedures (for example, dressing changes) performed in the same way can contribute to the patient's sense of security. He knows more about what to expect and how his behavior will be accepted when there are fewer people to deal with and fewer surprises when a treatment is performed.

Ego and self-esteem needs and the need to be loved and to have a sense of belonging are not always immediately recognized in the rush to meet physiologic needs. They are, however, no less important to the total well-being of the patient. Clues that these needs are not being met usually can be found in what the patient says and how he expresses himself nonverbally. Saying such things as, "I'm not worth all the trouble you're going to," or "I know you are busy and don't want to be bothered making this phone call for me," can tell a lot about a patient's frame of mind. A little time spent listening to the patient can give even more clues as to what is going on within him, as can such body language as staring out the window, averting the eyes, drooping shoulders, wringing hands, and tears coursing down the cheeks. Recording any of these statements and nonverbal clues can give others insight into what is happening to the patient and the kind of help he needs. Additionally, documenting those actions that have been helpful in satisfying a particular need tells his other nurses how they can be more effective in their care for him.

SOAP NURSE'S NOTES

This method is an integral part of the problem-oriented medical record keeping system discussed in the next section. The "S" stands for *subjective information*, particularly information that the patient has stated. "I need some pain medication" would be the type of statement that goes under the "S." "O" stands for *observations*. In this instance the nurse would chart her observations relative to the patient's pain status. "Tense facial expression, knees drawn up; abdomen tender to touch and slightly swollen; bowel sounds hyperactive; three loose stools last hour." The "A" stands for *assessment*, but it really means *analysis*. A statement about what the "S" and "O" data indicate goes here. For this patient it would be "Pain related to gastrointestinal infection or upset." "P" indicates plan. For this patient it might be "Give Lomotil (atropine sulfate and diphenoxylate hydrochloride) q 4 hours prn diarrhea." When only an action needs to be documented, it is placed under the "O": Lomotil 1 tab at 10:15; no further loose stools until 13:30." "P": Continue plan.

PROBLEM-ORIENTED RECORD KEEPING

Problem-oriented records are, as previously explained, focused on specific problems presented by a patient. The system of problem-oriented medical record keepting (POMR) is not used throughout the United States, but it is gaining acceptance, particularly in psychiatric settings, chiefly because it has several advantages over the more traditional source-oriented system.

In describing the advantages of POMR, Gloria Peterson writes:

> It provides a communication link between the doctors, nurses and other providers and the patient, who is the central figure in the development of his own problem list, plans and follow-up. The POMR enables us to improve staff and patient education; and it helps us measure the quality of care our patients receive.

In recent years, citizens, governmental agencies, and insurance companies who pay for health care have become increasingly interested in the evaluation of it. The advantages that POMR offers in providing quality assurance and a means of auditing the records of patient care cannot be ignored.

In regard to staff education, the establishment of criteria against which performance can be measured is extremely helpful. If the entire staff is allowed to participate in the establishment of standards by which performance and patient response can be measured, all the people involved have a much clearer idea of what is to be observed and how patient problems can be resolved.

Components of the POMR

There are four basic components of the problem-oriented system: (1) data base, (2) problem list, (3) initial plan, and (4) follow-up (progress notes) (Fig. 4–4).

An additional component might be the audit, which is a type of evaluation.

Data Base

The data base is the basic information that pertains to an individual in a particular setting. In the hospital, the data base can contain such information as the medical and nursing history, nursing observations, physical examination findings, vital signs, body measurements (height, weight, etc.), and results of routine laboratory tests. The data base functions as a kind of benchmark from which changes can be determined and measured. For example, if the patient's weight on admission is 198 pounds and he is suffering from edema, some of his weight can be attributed to the collection of fluid in his body. The use of diuretics can help eliminate some of this excess fluid and the patient will lose weight. If we know the intial weight was 198 pounds, we can determine how much fluid is lost by weighing the patient daily. The original information

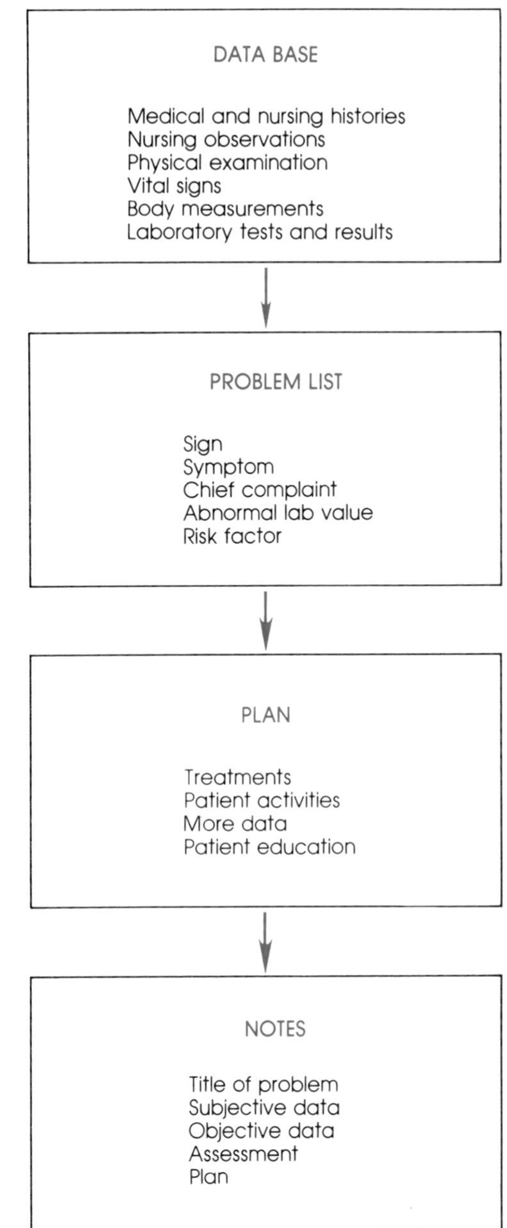

Figure 4–4 Components of the POMR system. Each component leads to the development of the next.

serves as a baseline against which we can measure weight loss.

As mentioned earlier, the information that forms the data base traditionally has been scattered throughout the patient's chart. In the POMR system, these data are all in one place, usually on special forms. It is recommended that the data base be revised as necessary and that a new "active" data base be completed and the older "inactive" data base be retired to an inactive file if there are extensive changes. The active data base should accompany the patient each time he is hospitalized, referred to an outpatient clinic, or treated by a community health agency. In this way communication and continuity of care are maintained.

Problem List

The problem list is developed from the information obtained during assessment and recorded in the data base. A problem can be a sign, syndrome, symptom, abnormal laboratory value, or risk factor, such as a strongly positive family history of a certain disease.

The problems presented by the patient might be numerous and should be placed in order of priority; those requiring immediate attention should be listed before those that are less urgent. The problem list should be a kind of index to the progress notes. Its purpose is to draw attention to a problem area so that it will not be overlooked when the patient's progress is being checked.

The problem list is of benefit to the nurse as she plans patient care. If she has a clear idea of what the problems are, she is in a much better position to know precisely what observations should be made. Another advantage to the problem list is that it provides part-time staff, newly hired personnel, and "floaters" with a brief and concise record of each patient's problems. They are much better prepared to render care to patients they have not seen before if they know what each patient's current and immediate problems are.

Initial Plan

The initial plan outlines specific actions that might be taken to (1) obtain more data (for example, from additional observation, interview, and diagnostic studies), (2) establish guidelines for treatment and patient activities, and (3) provide education for the patient and family. If the problem does not demand immediate action, the plan for its resolution might simply be to remain aware of it and to continue to gather more data related to it.

Physicians' and nurses' care plans should be completely integrated and communicated to everyone concerned. Goals and objectives of the plan should be clearly stated so that everyone understands what is expected from the various activities outlined in the plan. For example, if the goal is that a stroke victim with partial paralysis will be able to walk with a cane within 1 month of the time therapeutic exercises are started, this should be written in the plan for patient activities.

The plan of action for a specific problem should be listed under that problem in the progress notes. In this way it is possible to follow the progress that is made toward meeting the specific goals and objectives stated in the plan.

Progress Notes

The progress notes provide a single section in which each person participating in the care of the patient can document what is being done for him and how he is responding. This method of charting avoids duplication of notes and provides a means of communication among the various members of the patient care team (Fig. 4–5).

Each progress note has a heading that names the specific problem being dealt with. Plans or orders related to the problem are written on the notes along with physical findings; observations, and other data about the patient's progress. As stated earlier, the SOAP format gives organization to the writing of progress notes.

The POMR system is well organized, logical, and sensible. Each component leads to the next in a reasonable way. The data base provides information for the problem list. The problem list serves as an index for the progress notes. Each progress note is titled with one special problem. If an audit is performed to evaluate effectiveness of care, there is a logical progression that can be followed from identification of the problem to its eventual outcome.

The material presented here has only highlighted the important features of the system. The reader who is interested in pursuing the subject and studying it in greater depth is encouraged to look for additional information in periodicals and publications.

COMPUTERIZED NURSE'S NOTES

Several methods of documenting patient care directly on a computer are presently being researched. Some systems use a bedside terminal for the nurse to enter observations and tasks and treatments completed; others use a pocket terminal that is carried from room to room.

One of the problems with all of the systems is trying to devise security methods to keep each patient's records totally private. To date, no fail-safe system has been devised to ensure that only those health professionals who are working directly with the patient can access his medical

PROGRESS NOTES		ORDERS
3-4-85	New problem: Acute pericarditis	Stat portable EKG and chest x-ray.
S—	Reports chest pain aggravated by moving, coughing, taking deep breaths. Says she is very weak and tired.	Prednisone 40 mg p.o. daily.
O—	Tachycardia; intermittent precordial friction rub. Temp. 101.4°F.; mild dyspnea	Codeine 30 mg prn for pain.
A—	Pericarditis sec. to URI	
P—	Monitor progress, institute steroid therapy	
3-4-85	Pericarditis	
9:45 PM		
S—	States "pain almost gone; doesn't hurt so much when I move or cough." "Did I have a heart attack?"	Bed rest; assist with position changes, coughing. Adm. pain med. as needed. Instruct patient to ask for med. when pain first begins.
O—	Temp. 100°F; able to doze for 15–20 minutes at a time. Less anxious about chest pain.	
A—	Inflammation not progressing; chest pain relieved.	Check vital signs q 4 h. Reassure patient and family cause of chest pain was not a heart attack.
P—	Provide rest. Continue to monitor temp., pulse, heart and lung sounds.	

Figure 4–5 Sample problem-oriented progress notes by physician and nurse.

records. However, with time, a method should be devised that will make handwritten nurse's notes obsolete.

CHART REVIEW

The nurse assigned to a patient can best prepare herself to care for that patient by doing a quick, orderly chart review. The face sheet will provide information on marital status, age, insurance coverage, occupation, significant others, and location of home. The most current set of physician's orders provides a clue as to the plan for that day (i.e., tests or treatments). The physician's history and physical examination give an overview of the patient's total health status and provide a summary of his current health problems. This part of the chart can provide a great deal of information, including allergies. The admission nursing assessment form can also provide additional helpful data.

Skimming through current lab data can give an idea of any abnormal values and areas that need watching closely. Other test data can provide information on what might be in store for the patient and areas where teaching might be needed. The medication profile sheets tell what is currently ordered for the patient and what PRN (as needed) medications he has actually needed. Consultation sheets and dietitian's or respiratory therapist's notes are also helpful. Nurse's notes from the previous 24 hours should be read and all of the flow sheets should be skimmed (Fig. 4–6). The nurse who regularly skims all of this data will have a much better knowledge of her patient's needs and will be more comfortable and proficient in caring for him.

COMPUTERIZED CARE PLAN

Many hospitals now have available for each nurse a printed sheet of current data about the patient. This sheet usually contains a demographics line listing the room, name, date of admission, age, doctor, and admitting diagnosis. A list of nursing diagnoses is given. A list of nursing orders is included that tells when vital signs should be taken; flow of oxygen, if in use; need for safety devices; type of diet; schedule for turning, coughing and deep breathing; IV information, etc. A medication schedule will soon be incorporated into this data sheet.

This sheet can be used as a work sheet during the shift, and if notations are made on it as the nurse does her work, it provides an excellent guide for charting.

The only problem with this type of transfer of information is that the nurse must be certain that the data on it are current. This means that the nurse should update the computerized care plan, preferably during each shift, but most certainly at least once each 24 hours.

REPORT

Report is given by the departing staff to the arriving staff. There are many methods of giving and receiving report. A tape-recorded report is

	DATE:	NIGHTS TIME ______	DAYS TIME ______	EVENINGS TIME ______
DIET	TYPE OF DIET	NONE☐ TYPE______	NONE☐ TYPE______	NONE☐ TYPE______
	AMOUNT TAKEN	______	BREAKFAST ______ LUNCH ______	______
	DIETARY SUPPLEMENT AND SNACK	NONE☐ TYPE______	NONE☐ TYPE______	NONE☐ TYPE______
	CALORIE COUNT (SPECIFY)	YES☐ NO☐	YES☐ NO☐	YES☐ NO☐
	FOOD TAKEN PER	SELF☐ ASSIST☐ FED☐	SELF☐ ASSIST☐ FED☐	SELF☐ ASSIST☐ FED☐
	TUBE FEEDING	NA☐ SOLUTION______	NA☐ SOLUTION______	NA☐ SOLUTION______
	(INDICATE SOLUTION & RATE)	RATE ______	RATE ______	RATE ______
	FLUIDS	NA☐ ☐ENCOURAGED ☐RESTRICTED	NA☐ ☐ENCOURAGED ☐RESTRICTED	NA☐ ☐ENCOURAGED ☐RESTRICTED
SKIN HYGIENE	BED BATH, SPONGE BATH, TUB BATH SHOWER BATH, SITZ BATH (CIRCLE)	SELF☐ ASSIST☐ COMPLETE☐	SELF☐ ASSIST☐ COMPLETE☐	SELF☐ ASSIST☐ COMPLETE☐
	SHIFT CARE	AM☐ SHAVE☐	AM☐ SHAVE☐	PM☐ HS☐ SHAVE☐
	ORAL CARE	NA☐ SELF☐ ASSIST☐ COMPLETE☐	NA☐ SELF☐ ASSIST☐ COMPLETE☐	NA☐ SELF☐ ASSIST☐ COMPLETE☐
	PERI CARE	NA☐ SELF☐ ASSIST☐ COMPLETE☐	NA☐ SELF☐ ASSIST☐ COMPLETE☐	NA☐ SELF☐ ASSIST☐ COMPLETE☐
	SKIN CARE	NA☐ SELF☐ ASSIST☐ COMPLETE☐	NA☐ SELF☐ ASSIST☐ COMPLETE☐	NA☐ SELF☐ ASSIST☐ COMPLETE☐
	CONDITION	WARM☐ COLD☐ DIAPHORETIC☐ DRY☐ CLAMMY☐	WARM☐ COLD☐ DIAPHORETIC☐ DRY☐ CLAMMY☐	WARM☐ COLD☐ DIAPHORETIC☐ DRY☐ CLAMMY☐
	ABRASIONS/RASH/SKIN TEAR	NA☐ LOCATION ______	NA☐ LOCATION ______	NA☐ LOCATION ______
	EDEMA (LOCATION, EXTENT)	YES☐ NO☐ ______	YES☐ NO☐ ______	YES☐ NO☐ ______
	DECUBITUS (CIRCLE)	Y/N FLOW SHEET IN USE: Y/N TURN SHEET IN USE: Y/N	Y/N FLOW SHEET IN USE: Y/N TURN SHEET IN USE: Y/N	Y/N FLOW SHEET IN USE: Y/N TURN SHEET IN USE: Y/N
ACTIVITY	EQUIPMENT	NA☐ EGGCRATE☐ OTHER ______	NA☐ EGGCRATE☐ OTHER ______	NA☐ EGGCRATE☐ OTHER ______
	TYPE OF ACTIVITY	BED☐ CHAIR☐ AMB☐ BSC☐ DANGLE☐ BRP☐ ROM☐	BED☐ CHAIR☐ AMB☐ BSC☐ DANGLE☐ BRP☐ ROM☐	BED☐ CHAIR☐ AMB☐ BSC☐ DANGLE☐ BRP☐ ROM☐
	HOW ACCOMPLISHED	SELF☐ ASSIST☐ P.T.☐	SELF☐ ASSIST☐ P.T.☐	SELF☐ ASSIST☐ P.T.☐
	LENGTH OF TIME, DISTANCE TOLERANCE	______ ______	______ ______	______ ______
	DEEP BREATHE AND COUGH	NA☐ Q2H ASSISTED☐ Q2H SELF☐	NA☐ Q2H ASSISTED☐ Q2H SELF☐	NA☐ Q2H ASSISTED☐ Q2H SELF☐
	REPOSITION	NA☐ Q2H ASSISTED☐ Q2H SELF☐	NA☐ Q2H ASSISTED☐ Q2H SELF☐	NA☐ Q2H ASSISTED☐ Q2H SELF☐
SAFETY	UNIVERSAL PRECAUTIONS	IN USE______ INITIAL ______	IN USE______ INITIAL ______	IN USE______ INITIAL ______
	EQUIPMENT	NA☐ K-PAD☐ IVAC☐ TEDS☐ TIME ON ___ TIME OFF ___	NA☐ K-PAD☐ IVAC☐ TEDS☐ TIME ON ___ TIME OFF ___	NA☐ K-PAD☐ IVAC☐ TEDS☐ TIME ON ___ TIME OFF ___
	SIDERAILS (UP/DOWN)	HEAD ↑ ☐ ↓ ☐ FOOT ↑ ☐ ↓ ☐	HEAD ↑ ☐ ↓ ☐ FOOT ↑ ☐ ↓ ☐	HEAD ↑ ☐ ↓ ☐ FOOT ↑ ☐ ↓ ☐
	BED IN LOW POSITION	YES☐ NO☐	YES☐ NO☐	YES☐ NO☐
	CALL BUTTON WITHIN REACH	YES☐ NO☐ OTHER ______	YES☐ NO☐ OTHER ______	YES☐ NO☐ OTHER ______
	SEIZURE PRECAUTIONS	NA☐ YES☐ NO☐	NA☐ YES☐ NO☐	NA☐ YES☐ NO☐
	RESTRAINTS (ON/OFF)	NA☐ POSEY☐ WRIST☐ ANKLE☐ TIME ON:______ TIME OFF:______	NA☐ POSEY☐ WRIST☐ ANKLE☐ TIME ON:______ TIME OFF:______	NA☐ POSEY☐ WRIST☐ ANKLE☐ TIME ON:______ TIME OFF:______
	ISOLATION	NA☐ TYPE______	NA☐ TYPE______	NA☐ TYPE______
PAIN	LOCATION & INTENSITY/DESCRIBE	NA☐ ______	NA☐ ______	NA☐ ______
	MEDICATION GIVEN	NA☐ YES☐	NA☐ YES☐	NA☐ YES☐
	RESULTS	NO RELIEF☐ RELIEF: MILD☐	NO RELIEF☐ RELIEF: MILD☐	NO RELIEF☐ RELIEF: MILD☐
	NOTE ACTION TAKEN IN NRS DOC.	MOD☐ COMPLETE☐	MOD☐ COMPLETE☐	MOD☐ COMPLETE☐
MD. CALL	PHYSICIAN CALLED NAME:	______	______	______
	REASON FOR CALL:	______	______	______
	RESPONSE:	______	______	______
	SIGNATURES	11-7 ______	7-3 ______	3-11 ______
		11-7 ______	7-3 ______	3-11 ______

Figure 4–6 Portion of activity flow sheet and assessment record used to document routine nursing care for each patient. (Courtesy of Santa Ynez Valley Hospital, Inc., Solvang, California.)

probably the most efficient method, because only one nurse is occupied while giving report on her patients. When the arriving staff is getting the report from the tape, the departing staff can be on the floor providing attention to patient needs. The problem with a taped report is that often it is not clearly audible or well organized, and the listener cannot ask any questions of the patient's previous nurse. However, if the department staff remain on the unit until the arriving staff have finished listening to the report, questions can be asked and answered.

Oral report from one staff member to another is usually given by the charge nurse to all of the arriving staff members. The entire arriving staff listens to the report on all patients; in this way staff members are more knowledgeable about all patients and can assist each other by answering call lights, filling in during meal breaks, etc. This method is time consuming, as each arriving

TABLE 4–4 SHIFT REPORT DATA

1. Room number and bed designation, Patient name, age, sex, date of admission, medical diagnoses, primary physician.
2. Tests and treatments/therapies performed in past 24 hours and patient response to them (i.e., blood transfusion, blood gas analyses, surgery, arteriogram, etc.); intake and output.
3. Significant changes in patient condition (utilize nursing process to organize the data in systematic fashion—assessment data, nursing diagnosis [if appropriate], planning, intervention, and evaluation).
4. Scheduled tests; consults or surgery; current IV solution, flow rate, and amount remaining or when next bag is due to be hung; oxygen flow rate; equipment in use and current settings (gastric suction, ventilator, CPM, PCA pump, etc.).
5. Current problems (i.e., fever, draining wound, severe pain, depression, anxiety, insufficient rest, abnormal lab values or test results) and amount of assistance needed.
6. Scheduled treatments, status on PRN medications with times and amounts given, response to medications and treatments.
7. Concerns, need for order changes, teaching, pertinent family dynamics, emotional status.

CPM, Continuous passive motion; PCA, patient-controlled analgesia.

nurse stays for the entire report for every patient on the unit.

A focused report is a method whereby the department nurse gives a report on specific patients assigned to the arriving nurse and only to her. Thus each nurse is only occupied for the time it takes to listen to the reports on her 4 to 10 patients. However, with this method, the other nurses do not know much about other patients on the unit.

Walking rounds is another method of giving and receiving report. The departing and arriving nurses go to the various patient rooms, and the departing nurse, along with the patient, describes what has happened during the previous shift and what the patient and nurse see as current needs and priorities for the present shift. This method allows the patient a greater feeling of input and control over his care. It is more time consuming than other methods, as patients are not usually as concise as the nurse in communicating needs.

Traditionally, a format like that shown in Table 4–4 has been used to organize and give report (Table 4–5) on each patient. With the

TABLE 4–5 EXAMPLE OF REPORT

Room 728, bed A, Mr. Harold Donald, 48-year-old male patient of Dr. Hopwitz admitted on the 2nd with abdominal pain; had an appendectomy yesterday with the wound left open, because the appendix was ruptered.

No problems during surgery; continuous IVs and IVPB antibiotics, NPO with NG tube to Gomco with low suction, no bowel sounds, wound irrigations with antibiotic solution tid. Intake 2,550 mL, output 1,730 mL.

Temperature has risen to 100.8°F, skin flushed, given Tylenol suppository at 8:00 and 12:00; decreased temperature to 99.6°F, but it went right back up. Some purulent drainage noted on wound irrigation; Dr. Hopwitz notified.

Wound culture ordered before next irrigation; IV D5 ½ NS with 20 mEq KCl at 125 mL/h, count 675 mL remaining, PCA pump with Demerol; he's using it appropriately, and pain appears to be well controlled.

Vital signs q 4 h, but take temperature q 2 h until stable again; observe for changes in secretions in wound drainage or signs of abdominal abcess; watch his electrolyte values—they were within normal limits this morning. WBC count was 14,200. Needs help to stand to urinate and with turning, coughing, and deep breathing. He smokes, so encourage coughing and deep breathing; with that open wound, he doesn't like to cough.

The irrigation solution is in the medication refrigerator and needs to be allowed to warm up before you use it. The equipment is in his room. Irrigations are done at 10:00, 2:00, and 8:00. He has Montgomery straps to ease dressing changes. Dressing has needed changing every 2 hours. He's on Unasyn and Mefoxin piggybacks; we are waiting for culture results.

He is very worried about the wound being left open and just how long he will be off work. He works as a carpenter and doesn't get paid when he is off. He will need to be taught proper wound care before discharge. His wife visits, but they have three small children at home and she can't stay long.

need for conserving the nurse's time and the extensive documentation systems currently in use, perhaps a modified report format might be more workable and efficient. Certainly with computerized care plans in hand, the nurse does not need to repeat a lot of the same data orally.

FUTURE TRENDS

In this age of computerization, shortage of nurses, and need for time efficiency, many changes will be seen in the way documentation is performed. The key issues will still be the need for thorough, accurate communication of patient data, care given, response to that care, and documentation in some form that such care has been received. A record will still need to be available over time, even though it may be preserved on a computer disk of some sort rather than on paper.

BIBLIOGRAPHY

American Nurses' Association: Standards: Medical-Surgical Nursing Practice. Kansas City, American Nurses' Association, 1974.

Collins, H. L.: Legal risks of computer charting. RN, May, 1990, p. 81.

Eggland, E. T.: Documenting completely and fully. Nursing 88, Nov., 1988, p. 76.

Fish, S., and Shelley, J. A.: Spiritual Care: The Nurse's Role. Downers Grove, IL, Intervarsity Press, 1978.

Goodall, C.: How should we teach the nursing process? Nurs. Times, Nov. 30, 1988, p. 47.

Gordon, M.: The concept of nursing diagnosis. Nurs. Clin. North Am., Sept., 1979, p. 487.

Green, E., et al.: A quality assurance tool that works overtime. RN, Sept., 1989, p. 30.

Harrington, A. M.: 8 steps for evaluating a new long-term care patient. Nursing 89, May, 1989, p. 74.

Ignatavicius, D.D., and Bayne, M. V. Medical-Surgical Nursing: A Nursing Process Approach. Philadelphia, W. B. Saunders, 1991.

Iyer, P. W.: New trends in charting. Nursing 91, Jan., 1991, p. 48.

Iyer, P. W.: Thirteen charting rules to keep you legally safe. Nursing 91, June, 1991, p. 40.

Krohn, B.: Spiritual care: The forgotten need. Imprint, Feb./Mar., 1989, p. 95.

Lampe, S. S.: Nursing documentation. A new perspective. J. Nurs. Admin., March, 1989, p. 3.

Magliozzi, H. M.: Charting that makes it through the Medicare maze. RN, June, 1990, p. 75.

Montemuro, M. CORE documentation: A complete system for charting nursing care. Nurs. Management, Aug., 1988, p. 28.

Peterson, G.: POMR: the SOAP revolution. J. Pract. Nurs., Aug., 1977, p. 36.

Predd, C. S.: Great tips for setting priorities. Nursing 89, Oct., 1989, p. 120.

Ramdayal, I.: For smoother shift changes, try walking rounds. RN, Sept., 1990, p. 19.

Richard, J.: Walking rounds: A step in the right direction. Nursing 89, June, 1989, p. 63.

Smith, C. E.: Upgrade your shift report with the three R's. Nursing 86, Feb., 1986, p. 63.

Stoll, R. I.: Guidelines for spiritual assessment. Am. J. Nurs., Sept., 1979, p. 1574.

Taptich, B. J., et al.: Nursing Diagnosis and Care Planning. Philadelphia, W. B. Saunders, 1989.

Ulrich, S. P., et al.: Nursing Care Planning Guides: A Nursing Diagnosis Approach. Philadelphia, W. B. Saunders, 1990.

Yura, H., and Walsh, M. B.: The Nursing Process, 5th ed. East Norwalk, CT, Appleton-Lange, 1988.

Zimmer, E.: The nursing health history: A powerful tool. Adv. Clin. Care, May/June, 1990, p. 31.

STUDENT STUDY AIDS

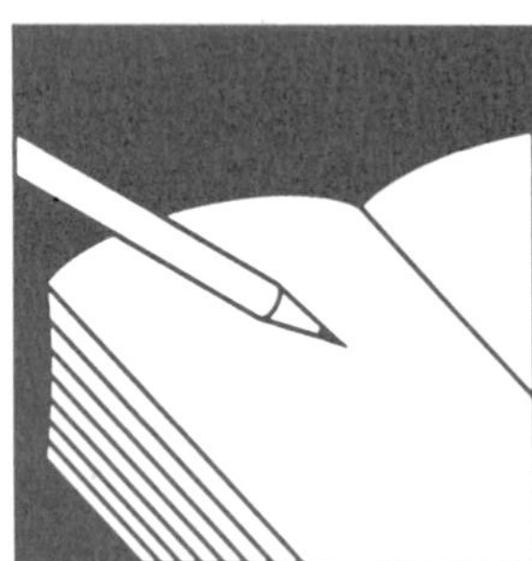

CLINICAL CASE PROBLEMS

Read each clinical situation and discuss the questions with your classmates.

1. Mrs. Farmer, age 48, is admitted to the Outpatient Surgery unit with abnormal menstrual bleeding. She is scheduled for a dilatation and curettage (D and C) for diagnostic purposes.

- What kinds of nursing assessment questions during the interview would you expect to ask when Mrs. Farmer is admitted?
- How could you contribute to the collection of data for assessment and identification of patient care problems Mrs. Farmer is likely to have?

2. Mrs. Farmer is very anxious about what the surgeon might find. She is especially concerned about malignancy. She also is worried about whether she will "wake up" from the anesthesia. Her nursing care plan includes nursing intervention to help minimize Mrs. Farmer's anxiety, as well as preoperative teaching in coughing and deep breathing.

- Using the components of the teaching-learning process, develop a simple plan for teaching Mrs. Farmer what she needs to know about coughing and deep breathing.
- What else might you talk with Mrs. Farmer about to help allay her fears and anxieties?

- How could you evaluate the effectiveness of the nurses' efforts to allay anxiety and your efforts to instruct Mrs. Farmer?

---

3. Mr. Johanssen has just been told by his physician that he has a chronic and incurable illness. He will be able to manage the illness if he is willing to learn about it and follow his physician's orders. Mr. Johanssen alternates between being very angry and very depressed and bewildered.

- Discuss with your classmates how a nurse might assess Mr. Johanssen's spiritual needs and what might be done to help him cope with his illness.

---

4. You have been caring for Mrs. Wolonski this shift. She is recovering from a fractured femur that is being treated with balanced traction. When you examine her pin sites, you notice a slight amount of bloody drainage around the pin on the left. Her pain is controlled for only 2 hours on the ordered oral analgesics, and she is complaining of a stuffy head and "sinus."

- Write out your nurse's note for her for this shift.
- Give a report to another nurse as if it is the end of the shift.

STUDY OUTLINE

I. Characteristics and goals of the nursing process

A. Process: a series of actions that move toward achievement of a goal.
B. Actions are carried out deliberately and systematically.
C. Nursing process: a goal-directed series of actions whereby nursing practice is approached.
D. Goal is to alleviate, minimize, or prevent real or potential health problems that a nurse is qualified to treat.
E. Nursing process is a deliberate, rational, and logical approach to the task of helping the patient deal with health problems.
F. Demands knowledge, skills, and belief in the worth of every person.

II. Differences in nursing roles

A. Based on differences in educational preparation and experience.
B. Minimal expectation for new graduates of various nursing programs have been defined by the NLN.
C. Essential tasks of beginning nurses are:
   1. Collecting specific kinds of information.
   2. Contributing to development of nursing care plans.
   3. Performing basic therapeutic and preventive nursing measures.
   4. Participating in evaluating outcomes of care.

III. Underlying assumptions

A. Fundamental beliefs about human life, role of nursing, and the delivery of health care.
B. Respect the worth, dignity, and individuality of each person.
C. Recognize common human needs and the fact that people must have help in meeting those needs.
D. Emphasize the right to patient-centered, high-quality health care and importance of patient input.
E. Focus on the role of nursing in health maintenance and care of the sick and injured.
F. Encourage self-fulfillment of the nurse.

IV. Nursing process and the scientific method

A. Nurses use the scientific method as framework for nursing practice.
B. Problem-solving approach to problems of health.
C. Physicians and nurses use the same methodology, but information needed and used and activities performed are different.

D. Nurse is aware of the rationale for medical treatment.
E. Actions of physician, nurse, and other health team members are complementary.

V. Components of the nursing process

A. Components: structural parts or elements.
  1. Components are interdependent and continuously interacting with one another.
  2. Components represent points in the system at which action can take place in response to feedback.

B. Assessment (data gathering).
  1. Purpose is to collect data about patient's health status in order to establish nursing diagnoses.
  2. Information should be relevant to the problem and of sufficient quantity to allow valid conclusions to be drawn.
  3. Assessment is ongoing; therefore, a plan of care can be revised when there is new information.
  4. Initial assessment made at the time of nurses's first encounter with the patient to provide a data base. Baseline information useful for later comparisons of patient's status.
  5. Sources of data include patient or client, his family members or significant others, findings of other health team members.
  6. Techniques for gathering information about the patient:
    a. Records: new admission records and old records from previous admissions.
    b. Interview: to obtain nursing history.
      (1) Purpose is explained to the patient.
      (2) Conversational tone using direct and indirect open-ended questions.
      (3) Summarizing at end of interview helps clarify and validate information.
      (4) Psychosocial assessment
        (a) Educational level, employment status, marital status, number of children, health insurance, type of household, hobbies, leisure activities, pets.
        (b) Significant relationships and support system.
        (c) Other problems that might impact health.
        (d) Cultural beliefs and values, especially regarding illness and health care.
        (e) How the patient perceives his state of health.
        (f) Coping patterns.
        (g) Level of self-esteem, perceived roles, dynamics of family relationships.
        (h) Signs of anxiety or depression.
      (5) Spiritual assessment:
        (a) Necessary for holistic care of the patient.
        (b) Can be done during initial assessment interview or at any time that seems appropriate.
        (c) Guidelines suggest four general areas of concern and pertinent questions (see Table 4–3).
        (d) Sources of spiritual help include use of self, prayer, Scripture, and referral to or consultation with clergy.
    c. Observation: perhaps most important of all techniques.
      (1) Includes subjective and objective symptoms.
      (2) Nurse uses all of her senses to assess patient's health status.

d. Physical examination: includes vital signs, inspection, auscultation, and palpation.
e. Laboratory data.
f. Consultation with people and with the written word.

C. Analysis and nursing diagnosis.
1. A nursing diagnosis is a concise statement of a patient's actual or potential health problem that nurses are able and licensed to treat.
2. Categories of nursing diagnoses currently being refined. First proposed in 1972 at National Conference on Classification of Nursing Diagnoses.
   a. Goal is to standardize nursing diagnoses so as to facilitate communication among nurses and identify specific outcome criteria and nursing interventions for resolution of patient care problems.
3. Nursing diagnoses are primarily concerned with
   a. Patient's comfort and sense of well-being.
   b. Prevention of complications.
   c. Patient education.
4. Medical diagnosis and nursing diagnosis complement one another.
5. Nursing diagnoses give direction to nursing care plan.

D. Planning.
1. Provides a blueprint for nursing interventions.
2. Requires input from patient and family.
3. Steps include:
   a. Determining priorities from problem list.
   b. Setting goals. Goals are broad statements describing restoration to, maintenance of, or promotion of health.
   c. Developing objectives or outcome criteria to reach goals. Outcome criteria are measurable and attainable steps toward accomplishment of overall goals. Elements include patient activity that can be observed or tested, conditions provided to help patient reach objective, and time objective will be met and quality of performance.
   d. Writing nursing orders. Nursing orders include actions of nurse and patient activities prescribed to help reach objectives and goals.
4. Plan is revised as problems are resolved and others arise, or when nursing intervention is changed.

E. Implementation.
1. The phase during which the plan is put into action.
2. Nursing actions are coordinated with other forms of therapy so that the total care given is beneficial to the patient.
3. Implementation concludes with documentation of care given and the patient's response to that care.

F. Evaluation.
1. The evaluation step of the nursing process is continuous and ongoing.
   a. Nursing interventions are evaluated to see whether they have been effective.
   b. Interventions are judged effective if outcome criteria are being met.
   c. If intervention seems ineffective, plan needs to be revised.
2. Quality assurance is aimed at evaluation of the hospital, unit, nursing care, and other aspects of hospital function.

a. Quality assurance audits scrutinize various aspects of hospital care to see if they are meeting standards.
b. The Joint Commission on Accreditation of Hospitals reviews care given by hospitals.
c. A chart audit is done after the patient is discharged to see if the care he received meets set standards for the type of problem he had.
d. Each hospital has a quality assurance committee or board that coordinates audit activities.
e. ANA Standards of Nursing Practice are used as criteria for process evaluation of nursing care.

3. Ultimate goal of all evaluation activities is improvement of nursing care.
4. Evaluation *not* done to find someone to blame. It *is* done to improve nursing care.

VI. Patient education

A. Overall goals are to:
1. Promote the health of the patient and his family.
2. Maintain or improve the patient's current health status.
3. Help the patient learn to help himself.

B. Components of the teaching-learning process:
1. Assessment: determining learning readiness and learning needs in three areas: cognitive (knowing), psychomotor (doing), and affective (feeling).
2. Planning: based on specific learning objectives; includes content (what is to be taught), method (how), resources and materials (who), time (when), and place (where).
3. Instruction: carrying out the plan for teaching.
4. Evaluation: measuring what the patient knows, what he is able to do, and what he values after he has been taught.

C. Patient education is essential to *total* patient care:
1. Provides a means by which the patient can participate in his own care.
2. Meets learning needs that directly affect his health status.

D. Documentation of the teaching process:
1. Teaching plan is detailed under the nursing diagnosis of "knowledge deficit" or is placed on a separate flow sheet.
2. The nurse records material taught, patient response and evaluation of the process, and the patient's progress for each teaching session.
3. The time spent doing patient teaching must be documented for insurance coverage of the cost.

VII. Documentation and interstaff communication

A. Documentation gives concrete evidence of the quality of care given.
B. Provides communication mode between shifts and between nurses and other health professionals.
C. Protects nurse and institution when legal action is taken against them.
D. Provides for verification of services rendered for Medicare and insurance payments.
E. Thorough documentation is essential to good communication and to continuity of care.

VIII. Source-oriented and problem-oriented record keeping

A. Source-oriented record keeping is traditional system. Data arranged according to source of information.

B. Problem-oriented record keeping focuses on specific problems presented by the patient.
C. Whatever the system in use, nurse's notes should include:
   1. Treatments and medications not charted elsewhere.
   2. Nursing observations and interventions.
   3. Patient response to treatment, nursing interventions, and diagnostic procedures.
   4. Symptoms and changes in patient's condition.
   5. Irregularities and unusual incidents.

IX. Charting formats

A. Documentation is placed on flow sheet and in nurse's notes.
B. Methods of documentation are undergoing considerable change at the present time.
C. Systems charting: the nurse charts pertinent data regarding each physical system of the patient and then adds psychosocial data.
D. PEMS format useful for source-oriented record keeping:
   P—physical problems.
   E—emotional needs.
   M—mental status.
   S—safety needs.
   1. Additional information also must be charted (e.g., physicians' visits, teaching and evidence of learning, discontinued treatments, and other significant data).
E. Focused charting: utilizes a narrative format for data about the "focus" of the patient's problem, and then other data is noted on flow sheets.
F. Hierarchy of human needs also helpful in organizing thinking about what to look for and what to chart:
   1. Acronym RN'S HOPE serves as a guide:
      R—rest and activity.
      N—nutrition.
      S—safety and self-care deficit.
      H—hygiene and skin.
      O—oxygenation.
      P—psychosocial assessment.
      E—elimination.
      a. Basic physical needs
      b. Safety and security needs
      c. Ego and self-esteem needs
      d. Need to be loved and to have a sense of belonging. Verbal and nonverbal clues can help nurse recognize unmet psychological and social needs.
G. SOAP nurses's notes: an integral part of the problem-oriented medical record keeping system.
   S—subjective symptoms and information.
   O—objective symptoms and observations.
   A—assessment (analysis), conclusion drawn: nursing diagnosis.
   P—plan: what will be done now or later

X. Problem-oriented medical record keeping (POMR).

A. More logical and better organized than traditional source-oriented record keeping.
B. Greatly improves communication and coordination of patient care.
C. Enables patient care managers to improve staff and patient education.
D. Provides a means for evaluating quality of patient care.

E. Components of POMR system:
1. Data base: basic information about patient's medical and nursing history, physical, mental, and psychosocial status.
2. Problem list: serves as an index to the progress notes.
3. Plan: proposed activities, treatments, etc., designed to help patient deal with each problem.
4. *Notes:* the section in which all persons participating in the care of the patient can document what is being done about each problem and how these activities are affecting the patient's progress.

UNIT TWO

DISEASE-PRODUCING FACTORS AND THE RESPONSES THEY EVOKE

In Unit 1 we discussed the concepts of health and illness and the goals of the human living system. We also discussed use of the nursing process as a systematic approach to the goals of maintaining and restoring health. To be well is to be able to maintain constancy in the internal environment and to live in harmony with the world (that is, with all the factors in the external environment). However, the environment in which humans live is a hostile one, and the body must have both external and internal defenses to protect itself and to recover from invasion of harmful agents once they gain access to the internal environment. Fortunately there are remarkable processes at work in the human body to ensure survival of the species, if not optimal health for every living person. One of the tasks of nursing is to strengthen the resources of each patient so that he can resist and overcome disease-producing factors in his environment.

Aging is a natural process in which individuals progress through the life span in stages. At each stage of development there are certain tasks that one must accomplish in order to advance to the next stage and to maintain an acceptable level of physical and mental health. The stage at which one is during a particular time of life is directly related to one's vulnerability to certain threats to health and welfare. Thus the first chapter of this unit gives an overview of the various stages of adult life and considers age as a factor in the maintenance of health and development of illness.

It is always wise, when preparing to engage in a battle against hostile forces of any kind, to do all that you can to "know your enemy." If we are to help our patients in their efforts to respond appropriately to harmful agents, we need to know what those enemy forces are and how best to deal with them. Chapter 6 discusses how to identify the major disease-producing factors that threaten health, utilize effective measures to contain and destroy them, and assist our patients in their recovery from illness and injury. This chapter also covers the first and second lines of defense against disease, which include both protective structures and organs as well as such internal mechanisms as inflammation, repair and healing. Chapter 7 discusses the immune response and the chemical and mechanical activities the body uses internally to protect against invading organisms and to attempt to eliminate them. In each chapter an attempt has been made to show the relationships between effective nursing actions and achievement of the goal of living in harmony with the outside world.

CHAPTER 5

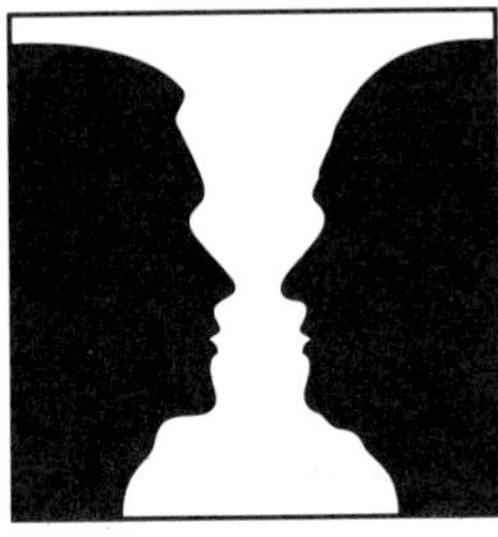

Age as a Factor in Illness

VOCABULARY

cirrhosis
disorientation
familial
flatulence
geriatric
gerontology
grimacing
hypertension
imperceptible
motility
philosophy
prophylactic
psychosocial
resilience

Upon completion of this chapter the student should be able to:

1. Discuss major sources of psychological and physiologic stress in persons between the ages of 20 and 70 years.
2. Identify lifestyle behaviors during young adulthood that can have an adverse effect on health status in later life.
3. List specific resources and interventions that can help young adults maintain health and avoid premature death.
4. Give three reasons why the period between 45 and 60 years of age is often called a time of the "change of life."
5. Identify some major sources of psychological and physiologic stress during the middle years.
6. List specific health care needs of persons in middle adulthood and interventions that can help meet those needs.
7. Discuss significant physiological changes and social factors that can adversely affect the physical and mental health of persons over 60 years of age.

In recent years many scholars and authorities in the life sciences have written about the various stages of life and how they affect physical and mental health. Statistics on morbidity and mortality rates for various age groups clearly show that the physiologic and psychological events occurring during the stages of life from birth to old age have an impact on an individual's health and survival. Table 5–1 shows the major causes of death by age group. Young adults, for example, face stresses and sometimes choose lifestyles that make them more susceptible to certain kinds of illness and injury and predispose them to the development of chronic illnesses later in life. Persons in middle age must deal with different kinds of stresses and life crises, and so must the elderly.

An important responsibility of nurses and others in the health care field is to recognize the relationships between an individual's age, his potential for certain kinds of health problems, and the health care he requires. Once these relationships are acknowledged and understood, the nurse is in a better position to help people

TABLE 5–1 FIFTEEN LEADING CAUSES OF DEATH, BY AGE GROUP, UNITED STATES, 1982

Cause of Death	All Ages*	Under 1 Year	1–14 Years	15–24 Years	25–34 Years	35–44 Years	45–54 Years	55–64 Years	65–74 Years	75–84 Years	85 Years and Over
1. Heart diseases	296.3	18.8	1.1	2.1	7.5	30.8	124.6	377.8	910.1	2,412.5	6,742.6
2. Malignant neoplasms	200.3	1.5	3.2	5.3	13.3	45.0	158.5	451.4	843.5	1,338.4	1,655.2
3. Cerebrovascular diseases	59.4	2.8	0.3	0.4	1.9	6.7	18.1	50.6	147.6	530.2	6,632.8
4. Accidents and adverse effects	38.2	28.4	13.3	47.7	36.1	29.9	29.8	34.1	49.1	108.9	277.1
5. Chronic obstructive pulmonary diseases and allied conditions	34.0	1.5	0.3	0.5	0.8	2.1	9.6	48.9	147.2	314.7	407.0
6. Pneumonia and influenza	30.3	12.7	0.6	0.8	1.7	3.6	6.1	18.0	55.5	242.5	1,082.5
7. Diabetes mellitus	18.8	—	0.0	0.3	1.7	4.1	11.2	30.9	70.3	143.2	263.0
8. Suicide	12.6	—	0.5	13.8	15.8	14.3	14.8	15.7	16.8	28.9	14.7
9. Chronic liver disease and cirrhosis	10.6	0.0	0.0	0.2	2.4	10.3	20.7	30.1	35.7	31.0	18.3
10. Atherosclerosis	7.7	—	—	—	0.0	0.1	0.9	3.8	16.2	74.1	428.8
11. Homicide and legal intervention	9.3	8.1	1.7	16.7	17.2	10.6	7.5	5.2	4.2	4.2	3.6
12. Certain conditions originating in the perinatal period	7.5	464.4	0.3	0.0	0.1	—	0.0	—	—	—	—
13. Nephritis, nephrotic syndrome, and nephrosis	8.6	5.6	0.1	0.3	0.6	1.2	2.9	8.7	24.0	71.9	204.8
14. Human immunodeficiency virus infection	8.6	0.5 (Under 1 Year and 1–14 Years combined)		1.4	16.9	23.6	12.0	3.0 (55 Years and Over combined)			
15. Septicemia	7.7	6.0	0.1	0.3	0.9	1.7	3.1	7.6	20.6	62.1	178.5

* Figures for age not stated included in "All Ages" but not distributed among age groups.

Data adapted from Hoffman, M.S.: The World Almanac and Book of Facts 1990. New York, Pharos Books, 1990. Rates per 100,000 population in specified group.

avoid or at least defer illness and death past the life stage at which they are most susceptible. In this way a nurse assists them in living their lives more fully and with a greater sense of well-being.

In this chapter we will briefly discuss several periods of life, beginning with early adulthood (20 to 29 years of age) and continuing through older adulthood (75 years of age and older). Each of these life periods is characterized by physical health problems, developmental tasks, psychosocial crises, and health care needs that are unique to and typical of each age group.

EARLY ADULTHOOD (20 TO 29 YEARS)

Persons in early adulthood have reached biologic maturity, and so their task is one of preservation and maintenance of health. However, they do face psychological stresses that can play havoc with their physical and mental well-being. This period of life is one of change and new beginnings: starting a new career, living away from home for the first time, and beginning serious and intimate relationships such as marriage. The demand for more and more education in our society has lengthened the time period for completion of schooling. Many people in this age group are spending these years pursuing further education and higher degrees.

HEALTH PROBLEMS

The four major causes of death in this age group are all violent in nature — vehicular or other accidents, suicide, or homicide.

Typical health problems are anxiety, depression, complications of pregnancy, cervical and breast cancer, and back, limb, and hip injuries. Factors that can create health problems are related to the physical and psychological pressures on young adults to establish their independence and "make it on their own." In pursuing their goals and striving to achieve useful employment, they often tend to work and play too hard. Such a busy lifestyle frequently leads young adults to rely heavily on fast-food restaurants for meals. Sleep and rest, good nutrition, and sensible exercise are sacrificed for activities that they think will satisfy their needs for security, self-esteem, and love. They might, for example, go on crash diets to lose weight in an effort to satisfy a need for acceptance by their peers.

Persons in this age group experience keen competition from their peers in the areas of employment and social relationships. Stress and the desire for acceptance coupled with the newfound freedom to experiment and try various lifestyles contribute to drug and alcohol abuse, dietary excesses, and smoking. Choices made during this stage of life before the age of 29 can have a direct bearing on one's health status later in life (Table 5–2).

HEALTH CARE NEEDS

The health service most needed during early adulthood is a thorough assessment of health status. This should include a physical examination; assistance with completion of developmental tasks; health education and individual counseling on nutrition and exercise; assistance and support in dealing with alcohol, drugs, and smoking; and counseling and guidance on sexual behavior, contraception, and marriage and family relationships. Blood pressure should be checked at least annually.

Because young adults are for the most part physically healthy, or at least like to think they are, it is important that they be encouraged to have at least one complete physical examination early in this period of their life. The examination should include tests for sexually transmitted diseases, hypertension, and cholesterol level. If the person has not had a tetanus booster in the previous 10 years, the booster should be given at this time. Young women should be encouraged to have a Pap smear done at least every 3 years and should be taught the technique and importance of breast self-examination. Young men should be taught and encouraged to do testicular examinations.

Developmental tasks that should be completed during this period of life to ensure continuing psychosocial growth and maturity include (1) accepting oneself and stabilizing self-concept and body image; (2) establishing a personal identity; (3) achieving independence from parental controls and establishing and maintaining a residence; (4) establishing intimate relationships outside the family; (5) becoming established in a career that provides personal satisfaction, economic security, and a feeling of contributing to the welfare of society; and (6) establishing a personal set of values and formulating a meaningful philosophy of life. Marriage, childbearing, and work are important areas in which the individual's developmental tasks are focused.

As a person enters young adulthood, his need for calcium and protein is slightly increased. Young women need more protein than men because of blood loss during menstruation. They also require almost twice as much iron (18 mg daily) to counteract anemia. About one third of American women between the ages of 10 and 55 years are anemic because of inadequate intake of iron. Exercise for 30 minutes three times a week, combined with adequate calcium intake at this age, is thought to help prevent osteoporosis in women later in life.

TABLE 5-2 HARMFUL HABITS OF LIFESTYLE AND THEIR EFFECTS ON HEALTH

Habit or Behavior	Possible Effect
Alcohol abuse	Cirrhosis of the liver, brain damage, malnutrition. Motor vehicle and other accidents.
Cigarette smoking	Chronic bronchitis, chronic obstructive lung disease, coronary artery disease, and lung cancer.
Drug abuse	Drug dependence and addiction, drug reactions, and mental changes leading to suicide, homicide, and accidents.
Overeating and crash diets	Obesity, diabetes mellitus, and malnutrition.
High fat intake	Atherosclerosis and coronary artery disease.
Lack of sensible exercise	Obesity, loss of physical fitness, and orthopedic injuries.
Lack of recreation and relief from work	Stress-related illnesses such as hypertension, coronary artery disease, gastrointestinal disorders.
Sexual carelessness and irresponsibility	Sexually transmitted diseases and unwanted pregnancies.

Young persons with a family history of diabetes or cardiovascular disease should be particularly careful to keep their body weight within the normal range. It is especially important for later health that eating nutritious, low-calorie meals and exercising sensibly be made a way of life during these years.

Health care providers should establish programs that are tailored to the needs, expectations, and lifestyles of young adults.

Programs of this kind might include weight control, problems related to human sexuality, family planning, the effects of drugs and alcohol, child care, and home management.

YOUNG ADULTHOOD (30 TO 44 YEARS)

When most people reach 30 years of age, they tend to evaluate where they are and where they wish to go with their lives. In our youth-oriented society, reaching age 30 can be very traumatic. However, for most it is a time to reset goals to be accomplished in adulthood.

These middle years are directed mainly toward raising a family and furthering a career. It is the "prime time" of adulthood, and these years are directed toward achievement. Toward the end of this period some females may experience the onset of menopause and the end of their childbearing years.

HEALTH PROBLEMS

In recent years many people have postponed marriage and beginning a family until this stage of their lives. One problem that has arisen is difficulty with conception, which can create considerable stress for a couple.

Major causes of death in this age group reflect the psychosocial stresses of this period and the impact of unhealthy lifestyles adopted earlier in life. Heart attack replaces motor vehicle accidents as the leading cause of death in white males between the ages of 30 and 44 years. Stroke and cirrhosis (degenerative disease) of the liver, both of which are related to lifestyle, first appears among the five major causes of death in males and females of this age group.

Factors that contribute to illness and death in those in this age group include such external environmental conditions as a stressful job or other occupational hazards and marital problems, including adjustment to the responsibilities of parenting. Other disease-producing factors are the stresses of managing a household, smoking, drug abuse, poor nutrition, and failure to acknowledge the benefit of changing lifestyle to avoid illness.

HEALTH CARE NEEDS

Health care for individuals in this age group should be directed toward the goal of helping them enjoy maximum physical energy for fulfillment of their emotional and social potential.

Another goal is to guard against the onset of chronic illnesses through good health habits, early detection of chronic disease such as cardiovascular disease and cancer, and prompt treatment to avoid long-term consequences.

During this age period the young adult should have periodic visits with a physician or nurse to evaluate his health status. These visits usually are recommended at age 30, age 35, and then every 3 years thereafter. The physical examination should include tests for hypertension, anemia, and cholesterol level, as well as a cervical smear for cancer in females and a baseline mammogram at age 35. Teaching should be reinforced on how to conduct monthly self-examination of the breasts and testes, periodic assessment of the skin for potentially malignant lesions, and inspection of the mouth for precancerous lesions.

Dental examinations, professional cleaning of the teeth, and any other necessary prophylactic (preventive) measures should be done at least once every 2 years and preferably every 6 months if there are any dental problems.

Developmental tasks for persons in this age group are related to managing a household, rearing children, and developing a career.

Some specific interventions to help accomplish the goals of promoting health and preventing or at least deferring the onset of chronic illness include (1) instruction and support in the management of stress; (2) utilization of resources and instructional courses in household management and effective parenting; (3) encouraging reduced intake of sodium, fat, and sugar and maintenance of normal body weight; (4) developing an awareness of the dangers of excessive alcohol intake and drug abuse and utilization of available self-help groups in dealing with these problems; (5) providing classes and support groups to help those who smoke or are overweight develop more healthful habits; and (6) encouraging a program of moderate exercise.

MIDDLE ADULTHOOD (45 TO 65 YEARS)

Middle age is truly the time of a "change of life." It is the time when one begins the task of reevaluation of the direction life is taking. There is a period of looking back over previous accomplishments, some regret for those things that have not been accomplished, and a setting of new goals for the later years. For many, this is a period of enjoying the benefits of the hard work done in earlier years.

During the middle years there is a change in one's self-image as the body begins to show external signs of aging.

The hair grays, the skin wrinkles and sags, the muscles lose some of their tone, and the waistline thickens. Less visible changes in the internal organs begin to take place, and the body that once seemed indestructible and tireless begins to develop aches and pains. If all these changes seem somewhat grim, that is in large part because our society values youth and aspires to the unattainable dream of staying young forever. However, it is possible to adopt values that transcend personal appearance and external beauty. People can and do grow old gracefully and learn to appreciate the advantages of being older, wiser, and at peace with themselves and with the society in which they live.

Crises during middle age, just as at any other time of life, can be accepted as challenges to individuals to change and to grow mentally and emotionally. Social changes that occur in the middle years center on role changes. If the person is married and has children who are grown and have achieved their independence, the role of parent must be exchanged for a return to the role of full-time husband or wife. If the person's mother or father is still living, sometimes the middle-aged offspring acts as a parent to his or her own parent. Roles are reversed in this situation, and the reversal demands adjustments that are not easy. Furthermore, as the costs of maintaining a separate residence increase, more parents are experiencing a return of grown children into their home for an extended interval. Considering the stress of dealing with their own aging parents, this can be an overwhelming burden. A new relationship, on an adult-to-adult level, must be developed. Illness can be precipitated if adjustments to these stresses are not managed well.

Death begins to claim parents, spouses, and friends during these years. Coping with such loss is never easy. The ability to resolve grief in a healthy way often depends on the number of other stressors the person is experiencing at the time and the availability of others for support.

When a middle-aged person becomes ill, the accompanying loss of some degree of independence may be difficult for him and his family members and friends to accept. Worries about job security and the welfare of those who have depended on him may create stress and emotional illness. Women who have devoted their earlier years to child-rearing and focused their time and energies on their children may face crises of identity once their adult children have left home. Some view the situation as a well-deserved freedom that allows them to seek opportunities for self-realization. A new career, completion of an education that was interrupted by marriage, and the opportunity to travel are all ways in which middle-aged women have met critical changes in their middle years. Others are frustrated or frightened by the changes imposed on them and are unable to embark on new activities that can give meaning and purpose to their lives. Males and females in middle adulthood often find satisfaction in community service projects and other activities that improve the quality of life for other members of their community.

Toward the end of this period, people begin to consider retiring from work and must plan for the reduction in income they will experience. However, there is a growing trend for more people to continue employment into late adulthood.

Many middle-aged adults are experiencing separation and divorce. This causes a significant blow to self-esteem and requires a restructuring of lifestyle—a task that does not come as easily as in younger years.

HEALTH PROBLEMS

Cardiovascular diseases such as heart attack and stroke become the major causes of death in both males and females as they reach their middle years. Among the top five causes of mortality are lung and breast cancer and cirrhosis of the liver. Chronic respiratory disease and hypertension (elevated blood pressure) also are major health problems that require continuous cooperative management on the part of the patient and health care providers. As life stresses and affluence have increased in our society, the use of alcohol has become more prevalent. Alcoholism is another major health problem in this age group.

External and internal factors that contribute to deterioration of health status in the middle-aged are similar to those of young adulthood.

HEALTH CARE NEEDS

As in young adulthood, the health goals of persons in middle adulthood should be related to preserving and prolonging the period of maximum energy and optimal mental and social activity. If good physical and emotional health has been maintained up to this stage in life, the middle-aged person can pursue the interests and activities that he or she might have postponed while child-rearing and career goals were being accomplished.

Regular assessment of health status is very important in maintaining good health during these years. Identification of illness in its earliest stage helps prevent complications. A complete physical examination is recommended at age 40 and every 3 years thereafter. Annual checkups for women that include breast examination can identify early breast cancer. Mammograms should be done every 2 to 3 years, depending on the risk factors of each woman. At age 50 and thereafter, annual physical examinations are recommended and should also include an examination for colon cancer. A baseline sigmoidoscopy should be performed at age 50, and if stool tests for occult blood are negative each year, the sigmoidoscopy should be repeated every 3 years.

Immunizations also should be reviewed at this time. During interviews for medical and nursing history one should be alert for problems related to nutrition, physical exercise, occupational hazards, sexual dysfunction and adjustment to menopause, marital and parenting difficulties, and the use of alcohol, tobacco, and drugs.

Nutrition counseling should encourage a diet in which there is a reduction in the daily intake of calories, saturated fats, and cholesterol. This is recommended because there is a gradual slowing of intestinal motility, with accompanying digestive impairment, during middle age. The metabolic rate declines, and the lungs become more rigid, causing a decrease in breathing capacity.

People at this age also have a tendency to use nonprescription drugs for their aches and pains and problems of sleep and rest. Drugs that are advertised to guarantee a good night's sleep tend to decrease the amount of deep, restful sleep needed to prepare for physical activities during the day. Prescription drugs also can be dangerous if the person is not informed about the purpose of the drug, its expected action, possible untoward reactions that should be reported to the nurse or physician, and the necessity of taking the drug exactly as prescribed.

Developmental tasks at this stage of life are related to management of the household, adjusting to changes in role, career management, and the dedication of resources, skill, and creativity toward improving the quality of life for the young.

Some specific developmental tasks are as follows:

1. Discovering and developing new satisfaction, if the person is married, by enjoying joint activities and developing an abiding sense of intimacy and unity with the marriage partner.
2. Helping growing and grown children become happy and responsible adults and freeing one-self from emotional dependence on children.
3. Creating a pleasant, hospitable, and comfortable home that is compatible with one's values and resources.
4. Balancing work with other roles and preparing for retirement.
5. Accepting role reversal with aging parents and preparing emotionally for the eventual death of living parents.
6. Coping with loss of parents, spouse, or friends as a result of death or divorce.
7. Achieving mature social and civic responsibility and involvement in altruistic activities and concerns.
8. Accepting and adjusting to the physical

changes of middle adulthood and maintaining healthful ways of living.

9. Continuing to formulate a philosophy of life (i.e., set of principles; ethics) and a religious or philosophical affiliation.

Suggestions for helping middle-aged persons improve their energy level and maintain health are summarized in Table 5-3.

LATE ADULTHOOD (66 TO 74 YEARS)

To someone in his late teens or early twenties a person over 65 years of age is "elderly" or "very old." But the person who is in late adulthood may not think of himself as old at all. So much depends on one's outlook and attitudes toward aging, and on one's physical condition and personal resources, that it is best not to make judgments about what all older and elderly people are like or what it means to grow old.

There are, however, some significant changes that occur at this time of life. These are related to aging and require a flexible response and adaptation to maintain good mental and physical health. It is during late adulthood that people retire from work, experience a reduction in income, and possibly suffer the loss of a spouse. In the United States the death rate for men is almost double that for women at this stage of life. This means that women in this age group substantially outnumber men.

During this life stage both men and women need to be able to adjust to physical as well as social changes. Sight and hearing begin to decline, and the senses of touch, taste, and smell become less acute. Reaction time slows down, and the muscles do not respond as readily as they did when the person was younger. As aging progresses there is less elasticity and more rigidity on all levels—physical, emotional, and social.

On the positive side, at this age one can enjoy freedom from career competition and from the responsibility of rearing and supporting children. There is time to develop new and stimulating interests and to use the knowledge and experience accumulated in earlier years to do the creative and self-satisfying things one really wants to do, and there is time to relax and enjoy the fruits of one's labors.

TABLE 5-3 SUGGESTIONS FOR IMPROVING ENERGY AND HEALTH DURING MIDDLE AGE

1. Eat nutritious foods that help you maintain normal weight, and get sufficient sleep and rest.
2. Sign up for an exercise class if you do not follow a regular exercise program.
3. Check and correct your posture for better chest and lung expansion.
4. Attend courses for weight control, stopping smoking, and management of alcohol intake if you have a problem in any of these areas.
5. Take vacations to recharge yourself physically and emotionally.
6. Check your environment at home and at work for too much noise, poor lighting, poor ventilation and temperature control, and safety hazards that could cause accidents.
7. Think positively. There are positive aspects to growing older.
8. Have regular physical assessments and appropriate testing.
9. Be active as a citizen; become involved in political and social issues that interest you.
10. Prepare physically, mentally, and emotionally for the coming years so you will remain as productive and live as purposefully as possible for as long as you can.

Data from Murray, R., and Zentner, J.: Nursing Assessment and Health Promotion Through the Life Span, 3rd ed. Englewood Cliffs, NJ, Prentice-Hall, 1985.

HEALTH PROBLEMS

As might be expected, the major causes of death in persons over the age of 65 are chronic conditions such as cardiovascular disease (including congestive heart failure and stroke), cancer, and diabetes.

Illnesses commonly found in this age group include gastrointestinal problems, such as peptic ulcer and constipation; acute and chronic respiratory diseases, such as influenza, pneumonia, and emphysema; and gallbladder disease. Prostatic enlargement, both benign and malignant, is commonly found in males, and breast cancer is found in females.

HEALTH CARE NEEDS

In addition to health care to help these patients manage their chronic illnesses, a major goal of health care should be to help them prolong the period of optimal physical, mental, and social activity.

If plans have not already been made for retirement, these should be discussed and formulated before the person reaches that milestone. An effort should be made to minimize the physical handicaps and discomforts of illnesses so that the older adult can continue to be active and feel useful. For example, there are many aids that can be used to help a person with arthritis perform self-care activities, do the daily cooking and laundry chores, and remain physically mobile and socially active.

An important goal for maintaining the physical and mental health of the older adult is to prolong their ability to live independently in their own homes and thus avoid institutionalization. The daily tasks of caring for oneself and a home, shopping, cooking, or caring for a yard largely contribute to the meaning of life for those in this age group.

Everyone over 65 years of age should have a physical examination that includes special tests similar to those for persons in their middle years. Immunization against influenza may be indicated. Dental examinations and prophylactic measures are necessary to preserve the teeth so that dental problems do not interfere with good nutrition. At this stage in life it also is recommended that the feet be periodically evaluated and treated by a podiatrist to preserve as much physical mobility as possible.

People in this age group should be counseled to eat a high-fiber diet, reduce sodium intake, and eat complex carbohydrates rather than simple sugars. Caloric needs will probably be less because of a decrease in physical activity.

Adequate daily exercise, such as walking for 20 to 30 minutes, will preserve coordination, improve mobility, and help prevent falls and consequent hip fracture. Exercise also has a positive effect on blood pressure, weight, heart function, and mental attitude and acuity.

Recognition of the social needs of people in late adulthood is especially important to their continued physical health and sense of worth. They have much to offer and need to feel needed for their wisdom and experience in life. They should be respected for their age and not subjected to prejudicial opinions about their worth and productivity. Much of what they can offer cannot be measured in terms of financial wealth, but their contributions are nonetheless valuable to the integrity and overall well-being of society.

Developmental tasks for those over 65 years of age include redirection of their energy and talents to new roles and activities, acceptance of one's life with its joys and limitations, and developing a personal view of death that prepares one for this final stage of life.

In the coming years more and more people needing health care will be 65 years of age or older. Currently there are 26.3 million Americans in the older adulthood stage of their lives.

SENIOR ADULTHOOD (75 TO DEATH)

More and more people are surviving past age 75 and even into the ninth decade. The Census Bureau predicts that during the 1990s there will be a 13% increase in the group aged 75 and over. This means that elderly patients will eventually be the rule, rather than the exception (Beare and Myers, 1990). The health status and degree of activity in this age group vary considerably. Many adults in this age group have suffered chronic health problems for many years and are confined to their home or a long-term care facility during this period of life. Many others are still very active. A small percentage are still working, and many more are involved in community, athletic, and travel activities.

The changes that began in late adulthood become more pronounced with increased problems of vision and hearing, decreased mobility as a result of arthritis and loss of muscle tone, and slowed reaction times.

HEALTH PROBLEMS

The major causes of death in the senior adult group are similar to those of late adulthood, with cardiovascular disease and cancer leading the list.

External factors that contribute to illness during this life stage are often related to negative attitudes toward older persons and society's uncaring treatment of them.

In many cases senior adults lose their purpose in life and become isolated, treated as dependent beings, and are removed from their homes and confined to long-term care facilities. Much of the attention they do receive is focused on their physical illnesses, giving them positive reinforcement for being ill.

HEALTH CARE NEEDS

In addition to assistance in managing their chronic diseases, a major health care goal for this age group should be to help them retain some purpose in life, which will aid in promoting optimal physical, mental, and social activity.

We have a tremendous untapped resource in the alert, healthy senior adults in this country. More attention needs to be directed toward assisting all of us to make the best use of this resource. Networking is active in every other age group and should be encouraged in this one. Just being supportive and helpful to each other can give added meaning to life. Allowing senior adults to perform whatever tasks they are capable of doing for family members can also lend more meaning to life. Young people are badly in need of mentors and tutors; certainly a percentage of those in the senior adult group are capable of handling these functions if approached and utilized properly.

Health care needs are similar but more pronounced for this group than for the late adults. Chapter 12 discusses these issues in more depth.

BIBLIOGRAPHY

Adams, B. N.: Adolescent health care: Needs, priorities and services. Nurs. Clin. North Am., June, 1983, p. 237.

Archibald, J. W., and Ullman, M. A.: Is it really senility—or just depression? RN, Nov., 1983, p. 49.

Beare, P. G., and Myers, J. L.: Principles and Practices of Adult Health Nursing. St. Louis, C. V. Mosby, 1990.

Burnside, I.: Nursing and the Aged: A Self-care Approach, 3rd ed. New York, McGraw-Hill, 1988.

Duffy, M. E.: Determinants of health promotion in midlife women. Nurs. Res., Nov.-Dec., 1988, p. 358.

Ellor, J. R., and Kurz, D. J.: Misuse and abuse of prescription and nonprescription drugs by the elderly. Nurs. Clin. North Am., June, 1982, p. 319.

Frielberg, K. L.: Human Development. New York, Duxbury Press, 1980.

Hayter, J.: Modifying the environment to help older persons. Nurs. Health Care, May, 1983, p. 265.

Hazard, M. P.: Keeping the well-elderly well. Am. J. Nurs., April, 1983, p. 567.

Levinson, D. J., et al.: The Season's of a Man's Life. New York, Alfred A. Knopf, 1978.

Lindberg, S. C.: Adult preventive health screening. Nurse Pract., May, 1987, p. 19.

Murray, R. B., and Zentner, J. P.: Nursing Assessment and Health Promotion Throughout the Life Span, 3rd ed. Englewood Cliffs, NJ, Prentice-Hall, 1985.

Neville, K.: Promoting health for seniors. Geriatr. Nurs., Jan.-Feb., 1988, p. 42.

Panicucci, C. L.: Functional assessment of the older adult in the acute care setting. Nurs. Clin. North Am., June, 1983, p. 355.

Sanders, F. M., and Plummer, E. M.: Assault on the aged—is your patient a secret victim? RN, July, 1983, p. 20.

Sanger, E., and Cassino, R.: Eating disorders: Avoiding the power struggle. Am. J. Nurs., Jan., 1984, p. 81.

Scarf, M.: Unfinished Business—Pressure Points in the Lives of Women. Garden City, N.Y., Doubleday & Co., 1980.

Smith, J. M., and Sorrell, V.: Developing wellness programs: A nurse-managed stay well center for senior citizens. Clin. Nurse Spec., Winter, 1989, p. 198.

STUDENT STUDY AIDS

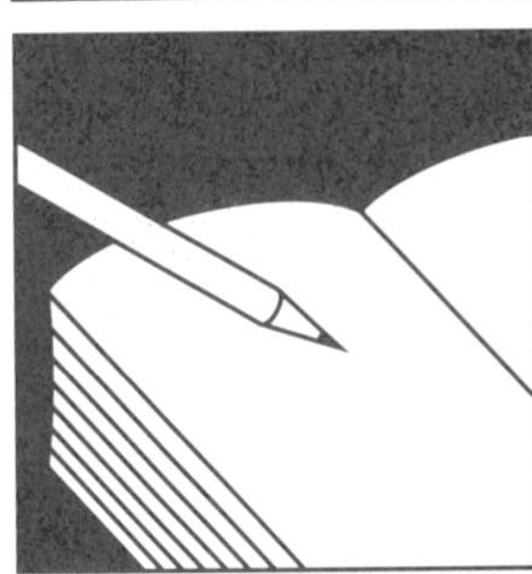

CLINICAL CASE PROBLEMS

Read each clinical situation and discuss the questions with your classmates.

1. Marcia Day, 20 years old, has just moved into your neighborhood. She has a child 18 months old and works at night. Her husband works during the day and is attending the local community college to get his degree in electrical engineering. They enjoy a fast-paced life, eat mostly "junk foods," and do not have any recreational outlets other than partying with their friends.

Lately, Marcia has complained to you that she is tired all the time and has difficulty "keeping up with the crowd." She says she has never been sick and hasn't seen a doctor since her baby was born. She is slightly overweight and frequently goes on some kind of fad diet to try to lose weight. Her husband admits to using marijuana as a recreational drug and sometimes uses cocaine. Marcia says she doesn't believe in using "the hard stuff" but doesn't see anything wrong with smoking pot. They seem to love their child, but he stays with his grandparents most of the time.

- What are the major causes of death in Marcia's age group?
- What developmental tasks must Marcia and her husband complete in order to become more mature?
- What health-related problems can you identify in these young people?
- What community resources are you aware of that could be recommended to Marcia and her husband?
- Identify some specific diseases that could occur later in life as a result of the lifestyle chosen by Marcia and her husband.

---

2. Mr. Brock, age 53, has been admitted to the hospital with a tentative diagnosis of diabetes mellitus. His nursing history shows that he drinks "about a six-pack of beer every day," smokes two packs of cigarettes daily, and enjoys gourmet cooking as a hobby. He says that now that his children are grown and no longer dependent on him he intends to really enjoy life to the fullest. He is very depressed about the possibility that he might have diabetes and boasts that he has not been to a doctor in "at least 15 years."

- What are the major causes of death in persons in their middle years of life?
- What should be the health-related goals of middle age?

- How often should a person have a thorough health assessment after the age of 50?
- What are the developmental tasks of middle adulthood?

STUDY OUTLINE

I. Introduction

A. Morbidity and mortality rates for various age groups show that physiologic and psychosocial events unique to each life stage have an impact on health and survival.

B. Nurses need to be aware of the relationship between age and the potential for specific kinds of illness and injury, including the general kinds of health care needed by people in each age group.

II. Early adulthood (20 to 29 years)

A. Biologic maturity has been reached; major task is preservation and maintenance of health.

B. This is a period of beginnings.

C. Health problems.

1. Major causes of death are vehicular and other accidents, suicide, and homicide.
2. Typical health problems are anxiety, depression, complications of pregnancy, cervical and breast cancer, and orthopedic injuries.
3. Factors contributing to health problems include physical and psychological pressures to establish independence and become self-supporting.
4. Harmful health habits and their effects are shown in Table 5–2.

D. Health care needs.

1. At least one thorough health status assessment during this period, including testing for sexually transmitted diseases, hypertension, and cholesterol level. Tetanus booster as indicated.
2. Teaching regarding regular breast self-examination and testicular examination.
3. Developmental tasks to be completed:
   a. Achieving independence from parental control.
   b. Establishing intimate relationships outside the family.
   c. Establishing set of personal values.
   d. Developing sense of personal identity.
4. Need for nutrition counseling to help maintain normal body weight, avoid iron-deficiency anemia, and ensure adequate protein intake.

III. Young adulthood (30 to 44 years)

A. Reaching the age of 30 can be traumatic for some.

B. There is a sense of urgency to reach goals they have set for themselves.

C. Health problems.

1. Major causes of death begin to include cardiovascular disease and other illnesses related to lifestyles adopted earlier.
2. Environmental factors contributing to illness include a stressful job, occupational hazards, and marital and parenting problems.

D. Health care needs.

1. At least two visits to a physician or nurse practitioner for health status assessment. This could be done at age 30 and again at 35.
2. Pap smear at least every 3 years.
3. Health education with instruction in self-examination of the

breasts and testes, skin assessment, and inspection of the mouth for precancerous lesions.

4. Baseline mammogram for females at age 35.
5. Dental health and preservation of the teeth. Both are important at this stage to avoid problems later in life.
6. Adequate exercise and calcium intake necessary to prevent osteoporosis in females later in life.
7. Developmental tasks include managing a household, rearing children, and managing a career.
8. Assistance with managing stress and utilizing resources to help with completion of developmental tasks.
9. Support and assistance in changing to and maintaining healthful lifestyles.
10. Assistance with issues of infertility as needed.

IV. Middle adulthood (45 to 65 years)

A. Time of change in self-image, gracefully giving up youthful goals.
B. External signs of aging begin to appear. Less visible internal changes also occur, affecting digestion, mobility, and comfort.
C. Need to adopt values that transcend external beauty and to appreciate the advantages of growing older.
D. Social changes center on role changes. Middle-aged offspring may need to act as parents of their own parents. This role reversal creates stress and can precipitate illness.
E. Adult children may return home, causing additional stressors.
F. Menopause may require adjustment.
G. May experience loss of parents, spouse, or friends by death.
H. Decreased self-esteem may occur with divorce.
I. Plan for retirement.
J. Health problems.
   1. Major causes of death are heart attack, stroke, lung and breast cancer, and cirrhosis of the liver.
   2. Major health problems are chronic respiratory disease, alcoholism, and hypertension.
   3. Contributing factors are similar to those for young adults.
K. Health care needs.
   1. Health goals related to preserving and prolonging period of maximum energy and optimal mental and social activity.
   2. Periodic health assessment and physical examination. Annual assessment for persons over age 50.
      a. Specific tests for hypertension, diabetes, respiratory disease, and cancer.
      b. Immunizations review.
      c. Problems related to nutrition, physical exercise, occupational hazards, sexual dysfunction and menopause, marital and parenting difficulties, and use of alcohol, tobacco, and drugs.
      d. Nutrition counseling.
      e. Instruction in proper use of nonprescription and prescription drugs.

V. Late and older adulthood (6 to 74 years)

A. Perception of what constitutes being "old" depends on the individual.
B. Best to withhold judgment about what elderly people are like and what it means to grow old.
C. Significant changes related to aging and ability to adapt.
D. During late adulthood changes involve retirement from work, reduction in income, possibly loss of spouse.

E. Sensory deficits become more common.
F. Positive aspects of growing older: freedom from competition at work and responsibilities of child rearing at home. Time to enjoy creative and self-satisfying pursuits.
G. Health problems.
   1. Major causes of death in persons over 69 are chronic cardiovascular disease, cancer, and complications of diabetes.
   2. Common illnesses include gastrointestinal disorders such as peptic ulcer and constipation, acute and chronic respiratory disease, and gallbladder disease. Prostatic enlargement common in males at this age.
   3. Depression is common in the later years.
   4. External factors contributing to illness include society's attitude toward and treatment of the elderly and the attention focused on their physical illness.
H. Health care needs.
   1. Major goals are to assist patients in managing their chronic illnesses and helping them remain physically, mentally, and socially active.
   2. Physical aids and equipment can help the elderly remain independent and able to perform self-care activities.
   3. Important to help elderly live independently in their own homes and avoid institutionalization as long as possible.
   4. Annual physical examination recommended. Dental care and immunizations also important.
   5. Nutrition counseling to encourage high-fiber, low-sodium diet; caloric intake adjusted according to physical exercise.
   6. Adequate daily walking can improve health and prolong productivity.
   7. Elderly have need to feel needed and respected.
   8. Developmental tasks for those over 60:
      a. Redirection of energy and talents to new roles and activities.
      b. Acceptance of one's life.
      c. Development of a personal view of death and preparation for it.

VI. Senior adulthood (75 to death)

A. In the 1990s there will be a 13% increase in the number of persons age 75 and older.
B. Changes apparent in late adulthood become more pronounced.
C. Health problems.
   1. Cardiovascular disease and cancer are leading causes of death in this age group.
   2. Many senior adults lose their purpose in life and become isolated.
D. Health care needs.
   1. Major health care goals include helping people in this age group retain some purpose in life and promoting optimal physical, mental, and social activity.
   2. Networking should be encouraged; skills of senior adults should be put to use within the community.

CHAPTER 6

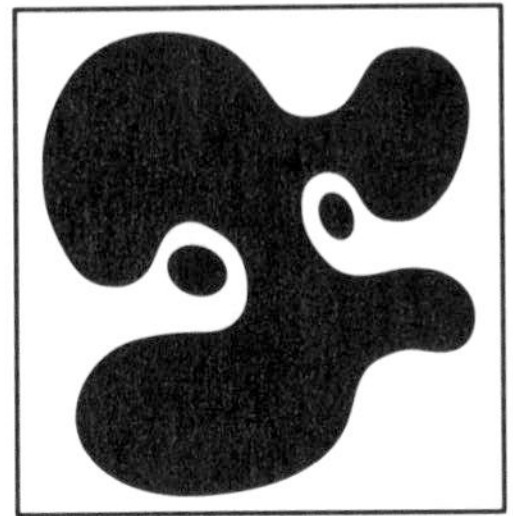

Disease-Producing Factors and Protective Mechanisms

VOCABULARY

aerobic
anaerobic
antibiotic
antimicrobial
antiseptic
asepsis
bacteria
carrier
contamination
detoxify
disinfectant
endemic
enzyme
epidemic
exudate
fungi
gram-negative
gram-positive
infection
inflammation
leukocytosis
microbe
nonpathogenic
nosocomial
objective
pathogenic
phagocytosis
prodromal
protozoa
rickettsiae
spores
sterilization
subjective
virus

Upon completion of this chapter the student should be able to:

1. List at least six nursing actions (assessment and intervention) that are related to prevention of disease and injury caused by mechanical and chemical factors.
2. Identify at least three major characteristics of bacteria.
3. Identify at least three major characteristics of viruses.
4. Discuss effective means for the removal or destruction of microbes on living and nonliving matter.
5. List the six links of the infectious process and give an example of each.
6. Devise a general nursing care plan for the patient hospitalized with a systemic infection.
7. Describe the method used for surveillance and reporting of infections in hospitalized patients.
8. Describe the measures to be taken for "universal precautions."
9. Write a teaching plan for home care that also includes family precautions for a patient who has a staphylococcal infection.
10. State specific tasks the nurse can perform to help patients maintain the protective structures and mechanisms of the body.
11. Identify the major defensive organs and a protective function of each.
12. List and briefly describe each of the five kinds of physiologic changes that occur in the inflammatory process.
13. Identify the factors that impede healing and repair.
14. List five nursing actions that specifically affect healing and repair.

MECHANICAL, CHEMICAL AND GENETIC FACTORS

MECHANICAL FACTORS

We are familiar with many of the external forces in our environment that can cause mechanical injury to the body. In fact, accidental injury is a major health concern in the modern world; accidental death ranks first among the causes of death occurring in the period between infancy and young adulthood. Physical blows such as those received in a fall or vehicular accident are examples of mechanical factors that cut, bruise, fracture, and otherwise harm body tissues.

Extremes of heat and cold are also mechanical factors that produce injury. Burns caused by flames, ultraviolet rays from the sun, or electrical energy can damage and destroy body cells. Extreme cold can produce localized cell death, as in frostbite, or a generalized chilling of the whole body, as in hypothermia, which threatens the life of all the body's cells. Other mechanical forces that are capable of causing serious damage to the cells and tissues are emissions from radioactive elements, high-voltage x-ray machines, and microwave ovens.

Internal mechanical forces in the body are not easily apparent, but they too can cause disease by affecting body structure and interfering with normal function. There might be partial or complete obstruction of the flow of air, food elements, blood, or lymph. An obstruction may be congenital (present at birth) or acquired. An example of a congenital deformity in which there is interference with the flow of blood is the narrowing of a portion of the aorta (coarctation of the aorta). An acquired obstruction of blood flow might be the formation of a blood clot in a vein or artery. Other examples of obstructive disorders are chronic obstructive pulmonary disease (COPD) and intestinal obstruction.

CHEMICAL FACTORS

When we think of chemicals in the environment, we often think of pollutants, poisonous insecticides, defoliants, and other industrial and agricultural products. These are real hazards to health, but so are the chemicals used to manufacture antiseptics, disinfectants, and cleaning compounds used in the care of the sick. Drugs that are made for oral and parenteral administration are chemicals and therefore must be considered potentially dangerous under certain circumstances. It is estimated that from 3% to 5% of all patients admitted to hospitals are suffering primarily from a drug reaction and that 30% of these patients experience a second reaction during their hospital stay.

Many of the substances found in the home are potentially fatal poisons. Even sugar, salt and other common minerals, and soap, although not customarily considered harmful agents, can be extremely dangerous if used in improper amounts or allowed to come into contact with cells that cannot adapt to their presence or are extremely sensitive to them.

Plant products, insect and snake venom, and a host of other natural substances are capable of triggering a protective inflammatory and immunologic response in a susceptible person. In some instances, these responses can be fatal, as, for example, in a severe allergic reaction to a bee sting.

Internally, the body's own chemical substances can be harmful to its cells if they leave their normal locale and enter the environment of cells that are not accustomed to contact with them, or if they are produced in either excessive or insufficient amounts.

Gastric juices containing hydrochloric acid and other caustic elements can produce ulcers in the lining of the stomach and duodenum if present in amounts and concentrations that are more than the cells lining the gastrointestinal tract can tolerate. At the other extreme, a deficiency of gastric juices and digestive enzymes can lead to inadequate nutrition, because they fail to break down food particles into chemical nutrients that the cells can use.

If digestive fluids leaking around a colostomy or an ileostomy are allowed to remain on the skin of the abdomen, the skin will become very irritated and inflamed.

Blood that has leaked from torn vessels and entered other body tissues can be a chemical source of pain, irritation, and cellular damage.

Hormones are chemical substances that are secreted by the endocrine glands. Each hormone has one or more specific functions that it is supposed to perform. If there is too much of the hormone or not enough of it, the body cells will be damaged and their physiologic functions impaired. A classic example is the hormone thyroxin, secreted by the thyroid gland. If an overactive thyroid gland produces excessive amounts of thyroxin, all the metabolic processes will be speeded up and cellular damage will occur.

The body carries on its physiologic functions within a very narrow range of adaptability. For example, the normal pH range for an acid-base balance in the internal environment is only from 7.35 to 7.45. (This is discussed in more detail in Chapter 8.) The normal temperature range of the body is also very narrow, compared with the extremes of external environmental temperature that can be tolerated. To illustrate, a body temperature of 110°F (43.3°C) usually is fatal, yet that is only about 11°F above normal body temperature. Outside the limits of 95°F (35°C) and

110°F (43.3°C), the body suffers cellular damage that can be fatal.

The two major components of the extracellular fluid are water and electrolytes. These will be discussed more fully in Chapter 8. At this point, however, it should be noted that either excessive amounts of water (edema) or an insufficient supply of water to the cells (dehydration) can have serious and even fatal consequences in a very short time.

Deficiencies or excesses in electrolytes also can quickly initiate a kind of chain reaction that profoundly affects the vital organs. In addition to electrolytes, the body needs vitamins to carry on its normal functions and to resist disease. A vitamin deficiency caused by insufficient intake or impaired absorption and utilization can be a major cause of cellular damage and loss of function. Table 6–1 summarizes the nursing actions that help to minimize opportunities for mechanical and chemical factors to induce disease.

TABLE 6–1 NURSING ACTIONS RELATED TO MECHANICAL AND CHEMICAL DISEASE-PRODUCING FACTORS

1. Education of the general public in the prevention of accidental injury, hazards of smoking and other harmful habits, and environmental pollution.
2. Attention to safety needs of high-risk patients (e.g., the elderly, the confused or delirious, and the patient likely to have seizures).
3. Proper positioning and support of body structures to aid respiration and circulation and to preserve integrity of the skin.
4. Caution in preparing solutions for irrigations of the skin and mucous membranes.
5. Strict adherence to rules for the safe administration of drugs.
6. Assessing patients for signs of side effects and adverse reactions to drugs, and promptly reporting them.
7. Protection of skin and mucous membranes from body secretions that are injurious to tissues not normally in contact with them.
8. Applications of cold to control bleeding into tissues adjacent to a ruptured blood vessel.
9. Monitoring body temperature: reporting extremes and implementing nursing measures to return temperature to normal range.
10. Promoting well-balanced diet and adequate intake of liquids.
11. Assessment of bowel and urinary elimination.
12. Accurate measurement of intake and output.
13. Teaching patient ways to prevent injury to and infection of wounds.

GENETIC FACTORS

Genes are the biologic units of heredity. They are themselves composed of chemicals (ribonucleic and deoxyribonucleic acids [RNA and DNA]) and in turn profoundly affect the chemical makeup of every cell in the human body. Genes are called *units of heredity*, because they carry the physical, biochemical, and physiologic traits that children inherit from their parents. Genetic disorders may or may not be present in the parents of the child who has inherited the disorder.

Diseases considered to be genetic disorders are sickle cell diseases, thalassemia, and other blood dyscrasias resulting from abnormalities in hemoglobin.

Other genetic disorders are inborn errors of metabolism in which there is faulty or incomplete metabolism of carbohydrates, proteins, or fats. There are at least 200 inborn errors of metabolism that have been recognized. *Galactosemia* and *phenylketonuria* (PKU) are examples of inborn errors of metabolism. In galactosemia, there is a lack of the enzyme that is necessary for proper metabolism of galactose (a sugar). This enzyme normally changes galactose, which cannot be utilized by the body, into glucose, which can be used. Because the galactose cannot be utilized, it accumulates in the blood. In PKU, there is a disturbance in the metabolism of an amino acid (phenylalanine). This results in a lack of tyrosine, a substance necessary for the production of the thyroid hormones and epinephrine. A deficiency of these hormones leads to severe mental retardation and severe physical symptoms, unless the condition is detected early in the infant's life and corrected.

In some genetic disorders there is an imbalance of genetic material; for example, there are too many or too few chromosomes. Such imbalances can lead to mental and physical defects. Down's syndrome (at one time called *mongolism*) is an example of this type of genetic disorder. The infant with Down's syndrome has 47 chromosomes instead of the normal 46.

Research into genetic disorders and an increasing awareness of the importance of early diagnosis and treatment have greatly improved patient prognosis and reduced the danger of permanent disability from such defects.

INFECTIOUS AGENTS

We are all aware that there are "germs" in our environment and that these agents can cause local and generalized infections. These infectious agents are sometimes called *biologic agents*, because they are living organisms that are either plants or animals and have a cellular structure similar to that of all living things.

Infectious agents include bacteria, viruses, protozoa, rickettsiae, and fungi.

BACTERIA

Bacteria are microscopically small organisms belonging to the plant kingdom. They can be classified into three major categories according to their Gram-staining properties, their shape, and their requirements for oxygen.

Bacteria in their natural state are seen under the microscope as tiny, colorless organisms. In order to make them more identifiable they can be stained with a dye, usually methylene blue. The procedure is called *Gram staining* after the scientist who first used this method. Organisms that will not retain the dye are called *gram-negative;* those that "take" the dye are called *gram-positive.* All streptococci and all staphylococci are gram-positive. The bacillus that causes tuberculosis is gram-negative, as are many of the organisms that cause hospital-acquired infections.

Classification of bacteria according to their shape, or morphology, is based on whether they belong to one of three main groups. *Cocci* are round, *bacilli* are rod-shaped, and *spirochetes* are spiral or corkscrew-shaped (Fig. 6–1).

Bacteria can be grown in the laboratory in a specially prepared broth or jelly called a *culture medium.* In this way the manner in which they arrange themselves in groups can be observed. This provides another means of classifying them. Some grow in chains *(streptococci),* some in pairs *(diplococci),* and some in clusters *(staphylococci).* Thus we can see that "strep" throat (short for streptococcal infection of the throat) is caused by round organisms that grow in chains.

Some bacteria must have oxygen in their environment in order to grow and thrive. These bacteria are classified as *obligate aerobes.* Others cannot tolerate the presence of oxygen and are called *obligate anaerobes.* A third group (for example, the streptococci) are adaptable and can thrive with or without oxygen. They are called *facultative anaerobes.*

The environment of bacteria is as important to their survival as our environment is to our own well-being. Some form spores (reproductive cells with a thick membrane) to protect themselves against destruction from heat, cold, lack of water, toxic chemicals, and radiation. Others thrive best in water. Still others, such as the bacterium that causes tuberculosis, can survive for years in dust. Temperature also is an important factor in the life of a microorganism. Rickettsiae do not flourish and lose their ability to cause disease when subjected to temperatures less than 36°C. However, *Staphylococcus aureus* can tolerate extremely high temperatures. The different factors affecting microorganisms pathogenic to humans are mentioned to emphasize the fact that harmful microorganisms are not all destroyed by any single method. Depending on the bacteria involved, different methods are necessary to rid animate and inanimate objects of these disease-producing agents.

When bacteria enter the body tissues, they trigger an immune response that includes the production of *antibodies.* These are capable of destroying the bacteria or rendering them harmless. Some bacteria produce poisonous substances called *endotoxins* and *exotoxins.* These toxins evoke the production of special kinds of antibodies called *antitoxins.* Antibodies and antitoxins are discussed more fully in Chapter 7. They are mentioned here because they play an important role in immunization for prevention of the spread of infectious diseases.

VIRUSES

The chief characteristics of viruses are: (1) they are extremely small (visible only with an electron microscope); (2) they are composed of particles of nucleic acids, either DNA or RNA (the "stuff" of which genes are made), with a coat of protein and, in some cases, carbohydrate and fatty material; and (3) they can grow and replicate only in a living cell.

These characteristics, while no doubt advantageous to the viruses, make them particularly dangerous to humans. Because of the way they are made, viruses can camouflage themselves and take up residence in the body's cells without calling attention to themselves. Once there, they can trigger an immune response that is harmful to the body's cells, or they can damage cells in other ways.

In some acute viral infections, such as measles and chickenpox, the viruses reproduce within the cells, causing them to burst. In more chronic viral infections, in which the disease is slower or is in remission, the viruses change the cells' membranes so that they are not recognized by the body as part of its "self." In this case the body's own cells are attacked and injured or destroyed by the body's immune system.

Many of the so-called "slow" viruses can reside in the body for years without producing symptoms and then suddenly cause an acute flare-up up of symptoms. Herpes viruses are examples of these kinds of viruses. Certain strains of influenza viruses also can lie dormant for years and then later attack cells of the central nervous system, the heart, and other tissues.

Destruction of Viruses

Viruses, like bacteria, vary in their resistance to destruction by chemical disinfectants. Most are easily inactivated by heat, but the hepatitis viruses can resist boiling for at least 30 minutes.

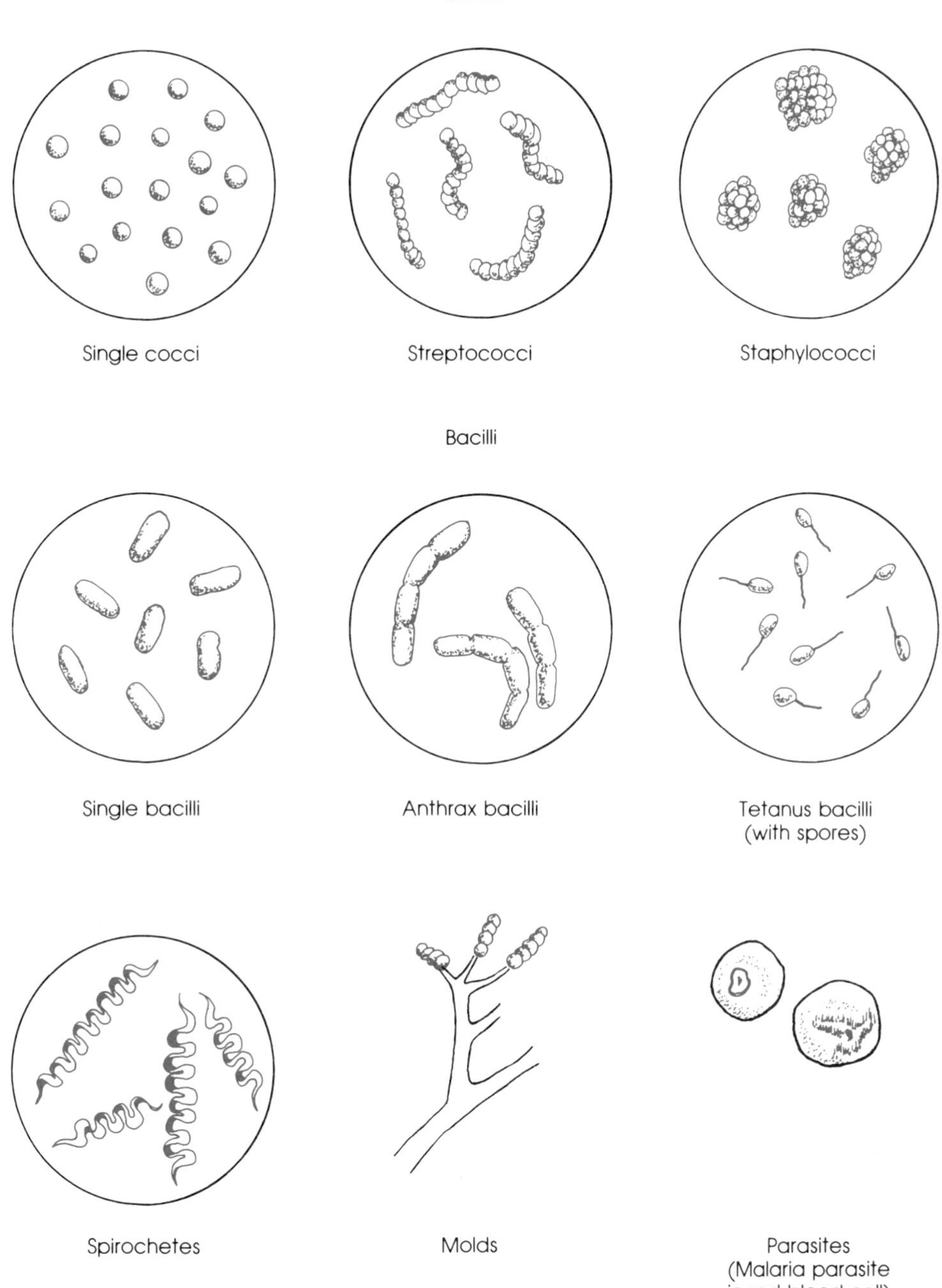

Figure 6-1 Drawings of various pathogenic microorganisms as they appear under the microscope. Their shape and groupings determine their classification.

The most effective means for destroying viruses and all other kinds of microbes is to expose them to moist heat at a temperature of 250°F (121°C) for 15 to 20 minutes.

Types of Viruses

There is still no universally accepted classification of viruses. Some authorities classify them on the basis of size and chemical composition, others on the type of tissues a particular kind of virus prefers to attack. You will notice in Figure 6-2 that viruses vary greatly in size and shape.

Response to Viruses

There are four general ways in which susceptible host cells may respond to invasion by viruses: (1) the host cell may allow the virus to live within its cytoplasm, but the virus lies dormant and does not reproduce; (2) the host cell may die without reproducing itself; (3) the host cell may

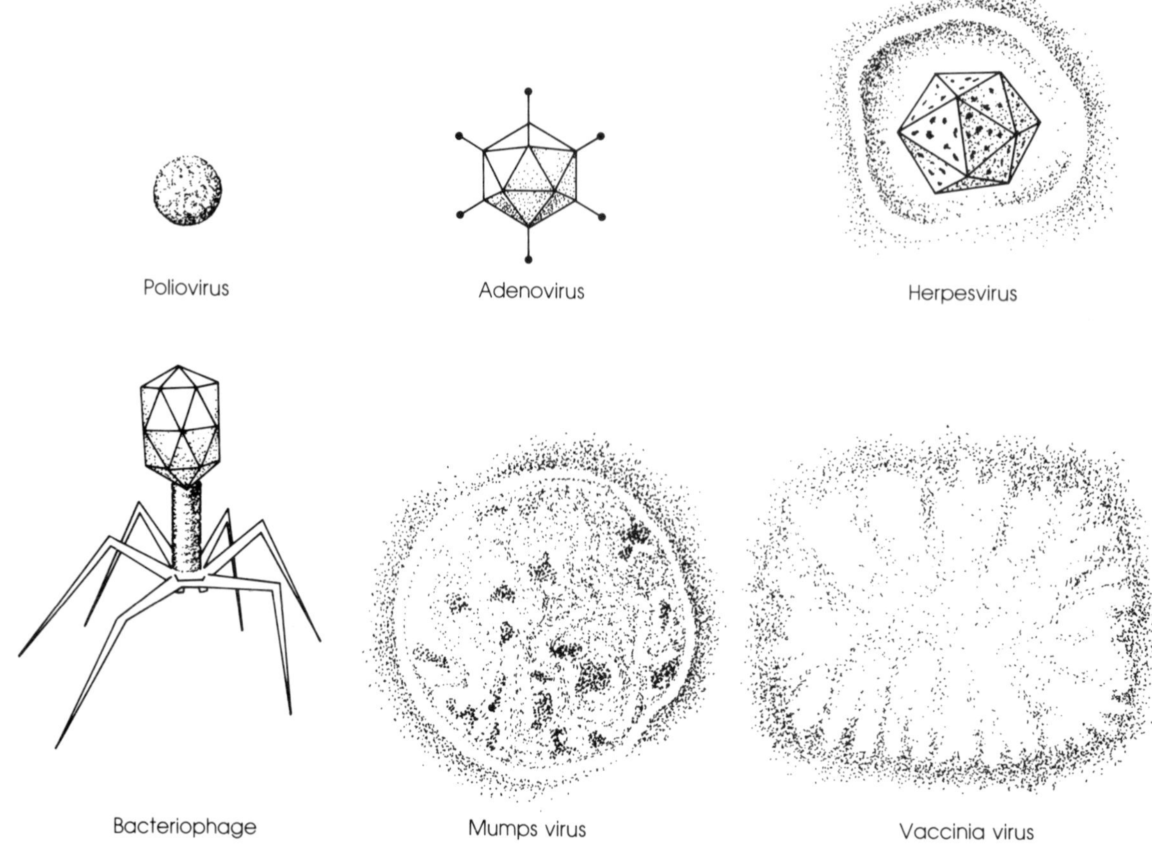

Figure 6–2 Comparison of shapes and sizes of viruses.

divide and then die; or (4) the host cell may be transformed in such a way that it divides and takes on abnormal growth patterns.

PROTOZOA

Protozoa are microscopic one-celled organisms belonging to the animal kingdom. (Bacteria, viruses, yeasts, and molds belong to the plant kingdom.) Protozoa that are pathogenic to man include the *Plasmodium* species that cause human malaria; *Entamoeba histolytica*, which causes amebic dysentery; and other strains capable of causing diarrhea.

RICKETTSIAE

Rickettsiae are small round or rod-shaped microorganisms that are transmitted by the bites of lice, ticks, fleas, and mites. Among the diseases caused by rickettsiae are Rocky Mountain spotted fever, typhus, and trench fever. Diseases of this kind are most likely to develop wherever sanitation standards are low and there is poor control of rodents and insects.

FUNGI

Fungi are very small, primitive organisms of the plant kingdom; yeasts and molds are also members of this group (Fig. 6–3). They feed on living plants and animals and decaying organic material and thrive in warm, moist environment. Fungal infections in humans are called *mycoses* and are classified into three main types: (1) systemic for deep mycoses involving internal organs, especially the lungs; (2) subcutaneous mycoses, which involve the deeper layers of the skin, subcutaneous tissues, and sometimes bone; and (3) superficial or cutaneous mycoses, which grow in the outer layer of the skin, hair, and nails.

Fungal infections are difficult to eradicate once they have invaded a human host, mainly because fungi tend to form spores that are resistant to ordinary antiseptics and disinfectants. The course of treatment must be carried out conscientiously and over a long period. In recent years, there has been an increase in the frequency of fungal infections of the oral and vaginal mucosa because of the widespread use of antibiotic drugs. These drugs destroy the normal bacterial flora of the mucosa, allowing the "weeds" of fungi to flourish

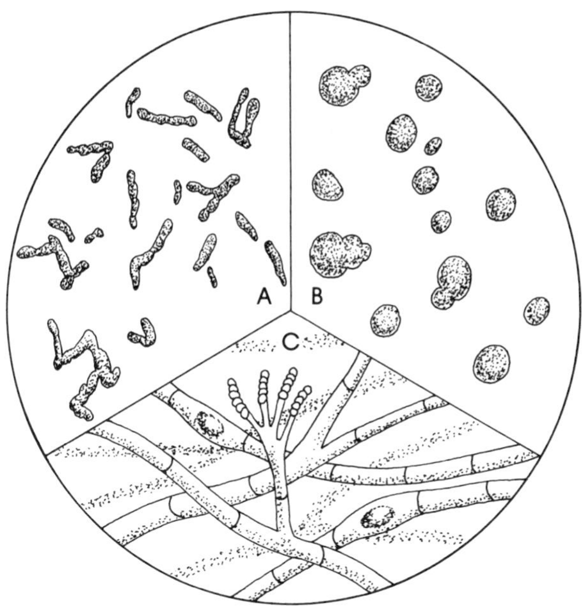

Figure 6-3 Fungal types: actinomycete (A), yeast (B), and mold (C).

and grow without competition. This occurs because many antibiotics are themselves derived from fungi, and their presence in the intestinal tract has an antibacterial but not an antifungal effect.

Fungi are so widespread in nature that it is all but impossible to eliminate them as sources of infection in humans. Control is aimed at changing the environment so that their numbers are decreased and they do not become numerous enough to constantly produce symptoms in humans. Among the more common superficial fungal infections are athlete's foot and ringworm of the scalp and nails. Vaginal fungal infections such as candidiasis are fairly common and particularly difficult to eliminate.

Systemic mycoses have become somewhat more frequent in recent years, probably because of increased use of antibiotics and the highly toxic drugs used in the treatment of cancer. Both of these kinds of drugs upset the normal balance of flora by destroying only the bacteria and allowing yeasts and molds to flourish. *Actinomycosis* is a relatively common systemic fungal infection that most frequently infects the head and neck. It usually starts as a swelling around the teeth and spreads to adjacent tissues. *Histoplasmosis* affects the lungs and is transmitted by the inhalation of spores.

Antifungal drugs that are effective in treating fungal infections include those applied topically to have a local effect and those taken orally to have a systemic effect.

THE INFECTIOUS PROCESS

The process by which an infectious disease is spread from one person to another can be thought of as a continuous chain. Each link must be present in its proper order for the chain to remain intact and for the infection to be passed on to someone else. Figure 6-4, which depicts the links in the unbroken chain, can be used as a guide to learning nursing responsibilities for preventing the spread of infectious diseases.

LINK ONE

Link one is the *causative organism*. In order to remove this link from the chain, the causative organisms must be destroyed or rendered relatively harmless whenever they are in the environment of a susceptible host. Disinfection and sterilization should be familiar to anyone working in the health field. Procedures for concurrent and terminal disinfection should be readily available in all areas in which patients with infectious disease are receiving treatment. The Centers for Disease Control (1600 Clifton Road, N.E., Atlanta, GA, 30333) provide a wealth of information on prevention of the spread of infectious disease.

LINK TWO

Reservoirs of causative organisms, which constitute link two, are places in which the organisms thrive and reproduce. These might include the body tissues and wastes of humans, animals, and insects. Reservoirs can also be food or water that is contaminated by the microorganism. In the hospital, the patient with an infectious disease is cared for under special precautions in an effort to remove this vital link from the chain. Also, the nurse must consider all the patients in

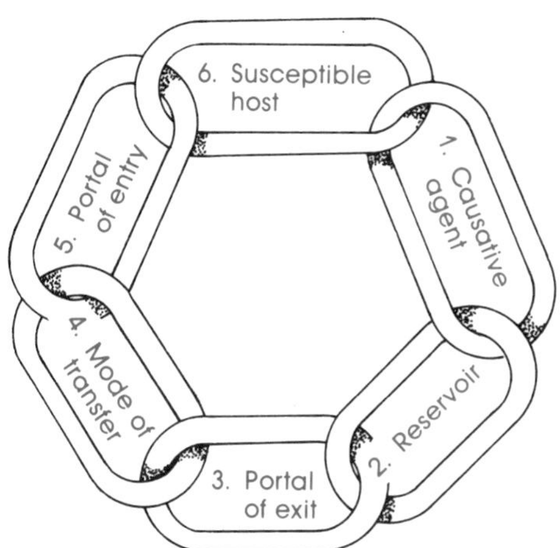

Figure 6-4 Each link of the infectious process must be present and in proper sequence to produce disease.

the hospital as possible sources of infection. That is why she is admonished over and over again to wash her hands after contact with each patient, regardless of his diagnosis.

All newly admitted patients should be observed for signs of infection, such as boils, infected wounds, or fever. If there is a sign of infection, it should be reported immediately so that proper precautions can be taken.

Every student nurse should know that hospital dust, insects, and vermin are all extremely likely to serve as reservoirs for infectious microorganisms. Do not, however, let familiarity breed complacency so that you become careless in maintaining an environment of cleanliness and order for patients and yourself.

LINKS THREE AND FIVE

The route by which a pathogen leaves the body of its host is called its *portal of exit* (link three), and the route by which it enters the body to establish infection is called the *portal of entry* (link five). An example of a portal of exit is the intestinal tract, through which the feces transport the typhoid bacillus. The digestive tract also serves as a portal of entry when one eats food or drinks water that contains pathogens. Another example of a body structure that serves as a means by which microorganisms enter and leave the body is the respiratory tract, which can admit and pass on a large number of different pathogens capable of causing diseases. These range from measles and mumps to tuberculosis and hepatitis. The skin and mucous membranes can also serve as portals of entry and exit if they are cut, torn, infected, or damaged in such a way that microorganisms can gain entry or leave.

LINK FOUR

Modes of transfer of pathogens (link four) include (1) direct personal contact with body excreta or drainage from an ulcer, infected wound, boil, or chancre; (2) indirect contact with inanimate objects (called *fomites*), such as contaminated needles and syringes, drinking and eating utensils, dressings, and hospital equipment; (3) vectors, such as fleas, flies, mosquitoes, and other insects that harbor infectious agents and transmit infection to man through bites and stings; (4) droplet infection, or contamination by the aerial route through sneezing and coughing; and (5) endogenous spread of infection from one part of a person's body to another.

LINK SIX

The sixth link in the chain is the *susceptible host.* This link presents a very real challenge to the nurse. Many people are susceptible by virtue of age, weak state of health, and poor living conditions. The nurse strives to protect these people from exposure to infectious agents and also endeavors to improve their state of health and living standards by encouraging good health habits. She also works to see that all people in need of immunization receive it.

CONTROLLING INFECTIOUS DISEASE

Controlling the spread of infectious diseases is a worldwide effort of public health officials. Their major goals and those of nurses who work with them are (1) promotion of sanitary standards in communities; (2) identification of persons who are highly susceptible to infection and reduction of their chances of developing an infectious disease, and (3) implementation of immunization programs to protect people against certain infectious diseases.

Sanitary living conditions have been the concern of authorities since biblical times. Many of the religious restrictions and rituals described in the Old Testament, when looked at as guidelines for healthful living, are as valid today as they were thousands of years ago. In our modern society governmental agencies have largely replaced religious leaders as the guardians of public health, but the problems remain almost the same. Substandard housing, rodents and insects, dust, human waste, contaminated food, and contaminated water supplies are all major sources of infections.

Nurses share the responsibility for educating the public and promoting sanitary living conditions in the communities in which they live and work. Each nurse also must be aware of what she is doing when working with her patients. She might be helping to contain and prevent the spread of infection, or she could actually be contributing to it. Table 6–2 lists definitions of terms commonly used in infectious disease nursing.

HOSPITAL-ACQUIRED (NOSOCOMIAL) INFECTIONS

The word *nosocomial* literally means hospital-acquired. A nosocomial infection occurs when a patient is infected while in a hospital. The term currently is used in a broader sense to include infections resulting from health services provided in all types of health care facilities.

There is a disturbing increase in the number of infections patients acquire during their stay in a hospital. Although inanimate objects such as needles, contaminated surgical instruments, and linen are major sources of infection in health care facilities, every patient is directly and indirectly in contact with untold numbers of persons,

TABLE 6-2 **TERMS FREQUENTLY USED IN INFECTIOUS DISEASE NURSING**

Term	Definition
Antibiotic	A chemical substance produced by a microorganism that has the capacity, in dilute solutions, to kill or inhibit the growth of other microorganisms.
Antimicrobial	An agent that kills microbes or suppresses their multiplication or growth.
Antiseptic	Any substance that inhibits the growth of microbes. The term includes disinfectants, although most disinfectants are too strong to be used on body tissues.
Carrier	An apparently healthy person who harbors living pathogenic microorganisms and can transmit them to other people.
Contamination	The presence or possible presence of living pathogenic microbes in or on an article, person, or matter.
Disinfectant	An agent that destroys infection-producing microbes. Disinfectants are usually applied to inanimate objects, because they are too strong to be used on living tissues.
Epidemic	A temporary and significant increase in the occurrence of disease in a specific area at any given time.
Endemic disease	One of low incidence that is constantly present in a community.
Infectious disease	One caused by a specific pathogenic microorganism.
Sterilization	The process of destroying all microorganisms and their pathogenic products.

each of whom could be responsible for infecting the patient.

Although emphasis has traditionally been placed on sterilization and thorough cleansing of inanimate objects, there is strong evidence that carelessness on the part of doctors, nurses, and other people in the patient's environment is primarily responsible for the unbelievably high incidence of hospital-acquired infections.

The true cost of nosocomial infections is not known. One study, completed in 1975, showed that the additional hospitalization needed to treat these infections cost more than $1.5 billion each year. Added to the dollar cost is the cost in human suffering that such infections entail. Nearly 3% of the estimated two million patients who acquire an infection in a hospital each year do not survive the infection.

The major sites of nosocomial infections, the infectious agent most often responsible, and some actions nurses may take to prevent infection at each site are presented in Table 6-3.

SIGNS AND SYMPTOMS OF INFECTION

Detection of infection in a patient requires a thorough nursing assessment that includes both subjective and objective data gathering. Subjective complaints that may indicate infection include fatigue, loss of appetite, headache, nausea, or general malaise or pain. Objective data often point to the specific body system affected by the infection, but also include systemic signs such as fever and increased pulse and respiratory rate. Other objective data could be vomiting, diarrhea, cough, decreased breath sounds, swollen lymph nodes, cloudy urine, and purulent sputum. Signs of local infection are redness, swelling, pain or tenderness on palpation or movement, heat in the affected area, and possibly loss of function of the body part affected.

Laboratory data that may indicate infection include an elevated white blood cell (WBC) count, changes in the distribution and number of the types of leukocytes on the differential WBC count, an elevated erythrocyte sedimentation rate (ESR), and cultures that test positive for microorganisms.

Any patient entering the hospital for surgery or an invasive procedure is at risk of a nosocomial infection, and "Potential for Infection" should be listed as a nursing diagnosis on his care plan.

NURSING INTERVENTIONS FOR PREVENTION OF INFECTION

Nurses can do many things to help in the prevention of infection. Careful attention to hand washing before and after any direct patient contact, before any invasive or sterile procedure, after contact with infectious materials (e.g., wound drainage, feces, urine, or sputum), and before contact with immunocompromised patients is the primary method by which infection

TABLE 6–3 **COMMON FEATURES OF NOSOCOMIAL INFECTIONS**

Most Common Sites	Most Frequent Causative Organism	Nursing Actions to Prevent Infection
Urinary tract	*Escherichia coli*, *Enterococcus*, *Klebsiella*, and *Proteus*, all from patient's own normal bowel flora. *Pseudomonas* and *Serratia* from other sources occur less frequently but often are resistant to antimicrobial drugs.	Observe sterile technique when catheterizing patients. Keep drainage system for indwelling catheter closed. Keep drainage bag below bladder level at all times to avoid reflux. Separate patients with known urinary tract infections. Catheterize only when absolutely necessary and folllow faithfully the procedure for catheter care.
Surgical wounds	*Staphylococcus aureus*, *Escherichia coli*, *Proteus*, and *Klebsiella*.	Administer prophylactic antibiotics as ordered. Follow strict aseptic technique during surgical procedures, whether minor or major and in whatever setting. Be sure patient's skin is correctly prepared for surgery. Use care in dressing and cleaning postoperative wounds. Ensure that patient has adequate nutrition and sufficient fluid intake, if he is able to eat and drink after surgery.
Respiratory tract	*Pseudomonas aeruginosa* and *Klebsiella*	Adequately decontaminate respiratory therapy equipment. Perform suctioning, tracheostomy care, and other procedures under aseptic technique.
Blood stream (bacteremia)	Secondary to infection elsewhere in the body or can be a primary infection caused by contamination of IV fluids, in which cases *Klebsiella*, *Enterobacter*, and *Serratia* are most common causative agents.	Scrupulous technique in the administration of IV fluids. Follow recommended procedure for daily care of insertion site and IV tubing, needles, and catheters.

can be prevented. Changing soiled dressings promptly and replacing soiled linens quickly prevents spread of infectious organisms. Disposal of infectious materials such as tissues, used dressings, and contaminated equipment in covered, moisture-resistant containers helps contain organisms. Such items should not be left to sit in uncovered trash baskets in the patient's room.

Insisting on sticking to strict aseptic technique for all invasive procedures (e.g., insertion of intravenous needles or bladder catheterization) can greatly reduce the incidence of nosocomial infection. Changing IV dressings, containers, and tubing according to hospital policy and maintaining sterility of closed drainage systems will also help.

Encouraging patients to move, cough, and deep breathe on a regular basis will decrease the chance of respiratory infection. Protecting patients from others with respiratory infections and from visitors with other communicable diseases is also appropriate. Administering prophylactic antibiotics as ordered is equally important in preventing postoperative infection. Encouraging adequate rest and nutritional and fluid intake will help the patient maintain the body in optimum condition to discourage infection.

Along with preventive interventions, the nurse must continuously assess the patient to detect early signs of infection so that treatment can begin immediately. The nurse also assesses every patient for appropriate immunization against infectious diseases such as tetanus, pertussis, diphtheria, polio, influenza, pneumococcal pneumonia, measles, mumps, and rubella.

NURSING INTERVENTIONS FOR CONTROLLING THE SPREAD OF INFECTION

Nursing responsibilities for controlling the spread of infectious diseases fall into four main categories: (1) surveillance for and reporting early signs of infection, (2) destroying and containing infectious agents, (3) promoting immunization against infectious diseases, and (4) supporting and strengthening each patient's capacity for recovery from infection.

Surveillance and Reporting

Surveillance demands that every nurse keep a watchful eye for signs of infection in every patient who is receiving health care.

In the hospital, this means always being alert for the signs and symptoms of infection. Each patient should be routinely assessed for unexpected elevation of temperature, malaise, loss of appetite, purulent or foul-smelling discharge, cough, diarrhea, and sores and skin lesions that are red, swollen, and painful and contain pus. The color of the purulent drainage is helpful in identifying the kind of organism causing an infection. For example, *Staphylococcus aureus* produces a golden color and *Pseudomonas* organisms a bluish green color.

In her surveillance of patients for signs of infection, the nurse should know which of her patients are especially susceptible to an attack by microbes and therefore in need of more frequent and thorough assessment. Patients at greater risk for infection are those who (1) are weakened by severe illness or injury; (2) have catheters, venipunctures, and other invasive techniques for treatment or monitoring; or (3) are very young or elderly, or are immunocompromised from chemotherapy or immunosuppression. Also, obese patients are particularly susceptible to infection of surgical wounds.

If any signs of infection are detected, they should be reported immediately to the patient's physician and to the infection control nurse of the institution.

It is also important that the subjective and objective signs presented by the patient be fully documented on his chart, along with information about who was notified and when. The infection control nurse is a member of the hospital infection control committee. The infection control committee establishes a system for reporting infections, keeps records of all hospital infections, analyses and makes recommendations about the hospital's aseptic practices, and provides an ongoing educational program in infection control for all hospital employees. Although the responsibilities of the infection control nurse vary from one institution to another, in general they include supporting positive attitudes toward infection control, reporting any problems in implementing infection control measures, presenting proposals for measures concerning infection control, carrying out the infection control education program for all hospital employees, collecting data regarding hospital infections among staff and patients, gathering statistical data regarding the incidence of hospital infections, and coordinating the hospital's infection control program with that of the community.

When a nurse suspects that a patient is developing an infection, she should be extra careful in handling and disposing of articles contaminated by the patient. Additionally, she should be especially careful and thorough when washing her hands after being in contact with the patient. The conscientious nurse does not wait until a diagnosis of infection has been established before she makes a special effort to avoid spreading an infection.

Destroying and Containing Infectious Agents

The environment in which each of us lives is teeming with organisms we cannot see without the aid of a microscope. Some are useful and are considered a part of the normal "flora" in and on our bodies. They usually are *nonpathogenic*, which means that they do not cause disease or pathologic conditions. However, if they migrate to parts of the body where they do not normally reside, or if the balance among all the microbes in their environment is upset, these, too, can become pathogenic. An example is the entrance of intestinal bacteria such as *Escherichia coli* into the urinary tract. The colon has an abundance of flora of many kinds, and the mouth, nose, throat, and skin contain a host of resident microbes. The stomach, urinary bladder, uterus, trachea, and lungs do not normally harbor microorganisms.

Health care givers must be especially careful to avoid infection in* all *of their patients, under* all *circumstances, and at* all *times.

The goals of destroying and containing infectious microorganisms are achieved by techniques and methods that (1) either kill the organisms or render them harmless by sterilization and disinfection and (2) separate the sources of infection, so that they are isolated or "contained" within a specific area and therefore cannot spread to others.

Universal Precautions

In the 1980s the spread of acquired immunodeficiency syndrome (AIDS) prompted the Centers for Disease Control to recommend the use of universal blood and body fluid precautions, or "universal precautions," for every patient as a means to prevent the spread of this lethal disease. The purpose of these precautions is to protect hospital personnel from exposure to human immunodeficiency virus (HIV), hepatitis B, and other blood-borne diseases. These universal precautions are listed in Table 6-4 and are recommended for use during care of *all* patients.

Surgical and Medical Asepsis

Two important kinds of techniques and procedures used to destroy and contain infectious agents are surgical and medical asepsis. *Surgical asepsis* is concerned with destroying infectious agents *before* they enter the body. *Medical asepsis* is concerned with destroying the infectious agents *after* they *leave* the body of a patient who is infected and containing or isolating them within an area that is already contaminated.

Surgical asepsis involves the sterilization of instruments, linens, and other articles used to treat the patient whenever his first lines of defense have been crossed. This compromise of defense occurs with surgical incisions, catheterization, and the puncture of blood vessels for intravenous therapy and monitoring devices. Hand washing for surgical asepsis must be done according to procedure. In a surgically aseptic environment, surgical gowns, masks, and gloves are necessary and must be put on and removed strictly according to procedure. Surgical asepsis at the bedside requires sterile gloves, draping the patient with sterile drapes, and using sterile equipment and supplies.

Medical asepsis includes hand washing, separation or isolation of the patient, precautions for handling and disposing of contaminated articles, and other techniques devised to destroy and contain infectious agents.

Hand washing, when done correctly, is the most effective of all the procedures recommended for prevention of the spread of infectious agents.

Although the procedure may vary slightly depending on the recommending authority, the essence of the recommendations is that the hands should be washed *before* the nurse starts procedures, handles clean supplies, touches equipment, or makes contact with a patient, and before the nurse eats, drinks, or smokes. Additionally, the hands should be washed *after* any

TABLE 6-4 UNIVERSAL PRECAUTIONS

1. Use barrier precautions such as gloves, mask, gown, and protective eyewear to prevent exposure of skin or mucous membranes to patient's blood and body fluid.
   a. Use gloves when likely to come in contact with blood, body fluids, mucous membranes, or broken skin or when handling items or surfaces that are soiled with blood or body fluids.
   b. Change gloves between contact with each patient.
   c. Wash hands immediately after removing gloves.
   d. Discard used gloves; do not wash and reuse them.
   e. Wear a gown, mask, and protective eyewear during any procedure that might generate droplets of blood or body fluid.
2. Prevent injury by needle-stick or cut from sharp instruments.
   a. Be cautious and attentive any time a needle is handled.
   b. Do not recap a used needle by hand; scoop the cap onto the needle on a flat surface.
   c. Immediately dispose of a contaminated needle or other sharp instrument puncture-resistant container provided for that purpose in the room.
   d. Replace full puncture-resistant containers as needed; do not attempt to push needles bulging from the container down into it.
3. Prevent possible self-contamination through broken skin.
   a. If you have open lesions or weeping dermatitis on the skin, do not give direct patient care or handle patient care equipment until the condition is corrected.
4. Prevent possible self-contamination during cardiopulmonary resuscitation.
   a. Use disposable mouthpiece or resuscitation bag for emergency mouth-to-mouth breathing.
5. Prevent transmission of HIV or other blood-borne disease to the fetus.
   a. If pregnant, be especially diligent in maintaining universal precautions at all times.

touching contact with the patient and the supplies and equipment in his room, and after personal use of the bathroom, blowing or wiping the nose, and eating, drinking, and smoking.

Hand washing is essential, regardless of whether a patient is known to have an infection and whether medical aseptic techniques are being enforced. If there is no evidence of infection and no special precautions are in effect, hand washing should be done *with an approved soap or detergent under running water, using friction, for at least 20 seconds.* When isolation and precautionary measures are in effect, hand washing must be done as recommended by the infection control committee of the institution.

Isolation and Other Precautions

Although universal precautions are used with all patients, the type of infectious disease a patient has will dictate what additional isolation measures are necessary to prevent the spread of his infection to others. Two systems are available for use as guidelines to be used for patients with an infectious disease. The two systems are called *category-specific isolation precautions* and *disease-specific isolation precautions.* The Centers for Disease Control has recommended seven categories of isolation precautions: (1) strict isolation, (2) respiratory isolation, (3) contact isolations, (4) acid-fast bacillus isolation, (5) enteric precautions, (6) drainage and secretion precautions, and (7) blood/body fluid precautions (Figs. 6–5 to 6–11). Guidelines for their use with patients who have relevant diagnoses are given for each category. In order to improve observance of these precautions by everyone having contact with the patient, there is a color-coded instruction card for each category. The appropriate card is placed on the door of the patient's room or at the head or foot of his bed as a reminder.

The card used for disease-specific isolation precautions is basically the same for all diseases.

Failure to abide by the recommended procedures and practices for infection control is not uncommon among doctors and nurses. Such ne-

STRICT ISOLATION

Visitors—Report to Nurses' Station Before Entering Room

1. Masks are indicated for all persons entering room
2. Gowns are indicated for all persons entering room.
3. Gloves are indicated for all persons entering room.
4. HANDS MUST BE WASHED AFTER TOUCHING THE PATIENT OR POTENTIALLY CONTAMINATED ARTICLES AND BEFORE TAKING CARE OF ANOTHER PATIENT.
5. Articles contaminated with infective material should be discarded or bagged and labeled before being sent for decontamination and reprocessing.

Diseases Requiring Strict Isolation*

Pharyngeal diphtheria

Lassa fever and other viral hemorrhagic fevers, such as Marburg virus disease†

Pneumonic plague

Smallpox†

Varicella (chickenpox)

Herpes zoster, either localized in an immunocompromised patient or disseminated

*A private room is indicated for strict isolation; in general, however, patients infected with the same organism may share a room. See *Guideline for Isolation Precautions in Hospitals* for details and for how long to apply precautions.

†A private room with special ventilation is indicated.

Figure 6–5 Instructions for strict isolation.
(Data courtesy of the Centers for Disease Control, Atlanta, GA. CDC Guidelines, Infection Control 4(4):284–290, 1983.)

RESPIRATORY ISOLATION

Visitors—Report to Nurses' Station Before Entering Room

1. Masks are indicated for those who come close to patient.
2. Gowns are not indicated.
3. Gloves are not indicated.
4. HANDS MUST BE WASHED AFTER TOUCHING THE PATIENT OR POTENTIALLY CONTAMINATED ARTICLES AND BEFORE TAKING CARE OF ANOTHER PATIENT.
5. Articles contaminated with infective material should be discarded or bagged and labeled before being sent for decontamination and reprocessing.

Diseases Requiring Respiratory Isolation*

Epiglottitis, *Haemophilus influenzae* infection

Erythema infectiosum

Measles

Meningitis
- Bacterial, origin unknown
- *H. influenzae* infection, known or suspected

Meningococcal pneumonia

Mumps

Pertussis (whooping cough)

Pneumonia, *H. influenzae* infection in children (any age)

*A private room is indicated for respiratory isolation; in general, however, patients infected with the same organism may share a room. See *Guideline for Isolation Precautions in Hospitals* for details and for how long to apply precautions.

Figure 6-6 Instructions for respiratory isolation.
(Data courtesy of the Centers for Disease Control, Atlanta, GA. CDC Guidelines, Infection Control 4(4):284-290, 1983.)

glect of the recommended procedures often derives from the belief that infectious diseases are no longer a serious threat because of the availability of so many antimicrobial drugs. However, it is simply not true that there is a drug that will cure every type of infection. As early as the 1950s, bacteria were developing strains resistant to penicillin. Since that time, many microbes have become resistant almost as fast as new drugs have been introduced. We need only look at the ever-increasing numbers of nosocomial infections to be reminded of the dangers of complacency in the battle against infectious agents.

Health Teaching

Nurses have an obligation to teach the patient how to care for himself and how to avoid infection by good personal hygiene and sanitation. If a patient already has an infection, he and his family will need to know (1) the ways in which the infection is transmitted, (2) proper hand-washing techniques, (3) the approved disinfectants for the microorganism causing his infection, (4) methods for proper handling and disposal of contaminated articles, and (5) other precautions indicated for the kind of infectious disease the patient has. This information should be given while the patient is hospitalized, so that he and his family will understand why precautions are necessary. Knowing why and how to take these precautions also prepares the patient to have optimal care once he returns home. The nurse can serve as a model by demonstrating good infection control behaviors such as careful hand washing and care in avoiding contamination of objects in the patient's room.

If a patient is to continue taking medications at home to control his infection, he must be taught how to take them. He must also be cautioned not to discontinue taking any prescribed medication, even when he begins to feel better. All antimicrobial drugs should be continued for as long as they are prescribed. To stop before the full amount has been taken can lead to a second outbreak of the infection and possibly to readmission to the hospital.

Other aspects of teaching will depend on each

CONTACT ISOLATION

Visitors—Report to Nurses' Station Before Entering Room

1. Masks are indicated for those who come close to patient.
2. Gowns are indicated if soiling is likely.
3. Gloves are indicated for touching infective material.
4. HANDS MUST BE WASHED AFTER TOUCHING THE PATIENT OR POTENTIALLY CONTAMINATED ARTICLES AND BEFORE TAKING CARE OF ANOTHER PATIENT.
5. Articles contaminated with infective material should be discarded or bagged and labeled before being sent for decontamination and reprocessing.

Diseases or Conditions Requiring Contact Isolation*

Acute respiratory tract infections in infants and young children, including croup, colds, bronchitis, and bronchiolitis caused by respiratory syncytial virus, adenovirus, coronavirus, influenza viruses, parainfluenza viruses, and rhinovirus

Gonococcal conjunctivitis in newborns

Cutaneous diphtheria

Group A endometritis

Streptococcus infection

Staphylococcal furunculosis in newborns

Disseminated herpes simplex infection, severe primary or neonatal

Impetigo

Influenza in infants and young children

Multiple-resistant bacteria, infection or colonization (any site), with any of the following:

- Gram-negative bacilli infection resistant to all aminoglycosides that are tested. (In general, such organisms should be resistant to gentamicin, tobramycin, and amikacin for these special precautions to be indicated.)
- *Staphylococcus aureus* infection resistant to methicillin (or nafcillin or oxacillin, if used instead of methicillin for testing.)
- *Pneumococcus* infection resistant to penicillin
- *Haemophilus influenzae* infection resistant to ampicillin (β-lactamase-positive) and chloramphenicol
- Other resistant bacterial infections may be included in this isolation category if they are judged by the infection control team to be of special clinical and epidemiologic significance

Pediculosis

Infectious pharyngitis in infants and young children

Viral pneumonia in infants and young children

Pneumonia, *S. aureus* infection, or group A *Streptococcus* infection

Rabies

Rubella, congenital and other

Scabies

Scalded skin syndrome (Ritter's disease)

Major skin, wound, or burn infection (draining and not covered by a dressing, or dressing does not adequately contain the purulent material), including infection with *S. aureus* or group A *Streptococcus*

Vaccinia (generalized and progressive eczema vaccinatum)

*A private room is indicated for contact isolation; in general, however, patients infected with the same organism may share a room.

During outbreaks, infants and young children with the same respiratory clinical syndrome may share a room. See *Guideline for Isolation Precautions in Hospitals* for details and for how long to apply precautions.

Figure 6-7 Instructions for contact isolation.
(Data courtesy of the Centers for Disease Control, Atlanta, GA. CDC Guidelines, Infection Control 4(4):284–290, 1983.)

ACID-FAST BACILLI (TUBERCULOSIS ISOLATION)

Visitors—Report to Nurses' Station Before Entering Room

1. Masks are indicated only when patient is coughing and does not reliably cover mouth.
2. Gowns are indicated only if needed to prevent gross contamination of clothing.
3. Gloves are not indicated.
4. HANDS MUST BE WASHED AFTER TOUCHING THE PATIENT OR POTENTIALLY CONTAMINATED ARTICLES AND BEFORE TAKING CARE OF ANOTHER PATIENT.
5. Articles contaminated with infective material should be discarded, cleaned, or sent for decontamination and reprocessing.

Diseases Requiring Acid-Fast Bacilli Isolation*

This isolation category is for patients with current pulmonary tuberculosis who have a positive sputum smear or a chest radiograph appearance that strongly suggests current (active) tuberculosis. Laryngeal tuberculosis is also included in this category. In general, infants and young children with pulmonary tuberculosis do not require isolation precautions, because they rarely cough and their bronchial secretions contain few acid-fast bacilli (AFB) when compared with adults with pulmonary tuberculosis. To protect the patient's privacy, this instruction care is labeled "AFB Isolation" rather than "Tuberculosis Isolation."

*A private room with special ventilation is indicated for AFB isolation. In general, patients infected with the same organism may share a room. See *Guidelines for Isolation Precautions in Hospitals* for details and for how long to apply precautions.

Figure 6-8 Instructions for AFB (tuberculosis) isolation.
(Data courtesy of the Centers for Disease Control, Atlanta, GA. CDC Guidelines, Infection Control 4(4):284-290, 1983.)

patient's learning needs. A patient may need to learn how to change dressings or handle secretions without spreading infection to others or reinfecting himself. Nurses may also need to teach patients how to dispose of contaminated articles and maintain a clean and sanitary environment, how to plan nutritious meals that provide adequate protein and vitamin intake, and how to ensure the rest and activity necessary to promote healing.

Strengthening the Patient's Capacity for Recovery from Infection

In her efforts to enhance and strengthen a patient's own resources for overcoming an infection, the nurse first assesses the patient's health status and the resources he has available. She then sets goals with him and plans and implements nursing measures to strengthen his capacity for recovery.

Assessment

In her assessment of the patient at the time of admission or when a diagnosis of infection has been verified, the nurse will need to consider the age of the patient and his nutritional status. She also will need to know his patterns of bladder and bowel elimination and the degree of physical activity he can tolerate. The results of laboratory tests, especially culture and sensitivity tests, will also be helpful in assessing the patient.

Cultures are grown from specimens collected at the site of infection. When obtaining a culture, the nurse must be careful to (1) collect fresh material from the site only, avoiding contamination by microbes from nearby tissues and fluids; (2) use sterile equipment and the appropriate container for the sample; and (3) be sure the container is tightly covered to avoid spilling and contamination during transport to the laboratory.

Sensitivity tests are performed to determine which drug or drugs a particular microbe is sensitive to, that is, which antimicrobials can most effectively destroy or inhibit the multiplication and growth of the infecting microbe. Once this has been determined, the drug of choice must be administered exactly as prescribed. As explained later, inadequate dosage or delay in administration can lead to genetic mutation and the development of a strain of microbe that is resistant to the drug.

Periodic reassessment of the patient's status

ENTERIC PRECAUTIONS

Visitors—Report to Nurses' Station Before Entering Room

1. Masks are not required.
2. Gowns are indicated if soiling is likely.
3. Gloves are indicated for touching infective material.
4. HANDS MUST BE WASHED AFTER TOUCHING THE PATIENT OR POTENTIALLY CONTAMINATED ARTICLES AND BEFORE TAKING CARE OF ANOTHER PATIENT.
5. Articles contaminated with infective material should be discarded or bagged and labeled before being sent for decontamination and reprocessing.

Diseases Requiring Enteric Precautions*

Amebic dysentery

Cholera

Coxsackievirus disease

Diarrhea in acute illness with suspected infectious origin

Echovirus disease

Encephalitis (unless known not to be caused by an enterovirus)

Enterocolitis caused by *Clostridium difficile or Staphylococcus aureus*

Enteroviral infection

Gastroenteritis caused by:
- *Campylobacter* organisms
- *Cryptosporidium* organisms
- *Escherichia coli* (enterotoxic, enteropathogenic, or enteroinvasive)
- *Giardia lamblia*
- *Salmonella* organisms
- *Shigella* organisms
- *Vibrio parahaemolyticus* infection viruses, including Norwalk and human rotavirus
- *Yersinia enterocolitica*
- An unknown agent, but presumed to be of infectious origin

Hand, foot, and mouth disease

Viral hepatitis, type A

Herpangina

Viral meningitis (unless known not to be caused by an enterovirus)

Necrotizing enterocolitis

Pleurodynia

Poliomyelitis

Typhoid fever (*Salmonella typhi* infection)

Viral pericarditis, myocarditis, or meningitis (unless known not to be caused by an enterovirus)

*A private room is indicated for enteric precautions if patient hygiene is poor. A patient with poor hygiene does not wash his hands after touching infective material, contaminates the environment with infective material, or shares contaminated articles with other patients. In general, patients infected with the same organism may share a room. See *Guideline for Isolation Precautions in Hospitals* for details and for how long to apply precautions.

Figure 6-9 Instructions for enteric precautions.
(Data courtesy of the Centers for Disease Control, Atlanta, GA. CDC Guidelines, Infection Control 4(4):284–290, 1983.)

during the course of his illness includes monitoring his vital signs for evidence of continued infection or signs of recovery, observing wounds or lesions (if any) for signs of healing or delay in healing, noting whether the patient is able to maintain adequate nutrition and hydration, and keeping track of the degree of activity he is able to tolerate.

Other needs that often occur when a person has an infectious disease are those related to feelings of being "unclean" or "dirty," worry and guilt about giving the infection to someone else, and loneliness resulting from being separated from other people.

Planning and Intervention

The goals of nursing intervention to enhance recovery from infection include measures to help the patient achieve optimal use of the body's defensive and healing processes. Adequate rest; freedom from physical discomfort, mental anxiety, and depression; adequate nutrition and hydration; and sufficient oxygen and blood supply

DRAINAGE/SECRETION PRECAUTIONS

Visitors—Report to Nurses' Station Before Entering Room

1. Masks are not indicated.
2. Gowns are indicated if soiling is likely.
3. Gloves are indicated for touching infective material.
4. HANDS MUST BE WASHED AFTER TOUCHING THE PATIENT OR POTENTIALLY CONTAMINATED ARTICLES AND BEFORE TAKING CARE OF ANOTHER PATIENT.
5. Articles contaminated with infective material should be discarded or bagged and labeled before being sent for decontamination and reprocessing.

Diseases Requiring Drainage/Secretion Precautions*

Infectious diseases included in this category are those that result in production of infective purulent material, drainage, or secretions, unless the disease is included in another isolation category that requires more rigorous precautions. (If you have questions about a specific disease, see the listing of infectious diseases in *Guideline for Isolation Precautions in Hospitals,* Table A, Disease-Specific Isolation Precautions.)

The following infections are examples of those included in this category, provided they are not (1) caused by multiple-resistant microorganisms, (2) major skin, wound, or burn infections (i.e., draining and not covered by a dressing or dressing does not adequately contain the drainage), including those caused by *Staphylococcus aureus* or group A *Streptococcus*, or (3) gonococcal eye infections in newborns (see "Contact Isolation" if the infection is one of these three):

Abscess, minor or limited	Infected decubitus ulcer, minor or limited
Burn infection, minor or limited	Skin infection, minor or limited
Conjunctivitis	Wound infection, minor or limited

*A private room is usually not indicated for drainage/secretion precautions. See *Guideline for Isolation Precautions in Hospitals* for details and for how long to apply precautions.

Figure 6-10 Instructions for drainage/secretion precautions.
(Data courtesy of the Centers for Disease Control, Atlanta, GA. CDC Guidelines, Infection Control 4(4):284-290, 1983.)

to the infected tissues are all a necessary part of a patient's recovery.

Among the specific goals that could be included in a nursing care plan for a patient with an infection are to ensure that

- Temperature, pulse, and respirations are nearing normal or within normal range.
- The patient is able to rest comfortably and reports absence of or decrease in severity of pain or discomfort.
- Total fluid intake is at least 2000 mL every 24 hours.
- Nutritional needs are met, weight loss gradually regained (if this is desired, depending on patient's weight status), and normal body weight maintained.
- The patient is able to explain the purposes of diagnostic tests, treatments, and special precautions.
- The patient and family are able to maintain medical asepsis at all times and prevent spread of infection.

Physiologic Support. Physiologic support of the patient is truly the domain of the nurse. It is through her nursing actions that the patient is able to marshal all his inner resources to overcome his illness. She makes sure that the patient gets adequate rest and nutrition so that the natural curative powers of the body can function effectively. The patient's need for rest is best met when he is in a quiet environment with minimal interruption and excitement.

Relief of Symptoms. Relief of symptoms from fever, muscle tension, and dehydration also is within the realm of nursing care. Cool sponge baths, ice bags, use of antipyretics, and other measures to reduce body temperature can help manage the symptoms associated with an elevated body temperature. Warm compresses and

BLOOD/BODY FLUID PRECAUTIONS

Visitors—Report to Nurses' Station Before Entering Room

1. Masks are not indicated.
2. Gowns are indicated if soiling is likely.
3. Gloves are indicated for touching blood or body fluids.
4. HANDS MUST BE WASHED IMMEDIATELY IF THEY ARE POTENTIALLY CONTAMINATED WITH BLOOD OR BODY FLUIDS AND BEFORE TAKING CARE OF ANOTHER PATIENT.
5. Articles contaminated with blood or body fluids should be discarded or bagged and labeled before being sent for decontamination and reprocessing.
6. Care should be taken to avoid needle-stick injuries. Used needles should not be recapped or bent; they should be placed in a prominently labeled, puncture-resistant container designated specifically for such disposal.
7. Blood spills should be cleaned up promptly with a solution of one part 5.25% sodium hypochlorite and 10 parts water.

Diseases Requiring Blood/Body Fluid Precautions*

Acquired immunodeficiency syndrome (AIDS)

Arthropodous viral fevers (e.g., dengue, yellow fever, and Colorado tick fever)

Babesiosis

Creutzfeldt-Jakob disease

Hepatitis B (including HBsAg antigen carrier)

Hepatitis C, non-A, non-B

Leptospirosis

Malaria

Rat-bite fever

Relapsing fever

Syphilis, both primary and secondary, with skin and mucous membrane lesions

*A private room is indicated for blood/body fluid precautions if patient hygiene is poor. A patient with poor hygiene does not wash his hands after touching infective material, contaminates the environment with infective material, or shares contaminated articles with other patients. In general, patients infected with the same organism may share a room. See *Guideline for Isolation Precautions in Hospitals* for details and for how long to apply precautions.

Figure 6-11 Instructions for blood/body fluid precautions.
(Data courtesy of the Centers for Disease Control, Atlanta, GA. CDC Guidelines, Infection Control 4(4):284-290, 1983.)

applications of heat, when appropriate, can promote relaxation and healing.

Such nursing actions as a back rub, assistance in moving to a comfortable position, and maintenance of good body alignment are comforting and conducive to rest and relaxation. Physical exercise also can promote rest if the patient is able to tolerate mild physical activity.

Adequate Hydration. An accurate record of the patient's intake and output can help the nurse determine whether he needs to be encouraged to increase his intake of fluids to combat dehydration. Remember that the internal environment is composed of fluids. Cellular dehydration can work against the adequate transport of nutrients to the cells and of waste products from the cells. It thus delays healing. An ideal intake would be at least 2,000 mL every 24 hours.

Psychological Support. A patient's acceptance of isolation precautions, uncomfortable treatments, and other unpleasant features of his illness can be greatly affected by his relationship with the nurses who care for him. If he is able to trust them, to know they are concerned about his welfare, and to realize that their goal is to help him cope with and recover from a difficult illness, he will be strengthened and supported in ways that perhaps cannot be measured precisely but are nonetheless effective.

The patient with an infectious disorder also is likely to worry about the spread of infection in his own body and to those around him. Some infections do tend to recur or to involve other systems of the body if they are not effectively eradicated. The patient should have opportunities to ask questions about the nature of his illness and to receive informative answers. He will probably be most concerned about diagnostic procedures and their results, special medications he is receiving, and treatments that are prescribed. Concerns about his family, finances, and other social problems can be referred to a medical social worker.

Drugs. A major supportive measure included in the total patient care plan is the administration of antiinfective or antimicrobial drugs. These drugs are given for the purpose of strengthening the patient's own defense mechanisms and supporting the body's natural healing powers. It is these natural defensive and healing activities that determine whether the patient will recover. The drugs merely assist the body by decreasing the number of microbes, either by destroying them or by inhibiting their growth. This is not to say that antimicrobials have not been of tremendous benefit to mankind. They have helped and will continue to help patients overcome many infectious diseases. Because they are so effective in preventing and treating infections, antimicrobial drugs are among the most frequently prescribed drugs.

However, we are reluctantly coming to realize that antibiotics and other antimicrobial drugs are not the "miracle drugs" we once thought them to be. Just as man has learned to adapt and become immune to harmful agents through successive generations, so, too, have bacteria been able to develop resistance to certain antibiotics. Bacteria, however, do not need to wait 20 to 25 years for a new generation to develop. They reproduce quite rapidly and therefore can produce, in a relatively short time, a new strain of organism that is able to survive in the presence of an antibiotic. When this happens, the antibiotic becomes all but useless in the fight against the infectious agent that has developed a resistance to it. Although we cannot completely control the evolution of resistant strains of bacteria, we can reduce the likelihood that resistance will develop.

The responsibility of the nurse lies in accurate administration of antibiotics so that neither too much nor too little is given.

Antibiotics must be given at the specific hours for which they are ordered; otherwise the level of drug in the blood and tissues fluctuates widely, and the bacteria have an opportunity to develop resistance.

The public needs to be aware of the fact that taking "most but not all" of the antibiotic prescribed for them or their children can actually help some bacteria to survive and live to produce resistant strains. Many people are tempted to stop taking a drug after the serious symptoms are relieved. They should be reminded of the importance of taking all of the drug in the exact manner in which it has been prescribed for them.

Another responsibility of the nurse is to discourage people from demanding "a shot of penicillin" for minor colds and sore throats. The indiscriminate use of an antibiotic for any and all ailments only serves to make it ineffective for more serious infections.

Nursing interventions for selected nursing diagnoses in a patient with a wound infection are summarized in Nursing Care Plan 6–1. General nursing measures for patients with an infection are listed in Table 6–5.

Immunization

Providing individuals with an active immunity so that the incidence of specific infectious diseases is reduced is an important part of disease control. The nurse should encourage childhood immunization programs that protect children against diphtheria, whooping cough (pertussis), tetanus, polio, measles, and mumps.

Identification of high-risk people who are particularly susceptible to infections is also necessary in order to reduce the suffering and possible death that infections can bring about. A person's defense mechanism might be lowered and his susceptibility to infections increased by burns, extensive surgery, and other kinds of trauma. Patients with chronic diseases are also at high

TABLE 6–5 GENERAL NURSING MEASURES FOR PATIENTS WITH AN INFECTION

- Ensure adequate rest.
- Provide good nutrition with sufficient protein and vitamin content to promote healing.
- Provide nonstressful environment.
- Administer antiinfectives on time as ordered.
- Encourage good hydration.
- Keep patient clean and dry.
- Provide comfort measures.
- Provide care to relieve or treat specific symptoms of infection such as fever, cough, diarrhea.
- Prevent exposure to additional infectious agents.
- Maintain asepsis to prevent spread of infection or reinfection.

NURSING CARE PLAN 6–1

Selected nursing diagnoses, goals/outcome criteria, nursing interventions, and evaluations for a patient with wound infection

Situation: Patient is a 28-year-old male with *Staphylococcus aureus* infection of a wound sustained during an automobile accident.

Nursing Diagnosis	Goals/Outcome Criteria	Nursing Interventions	Evaluation
Impaired skin integrity related to infected wound. SUPPORTING DATA Draining wound on right leg; positive culture for *Staphylococcus aureus*.	Staphylococcal infection will not be spread to others or other parts of patient's body.	Follow CDC's drainage/secretion precautions. Explain purpose of precautions to patient and visitors. Change wound dressing A.M. and P.M.; assist patient with bath to ensure skin has been cleaned and dressing does not become wet.	In drainage/secretion isolation; explanations given; dressings changed A.M. and P.M. using sterile technique; dressing remains dry. No evidence of spread of infection.
Knowledge deficit related to proper wound care at home. SUPPORTING DATA "I don't know how to change a dressing properly."	Patient will state reasons for using special precautions for dressing change. Patient and one family member will demonstrate dressing change, maintaining medical asepsis before discharge. Patient and family member will demonstrate proper hand-washing technique before discharge. Patient will list signs and symptoms that should be reported to physician. Patient will take full prescription of antibiotics exactly as directed.	Explain purpose of special precautions for dressing change and handling of soiled dressings. Demonstrate proper dressing change and wound cleansing procedure; obtain return demonstration from patient and family member before discharge. Demonstrate proper hand-washing technique; observe patient and family member perform hand washing. Instruct patient to watch for elevated temperature; increased redness, swelling, or pain; or purulent discharge from wound and to report such findings to the physician should they occur. Explain importance of taking medication exactly as prescribed and of finishing entire prescription.	Patient verbalizes reasons for special precautions; patient and family member demonstrate proper hand washing, wound cleansing, and dressing change using medical asepsis; patient verbalizes signs and symptoms to report to physician and states that he understands how to take medication and why he must finish the prescription.

risk, especially those who have either liver or kidney disease. The nursing care of all susceptible persons should take into consideration the special precautions needed to protect them.

Passive immunity is another way in which the patient's defenses against certain infectious diseases can be strengthened. Some, but not all, infections stimulate the production of antibodies, which are proteins capable of destroying the causative agent of the disease. When a patient does not have a sufficient supply of antibodies that he has produced himself, he can be given "ready-made" antibodies to help fight an infection. These antibodies are given by administering immune serum and gamma globulin. Passive immunity is discussed more fully in Chapter 7.

PROTECTIVE STRUCTURES AND MECHANISMS

Considering the great number and variety of agents, both living and nonliving, that can harm the human body, it is remarkable that any of us can survive in such a hostile environment. If the body was not so adaptable and resilient, human beings would have become extinct long ago. Inner resources, both physiologic and psychological, cause humans to survive and enable them to cope with such hostile agents.

There are many protective structures and mechanisms that the body uses to keep us well or, in the event of injury or illness, help us recover. Such external structures as the skin and mucous membranes and the substances they secrete are important parts of the natural or innate immunity of humans. Internally, the bones protect the more delicate and vital organs so that they are less likely to be injured. Even the blood itself contains certain chemical compounds that destroy foreign microorganisms and promote healing. Additionally, there are protective organs such as the liver, which filters out and detoxifies (i.e., makes harmless) poisons that enter the body.

PROTECTIVE ORGANS

The largest organ of the body, the skin, serves as a first line of defense against harmful agents in the environment. It functions as a protective covering for the more delicate and vulnerable underlying tissues. It also excretes, through the sweat and sebaceous glands, lactic acid and fatty acids that inhibit the growth of bacteria.

Secretions from the *mucous membranes* lining the respiratory, gastrointestinal, and reproductive tracts contain an abundance of the enzyme *lysozyme*, which is bactericidal. The same enzyme is also found in tears and saliva. Cilia, which line the respiratory tract, trap organisms and debris and propel them up and out of the body with a wavelike action.

Internally, the bones protect the more delicate and vital organs from outside blows. The bone marrow plays an important role in the production of defensive blood cells.

A major organ of defense is the liver, whose Kupffer's cells move and destroy bacteria that have found their way into the blood circulating through the portal system. No more than 1% of the bacteria that escape from the intestines and enter into the portal circulation pass through the liver into the general circulation. Because the intestinal tract is a major route for the entry of microorganisms into the blood and from there into other tissues of the body, the liver is essential to the body's system of defense.

The liver also detoxifies harmful chemicals by isolating the poisonous substances and facilitating their breakdown and excretion from the body.

NURSING ASSESSMENT AND INTERVENTIONS

Assessment of the patient for evidence of difficulty in maintaining the protective organs of the body begins with noting the condition of the patient's skin. Cuts, bruises, sores, and reddened areas should receive prompt attention. Nursing interventions to help preserve the skin and maintain its protective functions include (1) gentle handling of the patient when he is being positioned in bed, transported in a wheelchair or on a stretcher, or moved from chair to bed; (2) sensible use of lotions and lubricants that keep the skin soft and pliable, thereby avoiding drying and cracking that can lead to development of portals of entry for infectious organisms; and (3) cleansing the wound and promoting healing once the skin has been broken.

The mucous membranes require similar attention. Adequate hydration and regular mouth care can help keep the lips and mouth moist and free from drying and cracking. The nurse also should be alert to the dangers of frequent use of unprescribed and mildly antiseptic gargles, mouthwashes, eye drops, and vaginal douches that can remove the body's natural antiseptic secretions. Astringent and chemically strong solutions can make the body more, rather than less, susceptible to harm.

Mucous membranes should be protected from injury whenever a tube or instrument (e.g., a rectal tube) is introduced into a body opening. The tip of the object should be well-lubricated, and force must never be used. Care must be taken that the insertion is made in the proper direction and for no more than the proper distance.

Assessment of bone function and nursing intervention to maintain normal protective properties are discussed more fully in Chapter 26.

The liver is the largest gland in the body. Assessment of liver function involves laboratory testing, radiologic studies, and observation of the patient for jaundice and other outward signs and symptoms of liver disease. These and nursing interventions for patients with liver disorders are discussed in Chapter 24.

DEFENSIVE CELLS

In addition to the protective organs, the body has another system of defense that involves the blood cells and mononuclear phagocytes. These cells literally engulf or swallow up foreign organisms by a process called *phagocytosis*. They also release chemicals into the environment of damaged cells that are important to repair and healing.

LEUKOCYTES

The leukocytes might be thought of as the mobile units of the body's defense system. They increase in number as soon as injury occurs and are quickly transported to any part of the body where they are needed to destroy invading microorganisms and other harmful agents.

There are six different types of leukocytes. Three of these types have nuclei of many different shapes. For this reason they are called *polymorphonuclear leukocytes*, or "poly's" for short.

These cells have a granular appearance when viewed under a microscope and are thus sometimes called *granulocytes.* The most abundant kind of granulocytes are the *neutrophils,* which make up about 67% of the total number of leukocytes in the blood.

Other types of white blood cells include the *monocytes,* whose most important function is phagocytosis. This is also the major function of the neutrophils. Defensive cells that are phagocytes are able to surround or engulf foreign particles, including both living matter, such as bacteria, and nonliving matter, such as dust and carbon. Besides engulfing the foreign particles, the phagocytes also can digest some of them. This is possible because the defensive cells release enzymes specifically designed to destroy the substance of the particles by chemical action.

The neutrophils also play an important role in repair of damaged tissues because they remove debris from the battlefield. By clearing away dead bacterial and tissue cells, they leave a clean area in which the process of repair can begin.

Whenever the tissues of the body become inflamed, the number of leukocytes is greatly increased (i.e., leukocytosis). For example, at the time of a "heart attack," cells in the heart are deprived of oxygen and therefore are injured. An inflammatory response begins at the site of the damaged tissues, and the body increases its supply of neutrophils, a particular type of leukocyte. *Neutrophilia* is an important diagnostic sign that damage has been done to the heart muscle by a myocardial infarction. Table 6–6 lists the types of leukocytes and their functions.

THE MONONUCLEAR PHAGOCYTE SYSTEM

The mononuclear phagocyte system (formerly called the *reticuloendothelial system*) is a defense system made up of a network of specialized cells called *macrophages* that, although they are scattered around the body, share a common purpose in defense. These cells are found in many body organs and are strategically placed so they can trap and destroy foreign matter almost as soon as it has entered the body. They are both stationary and mobile and are found in lymphatic tissue, the alveoli of the lungs, the gastrointestinal system, the spleen, and the liver (Kupffer's cells). The macrophages remove cellular debris, engulf and destroy bacteria and viruses (thus preventing infection), and remove metabolic waste products.

Some of the mononuclear phagocytes are called *tissue macrophages;* others, which are concerned with immunity, are the *lymphocytic cells.* A macrophage is a very large (macro-) cell that is capable of phagocytosis. Some macrophages are in the alveoli of the lung, where they lie in wait for bacteria, dust particles, and any other foreign material that might threaten to damage the lung tissues. If the foreign particles are not digestible, the macrophages in the alveoli help wall them off, thereby preventing their spread to other tissues. An example of this process is the localizing of tubercle bacilli that have not been destroyed by the body's other defenses. Tuberculosis is controlled, if not cured, by walling off the bacilli.

Bacteria that attempt to enter the general cir-

TABLE 6–6 LEUKOCYTES AND THEIR FUNCTIONS

Cell Type	Function
Granulocytes (Polymorphonuclear, or "poly's")	
Neutrophils	Phagocytosis; clean site of inflammation; elevated by bacterial infection, inflammation, some tumors, and stress.
Eosinophils	Mild phagocytic action; elevated by allergic disorders, parasitic infections, certain skin disorders, and some cancers.
Basophils	Release histamine in presence of allergic reaction; release heparin into blood at site of inflammation; elevated by asthma, some cancers, blood disorders, and chronic inflammation.
Agranulocytes	
Lymphocytes	Phagocytosis; produce gamma globulin; cell-mediated reactions; elevated by viral infection and some cancers.
Monocytes	Phagocytosis; can ingest large numbers of bacteria; clean inflammatory site; elevated by chronic infection and liver disease.

culation must contend with reticulum cells in the liver (*Kupffer's cells*). They destroy the organisms being transported through the portal circulation.

Other cells of the mononuclear phagocyte system are located in the lymph nodes. If foreign particles escape destruction when they pass through the portals of entry, they are able to enter the lymphatic system. This would be an ideal means of transportation for the harmful agents were it not for the lymph nodes located along the way. The tissues of the lymph nodes are lined with macrophages that trap and engulf the foreign particles as they travel by.

Another location of macrophages is the spleen. Foreign substances that have managed to get by the liver, alveoli, and lymph nodes or have somehow entered the blood stream, are dealt with by the macrophages of the spleen.

The functions of the defensive cells just described are part of the inflammatory process. Nursing assessment and intervention related to this process are discussed below.

THE PROCESS OF INFLAMMATION

Inflammation is an immediate response of the body to any kind of injury to its cells and tissues.

Inflammation occurs at the cellular level where the injury has taken place and is the most common kind of response to damage to the cells. Almost all tissues of the body respond to injury by initiating the inflammatory process.

The inflammatory process can be induced by any of the mechanical, chemical, and infectious disease-producing factors described in the previous chapter. Although bacteria, viruses, and other infectious microorganisms evoke an inflammatory response, the terms *infection* and *inflammation* are not synonymous. The word *infection* means that the inflamed area has been invaded by infectious agents. *Inflammation* is a localized protective response brought on by injury or destruction of tissues. The injury can be caused by infectious agents, mechanical or chemical trauma, or any other abnormal condition affecting the tissues.

The basic purposes of the inflammatory response are to (1) neutralize and destroy harmful agents, (2) limit their spread to other tissues in the body, and (3) prepare the damaged tissues for repair (Fig. 6–12).

INFLAMMATORY CHANGES

Changes that are part of the inflammatory process can occur locally at the site of injury and also systemically. These changes involve (1) the cells of the damaged tissues and adjacent connective tissues; (2) the blood vessels in and near the site of injury; (3) the blood cells, particularly the leukocytes; (4) the macrophages of the mononuclear phagocyte system; (5) the immune system; and (6) the hormonal system.

Vascular Changes

As soon as injury occurs, the blood vessels in the injured area momentarily constrict and as histamine and serotonins are released, they dilate so that more blood is brought to the damaged cells. The walls of the capillaries become more permeable (i.e., their pores enlarge) so that water, proteins, and defensive cells can pass out of the blood and into the fluid surrounding the damaged cells. This leakage of fluid into the spaces around the cells produces a localized swelling, or edema, which is one of the classic outward signs of inflammation.

When the fluid and fibrinogen brought by the blood leak through the walls of the capillaries, they fill the tissue spaces and block the lymphatic vessels with fibrinogen clots. This results in a "walling off" of the area and delays the spread of bacteria, toxins, and other harmful agents to other parts of the body.

Leukocytosis

Another substance that is believed to be liberated from damaged cells is the *leukocytosis-promoting factor*. It acts on the bone marrow, which is stimulated to release granulocytes—especially neutrophils—that have been stored there. These defensive cells then enter the blood stream and are transported to the site of injury. The factor also increases the rate of production of granulocytes so that a supply of them is available as long as needed to inactivate and destroy harmful agents.

Reticulum Cells

Within the first few hours of the onset of the inflammatory process, the monocytes undergo drastic changes. They swell, becoming very large cells (macrophages) that then migrate to the inflammatory site. There they ingest foreign particles and necrotic (dead) tissue.

After the neutrophils and macrophages engulf and destroy bacteria and foreign matter, they themselves die, producing debris that is composed of tissue fluid, dead cells, and their products. This exudate is commonly known as pus. A yellow or greenish purulent drainage is a sign of infection.

Immune System

While the phagocytes are engulfing and destroying bacteria and other harmful agents, the immune response has elicited the production of

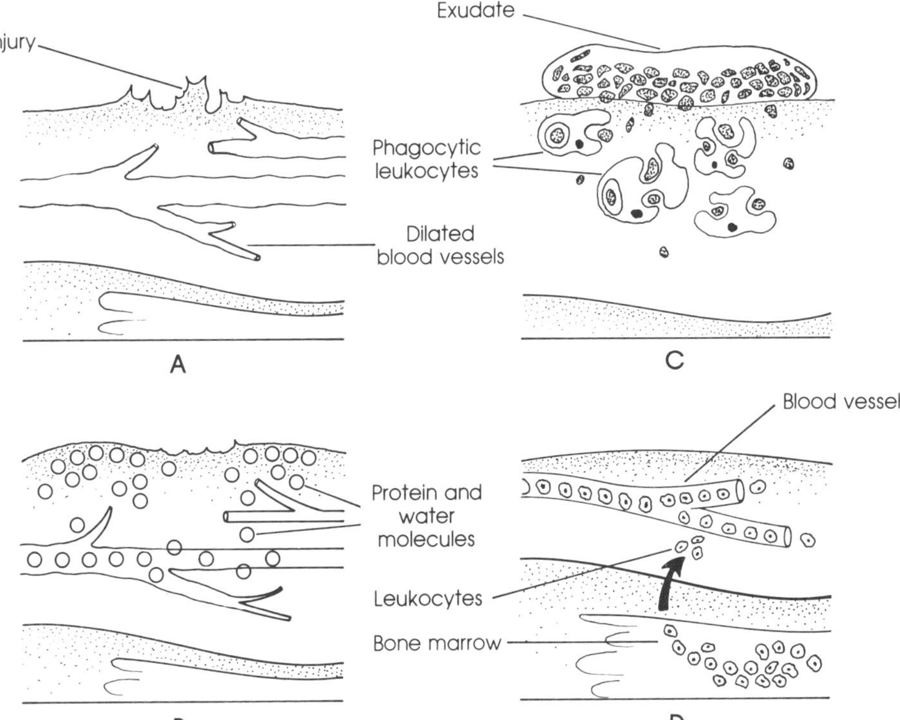

Figure 6–12 Inflammatory process resulting from trauma and introduction of bacteria. *A*, Injury to tissue stimulates release of histamine, which dilates blood vessels and produces increased blood flow and accompanying redness. *B*, Capillary walls become more permeable, allowing fluid and plasma proteins to move out of blood vessels and into tissue spaces, thus causing swelling. *C*, Leukocytes are transported to site of injury, where they destroy and ingest foreign agents and die. Dead phagocytes, cell debris, and tissue fluid form exudate. *D*, Dying leukocytes release pyrogens, which circulate to the brain, raising body temperature, and to the bone marrow, where they bring about release of more leukocytes.

specific antibodies and antitoxins. They are called *specific* because they are designed to attack only the infectious agent or harmful substance that triggers their production. These immune bodies are transported by the blood to the tissue spaces at the site of inflamm
they attack foreign cells and neutr
sons these cells produce. The imm
is discussed in greater detail in
chapter.

Hormonal Response

Some hormones, such as cortis
antiinflammatory action that limits
to the locally damaged tissues wh
needed. Other hormones, such a
are *proinflammatory* corticoids,
that they stimulate the body's pro
matory response. Thus the hormor
ulatory effect on the inflammatc
that it is well-balanced and provi
benefit. In some cases of severe
the physician may prescribe an ar
drug to relieve the symptoms of
However, hormones such as the
can interfere with healing.

SIGNS AND SYMPTOMS O
INFLAMMATION

Local Reactions

***The five** local **signs and sympt
inflammation are heat, rednes
pain, and limitation or loss of***

The increased blood flow to the affected area produces heat and redness. Swelling is the result of the increased permeability of the capillaries and the leakage of fluid from the blood into the tissue spaces around the cells. Blockage of lymphatic drainage from the site also contributes to muscle aches, and fever are common symptoms. Sweating and chills are sometimes experienced, as are anorexia and a sensation of "just feeling sick" and depressed. Laboratory tests will show that the white cell count is elevated; the leukocyte count can be as high as 30,000 per milliliter of blood.

Patient care problems associated with systemic inflammatory responses include those related to inadequate nutrition and fluid intake, discomfort, need for rest, and need for maintenance of normal body temperature and fluid balance.

If there is an inadequate inflammatory response, which sometimes occurs in patients receiving certain drugs or suffering from chronic illness, the patient may develop infections of the throat or colon, susceptibility to bacterial infections elsewhere in the body, and delayed tissue repair and wound healing.

REPAIR AND HEALING

Repair of the damage done to cells and tissues begins almost at the same time that the inflammatory process begins. When the body has been injured and responds by initiating the inflammatory and the repair process, there are three possible outcomes of its attempts toward healing: *recovery, regeneration,* and *replacement.*

If the cells are not damaged beyond recovery, they will restore themselves, and there will be no permanent evidence of injury. If an infection is present and is localized, the exudate is removed, and the tissues return to normal. This is called *localization* and *resolution.* The outcome is *recovery*—that is, restoration of the tissues to their former state.

A second possibility is that some of the cells
y be fatally injured (necrosis). The affected
then must heal by *regeneration,* which
hat new cells similar in structure and
the dead ones are produced as re-
This is not possible in all types of
ithelial, fibrous, bony, and lym-
enerate well, but the nervous,
tissues do not.
utcome is replacement of
fibrous scar tissue (scar-
d with the inflamma-
er) contains fibrin,
ands on which
ebris from the
leukocytes,
begin to
small
ation
oo

excessive granulation tissue is commonly called *proud flesh.* It occurs when wound infection or prolonged wet dressings overstimulate the production of granulation tissues. Proud flesh must be removed by cautery or by chemical or surgical débridement before the wound can heal properly.

Scar formation is a natural result of the process of repair. The capillaries and connective tissue cells in the wound shrink and become taut, appearing as hard reddish tissue and gradually becoming white and glossy to form the typical scar tissue with which we are all familiar. Collagen overgrowth results in a "keloid"-type scar, which occurs mostly in dark pigmented skin. Internally, the formation of scar tissue can create some difficulties. Adhesions may form and become troublesome when tough fibrous tissues interfere with the normal functions of the internal organs around which they form. If the scar tissue is very large, it may disable the organ affected, as, for example, a large area of scar tissue in the heart muscle after recovery from a myocardial infarction.

TYPES OF WOUND HEALING

There are two general types of wound healing: (1) healing by primary union, called *first intention,* and (2) healing by secondary union, called *second intention.* In the first type, the two edges of the wound are close together and a crust forms between them to seal the wound. A thin scar results (Fig. 6–13).

In healing by second intention, the edges of the wound are far apart and cannot be brought together (Fig. 6–14). Usually a large amount of tissue is lost because of necrosis or severe physical trauma. The ulcerated area in the middle fills with granulation tissue, and the wound heals from the edges inward. A decubitus ulcer is an example of a wound that must heal by second intention.

FACTORS THAT AFFECT WOUND HEALING AND RELATED NURSING ACTIONS

Rest

When appropriate, rest favors healing. It is not always possible to provide rest for an affected part, and continued immobility presents problems of its own (see Chapter 9). Some areas can be rested by immobilization rather easily; for example, a broken bone of a leg or arm can be splinted with a cast, or the limb can be placed in traction while healing takes place. The healing of joints affected by arthritis is facilitated by a combination of rest and mild exercise. The exercise is necessary to maintain mobility of the joint.

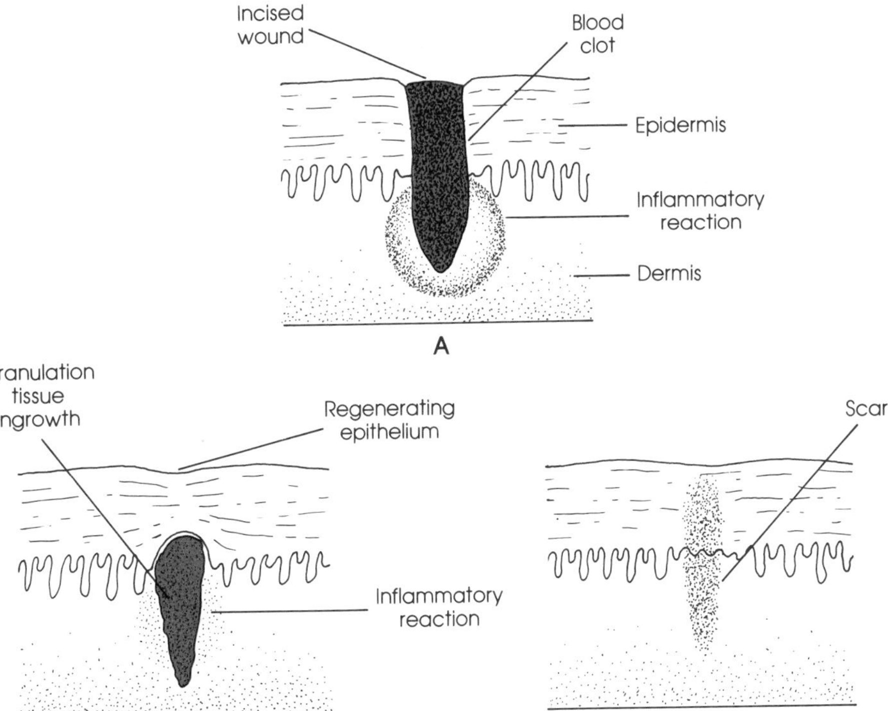

Figure 6-13 Wound healing by primary, or first, intention. In primary wound healing there is no tissue loss. *A*, Incised wound is held together by a blood clot and possibly by sutures or surgical clamps. An inflammatory process begins in adjacent tissue at the moment of injury. *B*, After several days, granulation tissue forms as a result of migration of fibroblasts to the area of injury and formation of new capillaries. Epithelial cells at the wound margin migrate to the clot and seal the wound. Regenerating epithelium covers the wound. *C*, Scarring occurs as granulation tissue matures and injured tissue is replaced with connective tissue.

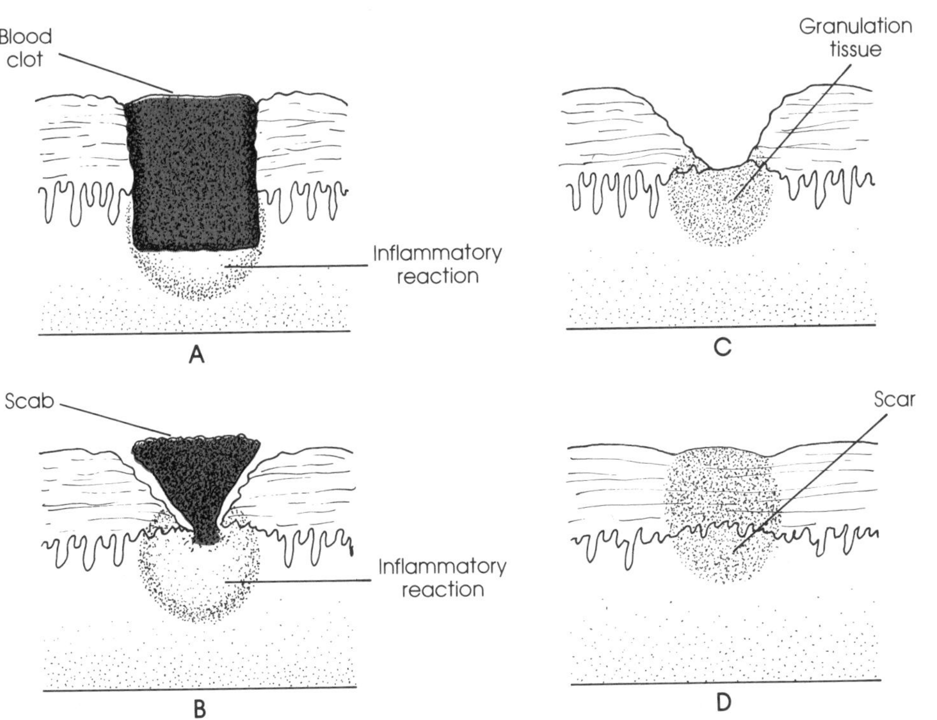

Figure 6-14 Healing by second intention occurs when there is tissue loss, as in extensive burns and deep ulcers. The healing process is more prolonged than in healing by primary intention, because large amounts of dead tissue must be removed and replaced with viable cells. *A*, Open area is more extensive; inflammatory reaction is more widespread and tends to become chronic. *B*, Healing may occur under a scab formed of dried exudate or dried plasma proteins and dead cells (eschar). *C*, Fibroblasts and capillary buds migrate toward the center of the wound to form granulation tissue, which becomes a translucent red color as the capillary network develops. Granulation tissue is fragile and bleeds easily. *D*, As granulation tissue matures, marginal epithelial cells migrate and proliferate over connective tissue base to form a scar. Contraction of skin around the scar is a result of movement of epithelial cells toward the center of the wound in an attempt to close the defect. The surrounding skin also moves toward the center of the wound in an effort to close the defect.

In other cases—for example, inflammation of the liver (hepatitis) or of the heart (myocarditis)—some rest can be provided, but the organ must continue to function or the patient will not survive. In cases of a generalized inflammation, as in influenza, bed rest can greatly facilitate recovery.

Adequate Blood Supply

It is obvious that a good supply of blood, which contains the amino acids and other elements needed for rebuilding tissue, is essential to healing. Good circulation of blood to an infected area also is necessary for the removal of waste products of metabolism and the inflammatory process.

Edema or tight bandages and dressings can restrict blood flow. Narrowing of the lumen of the arteries by atherosclerosis is also a common cause of inadequate circulation to the body's tissues. If a patient is confined to bed, lack of exercise can lead to poor circulation of blood to healing tissues. Patients who cannot move about in bed must have their body positions changed so that no part of the body is subjected to prolonged pressure, which decreases the blood supply to the affected part.

Age

Older people heal more slowly than do children and young adults and are more prone to infections. Many older people have chronic illnesses, such as diabetes, COPD, or atherosclerosis, that interfere with oxygenation and transport of nutrients to the cells and removal of wastes from the body cells. Nutritional deficiencies are frequent in the aged, and the nurse should pay special attention to this area.

Nutrition

Vitamins, minerals, and trace elements are essential for adequate wound healing. *Vitamin A* is needed for the synthesis (creation) of collagen for scar formation and for the growth of epithelial cells over denuded surfaces. The *vitamin B complex* is necessary for proper functioning of the enzyme system. *Vitamin C* is necessary for collagen synthesis, the formation of capillaries that bring blood to the healing tissues, and resistance to infection. *Vitamin K* plays an important role in normal clotting. The minerals zinc, copper, and iron assist in the synthesis of collagen.

Patients who are generally malnourished have difficulty maintaining a normally functioning immune system, because proteins are needed for the synthesis of antibodies, which are themselves made of proteins. In fact, protein deficiency can affect all of the processes involved in the healing of damaged tissues, because the amino acids of proteins are the building blocks of tissue.

Obesity is not indicative of a well-nourished body. The person who is obese is a poor candidate for rapid healing, because fatty tissue does not have an adequate blood supply, and resistance to infection is reduced. Additionally, fatty tissue is hard to sew together, and sutures placed in adipose tissue are likely to tear.

Drugs

As previously mentioned, there are some drugs that suppress the inflammatory process and the healing functions of the immune system. The most important of these drugs are the corticosteroids. Other drugs that can interfere with healing are those used for the treatment of cancer.

Smoking

Cigarette smoking produces a decrease in the amount of functional hemoglobin and therefore reduces the level of oxygen available to the tissues for healing. There also is evidence that chronic smokers have platelets that tend to clump together, which can result in excessive formation of clots.

Mechanical Injury

Friction, pressure, blows to the wound, and foreign objects in the wound will delay healing. Physical injury destroys granulation tissue, which is the framework on which new cells grow and mature to form a covering for the wound. All healing wounds should be handled gently and shielded from injury. When dressings are removed from wounded tissue, care must be taken that healing tissues are not ripped away from the wound.

Infection

The presence of pathogenic microorganisms in a wound prolongs the inflammatory process and delays healing. Sterile technique is used in the care of the wound so that no infectious agents are introduced. Antiinfective drugs should be administered conscientiously.

Foreign Bodies, Necrotic Tissue, and Debris

If the area of inflammation is not very large, the products of inflammation are eventually absorbed into the blood stream and disposed of. Severely infected wounds or those in which there is a large amount of dead cells and debris, pus, and blood clots must be cleansed in order to facilitate healing. Sutures and other foreign bodies—for example, slivers of glass and splinters of wood—also delay healing and serve as ideal vehicles for the entry of infectious agents.

Irrigations with saline, hydrogen peroxide, or a

mild antiseptic may be used to remove exudate, clots, and pus. These irrigations should be administered with just enough force to remove the purulent material but not so forcibly as to spread the infectious material to adjacent areas.

Hormones

As previously stated, some hormones from the cortex of the adrenal gland significantly suppress the inflammatory process, whereas others encourage it. In order to obtain the desired effect in the administration of corticoids, the nurse must adhere to the rules for safe administration of drugs and observation of their effects on the patient.

Stress

According to the theory of stress and disease, anxiety, apprehension, and other emotional disturbances can greatly affect an individual's progress toward recovery. Stress seems to make the body more vulnerable to invasion by foreign organisms by depressing the immune system. When under excessive stress, the body is also less able to mobilize the elements and cells that promote healing. The nurse should realize that her attitude toward a patient and the ways in which she strives to meet his needs can reduce stress and promote healing in ways that are not yet completely understood.

The manner in which a person is physically handled, the tone of voice used in speaking to him, and the availability of others to listen to him can have profound effects on his physical condition. We must not forget that nursing is a healing profession. Much of what is done to, for, and with a patient reflects a willingness (or a lack of it) to use one's self to heal another.

During her studies on "therapeutic touch," which attempted to measure in a scientific manner the effects of "laying-on of hands with the intent to heal," Dr. Dolores Krieger became convinced that the *intent to heal* another is a critical factor. Noting that even the most basic of nursing skills cannot be performed without the act of touching the patient, Dr. Krieger contends that

TABLE 6–7 FACTORS IN WOUND HEALING AND RELATED NURSING CARE

Factors Involved	Nursing Actions
Rest	Provide restful environment. Explain to patient the effects of rest on healing. Participate in care of splints, casts, and other devices employed for immobilization.
Blood supply	Avoid tight bandages or other sources of restriction of blood vessels in vicinity of wound. Observe for signs of circulatory stasis. Relieve edema by proper positioning and elevation of the affected part; apply, as prescribed, cold compresses, ice caps, etc. Apply heat, as prescribed, for improvement of circulation to and from the wounded area. Assist patient with ambulation and performance of prescribed exercises.
Nutrition	Encourage patient to eat high-protein foods and those rich in vitamins A, B, and K. Give citrus fruits and juices and other sources of vitamin C. Encourage weight loss, if indicated, and maintenance of normal body weight. Measure and record intake and output of fluids. Help maintain a normal fluid balance.
Mechanical injury	Protect wound from friction and direct blows. Handle affected part gently. Use great care in applying and removing dressings and bandages. Devise protective bandages and shields using foam rubber, plastic cups, tongue blades, and other supportive materials.
Foreign bodies	Assist in removal of foreign bodies imbedded in the wound. Use irrigations to remove exudate, pus, and clots. Irrigate only the affected area.
Infection	Observe patient for early signs of infection and report immediately. Wash hands thoroughly before and after each contact with patient. Use strict aseptic technique during dressing changes and wound cleansing. Administer antimicrobials as ordered. Observe patient for effects of drugs. Follow precautions and isolation procedures as indicated.
Hormones	Administer as prescribed. Provide rest; relieve anxiety that might stimulate release of adrenal hormones.
Stress	Handle patient gently. Evaluate personal feelings about desiring patient's recovery. Relieve anxiety, if possible. Relieve pain and promote comfort.

touch can be therapeutic when used appropriately.

Regardless of whether one is totally convinced of the effectiveness of touching, each of us can recall incidents when the touch of someone's hands affected us in a very personal way. These experiences should have special meaning for nurses. Nonverbal communication that involves touching is often as effective as the spoken word.

In regard to the intent on the part of the nurse to heal, we cannot ignore the strong evidence that the will of an individual to recover from his illness is somehow intricately bound to his ability to do so. If those who care for a patient share with him a strong desire for his recovery, his will to be healed is strengthened.

Table 6–7 summarizes the factors that affect wound healing and related nursing actions.

BIBLIOGRAPHY

American Hospital Association: Infection Control in Hospitals, 4th ed. Chicago, American Hospital Association, 1989.

Centers for Disease Control: Guidelines for the prevention of nosocomial infections. Atlanta, U.S. Department of Health and Human Services, 1989.

Centers for Disease Control: National nosocomial infections study report, annual summary, 1989. Atlanta, U.S. Department of Health and Human Services, 1990.

Centers for Disease Control: Recommendations for prevention of HIV transmission in health-care settings. Morbidity and Mortality Weekly Report vol. 36, no. 2S, August 21, 1987, p. 3.

Centers for Disease Control: Update: Universal precautions for prevention of transmission of human immunodeficiency virus, hepatitis B virus, and other bloodborne pathogens in health-care settings. Morbidity and Mortality Weekly Report, June, 1988, p. 377.

Coleman, D.: The when and how of isolation. RN, Oct., 1987, p. 5.

Garner, J. S., and Simmons, B. P.: CDC Guideline for Isolation Precautions in Hospitals. Atlanta, U.S. Department of Health and Human Services, 1989.

Guyton, A. C.: Textbook of Medical Physiology, 8th ed. Philadelphia, W. B. Saunders, 1991.

Krieger, D.: The Therapeutic Touch: How to Use Your Hands to Help or to Heal. Englewood Cliffs, N.J., Prentice Hall, 1979.

Luckmann, J, and Sorensen, K. C.: Medical-Surgical Nursing: A Psychophysiologic Approach, 3rd ed. Philadelphia, W. B. Saunders, 1987.

Mooney, R. B., and Armington, L. C.: Infection control: How to prevent nosocomial infections. RN, Aug., 1987, p. 21.

Pavel, J. N.: Hemotalogic problems: Blood cell abnormalities: Leukocyte disorders. *In* Nurse Review. Springhouse, PA, Springhouse Corporation, Edited by Goldberg, K. 1989.

Price, S. A., and Wilson, L. M.: Pathophysiology: Clinical Concepts of Disease Processes, 3rd ed. New York, McGraw-Hill, 1989.

Pritchard, V.: Preventing and treating geriatric infections. RN, March, 1988, p. 36.

STUDENT STUDY AIDS

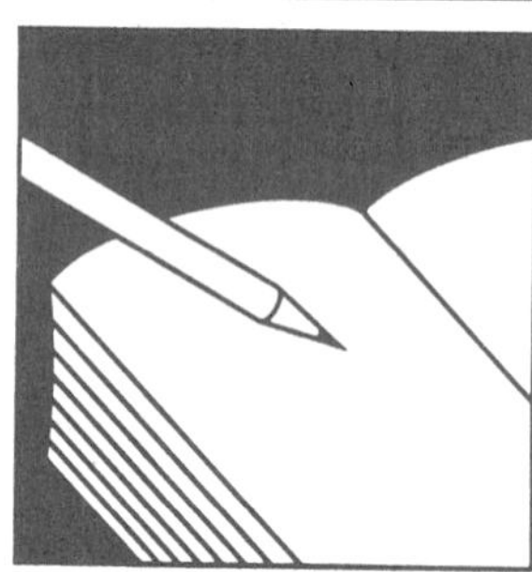

CLINICAL CASE PROBLEMS

Read each clinical situation and discuss the questions with your classmates.

1. You have been asked to speak to a group of sixth-grade students about the prevention of disease and promotion of health. The children are especially interested in "how people get sick" and how disease can be avoided.

- What kinds of disease-producing factors should you include in your discussion?
- Considering the age of your audience, what safety precautions might you stress?

---

2. Mrs. Chambers, aged 44, is admitted to the hospital for a hemorrhoidectomy. During the admission procedure, you notice a large, draining boil in her axillary region. She also has a temperature of 100°F and she tells you that she has not felt well for the past few days.

- What would be your course of action following this discovery?
- What specific nursing actions could be taken to eliminate links in the chain of the infectious process so that Mrs. Chambers' infection is not spread to others?

---

3. Conduct a survey in the clinical area in which you are practicing as a student nurse, observing ways in which infectious agents can be spread from one person to another through carelessness and poor sanitation practices. These might include failure to wash hands as often as needed, improper disposal of contaminated dressings and equipment, careless handling of soiled linens, and taking objects into a patient's room that are contaminated with infectious agents.

---

4. Martha Leander, 18 years of age, is admitted to the orthopedic unit following an automobile accident. She has sustained an open fracture of the femur and chest injuries. Her fractured leg has been placed in traction; the open wound is covered with a bandage.

- What protective body structures would be involved in Martha's injuries?
- What would be some expected signs and symptoms of inflammation that Martha might experience?
- What process would produce each of those signs and symptoms?
- What are some possible outcomes for each of her injuries?
- What specific problems might Martha's care present for the nurse?
- How would you determine whether these problems were present?
- What nursing actions should be planned and implemented to deal with each of the problems you have identified?

STUDY OUTLINE

I. Mechanical, chemical, and genetic factors

A. Mechanical:
1. Accidental injury from violent blows.
2. Extremes of heat and cold.
   a. Thermal burns, ultraviolet rays, electrical energy.
   b. Frostbite, hypothermia.
3. Internal obstructions in the respiratory tract, intestinal tract, and circulatory system.

B. Chemical:
1. Strong acids and alkalies; disinfectants and antiseptics.
2. Drugs administered orally and parenterally.
3. Common minerals, etc., normally found in the home.
4. Plant and animal products.
5. The body's own chemicals: hormones, digestive juices, blood.
6. Very narrow range of adaptability in the maintenance of balance of water and electrolytes, acids and bases.

C. Genetic:
1. Genes are biologic units of heredity.
   a. Genetic disorders include sickle cell disease and other hemoglobin abnormalities and inborn errors of metabolism.
   b. Prognosis for many genetic disorders has greatly improved.

II. Nursing activities related to mechanical and chemical factors (see Table 6-1)

III. Infectious agents

A. Bacteria: microscopically small organisms belonging to the plant family:
1. Classification:
   a. Gram-positive: those that "take" Gram stain. All streptococci and staphylococci are gram-positive.
   b. Gram-negative: those do not retain the stain. Tuberculosis bacillus and many hospital-acquired infectious agents are gram-negative.
   c. Morphology (shape):
      (1) Cocci: round.
      (2) Bacilli: rod-shaped.
      (3) Spirochetes: spiral.

d. Arrangement in cultures:
(1) Streptococci—grow in chains.
(2) Diplococci: grow in pairs.
(3) Staphylococci: grow in clusters.
e. Oxygen requirement:
(1) Obligate aerobes must have oxygen to survive.
(2) Obligate anerobes cannot tolerate oxygen.
(3) Facultative anaerobes can thrive with or without oxygen.
2. Control of bacteria: Destruction of harmful microbes is not simply a matter of using one method of sterilization or disinfection. Microbes vary in their ability to resist heat, cold, water, and chemical poisons.

B. Viruses: extremely small, cannot be seen with ordinary microscope. Made up of a core of nucleic acids (of RNA or DNA), contained within a coating of protein, carbohydrate, or fatty material. Cannot live or replicate outside a living cell.
1. Can camouflage themselves inside cells of the body. Once there, they can cause a cell to burst and die or to change its membrane so that it is attacked by the body's immune system.
2. Many of the "slow" viruses can live in cells for years without causing symptoms and then suddenly cause an acute illness.
3. Destruction of viruses:
a. Most are easily inactivated by heat. However, some (for example, the hepatitis viruses) can resist boiling for at least 30 minutes.
b. Most effective means of destroying viruses and all other microbes is by moist heat at 250°F (121°C) for 15 to 20 minutes.
4. Types of viruses: classified according to:
a. Whether core is RNA or DNA.
b. Size.
c. Tissues they prefer.
d. Types pathogenic to man.
5. Response of host cell to virus:
a. May allow it to live peaceably in dormant state.
b. Host cell may die without reproducing.
c. Host cell may divide and then die.
d. Host cell may be changed and take on abnormal growth pattern.

C. Protozoa: microscopic, one-celled organisms belonging to the animal kingdom.
1. Malaria is an example of a disease caused by protozoa.

D. Rickettsiae: small, round, rod-shaped, parasitic.

E. Fungi: members of a class of vegetable organisms, including yeasts and molds.
1. Diseases caused by fungi include athlete's foot and systemic mycoses.

IV. The infectious process

A. Each link in the circular chain must be present in order for the process to take place.

B. Links:
1. Causative organism.
2. Reservoir.
3. Portal of exit.
4. Modes of transfer.
5. Portal of entry.

6. Susceptible host.

C. Goal of preventing spread of infection is achieved by controlling the links of the process.

V. Controlling infectious disease

A. Major goals of public health officials and professionals:
1. Promotion of sanitary living conditions.
2. Identification of susceptible persons and reduction of their chances of developing an infectious disease.
3. Immunization programs.

B. Nosocomial infections:
1. Nosocomial literally translated means hospital-acquired. Now used to include all infections resulting from health care services in all kinds of agencies.
2. Nosocomial infections are becoming increasingly more costly in terms of dollars and human suffering and death.
3. Common features of nosocomial infections are summarized in Table 6–3.

VI. Signs and symptoms of infection

A. Detection of infection requires thorough nursing assessment.

B. Subjective signs include fatigue, loss of appetite, headache, nausea, general malaise, or pain.

C. Objective signs—fever, increased pulse and respiratory rate; vomiting, diarrhea, cough, decreased breath sounds, swollen lymph nodes, cloudy urine, purulent sputum—usually indicate the body system involved.

D. Signs of local infection are redness, swelling, pain, or limitation of movement caused by discomfort.

E. Laboratory data indicative of infection: elevated WBC count, changes in distribution of cells on differential count, elevated erythrocyte sedimentation rate, and positive culture result.

F. Any patient admitted for surgery or other invasive procedure is at risk of infection.

VII. Nursing interventions for prevention of infection

A. Close attention to hand washing is of primary importance.

B. Changing soiled dressings and linens promptly removes growth medium for bacteria.

C. Proper disposal of infectious materials and contaminated equipment decreases incidence of infection.

D. Use strict aseptic technique for all invasive procedures.

E. Encourage patients to move, cough, and deep breathe to prevent respiratory infection.

F. Protect patients from others with infections.

G. Administer prophylactic antibiotics as ordered.

H. Encourage adequate rest, nutrition, and fluid intake to increase resistance to infection.

I. Vigilantly assess for beginning signs of infection.

VIII. Nursing actions in controlling the spread of infection

A. Surveillance and reporting.
1. Every patient is assessed for signs and symptoms of infection.
2. If signs are detected, the patient's physician and the infection control officer of the institution are notified.
3. The infection control nurse is responsible for staff education regarding infection control, collection of statistical data on hospital infections, and making recommendations for changes in procedures.
4. Patients at risk who require careful watching are those already

weakened by severe illness, the very young, and the elderly. Obese patients are particularly at risk for infection of surgical wounds.

B. Destroying and containing infectious agents.
   1. Techniques and procedures used to destroy and contain infectious microbes:
      a. Surgical asepsis: The destruction of organisms *before* they enter the body. Procedures include sterilization of instruments and linens, surgical masks, gowns, and gloves, and draping the patient.
      b. Medical asepsis: The destruction of microbes *after* they leave the body of an infected person and separation of the sources of infection from other people.
      c. Hand washing is the single most important procedure for preventing the spread of infection.
      d. Universal precautions are taken by all health care workers with every patient: barriers are used for contact with blood and body fluids or broken or weeping skin, and when droplet contamination might occur (Table 6–4).
      e. Isolation and precautionary measures carried out according to type of infection presented by patient.
         (1) Strict isolation
         (2) Respiratory isolation
         (3) Enteric precautions
         (4) Contact isolation
         (5) Acid-fast bacillus (AFB) isolation
         (6) Drainage and secretion precautions
         (7) Body substance isolation

C. Health teaching as an integral part of nursing care.
   1. Learning needs of the patient are identified, and he is taught how to care for himself so that he does not spread infection to others or reinfect himself and is able to recover from the infection.

D. Strengthening the patient's capacity for recovery.
   1. Assessment:
      a. Considers the patient's age, nutritional and hydration status, patterns and habits of bowel and bladder elimination, and degree of physical activity tolerated.
      b. Culture and sensitivity testing part of overall assessment.
      c. Periodic reassessment of the patient during the course of his illness could include checking vital signs, observing wounds and lesions (if any), noting type of cough and characteristics of sputum, noting any drainage (amount and character), noting whether the patient is able to maintain adequate nutrition and hydration, and checking the degree of activity he is able to tolerate.
   2. Planning and intervention:
      a. Goals are that the patient will be able to achieve adequate rest, freedom from discomfort, adequate nutrition and hydration, and sufficient oxygen and blood supply to infected tissues.
      b. Specific goals in the care plan might include: adequate rest, total fluid intake of at least 2000 mL daily; nutritional needs met; able to explain purposes of diagnostic tests, treatments, and special precautions; able to maintain medical asepsis to prevent spread of infection.

c. Nursing interventions aimed at physiologic support, relief of symptoms, adequate hydration, and psychological support.
d. Drugs: All antimicrobial drugs must be given precisely as ordered to avoid development of resistant strains and to prevent recurrence of the infection.
e. Immunization: Passive immunity to provide "ready-made" antibodies against the infectious agents.

3. Evaluation must consider other variables beyond control of nurse. Outcome criteria related to patient's response to nursing interventions.

IX. Protective structures and mechanisms

A. Human body remarkably well equipped to defend itself against harmful agents in the environment.
B. External structures, internal organs, and protective mechanisms provide a natural or innate immunity.

X. Protective organs

A. The skin—excretes bactericidal and antiviral substances, serves as a shield.
B. Mucous membranes—secrete bactericidal substances.
C. Bony structures—protect deeper vital organs.
D. Liver cells—filter bacteria from blood; detoxify various poisons.
E. Nursing assessment and intervention.
   1. Assess status of skin.
   2. Protect skin and mucous membranes from trauma.
   3. Do not unnecessarily remove normal secretions from mucous membranes.

XI. Defensive cells

A. Leukocytes—increase in number as soon as injury occurs.
   1. Six different types; three types of granulocytes ("poly's").
   2. Neutrophils make up 67% of total number of leukocytes.
   3. Are capable of engulfing foreign particles. Contain enzymes that neutralize or destroy foreign agents.
   4. Clear inflamed area of debris in preparation for repair.
B. Mononuclear phagocytes.
   1. Located throughout the body: alveoli, liver, lymph nodes, and spleen.

XII. Process of inflammation

A. Induced by *any* disease-producing factor.
B. Important defense mechanism of the body.
C. Purposes of inflammatory process:
   1. Neutralize and destroy foreign agents.
   2. Limit their spread.
   3. Prepare damaged tissue for repair.
D. Inflammatory changes—local and systemic.
   1. Vascular changes—vasodilation and increased capillary permeability.
   2. Leukocytosis.
   3. Reticulum cells enlarge, migrate to inflamed site. Formation of exudate. Pus composed of dead bacteria, dead defensive cells, and tissue fluid.
   4. Immune system—formation of antibodies.
   5. Hormonal system—both pro- and antiinflammatory hormones involved; allows for a beneficial balance of defensive actions.
E. Signs and symptoms.
   1. Classic local signs of inflammation: heat, redness, swelling, pain, and limitation of motion.

a. Local symptoms can create problems related to need for rest and activity, protection from infection, and maintenance of fluid balance.

2. Systemic symptoms—fever, malaise, generalized aching, weakness, anorexia.

a. Nursing diagnoses commonly found include activity intolerance, sleep pattern disturbance, pain, self-care deficit and potential for or actual infection.

3. An inadequate inflammatory response makes patient more susceptible to infection.

XIII. Repair and healing

A. Begins almost at the same time inflammatory process begins.

1. Defensive cells brought to area; waste products and debris removed.

B. Possible outcomes.

1. Resolution and recovery.
2. Necrosis and degeneration.
3. Replacement and scarring.

C. Types of wound healing.

1. Primary union (first intention).
2. Secondary union (second intention).

D. Factors that affect wound healing and related nursing actions. Summarized in Table 6–7.

CHAPTER 7

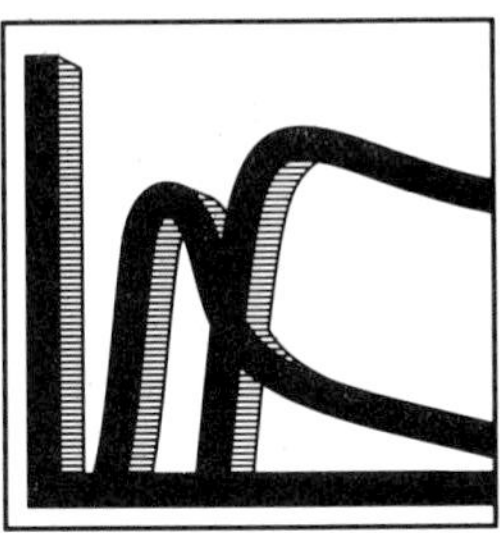

The Immune Response

VOCABULARY

agglutination
AIDS
allergen
anaphylaxis
antibody
antigen
antitoxin
ARC
autoimmune
humoral
immunity
lymphadenopathy
mediate

Upon completion of this chapter the student should be able to:

1. Describe three physiologic functions the body must perform in order for a normal immune response to occur.
2. Contrast the characteristics of humoral and cellular immunity.
3. Compare active and passive immunity and the immunizing agents used to provide each kind of immunity.
4. Summarize ways in which the nurse can increase public participation in immunization programs.
5. State the primary problems encountered when caring for a patient with an immune deficiency.
6. Describe AIDS and ARC and compare their characteristics.
7. List five ways to prevent the spread of AIDS.
8. Describe the treatment that is available for AIDS patients.
9. List the major goals in the management of hypersensitivity and allergic reactions.
10. List specific medical treatments and nursing actions helpful in the management of the symptoms of an allergy and the prevention of anaphylaxis.
11. Briefly describe desensitization, its purpose, and how it is done.

PHYSIOLOGY

The immune response is a remarkable series of complex chemical and mechanical activities that take place in the internal environment. These activities involve (1) constant surveillance to detect the entry of foreign agents as soon as they gain access to the body's cells, (2) immediate recognition of the agents as "nonself" (that is, foreign or alien), and (3) the ability to distinguish one kind of foreign agent from another and to "remember" that particular agent if it appears again at a later time.

TYPES OF IMMUNE RESPONSE

Once a particular kind of foreign substance has been detected and identified, the body responds in two general ways. It immediately produces a protein (called an *antibody*) that is specifically designed to do battle with the agent (called an *antigen*). There also is a delayed response that involves the use of sensitized lymphocytes to attack whole cells, such as those of bacteria and viruses, and malignant cells. This second kind of response is called a *cellular* or *cell-mediated response.*

HUMORAL (IMMEDIATE) RESPONSES

The immediate response to invasion by a foreign agent is called the *humoral response* because the action takes place in cell-free plasma *(humor)*. This is where the immune bodies that have been produced are circulating and where they react to the specific antigen for which they are formed. The immune bodies are called *antibodies* or *antibody*. The singular form, antibody, is often used to designate a group of antibodies, because all antibodies of a particular type are chemically the same. A rapid increase in the production of antibody takes place almost immediately after its antigen has entered the body.

The major function of the humoral (antigen-antibody) response is to provide protection against acute, rapidly developing bacterial and viral diseases. The antigen-antibody response also is involved in allergies and transfusion reactions.

Antigen

The word *antigen* is a combination of *anti-*, meaning "against," and *-gen*, meaning "generate" or "cause to be." Thus an antigen is any substance that can bring about or generate production of an antagonist. The most common response to the antigen is the production of antibody.

Each type of organism, toxin, or other foreign protein has a chemical structure that makes it different from any other. Because each kind of antigen is chemically unique, it evokes the synthesis of an antibody that is chemically different from any other kind of antibody. This principle of *specificity* is easily understood if we recall that having had chickenpox as children provides us with an immunity to chickenpox only. The antibodies produced as a response to chickenpox do not provide immunity against mumps or any other kind of bacterial or viral infection.

Examples of antigens include the cells of bacteria, viruses, fungi, and other infectious organisms, as well as the toxins they produce. Nonliving matter such as pollen, dust, and the chemicals in detergent also can be antigens. In fact, all the proteins and some of the polysaccharides (sugars) in nature can be interpreted by the body as foreign agents to be rejected. For example, the interpretation of the protein in milk as a harmful substance may trigger an allergic reaction to milk in some persons. The same is true of many other substances. Substances that have no harmful effect on some people may cause potentially fatal allergic reactions in others. This will be discussed more fully in the section on allergies.

In instances in which transplanted organs are rejected by the recipient, the cells of the transplanted organs are recognized by the body as foreign antigens. Red blood cells can become antigenic if they are mixed with cells of a different type, as in a transfusion of mismatched whole blood. The wrong type of red cells in the blood stream of the recipient can stimulate the production of antibody and result in the symptoms of a transfusion reaction.

Antibody

Just as almost all antigens are proteins, so are the antibodies that are produced in defense against them. Antibodies are a kind of protein synthesized by plasma cells. They are called *immunoglobulins. Globulins* are proteins that are soluble in moderately concentrated salt solutions. The prefix *immuno-* tells us that these kinds of globulins provide some kind of immunity.

There are five classes of immunoglobulins (Ig): IgA, IgD, IgE, IgG, and IgM. Each antibody is able to "stick to" the kind of antigen for which it is made. The number of sites at which an antibody can attach itself to its antigen depends on the class to which it belongs. This ability of an antibody to form a bond with its antigen is important to the destruction of the antigen, but it can sometimes result in damage to the body's own cells.

Antibodies are found in the serum of blood, of course, but they are also found in other body fluids and tissues, including the urine, spinal fluid, lymph nodes, and spleen.

Antibody can either destroy or inactivate its particular antigen by (1) mechanically harming it, (2) activating a "complement" system, and (3) causing the release of chemicals that affect the environment of the antigen and hasten its destruction and removal.

In some instances the antibody prepares the antigen for ingestion by phagocytes. It does this by a process called *lysis*, in which the antibody damages the membrane of the antigen's cell, causing it to rupture and making its contents accessible for digestion.

Another means by which antibody attacks antigen is through *agglutination*. This causes the antigens to lump together (agglutinate), forming a heavy, inactive mass. This is what sometimes happens in a transfusion reaction. When the mismatched red blood cells of the donor blood come into contact with the red cells of the recipient's blood, antibodies are attached to the recipient's red cells. These antibodies stick to the antigens, causing the blood cells to clump together. The clumps of cells then obstruct small blood vessels and thereby produce some of the symptoms of a transfusion reaction.

Some antibodies cause their antigens to form a heavy mass that is insoluble. This causes them to settle into an inactive deposit of solid particles called a *precipitate*. The process is called *precipitation*, and the antibodies are called *precipitins*.

If the antigen is a toxin (poison) produced by a bacterial or viral cell, the antibody produced is called the *antitoxin*. It is capable of neutralizing the poisonous chemical of the antigen by covering the toxic sites of the antigenic agent. An antitoxin is, therefore, a specific type of antibody that acts through the process of *neutralization*.

In the *complement* system, certain enzymes in the plasma that are normally inactive are stimulated by the antigen-antibody reaction. These enzymes not only attack the invading antigens, but also protect local body cells from damage by the foreign substances.

During the antigen-antibody reaction some of the antibodies attached to the tissue and blood cells cause these cells to rupture. This brings about the release of histamine and other substances that can be harmful to the body. If the reaction is extreme and widespread, the individual can die from circulatory shock and respiratory failure. This reaction is discussed more fully later in this chapter in the section on anaphylaxis.

CELLULAR (DELAYED) RESPONSE

The second type of immunologic response of the body involves various interactions with antigens by T lymphocytes. Unlike the humoral response, which takes place in cell-free plasma, the cellular response involves whole cells called *sensitized lymphocytes*. They are said to be *sensitized* because they have been made sensitive to a specific antigen after their first contact with it. They are "special troops" in the same sense that antibodies are "special troops." Subsequent exposure to the antigen to which they are sensitive triggers a host of chemical and mechanical activities, all of which are designed to either destroy or inactivate the offending antigen.

The T lymphocytes mediate (indirectly accomplish) the cellular response. When an antigen is complex (e.g., a bacteria or another type of living cell), T lymphocytes that are specifically reactive with the particular antigen mediate the cellular response in several ways. These specific T lymphocytes enter the circulating fluids of the body from the lymphoid tissues, migrate widely, and react anywhere in the body where they encounter the particular antigen. Destruction of the antigen may occur by release of chemicals into the membrane of the target cell, by secretion of lymphokines such as interleukin-2 or T-cell growth factor, or by other processes. This direct contact by the T lymphocytes with an antigen is called *killer activity* and such lymphocytes are named *killer T cells*. In the presence of an infectious disease, both humoral and cell-mediated immune responses occur.

Cellular immune response is often termed *delayed hypersensitivity*. The larger the amount of antigen present, the greater is the response of sensitized T lymphocytes. These T lymphocytes, along with migrating macrophages, are responsible for rejecting transplanted organs.

The T lymphocytes perform immune surveillance for the body by detecting cells that enter the host and have foreign antigens on their surface. They are defensive cells that patrol the blood and tissues. This is why transplanted tissue must have surface antigens that are very similar to those of the host tissue in order to be accepted by the host body.

Sensitized T lymphocytes are the cause of allergic reactions. T cells are also responsible for the inflammatory response present in people with a variety of autoimmune diseases. *Autoimmune* means that there is a defective cellular immune response and that antibodies are produced against normal parts of the person's body.

T LYMPHOCYTES AND B LYMPHOCYTES

Both humoral and cellular immunity originate in the lymphocytic stem cells found in the bone marrow of the developing fetus. Within a few months after birth those lymphocytes destined to provide cellular immunity have passed through the thymus and migrated to the lymph nodes throughout the body. These are called the *T lymphocytes.*

The second group of lymphocytes, the B cells, are involved in humoral immunity and the production of antibody. They are processed in another area of the body that is still unknown. Because early research in the immune response showed that the preprocessing of these cells takes place in the bursa of Fabricius in birds, they were given the name B lymphocytes. B lymphocytes are the prime movers in antibody production.

As shown in Figure 7–1, both T and B lymphocytes migrate to lymphoid tissue, where they wait in readiness to form either sensitized lymphocytes or antibodies.

The sensitized lymphocytes produced by tissue in the lymph nodes may remain in the lymphoid tissue for as long as 10 years, whereas humoral antibodies probably last no more than a few months. How is it, then, that there are always sufficient numbers of immune bodies (antibody) for resistance whenever a person is exposed to a disease to which he has been immunized? The answer is that some lymphocytes are stored as *memory cells.*

Some of the young B lymphocytes do not go on to form plasma cells that produce antibody. Instead, they lie dormant in the lymphoid tissue as memory cells. These cells are activated when a

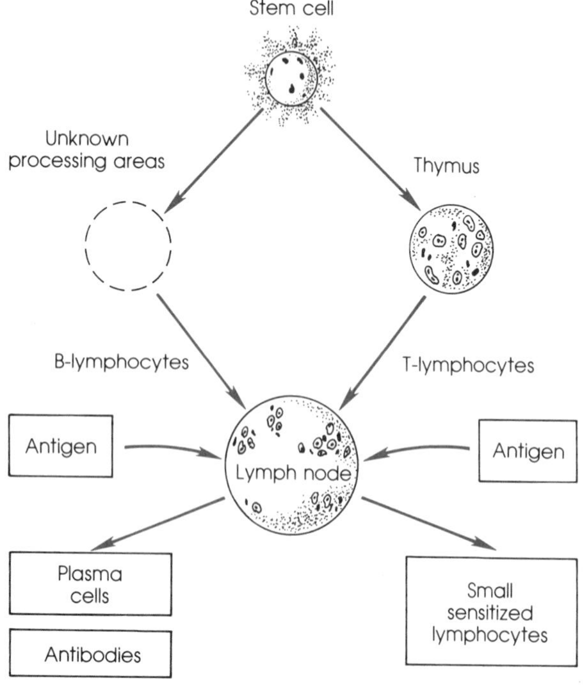

Figure 7–1 Origin of B and T lymphocytes responsible for cellular and humoral immunity. In response to antigens, B and T lymphocytes are sensitized by lymphoid tissue.

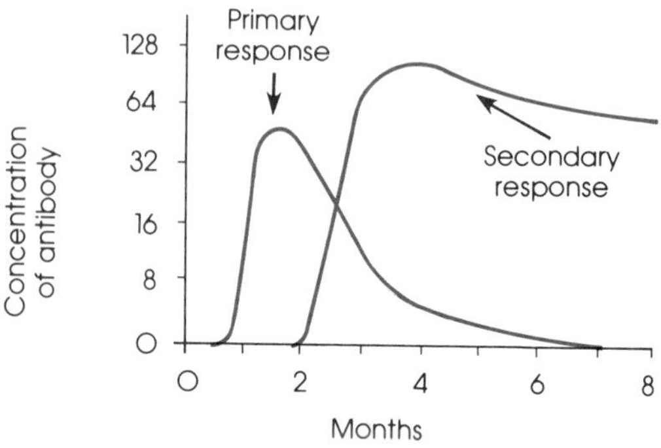

Figure 7–2 Time course of antibody responses to a primary injection of antigen and to a secondary injection 2 months later.

foreign substance reenters the body. They rapidly respond to its presence by producing large quantities of the specific type of antibody needed for defense against the particular type of antigen. This *secondary response* takes place only on second and subsequent exposures to the antigen. It is a potent immediate response, and antibodies continue to form for many months (Fig. 7–2). Because of this secondary response, vaccination usually is achieved by administration of the vaccine in divided doses over a period of weeks or months. This sets in motion the more powerful, longer-lasting secondary response. For example, infants are given vaccinations at age 2 months, 4 months, and 6 months and at regular intervals after that. Adults should have vaccinations against tetanus and diphtheria every 10 years (Table 7–1).

Memory cells are formed in the cellular immune response in the same way they are formed in the humoral antibody system. Thus when there is a second exposure to the foreign cell to which the lymphocytes are sensitized, the population of sensitized lymphocytes is greatly increased.

TABLE 7–1 RECOMMENDED VACCINATION SCHEDULE*

Age	Type of Vaccination
2 months	DTP-1: diphtheria, tetanus, and pertussis OPV-1: oral polio vaccine
4 months	DTP-2 and OPV-2
6 months	DTP-3
15 months	MMR: measles, mumps, and rubella
18 months	DTP-4 and OPV-3
4–6 years	DTP-5 and OPV-4
14–16 years	Adult tetanus and diphtheria, which should be repeated every 10 years through life

* Recommended by the American Academy of Pediatrics.

IMMUNITY AGAINST DISEASE

There are two major types of immunity to specific diseases: natural (innate) immunity and acquired (adaptive) immunity.

INNATE IMMUNITY

Certain innate, or inborn, features of human cells make a person naturally immune to certain diseases. Some of us are immune simply because we belong to a certain species, race, or gender or because we have a particular kind of constitution. Humans are not susceptible to the same diseases as are animals of lower orders. Some people are able to resist disease more easily than others because they are physically and mentally more healthy.

ACQUIRED IMMUNITY

In acquired immunity a person can either actively produce his own antibody or passively receive antibodies that have been produced by another person or animal. Table 7–2 shows some of the ways immunity can be attained by humans.

Naturally Acquired Active Immunity

Before vaccination and inoculation became commonplace, it was believed that the only way an individual could acquire immunity was to suffer an attack of the disease and, owing to a strong constitution and good fortune, manage to survive. Once he had survived this "trial by fire," he was immune and no longer needed to fear that particular disease.

Artificially Acquired Active Immunity

Establishment of immunity by vaccination became widely accepted through the efforts of an English country doctor, Edward Jenner. He had heard a milkmaid remark, "I cannot take the smallpox, for I have already had the cowpox." Dr. Jenner knew that this was a common belief among his patients, and in 1796 he set about to prove the theory. He performed the first crude form of vaccination on a boy 8 years of age by scratching the surface of the boy's skin and rubbing in some purulent material from the sore on the hand of a milkmaid infected with cowpox, which is closely related to smallpox but much less serious. Six weeks later, a potentially fatal amount of the deadly smallpox exudate was introduced into the boy's arm. The young man proved to be immune. He did not develop smallpox, and Dr. Jenner was hailed as the father of preventive medicine. The same method, with some refinements that include safety control for the dosage and strength of the cowpox organisms, is used in smallpox vaccinations today.

To provide active immunity to other diseases by artificial means, the actual pathogenic microorganisms are grown and cultured in the laboratory. They are divided into single doses under rigid controls and made into vaccines. These specially treated microorganisms are weakened so that they will stimulate the production of antibodies but will not cause the disease itself. Vaccines from cowpox viruses, tetanus, and tubercle bacilli, and more recently the polio, measles, and mumps vaccines, are all examples of agents used to produce an active immunity in humans (Table 7–2).

This method of stimulating the production of immunizing substances in the body is successful

TABLE 7–2 **TYPES OF IMMUNITY**

Type of Immunity	Means of Acquisition
Natural or innate	Species Race Sex Cell and tissue resistance Emotional state
Adaptive or acquired	
Active	Attack of the specific disease Artificial means: Vaccines—dead or harmless, weakened living organisms Toxoids—modified toxins
Passive	Passed from mother to fetus Artificial means: Immune serum—contains antibodies, some of which are antitoxins Gamma globulin—contains antibodies against several kinds of antigens Sensitized lymphocytes—given by transfusion Antivenin—for poisoning from animal venom

in situations in which there is time to wait for the person to build up his own defenses. However, what can be done if a person has no immunity and contracts the disease? Obviously there is no point to injecting more antigens into his body. He needs antibodies that can go to work immediately to destroy the harmful agents.

Artificially Acquired Passive Immunity

As the name implies, passive immunity is acquired through the efforts of someone else. Usually the "someone else" is a horse or a rabbit, although it may be a human. The serum from the blood of one of these animals contains ready-made antibodies that include antitoxins. It is prepared in a laboratory by increasing the strength of injections of specific antigens given to the animals over a period of time so that they build up the necesssary antibodies.

The most common diseases against which passive immunity is used effectively to bolster the patient's defenses are diphtheria, tetanus, scarlet fever, and gas gangrene. There also are *antisera* containing antibodies against snake venoms and the poisons produced by the black widow spider. These are called *antivenins*. It must be remembered, however, that injections that provide passive immunity should be given in the earliest stages of the disease, because they can only help prevent damage to tissues; they cannot repair damage already done.

Sometimes passive immunity is established before the disease is contracted. In instances of known contact with a disease such as measles, when the exposed person is considered too weak to withstand the rigors of a full-blown disease, gamma globulin is given to prepare the body in advance and to lessen the severity of the disease, should the person exposed actually contract it.

Gamma globulin, also called *pooled adult serum*, contains antibodies against not just one, but many infectious diseases. It is used for some of the so-called childhood diseases, because it is assumed that adults have been exposed to and developed antibodies against these diseases during their lifetime.

Naturally Acquired Passive Immunity

The fetus in the uterus can *passively* receive some natural immunity from its mother. Most antibodies in the mother's blood stream can pass through the placenta and become mixed with the blood of the fetus, so that they are present in the infant's blood at birth. Thus an expectant mother who has a high level of immunity to diphtheria, tetanus, and whooping cough can be assured that her newborn baby will have some immunity to these diseases. This is only a temporary arrangement, however, and the child must be immunized again when it has reached the age of 2 months.

Actually, all passive immunity is useful only as a temporary safety measure and cannot be expected to guarantee a permanent safeguard against attacks of a specific disease. In fact, for such diseases, the antibody content may drop to a very low level over a period of years, even with active immunity. It is then necessary that the body's immune system be reminded of the need to produce more antibodies. To achieve this, single doses of antigens are given. These are the "booster doses" that jog the memory of the specific immune cells and cause them to activate the production of antibodies.

IMMUNIZATION AND NURSING IMPLICATIONS

The nurse has three major goals in regard to immunization against specific diseases: (1) to increase public participation in immunization programs recommended by health officials, (2) to contribute to identification of persons in need of immunization, and (3) to prevent or mitigate sensitivity reactions to immunizing agents.

IMMUNIZATION PROGRAMS

An important aspect of health teaching is to improve the general public's awareness of the importance of immunization as a means of avoiding certain diseases and their consequences. In spite of the availability of vaccines against poliomyelitis, measles, rubella, and other potentially dangerous diseases, there still are many children who have not been adequately immunized.

In recent years the concern of public health officials has led to enactment of laws requiring children to be immunized before they are allowed to enter school. These laws are in effect in the 50 states and the District of Columbia of the United States, Puerto Rico, the Virgin Islands, and Guam. Because of enforcement of these laws, there are far fewer children who are not immunized, but those who are not still pose a danger to themselves, as well as to those around them.

Nurses have a responsibility to inform the public of the purpose of immunization in terms the lay person can understand.

Parents should be told why immunization is best for their children and warned of the dangers faced by children who are not immunized. This information must be presented in such a way that the parents do not feel threatened or badgered by the nurse.

Older adults and others who are particularly

susceptible to influenza also should be immunized according to the recommendations of public health officials. There are, however, some contraindications to immunization. In these cases immunization can be postponed until there is no danger to the patient.

Circumstances that require postponement of immunization include fevers, pregnancy, immune deficiency disease, immunosuppressive therapy, and administration of gamma globulin, plasma, or whole blood transfusion 6 to 8 weeks before the immunization. Immunization also is contraindicated when a person is taking certain drugs. Brochures accompanying these drugs will state whether they prohibit the administration of an immunizing agent.

Persons who have a history of sensitivity to any drug or other chemical or natural antigen may not be able to receive immunization as scheduled. When such a person is identified by the nurse, she should inform the physician of the patient's hypersensitivity.

SCREENING AND DIAGNOSTIC TESTING

The purpose of screening and testing is to identify persons who are in danger of contracting an infectious disease or who may have it without knowing it and therefore are likely to infect others. Persons in danger of contracting an infectious disease include all persons in an area in which there is an epidemic or where there is a polluted water supply.

Persons who live in substandard housing in crowded conditions, who are not well nourished, or who suffer from a chronic illness also are at high risk for developing an infectious disease. This is not to say that in her assessment of a patient the nurse should consider only these patients as possible candidates for immunization. Infectious disease organisms do not respect places or persons.

Most immunization programs use vaccines and other sera to provide active immunity. When active immunization is not possible and there is known contact with an infected person or with any other source, passive immunization is an alternative.

Skin testing is one of the most commonly used techniques to measure immunity and to identify people who may have a dormant infectious disease. These tests include the *Schick test* to determine susceptibility to diphtheria and the *tuberculin test* to identify those who might need treatment for tuberculosis. Skin tests also may be performed to establish the presence of circulating antibody against specific antigens that are infectious organisms (for example, fungi and parasites) and for those that produce an allergic reaction.

Testing for a reaction to tuberculin (a product of the organism that causes tuberculosis) can be done in several ways. These include the Mantoux test (intradermal injection), jet-gun injection, and multiple-puncture techniques. Interpretation of results will depend on the technique used. In general, a positive reaction means either that the person has had a tuberculosis infection somewhere in the body that has healed or that he has an infection that is currently active. It does not mean simply that the person has been exposed to someone who has active tuberculosis. Tuberculin testing alone does not confirm a diagnosis of tuberculosis. It is a screening device to detect those who need a more thorough workup to establish or rule out a diagnosis of tuberculosis.

PREVENTING OR MITIGATING SENSITIVITY REACTIONS

Whenever an immunizing agent is to be administered, precautions must be taken to ensure as far as possible that the patient is not hypersensitive to the components of the agent. Many times chick embryo, horse serum, and other substances are used to make the vaccine or immune serum. These substances can produce a serious allergic reaction in persons who are hypersensitive to them. Immunizing agents that are most often associated with anaphylaxis, a potentially fatal reaction, include tetanus antitoxin, diphtheria antitoxin, rabies antitoxin, and antilymphocytic globulin.

It is imperative that a history of allergies in the patient and his family be obtained before administration of an immunizing agent. It also should be determined whether the patient has an immune deficiency disease of any kind that would prevent a normal immune response to the immunizing agent. If a patient does have a history of allergies or an immune deficiency, the physician should be made aware of this fact before the immunizing agent is given. If the patient has had an allergic reaction to the specific agent he is supposed to receive, the drug must not be given.

There are times when a skin sensitivity test is indicated before any serum is administered to a patient. Skin testing for sensitivity should not be confused with skin testing for diagnostic purposes. Testing for sensitivity is done to determine whether a minute amount of the immunizing agent will produce a local reaction. If it does, chances are the patient will have a severe reaction if the agent is given systemically.

In spite of these precautions it is possible that a patient will suffer from hypersensitivity to an immunizing agent. To avoid serious problems, the nurse should always be prepared to act quickly and effectively in such an emergency. In all patient care areas where immunizing agents are administered, emergency equipment should be readily available. This includes epinephrine, aminophyllines, and other drugs as indicated; syringes and other equipment for administration; a tourniquet; an airway; oxygen; and equipment for intravenous infusion. As an extra precaution to ensure prompt treatment of a hypersensitivity reaction if one occurs, it is advisable for persons receiving immunizing agents to remain in the clinic or office for 15 to 20 minutes after an injection.

DISORDERS OF THE IMMUNE SYSTEM

Abnormal responses of the immune system are divided into four basic categories: (1) *immune deficiency*—that is, insufficient production of either antibodies or immune cells or both; (2) *excessive response*, which involves increased growth of the plasma cells and the synthesis of abnormal antibodies; (3) *overreaction* or *hypersensitivity* to antigens from the external environment (exogenous antigens); and (4) *autoimmune disease*, in which the immune system reacts against the body's own cells or a substance arising in the body (endogenous antigens) (Table 7–3).

IMMUNE DEFICIENCY

Inadequate function of the immune system can affect either the humoral or the cellular components of the system. Insufficient production of these components can be present at birth (congenital) or acquired during life. In some cases the acquired deficiency is a primary condition; in others it is secondary to some other disorder or treatment.

In all cases, a deficiency of immune bodies leaves its victims unable to resist foreign agents and therefore susceptible to overwhelming infection.

Primary congenital immune deficiency can range from a complete absence of immunoglobulins (*agammaglobulinemia*) to an inadequate level of immune bodies (*hypogammaglobulinemia*). Infants born with agammaglobulinemia have no B cells for the production of antibody. Prognosis depends on the severity of the deficiency and the infections the child develops. The life span of the infant with no immunoglobulins is extremely short, because he or she has no humoral defense against infectious agents.

Secondary acquired immune deficiency can result from any of a number of factors. Age is a factor because at birth the infant begins to lose some antibodies acquired from the maternal blood. Eventually the infant is able to produce his own, but for a time he has a deficiency of certain antibodies. With advancing age, when the physiologic processes of the body slow down, humoral immunity declines, leaving the aged person more susceptible to infection.

Malnutrition, malignancy, stress, and some drugs can suppress function of the immune system, as can liver disease, nephrosis, and lymphatic disorders.

Acquired Immunodeficiency Syndrome (AIDS)

AIDS is a relatively new disease first described in the early 1980s. It is believed that the disease came about by mutation of a virus that originally infected the African green monkey. AIDS is a fatal disease that mainly affects people during the most productive years of their lives. The

TABLE 7–3 MALADAPTIVE AND INAPPROPRIATE IMMUNE RESPONSES

Response	Example	Pathophysiology	Outcome
Inadequate	Congenital: Immune deficiency (hypogammaglobulinemia) Acquired: AIDS; severe combined immune deficiency (SCID) syndrome	Body produces too few or no immune cells	Patient requires immune cells and antibodies from a source other than himself Body unable to defend itself
Excessive	Myeloma (hypergammaglobulinemia)	Plasma cells multiply rapidly but produce abnormal, apparently ineffective antibodies	Body unable to defend itself against infection
Exaggerated	Allergy; hypersensitivity (anaphylaxis, serum sickness)	Antigen-antibody response causes cell rupture and release of histamine; excessive inflammatory response is damaging to body cells	Redness, heat, swelling, loss of motion; varies in severity
Inappropriate	Autoimmune disease (rheumatoid arthritis, systemic lupus, rheumatic fever)	Immune system fails to recognize body cells as "self"	Chronic inflammation, usually of collagenous connective tissue

incidence of AIDS in the United States is predicted by the U.S. Public Health Service to be about 365,000 cases by 1992.

The disease is caused by infection with the human immunodeficiency virus (HIV). HIV is a human retrovirus, which means it has the ability to integrate the viral genetic make-up into the cell it infects, causing an abnormal cell that can produce more virus.

HIV is transmitted by contact with blood or blood products, by sexual contact, and from mother to fetus. Any sexual contact with an HIV-infected person puts the uninfected partner at risk of acquiring the infection. The greatest incidence of HIV infection is traced to homosexual practices. A smaller number of cases results from sharing of needles (blood contact) by intravenous drug users. Unfortunately, a portion of the HIV-positive population received the virus via blood transfusion before March, 1985, when adequate testing of the blood supply for the virus became available. There is now a growing problem of children with AIDS who are born to HIV-infected mothers.

The HIV retrovirus attacks and cripples an important type of T lymphocyte, eventually destroying all of them. This seriously impairs the person's immune response. Some individuals have HIV infection but no symptoms. Others who are infected with HIV display two or more symptoms of AIDS and have at least two laboratory test results that indicate a state of immunodeficiency. This group of people is said to have *AIDS-related complex* (ARC). True AIDS is diagnosed when the individual is HIV positive and has the following signs and symptoms: swollen lymph nodes (lymphadenopathy), thrombocytopenia, persistent weight loss, fever, night sweats, diarrhea, fatigue, and immune abnormalities shown by laboratory tests. AIDS patients frequently develop *opportunistic infections*, which are caused by organisms that are usually not pathogenic in healthy people. If, however, there is an inadequate immune response and a resultant lowering of resistance, the infectious organisms take the opportunity to cause serious and often fatal infections. The current mortality rate is about 80%, with death occurring within 3 to 5 years from the time of diagnosis with AIDS.

It is evident that HIV can remain inactive inside a cell for a very long time. HIV then becomes active when the cell is stimulated. It is thought that HIV activity may be stimulated by other viral and parasitic infections that activate T cells. Possible culprits may be cytomegalovirus (CMV), Epstein-Barr virus, and hepatitis B virus.

The most common of the opportunistic infections associated with AIDS is a kind of pneumonia caused by *Pneumocystis carinii*, a protozoan that is found virtually everywhere. The organism, a parasite, enters the lungs in large numbers, proliferates, and forms cystic packs that gradually occupy all air space. The end result is gradual suffocation as the lungs are filled with the organisms. *P. carinii* pneumonia is contagious and is spread by the respiratory route. There is currently no drug or treatment that will cure the infection.

Kaposi's sarcoma is yet another disease related to AIDS. It has always been known as a rare malignant disease that produces tumors of cells derived from connective tissue, especially the skin and lymphoid tissue. The form of Kaposi's sarcoma seen today in increasing numbers produces tumors that are not restricted to the lower extremities, as in classic Kaposi's sarcoma. Lesions can occur in lymphoid tissue and are also found on internal organs. If lymphadenopathy is present, the patient may not live more than 3 years.

Assessment

Persons most at risk for AIDS are homosexual or bisexual men with many partners, intravenous drug users, and those who have received the HIV retrovirus from blood products. Exposure to the blood of infected persons is probably the one thing these persons have in common. Transfer of the virus among homosexuals is related to anal intercourse, which can bring about minimal bleeding from the lining of the anus. Intravenous drug users frequently share the same needles without sterilizing them.

Objective and subjective signs and symptoms of AIDS include swollen glands in the neck, armpits, and groin; rapid loss of weight; unexplained fever; chronic diarrhea; skin changes, especially the appearance of purplish spots similar to bruises; severe and prolonged fatigue; and cough or shortness of breath.

Preventing the Spread of AIDS

Until medical science develops some means for effectively treating patients with opportunistic infections associated with AIDS, it is imperative that measures be taken to limit its spread. So far, the measures suggested by public health officials can only be based on assumptions. There is no scientific evidence that these measures will be totally effective, but they are based on common sense and an understanding of how infectious diseases are transmitted. The recommended procedures and precautions are as follows:

- Those persons who are known to be at risk for developing AIDS should voluntarily refrain from donating blood. The Public Health Service includes in this category those with symptoms that suggest AIDS, sexual partners of AIDS victims, or persons at risk for AIDS;

sexually active homosexuals or bisexuals who have many partners; persons who are or have been abusers of intravenous drugs; and persons with hemophilia.
- Homosexual men should be encouraged to refrain from intercourse with many partners and to use barrier precautions during sexual contact.
- Intravenous drug users should be educated about the hazards of sharing contaminated needles and syringes.
- Doctors, nurses, and other health care personnel should use special precautions when handling the blood and blood-contaminated equipment of AIDS victims. Universal precautions are to be used with all patients.

No matter what the modes of transfer in any infectious disease, hand washing and careful handling of linens, soiled instruments, and contaminated equipment are essential.

Abstinence from sexual contact and from contact with blood and blood products is the most effective way to prevent infection with the HIV retrovirus. Maintaining a healthy body and immune system with adequate sleep, good nutrition, and appropriate exercise is the other way that each person can help prevent the spread of this fatal disease. Table 7-4 provides other suggestions for prevention of infection with HIV.

Treatment for AIDS

To date there is no known cure for AIDS. Treatment is aimed at preventing replication of the HIV and treating opportunistic infections. Zidovudine (formerly called AZT) is given to patients with AIDS or ARC to prevent the HIV from replicating. It improves the status of the immune system and helps decrease the number and severity of opportunistic infections. It is cytotoxic and nephrotoxic, and the patient's complete blood cell (CBC) count, blood urea nitrogen (BUN) levels, and serum creatinine levels should be checked periodically. Usual dosage is 200 mg by mouth every 6 hours. Side effects include nausea, headache, muscular pain, sleeplessness, anemia, and granulocytopenia.

Drugs used to treat *P. carinii* pneumonia (PCP) include trimethoprim-sulfamethoxazole (Bactrim; Septra), pentamidine (Pentam 300), and dapsone (Avlosulfon). Without these drugs, the patient with PCP often dies of respiratory failure. Trimethoprim-sulfamethoxazole is usually given intravenously for a 2-week period. Unfortunately many patients cannot tolerate the drug combination and develop severe reactions that require stopping the medications. In that event, pentamidine therapy is begun intravenously. Side effects include nausea, vomiting, hypoglycemia, hypotension, leukopenia, and sterile abscesses. Dapsone is used for acute PCP and is given orally. Side effects include peripheral neuropathy, hemolytic anemia, dermatitis, nausea, and vomiting (Porterfield, 1990).

Other treatment consists of attempts to boost the immune system through nutritional therapy, stress reduction, and imagery.

Nursing Intervention

Nursing intervention for the AIDS patient is complex and involves planning care for the problems the patient is experiencing at the time with various systems of the body. Prevention of infection and transfer of the AIDS virus is a high priority, and the nurse must keep in mind at all times that this patient is highly susceptible to

TABLE 7-4 WAYS TO PREVENT INFECTION WITH HIV

- Obtain regular medical evaluation to detect minor health problems
- Avoid sexual activity or maintain a totally monogamous relationship with an HIV-negative person
- Use a latex condom for oral sex and one lubricated with a spermicide containing nonoxynol-9 for intercourse; refrain from sexual practices such as anal intercourse that damage mucosal tissue
- Refrain from open-mouth, "French" kissing
- Don't share toothbrushes, razors, or other items that could be contaminated with blood
- If you use drugs, break the habit; never share drug equipment
- Obtain HIV testing if you have been sexually active with several people, have had a blood transfusion before March 1985, have been exposed to a known HIV-positive person on an intimate basis, or are especially concerned about the possibility of HIV infection
- Decrease the stress in your life; learn relaxation techniques (stress has an adverse effect on the immune system)
- Maintain healthy habits of nutrition, rest, and exercise, and avoid infection as much as possible

every infection. She must use vigilant aseptic technique in all aspects of care.

Psychosocial care is equally important for the AIDS patient, as he has a dreaded, fatal disease, eventually loses his health and independence, and often is treated badly by others in society. The nurse can do much to make him feel worthwhile, pointing out that he is still the same person he has always been and focusing on his strengths. Selected points of nursing care for the AIDS patient are presented in Nursing Care Plan 7-1.

Therapeutic Immunosuppression

Sometimes it is beneficial to the patient to have his immune response deliberately suppressed. To illustrate, the patient who has received an organ transplant may suffer from total rejection of the organ by his own body cells, which react to the organ as if it were a harmful agent. To avoid rejection of the transplanted organ, the patient may receive certain drugs that inhibit the action of his immune system. As previously explained, certain cytotoxic drugs, as well as x-rays used to produce radiographs, can be immunosuppressive. Hence these agents can be used to benefit the patient when immunosuppression is desirable. The use of immunosuppressive agents requires the maintenance of a delicate balance between control of the immune response and control of infections that occur when the immune response is suppressed.

In 1983 the Food and Drug Administration approved a new drug called *cyclosporine.* This drug acts as a selective immunosuppressant, leaving intact some of the body's defenses against infection. Cyclosporine has been approved for administration to patients who have kidney, liver, and heart transplants. There is evidence that use of the drug increases the survival rate of patients with certain organ transplants, but it does not completely eliminate the danger of organ rejection. Another problem is that the immunosuppression tends to allow growth of some cancers.

In addition to preventing the rejection of transplanted organs, immunosuppressive therapy also may be employed in the management of multiple myeloma, other kinds of neoplastic growths, and autoimmune diseases.

Whatever the reason for the immune deficiency, the patient will require special nursing care so that the possibility of an overwhelming infection is kept at a minimum.

Treatment of Immune Deficiencies

The management of immune deficiency depends on its degree of severity and its primary cause. Some patients have virtually no ability to synthesize antibodies or sensitized lymphocytes, whereas others experience only a temporary minor defect in humoral immune response and cell-mediated immunity.

Injections of human gamma globulin may be given on a regular basis to provide passive immunity for those who are unable to produce their own antibodies. Antibiotics are used in large doses as soon as an infection is evident, but these drugs are rarely used as a preventive measure, because antibiotics themselves can be immunosuppressive.

In some types of immune deficiency, passive immunization can be accomplished by transfusing specifically sensitized lymphocytes to help the patient resist an infection. When function of the bone marrow is involved, as in leukemia, the patient may receive a bone marrow transplant to provide the stem cells that will eventually become immune bodies.

Providing passive immunization through transplants, administration of gamma globulins, and transfusion of sensitized lymphocytes only temporarily relieves the situation by bolstering the patient's resistance; it does not cure the primary cause any more than a blood transfusion relieves the cause of anemia.

Whenever possible, treatment is aimed at controlling the disease or eliminating the condition that is the primary cause of an inadequately functioning immune system. Sometimes, as in cases of nephrosis, liver disease, drug toxicity, and viral infections, this may be possible. In other instances, however, treatment consists of minimizing the effects of the immune deficiency.

Experimental drugs are currently being used in the treatment of Kaposi's sarcoma, AIDS, and *P. carinii* pneumonia. Research also offers hope for infants with combined immune deficiencies through administration of specially treated bone marrow containing stem cells that mature into normally functioning T lymphocytes.

Nursing Intervention

The primary concerns of the nurse caring for a patient who has an immune deficiency are (1) protection of the patient from infection, (2) improvement of health status, and (3) maintenance of as high a degree of wellness as possible so that the immune system can function at optimal level.

The patient who is suffering from immune deficiency will present many nursing care problems. *Protective isolation* is implemented so that exposure of the patient to infectious agents is kept at a minimum. Meticulous hand washing is

NURSING CARE PLAN 7–1

Selected nursing diagnoses, goals/outcome criteria, nursing interventions, and evaluations for a patient who has just been diagnosed with AIDS

Situation: Tad Whipple, age 38, was admitted with chronic, severe diarrhea, weight loss, fatigue, and dehydration. He is homosexual and has lived with his partner for 5 years. He had had several other lovers before this alliance. His health has deteriorated over the past year, and he has experienced recurrent episodes of severe diarrhea, fatigue, respiratory infection, and dehydration. He has been HIV positive for 2 years, and he has just been diagnosed as having AIDS.

Nursing Diagnosis	Goals/Outcome Criteria	Nursing Intervention	Evaluation
Diarrhea related to overgrowth of colon bacteria and opportunistic infection. SUPPORTING DATA Having approximately 15 loose stools daily.	Normal bowel pattern by discharge. No more than eight loose stools per day within 48 hours.	Administer Lomotil as ordered. Monitor intake and output with stool count. Clear liquid diet, progressing to bland foods as diarrhea resolves; maintain IV flow rate as ordered. Check skin turgor and mucous membranes q shift. Perineal care after each bowel movement; apply Desitin ointment to protect and help heal mucosa.	Lomotil q 4 h $\times$ 6; BMs decreased to 8; I = 5,500 mL; 0 = 4,100. Skin turgor improved; mucous membranes more moist. Taking clear liquids only. Rectal mucosa inflamed and cracked; Desitin applied after perianal care.
Activity intolerance related to diarrhea, dehydration, electrolyte imbalance, and fatigue. SUPPORTING DATA Dehydrated; 15 loose BMs per day; electrolytes out of balance, complains of fatigue.	Patient will be able to perform self-care by discharge.	Assist with all activities of daily living (ADL). Monitor hydration status and electrolytes daily. Provide restful environment. Encourage him to participate in self-care as condition improves.	Assisted with ADL; K^+ back to 3.5; NA^+, 132. Skin turgor slightly improved; mucous membranes moist but "sticky."
Infection with HIV virus and excessive colon bacteria. SUPPORTING DATA HIV positive; stool culture positive for excessive growth of *Escherichia coli* and *Cryptosporidium.*	HIV will not be passed to any other person during hospitalization. Patient will not develop other nosocomial infections before discharge.	Universal precautions at all times, as well as body fluid precautions for handling and disposing of stool. Allow only visitors and personnel without evidence of infection to be in contact with patient. Monitor for signs of nosocomial infection: urine, respiratory, skin. Review precautions necessary to prevent transfer of HIV to others. Review measures to protect self against infections; avoid crowds, maintain nutrition, obtain sufficient rest, use stress reduction techniques.	Universal and body fluid precautions maintained. No sign of nosocomial infection. Continue plan.
Anticipatory grieving related to loss of health, potential loss of employment, and eventual loss of life. SUPPORTING DATA Diagnosed with AIDS and has opportunistic infection. States that he is afraid he will lose job and partner; is afraid of death.	Patient will identify specific fears by labeling them before discharge. Patient will establish contact with an AIDS support group before discharge.	Encourage verbalization of specific fears; facilitate grieving process. Give information on community resources and AIDS support group. Encourage him to be open with partner and share feelings. Explore spiritual beliefs and encourage spiritual growth in direction of his choosing. Encourage him to consider future plans regarding will, decisions about life support and resuscitation, etc.	Beginning to discuss feelings more; was raised in Methodist church; might consider pursuing that religion again if he is not shunned by minister. Is not comfortable with talking to partner yet. Continue plan.

NURSING CARE PLAN 7–1, *Continued*

Nursing Diagnosis	Goals/Outcome Criteria	Nursing Intervention	Evaluation
Self-esteem disturbance related to having AIDS, weight loss, and general appearance. SUPPORTING DATA HIV positive; diagnosed as having AIDS; has lost 25 lb., appears emaciated.	Patient will accept self as is before death. Patient will be able to list five positive points about self before discharge.	Encourage him to talk about personal skills, strengths, and positive points and contributions he has made. Encourage him to set small daily goals for self. Encourage him to seek validation of self from partner (after assessing partner's perception of patient and situation). Demonstrate warmth and caring; utilize touch. Seek patient's opinion on topics. Explore areas in which he can still make a contribution to his community.	Demonstrating caring; spending at least 20 min./day sitting and talking with him. Having difficulty listing positive points about self as yet; listed one only. Continue plan.

essential before and after each contact with the patient or any object that may serve as a source of infection. Strict observance of surgical aseptic technique is imperative during the performance of such nursing care procedures as catheterization, dressing changes, intravenous infusions, and all other activities that might lead to introduction of pathogenic microorganisms into the body tissues.

The patient and his family will need continued instruction and support in learning how infection is spread and how they can participate in the prevention and control of infection. Before planning their instruction, the nurse needs to find out how much the immune-deficient patient and his family know about his condition and the problems it can present. They will need to understand the importance of sufficient sleep and rest, good nutrition, and prompt attention to the most trivial infections. If they are unfamiliar with the purposes and techniques of protective isolation (most people understandably are), they must have adequate instruction in these areas.

The assessment phase of the nursing process should include gathering information about the current physical status of the patient—his general state of health, any infections he may have at the time, and how these infections are being manifested (that is, what symptoms pose a threat to his comfort and affect his ability to combat infection).

The planning phase of the nursing process should take into account the physical strength of the patient, his need for rest, and the psychological impact of isolation. Every effort should be made to maintain integrity of the skin and mucous membranes so that they continue to serve as effective barriers to infectious agents. This means planning and implementing good skin care, oral hygiene, and personal cleanliness. Sites of intravenous injections should be checked frequently for signs of inflammation and cleansed daily with an antiseptic followed by application of an antibiotic ointment.

Considering the many causes and varying degrees of immune deficiency, it is likely that the nurse working in a hospital or outpatient clinic will frequently encounter patients who are highly susceptible to infection because of abnormal function of the immune system. It is the responsibility of the nurse to identify such patients and to plan their care so that the goals of preventing infection and strengthening resistance are accomplished in cooperation with the patient and his family.

EXCESSIVE RESPONSE

In an excessive response of the immune system, the plasma cells of the bone marrow begin to multiply very rapidly, forming a tumor within the bone marrow (myeloma). These plasma cells do not function normally. They produce excessive amounts of gamma globulins that are unable to carry out their roles in immunity. Thus the patient has *hypergammaglobulinemia*, with a seriously impaired ability to resist infection.

Because of the activities that they normally carry out, plasma cells in the bone marrow can enter the blood stream without difficulty and be transported to other tissues of the body. The abnormal plasma cells enjoy the same advantage and therefore are spread to tissues elsewhere in the body. In this way, the malignancy is quickly spread, and the patient with a myeloma usually rapidly develops multiple myeloma, which is fatal in a very short time.

HYPERSENSITIVITY AND ALLERGY

Pathophysiology

An *allergy* is an abnormal, individual response to certain substances that normally do not trigger such an exaggerated response. Allergies are divided into three major groups: (1) delayed-reaction allergies involving sensitized lymphocytes; (2) antigen-antibody allergies caused by a reaction between IgG and antigen; and (3) atopic or inherited allergies, which are characterized by the presence of large amounts of IgE antibody.

Examples of *delayed-reaction, cell-mediated hypersensitivity* include contact dermatitis resulting from exposure to certain drugs, chemicals such as those in cosmetic and household cleaners, and the toxins of plants such as poison ivy. On contact with the allergen the sensitized lymphocytes diffuse into the skin and bring about an immune response. During this reaction the lymphocytes release toxins, and macrophages invade the tissues. If the process continues unchecked, there can be extensive damage to the tissues as a result of inflammatory changes.

Antigen-antibody allergies occur when a person has a high titer of antibodies, especially the IgG type, circulating in his blood. The reaction results in formation of an antigen-antibody complex that precipitates and deposits small granules on the walls of blood vessels. Enzymes released during the reaction cause inflammation of the small blood vessels, which are subsequently badly damaged or destroyed. Examples of antigen-antibody reactions are transfusion reactions and drug reactions.

Atopic allergies affect about 10% of the population. The hypersensitivity is inherited, and excessive amounts of IgE antibodies are produced. Allergens that react specifically with IgE antibody include house dust, foods, and the venom of bees, wasps, and hornets. During this reaction histamine and other chemicals toxic to the body's cells are released. The chemicals cause dilation of blood vessels (which increases the transport of antibody and chemicals to the site of battle) and the contraction of smooth muscle tissues in the bronchioles. These internal changes produce the symptoms of allergy, notably redness, swelling, increased exudate, and breathing difficulties such as wheezing and dyspnea.

As with all types of immune response, abnormal as well as normal, a full-blown reaction will not occur until an individual's immune cells have been sensitized to the specific substance that triggers the response. This means that on first contact with the allergen, there will be very little specific antibody in the circulating blood or in the lymphoid tissues. On second and subsequent contacts, however, the antibody specific to the allergen will be produced in large quantities and circulated in the body fluids, where it can be transported to the site of the allergic reaction.

Management of Hypersensitivity and Allergic Reactions

Major goals in the management of hypersensitivity and allergic reactions are (1) to assist in the diagnosis of hypersensitivity, (2) to help the patient identify the particular substance or substances that trigger an allergic response, (3) to assist the patient in devising ways to avoid or at least limit exposure to these allergens, (4) to relieve the symptoms of an allergy, and (5) to decrease the exaggerated response to the allergen(s).

Assessment

Objective and subjective data suggestive of an allergy are summarized in Table 7–5. Identification of the specific allergen or allergens causing the allergic reaction may be fairly easy or extremely difficult. Reaction to stings, drug allergies, and other conditions that are not routine occurrences in the life of the patient are readily noticed because the cause-effect relationship is apparent.

Types of Allergens. In an effort to help the patient recognize less obvious allergic substances, it is helpful to put these substances in some kind of category. Four broad types of allergens may be distinguished according to the way in which they gain access to the body. *Inhalants* enter the body through the nose and mouth; they include dust, molds, pollen, animal dander, and some chemicals. *Contactants* come in direct contact with the skin. These include detergents and soaps, cosmetics, plants such as poison ivy, and dyes such as those used in shoe leather. *Ingestants* are swallowed. They usually are foods and drugs. Citrus fruits, tomatoes, cow's milk, wheat, seafoods, chocolate, and colas are common food offenders. Among the drugs, the most likely to cause an allergic reaction are aspirin, barbiturates, and antibiotics. *Injectables* enter the body through hypodermic, intramuscular, and intravenous injections; by snake and other animal bites; and by insect stings. Immunizing agents such as vaccines, animal saliva, and venoms are the allergens that most commonly enter the body by this route.

Identification of Allergens. *Skin testing* to identify specific allergens can be done in a number of ways. In the *scratch test,* the skin is slightly scratched so that only its upper layer is broken and no blood appears. A sampling of the suspected allergen is applied to the scratched area. In the *intracutaneous* or *intradermal*

TABLE 7-5 ASSESSMENT GUIDE FOR ALLERGY

Location	Objective Data	Subjective Data
Skin	Dryness, scaling, irritations, inflammations, hives, rash (note symmetry and location), scratches, urticaria	Itching, burning
Eyes	Discoloration below eyes (allergic shiners); conjunctivitis; long, silky eyelashes; rubbing or excessive blinking	Burning, itching, tearing; history of styes
Nose	Allergic salute (pushing nose upward and backward with heel of hand), nasal polyps, nasal voice	Nose twitching, "stuffiness," recurring nosebleeds, sudden episodes of sneezing, snorting
Mouth and throat	Open-mouth breathing, continual throat clearing; shiny, bald patches on tongue with slightly elevated borders; mouth wrinkling with facial grimaces; redness of throat; swollen lips or tongue.	Ability to tolerate only moderate exertion without tiring, wheezing, or shortness of breath
Ears	Drainage	Hearing loss
Neck	Palpable lymph nodes	
General		History of food intolerances; colic; abdominal cramping; vomiting and diarrhea in absence of general illness; unusual reactions to drugs, insect stings, odors, or fumes; recurrent respiratory problems; seasonal flareups of any symptoms

method, the sample of allergen is injected just below the epidermis. In the *patch test* a small amount of the allergen is simply placed on the surface of the skin and covered with an airtight dressing (patch). A positive reaction to these tests is indicated by the appearance of a small (dime-sized) wheal at the site of contact with the allergen.

Another helpful tool for identifying suspected allergens in foods is the *elimination diet*. It usually starts with foods that are known to be frequent offenders. The patient is asked to eliminate one food at a time and to record in a food diary *all the foods eaten each day*. This includes additives and preservatives in processed foods that were eaten. If the patient's symptoms persist for a week to 10 days after eliminating one food (for example, milk and dairy products), he is allowed to resume his intake of that particular food, and another one is chosen.

Identification of allergens can be a tedious process. Many times it is more than one substance that produces the symptoms of an allergy. The patient and family will need continued support and encouragement to keep looking for the offending substance or substances.

Nursing Intervention

Goals for nursing intervention to assist the patient with an allergy are (1) to help the patient avoid exposure to known allergens, (2) to manage the symptoms of the allergy, (3) to participate in a program of hyposensitization or immunotherapy, and (4) to provide health teaching.

Avoiding Exposure to Allergens

Once the allergens are identified, the patient will need help in devising ways to avoid them or to limit his exposure to them. This, too, is not as easy as it may seem. In some cases, it may mean parting with a cherished family pet, overcoming the habit of smoking and asking others not to smoke in one's presence, or purchasing and expensive air-conditioning unit that effectively filters out airborne allergens.

House dust and pollens are common allergens that are not easily eliminated from the environment. Overstuffed furniture, heavy draperies, and thick carpets serve as excellent reservoirs for these substances. Other common allergens found in the home include cleaning compounds, cosmetics, and dyes in fabrics and common materials. Some patients may need to wear rubber gloves each time they wash dishes, launder clothes, or perform other chores requiring contact with cleansing agents.

Nurses and others who handle certain drugs may develop allergies to these drugs. For example, penicillin and streptomycin can cause contact dermatitis in some persons who are regularly exposed to them.

As with the control of the spread of infectious agents, avoiding exposure to allergens requires a knowledge of the nature of the allergen, how it is transmitted, its source or reservoir, and its portal of entry. Once these have been established, the nurse and the patient work together to eliminate the allergen from the patient's environment insofar as this is feasible (Nursing Care Plan 7–2).

Management of Symptoms. As previously stated, symptoms of an allergic response vary widely, depending on the severity of the attack and the site of the reaction. Relief from the potentially fatal symptoms of anaphylaxis is discussed later in this chapter. Other allergic symptoms, while less lifethreatening, can certainly cause much discomfort and inconvenience.

Drugs that play an important part in alleviating the systemic reactions to allergens include epinephrine, the antihistamines, bronchodilators, corticotropin (adrenocorticotropic hormone, or ACTH) and cortisone, tranquilizers, and sedatives.

The antihistamines are particularly useful in controlling the symptoms of hay fever, serum sickness, and hives. These drugs are histamine-blocking agents, which means that they prevent the histamine released during an allergic reaction from coming in contact with its specific receptors in the body cells. Thus a reaction within the tissues is avoided or at least greatly reduced. The result of this blocking action is relief from itching, swelling of mucous membranes, increased secretions, and other symptoms of an allergic reaction.

Patients requiring antihistamines are warned of the side effects of drowsiness and impaired coordination, both of which contraindicate driving an automobile and operating machinery during the initial phase of therapy. Other side effects, such as dryness of the mouth, weakness, and blurred vision, are not uncommon.

Antiinflammatory agents such as corticotropin and cortisone are administered to reduce the inflammatory response that occurs in an allergic reaction. The bronchodilators help relieve the respiratory distress that may be a symptom of involvement of the bronchioles and obstruction of the air passages. Tranquilizers and sedatives promote the rest needed for repair of body tissues and relieve the stress that aggravates an allergic reaction.

Local reactions involving widespread and deep skin lesions are treated with salves, wet compresses, and soothing baths. The patient also must be protected from a secondary bacterial infection. These aspects of nursing care are discussed more fully in Chapter 33.

The nurse should be aware that a warm environment and sweating increase the sensation of itching. The patient should be kept cool without chilling. Another important aspect of care for these patients is prevention of scratching and excoriation of the skin.

Those patients who suffer from respiratory distress as a symptom of an allergic reaction will require proper positioning for optimal breathing, administration of oxygen as ordered, and other nursing measures discussed in detail in Chapter 17.

NURSING CARE PLAN 7–2

Selected nursing diagnoses, goals/outcome criteria, nursing interventions, and evaluations for a patient with hypersensitivity to contactant—probably a dishwashing detergent

Situation: 34-year-old married female with a history of rash on both hands for several months that has become progressively worse. Improvement was noted during 1-week vacation when she did not do household chores. After returning to regular housework, symptoms worsened.

Nursing Diagnosis	Goals/Outcome Criteria	Nursing Intervention	Evaluation
Impaired skin integrity related to allergy to household cleaning products. SUPPORTING DATA Dry, scaling, cracking skin on hands and wrists with rash.	Skin on hands without rash, scaling or cracking within three weeks.	Attempt to identify contact allergen by instructing how to record all activities in which hands are used for three days and noting each morning specific condition of hands. Have change brands of dishwashing detergent. Have wear rubber gloves for any activity using soap or cleaning solution beginning on day four.	Activity record kept; hands worse after mopping with cleaning solution. Rubber gloves worn starting day four; hands improving.

Desensitization. When it is not possible for a patient to avoid exposure to allergens, or if the symptoms cannot be managed successfully, the physician may suggest desensitization. The purpose of this form of therapy is to render the patient less sensitive to the allergens. It is not possible to make the patient totally free from this sensitivity, but his reactions to specific allergens can be lessened. The program involves regular injections of minute quantities of selected antigens on a daily, weekly, or monthly schedule. The amount given is gradually increased until there is noticeable clinical improvement, and then a maintenance dose is given. The program may last for years, but improvement should be noted in about 6 to 12 months after it is begun.

The mechanism by which desensitization is accomplished is related to the production of immunoglobulins or gamma globulins in response to the presence of an allergen. Of the five groups of immunoglobulins, IgG is the most abundant. It also floats free in the blood stream, where it can attach itself to available antigen. However, IgE is the immunoglobulin that plays a major role in an anaphylactic reaction. IgE sets off the anaphylactic process by responding to the antigen and triggering the release of chemicals. If the body is exposed to small amounts of the allergy-producing antigen, however, the body will produce IgG. This immunoglobulin attaches itself to the available antigen and thus blocks the IgE from reacting with it. In this way anaphylaxis is prevented.

Health Teaching. Successful management of hypersensitivity depends in large measure on the ability of the patient to understand his allergy and to follow the prescribed regimen of treatment. Information intended to help with educating the lay person can be obtained from:

- National Institutes of Allergy and Infectious Disease
  National Institutes of Health
  Bldg. 10
  Bethesda, MD 20892
- Local chapter of the American Lung Association

Patients who have a food allergy should be instructed to read carefully the labels on all food products before purchasing them. Monosodium glutamate, other preservatives, and artificial food coloring can be potent allergens for some people.

Anaphylaxis

Anaphylaxis is a serious, dramatic allergic reaction. When it occurs, there is swelling and rupture of the affected cells, with the release of histamine. This chemical substance causes dilation of small blood vessels, a pooling of blood, and release of fluid into tissues. These changes in turn may produce circulatory collapse and profound shock. The patient also suffers from difficult breathing as a result of the narrowing of the air passages and accumulation of mucus. Another manifestation of anaphylaxis is the appearance of "hives" *(urticaria)*. These are sudden outbreaks of itching and burning wheals (small areas of swelling) on the skin.

The patient with an anaphylactic reaction is in a very serious condition and requires immediate attention. Circulatory collapse can very rapidly lead to fatal *anaphylactic shock*. The heart muscles do not function as they should. Thus there is a decreased output of blood and a drop in blood pressure. The patient also experiences dyspnea of increasing severity, and convulsions may occur. If these conditions are not relieved immediately, the patient can die within 5 to 10 minutes.

Treatment of anaphylaxis includes (1) administration of antihistamines to stop the effects of the histamine released by the body cells, thereby restoring the circulatory vessels and the bronchioles to a more normal state; (2) administration of aqueous epinephrine to counteract the effect of histamine, thereby causing relaxation of the bronchioles, an increase in cardiac output, and an elevation of the blood pressure; (3) establishment of a patent airway and administration of oxygen to relieve the symptoms of dyspnea and hypoxia; (4) measures to control shock; and (5) provision for psychological support.

Avoidance of anaphylaxis requires an awareness of previous allergic reactions in individuals and identification of those people who are likely to experience a serious reaction. It is extremely important that anyone who is about to receive drugs that are likely to produce an allergic reaction be questioned about allergies before any medication is given. An emergency tray should be readily available whenever vaccines, sera, and highly allergenic drugs are administered.

People who are aware of their extreme sensitivity to certain substances should wear an identification bracelet giving that information. In this way, any medical staff will be forewarned if the person requires emergency treatment and is unable to communicate with personnel. It is also advisable for individuals who are highly allergic to stings from bees, wasps, or other insects to carry with them a small kit containing diphenhydramine hydrochloride (Benadryl), epinephrine, syringe, needle, and tourniquet. These kits are available, by prescription, from a pharmacy and are recommended by allergists who realize the rapidity with which a bee sting or similar event can be fatal to someone who is highly sensitive.

Serum Sickness

Serum sickness is another type of generalized, widespread reaction to an antigenic substance.

Usually the antigen is a drug or a foreign serum such as the immunizing sera that confer passive immunity.

Serum sickness, in contrast to anaphylaxis, does not occur immediately after contact with the antigen. It usually develops slowly over a period of 2 to 3 weeks after injection of the drug. It presents less serious symptoms and usually is self-limiting. Symptoms commonly associated with serum sickness include skin rash, edema, joint pain and swelling, renal vasculitis, adenitis, and sometimes high fever and prostration. Treatment most often involves administration of antihistamine and aspirin, the latter being helpful in reducing the inflammatory reaction that often affects the joints. More serious symptoms require treatment similar to that for anaphylaxis.

AUTOIMMUNE DISEASE

Normally, the body is able to distinguish between substances that are part of its "self" and those that are foreign or "not self." Strange as it may seem, it is possible for the body to fail to recognize its own cells. When this happens, the immune system attacks and attempts to reject substances that have been mistakenly identified as foreign agents. This reaction against the body's own cells is called an *autoimmune reaction*.

There are many theories as to why there are cases of mistaken identity that result in the body's destruction of some of its own tissues. There also is no general agreement as to exactly which diseases are actually "autoimmune." Most of the diseases that are considered to be related to the mechanism of autoimmunity are those in which there is some involvement of collagenous connective tissue, a type of tissue that is found throughout the body.

Some fairly well known diseases that are often classified as autoimmune are rheumatoid arthritis, systemic lupus erythematosus, rheumatic fever, glomerulonephritis, and Hashimoto's disease.

Treatment

The treatment of autoimmune diseases is discussed in later chapters under the heading of the specific disease. In general, treatment is aimed at managing the excessive inflammatory responses common to almost all autoimmune diseases and relieving the patient's symptoms. This includes (1) administering such antiinflammatory agents as the corticosteroids or nonsteroidal antiinflammatory drugs, (2) suppressing the immune response (therapeutic immunosuppression) through radiation by x-ray or radioactive substances or through immunosuppressive drugs, and (3) administering aspirin and other salicylates to provide relief of pain.

BIBLIOGRAPHY

Boland, M. G., and Czarniecki, L.: Starting life with HIV. RN, Jan., 1991, p. 54.

Bullock, B. L., and Rosendalhl P. O.: Pathophysiology: Adaptations and Alterations in Function, 2nd ed. Boston, Scott, Foresman, 1988.

Centers for Disease Control: CDC Update. Universal precautions for prevention and transmission of human immunodeficiency virus, hepatitis B virus, and other bloodborne pathogens in health care settings. MMWR, 37, 1988, p. 377.

Fogel, C. I., and Lauver, D.: Sexual Health Promotion. Philadelphia, W. B. Saunders, 1990.

Grady, C.: HIV: Epidemiology, immunopathogenesis, and clinical consequences. Nurs. Clin. North Am., Dec., 1988, p. 683.

Gurevich, I.: How to handle blood and body fluids. Adv. Clin. Care, May/June, 1990, p. 11.

Guyton, A. C.: Textbook of Medical Physiology, 8th ed. Philadelphia, W. B. Saunders, 1991.

Henderson, D. J.: HIV infection: Risks to health care workers and infection control. Nurs. Clin. North Am., Dec., 1988, p. 767.

Ignatavicius, D. D., and Bayne, M. J.: Medical-Surgical Nursing. Philadelphia, W. B. Saunders, 1991.

Luckmann, J., and Sorensen, K. C.: Medical-Surgical Nursing: A Psychophysiologic Approach, 3rd ed. Philadelphia, W. B. Saunders, 1987.

Porterfield, L. M.: Drugs used for patients with AIDS. Adv. Clin. Care, Jan./Feb., 1990, p. 40.

Price, S., and Wilson, L.: Pathophysiology, 3rd ed. New York, McGraw-Hill, 1986.

Rakel, R. E., ed.: Conn's Current Therapy 1990. Philadelphia, W. B. Saunders, 1990.

Randall, B. J.: Reacting to anaphylaxis, 1987–1988. C. E. Test Handbook, vol. 3., Springhouse, PA, Springhouse Corp., p. 26.

Robertson, S.: Drugs that keep AIDS patients alive. RN, Feb., 1989, p. 35.

Ungvarski, P.: Coping with infections that AIDS patients develop. RN, Nov., 1988, p. 53.

STUDENT STUDY AIDS

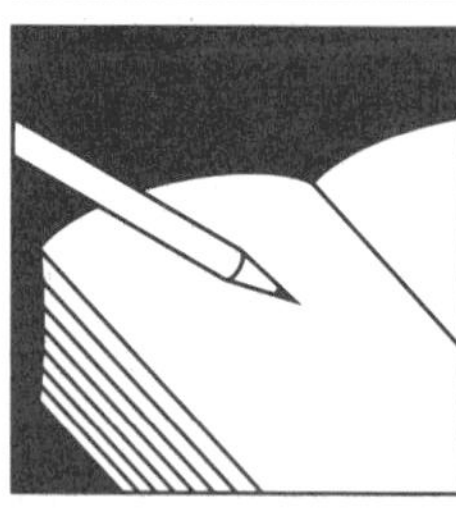

CLINICAL CASE PROBLEMS

Read each clinical situation and discuss the questions with your classmates.

1. Mrs. DeSilva is a young mother who has recently moved into your neighborhood. She has not had her children immunized against any diseases because she fears that "the shots will only make my healthy children sick." One of her children, aged 5, will need immunization before he can enter school. Mrs. DeSilva does not know whether her children received immunizations during infancy because she has moved from one community to another fairly regularly and has not taken them regularly to a pediatrician or to well-baby clinics.

Mrs. DeSilva is concerned about her children's health; she resists immunization only because she does not understand what these "shots" will do to the children and why they are necessary. She has also told you that she is worried about her children having tuberculosis because an aunt that once lived with them was diagnosed as having that disease.

- How would you explain active and passive immunization to Mrs. DeSilva?
- What would you say to try to convince her that her children should be immunized?
- How would you explain tuberculin testing to Mrs. DeSilva?
- How would you describe the benefits of skin testing for the members of her family?

---

2. Mr. Wooten is a 45-year-old patient who is admitted to the hospital for a hernia operation. You notice that he has the symptoms of a cold and you ask him about them. Mr. Wooten replies that he is "allergic to something" and often has these symptoms.

- How might you help Mr. Wooten determine the airborne substances to which he is allergic?
- What techniques are used to determine foods that may be allergens?
- What role does histamine play in the symptoms of an allergic reaction?
- Why are antihistamines helpful in the management of allergy symptoms?
- What measures should be taken to avoid a fatal allergic reaction to drugs that are administered in a hospital or clinic?

---

3. Mary Jo, aged 15, is a young friend of yours who is highly allergic to penicillin and bee stings. The last time she experienced a reaction to a bee sting on her leg, the entire limb became swollen. Mary Jo is active in the Girl Scouts and frequently goes on camping trips.

Her physician has suggested that she wear an identification bracelet stating her allergies and that she carry an emergency kit when she is on a camping trip. Mary Jo's mother sees no need for these precautions because "Mary Jo is a perfectly healthy girl." Mary Jo says she wouldn't know what to do with the kit if she did get stung by a bee or wasp.

- How would you explain to Mary Jo and her mother the need for the identification bracelet and the kit?
- How would you go about teaching Mary Jo to use the diphenhydramine hydrochloride (Benadryl), epinephrine, syringe, needle, and tourniquet in the kit?

STUDY OUTLINE

I. Physiology

A. Immune response is a series of complex mechanical activities involving (1) surveillance for and recognition of foreign agents and (2) the ability to distinguish foreign cells from "self."

II. Types of immune response

A. Humoral response:

1. Takes place in body fluids (humor).
2. Is an antigen-antibody response.
3. Provides protection against acute, rapidly developing bacterial and viral organisms.

a. Antigen: any substance capable of generating production of an antagonist.
b. Antibody: protein synthesized by plasma cells in response to a specific antigen.
(1) Five classes of antibodies (immunoglobulins). The number of sites where an antibody can attach itself to its antigen depends on the class to which it belongs.
(2) Chemical and mechanical actions by which antibody can attack antigen include lysis, agglutination, precipitation, formation of antitoxin, and use of the complement system in which certain enzymes attack the foreign agents and protect body cells.

B. Cellular (delayed) response:
1. Depends upon sensitized T lymphocytes.
2. Active against slowly developing bacterial infections. Also involved in autoimmune response, some allergic reactions, and rejection of foreign cells.
3. Sensitized lymphocytes have been sensitized to a specific antigen. Subsequent exposure triggers a host of chemical and mechanical activities.
a. Some sensitized lymphocytes are transformed into "killer" cells.
b. Chemicals involved include lymphokines, and macrophage-activating factor.
4. Cellular response is often termed *delayed hypersensitivity.*

C. T lymphocytes and B lymphocytes:
1. Originate in the lymphocytic cells of the developing fetus. T cells pass through the thymus gland. B cells are preprocessed in an area not yet known but similar to the bursa of Fabricius in birds; hence the name B cells.
2. Both T cells and B cells migrate to lymphoid tissue, where they wait to form either sensitized lymphocytes for cellular immunity or antibodies for humoral immunity.
3. Some young B cells do not go on to form plasma cells for the production of antibody. Instead, they lie dormant as memory cells. When a specific antigen enters the body, the memory cells greatly increase the number of sensitized lymphocytes available for defense.
4. T lymphocytes are responsible for rejection of transplanted tissue.

III. Immunity against disease

A. Two major types: (1) natural or innate and (2) acquired or adaptive:
1. Natural: based on sex, age, race, constitutional makeup, and other individual traits.
2. Acquired: person can actively produce his own antibody or can receive it passively. Means by which immunity can be acquired actively and passively as summarized in Table 7–2.

IV. Immunization and nursing implications

A. Immunization programs:
1. Nurse is responsible for encouraging public participation in programs to protect people from disease.
2. Recommended vaccination schedule shown in Table 7–1.
3. Contraindications to active immunization include fevers, pregnancy, immune deficiency disease, immunosuppressive therapy, administration of certain drugs, and a history of allergy or hypersensitivity to any drug, chemical, or natural antigen.

B. Screening and diagnostic testing:
   1. Part of assessment is to identify persons in need of immunization or treatment.
   2. Consideration of risk factors (e.g., inadequate housing, poor nutrition, age, chronic illness).
   3. Skin testing.

C. Preventing or mitigating sensitivity reactions to immunizing agents:
   1. History must be taken before administration.
   2. Findings of allergic reactions in the past must be reported to physician.
   3. Patient with an allergy to a specific immunizing agent must not be given the agent.
   4. If there is doubt about whether a reaction will occur, minute amount of the agent can be given intradermally to determine if there will be a local reaction.
   5. In all areas where immunizing agents are given there must be emergency equipment readily at hand in case a reaction occurs.

V. Disorders of the immune system

A. Immune deficiency: absence or inadequate synthesis of immune bodies. Can affect either humoral or cellular immunity or both.
   1. Congenital, primary immune deficiency can range from a complete absence (agammaglobulinemia) to an inadequate level (hypogammaglobulinemia). Prognosis depends on the available immune bodies and the kind of infections the child develops.
   2. Secondary acquired immune deficiency can result from a host of factors.
      a. Age: infants and the elderly have less resistance.
      b. Malnutrition, malignancy, stress, certain drugs, liver disease, and lymphatic disorders are also causative factors.
   3. Acquired immunodeficiency syndrome (AIDS) and associated immune disorders:
      a. Incidence of AIDS increasing yearly.
      b. AIDS is caused by human immunodeficiency virus (HIV).
      c. HIV is transmitted by blood products and sexual contact and from infected mother to fetus.
      d. Greatest incidence of AIDS found in homosexual males; smaller number of cases found among IV drug users who share needles.
      e. AIDS causes impairment of immune system; victims often die of opportunistic diseases such as *Pneumocystis carinii* pneumonia or Kaposi's sarcoma.
      f. Growing problem is birth of children with AIDS from mothers infected with virus.
      g. Aids-related complex (ARC) occurs in patients who are HIV positive and have two or more symptoms of AIDs and/or two laboratory test results that indicate a state of immunodeficiency.
      h. Symptoms of AIDS include swollen lymph nodes, thrombocytopenia, weight loss, fever, night sweats, diarrhea, or fatigue, along with HIV-positive state and laboratory tests indicating immunodeficiency.
      i. HIV retrovirus can remain inactive and undetectable inside a cell for a very long time.
      j. Cytomegalovirus (CMV), Epstein-Barr virus, and hepatitis B virus may possibly trigger activation of HIV virus within cells.

k. Ways to prevent spread of AIDS presented in Table 7–4.
l. No known cure for AIDS; treatment is drug therapy aimed at preventing replication of virus and treatment of opportunistic infections.
m. Zidovudine (formerly called *AZT*) is main drug used to prevent replication of HIV retrovirus.
n. Universal precautions are to be used by all health workers when caring for all patients.

4. Therapeutic immunosuppression is sometimes used to avoid total rejection of transplants, in the management of neoplastic growths, and in the treatment of autoimmune disorders.
5. Treatment of immune deficiency disorders depends on the degree of inadequacy of immune bodies and its primary cause.
   a. Passive immunization can provide some protection. This is accomplished through injections of human gamma globulin and transfusion of sensitized lymphocytes.
6. Nursing care is aimed at protecting the patient from infection and maintaining as high a degree of wellness as possible.

B. Excessive response: hypergammaglobulinemia, secondary to myeloma.

C. Hypersensitivity and allergy:
1. Three major groups of allergies:
   a. Delayed reaction is a cell-mediated hypersensitivity. Examples include contact dermatitis associated with cosmetics, plants, chemicals.
   b. Antigen-antibody allergy occurs when person has high titer of antibodies, particularly IgG. Examples are drug reactions and transfusion reactions.
   c. Atopic allergies affect about 10% of population. Characterized by excessive amounts of IgE antibodies. Allergens include house dust, foods, and the venom of bees and wasps.
2. In all types of allergies a reaction occurs only on second and subsequent contacts with the allergen.
3. Management of hypersensitivity and allergic reactions:
   a. Assessment: objective and subjective data summarized in Table 7–5.
      (1) Major goals are to assist with diagnosis of allergy and help patient identify particular allergen-causing problem.
      (2) Four broad types of allergens: Inhalants, contactants, ingestants, and injectables.
      (3) Skin testing to identify allergens.
      (4) Elimination diet to identify food allergens.
      (5) Identifying allergen is a slow and tedious process. Patient and family will need support and encouragement.
   b. Goals of intervention:
      (1) To help patient avoid exposure to known allergens.
         (a) Patient will need to know sources of allergens, how it comes into contact with body cells (inhalation, etc.).
         (b) Care must be taken not to make patient feel like an invalid or that his life must be completely disrupted.
      (2) To manage symptoms.
      (3) To participate in desensitization.
      (4) To provide health teaching.
4. Anaphylaxis: a serious and dramatic allergic reaction that can be fatal in a short time. Circulatory collapse can quickly lead to anaphylactic shock.

a. Treatment: administering antihistamines and epinephrine, establishing a patent airway, and providing measures to control shock.
b. Prevention: teaching hypersensitive persons how to avoid allergens, recommending identification bracelet to be worn at all times, and having person carry a kit for immediate treatment of reaction.

5. Serum sickness: delayed, generalized reaction to antigenic substances, often immunizing sera.
   a. Treatment often involves administration of antihistamines and aspirin.

D. Autoimmune disease:
   1. Body is unable to recognize its own cells as part of its "self."
   2. Primarily affects collagenous tissue.
   3. Treatment:
      a. Administration of antiinflammatory agents and nonsteroidal antiinflammatory drugs.
      b. Immunosuppression.
      c. Aspirin and other salicylates for pain.

UNIT THREE

BODY FLUIDS AND MOTION

Body fluids, which are made up of water and the substances dissolved and suspended in it, form the environment of each cell. They also move into and out of the cell, bringing in enzymes, hormones, and nutrients and taking out the end products of metabolism. The fluid in the blood and lymph vessels continually transports these substances to and from the cells. This continual movement of fluids is necessary to maintain stable or constant conditions in the internal environment. The maintenance of these constant and favorable conditions in the internal environment is called *homeostasis.*

Virtually every tissue and organ in the body takes an active part in maintaining homeostasis. Throughout this text we will be concerned with the ways in which the lungs, kidneys, intestines, and other organs work to keep the environment of the cells healthy and within safe limits. In the next two chapters we will take a closer look at the composition of body fluids, especially the electrolytes that are so essential to the life and function of each cell. And because many metabolic activities change the acidity and alkalinity of body fluids, we will also discuss the concept of acid-base balance.

The human body is designed for motion. Movement of fluids through blood and lymph vessels and into and out of each cell and its environment is essential. Lack of movement, including physical activity, exercise of the muscles, and frequent changes in posture and body position, threatens the stability of the internal environment. The effects of immobility, whatever its cause, are felt in the internal environment in a matter of hours, even in those persons who are healthy. In Chapter 9 we will discuss the impact of immobility on the major systems of the body.

CHAPTER 8

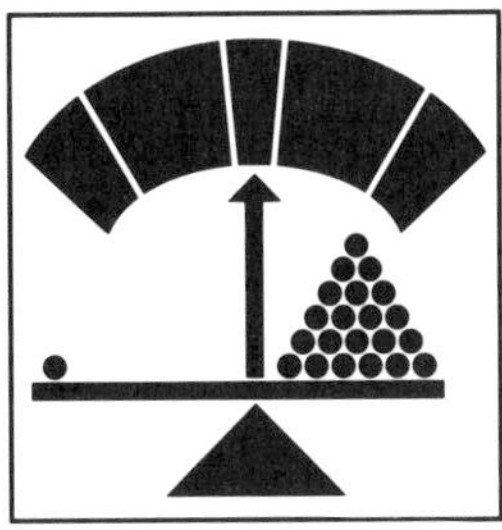

Fluid and Electrolyte Balance

VOCABULARY

acidosis
alkalosis
anions
deficit
diffusion
excess
homeostasis
hypercalcemia
hyperkalemia
hypernatremia
hypertonic
hyperventilation
hypocalcemia
hypokalemia
hyponatremia
hypotonic
hypoventilation
interstitial
isotonic
ketoacidosis
milliequivalent
osmosis
micron
turgor

Upon completion of this chapter the student should be able to:

1. List the various functions fluid performs in the body.
2. Describe three ways in which body fluids are continually being distributed among the fluid compartments.
3. Identify the relationship that exists between sodium and potassium.
4. List the major electrolytes and the function of each.
5. Describe the assessment factors for excess or deficit of sodium and potassium.
6. Prevent fluid and electrolyte imbalances in patients who are at risk.
7. Recognize the signs and symptoms of fluid and electrolyte imbalances and report them accurately.
8. State the major causes of acid-base imbalances.
9. List the major goals of nursing care of patients receiving intravenous therapy.
10. Recognize transfusion reactions and intervene appropriately when a reaction occurs.

PHYSIOLOGY

The fluid portion of the body accounts for about 56% of its total weight. The actual percentage depends on a number of factors: age, sex, nutritional status, and state of wellness. Figure 8–1 shows the differences in the average percentage of body water between the adult male and female and the infant. Throughout life there is a gradual decline in the amount of body water. The elderly and the very young are more likely to experience severe consequences with even minor changes in their fluid balance. However, persons of all ages and states of wellness need a normal fluid balance to survive.

Maintenance of body fluids within a normal range is necessary because the life processes of each cell of every organ take place in a fluid medium. The nutrients needed for life, reproduction, and the normal functioning of a cell must be dissolved or suspended in water. Moreover, the main constituent of each cell's own body is fluid. In order for all of the cell's life processes to take place there must be a continuous exchange of water, glucose, oxygen, nutrients, electrolytes, and waste products.

When a person becomes ill or suffers an injury, the symptoms he experiences are manifestations of changes within the cells and in the fluid that surrounds them. Just as the whole body cannot survive in an unhealthy and static environment, so, too, each cell requires a constant or stable and healthy environment in order to function normally.

The fluid outside each cell makes up its environment and is often called the body's *internal environment.* The term *homeostasis* is used by physiologists to refer to the maintenance of a constant or stable environment for the body's cells. Virtually every organ in the body is involved in the task of maintaining homeostasis so that the environment of every cell is essentially the same, that is homogeneous.

DISTRIBUTION OF BODY FLUIDS

FLUID COMPARTMENTS

Even though the body fluids are continually in motion—moving in and out of the blood and lymph vessels, the spaces surrounding the cells, and the bodies of the cells themselves—physi-

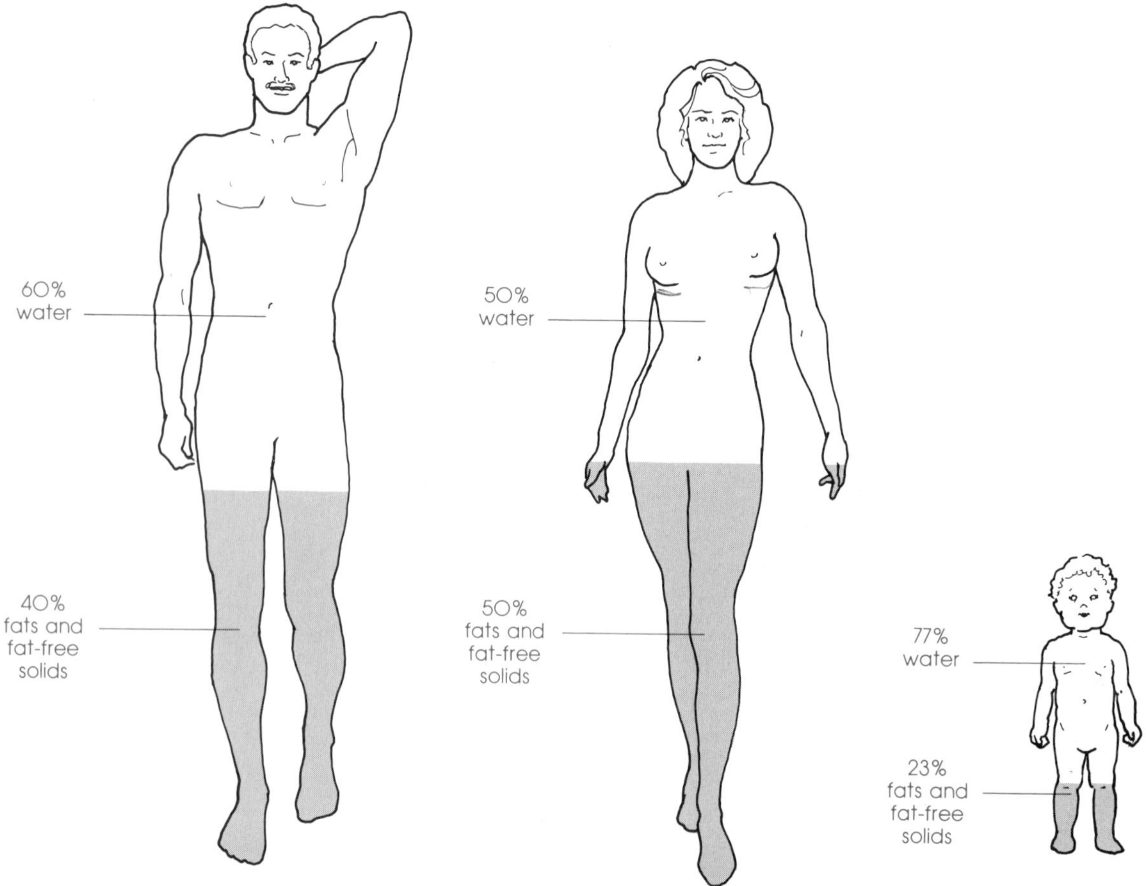

Figure 8–1 A comparison of the *average* percentage of body water in the total body weight of the adult male and female and the infant. The relationship of body water to fat varies in each person according to the amount of fatty tissue present.

ologists identify body fluid according to its location. That is, fluid within the cell is considered to be in one *compartment* and fluid outside the cell in another. As we shall see later when we discuss the composition of body fluids, fluid within the cell is not exactly the same as that which is outside the cell.

The prefix *intra-* means within; therefore, *intracellular fluid* is that which is within the cell walls. The prefix *extra-* means outside, and so *extracellular fluid* is outside the cell walls. The extracellular fluid is further divided into two other compartments. When fluid leaves a cell by passing through its outer membranes, it enters the spaces surrounding the cell. These spaces are called *interstitial spaces*, and the fluid in them is called *interstitial fluid*. When the fluid moves from these spaces into the blood and lymph vessels, it is called *intravascular fluid*.

A third major compartment for body fluids contains the so-called *transcellular fluid*. This fluid is composed of the secretions and excretions that move through the cell membranes (hence the prefix *trans-*) and eventually leave the body. Examples of transcellular fluid include urine, gastrointestinal secretions, saliva, and cerebrospinal fluid. Table 8–1 summarizes information about the fluids that are in the various compartments.

TABLE 8–1 **FLUID COMPARTMENTS**

Type of Fluid	Description
Extracellular fluid	That which is outside the cell. Constitutes the internal environment of the body. Transports water, nutrients, oxygen, waste, etc., to and from the cell.
Interstitial fluid	Extracellular fluid that is in the spaces surrounding the cell. Accounts for about 15% of total body weight.
Intravascular fluid	Extracellular fluid that is within the blood vessels. Blood cells do not normally pass in and out of the vascular compartment, and so the fluid is made up of plasma and the substances it transports. Accounts for about 5% of total body weight.
Intracellular fluid	That which is within the cell walls. Accounts for about 40% of total body weight. Most of the cell body is fluid.
Transcellular fluid	That which passes through cellular structures. Includes saliva, urine, gastrointestinal secretions, etc.

TRANSPORT OF FLUIDS AND THEIR CONSTITUENTS

The distribution and composition of body fluids depends on a dynamic movement of the fluids and the substances in them. Water and the molecules of the elements dissolved and suspended in it must move freely from one compartment to another so that they are uniformly distributed throughout the body. Many factors contribute to the continuous motion of body fluids. Among the more important are (1) the pumping action of the heart; (2) the spontaneous exchange of molecules, ions, cellular waste, and other substances *(diffusion)*; and (3) the movement of molecules of water across a semipermeable membrane *(osmosis)*.

Heart Action

The heart actually works as two pumps. One moves blood to the lungs and back to the heart through the pulmonary circulation to discard carbon dioxide and pick up a fresh supply of oxygen. The second pumping action moves blood through the general circulation to the rest of the body. As the blood moves through the large blood vessels and on to ever smaller ones, it eventually passes through the capillaries. These extremely small blood vessels are so abundantly scattered throughout the body tissues that there is not one cell that is more than 50 microns (μ) away from a capillary. (A micron is one one-thousandth of a millimeter.) Thus each cell in the body has access to the plasma in the intravascular fluid compartment once the plasma moves out of the capillary and into the interstitial spaces.

Diffusion

As the plasma moves along a capillary, large amounts of fluid pass through the large pores in the capillary walls. The fluid moves in both directions, that is, into and out of the capillaries. This movement is possible because of *kinetic motion*, which diffuses the molecules in both the intracellular fluid and the plasma. These molecules literally bounce off one another, mixing and stirring the body fluids. *Diffusion*, then, is a spontaneous mixing and moving that allows the exchange of molecules, ions, cellular nutrients, wastes, and other substances dissolved or suspended in body water. With diffusion, molecules and ions move from an area containing more particles (solute) or ions to an area where there are less. It is a process of equalization.

Osmosis

The principle of *osmosis* is related to the movement of molecules of water. The body does not tolerate differences in the concentrations (density) of fluids in the various compartments. It tends to equalize the concentrations by moving water from the less concentrated solution to the more concentrated until the solutions are of equal concentration.

In order for osmosis to occur, there must be a semipermeable membrane, that is, one that allows water and some other substances to pass through it and prohibits the passage of other substances. The membrane that makes up the cell wall is semipermeable, as are the walls of blood vessels. This is highly advantageous, of course, because such movement is essential to the survival of the cell and to the balance of water and electrolytes in the body fluids.

COMPOSITION OF BODY FLUIDS

BODY WATER

Of the two major constituents of the body fluids, water and electrolytes, water is, by far, in greater proportion and of greater importance. It is essential to normal functioning of the body because it is the medium in which the physiologic and chemical activities of the cells take place. Water serves as a vehicle for the transportation of substances to and from the cells. These include the gases oxygen and carbon dioxide, as well as the chemicals and nutrients that are used immediately by the cells and those that are stored for future use. The end products of cellular metabolism are diluted by water so that they are less injurious to the cells; they are excreted in water by the kidney.

In the body water (1) serves as a vehicle for the transportation of substances to and from the cells; (2) assists the body in heat regulation by the evaporation of perspiration; (3) helps maintain the delicate H^+ balance in the body; and (4) provides water to aid the enzymes of digestion.

ELECTROLYTES

Body fluid has been compared with sea water because both contain many of the same chemical compounds. Some of these substances remain intact and do not break up into atomic particles. Other molecules, when placed in solution, undergo a separation of their atoms into electrically charged *ions.* The electrolytes belong to the group of compounds whose molecules do break up into atomic particles that are either negatively charged *(anions)* or positively charged *(cations).* For example, when sodium chloride (table salt) is dissolved in body water, its molecules separate into sodium ions, which are positively charged (Na^+), and chloride ions, which are negatively charged (Cl^-).

The electrolytes derive their name from the fact that their atomic particles are capable of conducting an electric current. And because some are positively charged and some are negatively charged, they are chemically active. This chemical activity allows for the creation of an electrical impulse across the cell membrane, making possible the transmission of nerve impulses, contraction of muscles, and excretion of hormones and other substances from glandular cells. It is thus apparent that electrolytes are essential to the normal functioning of the body.

Although all of the electrolytes perform important functions, those of major significance to the nurse who is caring for patients with fluid and electrolyte imbalances and is concerned with maintaining normal balances are **sodium, calcium, potassium, magnesium,** *and* **phosphorus.** *There is scarcely a condition or illness that is not in some way affected by fluid and electrolyte balance.*

Sodium

Sodium is the most abundant electrolyte in *extracellular* fluid. It plays an important role in the movement of fluid back and forth between the intracellular and extracellular compartments. Sodium in the extracellular fluid is regulated by aldosterone, which is secreted by the adrenal cortex, through a feedback mechanism. Aldosterone signals the renal tubules to reabsorb sodium. As the extracellular fluid levels of sodium increase, the secretion of aldosterone decreases. Water imbalance, whether too much or too little, is always associated with sodium gain or loss. Whenever sodium is retained in the body, there will be a *retention of water* and an *increase in the extracellular volume.* That is why the intake of sodium is restricted in patients who have a heart condition, kidney disease, or liver disease in which there is retention of water in the spaces between the body cells (interstitial fluid). This condition is called *edema,* which is discussed in more detail later in this chapter.

Sodium influences the irritability of nerves and muscles and is an important factor in nerve conduction.

Calcium

Calcium does not greatly influence the movement of fluids in and out of their compartments, but it does have other functions of importance. Although about 99% of the calcium in the body is found in the bones, the remaining 1% in the blood is crucial to the normal functioning of the nerves and muscles. Calcium regulates neuromuscular activity, including that of the heart muscle. It also plays a role in the coagulation of blood and the formation of milk. Excess amounts of calcium *(hypocalcemia)* can cause cardiac arrest.

Potassium

Potassium is the most abundant electrolyte in *intracellular fluid* and is important for the maintenance of normal fluid volume within each cell and for the growth of cells. Like calcium, potassium is involved with regulating neuromuscular activity of heart, skeletal and smooth muscle. A drastic change in the level of potassium, either too much or too little, can affect the heart and bring about heart failure. Potassium also affects the hydrogen ion concentration in the blood, which is the determining factor in the maintenance of acid-base balance.

Magnesium

Magnesium in the intracellular fluid acts as a catalyst for many chemical reactions involving enzymes. It is particularly important in those reactions related to carbohydrate metabolism. In the extracellular fluid, magnesium is required for the transmission of nerve impulses, dilatation of peripheral blood vessels, and normal contractions of the heart muscle.

Phosphorus

Phosphorus is necessary for the metabolism of nutrients and is essential for the formation of bone. Intracellularly it acts as a cofactor in many enzyme systems active within the cells. Extracellularly it has a major effect on the regulation of calcium and phosphorus, and assists with acid-base balance.

Electrolyte Imbalances

Assessment and nursing interventions related to electrolyte imbalances are summarized in Table 8–2.

Nursing Diagnosis

Nursing diagnoses for problems of electrolyte imbalance are written to reflect the actual problem the imbalance is causing. For example, hypokalemia might cause muscle weakness or cardiac arrhythmias. Therefore appropriate nursing diagnoses might be:

- Impaired physical mobility related to muscle weakness.
- Decreased cardiac output related to arrhythmias.
- Self-care deficit related to muscle weakness and fatigue.

Nursing diagnoses for other electrolyte imbalances are determined in the same way. The nurse looks at the problems the imbalance causes and then formulates the nursing diagnosis.

FLUID IMBALANCES

The main source of water intake is, of course, simply the water that we drink. However, solid foods also contain water; some meats and vegetables are 60% to 97% water. The average amount of water taken in each day is about 1,500 mL as plain water or in liquids such as milk and juice; 700 mL in meats, vegetables, and fruits; and 250 mL produced during metabolism.

When it is not possible for a person to obtain an adequate intake of water through the gastrointestinal tract, fluids usually are given intravenously. It is also possible to ensure an adequate intake of fluid and nutritious elements by giving liquid feedings through a nasogastric tube.

Fluids are lost from the body through urine, feces, expired air, and perspiration. It is estimated that the internal secretions alone account for 8,200 mL of body fluid (Fig. 8–2). The total 24-hour output of fluid in urine and feces and through the lungs and skin is about 2,500 mL.

In a healthy person, balance between intake and output is maintained by drinking a sufficient amount of water each day and by having a diet that contains the essential substances needed to replace those lost through normal excretory functions. The excretion of fluids is regulated by hormonal mechanisms that affect the kidneys, lungs, and other excretory organs. The major organ involved in maintenance of fluid and electrolyte balance is the kidney, which regulates both the volume and the composition of extracellular fluid.

Illness can affect the fluid and electrolyte balance in many different ways. There may be an inability to ingest liquids or an impairment of absorption of liquids that enter the gastrointestinal tract. As expected, any illness that interferes with normal functioning of the kidney will affect fluid balance. Because circulation of fluids is important to maintenance of balance, any disease that affects circulation (e.g., congestive heart failure) will ultimately affect the distribution and composition of body fluids. Burns, in which large amounts of body fluid may be lost through the open wounds, also present problems of fluid balance. In fact, virtually every patient in a hospital is at risk for a fluid and electrolyte imbalance.

PATHOPHYSIOLOGY

A fluid imbalance exists when there is either a deficit (too little) or an excess (too much) of body water and one or more of the substances dis-

TABLE 8-2 ASSESSMENT AND NURSING INTERVENTIONS RELATED TO ELECTROLYTE IMBALANCES

Electrolyte and Imbalance	Serum Value	Risk Factors for Imbalance
SODIUM	Normal value: 135–145 mEq/L	
Hypernatremia	>147 mEq/L	Insufficient water intake, as in comatose, mentally confused, or debilitated patient. Excessive sweating, diarrhea, failure of kidney to reabsorb water from urine. Administration of high-protein, hyperosmotic tube feedings and osmotic diuretics.
Hyponatremia	<135 mEq/L	Inadequate sodium intake, as in patients on low-sodium diets. Excessive intake or retention of water (kidney failure and heart failure). Loss of bile, which is rich in sodium, as a result of fistulas, drainage, gastrointestinal surgery, and suction. Loss of sodium through burn wounds. Administration of IV fluids that do not contain electrolytes.
CALCIUM	Normal value: 4.5–5.5 mEq/L or 9–11 mg/100 mL	
Hypercalcemia	>11 mg/100 mL	Excess intake of calcium, as in taking antacids indiscriminately. Excess intake of vitamin D. Conditions that cause movement of calcium out of bones and into extracellular fluid, e.g., bone tumor, multiple fractures. Tumors of the lung, stomach, and kidney. Immobility and osteoporosis.
Hypocalcemia	<8.5 mg/100 mL	Inadequate dietary intake of calcium and vitamin D. Impaired absorption of calcium from intestinal tract, as in diarrhea, sprue, overuse of laxatives and enemas containing phosphates (phosphorus tends to be more readily absorbed from the intestinal tract than calcium and suppresses calcium retention in the body). The parathyroid regulates calcium and phosphorus levels. Hyposecretion of parathyroid hormone can result in hypocalcemia.
POTASSIUM	Normal value: 3.5–5.0 mEq/L	
Hyperkalemia	>5.5 mEq/L	Conditions that alter kidney function or decrease its ability to excrete potassium. Intestinal obstruction that prevents elimination of potassium in the feces. Addison's disease, chronic heparin therapy, lead poisoning, insulin deficit, crushing injuries, and burns.
Hypokalemia	<3.5 mEq/L	Inadequate intake of potassium-rich foods. Loss of potassium in urine when kidneys do not reabsorb the mineral. Loss of potassium from intestinal tract as a result of diarrhea or vomiting, drainage from fistulas, overuse of gastric suction. Improper use of diuretics.
MAGNESIUM	Normal value: 1.5–2.5 mEq/L	
Hypermagnesemia	>2.5 mEq/L	Overuse of antacids and cathartics containing magnesia; aspiration of sea water, as in near-drowning. Chronic kidney failure and adrenal insufficency.
Hypomagnesemia	<1.5 mEq/L	Chronic malnutrition; chronic diarrhea. Bowel resection with ileostomy or colostomy; chronic alcoholism; prolonged gastric suction; acute pancreatitis; biliary or intestinal fistula; diuretic therapy; diabetic ketoacidosis.
PHOSPHORUS	Normal value 2.5–4.5 mg/dL	
Hyperphosphatemia	>4.5 mg/dl	Occurs with renal insufficiency, hypoparathyroidism, or high phosphate intake.
Hypophosphatemia	<2.5 mg/dL	Increased urinary loss, decreased intestinal absorption, alcohol withdrawal, or diabetic ketoacidosis.

TABLE 8–2 **ASSESSMENT AND NURSING INTERVENTIONS RELATED TO ELECTROLYTE IMBALANCES** *Continued*

Subjective and Objective Data	Nursing Intervention
Dry mucous membranes, loss of skin turgor, intense thirst, flushed skin, oliguria, and possibly elevated temperature.	Encourage increased fluid intake; measure intake and output; give water between tube feedings; restrict sodium intake; monitor temperature.
Central nervous system and neuromuscular changes resulting from failure of swollen cells to transmit electrical impulses. Signs include mental confusion, altered levels of consciousness, anxiety, and coma. Muscular changes include weakness, abdominal cramping, muscle twitching, and eventually convulsions.	Restrict water intake as ordered for patients with congestive heart failure, kidney failure, and inadequate antidiuretic hormone production. Liberalize diet of patient on low-sodium diet. Closely monitor patient receiving intravenous solutions to correct hyponatremia.
Anorexia, abdominal pain, constipation, polyuria, confusion, renal calculi, pathologic fractures, cardiac arrest.	Health teaching in proper use and dose of supplemental vitamins. Encourage physical activity and weight bearing in patients with osteoporosis. Administer corticosteroids as prescribed. Administer diuretics as prescribed to increase urinary output and calcium excretion.
Muscular twitching and cramping, positive Chvostek's sign (spasm of cheek and corner of mouth in response to a tap on facial nerve in front of ear), Trousseau's sign (carpopedal spasm), convulsions, cardiac arrhythmias, cardiac arrest.	Instruct patient in careful use of laxatives, phosphate enemas, and antacids. Encourage adults to drink milk and to eat sufficient amounts of cheese, broccoli, shrimp, and other dietary sources of calcium. Have 10% calcium gluconate solution at bedside of patient having thyroid surgery in case of surgical damage to the parathyroid glands. Give all oral medicines containing calcium ½ hour before meals to facilitate absorption. Watch patients on digitalis when giving calcium solutions because their actions on the heart are similar.
Muscle weakness, hypotension, increasing and ascending paralysis leading to respiratory problems. When serum levels are more than 7 mEq/L cardiac abnormalities develop, and cardiac arrest can occur.	Monitor intravenous infusions of potassium closely; instruct patient in proper use of salt substitutes containing potassium; increase fluid intake to enhance urinary excretion of potassium; provide adequate carbohydrate intake to prevent use of body proteins for energy. Careful administration of proper dose of insulin to diabetic patients.
Abdominal pain; gaseous distention of intestines; generalized weakness; decrease or total absence of reflexes, beginning in lower extremities; cardiac arrhythmias.	Instruct patients (especially those taking diuretics) about foods high in potassium content, for example, meat, fish, fruit juices, bananas, tea, cola beverages. Observe closely for signs of digitalis toxicity in patients taking this drug. Teach patients to watch for signs of hypokalemia. Encourage patient to use potassium chloride as salt substitute.
Hypotension; sweating and flushing; respiratory depression; slow, weak pulse; cardiac arrhythmias.	Teach patients to avoid abuse of laxatives and antacids; instruct patients with renal problems to avoid over-the-counter drugs that contain magnesium. Encourage fluid intake to increase urinary excretion of magnesium.
Insomnia, hyperactive reflexes, leg and foot cramps, twitching, tremors, convulsions, positive Chvostek's sign, cardiac arrhythmias.	Diet counseling to help patients at risk increase level of magnesium to adequate level (for example, milk and cereals). Monitor closely intravenous infusions of magnesium.
Anorexia, nausea, vomiting, muscle weakness, hyperactive reflexes, tachycardia, and tetany may occur. Soft tissue calcification is common in the chronic state of hyperphosphatemia.	Check calcium levels and monitor for tetany. Monitor blood urea nitrogen and creatinine urine output, as hyperphosphatemia can interfere with kidney function.
Confusion, seizures, and neurologic abnormalities. Can cause changes in red blood cells, reducing oxygen-carrying capacity and thereby causing tissue anoxia.	Assess for restlessness, confusion, chest pain, and cyanosis. Monitor respirations. Check all electrolyte levels.

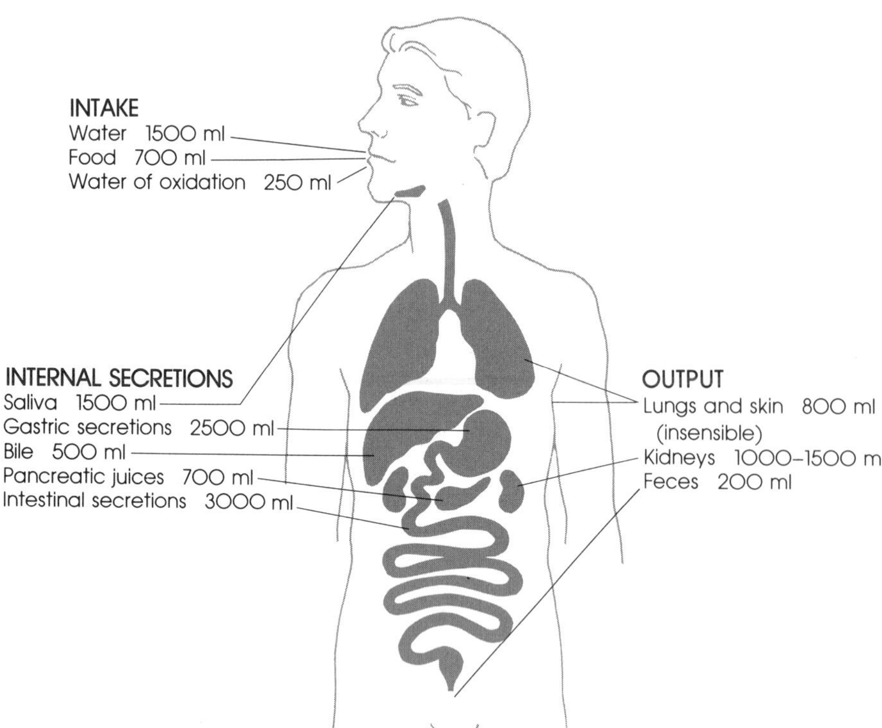

Figure 8–2 Balance between intake and output of fluid.
(Redrawn from Jacob, S. W., et al.: Structure and Function in Man, 5th ed. Philadelphia, W. B. Saunders, 1982.)

solved in it. Although it is possible for a person to suffer from an imbalance involving only one constituent of body fluids, it is more often the case that several substances are out of balance. Body water does not exist as pure water. It always has substances dissolved in it, and the concentration of these substances affects the shifting of fluid from one compartment to another and the eventual loss or retention of fluid.

Fluid Deficit

A fluid deficit occurs when there is either too little fluid taken into the body or too much lost without replacement. It is not always possible to prevent fluid deficit and dehydration, particularly in patients who are acutely ill, have undergone surgery, or suffer from kidney failure. However, many patients can be spared the harmful effects of a fluid deficit if the nurse is alert to its threat, especially to those who are most at risk. Assessment of the patient, identification of early signs of volume deficit, and appropriate nursing intervention often can prevent more serious problems of fluid imbalance.

Nursing Responsibilities in the Prevention of Fluid Deficit

Assessment. Patients most likely to suffer from fluid volume deficit that can be prevented or corrected relatively easily are (1) those who are unable to take in sufficient quantities of fluids because of difficulty in swallowing, extreme weakness, unavailability of water, confusion and disorientation, and coma; and (2) those who lose excessive amounts of fluid through prolonged vomiting, diarrhea, and copious drainage through operative wounds, burns, and fistulas.

Other factors that may contribute to fluid deficit are related to treatments for an underlying disorder, for example, the administration of diuretics and the continuous irrigation and suctioning of gastric contents.

The symptoms of fluid deficit are essentially the same as those of cellular dehydration; that is, loss of water from the cells. When there is not enough water in the plasma it becomes too concentrated, and so water is drawn out of the cells to equalize the concentrations. This causes the cells to shrivel from dehydration.

Subjective symptoms include thirst, complaints of dizziness and feeling faint upon standing up, recent history of weight loss, and weakness. Objective symptoms of fluid deficit are production of less than 20 mL of urine per hour; dark and concentrated urine; dry, cracked lips and tongue; thick, tenacious mucus that is difficult to cough up; dry, scaly skin that lacks turgor (elasticity or fullness); flat neck veins or collapse of neck veins with each inspiration of air; increased pulse rate and weak, thready pulse; and elevated temperature.

Medical Treatment and Nursing Intervention. Many times a fluid deficit occurs because the patient is unable to get a sufficient supply of water on his own, is too nauseated to keep it down, or is too confused and disoriented to recognize the need for fluids. The responsibility of the nurse in these instances is simply to provide an adequate intake for those who are unable to do this for themselves. An accurate record of intake and output must be maintained, and techniques must be employed to ensure that the patient drinks or receives sufficient fluids. Insertion of a nasogastric tube may be necessary if the patient is unable to swallow and will need continuous care over a long period of time. The newer small-bore feeding tubes, such as the Dobhoff, have allowed longer periods of enteral feeding (i.e., feeding via the gastrointestinal tract) with fewer complications such as esophageal-tracheal fistula. Many of the small-bore tubes are placed into the duodenum. Correct placement of these tubes is confirmed by radiograph. Presently there are formulas of various combinations of nutrients to meet the particular patient's nutritional needs.

Nursing interventions particular to these nasogastric tubes include ascertaining that the tube is in the proper position before beginning a feeding, checking for residual before the next feeding, irrigating the tube with 50 mL of tap water after the feeding to prevent clogging, and placing the patient in a semi-Fowler's position before beginning the feeding and for at least 30 minutes afterward.

For those patients who require only short-term feeding, intravenous therapy may be prescribed to ensure adequate fluid intake. Many times, however, intravenous administration of fluids to combat fluid deficit can be avoided through conscientious nursing care.

Included in the care plan should be the patient's preference in regard to temperature and taste of the liquids he is to drink. Some people do not like to drink ice water, whereas others do not like water that is room temperature. No one cares to drink water or any other liquid that has been left standing for a long time, nor would we expect anyone to want to drink from a water pitcher or glass that is dirty and quite possibly contaminated. The kinds of fluids that the patient drinks also should be planned. Water alone will not restore a fluid deficit. The patient also needs electrolytes and therefore should receive fruit juices, bouillon, and any other nutritious liquid he is able to tolerate.

The plan also should take into account the physical strength of the patient and his mental and emotional state. He may be totally dependent on the nurse to assist him in drinking the fluids he needs to avoid dehydration, or he may not fully understand the importance of an adequate fluid intake. (See Nursing Care Plan 8–1.)

If the patient's problem is not inadequate intake, but rather excessive loss of fluids, the nursing care is directed toward helping the patient cope with the specific condition that is contributing to a fluid imbalance. A frequent cause of excessive loss of fluids is abnormally rapid exretion of intestinal fluids, such as that which occurs in vomiting and diarrhea.

The Patient With Nausea and Vomiting

Nausea is a feeling of discomfort or an unpleasant sensation vaguely felt in the epigastrium and abdomen. It is accompanied by a tendency to vomit. Nausea usually is experienced when nerve endings in the stomach and other parts of the body are irritated. Usually the irritated nerve endings in the stomach send messages to the part of the brain that controls the vomiting reflex, but nerve cells in other parts of the body can trigger the same response. An example is intense pain in any part of the body. Pain can trigger the nausea-vomiting mechanism. The nausea and vomiting are an automatic response of the involuntary autonomic nervous system to unpleasant stimuli.

The *causes* of nausea and vomiting are many and varied. They include gastrointestinal irrigation from foods, viruses, radiation, and some drugs and other chemicals; certain types of anesthetics; and pregnancy.

Assessment. Subjective data indicating nausea and vomiting include complaints of nausea or feeling "sick to my stomach," queasiness, abdominal pain, epigastric discomfort or burning, and a history of vomiting. Objective data include pallor; mild diaphoresis; cold, clammy skin; excessive salivation; and attempts to remain quiet and motionless. If vomiting occurs, the vomitus should be observed for odor, color, contents (for example, undigested food), and amount. Noting and recording vomiting patterns, conditions that trigger vomiting, and quality of nausea as described by the patient can be helpful in planning treatment.

Medical Treatment and Nursing Intervention. Medical treatment most often consists of administration of one of the antiemetic drugs. These drugs usually are given to depress the vomiting reflex. Many also have a tranquilizing effect. Some must be used with caution, however, because they can produce oversedation and a lowering of blood pressure.

Antihistamines, sedatives and hypnotics, anticholinergics, phenothiazines, and other drugs have all been used to control nausea and vomiting. The variety of drugs that are tried attests to the difficulty of controlling nausea and vomiting, especially when these symptoms accompany long-term conditions that are themselves difficult to manage.

Nursing intervention during an episode of vomiting includes having the patient lie down and turn his head to one side so that vomitus is

NURSING CARE PLAN 8–1

Selected nursing diagnoses, goals/outcome criteria, nursing interventions, and evaluations for a patient with fluid volume deficit

Situation: A 79-year-old female is admitted to the hospital with a fractured femur. She is confused, disoriented, unable to feed herself, and extremely weak.

Nursing Diagnosis	Goals/Outcome Criteria	Nursing Intervention	Evaluation
Fluid volume deficit related to weakness, confusion, and lack of fluid intake. SUPPORTING DATA Found on floor at home 7 hours after injury; no oral intake for 11 hours. Too weak to drink by herself; 200 mL intake last shift.	The patient will have a normal fluid balance as evidenced by: 1. Normal skin turgor. 2. Moist mucous membranes. 3. B/P and pulse in normal range, stable with position change. 4. Balanced intake and output. 5. Urine specific gravity between 1.010 and 1.030.	Assess skin turgor and mucous membranes q shift. Measure specific gravity q 24 h. Record accurate intake and output. Offer fruit juices in small quantities totaling 8 oz. q 3 h. Offer sips of tap water in between juice. Give mouth care q 2 h. Apply lubricant to lips prn. Offer hard candy q 2 to 3 hr while awake to stimulate flow of saliva; stay with patient while candy is in mouth.	Taking 2 oz. of fluid per hour. Mucous membranes not as dry. Intake this shift, 495 mL; output, 320 mL. Urine specific gravity, 1.036. Patient improved; continue plan.

not aspirated into the respiratory tract. An emesis basin is held close to the side of the face. A cool, damp wash cloth can be used to wipe the patient's face and back of neck. After the episode is over, the patient may appreciate a mouthwash or cold water to rinse the mouth. Ice chips help reduce nausea in some patients.

Patients who are nauseated should be in a quiet, cool, odor-free environment. Physical activity and ingestion of food can trigger further attacks of vomiting. When a patient is able to resume eating and drinking, small meals of cold drinks and foods can be gradually added to his intake. Carbonated drinks are usually tolerated well at first. Foods and drinks that do not have a strong odor are less likely to bring on nausea and another episode of vomiting. Frequent oral hygiene is a must for patients who have prolonged periods of nausea.

If nausea and vomiting persist, the patient must be watched for early signs of dehydration. In some cases intravenous therapy is indicated to replace fluids and nutrients that have been lost because of vomiting and cannot be replaced because of nausea.

The Patient With Diarrhea

Diarrhea is defined as the rapid movement of fecal matter through the intestine. It results in poor absorption of water, nutritive elements, and electrolytes. These substances, especially the potassium needed by the body to prevent acidosis, are lost in large amounts.

Major *causes* of diarrhea are related to local irritation of the intestinal mucosa, especially that caused by infectious agents, such as *Salmonella* and *Escherichia coli*, and chemicals. Chronic and prolonged diarrhea is typical of such disorders as ulcerative colitis, irritable bowel syndrome, allergies, and nontropical sprue. Obstruction to the flow of intestinal contents, as from a tumor or a fecal impaction, also can produce diarrhea.

Assessment. The most outstanding subjective symptoms of diarrhea are a history of frequent bowel movements, abdominal cramping, and general weakness. Objective signs include frequent and watery stools that often contain mucus and are blood-streaked. It is the consistency rather than the number per day that is the hallmark of diarrhea. In some cases the number can be as high as 15 to 20 liquid stools. If the condition is chronic, the patient can suffer from anemia, malnutrition, and dehydration. Diarrhea is usually the result of increased peristaltic activity; hence bowel sounds heard through a stethoscope are likely to be loud gurgling and tinkling sounds that come in waves *(borborygmi)*.

In the assessment of diarrhea the nurse should clarify what the patient and family mean by diarrhea when they report this during an interview. For some people more than one stool a day constitutes diarrhea. When a nurse has direct responsibility for the care of a patient with diarrhea, she must note and record the number of stools during her shift and the characteristics of each stool, that is, color, consistency, unusual contents (for example, blood or mucus), any peculiar odor, and associated pain.

Medical Treatment and Nursing Intervention. The strength of the patient with diarrhea is rapidly spent. Nursing measures should be aimed at providing physical and mental rest, preventing unnecessary loss of water and nutrients, and eventually replacing fluids. Diarrhea is a symptom, rather than a disease, and it sometimes requires extensive testing to determine its cause. The nurse will need to explain the purpose of these tests to the patient, enlist his cooperation, and give him the support he needs to endure what could be trying and exhausting procedures.

In acute diarrhea the stomach and intestines are rested by limiting the intake of foods. The patient should avoid iced fluids, carbonated drinks, whole milk, roughage, raw fruits, and highly seasoned foods. Once oral feedings are allowed, they usually start with clear liquids and progress to bland liquids and then solid foods with increased calories, high protein, and high carbohydrate content.

Diarrhea can be and often is associated with nervous tension and anxiety. The patient often is embarrassed by his condition and inconvenienced by frequent trips to the bathroom or the need to request a bedpan. This emotional stress only serves to aggravate the condition and make it worse. The nurse can help break the vicious cycle by maintaining a calm and dignified manner, accepting and understanding the patient's behavior, and providing privacy and a restful environment for him.

An important goal in a plan of care for a patient with diarrhea is a return to normal patterns of bowel elimination. Other goals might be (1) fewer reports of abdominal cramping, (2) maintenance of the integrity of the skin around the anus, (3) adequate nutrition, (4) restoration and maintenance of fluid and electrolyte balance, (5) reduction of stress and tension through relaxation techniques, and (6) sufficient rest. If diet therapy is used to treat, minimize, or prevent a problem of chronic diarrhea, a major goal would be that the patient follow the prescribed dietary regimen.

Medications prescribed for diarrhea depend on the cause of the disorder and the length of time the condition has been present. Mild cases usually respond well to kaolin and bismuth preparations, (e.g., Kaopectate), which coat the intestinal tract and make the stools more firm. Antispasmodic drugs such as belladonna or paregoric reduce the number of stools by decreasing the peristaltic rate and relaxing the intestinal musculature. Bismuth subsalicylate (Pepto-Bismol) is helpful in that it soothes the mucosa and binds water. It is the recommended treatment for "traveler's diarrhea" and can also be used for prevention of this type of diarrhea. Codeine, diphenoxylate (Lomotil), or loperamide (Imodium) are useful for decreasing the peristaltic action that causes the frequency of stools. If the patient with diarrhea shows signs of nervous tension and anxiety, sedatives or tranquilizers may be prescribed. Diarrhea that is caused by infections may be treated with drugs that are specific for the causative organism.

Patients With Fluid Deficits From Other Causes

The improper use of gastric suction can rapidly deplete the level of body fluids. It is estimated that as much as 2,500 mL of gastric fluid and 1,500 mL of saliva can be removed from the body in a 24-hour period when there is continuous gastric suction.

It is essential, then, that an accurate record be kept of the amount of drainage removed by suction so that these fluids can be replaced and dehydration avoided.

Drainage fistulas and abscesses also can produce fluid deficit. These conditions require careful observation of the patient for signs of a fluid and electrolyte imbalance. An accurate recording of intake and output is essential, even though the amount of fluid lost by drainage onto dressings can only be estimated. One way in which estimates can be made with greater accuracy is to record *every* dressing change that is needed to keep the patient dry and comfortable.

Burn patients lose body fluids through the open wounds in the skin. To compensate for this loss, there is a shifting of fluids from one compartment to another. First the fluid leaves the plasma and moves into the interstitial spaces. Later the fluid moves in the opposite direction. These patients require careful monitoring of their fluid and electrolyte levels to avoid the serious consequences of fluid shift and fluid deficit. Burns are discussed more fully in Chapter 33.

Nursing Diagnosis

Nursing diagnoses for patients with fluid volume deficit could be:

- Fluid volume deficit related to loss of body fluids or electrolytes.
- Potential fluid volume deficit related to diarrhea.
- Potential fluid volume deficit related to nausea and vomiting.

Fluid Excess

An excessive amount of *body water* usually occurs first in the extracellular compartment, because the water enters and leaves the body from this compartment. When it is ingested or inhaled, water quickly moves into the circulatory system or intravascular compartment. When it is administered intravenously, it goes directly into the intravascular compartment.

Normally, an excess of water alone is not a problem. Healthy persons do not ordinarily drink too much water. When they become ill, however, they may take in more water than they excrete. This can happen if they receive too rapid an infusion of intravenous fluids, are given tap water enemas, or are persuaded to drink more fluids than they eliminate. The last situation can occur when there is inaccurate and inconsistent measurement of intake and output. When any of these conditions is present, the patient is likely to suffer from *water intoxication*.

A more common fluid imbalance is associated with the retention of water, sodium, and chloride, which produces *edema*. Edema is defined as an accumulation of freely moving interstitial fluid, that is, fluid in the spaces surrounding the cell. Edema also can occur in body cavities, as in the peritoneal cavity (ascites) and the cranial cavity. The accumulation of body fluids can affect almost all of the tissue spaces, in which case it is known as *generalized edema*, or it can affect a limited area, in which case it is called *localized edema*. Whenever sodium is retained in the body, there also is water retention. *Generalized edema* occurs when the body's mechanisms for eliminating excess sodium fail. The sodium, along with water, accumulates in the body. It becomes life-threatening when it overloads the circulatory system, as in congestive heart failure, and when it involves the lungs, as in pulmonary edema.

Generalized edema can occur as a result of (1) kidney failure and a resulting retention of sodium and water, (2) inadequate circulation of blood through the general circulation (heart failure) or through the portal circulation (liver failure), and (3) hormonal disorders. Hormonal disorders involve the overproduction of aldosterone and antidiuretic hormone (ADH). Thus the administration of large doses of hormones from the adrenal cortex (i.e., the adrenocortical hormones) may have a similar effect. Malnutrition, hypoalbuminemia, and anemia also can produce a generalized nonspecific edema.

Localized edema can be a sign of inflammation and increased permeability of the capillaries. This allows for the flow of unusual amounts of fluid out of the capillaries and into the tissue spaces. Localized edema usually is nonpitting, does not come and go, and is characterized by tight, shiny skin that is stretched over a hard and red area. Causes of localized edema include trauma, allergies, burns, obstruction of lymph flow, and liver failure.

Dependent edema is noted in the feet, ankles, and lower legs or in the sacral region of patients confined to bed or chair. It is an effect of gravity and therefore can be somewhat relieved by elevating the affected part when possible and repositioning the patient frequently.

Nursing Responsibilities in the Care of Patients With Fluid Excess

Assessment. Subjective and objective symptoms of fluid excess will depend on the kind of edema present, its location, its severity, and the extent of fluid shift from the plasma into the tissue spaces. The history given by the patient can be very significant. For example, consider the patient who states that he must sleep on several pillows or sitting up in a chair to breathe comfortably. Patients who have excess fluid trapped within a body cavity (for example, the abdominal cavity) will suffer from the effects of pressure against the abdominal and thoracic organs. The assessment of patients with specific kinds of edema is discussed in more detail in appropriate chapters.

If there is a possibility that fluid is seeping into the abdominal cavity forming *ascites*, the nurse should measure abdominal girth. Once every 24 hours, measure the abdomen at the level of the umbilicus. Mark where the tape is centered at the sides of the patient so that the next person will measure in exactly the same place. Chart the measurement.

An objective measure of water excess and circulatory overload is the hematocrit. This is a measurement of the volume percentage of red blood cells in whole blood. Normal hematocrit values range from 35 to 54 mL of red blood cells per 100 mL of whole blood, depending on age and sex. If there is an excess of water, the proportion of red blood cells to milliliters of blood will be lower, and the hematocrit will be below the normal values.

"Pitting edema" is common in patients with dependent edema. The name is derived from the fact that a pit or depression can be created by pressing a fingertip against the swollen tissue. To check for pitting edema the thumb is pressed into the patient's skin at a bony prominence, such as the tibia or malleolus, and held for 5 to 10 seconds. If the depression or "pit" remains for a while after the pressure is released, the patient has pitting edema. Assessment of the severity and progress of pitting edema in the feet and ankles (pedal edema) can be made more accurately by estimating the depth of tissue depression (Fig. 8-3).

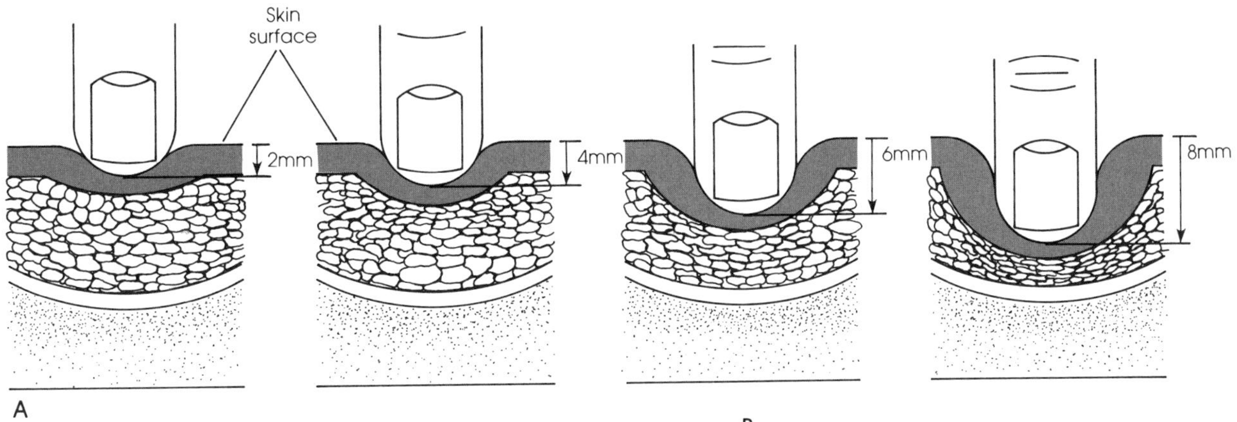

Figure 8–3 *A,* One method for a relatively accurate measurement of the progress of a patient with pedal edema is gently pressing the tissue and estimating the depth of tissue depression in millimeters. *B,* The progress of edema in the lower extremities can be assessed by using a measuring tape to measure in inches the circumference of the ankle or calf.

Ambulatory patients may say that their edema of the feet and ankles gets worse during the day but goes down at night. However, they also report an increasing need to get up during the night to urinate. This nocturia occurs because the fluid in the lower extremities is drained off during the night when the patient is lying down. The fluid is then excreted as urine.

The sacral region and buttocks of bedridden patients should be checked frequently for signs of edema. Frequent changes of position can help prevent accumulations in one area. For the patient who is able to sit up, exercises of the legs increase circulation, and periodic elevation of the feet and legs promotes removal of the excess fluid by the blood and lymph vessels. Lightweight elastic stockings, available from the hospital physical therapy department or a surgical supply house, can be used to counteract edema formation.

A common sign of edema, other than obvious swelling, is weight gain. Water is heavy, and therefore an accumulation of water in the tissues causes a gain in body weight. The physician usually requests that the patient be weighed daily when edema is present so that he or she can determine the amount of body fluid being lost or retained.

When daily weight measurement is indicated, the nurse must be careful to obtain as accurate a reading on the scales as possible. Ideally, the patient is weighed before breakfast and at exactly the same time every day. The same scales are used at each weighing, and the patient should be wearing the same type of clothing. *The loss or gain of 1 or 2 pounds of body weight can be quite significant in the course of a patient's illness.* For every pound of weight that is lost, about 1 pint (500 mL) of excess fluid is discarded.

Another symptom of fluid retention can be decreased urinary output. An accurate record must be kept of the fluid intake and output of the edematous patient. The intake reflects all fluids taken into the body, whether orally, intravenously, or any other way. Output includes all urine, vomitus, watery stools, and unusual sweating. Recording these measurements is a nursing responsibility and should not be delayed until a physician's order is written for an intake and output record.

Medical Treatment and Nursing Intervention. Strange as it may seem, edematous patients can suffer from dehydration. The fluid that has accumulated in one of the body cavities is trapped there and is therefore not available to other parts of the body. If the patient develops signs of dehydration, this should be reported immediately. The physician will assess the need for additional fluids and the method by which they are to be provided.

Sometimes the patient's fluid intake is *restricted* to a certain amount within a 24-hour period. The nursing care plan must then include a schedule of fluid intake arranged so that liquids are spaced evenly and the patient does *not* receive all of the allowed liquids in a short period of time, leaving many hours before he can again have something to drink. If they are not prohibited, hard candies and chewing gum can help relieve thirst. Frequent mouth care is essential.

Skin care is especially important in preventing a breakdown over the area of edema. The skin covering the edematous areas is extremely fragile. It has a decreased blood supply and is stretched beyond its normal limits so that it is no longer flexible. Care must be taken to preserve the skin as much as possible. Bed linens are kept dry and smooth, and the patient is turned frequently to relieve the pressure of the body's weight on susceptible areas. In turning and moving the patient, it is necessary to be as gentle as possible and to avoid friction against the skin. A break or abrasion of edematous skin can very rapidly develop into a decubitus ulcer. The use of a turning sheet for repositioning helps prevent abrasions from the sheets.

Because sodium retention is invariably accompanied by water retention, the patient with edema is placed on a low-sodium diet. Table salt is not allowed, and special attention must be paid to all foods and liquids consumed by the patient. There are many hidden sources of sodium in foods in their natural state as well as in those that are commercially prepared. The edematous patient should avoid any salted "snack" foods, delicatessen foods, preserved meats, all cheeses, dried fruits, canned soups and vegetables, and any foods preserved in brine.

Occasionally it is necessary for patients with edema to receive intravenous fluids. The administration of these fluids must be carefully monitored, particularly if the patient has or is likely to develop pulmonary edema. An infusion pump is used to prevent too much fluid from accidentally being infused over any one period of time. The nurse must still check on the IV frequently to see that is is patent and that the pump is functioning properly. Diuretics also are commonly prescribed for the control of generalized edema, especially when it is a manifestation of congestive heart failure.

When a patient with edema is to be discharged from the hospital, he should be instructed in the ways in which he can participate in the management of his illness, the control of his symptoms, and the prevention of complications.

Some outcome criteria that might be used for a patient with water and sodium retention related to congestive heart failure and those suitable for a patient with postmastectomy swelling are shown in Table 8–3.

Nursing Diagnosis

Some nursing diagnoses that may be appropriate for patients with fluid excess are:

- Fluid volume excess related to excessive fluid or sodium intake.
- Fluid volume excess related to compromised regulatory mechanisms.
- Fluid volume excess related to low protein intake or low serum protein levels.
- Potential fluid volume excess related to decreased heart function.
- Potential fluid volume excess related to decreased excretion by failing kidneys.

HYDROGEN ION CONCENTRATION (ACID-BASE BALANCE)

In order to understand the concept of acid-base balance and how it is maintained in the body fluids, one should be familiar with some basic facts about biochemistry and the terms commonly used in discussions of hydrogen ion concentration. These are summarized below.

Some of the more important facts about acid-base balance are:

- An acid is defined as a substance capable of giving up a hydrogen ion during chemical exchange.
- A base is a substance capable of accepting a hydrogen ion.
- Acids react with bases to form water and a salt.
- A reaction of an acid and a base to form water and a salt is a *neutralization* reaction, because both the acid and the base are neutralized.
- Acids react with carbonates and bicarbonates to form carbon dioxide gas.
- The term *pH* refers to the concentration of hydrogen (H) in a solution. The *p* represents a *negative* logarithm, which is an inverse proportion. Thus the higher the concentration of hydrogen ions in a solution, the lower the pH. A higher pH indicates the opposite, that is, a lower concentration of hydrogen ions.
- A chemically neutral solution has a pH of 7.00.
- The pH of the body's fluids is normally somewhat alkaline (between 7.35 and 7.45).
- A pH above 7.8 *(alkalosis)* or a pH below 6.8 *(acidosis)* usually is fatal.

TABLE 8-3 GOALS/OUTCOME CRITERIA FOR EVALUATING NURSING INTERVENTIONS TO MANAGE DIFFERENT TYPES OF EDEMA

Nursing Diagnosis	Goals/Outcome Criteria
Fluid volume excess related to inadequate heart action and resultant edema.	No evidence of skin breakdown. Lungs clear on radiograph and auscultation. Intake is balanced with output. Body weight returned to normal and maintained with no more than ½ lb. fluctuation.
Potential fluid volume excess related to surgical trauma of lymphatic system from radical mastectomy.	Minimal edema evident 24 hours after surgery and at discharge. Performs active range-of-motion exercises 24 hours after surgery. Able to perform postoperative exercises with affected arm by tenth postoperative day. At discharge can verbalize the "do's and don'ts" of arm and hand care that will help prevent lymphedema. Minimal edema present after wound is healed.

- A blood pH of 7.4 indicates a ratio of 1 part carbonic acid to 20 parts base bicarbonate.
- *Acidosis* is the result of either a loss of base or an accumulation of acid.
- *Alkalosis* is the result of either a loss of acid or an accumulation of base. (See Fig. 8-4 for an easy way to interpret blood gases.)

PATHOPHYSIOLOGY

Most of the body's metabolic activities produce carbon dioxide gas, which moves from the tissues into the blood, where it combines with water to form carbonic acid. The body deals with this constant manufacture of acid in a number of ways so that the ratio of carbonic acid to bicarbonate can be maintained and an alkaline environment provided for normal cellular activities. If the ratio is not maintained, the acid-base balance is upset. The pH will either fall below the normal range and acidosis will occur, or it will rise above normal range and alkalosis will be present (Fig. 8-5).

In general, there are two main types of mechanisms by which the pH is controlled: those concerned with respiration and those concerned with metabolism. As long as the ratio of carbonic acid to bicarbonate is maintained at 1:20, the pH remains within normal limits.

There are, therefore, four possible states of an acid-base imbalance: (1) respiratory acidosis, (2) respiratory alkalosis, (3) metabolic acidosis, and (4) metabolic alkalosis.

The progression of each of the four types of acid-base problems is depicted in Figure 8-6. The role played by the lungs in a respiratory imbalance is concerned with the "blowing off" or excretion of carbon dioxide (CO_2). In *hypoventilation*, the lungs do not eliminate enough CO_2, and it remains in the body, unites with water,

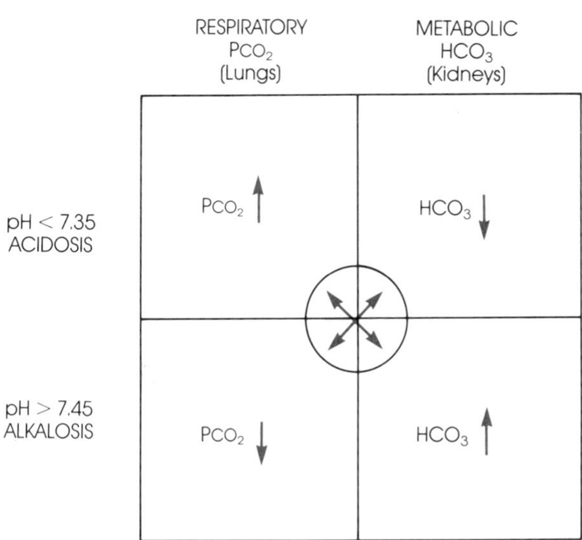

Figure 8-4 The boxes illustrate the four basic acid-base imbalances. The top left is respiratory acidosis, and the top right is metabolic acidosis; the bottom left is respiratory alkalosis, and the bottom right is metabolic alkalosis. The arrows show in which direction the components deviate from normal. The inner circle represents how the other system compensates for the primary abnormality.

(Courtesy of Kathleen M. White, RN, MS, CCRN.)

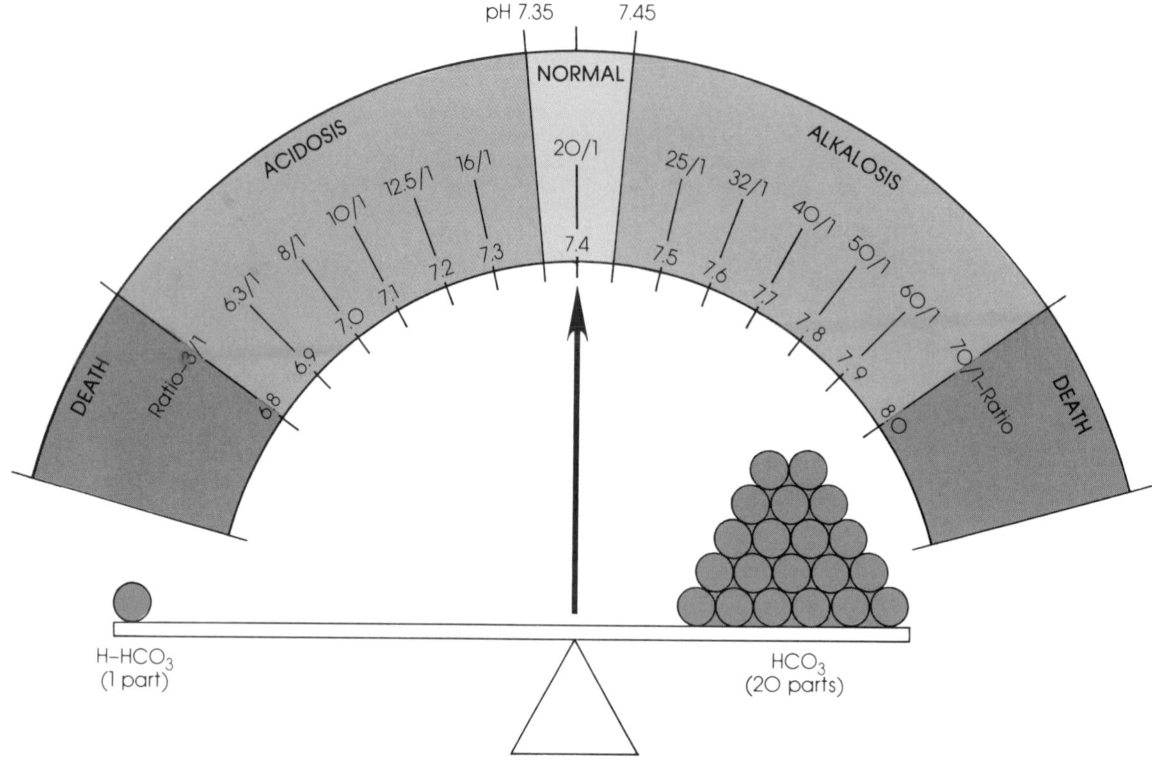

Figure 8-5 Acidosis and alkalosis. The narrow range of normal pH and the ratio of carbonic acid to bicarbonate ions are shown, along with the pH for states of alkalosis and acidosis. The ratio of one carbonic acid (H—HCO_3) molecule to 20 bicarbonate ions (HCO_3) is shown balanced on a fulcrum. Note that within the scale the number of bicarbonate ions in proportion to carbonic acid diminishes with acidosis and increases with alkalosis.

(From Jacob, S. W., et al.: Structure and Function in Man, 5th ed. Philadelphia, W. B. Saunders, 1982.)

and forms carbonic acid. The opposite is *hyperventilation*, in which too much CO_2 is excreted.

The kidneys are the principal organs of control in maintaining a normal pH during *metabolic* activities, because they either reabsorb or excrete bicarbonate. If they eliminate too much bicarbonate, acidosis will develop. Conversely, if they fail to eliminate enough bicarbonate and allow it to be reabsorbed into the blood stream, alkalosis will develop.

The last column of Figure 8-6 provides a brief summary of the body's attempts to compensate for an acid-base imbalance. In the presence of respiratory acidosis, the kidneys will retain and manufacture more bicarbonate than normal so that it is available for neutralization of the excess acid. However, this is a slow process that takes from a few hours to several days. In the presence of respiratory alkalosis, the kidneys will increase their excretion of bicarbonate. In response to metabolic acidosis, the patient will involuntarily hyperventilate in order to remove carbon dioxide so that it is not available for the production of carbonic acid. Should metabolic alkalosis develop, the patient will hypoventilate to retain the supply of carbon dioxide.

The foregoing information on acid-base balance, hydrogen ion concentration, and the carbon dioxide-bicarbonate ratio does not represent an in-depth explanation. Many complex chemical activities are involved in the maintenance of an internal environment that must be slightly alkaline for normal body function. For a more thorough study of the subject, the reader is referred to the bibliography at the end of this chapter.

It is important, however, that the nurse have some appreciation of the reasons for various metabolic and respiratory illnesses that are related to either acidosis or alkalosis. With an understanding of the rationale of medical management, the nurse will be better able to plan nursing care that is coordinated with and supportive of medical care. In the following pages, we will describe the kinds of acid-base problems patients are likely to encounter and discuss ways in which the nurse might help patients cope with these problems. Because acidosis and alkalosis are common to a great variety of medical and surgical conditions of illness, the chapters on specific illnesses will frequently refer to problems of this kind.

ARTERIAL BLOOD GAS ANALYSIS

Studies of the percentages of gases (oxygen and carbon dioxide) in the blood and the hydrogen ion concentration (pH) are useful in assessing the

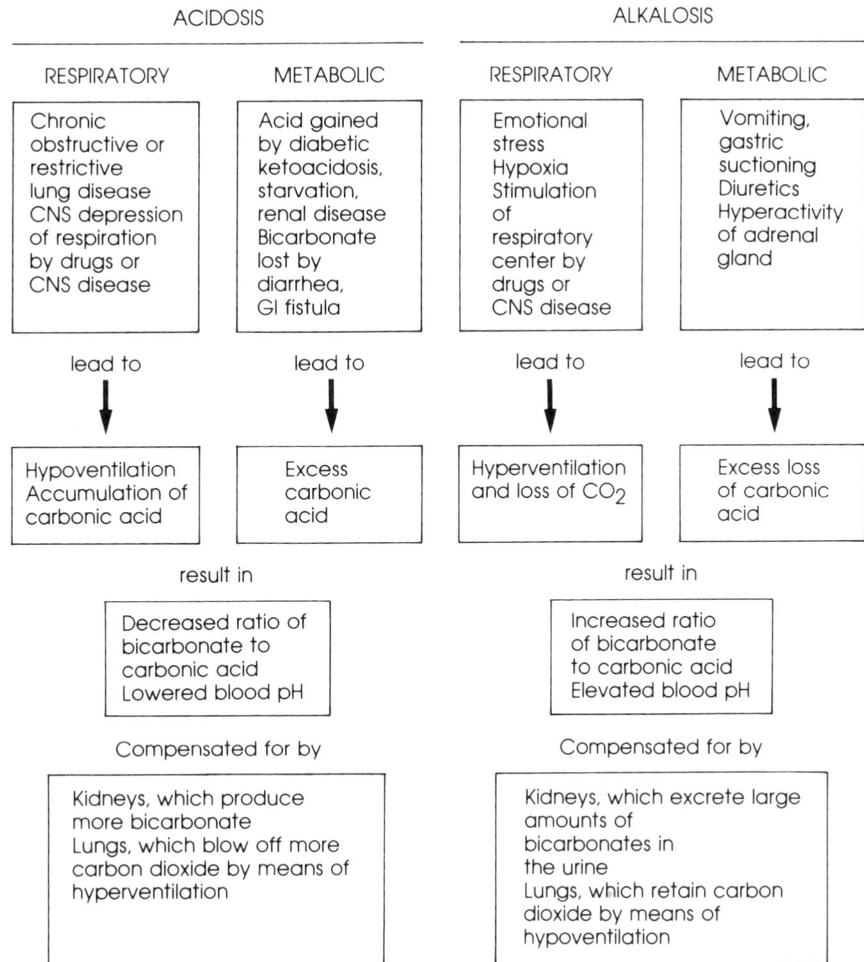

Figure 8-6 Causes, physiologic effects, and compensatory mechanisms in acidosis and alkalosis.

status of both respiratory and metabolic acid-base imbalances. They do not detect disease or distinguish the specific cause of the imbalance, but blood gas studies are valuable indicators of a patient's progress toward recovery or lack of it. They reflect the ability of the lungs to exchange oxygen and carbon dioxide, the effectiveness of the kidneys in balancing retention and elimination of bicarbonate, and the effectiveness of the heart as a pump.

The results of analyses of arterial blood gases (ABGs) are reported as follows:

- PaO_2—partial pressure (P) exerted by oxygen (O_2) in the arterial blood (a). Normal value is 75 to 100 mm Hg.
- $PaCO_2$—partial pressure of carbon dioxide in the arterial blood. Normal value is 35 to 45 mm Hg.
- pH—an expression of the extent to which the blood is alkaline or acid. Normal value is 7.35 to 7.45.
- SaO_2 (also abbreviated O_2Sat)—percentage of available hemoglobin that is saturated with oxygen, that is, combined to the total amount of oxygen the hemoglobin can carry. Normal value is 94% to 100%.
- HCO_3—the level of plasma bicarbonate; an indicator of the metabolic acid-base status. Normal value is 22 to 26 mEq/L.
- Base excess or deficit—indicates the amount of blood buffer present. Alkalosis is present when this value is abnormally high. Abnormally low values indicate acidosis. Measured in "+" or "−".

RESPIRATORY ACIDOSIS

Assessment

Patients most likely to suffer from respiratory acidosis are, of course, those whose respiratory functions are impaired so that the lungs are unable to remove sufficient amounts of carbon dioxide. *Acute* respiratory acidosis develops suddenly and occurs when an airway obstruction, acute respiratory infection, or acute pulmonary edema interferes with the normal exchange of oxygen and carbon dioxide, with a resulting accumulation of carbon dioxide in the blood.

Chronic respiratory acidosis is a slower process that accompanies the gradual loss of pulmonary function. The most common condition in which this is likely to occur is chronic obstructive pulmonary disease (COPD). This condition is explained in more detail in Chapter 17. A patient with COPD is most likely to develop acute acidosis when an infection of the respiratory tract further impairs his breathing capacity and the removal of carbon dioxide.

Subjective symptoms of respiratory acidosis include complaints of increasing difficulty in breathing, a history of respiratory obstruction (acute or chronic), weakness, dizziness, restlessness, sleepiness, and change in mental alertness. Objective data include increased levels of carbon dioxide in the blood, dyspnea, and obvious respiratory problems. Laboratory test results will show a blood pH of less than 7.35 and a PCO_2 above 45 mm Hg.

Nursing Diagnosis

Nursing diagnoses appropriate for the patient experiencing respiratory acidosis are:

- Impaired gas exchange related to airway obstruction, bronchoconstriction, acute respiratory infection, or pulmonary edema.
- Impaired gas exchange related to carbon dioxide retention secondary to COPD.

Medical Treatment and Nursing Intervention

The initial treatment for respiratory acidosis is immediate establishment of an airway if airway obstruction is at fault. This may involve the insertion of an endotracheal tube or a tracheostomy. Adequate ventilation is maintained through the administration of oxygen and possibly artificial ventilation using a ventilating machine. Conservative treatment in other patients is by intermittent positive-pressure breathing (IPPB) treatments, postural drainage, bronchodilators, or antibiotics if indicated.

Care must be taken in the administration of certain drugs that depress the respiratory center. These would include narcotics, hypnotics, and tranquilizers.

In patients with COPD, the respiratory drive mechanism is altered, and oxygen can act as a respiratory depressant. Oxygen should be administered with great care to these patients, because it can cause respiratory arrest.

Oxygen should be administered at a rate of 2 to 3 L per minute only in patients known to have chronic pulmonary disease. If a patient's history is unknown, oxygen is begun at a rate of 2 to 3 L per minute until it is determined that he can tolerate a higher flow rate.

The patient must be watched closely for respiratory and cardiac arrest. Should either occur, it will be necessary to maintain respiration and circulation artificially through cardiopulmonary resuscitation.

RESPIRATORY ALKALOSIS

Assessment

Respiratory alkalosis arises when hyperventilation results in excessive loss of carbon dioxide from the lungs. Patients hyperventilate for a variety of reasons; these include hypoxemia (insufficiency of oxygen, which triggers an automatic increase in respiration), fever, early stages of salicylate poisoning, reactions to certain drugs, pain, anxiety, and hysteria. The overzealous use of ventilating machines also can cause hyperventilation with too much CO_2 blown off.

Symptoms of respiratory alkalosis include deep, rapid breathing, tingling of the fingers, pallor around the mouth, dizziness, and spasms of the muscles of the hands. The pH will be greater than 7.45 with a PCO_2 less than 35.

Nursing Diagnosis

A nursing diagnosis appropriate for the patient experiencing respiratory alkalosis is:

- Ineffective breathing pattern related to hyperventilation.

Medical Treatment and Nursing Intervention

If the underlying cause of respiratory alkalosis is hysteria, treatment is aimed at preventing further hyperventilation and helping the patient reestablish a normal level of carbon dioxide in his blood. Sedatives may be given to calm the patient. To aid in the retention of carbon dioxide, the patient may be instructed to hold his breath or to breathe into a paper sack and rebreathe the carbon dioxide he has just exhaled. This recycling of the carbon dioxide can eventually restore normal carbonic acid levels in the blood.

Patients who develop respiratory alkalosis from causes other than hysteria or overzealous use of a ventilator will require treatment of the primary illness. If the cause is anxiety, a sedative may be given.

METABOLIC ACIDOSIS

Assessment

The usual causes of metabolic acidosis are (1) excessive burning of fats, such as occurs (a) when a diabetic patient does not metabolize carbohydrates because of insulin insufficiency and instead burns fat, the end products of which are fatty acids; and (b) in persons on low-carbohydrate, high-fat diets to lose weight; (2) abnormal carbohydrate metabolism in which, in the absence of oxygen, lactic acid accumulates in the blood; (3) failure of the kidneys to reabsorb bicarbonate; and (4) loss of bicarbonate through diarrhea or a gastrointestinal fistula.

The symptoms of metabolic acidosis include weakness, malaise, and headache. If the acidosis is not relieved, these symptoms progress to stupor, unconsciousness, coma, and death. The breath of the patient may have a fruity odor owing to the presence of ketone bodies (ketoacidosis). Vomiting and diarrhea may occur and aggravate the problem because of the loss of fluids and electrolytes, which are essential to restoring the acid-base balance. The pH will be less than 7.35 with an HCO_3 level less than 22 mEq/L.

Medical Treatment and Nursing Intervention

Prevention of acidosis is by far more desirable than treating the condition once it has developed. If the underlying cause is diabetic acidosis, it may be that the patient does not understand his role in managing the illness (see Chapter 28).

Another way in which metabolic acidosis can be prevented is by careful observation of patients receiving intravenous fluids that could upset the acid-base balance. Others who should be watched for early signs of acidosis are patients in shock, patients with hyperthyroidism, liver disease, and fluid-volume deficiency, and patients with continuous gastric or intestinal suction.

Treatment of metabolic acidosis is aimed at the underlying cause. Insulin is administered if the patient is in diabetic ketoacidosis. Dialysis may be necessary to correct the problem in the patient with kidney failure.

Immediate treatment of severe metabolic acidosis requires administration of bicarbonate or lactate by the intravenous route. When either of these drugs is administered, the patient should be watched closely, and vital signs should be recorded frequently. Careful measuring of intake and output helps determine how well the kidneys are able to regulate the acid-base balance.

As with any patient likely to develop disorientation or convulsions, safety precautions are taken to avoid injury. Mouth care using an alkaline mouthwash such as baking soda (sodium bicarbonate) will help reduce discomfort from acids in the mouth. Because these patients often breathe rapidly through their mouths, frequent mouth care is necessary.

METABOLIC ALKALOSIS

Assessment

There are three major causes of a shift toward the alkaline range of body fluids. These are (1) excessive loss of acid, (2) either excessive intake or retention of base, and (3) a low level of potassium in the blood (*hypokalemia*).

Loss of fluid from the gastrointestinal tract by gastric suction or emesis is the main cause of metabolic alkalosis. Other causes include drainage from intestinal fistula, diuresis resulting from potent diuretics that increase potassium loss in the urine, and steroid therapy, which causes retention of sodium and chloride and loss of potassium and hydrogen.

Symptoms of metabolic alkalosis include such neurologic signs as irritability, disorientation, lethargy, and convulsions; and respiratory manifestations such as slow, shallow respirations, decreased chest movements, and cyanosis. In addition, there may be symptoms of potassium and calcium depletion. The pH will be greater than 7.45 with the serum HCO_3 greater than 45 mEq/L.

Medical Treatment and Nursing Intervention

Because metabolic alkalosis often is associated with some form of medical treatment, the nurse is often able to detect it in its early stages and prevent more serious developments. However, once the condition is well established, the treatment is directed at correcting the underlying cause and attempting to restore the body fluids to a less alkaline state. Emergency measures include the administration of an acidifying solution such as ammonium chloride. Patients receiving this form of therapy must be watched carefully for signs of overcompensation and a resulting acidosis.

Again, it is necessary to take and record the vital signs frequently. If the pulse rate increases sharply and the blood pressure drops, the patient may be suffering from potassium depletion. (See Table 8–2 for symptoms). A record of intake and output is necessary so that replacement of lost fluids and electrolytes can be planned. Safety precautions are necessary, because the patient may experience mental confusion. If there are muscle spasms, they may be symptomatic of hypocalcemia.

THERAPY FOR FLUID/ELECTROLYTE IMBALANCES

INTRAVENOUS THERAPY

The administration of fluids through the veins is the most common means by which water, electrolytes, nutrients, and some drugs may be given when oral intake is not possible or must be supplemented. Medications may be administered in an intravenous solution when rapid action is required. A form of therapy called *total parenteral nutrition* also is used for the parenteral administration of all nutrients for patients with gastrointestinal problems. This form of therapy will be discussed in more detail in Chapter 23.

Some terms related to the concentration of an

intravenous fluid and the effect this has on cells are:

- *isotonic*—a solution that has the same osmotic pressure as intracellular fluid. Body cells can be bathed in an isotonic solution without net flow of water across the cell membrane.
- *hypotonic*—a solution that has a lower osmotic pressure (is less concentrated) than that of body fluids. Cells bathed in a hypotonic solution will swell as water passes from the less concentrated solution across the cell membrane and into the cell. *Note:* Sterile distilled water is hypotonic and is never added to an intravenous solution.
- *hypertonic*—a solution that has a higher osmotic pressure than that of body fluids. Cells bathed in a hypertonic solution will shrink as water passes out of the cell into the fluid surrounding it.

An example of an isotonic solution is 0.9% normal saline. Hypotonic solutions are those with less than 5% glucose or with anions less than 150 mEq/L.

Some fluids commonly used in intravenous therapy include:

- *Normal saline* (0.9%), which contains sodium and chloride ions in water.
- *Dextrose* or *glucose* solution, which contains water and carbohydrate for calories.
- *Lactated Ringer's* solution, which contains water, sodium, potassium, chloride, calcium, and lactate.

Blood-related fluids that are given intravenously include whole blood, packed cells from which the plasma has been removed, and plasma. Whole blood is given to replace that which has been lost through hemorrhage. Packed cells may be administered to patients with anemia or some other blood disorder or to patients who cannot tolerate a large volume of fluid very well, such as those with renal disease or congestive heart failure. Plasma is given to increase blood volume (as in shock), to provide protein, and to treat disorders of coagulation.

In the treatment of shock, fluids called *plasma expanders* are administered to increase the volume of plasma. Examples of plasma expanders are low-molecular-weight dextran, albumin, and plasminate.

Nursing Responsibilities in Administration of IV Fluids

Responsibility for the safe and effective administration of IV fluids rests with every member of the nursing staff. As with any therapeutic measure, intravenous therapy is not without its hazards to the patient. Many complications can be avoided through careful handling of equipment and meticulous monitoring of the patient's reaction to the fluids he is receiving.

The four goals of nursing care for a patient receiving an IV infusion are (1) preventing infection, (2) minimizing physical injury to the veins and surrounding tissues, (3) administering the correct fluid at the prescribed time and at a safe rate of flow, and (4) observing the patient's reaction to the fluid and medications being administered.

All equipment and fluids used for intravenous therapy must be sterile and safe for administration. Before any bottle or plastic bag of solution is added to an IV set, it must be checked for leaks and possible contamination. A plastic bag of solution may be squeezed to check for leaks. Any solution that is discolored or has small particles, a white cloud, or film in it should not be used. If there is no vacuum in the bottle when it is opened, the solution may be contaminated.

When a new bottle of fluid or additional medication is added to an IV already in progress, strict surgical asepsis must be observed. Because of the danger of incompatibility, it is recommended that the admixing of drugs in an intravenous solution be done by a clinical pharmacologist. Each time a new unit of solution or medication is added to an intravenous setup, there is danger of introducing bacteria into the patient's blood system.

The site of venipuncture should be watched closely for signs of inflammation. Redness, swelling, and heat in the area should be reported as possible signs of phlebitis. An elevation of body temperature and chills may indicate a bacterial infection.

When an IV is discontinued, the tubing is clamped, all tape is removed, and the needle or catheter is gently but quickly withdrawn using universal precautions. It should be removed from the vein in the direction in which it was inserted, avoiding an upward movement, which may traumatize the vein and tissues. A dry sterile gauze is held on the site with enough pressure to control the leakage of blood and to avoid the formation of a hematoma. If possible, raising the patient's limb for a minute or two to drain blood from the site of insertion will help prevent leakage of blood from the punctured vein.

The intravenous administration of fluids requires the same safety precautions that any other medication does. The label must be read several times to ensure that the correct solution is being given to the correct patient.

Rate of flow is an important factor in safe and effective IV therapy. In some hospitals, it is a general practice to ask the patient or a visitor to watch the IV bottle and, when it is nearly empty, to call the nurse. This is not safe, nor is it fair to delegate this responsibility to a patient who may or may not be physically able or mentally alert. Family members and visitors also should not be expected to understand the intricacies and hazards of IV therapy or to recognize situations that demand immediate attention. These are the duties and responsibilities of the nursing staff.

Principles that affect the rate of flow are:

- The higher the container is placed above the level of the patient's heart, the faster the rate of flow.
- The fuller the container, the faster the rate of flow.
- The more viscous the fluid, the slower the flow; for example, whole blood will flow more slowly than 5% dextrose in water.
- The larger the diameter of the needle and tubing, the faster the flow. IV sets usually indicate the number of drops per milliliter delivered by the set.
- The higher the pressure within the vein, the slower the flow. As an infusion progresses and the veins become fuller, the IV solution may drip more slowly.
- Fluid will pass through a straight tube faster than through one that is coiled.

There usually is a chart available to the nurse who needs to determine the number of drops that should be given per minute to administer a given amount of fluid in a specified period of time. The IV package will contain information about the number of drops the set will deliver per milliliter. If a chart is not available, the number of *drops per minute* can be calculated using a simple proportion and solving for x. Bear in mind that the set gives information about *drops per milliliter*. In order to check the rate of flow, the nurse must know how many drops should pass through the drip chamber in *one minute*.

Example: The patient is to receive 1,000 mL (1L) of fluid in 8 hours (480 minutes). The IV set states that the equipment will deliver 10 drops per milliliter. This would be a total of 10,000 drops because the bottle contains 1,000 mL. The ratio of drops to minutes is 10,000 drops in 480 minutes. The problem is written:

$$\frac{\text{Total infusion volume} \times \text{drops/mL}}{\text{Total time of infusion in minutes}} = \frac{1{,}000\ \text{mL} \times 10\ \text{drops/mL}}{480\ \text{minutes}} = \frac{10{,}000\ \text{drops}}{480\ \text{minutes}} = 20.8\ \text{drops/minute.}$$

Once the number of drops per minute has been determined, the IV set must be checked at 30-minute intervals to be sure that it continues to flow at the prescribed rate. As explained in the list of principles that affect the rate of flow, any number of factors can speed up or slow down the infusion.

If the IV slows down and has not been checked and readjusted for a period of time, *no attempt should be made to "catch up"* a large volume of fluid by speeding up the rate of flow. This can lead to circulatory overload and a volume excess that may produce pulmonary edema in susceptible persons. Remember that elderly persons and those with either renal or cardiac conditions cannot tolerate rapid administration of fluids. The symptoms of circulatory overload and other possible complications of intravenous therapy are shown in Table 8-4.

Intravenous therapy may become such a commonplace procedure to nurses that they are tempted to be complacent about it. However, it should never be thought of as a routine procedure that requires little attention. Any fluid or medication that enters a vein has an immediate effect. There is no margin for error in its administration.

TRANSFUSION OF WHOLE BLOOD AND BLOOD COMPONENTS

A transfusion is the intravenous administration of whole blood or one or more of its components. Among the components frequently transfused are plasma, packed red blood cells, granulocytes, platelets, and leukocytes. Table 8-5 shows some commonly used blood products, the usual amount given per transfusion, and reasons why each is used.

Special precautions are always taken when whole blood or any of its components are given. Blood banks have written procedures and policies for withdrawing and dispensing blood for transfusion. These procedures must be followed to minimize the possibility of an adverse reaction or administration of the wrong blood type to a recipient. Although many reactions and complications cannot be anticipated, carelessness in the handling of transfusion products cannot be excused.

Nursing Intervention

The nurse checks to see that a blood administration consent form has been signed by the patient. Next she determines whether the patient has an IV site already established and what size catheter is in place. Blood should be given through an 18-gauge or larger catheter.

Blood is given with a blood administration set with a filter, preferably a Y-set. This allows one arm of the Y to be used for the blood and the other to be used for normal saline. If a reaction to the blood occurs, the blood can be quickly

TABLE 8-4 **PROBLEMS, ASSESSMENT, AND NURSING INTERVENTIONS FOR IV THERAPY**

Problem	Assessment Data	Nursing Interventions
Infiltration caused by needle or catheter displacement or leakage of blood from vein.	Pain, redness, swelling around site, absence of backflow of blood, diminished rate or complete cessation of flow.	Stop flow of fluid and remove needle or catheter. Split arm to stabilize it when site is over a joint. If noticed within 30 minutes of onset, apply ice to swelling. If noted later than 30 minutes, apply warm compresses to encourage absorption.
Air embolism caused by air in tubing, allowing container to run dry.	Cyanosis, drop in BP, weak and rapid pulse.	Make sure all connections are airtight. Clear air from tubing before attaching to needle. Monitor and change containers promptly.
Circulatory overload caused by inability of cardiovascular system to handle fluids at current rate of flow and volume.	Rise in BP, headache, dyspnea, flushed skin, discrepancy between fluid intake and urinary output.	Note patient's cardiovascular status. Monitor urinary output. Slow infusion rate to keep vein open. Elevate head of bed. Monitor vital signs. Administer oxygen as prescribed. Change IV site.
Thrombophlebitis caused by injury to vein from movement, irritating additive, overuse of vein; too-slow flow rate that allows clot to form at end of needle.	Pain, redness, hardness along vein site. Sluggish flow rate. Swelling of limb.	Stabilize needle or catheter to minimize trauma to vein. Select large vein to help dilute additive. Alternate sites. Maintain desired flow rate.
Infected venipuncture site.	Swelling and soreness, yellow and foul-smelling discharge.	Use aseptic technique during venipuncture. Discontinue IV. Notify infection control officer so culture can be taken. Notify physician; apply antimicrobial ointment and dressing as prescribed.
Pyrogenic reaction caused by inadequate sterile technique, improper handling of tubing.	Rapid rise in temperature; severe chill 30 minutes after infusion started.	Check sterile technique when doing venipuncture. Avoid contamination of system when it is accidentally disconnected. Notify physician and administer prescribed therapy for infection.
Allergic reaction caused by hypersensitivity to additive.	Itching, rash, dyspnea.	Stop flow immediately; keep IV open with normal saline. Notify physician.

shut off and the normal saline opened to maintain patency of the IV site.

Before the blood is started, two nurses (many hospitals require registered nurses) verify the patient's name and identification number, the number on the blood bag label, and the ABO group and RH type on the blood bag label with the corresponding information on the patient's identification band and blood bank band on his wrist. Both nurses sign the blood bank form if everything is correct. The blood must be started within 30 minutes of arrival on the unit, as it should never be left at room temperature for more than 2 hours, and it takes about 1½ hours for a unit to run into the patient.

A set of baseline vital signs is taken just before the blood is administered to the patient. For the first 15 minutes of the transfusion, the blood is run at 20 drops per minute and the patient is observed for signs of reaction such as chills, nausea, vomiting, skin rash, back pain, or tachycardia. If any of these occur, the transfusion is

TABLE 8-5 INDICATIONS FOR USE OF BLOOD AND BLOOD COMPONENTS

Product	Volume	Indications and Rationale for Use
Whole blood	450–500 mL	Massive, acute blood loss, such as occurs with accidental injury and surgery
Packed red blood cells	300 mL	Moderate blood loss; anemia; less likely than whole blood to cause circulatory overload and reactions to antigens in plasma
Granulocytes	500–675 mL	Granulocytopenia, especially in association with infection
Albumin	500 mL	Blood volume expansion; decreased plasma protein
Plasma, fresh or frozen	250 mL	Clotting deficiencies; hypovolemia
Platelets: pheresis pack	300 mL	Platelet deficiency
Cells	250 mL	Patients with histories of transfusion reactions secondary to platelet, leukocyte, or plasma antibodies
Cryoprecipitate	5–10 mL per unit (10 units given per transfusion)	Hemophilia A (factor VIII deficiency); fibrinogen

Adapted from Woods, M. E., and Mazza, I.: Blood and component therapy. Nurs. Clin. North Am., Sept., 1980, p. 629.

stopped immediately and the charge nurse is notified at once. If no signs of reaction occur during the first 15 minutes, the infusion may be set to run at the ordered rate. Assess the patient again 15 minutes after the rate has been increased. As long as there are no signs of adverse reaction, the patient is assessed and vital signs are taken every 30 minutes until the transfusion is completed.

The word *reaction*, when used in reference to the transfusion of blood or the infusion of fluids, means a sensitivity to the blood itself or to the preservatives or other substances that have been added to a solution. Reactions to whole blood are the result of incompatibility between blood types. There are antigens on the surfaces of red blood cells that can bring about a reaction if exposed to blood that is not the same type and is incompatible. The antigen-antibody reaction causes the cells to clump together and obstruct the flow of blood through the capillaries.

The symptoms of a reaction may be so mild as to go unnoticed or so severe that death is the eventual outcome. In milder cases the patient may develop a rash, hives, itching, or facial flushing. In more severe reactions the patient may experience dyspnea, sudden chills and fever, chest pains or tightness, low back pain, and shock. A delayed reaction due to hepatitis, syphilis, or malaria might not be evident until 4 to 6 weeks after the blood has been given.

Treatment of a reaction depends on its cause and severity. If it is a mild allergic reaction, the physician may order antihistamines to relieve the symptoms. In severe anaphylactic reactions the treatment is the same as for anaphylaxis due to any extreme hypersensitivity.

Hospitals and other health care facilities in which blood transfusions are administered have written policies and procedures to guide the nursing staff when a patient shows signs of an adverse reaction. It is common practice to stop a transfusion immediately and notify the physician when early signs and symptoms of a reaction appear. The intravenous line usually is kept open with normal saline until further orders are obtained from the physician.

TOTAL PARENTERAL NUTRITION

Many patients with fluid and electrolyte imbalances are nutritionally depleted. If sufficient nutrition cannot be delivered by the oral route or by enteral hyperalimentation, total parental nutrition (TPN) is begun. TPN solution is made up of a nitrogen (protein) source, hypertonic dextrose, and supplementary vitamins and minerals. Because of its degree of concentration, it must be infused to a central vein, usually the subclavian, where the high rate of blood flow quickly dilutes it. The Hickman, Broviac, and Groshong are the most frequently used central line catheters and can be used for long-term therapy.

TPN solutions and catheters must be handled

with strict asepsis, as the solution is an ideal medium for bacterial growth. There are many complications of TPN in addition to infection, including glucose intolerance and other metabolic imbalances. The patient must be carefully monitored.

Concerns for the Elderly

Fluid volume deficit is a very common problem in the elderly. This is especially true of persons who are in long-term care facilities and are not totally capable of self-care. Because there is an age-related decline in total body water and a decrease in thirst sensation, people in this age group tend to skimp on fluids and easily become dehydrated. Fluid volume deficit contributes to constipation and orthostatic hypotension with related dizziness and falls and makes the person more susceptible to infection.

Skin turgor is altered in the elderly. As a result, when assessing for dehydration, the nurse should use the skin on the forehead or sternum to check turgor. The condition of the tongue and oral mucosa is a more useful indicator of fluid status in this age group. A furrowed, dry tongue that is not the result of drug therapy indicates a fluid deficit.

Elderly patients who have cardiac problems are at risk for fluid overload from IV infusions. Allowing a liter of fluid to infuse too fast can sometimes cause the patient to go into congestive heart failure. If an IV infusion falls behind, it should not be regulated to make up for lost time by infusing fluid at a rate faster than ordered.

Many elderly people rely on the use of laxatives and enemas to clear the bowel. This practice can cause fluid deficit along with sodium and potassium loss.

Any time an elderly patient has a change in mental status from alert to confused that cannot be linked to obvious physical problems, the nurse should carefully look for indications of fluid and electrolyte problems. Even slight alterations in electrolytes can cause confusion in this age group.

Dehydration and hyponatremia account for the majority of hospital admissions of patients from nursing homes. It takes a caring, skillful nurse to see that long-term-care patients take in enough fluids without interfering with their nutritional intake.

BIBLIOGRAPHY

Andreoli, T. E., et al.: Cecil Essentials of Medicine, 2nd ed. Philadelphia, W. B. Saunders, 1990.

Aspinall, M.: A simplified guide to managing patients with hyponatremia. Nursing 87, Dec., 1987, p. 32.

Beare, P. G., and Myers, J. L.: Principles and Practices of Adult Health Nursing. St. Louis, C. V. Mosby, 1990.

Chambers, J.: Metabolic bone disorders: Imbalances of calcium and phosphorus. Nurs. Clin. North Am., Dec., 1987, p. 861.

Chenevey, B.: Overview of fluids and electrolytes. Nurs. Clin. North Am., Dec., 1987, p. 749.

Guyton, A. C.: Textbook of Medical Physiology, 8th ed. Philadelphia, W. B. Saunders, 1991.

Holder, C., and Alexander, J.: A new and improved guide to IV therapy. Am. J. Nurs., Feb., 1990, p. 43.

Ignatavicius, D. D., and Bayne, M. J.: Medical-Surgical Nursing. Philadelphia, W. B. Saunders, 1991.

Janusek, L. W.: Metabolic acidosis. Nursing 90, July, 1990, p. 52.

Janusek, L. W.: Metabolic alkalosis. Nursing 90, June, 1990, p. 52.

Lenox, A. C.: IV therapy—reducing the risk of infection. Nursing 90, March, 1990, p. 60.

Lorenz, B. L.: Are you using the right IV pump? RN, May, 1990, p. 31.

Metheny, N. M.: Why worry about IV Fluids? Am. J. Nurs., June, 1990, p. 50.

Mueller, K. D., and Boises, A. M.: Keeping your patient's water level up. RN, July, 1989, p. 65.

Plumer, A., and Cosentino, F.: Principles and Practice of Intravenous Therapy, 4th ed. Boston, Little, Brown, 1987.

Poyss, A.: Assessment and nursing diagnosis in fluid and electrolyte disorders. Nurs. Clin. North Am., Dec., 1987, p. 773.

Price, S., and Wilson, L.: Pathophysiology, 3rd ed. New York, McGraw-Hill, 1986.

Querin, J. J., and Stahl, L. D.: 12 simple sensible steps for successful blood transfusions. Nursing 90, Oct., 1990, p. 68.

Reedy, D. F.: Fluid intake: How can you prevent dehydration? Geriatr. Nurs., July/Aug., 1988, p. 224.

Sommers, J.: Rapid fluid resuscitation—how to correct dangerous deficits. Nursing 90, Jan., 1990, p. 52.

Stroot, V. R., et al.: Fluids and Electrolytes: A Practical Approach, 3rd ed. Philadelphia, F. A. Davis, 1984.

Ward, L.: Home care: Patient teaching for home IV therapy. RN, April, 1990, p. 86.

Watson, J.: Fluid and electrolyte disorders in cardiovascular patients. Nurs. Clin. North Am., Dec., 1987, p. 797.

York, K.: The lung and fluid-electrolyte and acid-base imbalances. Nurs. Clin. North Am., Dec., 1987, p. 805.

Young, M. E., and Flynn, K. T.: Third-spacing: When the body conceals fluid loss. RN, Aug., 1988, p. 46.

STUDENT STUDY AIDS

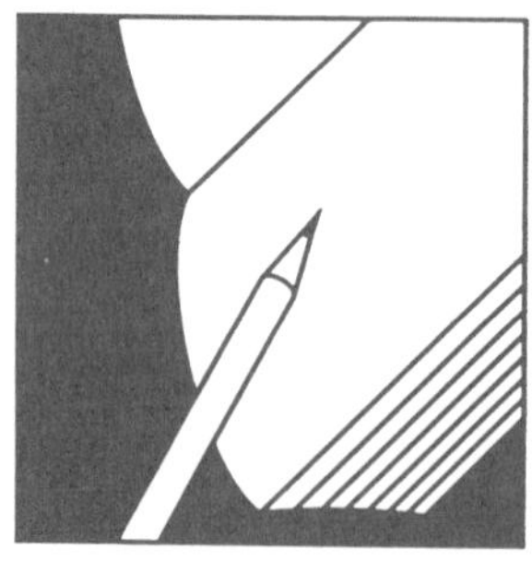

CLINICAL CASE PROBLEMS

Read each clinical situation and discuss the questions with your classmates.

1. Mrs. Carlos, age 61, is admitted to the hospital with congestive heart failure. She is extremely edematous and obese. Mrs. Carlos is slightly confused upon admission, and though she is not on absolute bed rest, she tells you that she cannot get out of bed. She continues to refuse to get up or move about in bed the next morning when you are assigned to care for her.

- What type of diet would you expect Mrs. Carlos' physician to prescribe for her? How would you explain to her the restrictions of her diet and the need for her to follow it?
- How might you encourage Mrs. Carlos to get out of bed for her daily weighing?
- If Mrs. Carlos' fluid intake is restricted, how would you schedule her fluid intake?
- What problems might be presented by Mrs. Carlos' obesity and her inactivity?

---

2. Mr. Wong is a 35-year-old patient who has suffered a severe gastrointestinal upset producing nausea, vomiting, and diarrhea. His physician has prescribed intravenous fluids.

- List the observations you should make while caring for Mr. Wong.
- What nursing measures might be taken to relieve his symptoms? What medications might you expect him to receive?
- What are your responsibilities regarding Mr. Wong's intravenous therapy? Why is it necessary to check the infusion frequently? Would you measure his intake and output? In what electrolytes might he be deficient?

STUDY OUTLINE

I. Physiology

A. Fluids account for about 56% of total body weight.
B. Differences depend on age, sex, state of hydration.
C. There is a gradual decline of body fluids with age.
D. Maintenance of normal fluid balance is necessary in all ages, because all cell processes take place in a fluid medium.
E. When a person becomes ill or injured, his symptoms are manifestations of changes on a cellular level.
F. The internal environment of the body is the fluid that surrounds and bathes each cell.
G. Homeostasis is the maintenance of a constant, stable environment for the cells.

II. Distribution of body fluids

A. Compartments of body fluids summarized in Table 8–1.
B. Transport: movement of fluids to assure normal distribution of fluids.
   1. Heart action necessary to pump intravascular fluid.
   2. Diffusion: the spontaneous mixing and moving of molecules.
   3. Osmosis: the passage of water molecules across a semipermeable membrane. Movement is from the less concentrated solution to the more concentrated, so that solutions on both sides of the membrane are made equally concentrated.

III. Composition of body fluids

A. Water is in greatest proportion.
   1. Serves as the medium in which physiologic and chemical activities occur.
   2. Transports essential nutrients.
   3. Dilutes toxins of waste.
   4. Allows electrolytes to become active by being in solution.
B. Electrolytes:
   1. Break into small atomic particles when placed in solution.
   2. Some particles are negatively charged (anions), and some are positively charged (cations).

3. Difference in electric charge creates an electrical impulse across membranes.
4. Important to contraction of muscles, nerve activity, and glandular secretions.
5. Important electrolytes and their relationship to the nursing process summarized in Table 8–2.

IV. Fluid imbalances

A. Main source of gain of body fluids is by ingestion and absorption from the digestive tract.

B. Average amount of water taken in each day is 2,500 mL. Source is water, liquids, fruits, vegetables, and meat. 250 mL produced during metabolism.

C. Normal output for a 24-hour period is about 2,500 mL.

D. Pathophysiology: fluid imbalance exists when there is either a deficit or excess of body water and the solutes it contains.

E. Fluid deficit:

1. Too little fluid taken in or too much lost without replacement.
2. Many patients can be spared the effects of fluid deficit if they receive planned and effective nursing care.
3. Nursing responsibilities in the prevention of fluid deficit:
   a. Assessment:
      (1) Patients at risk: those who are unable to drink sufficient quantities, and those with excessive loss through prolonged vomiting, diarrhea, draining fistulas and operative wounds, and burns.
      (2) Treatments such as gastric suction, diuretic therapy, and tap water enemas also predispose patients to fluid deficit.
      (3) Subjective symptoms: thirst, dizziness, feeling faint upon standing up (postural hypotension), weakness, and weight loss.
      (4) Objective symptoms: oliguria, dry mucous membranes, dry skin with poor turgor, and flat neck veins.
   b. Medical treatment and nursing intervention:
      (1) Measures to ensure adequate oral intake if at all possible.
      (2) Help control underlying disorder.
   c. Evaluation: see Nursing Care Plan 8–1.
4. The patient with nausea and vomiting.
   a. Nausea: feeling of discomfort in epigastrium and abdomen with tendency to vomit.
   b. Assessment:
      (1) Subjective symptoms: complaint of feeling nauseated or "sick to my stomach," queasiness, abdominal pain, epigastric discomfort or burning, history of vomiting.
      (2) Objective symptoms: pallor; mild diaphoresis; cold, clammy skin; attempts to remain motionless. Vomitus observed for amount, odor, color, and contents. Note and record patterns of vomiting and conditions that trigger it.
   c. Medical treatment and nursing intervention:
      (1) Administer medication ordered, position patient to prevent aspiration of vomitus, and wipe patient's face with cool, damp cloth during vomiting episodes.
      (2) Give ice chips and provide frequent oral hygiene.
      (3) Provide quiet and odor-free environment.
      (4) Reinstate diet slowly, beginning with clear liquids and gradually adding foods.
      (5) Goals usually appropriate for a nursing care plan for a patient with nausea and vomiting include:

(a) Patient is able to renew intake of fluids and food; no episodes of vomiting.
(b) Fluid intake and output balanced.
(c) Electrolytes restored to normal values.

5. The patient with diarrhea.
   a. Diarrhea: the frequent passage of watery stools; results in rapid loss of water, nutritive elements, and electrolytes.
   b. Assessment:
      (1) Patients at risk: likely to be those with intestinal infections, colitis, irritable bowel syndrome, and allergies. Also can occur with obstruction of bowel due to tumor or fecal impaction.
      (2) Subjective symptoms: history of frequent, watery stools, abdominal cramping, general weakness.
      (3) Objective symptoms: loose, watery stools; active bowel sounds. Stools observed for number and characteristics (e.g., color, consistency, unusual contents, and peculiar odor).
   c. Nursing intervention and medical treatment:
      (1) Provide rest and privacy.
      (2) Explain diagnostic procedures and give patient support and encouragement.
      (3) Limit intake of foods at first, then gradually add clear liquids and then more solid foods.
      (4) Assist patient by maintaining calm, understanding approach.
      (5) Administer antidiarrheic drugs as ordered.
   d. Goals in a plan of care might include:
      (1) Return to normal pattern of bowel elimination.
      (2) Reduction in complaints of discomfort.
      (3) Maintenance of integrity of perianal skin.
      (4) Adequate nutrition; cessation of weight loss.
      (5) Able to get sufficient rest.
6. Fluid deficits from other causes.
   a. Improper use of gastric and intestinal suction. As much as 2,500 mL of gastric fluid and 1,500 mL of saliva can be removed in a 24-hour period by continuous suction.
   b. Observe and note fluid loss from draining fistulas.
   c. Measure fluid intake and output of surgical patient.
   d. Be especially alert to fluid loss in severely burned patients.

F. Fluid excess.
   1. Excessive amount of body *water* alone is rare. Can occur, however, if patient drinks more water than needed, intravenous fluids administered too rapidly or in excess, and tap water enemas given.
   2. Edema more common problem. Edema: the excessive accumulation of freely moving interstitial fluid. Can be either generalized or localized.
      a. Generalized edema—occurs when body fails to eliminate sodium and water. Can be result of:
         (1) Kidney failure.
         (2) Heart failure.
         (3) Hormonal disorder with excess of aldosterone and ADH.
         (4) Malnutrition.
      b. Localized edema can occur as a result of trauma, allergies, burns, obstruction of lymph flow, and liver failure.
      c. Dependent edema is an effect of gravity. Especially noticeable in feet and ankles and in sacral region of bedridden patients.

d. Nursing responsibilities:
   (1) Assessment
      (a) Subjective symptoms: history can be very significant (e.g., whether patient needs more than one pillow to sleep, gets up frequently during the night to urinate, has shortness of breath from pressure of fluid in abdominal cavity). History of weight gain.
      (b) Objective symptoms: obvious edema of feet and ankles, sacral region, etc. Lab analysis of blood usually shows a low hematocrit. Patient may have pitting edema of body parts that are below the level of the heart.
   (2) Medical treatment and nursing intervention:
      (a) Weigh patient daily.
      (b) Measure intake and output; restrict fluid intake as ordered.
      (c) Exercise legs; periodically elevate feet and legs.
      (d) Give meticulous skin care to avoid breakdown of fragile edematous tissue.
      (e) Limit sodium and fluid intake as prescribed.
      (f) Carefully monitor intravenous fluids.
      (g) Prepare patient for discharge by teaching self-care.
      (h) Suggested outcome criteria for sample case of generalized edema and case of localized edema presented in Table 8–3.

V. Hydrogen ion concentration (acid-base balance)
- A. Definition of terms.
- B. Pathophysiology.
  1. Body fluids normally are slightly alkaline, even though metabolic activities produce acids.
  2. Two types of activities maintain normal pH.
     a. Respiratory activities in which carbon dioxide is exchanged for oxygen.
     b. Metabolic activities involving retention and excretion of bicarbonate by the kidney.
- C. Arterial blood gas analysis: useful in assessing status of imbalances related to both respiration and metabolism.
- D. Respiratory acidosis.
  1. Assessment:
     a. Patients at risk are those with acute or chronic impairment of respiration that causes accumulation of carbon dioxide in the blood.
     b. Subjective symptoms: complaints of increasing difficulty breathing, history of respiratory obstruction, weakness, dizziness, sleepiness, change in mental alertness, and restlessness.
     c. Objective symptoms: increased levels of carbon dioxide in the blood (noted in blood gas analysis), dyspnea, and obvious respiratory problems.
  2. Intervention:
     a. For acute respiratory acidosis, establish airway, administer oxygen with great caution; 2 to 3 L/min for patients with COPD.
     b. IPPB treatments, postural drainage, bronchodilators, or antibiotics if indicated.
     c. Prevention includes cautious administration of drugs that depress respiration.
- E. Respiratory alkalosis.
  1. Assessment: common in those who hyperventilate.

a. Subjective symptoms: complaints of dizziness and tingling of fingers.
b. Objective symptoms: pallor around mouth, rapid and deep breathing, spasms of hands and feet.

2. Intervention:
   a. Treat hysteria, if present; may require sedation.
   b. Have patient rebreathe exhaled air.
   c. Avoid overzealous use of ventilator.

F. Metabolic acidosis.
1. Likely to occur in those who have poor carbohydrate metabolism and burn fats for energy (e.g., those with uncontrolled diabetes, persons on low-carbohydrate, high-fat diet to lose weight, and those with kidney failure, diarrhea, and gastrointestinal fistula.
2. Assessment:
   a. Subjective symptoms: history of inadequate carbohydrate metabolism or intake (fad diets); weakness, malaise, headache.
   b. Objective symptoms: fruity odor to breath, vomiting and diarrhea, stupor, loss of consciousness.
3. Intervention:
   a. Help diabetic patient maintain control of illness.
   b. Teach public about hazards of fad diets.
   c. Carefully monitor patients receiving intravenous fluid therapy.
   d. Administer bicarbonate or lactate as ordered.
   e. Measure intake and output.
   f. Implement safety precautions for disoriented and those subject to altered levels of consciousness.
   g. Frequent mouth care.

G. Metabolic alkalosis.
1. Assessment: patients at risk include those with severe vomiting, gastric suction, intestinal fistulas, diuresis, steroid therapy.
2. Intervention:
   a. Observe for signs of potassium depletion.
   b. Measure and record intake and output.
   c. Institute safety precautions.
   d. Monitor vital signs.
   e. Watch for signs of calcium depletion.

VI. Therapy for fluid/electrolyte imbalances.

A. Intravenous therapy.
1. Purpose: administration of electrolytes, nutrients, water, etc.; rapid administration of drugs.
2. Concentration (osmotic pressure) of IV fluid has direct influence on hydration of cells.
3. Nursing responsibilities.
   a. Goals of care:
      (1) Preventing infection.
      (2) Minimizing trauma to veins and adjacent tissue.
      (3) Administering correct fluid at prescribed rate of flow.
      (4) Observing patient response.

B. Transfusion of whole blood and blood components.
1. Special precautions always indicated.
2. Transfusion reaction can be mild or fatal.
3. Usual procedure is to stop transfusion and notify physician when signs of reaction occur.
4. Nursing interventions
   a. Patient data checked with data on blood bank slips by two nurses.
   b. Baseline vital signs taken before blood is started.

c. Blood administration set used with filter and Y lines with normal saline and blood bag.
d. Begin blood at 20 drops per minute for first 15 minutes.
e. If no signs of reaction, increase flow to ordered rate.
f. Signs of reaction include fever, chills, nausea, vomiting, skin rash, back pain, or tachycardia.

C. Total parenteral nutrition
1. Provides long-term nutritional therapy for patients with fluid and electrolyte imbalances who cannot be fed orally or enterally.
2. Must be given by central line, usually in the subclavian vein, so that it will be immediately diluted by high blood flow. Types of central line catheters include the Hickman, Broviac, and Groshong.
3. Solution provides protein, glucose, vitamins, and minerals.
4. TPN can cause many complications such as infection and metabolic imbalances.
5. Patients receiving TPN must be monitored closely.

VII. Concerns for the elderly

A. Fluid volume deficit is a very common problem in the elderly.
B. The elderly become dehydrated easily.
C. Fluid volume deficit causes constipation, orthostatic hypotension, and dizziness, which can contribute to falls.
D. Mucous membrane and tongue condition are more reliable for assessment of fluid status in the elderly than skin turgor.
E. If skin is assessed, use the skin of the forehead or sternum.
F. Elderly with cardiac conditions are at risk for heart failure if they become overloaded with fluid; IV fluids must be very carefully regulated.
G. Laxative and enema use among the elderly often lead to fluid, potassium, and sodium loss.
H. If an elderly patient becomes confused for no obvious reason, suspect fluid and electrolyte imbalance.
I. Fluid and electrolyte imbalances often lead to need for hospitalization among long-term care facility residents.

CHAPTER 9

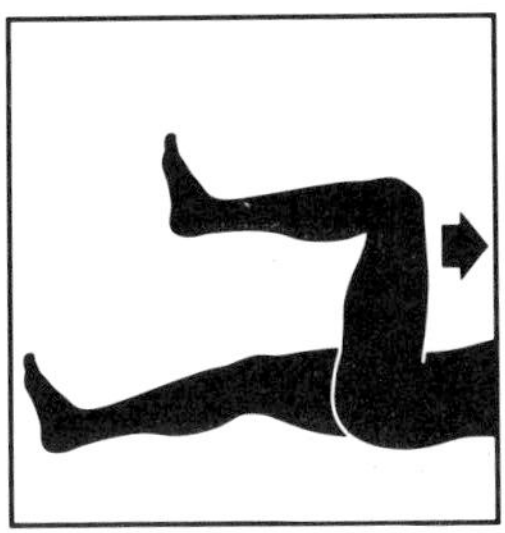

Problems of Immobility

VOCABULARY

contracture
decubitus ulcer
digital
erythema
orthostatic hypotension
osteoporosis
thrombus
Valsalva maneuver

Upon completion of this chapter the student should be able to:

1. Identify patients at risk for problems associated with immobility.
2. Describe in his or her own words the impact of immobility on each of the major systems of the body.
3. Assess the status of patients to identify potential or actual problems secondary to immobility.
4. Develop and implement plans for nursing interventions to prevent the adverse effects of immobility.
5. List nursing diagnoses and appropriate interventions to alleviate the problems associated with immobility.
6. Evaluate the effectiveness of nursing interventions to alleviate or prevent the problems associated with immobility for a clinical patient.

If we accept the statement that the human body is designed for motion, it follows that immobility, which is the lack of motion, will have harmful effects. Disabilities arising from immobility are a major health problem in this country, yet many of these disabilities can be prevented. Whether a patient suffers a permanent handicap from lying motionless in bed or sitting in a chair for prolonged periods *depends in large measure on the nursing care that is provided.*

The prevention of dependent disabilities begins the moment a patient first becomes ill or injured. It must continue as long as the patient needs health care, and this may be for the rest of his life if he has a chronic illness or a permanent injury.

There are many reasons why a person's ability to move is restricted. Paralysis may limit voluntary motion, as in physical injury to the spinal cord or brain damage from stroke. Pain or the fear of pain from arthritis, surgery, or physical trauma may also cause a person to avoid moving about. Weakness and extreme fatigue from a debilitating disease can encourage immobility. In this chapter, we discuss the effects of immobility that result from illness, injury, or enforced rest as treatment.

Some *therapeutic* purposes of rest and immobility include (1) relief from pain and further injury of a part, as in a fractured bone, (2) reduction of the work load of the heart in a cardiac or renal condition, (3) promotion of healing and repair, and (4) reversal of the effects of gravity, as in abdominal hernias and prolapsed organs.

Whatever the reason for resting a part or all of the body, some effort must be made to allow for the needed rest and at the same time prevent insofar as possible the adverse effects of immobility.

The systems of the body work together as parts of an integrated and interdependent whole. Immobility does not affect only one system, but for the sake of clarity we will consider each of the major systems separately. In this way, it may be easier to understand how lack of motion begins a vicious circle that can lead only to an ever-increasing loss of independence for the patient. As he becomes less able to move, he becomes more dependent, and as he becomes more dependent, he is less able to care for himself—which in turn leads to even more adverse effects from immobility. It is the responsibility of the nurse to avoid the beginning of such a cycle by helping the patient maintain normal functioning of each bodily system as much and for as long as possible.

CARDIOVASCULAR SYSTEM

PATHOPHYSIOLOGY

Inactivity of the body affects (1) the structure and function of the blood vessels, particularly the veins; (2) the work load of the heart; and (3) the level of blood pressure.

Blood Vessels

Blood flows from the heart through the arteries to the capillaries, where nutrients and waste products in the body are exchanged across the capillary membrane. The blood travels from the capillaries through the veins to the heart. This venous return of blood depends in part on the contraction and relaxation of muscles surrounding the veins. Muscular activity moves the blood in the direction of the heart by (1) pressing against the walls of the veins each time the muscle contracts, thereby "squeezing" the vessels and pushing the blood along; and (2) closing the one-way valves in the veins so that the blood will not flow backward or remain static and engorge the veins. When there is little or no muscle activity, the blood flow becomes sluggish, and there is inadequate circulation of blood to cells and tissues.

Decreased blood flow also predisposes the body to clot *(thrombus)* formation. The coagulation of blood to form a clot is directly related to the presence of platelets and the rate of blood flow. Pressure against the blood vessel damages its inner lining *(intima),* causing irritation and a "rough spot" on the lining. Platelets accumulate at the area and cover the injured tissues. This is the beginning of a blood clot, which grows larger as the blood slowly flows past and provides additional material for the formation of the clot. Eventually the walls of the vessel become inflamed, producing thrombophlebitis.

Pressure against a blood vessel and the resultant damage to the vessel wall can be caused by (1) allowing the patient to sit or lie in one position too long, (2) placing a pillow under the knees of a patient who is lying on his back, and (3) raising the foot of the bed so that it is bent under the patient's knees.

Assessment and nursing intervention for the patient with thrombophlebitis are discussed in Chapter 21.

Work Load of the Heart

There is evidence to support the belief that the heart works harder when the body is in a resting, supine position. Normally, the fluid in the intravascular compartment is distributed throughout the legs as well as the other parts of the body.

This distribution depends on gravity flow. When one lies down, a large portion of the blood usually located in the legs must be distributed to other parts of the body. This is accomplished by the pumping action of the heart. Because the heart must pump more blood than it would if the person were standing or sitting, its work load is increased.

Another situation that increases the amount of blood the heart must deal with at any given time is that which occurs during the *Valsalva maneuver*—a physical activity that involves holding the breath while exerting oneself and then releasing the breath suddenly. Patients who are confined to bed do this when they use their arms and upper trunk muscles to move themselves up in bed. This maneuver also is done when one strains at the stool while defecating.

When the breath is held by holding the chest muscles tense and pushing exhaled air against the closed glottis, the flow of blood in the large veins is stopped. As soon as the muscles are relaxed and the air is expired, the blood that has been dammed up in the large veins is suddenly delivered to the heart. In this way, the work load of the heart is suddenly increased. If the heart is weak and unable to deal with this rush of blood into its chambers, the heart muscle may fail, and the patient suffers cardiac arrest.

Authorities estimate that a patient confined to bed may perform the Valsalva maneuver many times per hour.

Blood Pressure

We all probably have experienced weakness and possibly fainting the first time we stood up after having been in bed for several days. The weakness, dizziness, and fainting that may occur is a result of a drop in blood pressure. This condition is called *orthostatic hypotension*, or low blood pressure from standing up straight.

The danger of this situation lies in the possibility that the patient may fall and sustain injuries if there is not sufficient help to support him when he first attempts to get out of bed after prolonged rest.

NURSING INTERVENTION

The responsibility of the nurse lies in being aware of the effects of immobility on the heart and blood vessels and in planning and carrying out nursing measures that will help avoid or mitigate these effects. These measures include (1) exercises, (2) frequent turning and proper positioning, (3) teaching the patient to avoid using the Valsalva maneuver, and (4) increasing fluid intake to enhance blood flow.

Exercises

In order to maintain adequate circulation through muscular activity, it may be necessary to plan a schedule of exercises for the patient who is confined to bed. Although the instruction of the patient in the performance of special exercises may be done by a physical therapist, the nurse must recognize the need for these exercises, encourage the patient to perform them and assist him as necessary, and accept responsibility for seeing to it that the exercises are included as part of the nursing care plan for the patient. In the absence of the physical therapist, the nurse will need to know how to instruct the patient.

Therapeutic exercises may be *active*—that is, carried out by the patient—or *passive*—that is, carried out by the therapist or nurse without assistance from the patient. *Range-of-motion (ROM) exercises*, shown in Figure 9–1, are effective in preventing disabilities of the musculoskeletal system and other systems as well. They are explained in more detail later in this chapter. *Isometric exercises* are performed to maintain muscle tone without moving the joint. In these exercises, the muscle is contracted and held in that position for several seconds. The muscle is then relaxed for a few seconds and contracted again.

The exercise best suited for each patient must be prescribed by the physician so that no harm is done and the beneficial effects are accomplished. In most instances, the physician and physical therapist work together to determine the kind of exercises needed. This does not mean, however, that the nurse has no responsibility for recognizing the need for exercise and initiating an exercise program after she has obtained a physician's written order. Encouraging the patient to rotate the feet and ankles and to dorsiflex the feet, for example, during each commercial break on television, can help blood flow considerably.

Through observation and knowledge of the patient's specific health problems, the nurse plans a *preventive*, as well as a *therapeutic*, program for each patient. If a patient is immobilized for any reason, the nurse recognizes the need to work cooperatively with the physician and other members of the health care team to develop a plan of exercises so that cardiovascular disabilities associated with immobility can be avoided.

Position Changes

If the patient is able to help himself move about in bed, he should be taught how to change position without using the Valsalva maneuver. He should be told to exhale when he moves up in bed, and if a trapeze bar is not contraindicated, he should be told how to use it.

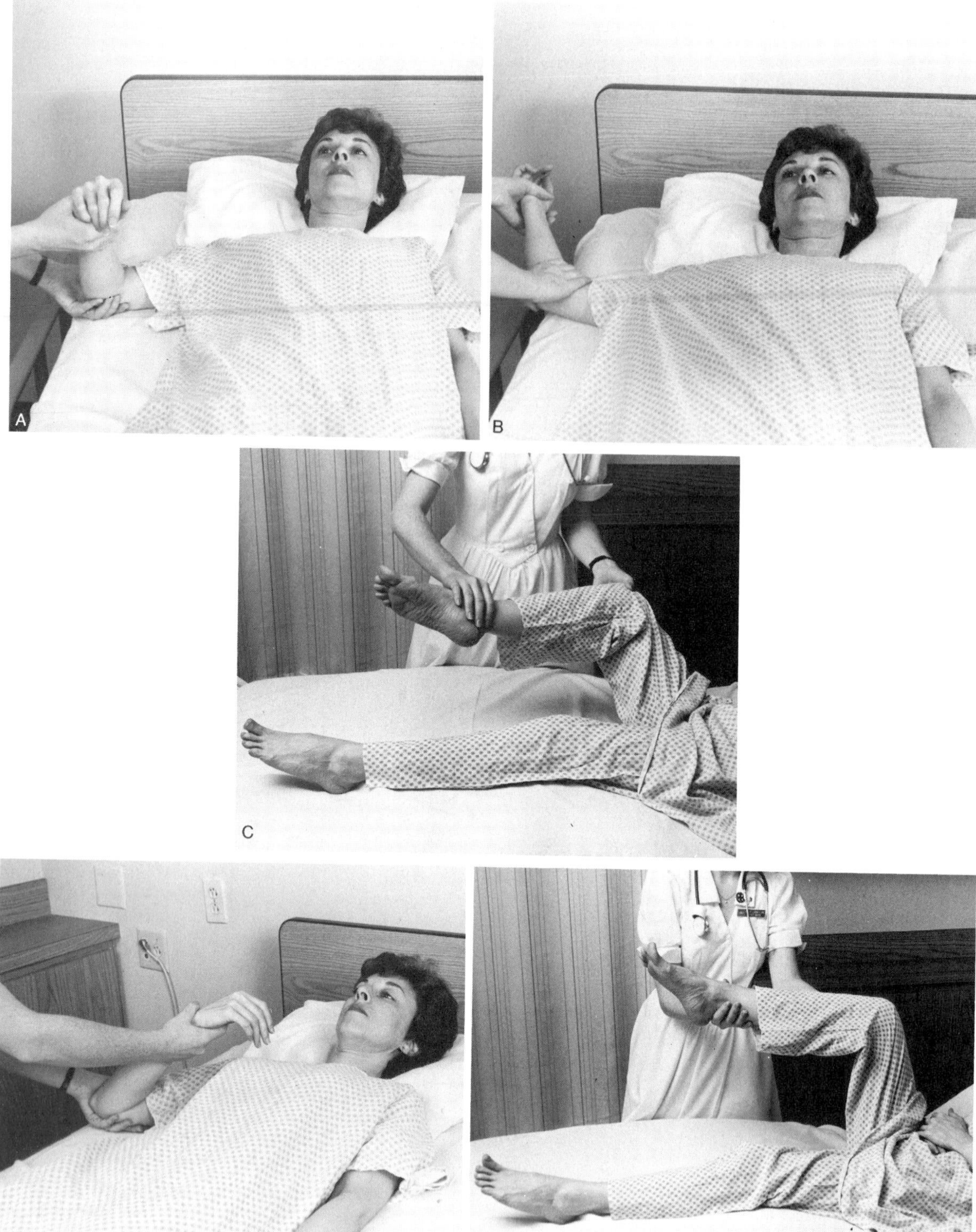

Figure 9-1 Range-of-motion exercises: rotation (*A* to *C*), flexion (*D* and *E*), extension (*F*), abduction and adduction (*G*), and hyperextension (*H*). *A*, Rotation of shoulder. *B*, External rotation of the shoulder. *C*, Rotation of the hip. Internal rotation. *D*, Flexion of elbow. *E*, Flexion of hip and knee.

Another way in which the Valsalva maneuver can be avoided is by helping the patient confined to bed to move into a sitting or squatting position when using the bed pan. A better alternative is to provide a commode chair or to help the patient to the bathroom if this is allowed by the physician in charge. Because constipation contributes to straining at the stool, measures should be taken to prevent this condition from developing. Stool softeners are preferred to harsh laxa-

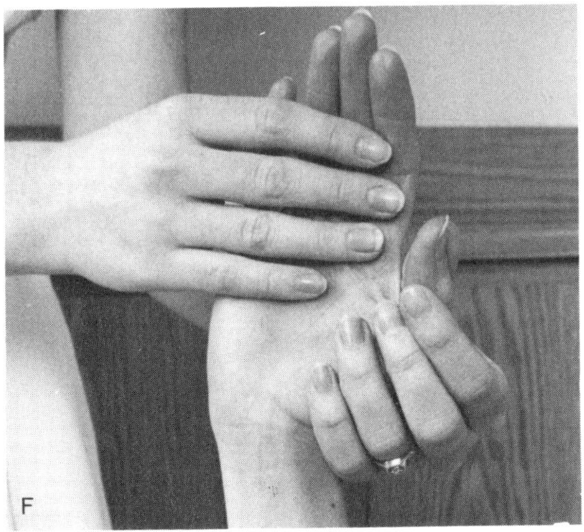

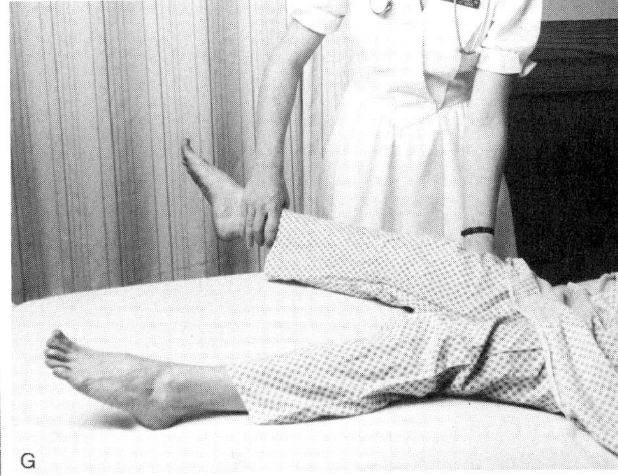

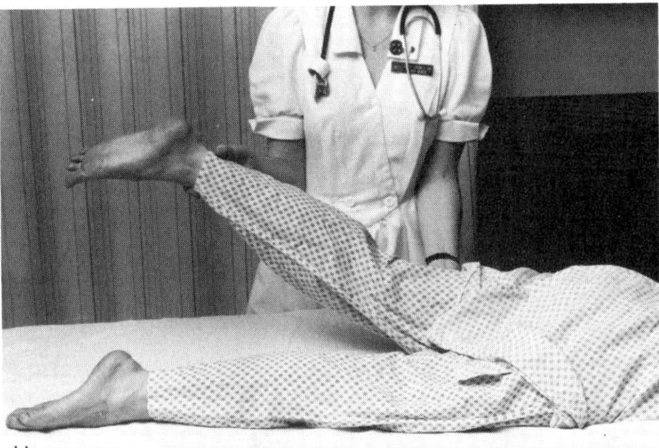

Figure 9-1 *Continued F,* Extension of fingers. *G,* Abduction and adduction of hip. *H,* Hyperextension of hip.
(Photos by Ken Kasper.)

tives. The effects of immobility on the gastrointestinal tract are discussed later in this chapter.

When a patient cannot change position because of weakness or paralysis, a schedule must be set up so that he is not allowed to lie in one position for too long. The usual period of time between changes of position is 2 hours, but the normal person moves about every few minutes, even when sleeping. If at all possible, some effort should be made to move the patient and change his position at least every hour and each time a medication is given or some other treatment is required.

It should be pointed out that turning a patient on his side will not prevent pressure on the blood vessels unless the uppermost leg is supported so that it does not rest on the other leg.

Injury from falling or fainting as a result of orthostatic hypotension can be prevented by raising the head of the bed and allowing the patient to sit up for a few minutes before moving him to a standing position. This change of position will help to overcome the effects of sudden drops in blood pressure when the patient is allowed to stand. Remember to move slowly and deliberately, and be sure there is sufficient help to support the patient if fainting occurs.

Elevating the head of the bed also is helpful, even though the patient may not be allowed to stand or to sit in a chair. This change of position will help to overcome the effects of sudden drops in blood pressure when the patient is allowed to stand.

RESPIRATORY SYSTEM

PATHOPHYSIOLOGY

The classic example of an automatic activity that is vital to life and health but nevertheless taken very much for granted is the act of breathing. Until something goes wrong, most of us do not think about the number of times we breathe per minute, how deeply we breathe, or what might happen if our breathing became abnormal.

The major function of the respiratory system is the exchange of oxygen and carbon dioxide. In order for this exchange to take place there must be thin, moist, mucous membrane along the airway passages and alveoli of the lung. The exchange of gases is impeded by accumulation of thick secretions, which have a tendency to pool in the lower respiratory structures when a person remains immobile or does not take deep breaths periodically. Healthy, normally active persons may not realize it, but they take about six to eight deep, sighing breaths every hour. These breaths help keep the lungs expanded and move secretions upward along the air passages. They also improve venous return of blood to the heart by way of the venae cavae and pulmonary veins. Thus they facilitate the transport of carbon dioxide from the tissues to the lungs for elimination.

ASSESSMENT

The nurse should be alert for respiratory problems in patients who are most at risk for such difficulties because of decreased motion of the organs of respiration. These include those who have been given a general anesthesia or are receiving sedatives, especially the sedative drugs that depress respiration. Other patients at risk are those who have tight bandages or binders that interfere with expansion of the chest; have abdominal distention from gas, fluid, or fecal material; or lie in one position for extended periods of time.

In assessing the respiratory status of a patient and determining the need for preventive and therapeutic measures, the nurse gathers both objective and subjective data. These are summarized in Table 9–1.

Additional assessment might include checking bandages and binders to be sure they are not restricting movement of the chest muscles, noting whether abdominal distention is causing pressure against the diaphragm, and determining whether sedatives and other drugs that depress respiration are interfering with normal breathing patterns.

NURSING INTERVENTION

Nursing measures to prevent respiratory problems related to immobility include frequent turning, coughing and deep breathing exercises, adequate fluid intake, and ambulation as soon as and whenever possible. When it is not possible for the patient to ambulate or sit up in a chair, changing his position to the semi-Fowler's or Fowler's position and from side to side can facilitate the movement of secretions in the air passages.

Controlled, deep-breathing patterns usually must be taught to the patient who is likely to have decreased respiratory function. He is taught to expand his lower chest and to use his abdominal muscles and diaphragm to improve aeration of the lungs. He is told to concentrate on exhaling the air slowly, to purse his lips, and to be more concerned with the *volume* of air being exhaled rather than the force with which he exhales it.

Effective coughing may not come naturally to the patient. He might be afraid that coughing will cause pain, and sometimes it is uncomfortable, especially when there is a surgical incision. Patients with a chronic cough often are fearful of triggering an exhausting episode of coughing, and some patients simply may not know that it is important to cough up secretions. When teaching a patient to cough effectively, the nurse should explain that the objective of coughing is to gradually move the secretions upward and to cough them out a little at a time. He is told to avoid a very large, explosive cough that can be painful or cause exhaustion.

The most effective technique for clearing secretions from the lower parts of the air passages

TABLE 9–1 ASSESSMENT AND NURSING INTERVENTIONS TO PREVENT OR ALLEVIATE RESPIRATORY PROBLEMS RELATED TO IMMOBILITY

Nursing Diagnosis	Assessment Data	Nursing Interventions
Potential for impaired gas exchange related to pulmonary stasis and accumulation of tracheobronchial secretions	Objective data: wheezing, rattling sounds in chest and throat; cough, productive or nonproductive; frequency of cough; characteristics of sputum; respiratory rate, patterns; characteristics of respiration—deep, shallow, rapid, slow; skin color; diaphoresis Subjective data: feeling of tightness in chest; shortness of breath; pain or discomfort on inhaling or exhaling; location and degree of pain	Instruct patient in deep breathing and coughing techniques Turn and change position at least q 2 h Support incision site during coughing exercises if surgical patient Give mouth care after coughing episodes Provide periods of rest Encourage ambulation when allowed Increase fluid intake unless contraindicated

is taking a single deep breath and following it with three consecutive coughs, trying to clear all the air from the lungs with each cough. This is most effective when the patient is in a sitting position while doing the coughing and deep breathing. Discomfort can be minimized by supporting the abdomen while the procedures are being done, especially if there is an incision and sutures.

Coughing and deep breathing exercises are done at the same time to allow for periods of rest and to obtain the best results. They usually are done every 2 hours until the patient is able to ambulate.

Adequate fluid intake is necessary so that the secretions in the air passages will not become too dry, thick, and difficult to remove by coughing. When the patient has abdominal distention or nausea or is otherwise not inclined to drink fluids, it is better to have him drink small amounts at frequent intervals rather than forcing down large quantities at a time.

Frequent changes of position help prevent pooling of bronchial and tracheal secretions and allow for easier removal by coughing and deep breathing exercises.

Although artificial ventilation that assists the patient's breathing may be indicated in some cases, this procedure is not a substitute for simpler, less hazardous, and sometimes equally effective nursing measures.

GASTROINTESTINAL TRACT

PATHOPHYSIOLOGY

Immobility from causes other than paralysis does not directly affect either the structure or the function of the gastrointestinal tract. However, it does have an *indirect* effect on the intake (ingestion) of food and elimination of waste.

Ingestion

Perhaps the most common difficulty experienced by a patient who is immobilized and unable to carry out the usual activities of daily life is that of loss of appetite. Worry, depression, anxiety about dependence on others, and decreased metabolic needs due to inactivity all contribute to anorexia.

As the food intake decreases, there is a possibility that the patient will develop a protein deficiency. *Hypoproteinemia* is a common disorder in immobilized patients. It can usually be avoided if measures are taken to guarantee a sufficient dietary intake of protein.

Elimination

Constipation is the most common gastrointestinal disorder likely to occur in a bedridden, extremely weak, or physically inactive person. Another, less common problem is diarrhea, which often occurs as a result of fecal impaction from constipation.

Many factors contribute to constipation in the patient who is physically inactive, not the least of which is a change in his usual routine and environment. Because of embarrassment, inability to defecate while lying on a bedpan, and weakened muscle tone, the patient unconsciously ignores the normal urge to have a bowel movement. If the impulse is ignored for a considerable time, the natural urge to defecate is diminished and eventually disappears.

> ***A fecal impaction** is the presence of either hardened or puttylike feces in the rectum and sigmoid colon. If the condition is not relieved, intestinal obstruction can occur. Symptoms of a fecal impaction include painful defecation, feeling of fullness in the rectum, abdominal distention, and sometimes cramps and watery stools.*

Diarrheic stools do *not* mean that the fecal impaction has been relieved; the liquid fecal material may bypass the hardened mass.

In order to allow early treatment to prevent chronic constipation and subsequent fecal impaction, it is important to keep an accurate record of each patient's bowel movements. It is not necessary for the patient to have a bowel movement each day, but the absence of stools for more than 3 days should be noted and the rectum examined for possible fecal impaction. Size of the stool also is important, because small amounts of stool may be passing without emptying the rectum and colon, allowing the fecal mass to become increasingly large.

Once an impaction has developed, the mass of feces must be broken up with a gloved finger. Before digital removal of the mass, it is sometimes helpful to give an oil retention enema to soften the mass. It is best to give an analgesic 1 hour before digital removal of an impaction.

NURSING ASSESSMENT AND INTERVENTION

Patients who are inactive for whatever reason require continual assessment in order to determine their specific nursing care needs. The care plan should include a schedule for checking the patient's dietary intake and accurately recording the exact amounts and types of food eaten. It also should note a patient's preference for certain foods and liquids and plans for providing a well-balanced diet based on the patient's particular likes and dislikes.

Because embarrassment and inability to use a bedpan with ease are major factors in the development of constipation, every effort should be made to provide privacy and to help the patient overcome these obstacles to normal elimination. Whenever possible, a commode chair at the bedside or transportation to a bathroom is preferred to the use of a bedpan in bed. When the patient must remain in bed, he may have less difficulty if he can be helped to a sitting or squatting position on the bedpan.

During the assessment phase of the nursing process, questions are asked to determine the patient's usual habits of elimination. How often during the week does the patient usually have a bowel movement? What time of day? Is he in the habit of taking laxatives or enemas? How frequently? What facilitates his bowel movement?

The prevention of constipation should not depend on such extreme measures as laxatives and enemas. Increased fluids and added roughage in the diet can help alleviate the problem. If the stools are hard and difficult to pass, stool softeners are indicated. These drugs do not increase the bulk in the intestine and are not irritating to the intestinal tract. Their action is primarily that of emulsifiying and softening fecal material so it is more easily eliminated. Examples of fecal softeners include docusate sodium (Colace and Doxinate) and docusate calcium (Surfak).

A *bowel training program* should be designed according to each patient's needs (see Chapter 15). The plan of care will depend on the cause of the difficulty in elimination and the patient's physical and mental capacities for cooperation. Adequate fluid intake should be considered as well as the time and location for elimination. In some cases, exercises to strengthen the abdominal muscles can be employed if the patient's physical condition permits. Patients also need to be informed of the importance of heeding the impulse to defecate so that this normal reflexive action can be preserved and chronic constipation avoided.

MUSCULOSKELETAL SYSTEM

PATHOPHYSIOLOGY

The muscles and bones of an immobile patient are likely to deteriorate very rapidly. Even in normal, healthy individuals, confinement to bed for only a few days results in muscle weakness and joint stiffness. The everyday activities of walking and lifting and otherwise exercising the muscles and joints are necessary for maintaining muscle tone and coordination and bone solidity, and for promoting circulation.

The adverse effects of immobility on the muscles and bones include loss of elasticity and range of motion and demineralization of bone *(osteoporosis).*

Range of Motion

Each of the joints of the body has a range of motion—that is, the extremes to which the joint may be moved in various directions. Muscular activity maintains that range of motion by allowing the joint to remain flexible and functional.

The purpose of ROM exercises is to put each joint that is at risk for loss of motion through its full range of motion during the exercises. The major motions are rotation, flexion, extension, abduction, adduction, and hyperextension. For the shoulder, internal rotation involves placing the arm at shoulder height, bending the elbow to a 90-degree angle, and turning the upper arm until the palm of the hand and inner arm face backward; for external rotation of the shoulder, turn the flexed arm until the palm and inner arm face forward. To exercise the hip joint, internal rotation is done by turning the leg inward so that the toes point in the direction of the opposite leg; external rotation involves turning the leg so that the toes point away from the opposite leg. To exercise the elbow, bend the elbow and bring the forearm and hand toward the shoulder; then straighten the arm. Flexion of the hip and knee is performed by flexing the knee and bending the leg toward the hip as far as possible. Abduction of the hip is performed by moving the straightened leg outward from the body as far as possible; for adduction, move the leg toward the body to neutral position next to the other leg and then move it across the other leg as far as possible. To hyperextend the hip, place the patient prone and move the straightened leg upward away from the mattress as far as possible. For the hand, extend each finger so that it can lie flat against a surface such as your own finger. Flex by gently curling each finger to the palm (see Fig. 9–1).

When there is little or no motion of a joint, its structures change. The muscles lose their elasticity and become shorter. Normal tissue is replaced by fibrous tissue. This adaptive shortening of the muscles and tendons is called a *contracture.*

Osteoporosis

Although we often think of bone as being a very dense, lifeless kind of structure, it actually is a living tissue in which there is a continual exchange of materials and a breaking down and building up of cells. Normally the replacing of old bone cells with new, stronger ones takes place because of the stress and strain that standing and walking place on the bone tissue.

Inactivity interferes with the process of building up the bone, causing a depletion of the supply of calcium, phosphorus, and nitrogen in bone. As a result of this demineralization, the bone becomes porous, hence the name *osteo* (bone) *porosis* (a state of being porous). The soft, spongy bones of osteoporosis are easily deformed or broken.

NURSING INTERVENTION

One of the first concerns of the nurse should be to maintain joints in their functional positions so that they are not abnormally flexed or extended.

Position maintenance can be accomplished by using a foot board that keeps the feet at right angles to the legs so that foot drop is avoided; by splinting limbs so that they are kept straight; by using a bed board to prevent curvature of the spine; and by placing a firm splint in the hands to keep the fingers from drawing up into a tight fist. The patient also should not be positioned with pillow and mattress supports that cause the knees and hips to remain flexed.

ROM exercises will help the patient maintain optimal function of his joints. If at all possible, the patient should be taught to do these exercises himself or at least to participate in them insofar as he is able.

Standing the patient on his feet and having him bear his weight on his legs is the best prevention of osteoporosis. If this is not possible, exercises in bed, in which he pushes his feet against a foot board, and isometric exercises to maintain muscle tone are helpful.

An increase in dietary and supplemental calcium may help prevent osteoporosis, but there is the possibility that in an immobilized patient the increased calcium intake can predispose him to the formation of stones in the urinary system. The calcium content of selected foods is shown in Table 9–2.

TABLE 9–2 CALCIUM CONTENT OF SELECTED FOODS

Food	Amount	Calcium Content (mg)
Low-fat yogurt, plain	1 cup	415
Sardines (with bones)	3 oz	372
Collard greens	1 cup	357
Skim milk	1 cup	302
Low-fat milk (2%)	1 cup	297
Whole milk	1 cup	291
Turnip greens	1 cup	287
Salmon (canned)	3 oz	285
Swiss cheese	1 oz	272
Oysters	1 cup	226
Kale	1 cup	206
Cheddar cheese	1 oz	204
Mustard greens	1 cup	193
American cheese	1 oz	174
Bean curd (tofu)	4 oz	154
Low-fat cottage cheese	1 cup	138
Broccoli	1 cup	136

SKIN

PATHOPHYSIOLOGY

Skin health depends on adequate circulation, cleanliness, and the exchange of nutrients and waste products in the environment of the cells of the skin. Pressure against the skin interferes with circulation, and because cells die very quickly without adequate blood supply, a *pressure sore* or "bed sore" can begin to develop within hours after a person is immobilized. The major effect of immobility as far as the skin is concerned is the development of bed sores or *decubitus ulcers*.

Decubitus Ulcer

The medical term for a pressure sore is *decubitus ulcer*. The word *decubitus* means "lying down," and an ulcer is a lesion produced by the sloughing of necrotic, inflammatory tissue (Fig. 9–2). Thus a decubitus ulcer is an open wound that is associated with lying in bed; however, lesions of this kind also can develop in patients who sit in one position for long periods.

Many different factors contribute to the development of decubitus ulcers, but the two major causes are prolonged pressure on a specific part of the body, and a *shearing force*, which exerts a downward and forward pressure on tissues underlying the skin. This shearing action takes place when a patient slumps down while sitting in bed or in a chair.

Decubitus ulcers are also called pressure sores because they result from pressure against the blood vessels that supply the affected area of skin. If you have ever sat with your legs pressing against the edge of a chair or crossed one leg over the other for an extended period of time, you may have noticed that an area of redness (erythema) appeared at the points of pressure. This erythema is the beginning of a pressure sore and is a sign that the capillaries in the area have become congested because of impaired blood flow.

The reddened area can occur within an hour or two in a person with healthy skin and adequate circulation. It is even more likely to develop and rapidly progress to an ulcerated stage in persons who are malnourished, obese, aged, or

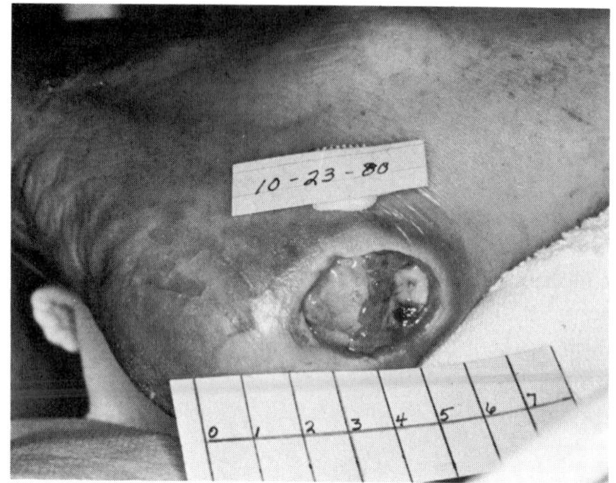

Figure 9-2 Decubitus ulcer.

suffering from circulatory disease. Breakdown of the skin is also more likely to occur if, in addition to continued pressure, the skin is subjected to heat, moisture, and irritating substances such as those present in decomposing urine, feces, perspiration, and vaginal discharge.

ASSESSMENT

Several kinds of preprinted forms for assessment of the skin for potential development of pressure sores are available. These assessment tools take into account the general condition of the skin, control of urination and defecation, mobility, mental status, and nutritional status (Fig. 9-3). Tools such as these provide for a more

SKIN CARE ASSESSMENT GUIDELINE

GENERAL INFORMATION

Prevention of decubitus ulcers is a vital part of long term patient care. It is important to evaluate your patient's condition by looking for factors that may lead to the formation of decubitus ulcers, i.e., immobility, skin debility, poor nutrition, apathy, or incontinence.

Evaluate each of your patients on the following scale, and select the one number in each category which best describes your patient's status. Add the numbers checked to obtain the total. A score of 10 or greater indicates a high probability of decubitus ulcer development.

If your patient does develop a decubitus ulcer, utilize the reverse side of this form to properly analyze your patient's condition.

PATIENT'S NAME________________ DATE________

(CHECK THE DESCRIPTION THAT BEST DESCRIBES YOUR PATIENT)

OVERALL SKIN CONDITION

	Grade	
	1	Turgor (elasticity) adequate, skin moist and warm
	2	Poor turgor, skin cold and dry
	3	Areas mottled, red or denuded

BOWEL AND BLADDER CONTROL

	Grade	
	1	Always able to ask for bedpan
	2	Incontinence of urine
	3	Incontinence of feces
	4	Totally incontinent

REHABILITATIVE STATE

	Grade	
	1	Ambulated with assistance
	2	Chair to bed ambulation only
	3	Confined to bed
	4	Immobile in bed

MENTAL STATE

	Grade	
	1	Alert and clear
	2	Confused
	3	Disoriented & senile
	4	Stuporous
	5	Unconscious

NUTRITIONAL STATE

	Grade	
	1	Eats all offered
	2	Eats very little offered
	3	Refuses food often
	4	Tube feeding
	5	Intravenous feeding

☐ Total Score (scale: 5-9 — low risk of decubitus ulcer development
10 and greater — high risk of decubitus ulcer development)

Figure 9-3 Sample form for assessment of skin care. (Courtesy of Dow B. Hickam, Inc.)

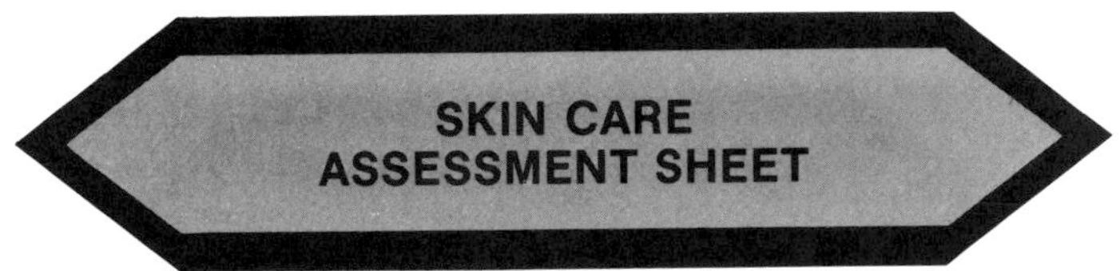

PATIENT'S NAME ______________________ DATE ______________________

SIZE OF ULCER ______________________ LOCATION OF ULCER ______________________
(Indicate on diagram below)

ADDITIONAL INFORMATION ______________________

Figure 9–3 *Continued*

systematic approach to assessment of a patient's potential for decubitus ulcer development and serve as a guide for a plan of nursing care.

In spite of all efforts to prevent them, pressure sores can develop in patient of all ages and states of health, or a patient can be admitted to the hospital or long-term-care facility with an existing ulcer. Assessment of the stage of ulceration can be useful in accurately documenting that an ulcer was present on admission. Classifying an ulceration also can be helpful in evaluating the effectiveness of treatment and progress toward healing and repair.

Stage I. The area of skin is deep pink, red, or mottled. Digital pressure on the area will cause temporary blanching for up to 15 minutes after pressure is released. The skin will feel very warm and firm or tightly stretched across the area. At this stage no destruction of tissue has occurred, and the condition is reversible.

Stage II. The skin appears blistered, cracked, or abraded. The area surrounding the damaged skin is reddened and probably will feel hot or warmer than normal.

Stage III. The skin is ulcerated. There is a craterlike sore, and the underlying tissues are becoming involved in the destructive process. The ulcer may or may not be infected. Bacterial infection is almost always present at this stage, however, and accounts for continued erosion of the ulcer and the production of drainage.

Stage IV. There is deep ulceration and necrosis

involving deeper underlying muscle and possibly bone tissue. At this point the ulcer usually is extensively infected. The ulcer can be dry, black in color, and covered with a tough accumulation of necrotic tissue, or it can be wet and oozing dead cells and purulent exudate.

NURSING INTERVENTION

Prevention of decubitus ulcers is far more desirable and less time consuming than treatment. Efforts to preserve the integrity of the skin must be the responsibility of the nursing staff, as well as the patient himself if he is able to participate in his care.

Frequent changes in position and proper alignment and support of body structures are essential to prevention of pressure sores. It is normal and natural for one to move about every few minutes, even in one's sleep. Patients who are not able to change their positions or are not mentally alert enough to relieve continuous pressure against a part of the body must be turned a minimum of every 2 hours. However, this is barely adequate for most patients and not nearly often enough for some. Those who are obese, malnourished, or suffering from diminished circulation will need to be turned and repositioned more often than every 2 hours.

The plan of care for prevention of pressure sores must take into account the *area* of pressure as well as the *amount* of pressure being exerted. Underlying bones such as those in the sacral area, buttocks, heels, hip, and ankle contribute to the interference of blood flow (Fig. 9–4).

Seventeen percent of all pressure sores occur over the trochanter. When patients are turned onto their sides to relieve pressure on the back, the practice has been to put the leg that rests on the mattress in a neutral position and to flex the uppermost leg across the body. In this position the hip is flexed at 55 to 60 degrees and the knee is flexed at 80 degrees. However, a study of paraplegic and quadriplegic persons has shown that pressure on the trochanter *can be reduced* by positioning the upper leg *behind* the midline of the body and supporting the lower part of this leg with a pillow. In this position the upper leg is flexed 30 degrees at the hip and 35 degrees at the knee. The authors of the study do not claim that positioning alone will prevent pressure sores over the trochanter, only that the recommended position will lessen the potential for skin breakdown in that area.

In addition to frequent changing of position, an effort must be made to keep the bed linens dry, smooth, and free of wrinkles. The same is true of any part of the patient's clothing that he is lying

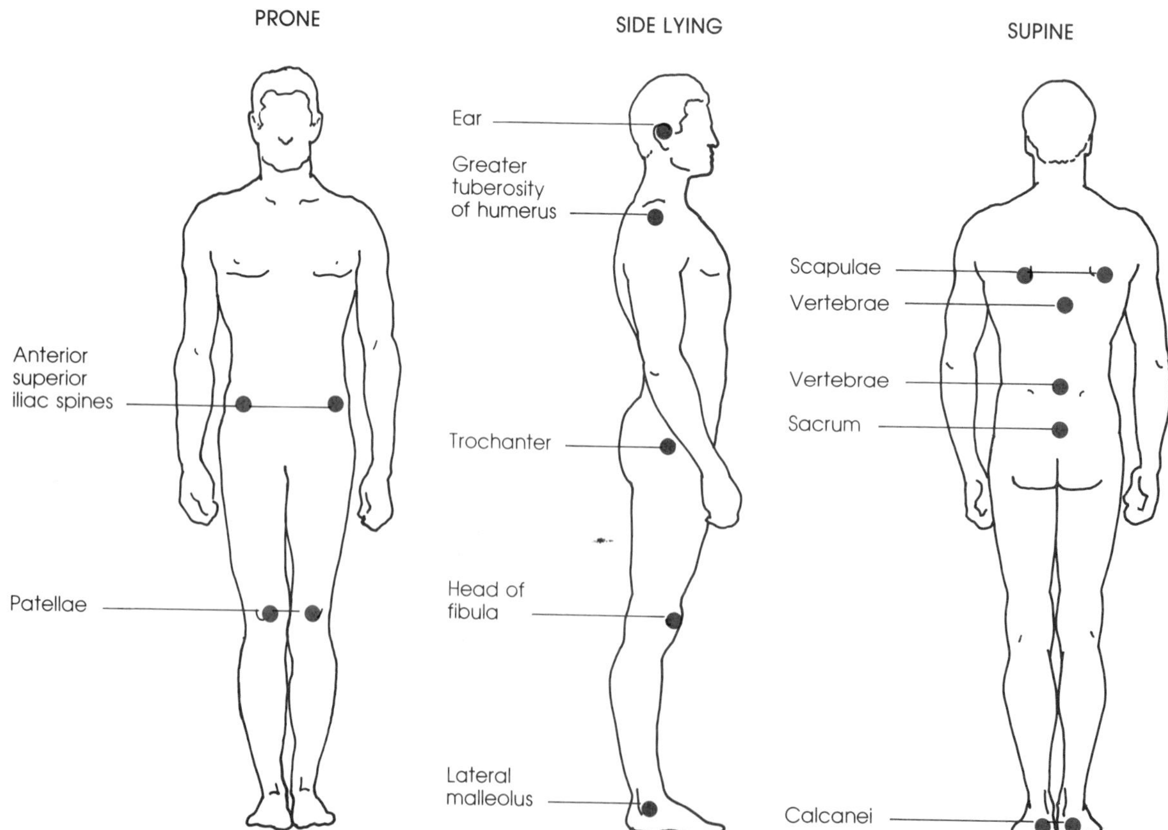

Figure 9–4 Bony prominences most susceptible to skin breakdown according to position.

on. Cleanliness, especially the removal of urine, feces, perspiration, and vaginal discharge, is extremely important in prevention of skin breakdown. Care should be used to remove all soap from the skin after bathing so that excessive drying and irritation of the skin is avoided.

A third component of prevention is gentle massage of areas in which ulcers are likely to develop. Massage is recommended at least once every 8 hours. A nonalcoholic lotion can be used to lubricate and strengthen the skin. The massaging should be done lightly with the tips of the fingers and in a circular motion in the direction around, but at least an inch from, the reddened area or ulcer.

Adequate nutrition, exercise when possible, and getting the patient out of bed when feasible are all important to prevention of skin breakdown. Additionally, the patient who is able to do so should be encouraged to accept some responsibility for skin care and decubitus ulcer prevention. He will need instruction in the causes of pressure sores, the areas most susceptible to pressure, and the techniques that are effective in maintaining the integrity of the skin.

Friction can contribute to damage to the uppermost layers of the skin and predispose it to ulceration. There are many ways in which friction and pressure can be avoided. First, it is imperative that the patient's body not be dragged over sheets when he is being repositioned or transferred from bed to chair. Gentle handling is essential to preservation of the skin and underlying tissues. A draw sheet should be used for every bedridden patient. With two people the sheet and patient can be lifted and repositioned or lifted and turned without endangering the patient's skin. There must be sufficient help available to move the patient who is unable to move himself.

Devices to relieve pressure and distribute it more evenly include a bed cradle to relieve the weight of top covers on the feet, specially designed socks, bootees, padding for the elbows and wrists, and pneumatic or fluid-filled flotation pads. Sheepskin and puff-packs are also used to avoid skin breakdown. Rubber rings and doughnuts made of gauze and cotton are not advised, because although they might reduce pressure in the area that is not in direct contact with them, they allow pressure to be applied to an even larger area, thereby causing larger areas of ulceration.

Prevention and treatment of pressure sores and other problems of immobility can be greatly facilitated by placing the patient on a special bed such as the Clinitron bed shown in Figure 9–5. The bed is designed to provide support for patients who must not move, such as the patient with a fractured spine; those who cannot move; and those whose handling, turning, and positioning is painful or difficult, such as a burn patient.

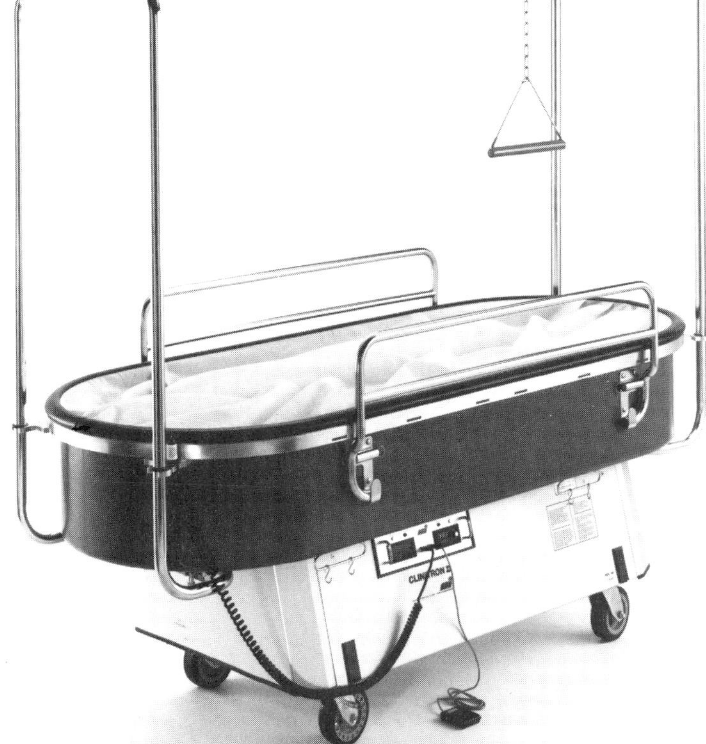

Figure 9–5 CLINITRON Air fluidized therapy for treatment of stage III and IV pressure ulcers, multiple stage II ulcers, or stage II ulcers where coexisting risk factors are present; posterior and lateral flaps and grafts; second- and third-degree burns; and intractable pain. This therapy is ideal for the patient who is nonambulatory and does not require frequent transfers. Therapy unit accessories allow for head elevation, which may be essential for concomitant treatments. This therapy unit provides pressure relief and reduces shear, friction, and maceration—all factors that contribute to the formation and degradation of pressure ulcers.

(Courtesy of Support Systems International, Inc., Charleston, SC.)

Treatment of decubitus ulcers varies widely from one institution to another and even from one patient care area to another. Generally, nursing intervention includes wound culture if the involved area has signs of infection. The ulcer is cleansed with an antimicrobial agent such as povidone iodine (Betadine) and then irrigated with normal saline. When further débridement is needed, the patient may have whirlpool baths prescribed along with enzymatic débriding agents and wet-to-dry dressing. Débridement is sufficient when the ulcer bed appears pink, indicating healthy granulation tissue.

The dressing should provide a clean, moist environment to promote healing. Occlusive dressings such as Duoderm or semipermeable films like Opsite are often used. For deep ulcers that are producing a large amount of exudate, karaya powder, Debrisan, or Bard absorptive materials are used. Applying a film dressing over a reddened area *before* the skin has broken has proved effective in preventing many pressure ulcers.

Perhaps the most important factor is the commitment of those who favor one method of therapy over another. Whatever the treatment prescribed, it must be followed *diligently* by everyone responsible for the care of the patient. If any aspect of the care is neglected for even 4 to 8 hours, deterioration of tissue will progress more rapidly than healing.

URINARY SYSTEM

PATHOPHYSIOLOGY

The urinary system is designed so that it functions best when the body is upright. Urine flows from the kidney downward in the direction of the pull of gravity. When the body is in a reclining position, the hilus of the kidney must force urine into the ureters against the pull of gravity. Urine is continually being formed in the kidney, but the peristaltic action of the kidney and ureters is not sufficient to maintain a constant flow of urine. If the body remains in a supine position, even for a few days, the flow becomes sluggish and there is a pooling of urine. This sets the stage for the formation of stones (calculi) and the development of infection.

Another effect that lying in bed has on the urinary system is the loss of control of the urinary sphincter muscles and resultant incontinence. Without the downward pressure of the full bladder against the sphincter muscles, there is less awareness of the need to void. The result is bladder distention and an overflow or dribbling of urine without the patient's awareness of it.

In the introduction to this chapter, we spoke of the interdependence of the various systems of the body. The urinary system, being a system of excretion, must work harder to eliminate the excess amounts of calcium, nitrogen, phosphorus, sodium, and other products of protein breakdown that build up with bed rest. Of these substances, the most troublesome is calcium, the mineral of which most urinary calculi are composed.

NURSING ASSESSMENT AND INTERVENTION

As for all other preventive measures previously discussed, a schedule of checking for early signs of urinary complications and a plan of prevention are essential.

The number of times a patient voids and the characteristics of the urine should be accurately recorded. Bladder distention should be watched for, and if possible, the bladder should be emptied at each voiding. For a male patient, this may necessitate having him stand and void. If this is not possible, he should be helped to sit upright. Women also should be helped to a sitting position when voiding. Moderate pressure of the hand against the lower pelvic region will facilitate emptying of the bladder and may be all that is needed to prevent bladder distention.

Adequate fluid intake is obviously an important factor in the prevention of urinary complications. Ideally, the patient should drink 8 ounces of fluid every hour when awake. The patient's intake of calcium may be restricted, and because most stones are formed in an alkaline environment, the physician may prescribe an acid-ash diet, which is a diet composed of foods and liquids that have an acid residue. Foods of this type include cereals, meat, and fish. Contrary to popular belief, citrus fruits such as lemons and oranges do not make the urine acidic.

Infections as well as calculi can be prevented best by keeping the urine dilute and flowing normally. Catheterization should be used only as a last resort because of the ever-present danger of introducing infectious organisms into the urinary tract.

Nursing interventions for selected problems in an immobilized patient are summarized in Nursing Care Plan 9–1.

PSYCHOSOCIAL EFFECTS OF IMMOBILIZATION

Perhaps more than any other consequence of illness and injury, being immobilized and unable to attend to one's own personal needs has the most profound and far-reaching effect on mental outlook and social adaptation. It is not hard to imagine the anxieties, fears, and sense of hopelessness one might feel when faced with the reality that he is dependent on others for help in meeting the most basic human needs.

NURSING CARE PLAN 9–1

Selected nursing diagnoses, goals/outcome criteria, nursing interventions, and evaluations for an immobilized patient

Situation: Patient is an 83-year-old male with extreme weakness and debilitation and with several chronic diseases. He was transferred from a convalescent center with pneumonia, which has now almost completely resolved.

Nursing Diagnosis	Goals/Outcome Criteria	Nursing Intervention	Evaluation
Impaired physical mobility related to weakness, debility, illness, and age. SUPPORTING DATA Unable to turn or reposition self unaided; cannot walk.	Patient will maintain present joint mobility. Patient will do active ROM of arms by discharge.	Perform ROM on all joints tid. Assist to turn and reposition q 2 h round the clock. Place in high Fowler's position for meals; assist to chair for lunch.	ROM: 10, 1, and 5 o'clock; turned: 8, 10, 12, and 2 o'clock; up in chair for lunch; continue plan.
Impaired skin integrity related to immobility and pressure over left trochanter. SUPPORTING DATA Pressure area, stage I, over left trochanter. History of previous pressure ulcers.	No further evidence of pressure damage to skin before discharge.	Position in bed so that one leg is not pressing on the other when patient is on his side; properly support with pillows. Turn more frequently than q 2 h if possible. Keep reddened area clean, clear dressing in place; inspect q shift. Inspect all pressure points q 4 h to identify problems early. Use turning sheet to turn patient.	Turned q 1 h; Tegoderm in place; redness decreasing; other pressure points clear; positioned with pillows.
Alteration in bowel elimination: constipation related to immobility. SUPPORTING DATA Has passed only small amount of hard, dry stool in past four days.	Normal bowel pattern by discharge.	Administer oil retention enema as ordered, followed by suppository; monitor results. Give stool softener daily as ordered. Increase fluids to 4 oz every hour while awake. Assist to bedside commode after breakfast each day. Provide privacy. Add bran muffin to breakfast. Offer prune juice nightly.	Taking 4 oz q h; small BM after breakfast; stool softener, prune juice, and bran muffin taken. Continue plan.
Potential for injury related to possible falls. SUPPORTING DATA Very weak and debilitated; cannot walk. Tends to be confused after sundown.	Patient will not sustain fall in hospital.	Keep siderails up at all times when not at bedside. Place call light and personal items within reach. Answer call light promptly. Frequently reinforce instructions not to get up without assistance. Assist to bedside commode with two people. Keep low light on in room at night to decrease confusion. Check on patient frequently; anticipate needs.	Siderails up; asking for assistance to get up; night light on during night; less confused.

Nursing Care Plan continued on following page

In addition to the loss of independence, there is worry over financial matters and concern for family members and friends and how their lives are affected. The immobilized patient also experiences isolation and depression, because he is no longer able to go to others to find comp and social interaction but must wait fc come to him.

The list of psychological and socia associated with immobility is almost

NURSING CARE PLAN 9–1, *Continued*

Nursing Diagnosis	Goals/Outcome Criteria	Nursing Intervention	Evaluation
Potential impaired gas exchange related to immobility and resolving pneumonia. SUPPORTING DATA Impaired mobility; weakness and debility; lungs just cleared from pneumonia; breathes shallowly naturally.	Patient will perform breathing exercises q 2 h while awake. Lung fields will remain clear.	Auscultate lungs q shift. Assist with sitting position for deep breathing and coughing exercises q 2 h. Encourage adequate fluid intake. Administer remaining doses of antibiotics as ordered. Encourage him to take deeper breaths during each commercial break when watching television.	Turn, cough, deep breathe: 8, 10, and 2; lungs clear to auscultation; intake 1,500 mL this shift. Taking antibiotics. Continue plan.
Potential for infection, urinary tract, related to immobility. SUPPORTING DATA Immobility causes stasis of urine; debilitated state makes patient more susceptible to infection; has history of urinary tract infections.	No urinary tract infection, as evidenced by clear urine, no dysuria, no fever. Patient will have fluid intake of at least 2,000 mL per day.	Assess for bladder distention q 4 h; observe characteristics of urine for signs of infection. Measure fluid I and O; encourage fluids every hour while awake.	Urine clear amber; I = 2,650 mL, O = 2020 mL; taking fluids q h; no bladder distention; continue plan.
Potential alteration in tissue perfusion related to possible thrombophlebitis from immobility. SUPPORTING DATA Immobile, debilitated, unable to walk. Has moderate peripheral vascular disease.	No evidence of thrombophlebitis or deep vein thrombosis; negative Homans' sign, no swelling of legs.	Encourage active ROM of legs, feet and ankles q 2 h while awake. Keep TED hose smoothly in place except for 30 min while bathing. Encourage extra fluid intake. Assess for Homans' sign q shift; visually inspect legs for reddening or swelling.	Homans' sign negative; leg exercises: 8, 10, 12, and 2; TEDs in place; taking adequate fluids.

are the activities that might be planned to help the patient deal with his problems. These activities are best planned and coordinated by utilizing the entire health care team, including the social worker, psychologist, occupational therapist, and others.

The primary responsibilities of the nurse in meeting the psychosocial needs of an immobilized patient, no matter what the cause of this immobility, center on doing that which she knows best; that is, (1) preventing the serious physiologic consequences that prohibit the patient from regaining some degree of independence, (2) attending to the patient's psychosocial concerns and needs, and (3) relating to the patient as a whole person so that he sees himself as a person of dignity and worth.

Negative attitudes toward the dependent and disabled are not uncommon, even among health care professionals. Our society as a whole places a high value on youth, productivity, and physical beauty. The goals are instant gratification and quick cures. Most of us are aware of this value system; the immobilized patient is no exception. Volumes have been written about the psychological impact of disability and disfigurement and how the way others feel about us affects the way we feel about ourselves. The complexities of these kinds of interpersonal reactions and interactions cannot be explored in the pages of this text, but perhaps the following quotation will give the reader some insight into dealing with these problems:

> If I am ugly, I am not ugly only in my own eyes, I see myself in the looking-glass of your eyes as ugly too. You are the witness of my ugliness. In fact, insofar as ugliness is relative, if you and everyone else saw me as beautiful, I might be ugly no more (Laing, 1966).

CONCERNS FOR THE ELDERLY

The elderly frequently have chronic disorders that augment the damaging effects of immobility. Muscle tone is decreased, which tends to increase urinary retention and constipation. The skin is more fragile and consequently is easily damaged with turning or pulling up in bed. The older patient is much more prone to orthostatic hypotension since the vascular system does not respond to position changes as effectively as in younger years.

A poor nutritional state is often found in the elderly. This predisposes to all types of infection that accompany immobility. Respiratory infection is particularly dangerous, as it can quickly progress to pneumonia.

The nurse must perform thorough assessment of the elderly immobile patient in order to prevent the various complications of immobility.

BIBLIOGRAPHY

Braden, B., and Bryant, R.: Innovations to prevent and treat pressure ulcers. Geriatr. Nurs., July/Aug., 1990, p. 182.

Chagares, R., and Jackson, B.: Sitting easy: How six pressure-relieving devices stack up. Am. J. Nurs., Feb., 1987, p. 191.

Colburn, L.: Preventing pressure ulcers. Nursing 90, Dec., 1990, p. 60.

Fowler, E. M.: Equipment and products used in management and treatment of pressure ulcers. Nurs. Clin. North Am., June, 1987, p. 449.

Gosnell, D. J.: Assessment and evaluation of pressure sores. Nurs. Clin. North Am., June, 1987, p. 399.

Holm, K., and Hedricks, C.: Immobility and bone loss in the aging adult. Crit. Care Nurs. Q., June, 1989, p. 46.

Holm, K., and Walker, D.: Osteoporosis: Treatment and prevention update. Geriatr. Nurs., July/Aug., 1990, p. 182.

Homes, R., et al.: Combating pressure sores—nutritionally. Am. J. Nurs., Oct., 1987, p. 1301.

Laing, R. D., et al.: Interpersonal Perception. New York, Springer Publ. Co., 1966.

Lovell, H., and Anderson, C.: Put your patient on the right bed. RN, May, 1990, p. 66.

Maklebust, J.: Pressure ulcers: Etiology and prevention. Nurs. Clin. North Am., June, 1987, p. 359.

Murray, S.M., and Thompson, R.: We've organized our approach to pressure sores. RN, Jan., 1991, p. 42.

Olson, E. V., et al.: The hazards of immobility. Am J. Nurs., March, 1990, p. 43.

Rubin, M.: The physiology of bedrest. Am. J. Nurs., Jan., 1987, p. 50.

Sebern, M.: Home team strategies for treating pressure sores. Nursing 87, April, 1987, p. 50.

Wells, T.: Conquering incontinence. Geriatr. Nurs., May/June, 1990, p. 133.

STUDENT STUDY AIDS

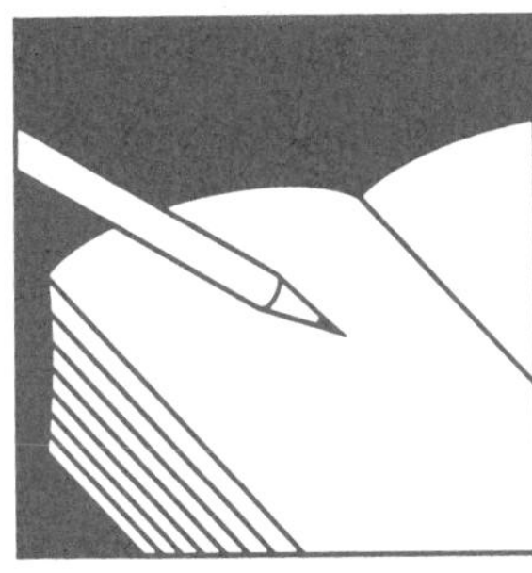

CLINICAL CASE PROBLEMS

Read each clinical situation and discuss the questions with your classmates.

1. Mark Hansen, age 26, has had skin grafting done to his abdomen and left leg to treat injuries from a motorcycle accident. He will be on bed rest for at least 10 days. He must be kept flat in bed with the head elevated no more than 20 degrees.

- Write a nursing care plan for Mark that will help prevent disabilities from inactivity.

2. Mr. Cobb is admitted to the hospital with a medical diagnosis of cerebral vascular accident (stroke). He has paralysis of his right arm and slight difficulty in moving his right leg. The physician has written an order saying that Mr. Cobb may be out of bed twice a day.

- Taking each system of the body, list nursing activities that should be included in a care plan that is designed to prevent disabilities from inactivity.

STUDY OUTLINE

I. Introduction

A. Human body is designed for motion.

B. Many disabilities arising from immobility can be prevented.

C. Prevention of disabilities caused by immobility is primarily a nursing responsibility.

D. Causes of immobility include paralysis, pain or fear of pain, surgery, physical trauma, weakness.

E. Therapeutic rest is prescribed for cardiac conditions, relief from pain, rest for healing of injury, reversal of effects of gravity.
F. Systems of body are affected singly and in relation to other systems.

II. Cardiovascular system

A. Blood vessels.
1. Major dangers are decreased blood supply to tissues and formation of a thrombus, caused by:
a. Allowing body to lie in one position too long.
b. Placing pillow under patient's knees.
c. Arranging bed so that it is bent under the knees.

B. Work load of the heart.
1. Heart works harder when the body is in a reclining position.
2. Valsalva maneuver produces a sudden increase in blood volume in the heart chambers, thereby increasing its work load.

C. Orthostatic hypotension: drop in blood pressure occurring when one stands for the first time after having been in bed for several days or longer.

D. Nursing intervention.
1. Exercises to maintain adequate circulation.
a. Active exercises are those carried out by the patient.
b. Passive exercises are those carried out by someone else.
c. Isometric exercises done to maintain muscle tone without moving the joint.
d. Type of exercise beneficial to the patient is prescribed by the physician or physical therapist.
2. Position changes.
a. Teach patient how to move himself in bed safely.
b. Every 2 hours is much less often than normal person changes position.
c. When patient is on his side, support upper leg so it is not resting on the lower.
3. Orthostatic hypotension presents danger of patient's falling and hurting himself. Have sufficient help and support for the patient when he first tries to stand after having been in bed for a period of time.

III. Respiratory system

A. Immobility restricts exchange of oxygen and carbon dioxide.
1. Limits movement of the lungs and muscles of respiration.
2. Decreases normal movement of secretions in tracheobronchial tree.

B. Nursing assessment: patients most likely to suffer from respiratory difficulties arising from immobility are:
1. Those who are heavily sedated, particularly with respiratory depressants.
2. Those having tight bandages or binders.
3. Those with abdominal distention.
4. Those who remain in a supine position for long periods of time.

C. Nursing intervention.
1. Proper positioning and frequent turning.
2. Teach patient coughing and deep breathing exercises.
3. Postural drainage.
4. Ensure adequate fluid intake.
5. Assessment of patient's respiratory status includes rate and depth of respirations; listening for moist, bubbling sounds or wheezing; color of skin.

6. Eventual outcome of unrelieved respiratory depression is hypostatic pneumonia.
7. Eventual outcome of hypoventilation may be cardiac arrest from severe respiratory acidosis.

IV. Gastrointestinal tract

A. Anorexia one of most common difficulties.
  1. Patients often suffer from hypoproteinemia.

B. Elimination of fecal material difficult because of embarrassment and inability to use bedpan.
  1. Chronic constipation likely to lead to fecal impaction.
  2. Unrelieved fecal impaction can lead to intestinal obstruction.
  3. Fecal impaction removed digitally; oil retention enema may facilitate removal.

C. Nursing assessment and intervention.
  1. Care plan should include schedule for checking dietary intake, noting patient's preferences in foods and liquids.
  2. Whenever possible, patient should be allowed to use commode chair at bedside or taken to the bathroom.
  3. Prevention of constipation should not depend on laxatives and enemas.
  4. Fecal softeners include Surfak and Colace.
  5. Bowel training program designed to meet individual patient's needs includes adequate fluid intake, time and location best for elimination, exercises to strengthen abdominal muscles.

V. Musculoskeletal system

A. Confinement to bed for even a few days can result in muscle weakness in normal, healthy person.

B. Range of motion lost when there is little or no motion of a joint; consequence of inactivity is *contractures.*

C. Osteoporosis occurs as result of decrease in normal stress on bones that occurs with standing and walking.
  1. Bones lose their minerals and become porous, easily deformed, and broken.

D. Nursing intervention.
  1. Keep joints in their functional position, using foot board, splints, bed board, rolled gauze in hands.
  2. Range-of-motion exercises.
  3. Stand patient up on his feet if at all possible.
  4. High calcium diet may lead to formation of urinary calculi.

VI. The skin

A. Decubitus ulcer most common consequence of prolonged pressure from lying or sitting in one position.
  1. Pressure against blood vessels deprives tissues of adequate blood supply.
  2. "Shearing" action forces a downward and forward pressure on tissues underlying the skin when patient sits in bed or chair and slumps down.

B. Assessment and prevention of pressure sores.
  1. Factors placing a patient at risk include:
    a. Altered mental status.
    b. Incontinence.
    c. Paralysis.
    d. Nutritional status.
  2. Systematically assess patients for skin changes.

C. Nursing intervention.

1. Institute a plan of care including schedule for changing position, massaging areas likely to break down.
2. Avoid friction against skin, wrinkles in bed clothes.
3. Use bed cradle to support weight of top covers.
4. Socks and foam rubber bootees preferred to rubber rings and doughnuts.
5. Flotation pads allow for even distribution of body weight.
6. Major factors in success of treatment of decubitus ulcers are commitment of nursing staff members and diligence with which they follow program of care.

VII. Urinary system

A. System designed so that it functions best when the body is in an upright position.

B. When body remains in supine position, there is a pooling of urine and sluggish flow.

C. Distended bladder leads to loss of control of external sphincter muscle.

D. Nursing assessment and intervention.

1. Observation for early signs of decreased urinary flow.
   a. Check and record number of times patient voids and characteristics of urine.
   b. Check for bladder distention.
   c. Have male patients stand to void whenever possible; if not, have them sit up to void. Females also should void while sitting up rather than while lying on bedpan.
   d. Moderate pressure of the hand on the lower pelvic region will help emptying of bladder.
2. Adequate fluid intake important in prevention of stones and infection.
3. Calcium intake may be limited.
4. Acid-ash diet may be prescribed.
5. Catheterization used only as a last resort because of danger of urinary infection.

VIII. Psychosocial effects

A. Effects on mental state include depression, anxiety, feeling of worthlessness.

B. Social effects include lack of social interaction because of isolation, inability to be physically active.

C. Therapeutic activities may be coordinated by many different members of the health care team.

D. Nurse's responsibilities primarily are:

1. Preventing physiologic disabilities that prohibit successful rehabilitation.
2. Helping patient see himself as a person of dignity and worth.

IX. Concerns for the elderly

A. Other chronic diseases among the elderly augment the effects of immobility.

B. Decreased muscle tone increases likelihood of urinary retention and constipation.

C. Elderly are especially prone to orthostatic hypotension.

D. Elderly often suffer from poor nutrition and are more susceptible to infection.

UNIT FOUR

MEDICAL-SURGICAL PATIENT CARE PROBLEMS

In the preceding units we have talked about some of the problems common to a variety of disorders. Regardless of the patient's medical diagnosis, it is essential that the fluid and electrolyte balance be maintained, that healing be promoted, that the hazards of immobility be prevented, and that infection be prevented or, if this is not possible, that the infectious process be halted.

All the information presented in earlier chapters is intended to serve as a foundation for competent and individualized nursing care of adult patients with medical-surgical conditions. In the following chapters, the reader frequently will encounter references to this basic information precisely because it is fundamental to effectively carrying out all phases of the nursing process.

This last unit begins with a discussion of pain, a universal problem that nurses deal with daily. Following the problem of pain is a discussion of the surgical patient, which includes the nursing implications of anesthesia and patients' response to the surgical procedures commonly performed in a general hospital. Recognizing that an informed patient is as important to recovery as an informed nurse, psychological preparation of the surgical patient and attendance to his learning needs are emphasized.

A major change in the makeup of the American population has been the increasing number of elderly persons who are and will continue to be in need of special health care. Attitudes toward and health care for older adults in this country have not always been what they should be. Nurses are obligated to become better informed about the process of aging and its impact on physical and mental health. Being old is not the same as being sick, but older persons are more likely to suffer from chronic illnesses. The health care needs of the elderly can be very complex and require continued support and nursing intervention to help these patients manage their illnesses and maintain as high a level of physical and mental wellness as possible. Chapter 12 discusses some of the special nursing care needs of older adults.

Another major area of medical-surgical nursing is that of oncologic or cancer nursing. Cancer is not a single disease. Rather, it is a group of diverse disorders that have in common the growth and spread of malignant cells. Malignant growths afflict a large segment of our population, but most types of cancer can be treated successfully if detected in their earliest stages. All of these facts mandate a thorough knowledge of preventive and therapeutic measures for combating cancer. Although it is true that the study of malignancy and its treatment has become a highly developed specialty in the fields of medicine and nursing, the widespread incidence of cancer requires that all practicing nurses have a basic understanding of its physiologic and psychological effects, preventive measures that can be employed, and current modes of therapy. These aspects of care of the patient with cancer and his response to his illness and its treatment are presented in Chapter 13.

Compassionate and knowledgeable care of terminally ill and dying patients is an integral and pervasive part of nursing. Chapter 14 covers this aspect of nursing. Chapters 15 to 35 are concerned with specialized care that is needed when a person suffers from a disorder affecting one of the major anatomic systems of the body. There are many ways in which information about illness, injury, and nursing care can be classified and organized. One of the more traditional ways is to consider each of the major anatomic systems as separate and distinct from the others. In fact, most textbooks of anatomy and physiology are organized in this manner, each section being devoted to a group of organs that make up one system. Although we are aware that the body functions as a whole, with each of its parts working interdependently within the body, there are certain advantages to studying disorders that affect one particular system. Specialties within the practice of medicine are, for the most part, based on specific groups of organs, and patient care units and clinics are organized similarly. The specialties of neurology, gynecology, urology, and gastroenterology are examples of this method of classification.

In each of the specialties, there are certain health maintenance problems that are common to disorders of that system. For example, the patient with respiratory disease will be most likely to have problems associated with an inadequate exchange of oxygen and carbon dioxide, whereas the most pressing needs of a patient with a urologic disorder probably will be related to the establishment and maintenance of urinary flow.

The problems common to each system and the nursing skills and competencies needed to help the patient cope with these problems are presented at the beginning of each chapter. This information is followed by a discussion of the more specific diseases that primarily affect the organs of that system. This includes an explanation of the disease process, various forms of therapy, and nursing care required by the individual patient.

Immediately following the chapters on the urinary system and the digestive system, there is a chapter on the care of the ostomy patient. This information has been inserted in this particular place because the types of ostomies discussed are those that provide for the diversion of either the wastes passing through the intestines or urine from the kidneys.

The last chapter of the text is devoted to care of the patient with a medical or surgical emergency who is likely to be encountered outside of the hospital setting.

It is hoped that the sequence of material in this text will seem logical to the reader. There is no reason, however, why the instructor and the students may not rearrange the material to suit their own needs and capabilities.

CHAPTER 10

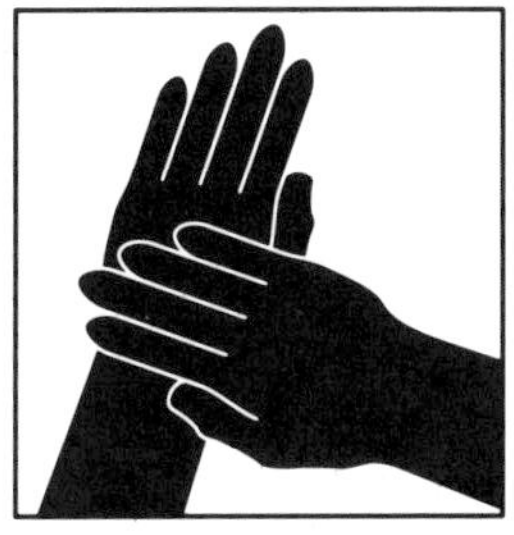

Care of Patients With Pain

VOCABULARY

abduction
addiction
aversion
endogenous
endorphin
enkephalin
euphoria
polypeptide
receptor

Upon completion of this chapter the student should be able to:

1. Define pain.
2. Describe physiologic and psychological reactions to pain stimuli.
3. Compare and contrast three different types of pain.
4. Describe common biases and myths about pain.
5. Assess pain in assigned patients, fully appreciating the subjective nature of pain.
6. List at least seven nursing interventions other than the administration of analgesics for the relief of pain.
7. Select nursing interventions appropriate for each type of pain experience.
8. Evaluate the effectiveness of measures used for the management of pain in assigned patients.

PHYSIOLOGY OF PAIN

Dictionary definitions of pain usually describe it as a feeling of distress, suffering, or agony that is caused by stimulation of specialized nerve endings scattered throughout the body. Pain is a universal symptom, which means that it is not specific to any one disease or type of injury. Its purpose is to act as a warning that tissues are being damaged and to motivate the sufferer to remove or withdraw from the source of the pain or otherwise seek relief.

Anyone who is trying to help a person cope with pain must be careful not to be judgmental and decide whether the pain actually exists. We can define pain in a somewhat detached and limited way for the purposes of study and communication, but the person experiencing pain is the most reliable source of information about how it feels, where it is located, and what provides relief.

McCaffrey says that pain is whatever the person who is experiencing it says it is, and it exists and is real whenever he says so McCaffrey (1989).

RECEPTION AND TRANSMISSION OF PAIN SIGNALS

All receptors for painful stimuli are free nerve endings that are specially designed to perform their function of receiving and relaying pain impulses. Pain receptors are abundantly distributed throughout the skin, as well as in deeper structures such as the peritoneum, the surfaces of joints, walls of arteries, and in parts of the cranial cavity. Mucous membranes lining the gastrointestinal tract also contain an abundant supply of pain receptors, as do the bile ducts, bronchi, and parietal pleura of the respiratory system. The eye has more pain receptors than any other body structure, because it is the most vulnerable and sensitive of all external organs.

Pain receptors do not adapt or become less sensitive to repeated stimulation as do other kinds of receptors. In fact, under some conditions the receptors become even more sensitive over a period of time.

This concept is important to an understanding of the assessment and management of chronic pain. The assumption that a person gets used to having continued pain simply is not true. Specialists who work with those suffering chronic pain almost all agree that instead of becoming accustomed to long-standing pain, patients seem, if anything, to become more sensitive and to suffer more as time passes.

A few pain receptors are so specialized they respond only to a specific stimulus (for example, histamine); however, most are sensitive to more than one kind of excitation. Pain is felt when tissues are damaged, because the hurt cells release chemicals such as histamine, potassium ions, acids, prostaglandins, and acetylcholine. These chemicals stimulate the chemosensitive pain receptors and also can damage the nerve endings themselves. If there is an inadequate supply of oxygen to a group of cells *(ischemia)*—as, for example, in coronary occlusion ("heart attack")—the ischemic tissue releases chemicals that stimulate the pain receptors, and the patient feels intense pain. Muscle spasm is another cause of pain, probably because it has the indirect effect of causing ischemia and stimulation of chemosensitive pain receptors.

Once pain stimuli have been recognized by the specialized nerve cells, the impulses travel to the spinal cord and then go upward along thin nerve fibers to the brain. Some go directly to the posterior part of the thalamus, which is the sensory relay station of the brain. Others go to the brain stem and from there are sent along to the thalamus.

Because of its role in recognizing pain impulses, the thalamus is sometimes called the *pain center.* However, the thalamus can only recognize the impulse as uncomfortable or disagreeable. It cannot tell where the pain is coming from. This must be done by the cerebral cortex, whose role is to "decide" where the pain is and how intensely it will be felt. Hence if the connections between the thalamus and cerebral cortex are broken, as in a frontal lobotomy, the person may report pain but will not feel it to an intense degree or be able to tell exactly where it is.

PERCEPTION OF AND REACTION TO PAIN

The *physiologic recognition* or *biologic perception* of stimuli by pain receptors is essentially the same for all persons with an intact and normally functioning nervous system. However, the reaction to the sensation of pain is highly individualized and depends on a number of factors within and outside of the individual. *Reaction* is used here in the sense of what the total person thinks, feels, and does when he is experiencing injury or any other stimulus to the pain receptors.

The way in which humans react to pain can vary widely from person to person and in the same individual under different circumstances.

There are many stories of people who have been severely injured but have not been aware of pain or complained of feeling distress. Soldiers injured in battle, young men undergoing unbelievably painful rituals during tribal initiations, and seriously injured athletes caught up in the excitement of a game have all provided examples of unusual or unexpected reactions to pain.

There are two major kinds of reaction to pain: physiologic and psychological. *Physiologic reactions* usually are automatic, involuntary responses that result from stimulation of the sympathetic and parasympathetic nervous systems. Objective signs of pain that are manifestations of physiologic reactions are presented in the section on assessment of pain later in this chapter.

Psychological reactions to pain are extremely complex. As mentioned previously, one can be so distracted by an external event or concentrate so completely on what he is doing that he does not seem to be aware of the pain and does not react to it as would be expected. On the other hand, fear and anxiety can make a person more sensitive to pain, thereby increasing his suffering.

Some psychological factors that are believed to influence an individual's reaction to pain are (1) his previous experience with pain, (2) the coping mechanisms he has developed, (3) training and cultural guidelines for acceptable responses to pain and discomfort, (4) his state of mental and physical health, and (5) his level of fatigue. As previously mentioned, distracting a person's attention from the pain also can influence how he reacts to it.

A person does not "get used to" pain, at least not in a purely biologic sense. As was stated earlier, pain receptors are the only receptors in the body that do not adapt or become less responsive to repeated stimulation. However, a person's experience with personal suffering can affect his attitude toward it and his ability to handle it. For some of us, memories of a previous pain experience trigger feelings of fear and anxiety, which make the current experience of pain more intense. Anyone who has been to a dentist and felt pain can appreciate how much the experience influences his attitude toward future visits to the dentist and his reaction to even mild discomfort while in the dentist's chair.

Some patients with chronic pain have learned to live with it and find ways to have some control over it. In other words, they have developed coping mechanisms and adapted to the pain in such a way that they have some measure of relief. Two important therapeutic goals for the person who has continuous or repeated experience with pain are to maintain some control over it and to find some meaning in their suffering.

A person's cultural background influences his feelings about pain and his overt reaction to it. In various cultures it is acceptable to complain bitterly, moan, thrash about, or otherwise bring attention to the fact that one is experiencing pain. In other cultures the admirable attitude is one of stoic and uncomplaining acceptance. A person with this cultural background and training may often be reluctant to talk about his pain and embarrassed to ask for relief lest it indicate a personal weakness or a flaw in his character. A high tolerance for pain is valued in Western culture, and this value often is expressed in a nurse's reluctance to give medication for relief and in her disapproval of patients who complain of pain.

Coping with pain and trying to find some relief so that it is at least tolerable takes a lot of energy. Patients who are debilitated are less able to withstand pain than are healthy, robust people. However, even those who are physically strong can become fatigued with the struggle and therefore likely to react more intensely to pain.

PHYSIOLOGIC CONTROL OF PAIN

Pain is a highly complex phenomenon and remains for the most part a mystery to those who study it. Nevertheless, in recent years there has been intense research to try to unravel the mystery. The results of research have given us a better understanding of pain and have contributed to more effective ways to manage it.

Among the most widely known theories is the *gate-control* theory proposed by Melzack and Wall in the early 1970s. They assumed that pain impulses travel along thin nerve fibers that convey the message to synapses in the dorsal horn of the spinal cord. The synapses act as gates that open and close and in so doing allow some impulses to pass through while others are prevented from entering the gate and going on to the brain. Signals for other kinds of stimulation, especially touch and pressure, travel along larger nerve fibers and compete with pain signals for passage through the gate.

If there are more tactile impulses than pain signals arriving at the gate at the same time, the tactile impulses will prevail and pass through. Thus the pain signals are prevented from getting through and ascending the spinal cord to the thalamus. When this occurs, the person is not aware that the pain receptors have been stimulated. However, if there are many more pain impulses than tactile signals arriving at the gate, the gates will allow them to pass through, and the person will feel pain. Tactile signals can be created by massage, contrastimulation, acupressure, and other noninvasive techniques used for the management of pain.

Although the above explanation is a vast simplification of the gate-control theory, it does help explain the effectiveness of measures that have been used for centuries and with varying degrees of success in the relief of pain.

Those who study pain also believe that the brain plays some role in mediating pain impulses that do manage to pass through the gates and ascend the spinal cord. It is thought that signals arising in the brain can travel downward toward the dorsal horn of the spinal cord and block or significantly reduce upward progress of pain signals on their way to the thalamus. This could account for the effectiveness of mental imagery, distraction, and other techniques that require activity of the cerebral cortex to mitigate awareness of the sensation of pain.

A third means by which pain might be controlled is by signals from the cerebral cortex. For example, simply knowing when pain will end or how it can be relieved can inhibit full transmission of the pain impulses and awareness of the presence of pain.

Enkephalins and Endorphins

In their research on pain, scientists found that certain neural tissues in laboratory animals contain receptor sites for opiates such as morphine. They concluded that these sites would not be present unless there were some endogenous chemical (i.e., one that is produced internally) in the tissues of the animals' bodies. In other words, why would there be receptor cells for something that would not naturally be present in the body and for which there would be no use?

The first endogenous chemical found to attach itself to the opiate receptors was a large polypeptide called *enkephalin,* which means "substance in the brain." Later, larger polypeptides having similar properties were found. These were called *endorphins,* a combination of the words *endogenous* and *morphine.*

The discovery of endorphins raised many more questions than it answered. However, researchers suspect that they modify and inhibit unpleasant stimuli, reduce anxiety, relieve pain, and sometimes produce euphoria and a feeling of well-being.

ASSESSMENT OF PAIN

As you know, assessing involves the gathering of subjective and objective data. In assessing the problem of pain, the subjective data far outweigh the objective data in importance and significance. You cannot see pain, and you cannot feel the pain of someone else.

Because pain is a subjective phenomenon, you must rely on the person who has the pain to tell you where it is, what it feels like, what makes it worse, and what gives him relief.

The more you know about a patient, the better able you will be to assess his pain. His beliefs, values, and attitudes will influence his behavior and his ability to communicate to you what you need to know to make a more accurate assessment. You also need to examine your own biases and personal feelings about complaints of pain and how you deal with the problem of pain in others.

BIASES AND MYTHS ABOUT PAIN

Since the attitudes of nurses and doctors are basic to the way in which they treat patients who say they have pain, it might be well to look at some values, misconceptions, and biases that have been identified through research. Not all nurses and physicians have these biases and counterproductive attitudes, of course, but perhaps by reviewing them you might avoid some of the more common pitfalls that prevent accurate assessment and effective management of pain.

Myth: If pain is really present, there must be a demonstrable cause.

Fact: *Pain can be very real to the patient even though no cause can be found. Cellular damage need not be present for pain to occur.* Although damage to the cells does lead to the release of chemicals that stimulate the pain receptors, in many cases no cellular abnormality can be found, but there is, nevertheless, pain. There is as yet no test or instrument that can precisely and objectively measure the degree of pain that is being felt. The search for evidence that pain exists is, in the words of Hackett, "fruitless and irrelevant." The patient with a tension headache may or may not suffer less than one with a brain tumor. We cannot say that just because the brain tumor can be shown on a brain scan and the tension headache cannot, the person with the brain tumor has pain and the person with the tension headache does not.

Myth: The person who has a low tolerance for pain has no self-control and probably is emotionally immature or childish.

Fact: *Pain tolerance is a physiologic response to pain that is made more complex by psychosocial factors, many of which can be beyond the control of the patient.* Tolerance for pain is defined as that duration or intensity of pain the person is *willing* to endure without seeking relief.

Pain tolerance varies greatly from one individual to another and in the same individual from time to time. Nurses often place a high value on a patient's ability to feel pain without complaining or asking for relief, and those who value a high pain tolerance usually impose their own values on their patients by ignoring or belittling their reports of pain. The person who should decide how willing he ought to be to tolerate pain is the one who is suffering.

Myth: Reactions to acute pain and chronic pain are the same.

Fact: *In general, acute pain is more often associated with anxiety and chronic pain with reactive depression.* This does not mean that the emotional reaction is the cause of the pain but that it often occurs with and intensifies pain. Physiologic reactions to acute and chronic pain also can differ; therefore management of acute and chronic pain is not the same. The differences between acute and chronic pain are explained further under Planning and Intervention later in this chapter.

Myth: Addiction to pain-relieving drugs is always a hazard, and for the sake of the patient, nurses often must withhold a drug even though the patient asks for it.

Fact: In spite of an abundance of evidence to the contrary, this mistaken belief about the dangers of addiction persists. Studies have repeatedly shown that *a very small percentage of patients (roughly 1% to 3%) become addicted to drugs administered for the purpose of relieving acute pain.*

Myth: Placebos are very useful in assessing whether a patient actually has pain.

Fact: The relationships of placebos and pain relief are perhaps the most misunderstood of all concepts related to the problem of pain. The question of how placebos affect people and why they have a positive response in some and not in others is still not completely understood. However, there has been sufficient study of the subject to show that *there is no basis for believing that a patient who finds relief from pain after receiving a placebo is pretending to have pain or that it is "all in his mind."* Because placebos and the placebo response are so relevant to the management of pain, a more detailed discussion of the topic is presented later under Selecting Measures for Pain Relief (McCaffrey, 1989).

SUBJECTIVE DATA

Although there is a wide variation in how individuals react to pain and the ways in which it is reported when it occurs, there are some specific questions one can ask to help a patient communicate more effectively when he reports pain. Assessment tools developed by nurses for more accurate evaluation of pain usually include information about location, quality, intensity, onset and precipitating or aggravating factors, and measures that bring relief.

Location

Perhaps the question most frequently asked about pain is, "Where does it hurt?" Sometimes the patient can answer this question without hesitation. If not, he might be able to point to the area that is painful. There is, however, the problem of *referred pain,* which means that the pain is felt at a distance from its source. This could be because branches of pain fibers leading from the viscera (large interior organs in the body cavities) enter the spinal cord at the same point as do neurons that receive pain sensations from the skin. When pain sensations from the viscera spread to the neurons that normally conduct only cutaneous pain sensations, the brain interprets sensations from the viscera as being from the skin, and the person has the feeling that the pain is originating in the skin itself.

There are many examples of referred pain. Kidney stones that have traveled down a ureter and become trapped there cause a sensation of pain in the flank above the ureter, and the pain "radiates" down the thigh to the groin or scrotum. Cardiac pain is referred to the neck and jaw, over the shoulders, to chest muscles, and down the arms. Gastric pain is usually felt in the front of the chest or upper abdomen. Liver and gallbladder pain might be felt at the shoulder under the tip of the right scapula (Fig. 10–1).

When assessing referred pain, it is sometimes helpful to have the patient trace the course of his pain or point to the areas where the pain is localized.

Quality

Patients do not always describe their pain in the same way, nor do they use the words nurses often use to describe pain. In answer to the question, "How does it feel?" they might say "crushing," "throbbing," "stabbing," "gnawing," "cramping," or any of a number of descriptive words or phrases.

Knowing the quality of a patient's pain can help in identifying its cause and can provide a sounder basis for effective management. Cardiac pain often is described as "crushing," "suffocating," "like a vise," or "like a steel band." Gastric pain related to ulcers or hyperacidity usually causes a burning or gnawing sensation. Muscle pain is typically called cramping, while pain in the viscera is described as dull and aching. Whatever words the patient uses to describe his pain, his exact words should be recorded.

Intensity

A common practice in recording a patient's report of pain is the nurse's use of words like "mild," "moderate," and "severe." These terms really don't mean very much in an in-depth assessment, because they are subject to a variety of interpretations. The nurse might evaluate a patient's pain as mild because he does not exhibit outward behavior indicative of extreme discomfort. However, if the patient were asked to evaluate the pain on a scale of 0 to 10, he might rank the pain as a 7 and want very much to have

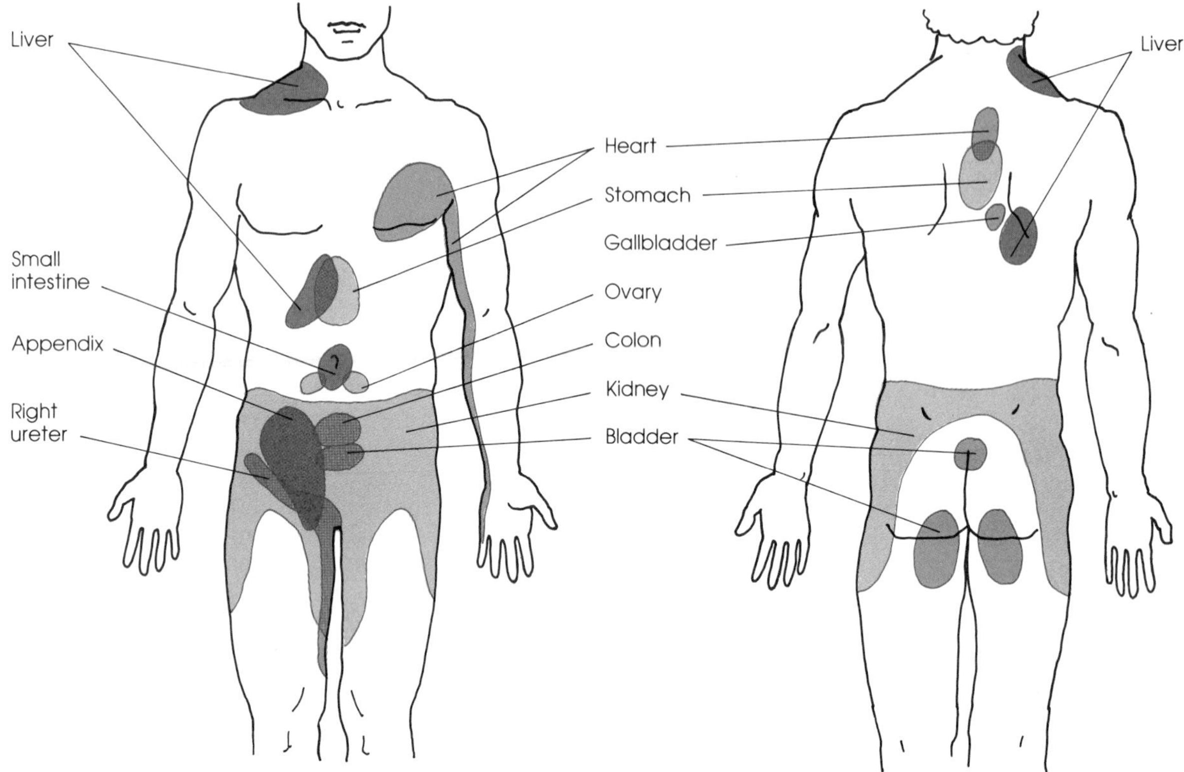

Figure 10-1 Referred pain, anterior and posterior views.

something for relief, even though he has not explicitly asked for it.

Although we continue to use the terms *mild, moderate,* and *severe* when writing or talking about the intensity of pain, a thorough assessment should go beyond these general terms to more specific measurements such as the scale mentioned above.

Onset and Precipitating or Aggravating Factors

There are several reasons why the nurse should know when pain is first noted by the patient and whether there are any precipitating or aggravating factors that he is aware of. In acute pain assessment, information about onset can help determine the cause of the pain and assist in surgical diagnosis. For example, if the pain occurs after the patient eats a meal with a high fat content, this could indicate gallbladder disease. Severe muscle pain in the legs after the patient walks a short distance could mean that he has a circulatory disorder affecting the blood vessels supplying the leg muscles.

In the management of chronic pain it is helpful to know what time of day the pain usually recurs or is noticed, whether there are any physical activities or emotional upsets that seem to bring it on or make it worse, and how long the pain usually lasts.

Nurses should not assume that if a patient needs relief from pain he will ask for it. The nurse must be actively involved in assessing the patient's pain and in helping him decide when he needs relief. Sometimes the nurse may need to intervene, take an authoritative approach, and administer a prescribed analgesic when objective data indicate the patient is indeed having pain that is interfering with rest and healing.

Measures That Bring Relief

Information from a patient or relative about the effectiveness of drugs, rest and relaxation techniques, massage, and any other activity that gives relief can provide significant help in determining the cause of the pain, as well as in planning for its control. For example, if rest reduces the pain, this could mean that the heart or blood vessels or both are not functioning properly. Cardiac pain (angina) typically is relieved by rest, as are muscle cramps resulting from poor blood supply.

In the case of acute pain related to surgical disorders, it is important that the nurse know whether the analgesic a patient is receiving is actually providing relief and allowing the patient to achieve as much rest as he needs for healing and recovery. Drugs affect people differently. Giving a patient an analgesic does not always guarantee removal of pain. The best way to find out if a drug has provided relief is to ask the patient. The second best is to observe him closely for objective signs of pain.

OBJECTIVE DATA

Objective signs of pain should* not *be used to "prove" that a patient does or does not have pain.

Objective signs are valuable additions to subjective data from the patient, and they are helpful when a patient is either unwilling or unable to report his pain. Hospitalized patients most often are in acute pain. However, often a patient with chronic pain is admitted to a hospital, where the pain continues or is made worse by hospitalization and by the condition that required his admission.

Objective signs of acute pain include some but not necessarily all of the following physiologic and behavioral indicators. *Physiologic signs* of low to moderate or superficial pain are related to response of the sympathetic nervous system. They include rapid, shallow, or guarded respirations, pallor, diaphoresis, increased pulse, elevated blood pressure, dilated pupils, and tenseness of the skeletal muscles.

When pain is severe or when it is located deep in the body cavities, stimulation of the parasympathetic neurons can produce a drop in blood pressure, slowing of the pulse, pallor, nausea and vomiting, weakness, and even loss of consiousness.

Behavioral signs of pain might include crying, moaning, tossing about in bed, lying quietly but tensely in one position, drawing up the knees (as with pain in the groin), rubbing the painful part (for example, a cramping muscle), and a pinched facial expression, or grimacing. The person in pain also might have difficulty concentrating and remembering or might become self-centered and preoccupied with his pain.

Elderly patients are particularly in need of a thorough and accurate assessment of their pain. Older adults often have a diminished sense of touch (tactile loss), in which case the protective mechanisms of pain are not fully operative. In her assessment of the elderly person, the nurse may notice bruises and cuts or pressure sores that the patient has not mentioned because the injury is not accompanied by the expected discomfort or pain.

Pain is very complex, and it is difficult to separate organic pain from emotional pain. Contrary to popular belief, many older patients have never been hospitalized before, and when they are admitted to an acute-care setting they experience fear, anxiety, and a sense of losing control. Although they could manage fairly well at home, the strange environment in the hospital threatens their sense of independence. In her assessment of the elderly patient, it is extremely important that the nurse find out what the patient was able to do for himself at home, how he coped with pain, and the measures that he used to find relief. This will help avoid erroneous assumptions about an elderly patient's physical and mental health status that are based solely on his appearance and behaviors while he is in the hospital.

Admission to a strange and fast-paced acute-care setting can cause the elderly person to become confused and disoriented; thus he has difficulty describing his pain accurately and specifically. Some older patients may not report their pain because they have mistakenly accepted it as a part of growing old or are afraid to admit they are not doing well enough to go home. Elderly patients in hospitals also are sometimes afraid they are going to die, and so their physical pain is intensified by their fear of death.

Whatever the reason for the difficulty in accurately assessing pain in the elderly person, the nurse is obligated to look for objective and subjective signs that indicate a problem of pain or discomfort. The patient might become noticeably more irritable, short-tempered, or uncooperative. He may resist or be unable to do some things for himself that he was previously able to do either at home or in the hospital. Depression can intensify pain, but it also can be a sign of unreported pain. If the patient becomes less inclined to communicate with the nurse, this could mean that he is withdrawing and using his available energy to try to cope with his pain.

PLANNING AND INTERVENTION

Acute and chronic pain differ in their causes and the reactions they can produce, and so measures employed for the management of acute and chronic pain are not always the same.

Acute pain is usually of short duration, has a sudden onset, is intense or severe, and eventually will subside with, or sometimes without, treatment. *Chronic pain* has a gradual onset, is prolonged and continuous, persists or recurs for an indefinite period, and is more difficult to manage successfully. Because of the nature of chronic pain, those who have it and those who try to relieve it are often frustrated in their attempts to control it.

A comparison of the characteristics of acute and chronic pain is shown in Table 10–1.

Among the measures employed for the relief, management, or control of pain are surgical and medical interventions and general nursing measures, including noninvasive techniques.

TABLE 10-1 **ACUTE AND CHRONIC PAIN**

	Acute	Chronic
Duration	Hours to days	Months to years
Prognosis for relief	Good; may occur spontaneously or in response to routine analgesic therapy.	Poor unless complicating factors are removed; spontaneous relief rarely occurs.
Cause	Relatively easy to identify.	Sometimes easy to find but diagnosis usually complex.
Psychosocial effects	Usually transient or none. Sometines interferes with social activities but only temporarily.	Can affect ability to earn a living, enjoy social interactions, maintain self-esteem.
Effect of therapy	Medication usually beneficial. Surgery often helpful.	Medication may be addictive. Surgery can worsen condition but is sometimes helpful.

MEDICAL AND SURGICAL TREATMENT

Medical and surgical treatments for relief of pain are usually done either (1) to remove the cause of pain or if that is not possible (2) to decrease sensibility to pain. In the first category are drugs that act on the injured tissues producing the pain. For example, an antiinfective is given to reduce infection in a person with bacterial pneumonia, thereby making it easier and less painful for him to breathe, or a muscle relaxant is prescribed to relieve spasms, thereby relieving muscle pain. These drugs are *not* analgesics. They act at the source of the pain rather than in the brain and other tissues removed from the source.

Surgical procedures to treat the cause of pain involve removal of tumors, diseased organs, and other abnormal tissues that either cause pressure on pain receptors or release pain-producing chemicals. Of course, surgical intervention itself can be a cause of pain during the operative and postoperative periods. Another cause of pain that often is overlooked is that which accompanies diagnostic tests performed for medical and surgical purposes.

Some surgical procedures are designed to decrease sensibility to pain and thus belong to the second category of pain treatment. These procedures are done to interrupt transmission of pain impulses so that the person is not aware that pain receptors are being stimulated. Procedures of this kind (for example, vagotomy) are discussed later and in more detail in appropriate sections in this text.

Analgesics

Also in the second category of interventions are analgesics, which are drugs that decrease sensibility to pain. The mechanisms by which analgesics bring about their effect are very complex and not completely understood. It is known, however, that narcotic and non-narcotic analgesics relieve pain in completely different ways. There also are drugs that enhance the pain-relieving effect of analgesics. That is why combinations of drugs often work better than any one drug alone.

In the administration of injectable analgesics, McCaffrey (1989) suggests two general guidelines for nurses: First, select the drug and dosage on the basis of each patient's *individual needs;* and second, practice *preventive* treatment, rather than crisis management of pain. These guidelines can apply to administration of analgesics by oral and other means, as well as to injectables.

Individualize Drug and Dose

Although the physician is responsible for prescribing analgesic drugs, his choice of drugs for a particular patient can be made more wisely if the nurse provides information about the effects of the drug and the patient's response to it. First of all, does the drug relieve pain so that the patient has adequate rest and also is able to perform some necessary activities? Coughing, ambulating, and exercise are important activities for the prevention of problems and promotion of recovery from surgery. If these activities cause pain that is not relieved, the patient will not be inclined to do them.

Failure of an analgesic to work as expected could be due to too low a dose or too long an interval between doses. If the pain is not sufficiently relieved but the patient seems oversedated, increasing the dosage probably isn't the answer. Another drug or combination of drugs probably should be tried.

On the other hand, the dose may be too high. The nurse should note whether the patient is so sedated that he is drowsy and unable to participate in his care. The drug could depress respirations to a potentially dangerous level. The physician should be notified if there is a drop of more than four or five respirations per minute after a patient has been given an analgesic.

Patient-Controlled Analgesia

Intravenous patient-controlled analgesia (PCA) machines are a common site in most hospitals today. The PCA pump is programmed to allow the patient to control administration of a narcotic analgesic with the push of a button. The physician writes his orders so that a bolus of the medication may be given at set intervals. The machine is designed so that no more than the physician-ordered amount may be given within a particular time period. This prevents the possibility of overdosage. Research has shown that most patients use less narcotic analgesic with this method than when the medication is ordered by "prn" intramuscular injection.

Epidural or Intrathecal Analgesia

Administration of narcotics such as morphine or fentanyl via a catheter that is placed into the epidural or intrathecal (subarachnoid) space is another new approach to pain control. The medication can be given by intermittent bolus or continuous infusion pump. Duration of pain relief by this method is quite long: about 5 to 15 hours with the epidural route and up to 36 hours for the intrathecal route.

Practice Preventive Pain Control

Practicing preventive pain management is primarily the responsibility of the nurse. This means treating acute pain before it becomes so severe that no analgesic will safely and completely relieve it. (Note that this practice may not be effective in the relief of chronic pain, which requires a different approach.) Patients should not have to wait until they are in trouble before something is done to help them. Perhaps the patient needs to be told to ask for medication when his pain first returns, or if he is hesitant to "bother the nurse," he should be looked in on frequently and asked if he feels the need for something before his pain gets too bad.

Nurses frequently hesitate to offer pain medication when a patient does not ask for it or try to stretch out the intervals between doses because they are afraid the patient will become addicted. As previously stated, the chances for creating addiction in patients who receive narcotics for short-term acute pain are very remote. Larkins presents two reasons why addiction is not likely to develop:

- The patient receiving the narcotic experiences *pain relief*, which is not the reinforcement ordinarily associated with addiction. The sensation that usually is responsible for addiction is euphoria due to a decrease in ungratified drives.
- The person who is *given* a narcotic has less control over reinforcement and is less apt to become addicted than the person who has possession of the narcotic and can inject himself whenever he wants to do so (Larkins, 1977).

GENERAL NURSING MEASURES: PLANNING AND INTERVENTION

Since before the time of Florence Nightingale, nurses have used positioning, back rubs, applications of heat and cold, and similar measures to relieve pain and discomfort (Fig. 10–2). It is only since the discovery of endorphins that a physiologic basis for the effectiveness of these measures has been suggested. However, regardless of whether endorphins are responsible for relief of pain and discomfort when nursing measures are employed, experience has shown that the nurse

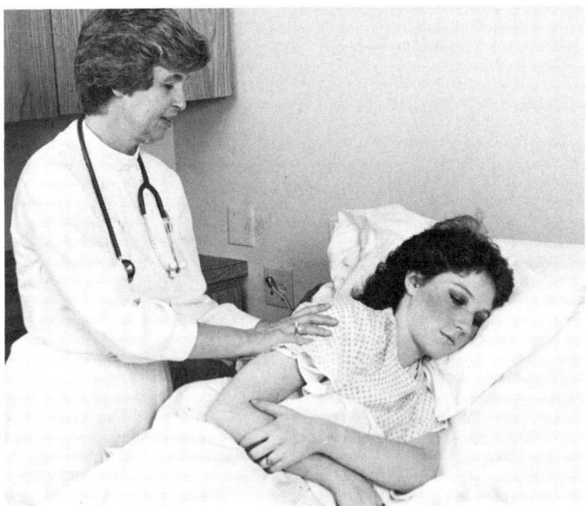

Figure 10–2 Gentle massage, back rubs, and other noninvasive techniques traditionally used by nurses can provide relaxation and relief from discomfort.
(Photo by Ken Kasper.)

can do much in addition to administering drugs to help her patient in pain.

An important aspect of any pain-relieving measures employed by the nurse is the use of her "self" to reduce or relieve the anxiety associated with pain or the anticipation of pain. She can be with the patient, listen to him, assure him that everything possible is being done, and teach him ways to relax, divert his attention from the pain, or otherwise control it.

Nursing care plans for the management of pain should, whenever possible, be developed *with* the patient rather than *for* him. Once the plan has been developed, it must be communicated and followed by everyone involved in implementing it. In the case of chronic pain, persistence in looking for the most effective therapies, in spite of frustration and failures, is probably the most important factor. The patient needs to feel that whatever his problem with pain, he will not be abandoned to deal with it alone, and if he needs encouragement or instruction in accepting and carrying out his plan of care, he must know that that, too, will be provided (see Nursing Care Plan 10–1).

Selecting Measures for Pain Relief

The specific measures chosen to help a patient deal with his problem of pain are selected according to the type of pain he is experiencing, his medical diagnosis or mode of surgical intervention, his experience with pain and knowledge of measures that work well for him, and the nurse's knowledge of and ability to use a particular measure effectively. Some techniques require more experience and expertise than others. Repositioning, back rubs, applications of heat and cold, and use of self (*being there* with the patient) are familiar to the average staff nurse. Relaxation techniques, meditation, mental imagery, and acupressure require more knowledge and skills than would be expected for one who has not specialized in pain control. Some of the more commonly used measures for pain management and some additional information about each are summarized in Table 10–2.

Managing Cancer Pain

The management of pain for the cancer patient requires a team approach. A combination of narcotic and non-narcotic drugs may work the best. It is very important that the nurse develop a trusting relationship with the patient in order for pain control measures to be maximally effective. There is a fine line between providing sufficient pain control and preventing severe side effects such as a decreased level of consciousness, respiratory depression, and constipation. Often, combining antidepressants, sedatives, or tranquilizers with the pain medications makes pain control more effective. Patient-controlled analgesia gives the patient a feeling of control over his pain. Whatever type of delivery system of pain medication is used, medication should be scheduled at regular intervals and not just given on an as-needed basis.

Whatever chemical means of pain control are utilized for the cancer patient, the nurse must also employ all of the nonchemical interventions she can. Relaxation, music distraction, imagery, and humor therapy can be most beneficial.

Pain-inducing activities or procedures should be scheduled during peak analgesic effect. Rest periods after such activities are vitally important.

Managing Other Chronic Pain

The patient who has chronic pain should become familiar with all the nonchemical methods for pain control that are available. Electrical stimulation devices, massage, whirlpool baths, applications of alternating heat and cold, yoga, meditation, distraction, imagery, relaxation, and music therapy can all be helpful. Biofeedback techniques help many patients.

Physicians hesitate to heavily medicate the chronic pain patient with narcotics because of the addictive nature of most of these medications. The chronic pain patient is not going to die of his condition; he needs pain control that will not cease to work over time.

Stress reduction and regular exercise can be very beneficial to improvement of pain management in these patients. If the patient is obese, weight loss can be very beneficial in reducing certain types of pain. Weight loss can improve the patient's self-image, thereby giving him a new outlook on life that might decrease his chronic pain.

Acupressure and acupuncture are other effective therapies for some patients with chronic pain. Therapeutic touch is also proving to be beneficial to many.

Whatever the type of pain, a thorough, detailed nursing assessment of the pain and the patient's habits is essential in providing the best pain control plan.

Placebos

The word *placebo* is taken from the Latin word meaning "I will please." The term was once used in reference to inert or inactive substance only —for example, a "sugar pill" or an injection of normal saline. This limited definition of a placebo has undergone significant change in recent years because of extensive drug research that was begun in the 1940s. During their research scientists needed to know whether it was the actual pharmacologic effect of the drug being

NURSING CARE PLAN 10–1

Selected nursing diagnoses, goals/outcome criteria, nursing interventions, and evaluations for a patient with pain

Situation: Patient is a 58-year-old black female admitted for bilateral total hip replacement. She is hesitant to ask for pain relief and frequently denies pain altogether, even though it is apparent that she is having moderate to severe pain. She has voiced her concern about becoming addicted to pain medication (Demerol).

Nursing Diagnosis	Goals/Outcome Criteria	Nursing Intervention	Evaluation
Ineffective individual coping related to cultural taboos about asking for something for pain. SUPPORTING DATA Black female; states that she feels that it's better to "tough it out."	Patient will accept analgesics when needed. Patient will ask for pain medication before pain becomes intense.	Establish trusting relationship. Encourage discussion of beliefs about pain and medication for control of pain. Explain that she must move about, cough, and deep breathe in order to prevent complications and that these activities will be easier if she is not in pain. Explain that she needs pain medication for a few days in order to hasten healing by preventing complications. Use alternative methods of pain relief as much as possible: positioning, music, relaxation exercises, heat and cold.	Discussed how decreasing her pain will allow her to move, cough, and deep breathe better, promoting quicker healing; taught relaxation exercise; she is practicing; had pain med at 8 and 1; continue plan.
Fear related to belief that narcotics are addicting. SUPPORTING DATA States that she has a brother who got hooked on drugs when he was treated with narcotics for back pain. "I don't want that to happen to me."	Patient will verbalize acceptance of analgesics as appropriate after surgery.	Encourage verbalization of beliefs about addiction. Explain that addiction to the small amounts of pain medication needed for a few days after surgery is unlikely. Observe nonverbal signs of pain: facial expressions, body tension, mood changes, etc. Encourage to take pain medication before pain becomes severe. Utilize distraction and diversion to ease pain. Reinforce need for pain medication after surgery.	Discussed narcotics and addiction; expresses more willingness to take medication for a few days postop; had pain med at 8 and 1; continue plan.

studied or psychological reactions that produced the beneficial effects they observed. This led to studies of how and under what conditions a placebo effect takes place. There still are no concrete answers to these questions, but the research has shown that there are many misconceptions of the phenomenon known as the *placebo effect* or response. Because this is true, there are many abuses of the placebo in the practice of medicine and nursing.

Placebos can have both positive and negative effects. They can be addictive, produce pronounced physical and psychological side effects, mimic the action of a drug, and even reverse the action of potent drugs. Additionally, placebos have been shown to change brain chemistry and alter the physiology of bodily organs.

A study completed in 1978 led researchers to the conclusion that placebo-positive responders—those who benefit from placebos—release endorphins in response to the placebo. These endorphins are believed to account for the pain relief placebo-positive persons report when they are given a placebo for pain (Beyerman, 1982).

Nurses should be aware of both positive and negative effects of the placebo response. Negative effects could account for the unpleasant side effects patients report after receiving a drug. In other words, administration of the drug not only produces the expected effect of the drug but also

TABLE 10-2 **INTERVENTIONS FOR THE MANAGEMENT OF PAIN**

Measure	When appropriate/General effects
Narcotic analgesics—e.g., morphine, codeine, meperidine (Demerol), oxycodone (in Percodan, Tylox)	Moderate to severe pain; acute or chronic. Postoperative pain.
Non-narcotic analgesics—e.g., aspirin, acetaminophen, ibuprofen (Datril, Tylenol, Motrin)	Mild to moderate pain. In combination with narcotics or alone. Oral medications act less quickly but are appropriate when injections are to be avoided because of age, emaciation, hemophilia, etc.
Combinations of tranquilizers, antidepressants, and narcotics	Chronic pain.
Cold packs	Reduce swelling, relieve pressure, provide cutaneous stimulation.
Menthol ointments	Probably provide cutaneous stimulation; could have some positive placebo effect.
Positioning and repositioning	Reduce muscle tension and fatigue from immobility; increase blood supply; relieve pressure on body parts.
Massage	Promotes relaxation, relieves muscle cramps.
Contralateral stimulation: stimulation of skin in area opposite area of pain or itching	When painful or itching area cannot be reached—e.g., when under a dressing or cast.
Relaxation techniques—e.g., Lamaze, rhythmic breathing	Particularly suited for ongoing pain. Provide relief of muscle tension and fatigue; reduce anxiety. Can give patient periods of rest, increase effectiveness of analgesics.
Distraction	Brief periods of acute pain.
Talk, conscious suggestion, conversation	A form of distraction; allays fright, can provide assurance in emergency situation; relieves loneliness.
Biofeedback	Helpful for coping with chronic pain to promote relaxation, relieve anxiety. Usually used with other pain-relief methods.
Hypnosis	Acute, short-term pain.
Transcutaneous electrical nerve stimulator (TENS)	Can relieve both acute and chronic pain. Enhances healing, increases blood flow, reduces muscle spasm.

an accompanying placebo response to its administration. Whether they realize it or not, nurses use the placebo response almost daily in their interaction with their patients. When a nurse says with honesty and conviction, "This will make you feel better," or "This lotion will clear up your rash," she is using the placebo effect.

Research indicates that between 30% and 40% of patients given placebos will consistently react to them. However, there is no group of people with certain personality traits who consistently react to placebos. Those who have a placebo response are no more gullible, suggestible, or emotionally unstable than those who do not react to placebos. Additionally, reactions to placebos can vary in an individual person, depending on the conditions under which they are given.

Another interesting result of placebo research that has great significance for the nurse is the conclusion that *how* the placebo is given and *by whom* has more influence on the outcome than the personality traits of the person receiving it. In other words, if the nurse truly believes that what she is doing will make a patient feel better and improve his condition, then the patient will usually have a favorable response to her actions. By her verbal and nonverbal behavior she tells the patient that she has faith in what she is doing for him. When that faith is conveyed to the patient he does indeed benefit from what she does. This is true of a back rub, repositioning, lowering the blinds, administering a drug, or whatever else the nurse does when she intervenes on her patient's behalf.

There are some complex and difficult moral and ethical issues associated with the administration of placebos, especially those intended to "trick" or "fool" the patient. The nurse must look at her own attitudes toward the use and abuse of placebos and learn more about them so as to correct any misconceptions she might have. Then she must make decisions from day to day about how she will use the placebo effect. Guidelines for the use of the placebo response are as follows:

- Always try to be honest in your dealings with patients. If you are uncomfortable with lying, deceiving, or "tricking" your patient into thinking he is receiving a drug when he is actually being given an injection of normal saline, your basic instincts are correct. You should do what you know and feel is the right thing to do. However, you should *never* tell him he is receiving a placebo.
- Do not use placebos to assess the severity of a patient's pain or to find out if the pain is real or imaginary. The issue is not that simple. A patient can have very real and intense pain and get relief from a placebo if he happens to be placebo-positive.
- Remember that being placebo-positive is not the same as being suggestible or having some personality defect or psychiatric disorder.
- Use the placebo effect for the benefit of your patients. When you are doing something that you honestly believe will help, say so. Be sincere and communicate to your patient your faith in the nursing measure, drug, or procedure. Help the patient use the healer that is in him and in you.

Concerns for the Elderly

Pain is not an inevitable part of aging, as was once thought. However, the elderly are at risk for many chronic disorders that result in pain, such as arthritis, osteoporosis, cardiovascular disease, and cancer. Research has failed to show any age-related difference in pain perception. Lack of pain expression in the elderly patient does not necessarily mean lack of pain. Many older people have experienced pain for a long time and have learned to minimize the expression of that pain for various reasons.

Narcotics can be effectively and safely used in the elderly if the person's response to the medication is evaluated closely and dosages are adjusted as needed.

Several factors affect the distribution of drugs in the elderly patient. Changes in the proportion of body fat may affect the way fat-soluble drugs are handled by the body. Heart, kidney, and muscle mass decrease with age, and elderly patients need to be monitored more closely for signs of drug toxicity. If the patient is protein deficient, which is common in the elderly, many drugs may build to higher than usual concentrations because of lack of protein binding, thereby causing toxicity.

The elderly do metabolize acetaminophen much more slowly than younger patients, and there should be longer intervals between doses in this age group to prevent toxic damage to the liver. Drugs that are excreted unchanged by the kidneys may also remain in the body longer than usual because of the decreased glomerular filtration rate that occurs with advanced age. Meperidine (Demerol) may quickly accumulate in the patient with renal insufficiency, causing central nervous system excitation. Morphine remains in the body longer in the elderly, and therefore its effects may be greater and will last longer than in the younger patient.

After surgery, narcotics should be used carefully in the early postoperative period and should be given orally or intravenously, as slowed circulation makes intramuscular or subcutaneous injection absorption erratic. Quality of perfusion should be kept in mind any time an intramuscular or subcutaneous injection is to be given to an elderly patient.

Chronic pain can best be handled by around-the-clock dosage schedules. It may be helpful to schedule the doses in relation to daily activities, rather than by specific hours of the clock, as this makes it easier to remember for most elderly patients.

Constipation and confusion are often caused by the total combination of drugs an elderly patient is taking, rather than by analgesics alone. Many experience considerable pain on a daily basis from chronic disease, and it is up to the nurse to see that comfort is obtained for these patients. Safe pain control means medicating before the pain becomes severe, using an around-the-clock dosage schedule, monitoring very closely for effect and signs of toxicity, and titrating the dosage as needed.

BIBLIOGRAPHY

Baquil, M. L.: What matters most in chronic pain management? RN, March, 1989, p. 46.

Beare, P. G., and Myers, J. L.: Principles and Practice of Adult Health Nursing. St. Louis, C. V. Mosby, 1990.

Beyerman, K.: Flawed perceptions about pain. Am. J. Nurs., Feb., 1982, p. 302.

Chalupka, S., and Gillon-Allard, B. Home care: When your patient has an epidural catheter. RN, Dec., 1989, p. 70.

Doehring, K. M.: Relieving pain through touch. Adv. Clin. Care, Sept./Oct., 1989, p. 32.

Empting-Koschorke, L. D., et al.: When pain is intractable. Patient Care, June, 1989, p. 107.
Gropper, E. I.: Your Jewish patients in pain. Adv. Clin. Care, Sept./Oct., 1990, p. 39.
Guyton, A. C.: Human Physiology and Mechanisms of Disease, 8th ed. Philadelphia, W. B. Saunders, 1991.
Hansberry, J. L., et al.: Managing chronic pain with a permanent epidural catheter. Nursing 90, Oct., 1990, p. 53.
Jones, J., and Brooks, J. The ABCs of PCA. RN, May, 1990, p. 54.
Larkins, F. R.: The influence of one's culture on pain response. Nurs. Clin. North Am., Dec., 1977, p. 663.
Mast, D., et al.: Relaxation techniques: A self-learning module for nurses. Cancer Nurs., June, 1987, p. 141.
McCaffrey, M.: Nursing Management of the Patient with Pain, 4th ed. Philadelphia, J. B. Lippincott, 1989.
McCaffrey, M. Would you administer placebos for pain? Nursing 82, Feb., 1982, p. 80.
McCaffrey, M., et al.: Giving narcotics for pain: The secrets to giving equianalgesic doses. Nursing 89, Oct., 1989, p. 68.
McGuire, D. B., and Yarbro, C. H., eds.: Cancer Pain Management. Orlando, Grune & Stratton, 1987.
McGuire, L., et al. Managing pain: In the young patient . . . in the elderly patient. Nursing 82, Aug., 1982, p. 52.
McGuire, L.: The power of non-narcotic pain relievers. RN, April, 1990, p. 28.
Meyer, T. M.: TENS—relieving pain through electricity. Nursing 82, Sept., 1982, p. 57.
Porterfield, L. M.: Narcotic analgesics. Adv. Clin. Care, July/Aug., 1990, p. 30.
Powell, A. H., et al.: How do you give continuous epidural fentanyl? Am. J. Nurs., Sept., 1989, p. 1197.
Thiederman, S.: Stoic or shouter, the pain is real. RN, June, 1989, p. 49.
Witte, M.: Pain control. J. Gerontol. Nurs., March, 1989, p. 32.

STUDENT STUDY AIDS

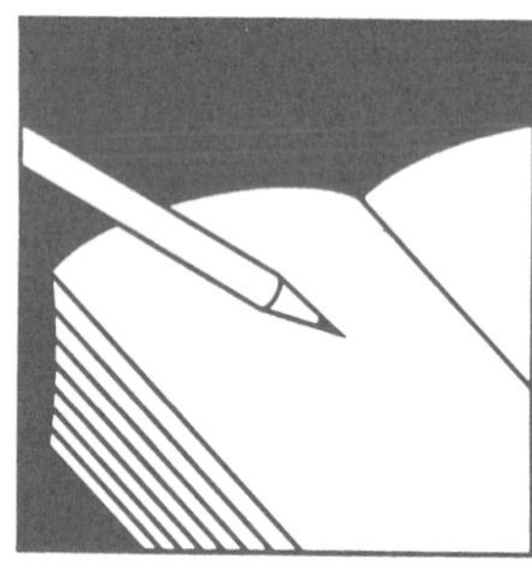

CLINICAL CASE PROBLEMS

Read each clinical situation and discuss the questions with your classmates.

1. Anne Mays, age 27, has suffered from muscle tension pain in her neck and shoulders for several years. Her physician has prescribed a muscle relaxant for her when the pain becomes particularly severe, but Anne does not want to continue taking "drugs that I might become addicted to."

- What is the intended action of a muscle relaxant?
- How would you respond to Anne's statement regarding her fear of addiction to a muscle relaxant?
- What other measures could you suggest for management of Anne's problem with pain?
- If you did not know how to teach these techniques to Anne, where would you go for the information you need?

2. At the change of shift the nurse going off duty says, "Mr Abernathy was given two placebos of normal saline during the day and slept for a couple of hours after each injection. It is obvious that he doesn't have pain. Mr. Davis probably could use the same kind of treatment for his pain, too. If he complains, I'm sure Dr. Evans will order a placebo if you just ask him."

- What do you think is the best response to the nurse's statements?
- Would you ask Dr. Evans for an order for a placebo for Mr. Davis?
- How could you use the placebo response to help Mr. Davis while giving him a back rub and preparing him for sleep?
- What are some other ways you could stimulate endorphin release for your patients?

STUDY OUTLINE

I. Physiology of pain

A. Pain is a feeling of distress, suffering, or agony resulting from stimulation of pain receptors.

B. The person experiencing pain is the most reliable source of information about whether pain exists and what it means.

C. Reception and transmission of pain signals.

1. All pain receptors are specialized nerve endings abundantly distributed throughout the skin, mucous membranes, peritoneum, coverings of joints, eye, and other structures.

2. Pain receptors do not become less sensitive to repeated stimulation.
3. Damaged tissues release chemicals that stimulate chemosensitive receptors. Resulting pain serves as a warning that the body is injured.
4. Pain impulses travel upward along the spinal cord from the source to the thalamus, the so-called pain center.
5. The cerebral cortex interprets pain signals.

D. Perception of and reaction to pain.
1. Physiologic recognition (biologic perception) of stimuli by pain receptors is essentially the same for all persons.
2. Reaction to sensation of pain is highly individualized.
3. *Reaction* refers to what the total person thinks, feels, and does when he feels pain.
4. Physiologic reactions are automatic responses to stimulation of the sympathetic and parasympathetic nervous systems.
5. Psychological reactions are extremely complex. They include:
   a. Previous experiences with pain.
   b. Coping mechanisms the person has developed.
   c. Cultural background and training.
   d. State of health.
   e. Level of fatigue.
6. A person does not "get used to" pain.
7. Two important goals for the person with chronic pain:
   a. To maintain control over it.
   b. To find some meaning in suffering.

II. Physiologic control of pain

A. Gate-control theory.
1. Pain impulses do not travel along the same nerve fibers as other signals.
2. Synapses between neurons act as "gates" to admit or prohibit passage of signals.
3. When tactile signals predominate at the "gate," they are allowed to pass through, while pain impulses are not.

B. Brain also plays some role in mediating pain impulses, possibly by blocking their transmission to the thalamus.

C. Enkephalins and endorphins: endogenous morphinelike polypeptides that modify and inhibit unpleasant stimuli, reduce anxiety, relieve pain, and produce a sense of well-being.

III. Assessment of pain

A. Biases and myths influence assessment. The *facts* are that:
1. Cellular damage need not be present for pain to occur.
2. Pain tolerance is a physiologic and psychosocial response; it may or may not be under the person's control.
3. There are differences between acute and chronic pain.
4. Placebos can be effective even though the patient's pain is real.

B. Subjective data:
1. Location: Where is the pain? Is it referred pain?
2. Quality: How does it feel? What does it feel like?
3. Intensity: More accurately measured on a scale of 1 to 10.
4. Onset and precipitating or aggravating conditions that bring on pain.
5. Measures that bring relief: What, if anything, helps the person find relief?

C. Objective data:
1. Physiologic signs:

a. Low to moderate pain produces symptoms of rapid, shallow, or guarded respirations, pallor, diaphoresis, increased pulse, elevated blood pressure, dilated pupils, tenseness of skeletal muscles.
b. Severe pain or pain located in deeper structures can produce drop in blood pressure, slowing of pulse, pallor, nausea and vomiting, weakness, loss of consciousness.

2. Behavioral signs: crying, moaning, tossing about in bed, lying quietly but tensely in one position, drawing up knees (groin or abdominal pain), rubbing the painful part. Patient also may have difficulty in concentrating and remembering or may become preoccupied with pain.
3. Elderly persons require a more in-depth assessment to determine behaviors prior to hospitalization. Fear, anxiety, and threats to their independence can intensify pain. New environment can cause confusion and difficulty in describing pain.

IV. Planning and intervention

A. Acute and chronic pain require different approaches.
   1. Comparison of acute and chronic pain shown in Table 10–1.

B. Medical and surgical treatment.
   1. Done for one of two reasons:
      a. To remove cause of pain by treating injured tissues with drugs or removing them surgically.
      b. To decrease sensibility to pain through surgical interruption of pain impulses.
   2. Analgesics: drugs that decrease sensitivity to pain. Narcotic and non-narcotic analgesics do not have the same action.
      a. Guidelines for giving analgesics:
         (1) Individualize drug and dose to meet patient's needs.
            (a) Evaluate effectiveness on basis of whether patient has relief and is able to rest and also can perform necessary activities to avoid problems of immobility.
            (b) Dose may be too high, causing drowsiness or lowering respiratory rate to dangerous levels. Notify physician if respiratory rate drops by more than four or five per minute after drug is administered.
         (2) Patient-controlled analgesia given intravenously allows the patient control over his pain.
         (3) Epidural or intrathecal analgesia provides much longer pain relief.
         (4) Practice preventive pain control, especially for acute pain. Treat pain before it becomes severe.
            (a) Patients should be assessed frequently for need for pain relief.
            (b) Nurse may need to take authoritative approach if patient shows objective signs of pain but does not ask for medication.
         (5) Addiction to drug given for relief of acute pain likely in only 1% to 3% of patients.
            (a) Pain relief not the reinforcement ordinarily associated with addiction.
            (b) Person who is given a narcotic has less control over reinforcement than one who can take the drug whenever he wants to.

C. General nursing measures: planning and intervention.
   1. Nurses can do much besides administer analgesics for pain relief.

2. Nurse uses her "self" to:
   a. Be with the patient, and check on him frequently.
   b. Listen to him.
   c. Assure him everything possible is being or will be done.
   d. Teach him ways to deal with his pain.
3. Care plans must be developed *with* the patient whenever possible.
   a. Plan is communicated to everyone responsible for implementing it.
   b. Patient must know he will not be abandoned to deal with his pain alone, that others have not given up on him. Most important factor in dealing with chronic pain is persistence in looking for most effective therapies.
   c. Sample care plan for patient with cultural biases in regard to pain.
4. Selecting measures for pain relief (see Table 10–2).
5. Managing cancer pain requires a team effort.
   a. Use combination of narcotic and non-narcotic medications.
   b. Adding antidepressants, sedatives, or tranquilizers with pain medications provides more effective relief.
   c. Pain medication should be given on a regular schedule, rather than "prn", for the cancer patient.
   d. All nonmedication methods of pain relief—relaxation, music, distraction, imagery, humor, biofeedback—should be combined with pain medication also.
6. Managing other chronic pain requires diligent use of nonchemical methods.
   a. Electrical stimulation devices, massage, whirlpool baths, applications of heat and cold, yoga, meditation, distraction, imagery, relaxation, and music therapy can all help.
   b. Stress reduction and regular exercise are also beneficial.
   c. Weight loss may be beneficial for the obese chronic pain patient, as it can improve self-esteem and well-being.
   d. Acupressure and acupuncture are effective therapies for some patients with chronic pain; therapeutic touch helps others.
7. Placebos:
   a. Word means "I will please."
   b. Placebos can have both positive and negative effects.
      (1) Can be addictive.
      (2) Produce pronounced physical and psychological side effects.
      (3) Mimic the action of a drug.
      (4) Reverse the action of potent drugs.
   c. Placebo-positive persons (those who have positive effects) are believed to produce endorphins that are responsible for positive effects.
   d. Between 30% and 40% of persons will consistently react to them.
   e. How and by whom a placebo is given has *more* influence on the outcome than the personality traits of the person receiving it.
   f. Guidelines for use of placebo effect:
      (1) Always try to be honest in your dealings with patients. Do what you know and feel is the right thing to do.
      (2) Do *not* use placebos to assess the severity of pain or determine whether it actually exists.
      (3) Being placebo-positive is not the same as being suggestible or gullible.

(4) Use the placebo effect for the benefit of your patient whenever you do something you honestly believe will help.

D. Concerns for the elderly
1. Pain is not an inevitable part of aging.
2. No difference in pain perception between elderly and young patients.
3. Chronic diseases often cause pain in the elderly.
4. Lack of pain expression does not necessarily mean lack of pain.
5. Narcotics can be safely and effectively used in the elderly.
6. Factors that may affect distribution of drugs in the elderly: proportion of body fat; decreased heart, kidney, and muscle mass; decreased kidney function; and decreased protein levels.
7. Elderly metabolize acetaminophen more slowly.
8. Meperidine (Demerol) may quickly accumulate in the patient with decreased renal function and cause CNS excitability.
9. For safe pain control, medicate before pain becomes severe, monitor side effects closely, use round-the-clock scheduling, and titrate dosage as needed.

CHAPTER 11

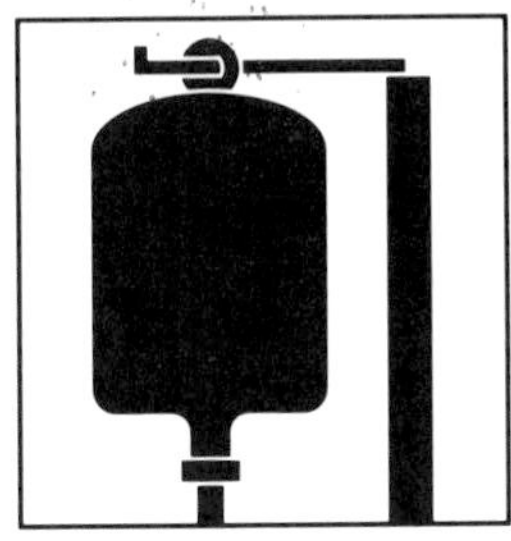

Care of Surgical Patients

VOCABULARY

anaphylaxis
atelectasis
dehiscence
emesis
evisceration
extracorporeal
hematoma
hypothermia
hypovolemia
hypoxemia
idiosyncrasy
ileus
oximetry
patent
serosanguinous
thrombus
viscera

Upon completion of this chapter the student should be able to:

1. Identify the types of patients most at risk for surgery and state why each type is at risk.
2. Prepare patients physically, emotionally, and psychologically for surgical procedures.
3. Plan and implement patient and family teaching to prevent postoperative complications.
4. Compare and contrast various types of anesthesia and the nursing care that is unique to each type.
5. Assess the status of patients during the immediate postoperative period while they are in the recovery room.
6. Provide routine postoperative care for patients who have had various types of surgery.
7. Discuss assessment and care of surgical wounds and drains.
8. Identify signs and symptoms of common postoperative complications.
9. Itemize the points to be covered in discharge planning.

Not as many patients are hospitalized for surgery today as in the past. To prevent added expense, many common surgeries such as cataract extraction, simple hernia repair, arthroscopy, and hemorrhoidectomy are done on an outpatient basis. Independent surgery day centers are increasing in numbers to fill this need. However, most large hospitals have an outpatient surgery unit where the patient is admitted the morning of surgery, prepared for surgery, and given post-recovery room care before discharge that afternoon. Diagnostic testing is done on the 2 days before surgery. The nurse cares for these patients before and after the surgical procedure, and she is the one who determines that the patient is stable and may be discharged.

For patients who are hospitalized for surgery, the preparation is begun on admission. The nurse performs much of the preoperative teaching and procedures. Her vigilance in the postoperative period can prevent the patient from experiencing a serious emergency or complication. The nurse is also the one who ensures that the patient leaves for home confident that he can manage with the help of his family or significant others.

PREOPERATIVE PERIOD

ASSESSMENT

Before surgery is undertaken, the patient should be in the best possible physical condition. In emergencies, of course, this cannot be controlled, but planned surgery might be postponed for days or weeks until the patient is physically able to withstand the rigors of anesthesia and major surgery. In order to determine the patient's readiness for surgery, a thorough assessment of his health status and risk factors is conducted.

Laboratory Data

Required tests before surgery include a complete blood cell (CBC) count and urinalysis. A chest radiograph is usually performed, and an EKG is ordered for any patient over 40 years of age. Other tests commonly ordered include tests to determine electrolyte and blood glucose levels, prothrombin time (PT), and partial thromboplastin time (PTT) (which indicate blood clotting ability, blood type, and cross-match for transfusion), and a profile that gives data about liver and kidney function. If the laboratory reports indicate any abnormal values, measures will be taken by the physician to improve the general health of the patient before surgery is scheduled. Most surgeons prefer to postpone surgery if a patient's hemoglobin level is below 10 gm per 100 mL.

Surgery puts a strain on the cardiovascular, urinary, and respiratory systems. Liver function also is important, because this organ is involved in synthesizing clotting factors, producing albumin, and metabolizing and detoxifying drugs.

Requesting preoperative diagnostic tests is the responsibility of the physician, but the nurse will need to explain to the patient why these tests have been ordered.

Nursing Assessment

The nurse's assessment of the patient's health status prior to surgery facilitates planning of his care during and after surgery. During assessment the nurse will check the patient's temperature, pulse, respiratory rate, and blood pressure. Any significant deviations from normal range should be brought to the attention of the surgeon. For example, an elevated temperature might indicate an infection that would need to be brought under control before surgery could be done. Knowing the patient's usual blood pressure reading is necessary for comparison later when postoperative shock is a concern. Height and weight are measured and charted so the anesthesiologist can accurately calculate anesthetic dosages.

Allergies must be identified and noted in a conspicuous place on the patient's chart. *All* allergies should be documented. Because the surgical patient is frequently exposed to iodine antiseptics used preoperatively to cleanse the skin (e.g., povidone-iodine [Betadine]), it is especially important to note any allergy to iodine or shellfish (which contain iodine) on the front of the chart, in the chart, and on the preoperative check list. An allergy to adhesive or paper tape must also be noted.

Nutritional status and *body weight* are significant factors in healing and repair of the surgical site. Obese persons present problems related to such routine procedures as venipuncture, intubation for general anesthesia, and prolonged uptake of anesthetic drugs. These patients also do not breathe as deeply and effectively as they should to avoid respiratory complications. Preoperative instruction must be tailored to meet the obese person's special needs, because there is more danger of strain on the surgical wound and greater demand for oxygen in these patients.

Obesity often prolongs surgery and increases tissue trauma, especially when the surgical site is the abdominal or thoracic cavity. Healing is slower and infection more of a threat, because adipose tissue contains fewer blood vessels. This limits the availability of nutritional elements for repair and defensive elements to fight infection. Obese patients also dehydrate more easily, because there is less body fluid in adipose tissue than in other tissues.

The malnourished or emaciated patient is also

at risk because of the need for protein to replace blood cells and serum lost during surgery. Protein is also needed for the formation of antibodies and defensive cells and for the repair of damaged cells. After surgery there is a metabolic change in which the catabolic (destructive) phase predominates. This results in a *negative protein balance*, which the emaciated patient can ill afford. Vitamins and other food elements necessary for tissue healing and repair are discussed in more detail in Chapter 6.

Nursing History

Assessment for factors that place the patient at risk for complications of surgery should be carefully completed. Elderly patients are at greater risk, because they often have chronic illnesses. People with respiratory, cardiac, or liver disorders or diabetes likewise have an increased risk.

Smoking has a negative effect on wound healing and on pulmonary function. It alters platelet function so that there is greater risk for abnormal clot formation and obstruction of blood vessels, particularly the small vessels that nourish tissue cells. Respiratory problems during the postoperative period are related to the reduced level of functional hemoglobin for the transport of oxygen, decreased lung expansion, inadequate oxygenation of the blood, and possibly acid-base imbalance.

The *diabetic* person is more at risk during and after surgical procedures. Stress and other factors can upset the blood glucose level and predispose the patient to either hypo- or hyperglycemic reactions. In the poorly controlled diabetic person there is greater chance for delayed healing, because high blood sugar levels impede the release of oxygen to the cells. Infection is also a potential problem, because poorly controlled diabetes inhibits the action of phagocytes, which are necessary for the body's defense against infectious agents.

Liver disease patients are at added risk, as impaired liver function interferes with normal clotting of blood, and the liver cannot properly detoxify anesthetics and other drugs.

Respiratory disease is an important risk factor during the surgery as well as the postoperative period. Many anesthetics are given by inhalation, and some of these irritate the respiratory mucosa, creating more secretions. Additionally, the immobility imposed by surgery increases the possibility of accumulated secretions and inflammation of the lungs and bronchial tree. Impaired respiration slows down oxygen and carbon dioxide exchange and predisposes the patient to delayed wound healing and possibly acid-base imbalance.

Psychological Assessment

The news that surgery is needed usually comes as an emotional shock to the patient and his family. The changes it brings about in the routine of their lives will naturally place some personal and financial burdens on them. For some patients the surgery will alter their lives permanently and possibly leave them handicapped in some way. Others might expect to be greatly helped by the surgical procedure. In any event, there will be some fears and misgivings about the prospect of having anesthesia and surgery.

During her assessment of the patient's level of anxiety and emotional readiness for surgery the nurse might seek answers to the following questions:

- What does the patient know about the surgical procedure to be done? What questions does he have about the procedure? What misinformation might he have that could cause needless worry?
- Has he ever had surgery before? What was done then? What experiences does he remember, and were they good or unpleasant?
- Does he have any particular concerns or fears now?
- Is he especially fearful of any medical problems that might affect his recovery from surgery? What can be done to help allay his fears?

Spiritual Assessment

Most people are concerned about whether they will "wake up" or survive the anesthesia and surgical procedure. Some patients have the strong spiritual beliefs they need to cope with sickness, suffering, and death. Others may need help in finding the spiritual support they need, and still others do not want to discuss this particular facet of their lives.

If a patient does not seem to have spiritual support, the nurse should help him find and use the available resources. The resource could be herself or another person, such as a special friend, family member, minister, or hospital chaplain. Table 4–3 summarizes the kinds of questions the nurse might ask during her assessment of the patient's spiritual needs.

Assessment of Learning Needs

There is some general information the surgical patient should have about what will be happening to him immediately before, during, and after surgery. There also are specific preventive measures he might need to learn to perform. Instruction in these and other pre- and postoperative procedures are discussed later under Intervention.

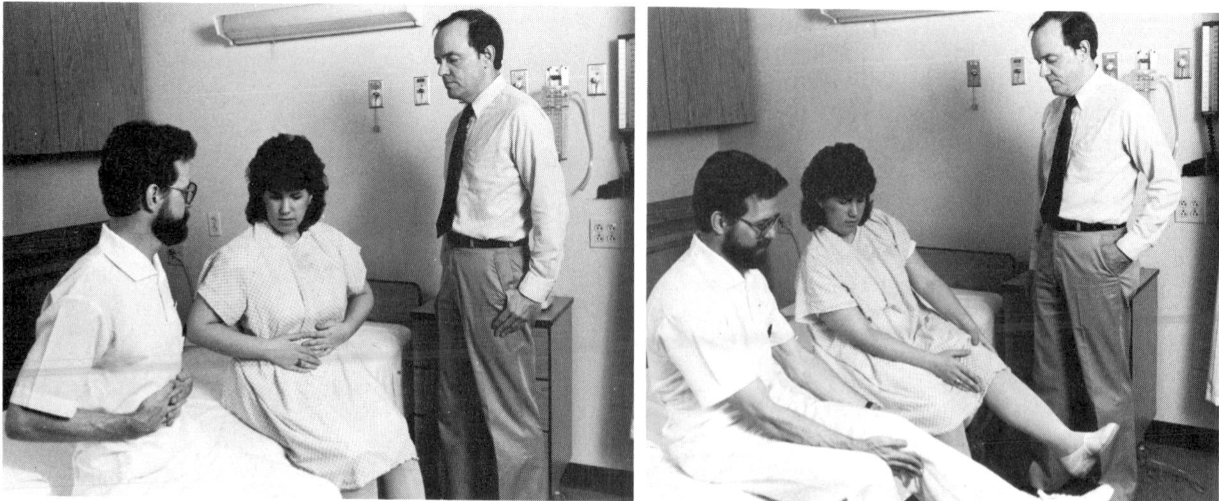

Figure 11-1 Deep breathing and leg exercises demonstrated by nurse and practiced by patient. Spouse will help in postoperative care. (Photos by Ken Kasper.)

If it is expected that members of the family will assist the patient during the postoperative period, they should be included in teaching sessions (Figs. 11-1 and 11-2).

INTERVENTION

Informing the Patient and His Family

In most hospitals it is the nurse's job to provide the patient the information he needs to help him feel less anxious and better prepared to undergo surgery. Explanation of what can be expected before, during, and after surgery is begun when the operation is scheduled. This can be valuable reinforcement for the anxious patient who can't take in all the information at one time. Some hospitals also make available pamphlets, filmstrips, and other teaching aids to instruct preoperative patients.

General Information About Surgery

General information that almost all surgical patients should receive includes information related to:

- *Preoperative procedures:* enemas, skin preparation, care of belongings, restriction of food and liquids, and administration of bedtime sedatives and preoperative medication.
- *Technical information:* anticipated surgical procedure; location of incisions; and dressings, tubes, drains, or catheters that are expected.
- *Day of surgery:* time surgery is scheduled,

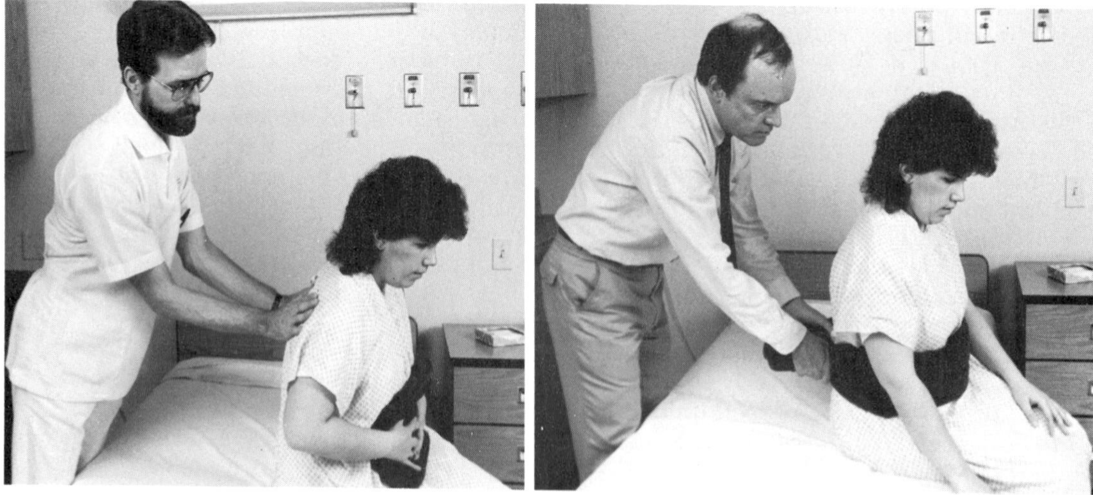

Figure 11-2 Coughing is more effective and less painful when the patient splints the operative site with a towel or pillow and the nurse gives firm support to the patient's back. Bracing with a towel pulled snug on the side opposite the operative site during cough is another way to provide support.
(Photos by Ken Kasper.)

time he is to leave his room, probable length of procedure, effects of preoperative medications, where family will wait, when and where they can see the patient after surgery, pain control, and postoperative routine.

- *Recovery room:* general environment (noise, lights, equipment), frequent taking of vital signs, and administration of oxygen.
- *Intensive Care Unit (Surgical ICU)* (if patient is to go there from recovery room): location of the unit, expected length of stay, and visiting privileges.

Special Information

The specific kinds of information a surgical patient needs will depend on the surgical procedure planned and anticipated length of recovery. There are distinct advantages to teaching the patient certain procedures and practices that will benefit him postoperatively. Such instruction gives the patient an opportunity to participate in his care insofar as he is able, obtains his cooperation in preventing postoperative complications, and works to reduce his anxiety and that of his family members.

Specific preoperative instruction varies from one institution to another but usually includes deep breathing and coughing techniques, use of an incentive spirometer, leg exercises, and practice in moving about in bed and getting in and out of bed. Figure 11–3 shows the kind of instruction sheet that can be used to instruct the patient during the preoperative period.

Instruction Techniques. The *how* of teaching might include (1) giving the patient a pamphlet to read or a filmstrip to view and returning later to answer his questions and clarify what he has read or seen; (2) demonstrating the use of special equipment (for example, an incentive spirometer) that he will be expected to use after surgery; (3) having the patient read about specific exercises he will need to perform after surgery, demonstrating them for him, and then having him practice them under your guidance; and (4) calling in such resource personnel as the physical therapist to teach specific exercises, the respiratory therapist, recovery room nurse, and any others who are in a better position to explain certain aspects of the patient's surgery and recovery period.

Informing the surgical patient is a continuous process during the preoperative period. The purpose is to let him absorb information at his own pace and provide an atmosphere in which he feels free to ask questions.

The family should be advised to come to the hospital 1 to 1½ hours before surgery. They should be told about the usual routines, the approximate time the patient may be expected to return to his room, and what to anticipate in the way of tubes, equipment, and patient appearance after surgery. This knowledge keeps them from thinking the patient has "taken a turn for the worse" when they see the extra equipment for suction, oxygen, or intravenous therapy in use after surgery. A warning about the occasional delays in starting surgery can keep the family from becoming excessively anxious if the patient is not back in his room at the expected time.

Preparation of the Skin

Scrubbing and shaving the operative site is most often done just before surgery. Hair may be shaved, clipped, or removed with a depilatory cream according to the surgeon's preference. For some types of surgery (i.e., bone and heart surgery and some plastic reconstructions), preoperative skin preparation may be started 24 to 72 hours beforehand. The patient is given a bacteriostatic cleansing solution (e.g., Hibiclens or pHisoHex) to use in the shower or on a designated body part.

Restriction of Oral Intake

The surgeon will leave written orders regarding restriction of food and drink before surgery. It may be necessary for the nurse to explain to the patient that he is not allowed anything by mouth because of the danger of vomiting with subsequent aspiration of the vomitus into the air passages during or immediately after surgery. Patients who smoke are asked to stop 24 hours before surgery. In some cases, a gastric tube may be inserted into the stomach by way of a nostril and gastric suction started the evening or morning before surgery. This tube is to be clamped off and left in place just before the patient is taken to the operating room. It may reassure the patient if he understands that gastric suction eliminates much unnecessary distention, nausea and vomiting, and consequent pain postoperatively. The nurse should clarify with the surgeon which, if any, routine medications should be administered (e.g., glaucoma, heart, or diabetic medications). Medications can be given with just a sip of water.

Elimination

Surgery involving the abdominal cavity, rectum, or perineum usually requires a cleansing of the lower intestinal tract by catharsis and/or enemas. This preparation will reduce the possibility of contamination of the operative area during surgery, when the sphincter muscles are relaxed and will also help to eliminate distention following surgery. "Enemas until clear" may be ordered for patients having rectal surgery or other operative procedures in which the surgeon

After your surgery, it is extremely important to breathe deeply, cough, change positions, and exercise your legs every 2 hours. These exercises may be uncomfortable but they are necessary to prevent complications.

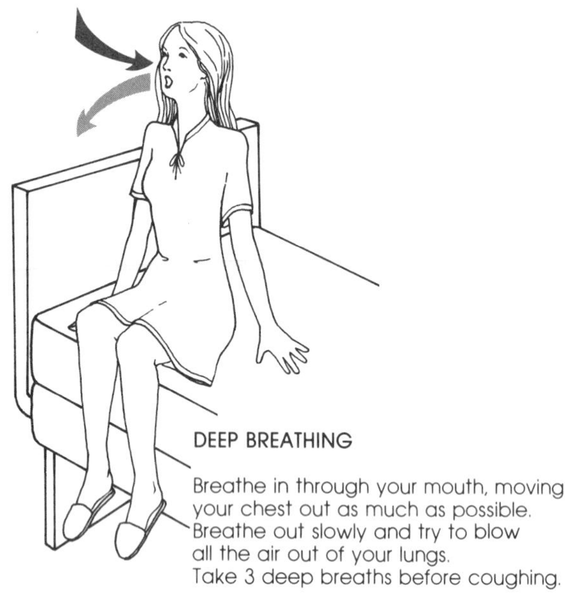

DEEP BREATHING
Breathe in through your mouth, moving your chest out as much as possible.
Breathe out slowly and try to blow all the air out of your lungs.
Take 3 deep breaths before coughing.

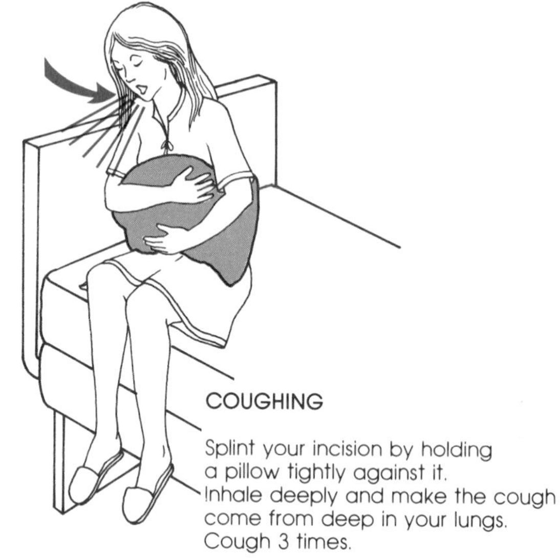

COUGHING
Splint your incision by holding a pillow tightly against it.
Inhale deeply and make the cough come from deep in your lungs.
Cough 3 times.

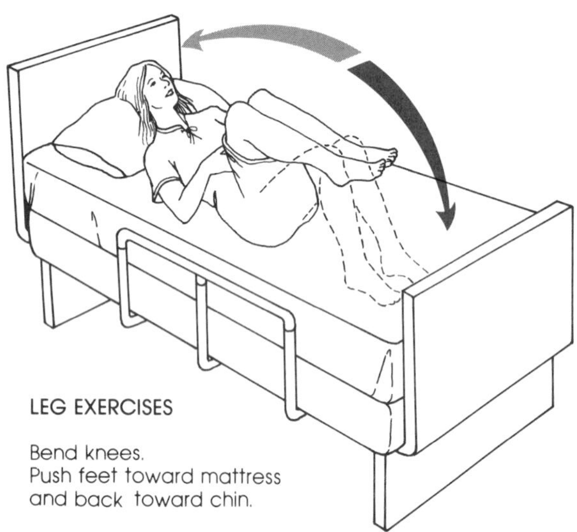

LEG EXERCISES
Bend knees.
Push feet toward mattress and back toward chin.

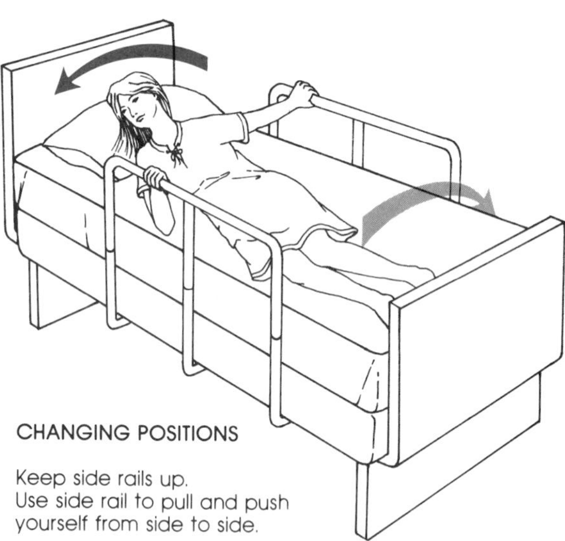

CHANGING POSITIONS
Keep side rails up.
Use side rail to pull and push yourself from side to side.

Figure 11-3 Postsurgery exercises.

does not wish the patient to have a bowel movement for several days after surgery. These can be exhausting and should be given slowly and with care, allowing the patient to rest between enemas.

Rest and Sedation

The body needs all its strength and physical resources when coping with surgical procedures. Thus the patient should have adequate sleep the night before surgery. A barbiturate is usually ordered, but this does not always guarantee that the patient will sleep well. He should be checked on frequently. If he is awake and restless, the nurse should take time to talk with him, allay fears, offer a soothing back rub, and repeat the sedation if necessary. If the patient is sleeping well, he should not be disturbed for routine procedures during the night and morning of surgery.

Consent for Surgery

Before the surgeon can perform an operation, he must have written permission signed by either the patient or his guardian. This written consent protects the surgeon against claims of unauthorized surgery and provides the patient an opportunity to exercise his right of informed consent. In most hospitals, the "contract" is a printed form that the patient signs before surgery. The consent form is then attached to the patient's chart and is sent to the operating room with the patient. The patient has the right to change his mind and revoke his consent up until the time of surgery. The nurse must always check to see that a consent form has been signed before giving the preoperative medication. Figure 11-4 shows an example of a standard consent form.

Immediate Preoperative Care

The patient must wear only a hospital gown to the operating room. The hair should be covered with a towel or cap, and in some hospitals, surgical boots are put on the patient. Women with very long hair should have it combed and plaited into braids, and all hairpins must be removed from the hair. If the patient wishes to wear a wedding ring, it should be secured in place with tape. Watches and other valuables must be removed from the bedside table and placed under lock and key according to hospital policy. Dentures are usually removed, placed in a labeled denture cup, and kept in a designated place according to hospital policy. Sometimes the anesthesiologist will request that the dentures be left in place, because they help maintain the contour of the face and facilitate the administration of inhalation anesthesia.

The patient's identification bracelet or tag is

CONSENT TO OPERATION

Date ______________________ Time a.m. p.m.

1. I hereby authorize Dr. ______________________ and whomever he may designate as his assistants, to perform upon ______________________ (Name of Patient or "Myself")

the following operation: ______________________ (Nature of Procedure(s) to be Performed)

and if any unforeseen condition arises in the course of the operation in his judgement for procedures in addition to or different from those now contemplated, I further request and authorize him to do whatever he deems advisable.

2. The nature and purpose of the operation, possible alternative methods of treatment, the risks involved, and the possibility of complications have been fully explained to me. I acknowledge that no guarantee or assurance has been made as to the results that may be obtained.

3. I consent to the administration of anesthesia to be applied by or under the direction of ______________________

______________________ or ______________________, and to the use of such anesthetics as may be deemed by any of them advisable with the exception of ______________________ ("None", "Spinal Anesthesia", etc.)

4. I am aware that sterility may result from this operation although such result has not been guaranteed. I know that a sterile person is incapable of parenthood.

5. I consent to the disposal by authorities of the ____________ Hospital of any tissues or parts which may be removed.

I CERTIFY THAT I HAVE READ AND FULLY UNDERSTAND THE ABOVE CONSENT TO OPERATION, THAT THE EXPLANATIONS THEREIN REFERRED TO WERE MADE, AND THAT ALL BLANKS OR STATEMENTS REQUIRING INSERTION OR COMPLETION WERE FILLED IN AND INAPPLICABLE PARAGRAPHS IF ANY, WERE STRICKEN BEFORE I SIGNED.

Signature of patient ______________________

Signature of patient's husband or wife ______________________

Signature of person authorized to consent for patient when a patient is a minor or incompetent to give consent ______________________

Witness: ______________________ Relationship to patient ______________________

Figure 11-4 Sample consent form for surgery.

checked with the chart for accuracy to avoid any error or mix-up of patients in the operating room.

Unless there is a urinary catheter in place, preoperative patients are asked to empty the bladder before administration of the preoperative medication.

A delay in the preoperative medication may cause difficulties for the patient and a great inconvenience to the person administering the anesthesia. All preliminary preparations should be done before the medication is given so that it will have maximum effect.

The preoperative medication must be administered at exactly the time ordered by the surgeon or anesthesiologist. This is essential because the amount of anesthesia and time of induction have been calculated according to the hour the premedication was expected to be given.

Preoperative medications are given to (1) reduce anxiety and promote rest, (2) decrease secretion of mucus and other body fluids, (3) counteract nausea and reduce emesis, and (4) enhance the effects of the anesthetic. The sedatives usually given include secobarbital (Seconal) and pentobarbital (Nembutal). Drying agents include atropine and scopolamine. Narcotics such as morphine and meperidine hydrochloride (Demerol) are given to supplement the anesthetic (Table 11–1).

Other agents commonly administered immediately prior to surgery are promethezine hydrochloride (Phenergan), hydroxyzine hydrochloride (Vistaril), or chlorpromazine hydrochloride (Thorazine), all of which produce sedative, antihistaminic, and antiemetic effects; and diazepam (Valium) or midazolam hydrochloride (Versed), which calm the patient.

It is important to attend to all the items on the checklist that can be handled ahead of time early in the morning. This avoids last-minute haste, prevents mistakes, and makes it easier to give the preoperative medication on time. After the preoperative medication is given, the patient is told not to get out of bed without assistance, siderails are raised, and the call bell is placed within reach.

Many hospitals have a preoperative checklist to be filled out by the nurse in charge before the patient is taken to the operating room. This eliminates the danger of omitting any part of the preoperative preparation (Fig. 11–5).

ANESTHESIA

Anesthesia (the loss of sensory perception) came into use as an accepted part of surgical procedure in the 1840s. With the advent of drugs that safely produced anesthesia, the performance of surgical operations became a more widely accepted and successful means of treating disease and injury. Few of us would accept surgery with out the advantage of being insensible to pain

TABLE 11–1 COMMONLY PRESCRIBED PREOPERATIVE MEDICATIONS

Drugs	Average Doses	Purposes	Nursing Implications
Sedatives:			
Nembutal sodium Seconal sodium	100 mg IM 90 minutes before surgery	Decrease anxiety; lower blood pressure and pulse; enhance action of anesthetic.	Be alert for opposite effect in certain patients, particularly the elderly, who may become restless and confused. Must be given at precise time ordered.
Tranquilizers:			
Thorazine Phenergan	12.5 to 25 mg IM—to 2 hours before surgery	Reduce anxiety; promote relaxation. NOTE: Can cause severe hypotension	Patient should be confined to bed after injection because of danger of fainting. Sensitive children and adults may exhibit motor restlessness and opisthotonos. Check blood pressure for signs of extreme hypotension.
Hydroxyzine pamoate (Vistaril)	25 to 50 mg IM	Reduce anxiety and tension; promote relaxation.	Raise side rails. Give IM Z-track.

TABLE 11-1 **COMMONLY PRESCRIBED PREOPERATIVE MEDICATIONS** *Continued*

Drugs	Average Doses	Purposes	Nursing Implications
Diazepam (Valium)	5 to 10 mg IM	Reduce tension and anxiety; promote relaxation; decrease muscle spasm.	Reduce dosage of narcotics. Monitor respirations.
Midazolam hydrochloride (Versed)	0.07 to 0.08 mg/kg IM	Induce drowsiness and relieve apprehension.	Conscious sedation; sedation before short-term diagnostic or endoscopic procedures; amnesic effect.
Drying agents:			
Atropine sulfate Scopolamine (Hyoscine)	0.3 to 0.6 mg IM 0.3 to 0.6 mg SQ	Inhibit secretions from mucous membranes of mouth and respiratory tract.	Do not give to patients with glaucoma. Observe for rash, flushing of skin, and elevated temperature, which are common side effects, particularly in children. Bed rails and close supervision of patient who has received scopolamine; may become very drowsy and injure self.
Glycopyrrolate (Robinul)	0.004 mg/kg IM	Diminish secretions; block cardiac vagal reflexes.	Contraindicated in glaucoma. Check dosage carefully. Use smaller doses in elderly. Watch for adverse reaction in elderly patients. Monitor for urinary hesitancy.
Analgesics:			
Morphine sulfate Meperidine (Demerol)	8 to 15 mg SQ 50 to 100 mg IM	Reduce anxiety; promote relaxation; not necessarily to relieve pain when given preoperatively.	Check respiratory rate before giving. Nausea, vomiting, and constipation may result. Observe patient for increased restlessness, tremors, and delirium, which may occur as side effects.
Hydromorphone hydrochloride (Dilaudid)		Reduce anxiety; promote relaxation.	Check vital signs before giving. Raise side rails.

during the operation, and modern surgical procedures requiring several hours would be impossible without adequate anesthesia.

The first anesthetics used were ether and nitrous oxide. It is interesting to note that these drugs were used as a source of entertainment and amusement before anyone considered using them in medical practice. Nitrous oxide, commonly called "laughing gas," was sometimes administered to a volunteer from the audience of a side show for the purpose of watching the antics of the victim as he was transported into a state of euphoria and became hysterical with laughter. Today, ether is rarely used, because it is highly explosive; however, nitrous oxide remains a frequently administered anesthetic.

ALLERGIES:

FLOOR CHECK LIST

1. Consent for surgery form signed __Yes __No
2. Special Consent form signed __Yes __No
Sterilization___Abortion___Disposal___
3. History & Physical ___Yes ___No
4. Doctors orders __Yes ___No
**5. Consultation ___Yes ___No
6. Urinalysis ___Yes ___No
*7. C.B.C. ___Yes ___No
8. Type & Cross match __Yes __No __Number
***9. Preoperative profile ___Yes ___No
10. Prep done by________
11. Patient dressed ___Yes ___No
12. T.P.R. ________Time________
13. B/P ________Time________
14. Oral Hygiene done ___Yes ___No
15. Voided________Time________
16. Retention Catheter ___Yes ___No
17. PROSTHESES:

	NONE	REMOVED	DISPOSITION	LEFT IN
Bridges				
Partials				
Plates				
Artifical Limbs				
Artifical Eyes				
Contact Lenses				
Hearing Aid				
Wig				

18. VALUABLES:

	REMOVED YES	REMOVED NO	DISPOSITION, IF REMOVED
Rings			
Watch			
Medal & Chains			
Glasses			

19. Identification band checked with chart ___Yes ___No
20. Pre-op medications and times ________

By________

Signature of Charge Nurse

Date

OPERATING ROOM CHECK LIST

	CHECK	COMMENT
1.		
2.		
3.		
4.		
5.		
6.		
7.		
8.		
9.		
10.		
11.		
12.		
13.		
14.		
15.		
16.		
17.		
18.		
19.		
20.		

POSTOPERATIVE

Sponge Count Correct ___Yes ___No
Specimen to Lab ___Yes ___No
Culture Done ___Yes ___No
Packing in Place ___Yes ___No
Procedure Done________

Signature of Circulating Nurse

Drains Left In________
Catheter In________

*NOTIFY DR. AND O.R. IF HEMOGLOBIN BELOW 11 Grams
** CONSULTATION ON ALL FIRST CAESAREAN SECTIONS
CONSULTATION ON ALL HYSTERECTOMIES 35 YEARS OLD AND YOUNGER
*** FOR ALL PATIENTS 35 YEARS OLD OR OLDER
CBC AND URINALYSIS MUST BE REPEATED IF OVER 48 HOURS.

Figure 11-5 Sample preoperative checklist.

There are three main objectives in the administration of an anesthetic: (1) to prevent pain, (2) to achieve adequate muscle relaxation, and (3) to calm fear, allay anxiety, and induce forgetfulness.

TYPES OF ANESTHESIA

In order to achieve the aforementioned objectives, anesthetics can be administered in a number of ways. The choice of anesthesia and route of administration rests with the anesthesiologist and depends on the type of surgery to be performed, the age and physical condition of the patient, and the patient's ability to tolerate the anesthetic and the surgical procedure.

Inhalants

Inhalation is the oldest, most easily controlled, and most frequently used method of administering anesthesia. Halothane (Fluothane) may be administered by the nonrebreathing, partial rebreathing, or closed technique. It is often given in combination with nitrous oxide. Because of its potential for damage to the liver, it is not given to patients with hepatic or biliary disease. Adverse reactions, in addition to liver toxicity, include hyperpyrexia, shivering, nausea, and emesis.

Methoxyflurane (Penthrane) is a form of ether that has been altered chemically so that it is not highly volatile. Analgesia and drowsiness from the effects of Penthrane may persist after the patient has regained consciousness and thus minimize the need for narcotics immediately after surgery. Renal toxicity associated with Penthrane seems to be related to the total amount given and the length of time it is administered. It is not recommended for diabetic patients and others with existing or potential kidney disease.

Intravenous Anesthesia

The administration of anesthetic by vein has as its major advantages (1) a rapid induction in which the patient quickly goes to sleep and (2) the absence of nausea and vomiting during the postoperative period. However, drugs administered intravenously are usually barbiturates, which are comparatively poor anesthetics and present problems of asphyxiation from laryngospasm and bronchospasm. The drug most commonly used as an IV anesthetic is *thiopental sodium* (Pentothal).

Thiopental sodium used in combination with fentanyl-droperidol (Innovar) is another popular anesthetic. It may also be used with fentanyl (Sublimaze) only. In recent years, morphine has been considered the agent of choice for open heart and vascular surgery.

Another drug, *ketamine* (Ketalar), also may be administered alone or in combination with nitrous oxide. The patient who has been given ketamine may be delirious, have disturbed dreams, or possibly hallucinate. The nurse should provide a quiet, nonstimulating environment while the patient is emerging from the effects of the anesthetic.

Regional Anesthesia

In this type of anesthesia, only one area of the body is deadened to pain; the patient remains conscious. Because the patient is awake, there are fewer respiratory difficulties due to pooling of mucus in the air passages.

Regional anesthetics may be administered *topically* (directly on the surface of the area to be treated), and by *injection*, either into the skin and subcutaneous tissues or into the spinal column. Drugs commonly used for regional anesthesia include *butacaine*, *tetracaine* (Pontocaine), *lidocaine* (Xylocaine), and *cocaine*.

Whenever a local anesthetic is administered, there is the potential for* anaphylaxis *due to hypersensitivity to the drug if it accidentally enters the blood stream. Precautions are the same as for any highly allergenic drug, and emergency equipment should be readily available.

These aspects of patient care are discussed in Chapter 6.

Spinal anesthesia, which is a form of regional anesthesia, can be used only for surgery below the diaphragm, but it is very effective and produces complete muscular relaxation even though the patient remains awake during the operation.

The postoperative care of the patient receiving spinal anesthesia is basically the same as for general anesthesia, although there are usually fewer gastrointestinal and respiratory complications to be guarded against following spinal anesthesia. On the other hand, the nurse must realize that respiratory difficulties and cardiovascular complications can develop when spinal anesthesia is given. If the anesthesia ascends beyond the point of injection, innervation of the respiratory muscles and blood vessels is affected. This produces depression of respiration and a lowering of the blood pressure.

As the anesthesia wears off, the patient may complain that he cannot move his legs and that they feel numb and heavy. This is to be expected at first and will gradually subside. The patient is kept flat in bed for 6 to 12 hours. He may be turned from side to side unless there are specific orders to the contrary.

The patient may experience spinal headache. Nursing intervention includes restricting him to bed rest; maintaining a quiet, darkened room; maintaining hydration orally or with IV fluids; and administering analgesics as needed.

Epidural or caudal anesthesia is used primarily in obstetric procedures. The anesthetic is injected into the epidural space rather than the subarachnoid space.

TABLE 11-2 **TYPES OF ANESTHESIA: USES, ADVANTAGES, AND DISADVANTAGES**

Route of Administration	Agents Commonly Used	Advantages and Disadvantages	Nursing Implications
General anesthesia			
Inhalation	Methoxyflurane (Penthrane)	Renal toxicity: related to total dose.	Contraindicated in patients with actual or potential kidney disease.
			Can reduce need for narcotics during immediate postoperative period.
	Halothane	Possible liver damage.	Monitor respiratory rate and pulse for signs of respiratory and circulatory depression.
	Nitrous oxide (laughing gas)	Relatively nontoxic; can cause hallucinations and dreams.	None
	Ethrane	Rapid induction, possible respiratory depression and cardiac arrythmia; similar to halothane, but does not cause kidney or liver damage.	Monitor for possible seizure activity.
	Isoflurane (Forane)	Rapid induction and recovery; enhances muscle relaxants; does not depress myocardium; causes respiratory depression.	Monitor respiration and blood pressure.
Intravenous	Combination of fentanyl and droperidol (Innovar), and thiopental Fentanyl (Sublimaze)	Not as easily controlled as inhalation anesthesia.	Do not give in combination with other sedatives, hypnotics, or other strong analgesics because of possible additive effects, chiefly hypotension and respiratory depression.
		Major dangers are laryngospasm and bronchospasm.	Monitor closely for signs of laryngospasm.
	Morphine sulfate	Increases cardiac output. Agent of choice for open heart surgery and vascular surgery.	Observe for respiratory depression.
	Ketamine (Ketalar) used alone or with nitrous oxide	Onset brief, suitable for short procedures.	Given with caution to elderly patients with atherosclerosis and contraindicated in patients with hypertension because of increased cardiac output and elevation of blood pressure.
		Postoperative hallucinations in adults.	Protective safety measures to prevent injury during irrational behavior, excitement, and confusion.
		Airway obstruction and vomiting may occur.	Provide quiet environment; avoid visual, auditory, and tactile stimulation.

TABLE 11-2 TYPES OF ANESTHESIA: USES, ADVANTAGES, AND DISADVANTAGES *Continued*

Route of Administration	Agents Commonly Used	Advantages and Disadvantages	Nursing Implications
	Methohexital sodium (Brevital)	Very short acting; five times stronger than sodium pentothal; less likely to cause bronchospasm.	Monitor respiration closely.
Regional anesthesia			
Topical anesthesia	Cocaine Tetracaine (Pontocaine)	Immediate effect, generally nontoxic.	Check for history of drug sensitivity or other allergies.
	Lidocaine (Xylocaine)	Major disadvantage is possibilty of drug sensitivity and anaphylactic shock.	Have emergency equipment and drugs for treatment of anaphylactic shock readily available.
Local block	Procaine hydrochloride (Novocain)	Danger of anaphylactic shock if drug is accidentally injected into a vein.	Same as for topical anesthesia. Protect involved part from injury during period of insensitivity after local anesthesia. Do not allow patient to rub eyes, caution about biting inside of mouth, withhold food and fluids until return of tissue sensitivity.
	Mepivacaine (Carbocaine)	Absorbs into blood stream; can cause cardiac depression.	Contraindicated if patient has been taking MAO inhibitors. Monitors blood pressure.
Spinal anesthesia	Procaine hydrochloride Tetracaine (Pontocaine)	Relatively safe method. May produce nausea, vomiting, pain during surgery.	Position patient only as directed during administration of anesthetic.
		Headache not uncommon, may last for days after surgery.	Assess neurologic status of patient during recovery period.
		Respiratory paralysis can occur if drug reaches upper levels of spinal column.	Keep patient lying down to decrease possibility of headache and auditory and visual problems related to increased intracranial pressure.
		Neurologic complications include muscle weakness and paraplegia	Patient allowed to sit up when spinal fluid pressure returns to normal. Numbing and tingling are expected, will abate after short period of time; reassure patient.

The first few times the patient is allowed out of bed, there must be someone in attendance to protect him from falls and injury because he may experience some difficulty in maintaining his balance.

A comparative summary of the types of anesthesia, their uses, advantages and disadvantages, and nursing implications can be found in Table 11-2.

HYPOTHERMIA

The term *hypothermia* refers to a reduction of body temperature. Its purpose in surgery is to lower metabolism and thereby decrease the need for oxygen. In many types of surgery involving the heart, blood vessels, or brain, it is necessary to interrupt the flow of blood through the body. Lowering the body temperature to between 32°C (89.6°F) and 26°C (78.8°F) reduces the metabolic needs of the vital organs so that they are less likely to be damaged by a decreased supply of blood and oxygen.

There are several ways in which hypothermia can be achieved. In *external hypothermia*, the patient's body is wrapped in a cooling blanket, packed in ice, or submerged in a tub of ice water. This is done after the patient has been anesthetized and immediately before the surgical procedure is performed.

In *extracorporeal* cooling, the patient's blood is cooled outside the body. It is removed from a major vessel, circulated through a refrigerant unit for cooling, and returned to the body by the way of another large blood vessel. This is the quickest way to achieve hypothermia and is usually the method used for patients undergoing open heart surgery.

During the rewarming process, the patient's temperature is raised gradually. Care must be taken to avoid burns if warm baths or heating blankets are used. The rewarming procedure is discontinued when the body temperature is within 1° or 2° of normal.

Observations during the rewarming include checking the pulse, blood pressure, and respiration as well as the temperature. Any sudden change must be reported immediately.

POSTOPERATIVE PERIOD

DURING RECOVERY FROM ANESTHESIA

The period immediately following surgery is a critical one for the patient and demands close and constant observation by specially trained nurses. The recovery room routine care plan is usually designed so that all aspects of patient care receive attention. An example of routine immediate postoperative care is given in Figure 11–6.

Nursing Assessment and Intervention

While the patient is still under anesthesia, the recovery room staff should be careful in their conversations. Talking should be limited to reassuring the patient that his surgery is over and telling him where he is. Communication with staff members should be done in a low voice. Whispering is inappropriate, as the patient may misinterpret what is said and become alarmed.

During the time that the patient is recovering from the effects of anesthesia, the nurse must provide simple nursing measures to relieve some of his discomfort. Because the patient has had nothing by mouth for 8 hours or more, he may experience severe thirst. If not contraindicated, a few ice chips may be offered; otherwise his lips can be moistened with a gauze square dipped in ice water. If he is receiving intravenous fluids, it is wise to stabilize the arm with an armboard so he will not dislodge the needle as he arouses. The bony prominences should be padded and the hand supported on the armboard.

Many surgical procedures extend over a period of hours, which means that the patient has been lying motionless, in a fixed position, on a hard table for that length of time. No wonder, therefore, that the patient often complains of backache when he first wakes up. Turning the patient on his side and administering a gentle back rub will help. If he cannot be turned, the lumbar region may be supported with a small pillow or folded bath towel.

Pain is an important factor in the care of the patient who is recovering from anesthesia. Before resorting to analgesic medications, which may not be allowed so near to the time an anesthetic has been given, the nurse should try to determine the cause of the pain. Perhaps the dressings are too tight, the bladder is distended, or the patient has abdominal distention from swallowing air. If the patient complains of chest pain or pain either on inhaling or exhaling, this should be reported to the anesthesiologist.

Operating rooms are kept very cool so that the staff members working under the bright lights do not become overheated. The patient's temperature in this environment often decreases, especially during prolonged abdominal surgery where the peritoneal cavity has been open for hours. His temperature should be checked frequently, and if there is an indication that hypothermia is present or developing, a warm blanket should be used to help maintain normal body temperature. The shivering that accompanies hypothermia produces an early need for analgesics, as these patients experience additional pain caused by uncontrollable shivering.

Nausea and vomiting following anesthesia are not uncommon. Supportive measures such as holding the patient's head or turning it to the side to prevent aspiration of the vomitus if he is not fully awake are most helpful and reassuring to the patient. He will also appreciate a few sips of water to rinse his mouth after the siege of vomiting is over.

AFTER RECOVERY FROM ANESTHESIA

Nursing Assessment and Intervention

Vital Signs

Vital signs are monitored as frequently as indicated by the physician's orders. By the time the patient has been returned to his room his vital signs should have stabilized. The purpose of continued monitoring is to note and report any significant changes that could indicate such complications as hypovolemic shock from bleeding and fluid loss, infection, hyperthermia (high temperature), and cardiac and respiratory problems.

Shock

The two most common complications of anesthesia and surgery are shock and infection. Of these, shock presents the most immediate danger to the patient, as it can quickly develop into a

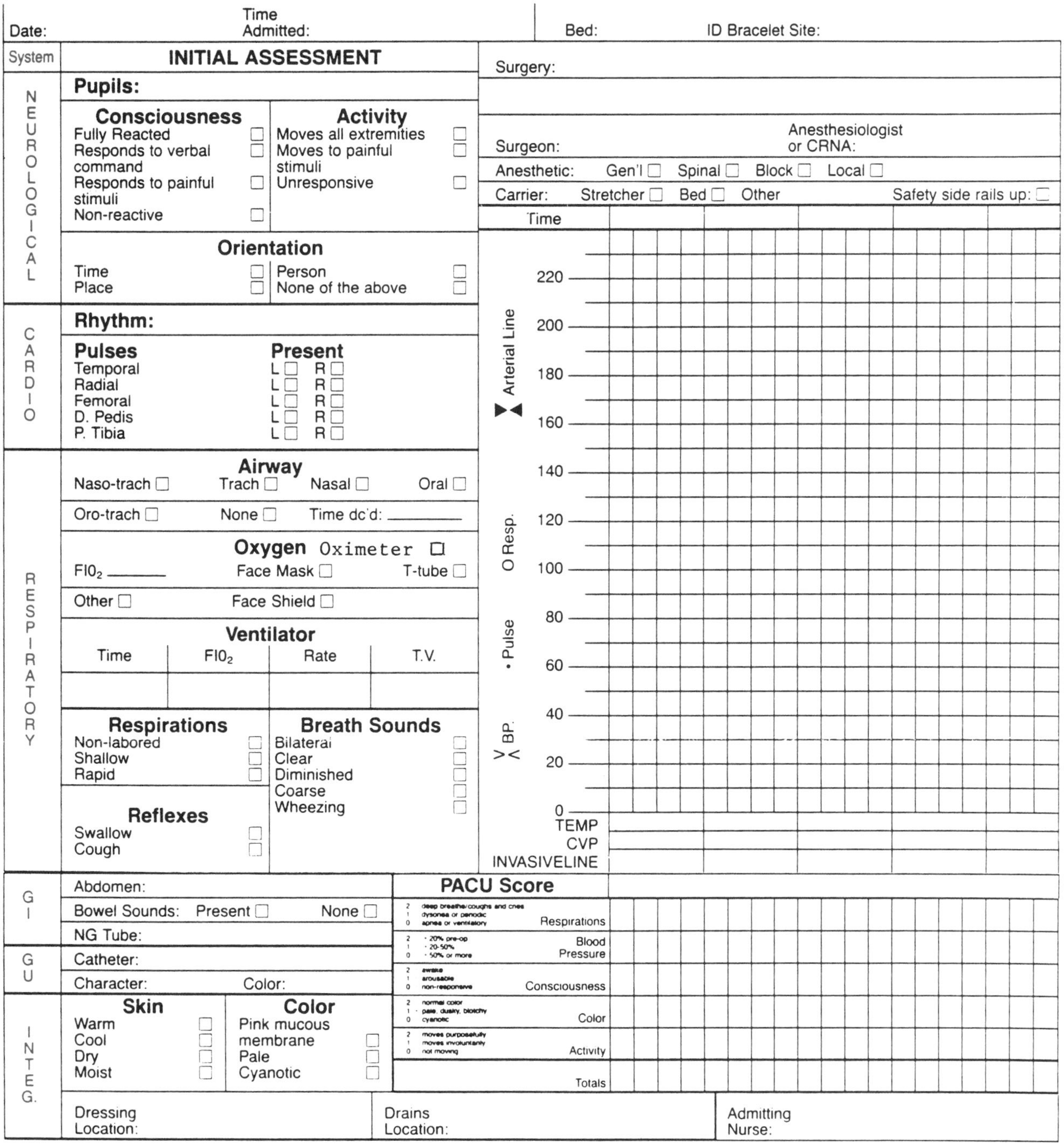

Date: Time Admitted: Bed: ID Bracelet Site:

System | INITIAL ASSESSMENT

NEUROLOGICAL

Pupils:

Consciousness
Fully Reacted ☐
Responds to verbal command ☐
Responds to painful stimuli ☐
Non-reactive ☐

Activity
Moves all extremities ☐
Moves to painful stimuli ☐
Unresponsive ☐

Orientation
Time ☐ Person ☐
Place ☐ None of the above ☐

CARDIO

Rhythm:

Pulses | **Present**
Temporal L ☐ R ☐
Radial L ☐ R ☐
Femoral L ☐ R ☐
D. Pedis L ☐ R ☐
P. Tibia L ☐ R ☐

RESPIRATORY

Airway
Naso-trach ☐ Trach ☐ Nasal ☐ Oral ☐
Oro-trach ☐ None ☐ Time dc'd: ________

Oxygen Oximeter ☐
FIO_2 ______ Face Mask ☐ T-tube ☐
Other ☐ Face Shield ☐

Ventilator

Time	FIO_2	Rate	T.V.

Respirations
Non-labored ☐
Shallow ☐
Rapid ☐

Breath Sounds
Bilateral ☐
Clear ☐
Diminished ☐
Coarse ☐
Wheezing ☐

Reflexes
Swallow ☐
Cough ☐

GI

Abdomen:
Bowel Sounds: Present ☐ None ☐
NG Tube:

GU

Catheter:
Character: Color:

INTEG.

Skin
Warm ☐
Cool ☐
Dry ☐
Moist ☐

Color
Pink mucous membrane ☐
Pale ☐
Cyanotic ☐

Surgery:

Surgeon: Anesthesiologist or CRNA:

Anesthetic: Gen'l ☐ Spinal ☐ Block ☐ Local ☐

Carrier: Stretcher ☐ Bed ☐ Other Safety side rails up: ☐

Time

▼▲ Arterial Line
O Resp.
• Pulse
∨∧ BP.

220
200
180
160
140
120
100
80
60
40
20
0

TEMP
CVP
INVASIVELINE

PACU Score

2 deep breathe/coughs and cries 1 dyspnea or periodic 0 apnea or ventilatory	Respirations	
2 · 20% pre-op 1 · 20-50% 0 · 50% or more	Blood Pressure	
2 awake 1 arousable 0 non-responsive	Consciousness	
2 normal color 1 · pale, dusky, blotchy 0 cyanotic	Color	
2 moves purposefully 1 moves involuntarily 0 not moving	Activity	
	Totals	

Dressing Location: Drains Location: Admitting Nurse:

Figure 11-6 Flow sheet used for charting nurses' observations in the postanesthesia recovery area.

Illustration continued on following page

Discharge Criteria Met ☐

TIME

Discharge Assessment

NEUROLOGICAL

Pupils:

Consciousness		**Activity**	
Fully Reacted	☐	Moves all extremities	☐
Responds to verbal command	☐	Moves to painful stimuli	☐
Responds to painful stimuli	☐	Unreactive	☐
Non-reactive	☐		

Orientation

Time	☐	Person	☐
Place	☐	None of the above	☐

CARDIO

Rhythm:

Pulses	**Present**
Temporal	L☐ R☐
Radial	L☐ R☐
Femoral	L☐ R☐
D. Pedis	L☐ R☐
P. Tibia	L☐ R☐

RESPIRATORY

Airway

Naso-trach ☐ Trach ☐ Nasal ☐ Oral ☐

Oro-trach ☐ None ☐ Time dc'd: ______

Oxygen Oximeter ☐

FI 0_2 ______ Face Mask ☐ T-tube ☐

Other Face Shield ☐

Ventilator

Time	FI 0_2	Rate	T.V.

Respirations		**Breath Sounds**	
Non-labored	☐	Bilateral	☐
Shallow	☐	Clear	☐
Rapid	☐	Diminished	☐
		Coarse	☐
		Wheezing	☐

Reflexes

Swallow	☐
Cough	☐

GI

Abdomen:

Bowel Sounds: Present ☐ None ☐

NG Tube:

GU

Catheter:

Character: Color:

INTEG

Skin		**Color**	
Warm	☐	Pink mucous membrane	☐
Cool	☐	Pale	☐
Dry	☐	Cyanotic	☐
Moist	☐		

Dressing Location:

Drains Location:

Date:

Allergies:

Time	Medication	Route	Site	Signature

Time	System	Assessment

Diagnostic Tests

Time	Tests	Results

I & O

	Time	Fluids	**Intake** I.V.	Blood	Other	Total	**Output** Time	Urine	NG	EBL	Total
OR							OR				
PACU		Fluids	I.V.	Blood	Other	Total	PACU	Urine	NG	Other	Total
		PACU Total					Output				

Disposition: I.C.U. ☐ D.S.U. ☐ NSG Unit ☐ ☐

Discharge Nurse: Report To:

PACU B.P. P. R. on unit

Received B.P. P. R. on unit

Discharged By:

Released By:

Figure 11–6 *Continued*

life-threatening emergency condition. The person in shock is suffering from a disruption of the circulation of blood. This disruption can result from (1) failure of the heart to function as a pump (cardiogenic shock), as in cardiac arrest; (2) a low volume of blood (hypovolemia), as in hemorrhage; (3) collapse of the blood vessels as a result of faulty nervous system regulation (neurogenic shock); (4) anaphylaxis (severe, allergic reaction), as in hypersensitivity to a drug or other allergen; and (5) sepsis, occurring when the toxins from bacteria bring about an expansion of blood vessels and a resultant drop in blood pressure.

In the immediate postoperative period the patient is most likely to suffer from cardiogenic, hypovolemic, or neurogenic shock. However, any of the five kinds of shock are a possibility after anesthesia and surgery. The symptoms of shock depend to some degree on the cause of circulatory failure. With hemorrhagic shock the patient may complain of thirst, restlessness, and blurred vision. Patients with neurogenic and cardiac shock may not present any warning signs of impending shock other than changes in the vital signs.

As the shock progresses, the blood pressure begins to drop. The pulse rate increases and may be bounding at first, but becomes thready and indistinct as circulatory collapse occurs. The skin becomes cold and clammy, and pallor becomes evident. There may be air hunger, with cyanosis of the lips and nail beds as a result of tissue hypoxia. As shock deepens, the blood pressure continues to fail, and the patient loses consciousness and eventually is comatose. Unrelieved shock ultimately is fatal.

Assessment of the postoperative patient must include frequent monitoring for the signs and symptoms of shock. Vital signs must be monitored frequently regardless of the type of anesthesia used during the operation. Urine output should be assessed frequently. Output should be more than 30 mL per hour. Less than this amount may indicate inadequate blood circulation to the kidneys and can be a sign of beginning shock. Both general and local anesthesia can bring about circulatory collapse. If there is evidence that the patient is in the early stage of shock, he should be placed in supine position with the lower extremities elevated to add blood volume to the vital organs. *Patients in cardiogenic shock are placed in an upright position* to lower the diaphragm and increase oxygenation as long as they do not become too hypotensive. Pain contributes to the progression of shock, but large doses of narcotics can add to the problem of low blood pressure.

Intravenous fluids and medications are an important part of the prevention and treatment of shock. They must be given as ordered, and the patient's response to them must be observed and recorded. Supplemental oxygen also is usually given to combat tissue hypoxia and cardiac response.

Report and Immediate Assessment

The recovery room nurse gives a report to the staff nurse caring for the patient. This includes the type of surgery and anesthesia, amount of blood loss, presence of all tubes and drains, IV fluids infused and currently hanging, urine and other output, medications given, any problems the patient experienced, current vital signs, and general condition.

The staff nurse then performs her own assessment, which should include measurement of all vital signs, inspection of the surgical dressing or wound area, location and function of each tube, auscultation of the lungs, and assessment of the patient's degree of arousal and pain level. If the patient has no indwelling urinary catheter and has not voided since before surgery, the bladder should be assessed for distention and an opportunity to void given. Pain medication may be needed.

Tubes and Drains

Tubes and drains are used to remove fluid and air from around the operative site or from a body structure such as the stomach, intestine, or urinary bladder. Each tube must be kept open *(patent)*, and there should be some evidence of the expected drainage—urine, bile, stomach contents, serosanguinous fluid—coming through it.

Although the specific purpose of a tube inserted during surgery will be discussed in more detail in appropriate chapters throughout this text, the importance of monitoring tubes and drains cannot be emphasized enough. In general, tubes are inserted into the stomach (nasogastric [NG] tubes), intestines (Cantor and Miller-Abbott tubes), chest cavity (thoracotomy or chest tube), and bladder or ureter (urinary catheters).

Drains are used to (1) prevent accumulation of fluids or air at the operative site, (2) protect suture lines, and (3) remove specific fluids such as bile, cerebrospinal fluid, or drainage from an abscess. Some drains require continuous suction and are therefore connected to some type of apparatus that creates suction to facilitate removal of drainage. If a drain is kinked, the accumulated fluid and gas can cause pain, create dead air space (which delays healing), damage the integrity of the suture lines, and delay healing by compressing surrounding capillaries and cutting off oxygen supply to the cells.

Another kind of drain system is the closed-wound suction device (e.g., Hemovac). The drainage catheter is connected to a spring-loaded drum, which must be collapsed periodically to create the desired suction, which pulls fluid into a collection area of the device. Jackson-Pratt suction devices are about the size of the bulb on a blood pressure cuff. They have a valve on top that is opened to allow removal of fluid and collapse of the bulb and then is closed to create negative pressure, which provides the suction. As drainage accumulates in the bulb, it is emptied and recompressed.

Nursing responsibilities in the care of drains include the following:

- Frequent monitoring to ensure that the drain is open and working as it should.
- Keeping the suction device functioning by checking it frequently and recollapsing it as necessary.
- Strict aseptic technique when changing dressings or emptying the drainage.
- Changing the dressings around the drain site at least every 8 hours, or more often if so ordered by the physician.
- Measuring amount of drainage in the collection device and recording it as output. Sometimes, when there is a significant amount of drainage oozing from around the drain and onto the dressings, it is important to estimate the amount, especially if it is bright red from blood.
- Assessing the skin around the area where the drain exits from the body and documenting the status of the skin and cleansing the area.

Drains that do not attach to a suction device either are attached to a drainage bag or have dressings placed to catch the fluid. Examples of drains include the Penrose, which is inserted into the abdominal cavity or any other area where an abscess, fistula, or other condition requires drainage, and other drains inserted into "ostomies" such as a colostomy. (Ostomy care is covered in Chapter 25).

Dressings

Surgical dressings should be checked each time vital signs are taken for the first 24 hours after surgery, every few hours during the next 24 hours, and then at least every 8 hours as long as the surgical wound is covered with a dressing. The surgeon usually does the first dressing change. If the dressing becomes saturated before this, it should be reinforced. The outer dressings are removed, leaving those in direct contact with the wound, and new dressings are secured in place. When there is excessive drainage, the dressing probably will require reinforcing or changing every 4 hours. Changing the dressing more often than this is not recommended because of the danger of introducing infectious agents, traumatizing the wound, and interfering with the regeneration of tissue.

Each time the dressing is changed, the amount and characteristics of drainage on it should be noted and documented. If the wound is infected, the odor of the drainage can give a clue as to the kind of organism causing the infection. A musty odor is characteristic of aerobic organisms. An acrid or putrid odor is characteristic of anaerobes. Anaerobic infections are frequently seen in colorectal and vaginal surgery.

Wound Care

The surgical wound should be inspected at least daily and more often if dressings are changed more than once a day. Assessment includes observing the incision line for signs of excessive swelling, formation of a *hematoma* (blood-filled swelling), *seroma* (serum-filled swelling), redness, and tearing of the skin or other signs of separation of the edges of the skin that have been sutured together. Normally, a surgical wound is sealed within hours and drainage is not expected. If there is evidence of bleeding, purulent drainage, or any other sign that the wound is not healing as it should, this should be reported and documented.

Factors that retard wound healing in a postoperative patient include vomiting, abdominal distention, and strenuous respiratory efforts such as coughing and forcefully exhaling breaths of air. Other factors that affect wound healing, such as age and nutrition, are summarized in Table 6–1. Nursing interventions for the patient with nausea and vomiting are covered in Chapter 8. Abdominal distention usually is relieved by insertion of a nasogastric tube and attachment to a suction device. Care of a patient with a tube of this kind is discussed in Chapter 23. Proper techniques for coughing and deep breathing that will minimize stress on the operative wound are discussed below.

Wound Infection. Infection of a wound can occur in any surgical procedure, but it is more common in old wounds caused by accidental injury and in those that were infected at the time of surgery. The nurse should assess for signs and symptoms of wound infection by looking for pain, redness, swelling and hardness in the area, purulent drainage, fever, and an elevated white blood cell (WBC) count. If an infection is going to develop, it usually becomes apparent 2 to 7 days postoperatively. For most patients this means that they will already be at home when postoperative infection becomes apparent. A few doses of antibiotics are usually ordered to prevent the occurrence of wound infection.

If the wound is infected, special wound and skin precautions should be followed so as to

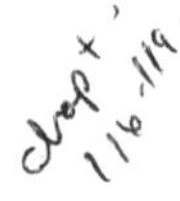

avoid spread of the infectious agent. Even if there is no evidence of infection, cleanliness, frequent handwashing, and proper disposal of soiled dressings are essential in the care of surgical wounds.

Discharge teaching for the patient and family should include assessing for these signs and symptoms and reporting them to the surgeon.

Dehiscence and Evisceration. Throughout the period following abdominal surgery, the nurse must be alert for possible disruption or separation of some or all the layers of the surgical wound. This is called *dehiscence*. If the wound completely separates and the contents of the abdominal cavity (viscera) protrude through the incision, the condition is called *evisceration*.

Dehiscence can occur at any time during the postoperative period, but it most commonly occurs between the 5th and 12th postoperative day. The separation or disruption usually is brought on by a sudden strain or stress on the suture lines, as for example when the patient sneezes, coughs, or has an episode of retching and vomiting.

Patients who are most at risk for dehiscence and evisceration are those who are obese, malnourished, or dehydrated, have a malignancy or have experienced multiple trauma to the abdomen, or have an infected wound. Abdominal distention, strenuous coughing, and broken sutures also are factors in wound disruption.

When the nurse checks an abdominal surgical wound, she should be particularly aware of any drainage on the dressing. In about half the cases of dehiscence, there is a noticeable increase in the amount of serosanguinous (i.e., composed of serum and blood) drainage on the wound dressing before the separation of the wound layers becomes apparent. Subjectively, the patient may not notice any symptoms until he feels something "give way" in the wound.

Needless to say, wound dehiscence and evisceration can be upsetting events for the patient and his nurse. They create an emergency that requires immediate surgery and are very serious complications. Between the time the dehiscence and evisceration occur and surgery is done, the wound should be covered with either a dry sterile towel or dressing or one that has been wet with sterile normal saline.

Respiratory Function

Healing wounds must have an adequate supply of oxygen at all times, which means that normal respiratory function has a direct bearing on the rate of repair and healing. The postoperative patient also is at risk for respiratory problems because of anesthesia and immobility. One fourth to one half of all patients having either abdominal or thoracic surgery suffer from such pulmonary complications as atelectasis (collapse of lung tissue) and pneumonitis.

Assessment of the patient for adequate respiratory function requires listening to the lungs through a stethoscope, observing the patient's rate and depth of breathing, noting any cough and whether it is productive, and noting wheezing or moist "bubbling" sounds when the patient breathes. Subjective data include complaints of shortness of breath, pain on inspiration, and extreme fatigue due to hypoxemia (insufficient oxygen supply in the blood).

Circulatory Function

If considerable blood is lost during surgery, the patient may receive blood transfusions. If the surgery is elective, the patient may donate some of his blood several weeks before surgery and have it held for him. This decreases the risk of AIDS and transfusion reaction. Autologous transfusion of the patient's blood lost during surgery may also be done.

Movement of the extremities and leg exercises encourage venous return to the heart and help prevent thrombus formation. Elastic stockings, TED or Jobst hose, are sometimes also ordered. They should be checked frequently to see that they fit smoothly. They may be removed for 15 to 30 minutes per shift for bathing and to allow air circulation to the skin. Thromboguards are devices that alternately inflate and deflate, putting pressure on the legs to encourage venous return. Low-dose subcutaneous heparin injections are commonly ordered for any patient who has a history of thrombophlebitis. Thrombophlebitis does not usually occur until after the fifth day of bed rest. The vigilant nurse will question the patient about pain or tenderness in the legs. She should assess for Homans' sign (pain in the calf when the leg is raised with knee bent and then straightened while dorsiflexing the foot).

If the patient complains of leg pain, the area should be gently felt for increased warmth, and the physician must be notified. The leg should *never* be massaged, as this might dislodge a blood clot and cause an embolus that could lodge in the lungs.

Turning, Coughing, and Deep Breathing. Preventive measures include assisting the patient in turning, coughing, and deep breathing. Because moving about and turning in the bed can put a strain on healing wounds, the patient should be assisted in turning when he is still drowsy from anesthesia or physically weak and unable to move himself without great effort. Overhead trapeze bars should *not* be used by patients who have had abdominal surgery, because this causes the Valsalva maneuver, which increases pressure within the abdominal cavity. When the surgical patient is able to get up on his own, he should be taught to roll to one side and push himself up on his elbow when getting out of bed.

The purpose of *deep breathing* is to expand and aerate the lungs. To accomplish this the patient should concentrate on inhaling deeply and holding the inhaled breath for a period of time. This is called *sustained maximal inspiration* (SMI). Some respiratory maneuvers that can be taught the patient include: (1) sighing or yawning; (2) drawing one deep breath and then drawing a second breath before exhaling the first; and (3) drawing in five, slow, deep breaths, holding the breath each time until the lungs are filled.

Another procedure for SMI involves using an *incentive spirometer*, which some authorities feel is the most effective way to avoid postoperative pulmonary problems (Figs. 11–7 and 11–8). Maximum benefit from this instrument can be obtained if the patient has been taught to use it before surgery.

Incentive spirometers are so called because the patient is encouraged to inhale deeply by watching the movement of one or more balls or lights in response to his efforts. As the patient inhales, these balls move upward in a cylinder. The spirometer must be held upright to obtain maximum therapeutic value. By tilting the spirometer toward his chest, the patient can reduce the amount of effort needed to move the balls. The nurse should monitor the patient's use of the incentive spirometer initially.

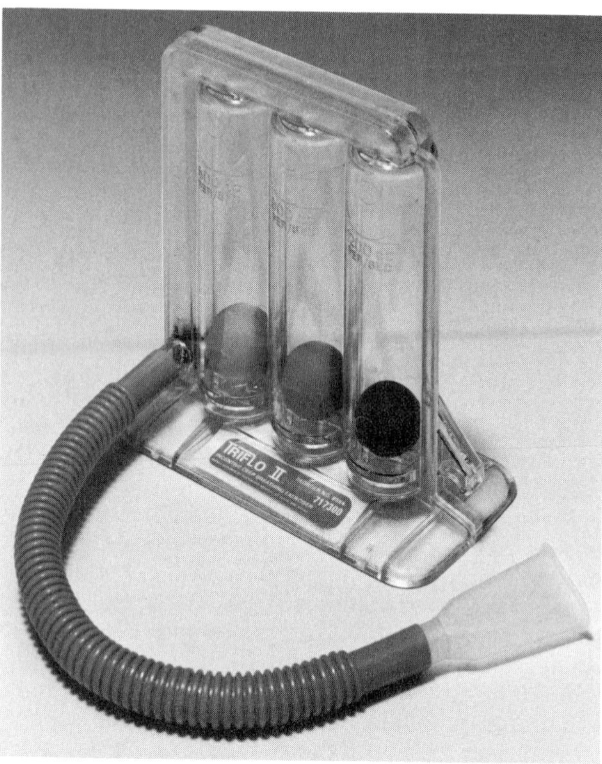

Figure 11–8 Triflo II incentive deep-breathing exerciser. (Courtesy of Sherwood Medical Company. Triflo II™ is a trademark of Sherwood Medical Company.)

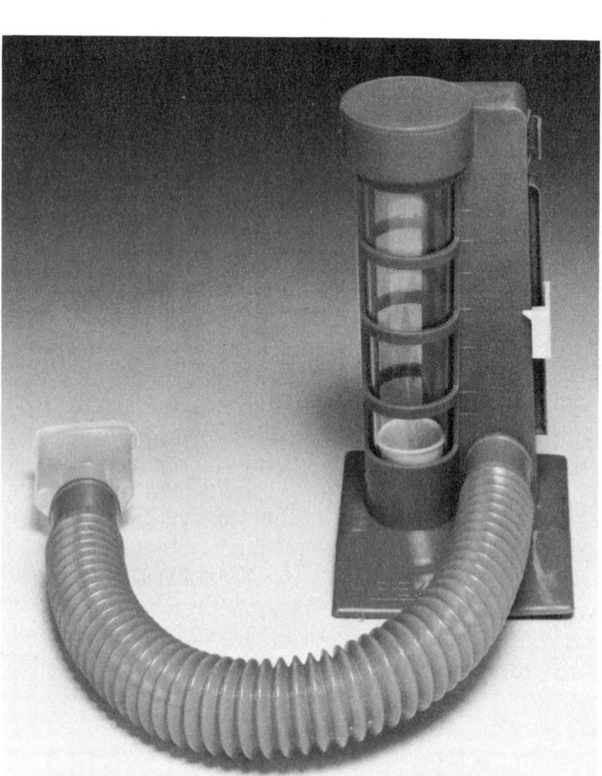
Figure 11–7 Air-Eze incentive deep-breathing exerciser. (Courtesy of Sherwood Medical Company. Air-Eze® is a trademark of Sherwood Medical Company.)

Coughing is encouraged for the purpose of removing secretions that have accumulated in the air passages. Although it is a forced expiratory movement that causes discomfort in abdominal and thoracic surgical wounds, it can help prevent pulmonary complications. When it is appropriate and done properly, coughing usually is effective in removing these secretions, thereby minimizing or eliminating the need for suctioning. The area of the surgical incision should be splinted with a small pillow or with the nurse's or the patient's hands.

The patient is taught to take a deep breath and then to cough strongly enough to move the secretions up from the lungs to the larger air passages. Several successive small coughs will then bring up secretions so they can be expectorated.

Coughing is contraindicated in some kinds of abdominal surgery (for example, hernia repair), following cataract extraction, and after most types of brain surgery when it is dangerous to increase intracranial pressure.

Intestinal Function

Nausea and vomiting are common in the early postoperative period. An emesis basin should be placed close to the patient. Medication is usually ordered for nausea, and the nurse should administer it *before* the patient starts vomiting. A cool cloth applied to the forehead and neck, rinsing the mouth, ridding the room of odors, and a quiet environment also help reduce nausea.

Patients who have had trauma to the abdomen, experience shock, or have respiratory problems or a metabolic disturbance are at great risk for intestinal problems related to inadequate peristalsis. Such a condition is termed *adynamic ileus, paralytic ileus,* or simply *ileus.*

Because there is little or no peristaltic action, fluids and gas accumulate in the intestine and cause distention. If the condition continues unchecked, the enlarged abdomen causes difficulty in breathing, while at the same time the fluids press against blood vessels and impede venous return of blood. The patient is in danger of developing atelectasis and pneumonia, hypovolemia due to escape of fluids from the blood into the intestinal tract, and metabolic alkalosis.

Adynamic ileus quickly leads to distention of the intestinal tract and abdominal cavity. Subjective signs include complaints of abdominal pain and tenderness and later nausea and vomiting. Objective signs include increasing expansion of the abdominal girth due to abdominal distention, the absence of bowel sounds, and no passage of either feces or gas rectally. Because of upward pressure against the diaphragm, the patient has increasing difficulty breathing and is subject to atelectasis and pneumonia. Impairment of venous return can lead to decreased cardiac output, diminished flow of urine (oliguria), and a decrease in blood pressure. If the buildup of gas and fluid in the intestine is not relieved, there is a potential for wound dehiscence and evisceration. Regular ambulation and abdominal effleurage are helpful in encouraging the passage of gas.

Any and all symptoms of adynamic ileus should be reported and well documented. The diagnosis is confirmed by radiograph, which shows a dilated bowel with accumulations of gas throughout the intestinal tract.

The condition is usually relieved by insertion of a nasogastric tube or Miller-Abbott tube and decompression. This removes the accumulated fluids and gas and often allows the bowel to return to normal position and function. The passage of flatus and fecal material and the return of bowel sounds indicate that persistalsis has returned. If intubation and decompression do not relieve the distention, surgery may be necessary to relieve an intestinal obstruction.

Urinary Function

Patients need to void within 8 to 10 hours of surgery. A common problem following surgery is retention of urine in the bladder. It can occur as a result of anesthetic medication, narcotics, trauma to the bladder or urethra during the operation, or anxiety and fear of pain.

Subjective data include complaints of feeling fullness and pressure in the bladder region. Objective signs include distention of the bladder, which can be noted by palpation and observation, and either total absence of urinary output or dribbling of small amounts of urine (not more than 50 mL), which indicates retention with overflow. When a patient cannot void after surgery, this must be stated at the change-of-shift report.

The nurse can utilize any of a number of methods to induce voiding; catheterization is used only when other measures fail. Some nursing actions that do not require a physician's order include providing privacy for the patient, warming the bedpan before placing it in position, helping the patient to stand or sit to void, and applying gentle but firm pressure over the bladder. Hearing the sound of running water or placing the hands in water also helps some patients, as does pouring warm water over the perineum, which has the effect of relaxing the muscles and thereby encouraging urination. Blowing through a straw into a glass of water while on the commode or bedpan is sometimes effective for female patients.

The postoperative complication of renal failure is not nearly so common as urinary retention. It is, however, a very serious condition that requires extensive treatment. Renal failure is discussed in more detail in Chapter 22.

Hiccoughs

This condition usually is a minor discomfort that disappears in a few minutes or, at the most, several hours. Sometimes, however, the spasms of the diaphragm persist for days or weeks, causing serious problems of discomfort, stress on the suture line, and interference with eating and rest.

Treatment usually involves administering carbon dioxide by having the patient rebreathe exhaled air in a paper bag or inhale the gas through a mask. Sedatives and tranquilizers are sometimes prescribed to promote relaxation and reduce irritation of the phrenic nerve. Intractable cases may require surgical interruption of impulses along the nerve pathways so as to remove the cause of the spasms of the diaphragm.

thorazine or tranquilizers

NURSING CARE PLAN 11–1

Selected nursing diagnoses, goals/outcome criteria, nursing interventions, and evaluations for a patient undergoing a mastectomy

Situation: Patient is a married 38-year-old female and the mother of two children ages 16 and 14. She is scheduled for simple mastectomy as treatment for a localized malignant tumor, detected early by self-examination of her breasts.

Nursing Diagnosis	Goals/Outcome Criteria	Nursing Interventions	Evaluation
Fear related to cancer, disfigurement, death. SUPPORTING DATA Malignant tumor by biopsy; grandmother died of breast cancer; is crying at intervals and is worried about husband's reaction to loss of breast.	Patient will discuss fears openly. Patient will look at incisional area before discharge. Patient will talk about having cancer. Patient will join support group for cancer patients. Patient will identify spiritual support. Patient will utilize community resources.	Establish rapport and trust. Encourage her to discuss fears with nurse and family. Help her to identify specific fears and deal with each one separately. Encourage her to think of cancer as a challenge. Teach relaxation exercises to decrease anxiety. Do preoperative teaching for patient and family: routine procedures, NPO, expected tubes and drains, equipment to expect in room, probable length of surgery, where family will wait, pain relief measures, handling of arm on operative side, coughing, deep breathing and leg exercises, ambulation, diet, daily postoperative routine. Call pastor/chaplain if patient desires to see him or her. Provide private time for patient and husband and patient and family. Seek physician's order for Reach to Recovery program.	Preop teaching done; states she is "afraid to die of cancer"; minister visited; relaxation exercise taught and practiced; continue plan.
Impaired skin integrity related to surgical wound. SUPPORTING DATA Right mastectomy	Wound will be free of signs of infection. Wound will heal completely.	Keep Jackson-Pratt suction functioning properly. Note character and amount of drainage; document. Reinforce dressing as needed. Assess for excessive bleeding q h for 4 h, then q 2 h for first 24 h. Assess pulses in arm q 2 h to detect excessive swelling in arm. Monitor temperature and WBCs. Assess wound for signs of infection with each dressing change. Change dressing q 8 to 24 h as needed.	Serosanguinous drainage in J-P; dressing dry and intact; brachial and radial pulses equal at 3+; Temp, 99.8° F; WBCs, 10,800; no signs of infection; continue plan.
Pain related to surgical incision SUPPORTING DATA Right mastectomy Rigid in bed Complains of incisional pain	Pain is controlled by analgesia as noted by patient. Patient appears relaxed. Pain is controlled by oral analgesia by discharge.	Assess need for pain measures q 3 to 4 h. Provide comfort measures. Administer analgesics as ordered; note response and assess for side effects. Refrain from giving injections in right arm (side of surgery).	Demerol per PCA pump—dosage adequate for control; repositioned q 2 h; states she is reasonably comfortable; pain controlled.

NURSING CARE PLAN 11–1, *Continued*

Nursing Diagnosis	Goals/Outcome Criteria	Nursing Interventions	Evaluation
Impaired gas exchange related to residual effects of anesthesia, immobility, and incisional pain. SUPPORTING DATA Inhalation anesthesia Right mastectomy Bed rest with BRP only	No atelectasis Lung sounds clear	Have patient deep breathe and cough q 2 h. Auscultate lungs q 8 h. Encourage ambulation when ordered. Monitor temperature and respirations.	Deep breathed and coughed at 8, 10, 12, and 2 o'clock; lungs clear to auscultation bilaterally; resp. 22; continue plan.
Potential for grieving related to loss of body part and perception of feminity. SUPPORTING DATA Right mastectomy Concern about husband's reaction to surgery and loss of breast.	Patient will verbalize feelings of self-worth and confidence. Patient will discuss sadness over loss of breast. Patient will develop new positive body image.	Have patient list her strengths and positive attributes. Encourage sharing of sad feelings and fears with husband. Talk with husband privately about his feelings. Involve husband in patient's care. Encourage daughters to discuss their feelings and fears with patient. Encourage independence in patient.	Husband appears supportive but scared: "I don't want to talk about it until the final report is in." Will wait 2 days postop before speaking to daughters about their fears. Patient assisted with own bath this A.M.

Pain

After the stress of surgery, the patient needs all his resources to recover. Pain and discomfort interfere with rest and inhibit the processes of healing and repair. Although analgesic drugs are almost always prescribed for the postoperative patient, comfort measures should be tried first. Narcotics tend to depress respirations and the cough reflex and therefore may contribute to the development of pulmonary problems. They also can increase the possibility of nausea and vomiting.

Before administering any analgesic drug, it is best to try to determine whether a distended bladder, abdominal distention, tight dressings or cast, or some other condition is interfering with the patient's comfort. A change of position, soothing back rub, or quiet environment may be all that is needed to relieve discomfort. If an analgesic medication is given, comfort measures used before the drug is administered will serve to enhance and prolong its effect.

The use of comfort measures and prompt attention to expressions of pain and discomfort can be reassuring to the patient. The knowledge that something is being done and the belief that it will be effective can have a placebo effect and thereby relieve discomfort and promote relaxation. Once the patient has been attended to and is resting comfortably, every effort should be made not to disturb him any more than is absolutely necessary to monitor his status and carry out prescribed treatments.

The problem of pain is discussed in greater detail in Chapter 10. Nursing interventions for pain and for other selected problems in a patient undergoing surgery are summarized in Nursing Care Plan 11–1.

Concerns for the Elderly

As mentioned in Chapter 8, fluid and electrolyte balance is more easily upset in the older patient. The stress of surgery and anesthesia has a more profound impact on patients over 65 years of age. The older the patient, the less blood loss he can tolerate, because the body's compensatory mechanisms do not work as well as in a younger patient. Hydration status must be carefully assessed, as this patient can become quickly dehydrated from vomiting. He can also suffer circulatory overload from too much, or too rapid, administration of IV fluid. Mild to moderate confusion from fluid and electrolyte shifts is not uncommon in the early postoperative period. Family members need to be assured that this is most likely a temporary state.

DISCHARGE PLANNING

When the patient is discharged, the nurse reviews specific instructions regarding care at home. This includes care of incision or wound, diet, activity level, medications, and signs and symptoms of complications to report. The nurse makes certain the patient understands when he is next to see the doctor. Sufficient supplies of items needed for dressing changes are sent home with the patient, and he is told where such items can be obtained. The nurse makes every attempt to see that the patient does not go home with unanswered questions concerning his care.

BIBLIOGRAPHY

Birdsall, C., et al.: How is autotransfusion done? Am. J. Nurs., Jan., 1988, p. 108.

Blackwood, S.: Back to basics: The preop exam. Am. J. Nurs., Jan., 1986, p. 39.

Burden, N.: Regional anesthesia: What patients—and nurses—need to know. RN, May, 1988, p. 56.

Chitwood, L. B.: Unveiling the mysteries of anesthesia. Nursing 87, Feb., 1987, p. 53.

Deters, G. E.: Managing complications after abdominal surgery. RN, March, 1987, p. 27.

Flynn, M. E., and Rovee, D. T.: Influencing repair and recovery. Am. J. Nurs., Oct., 1982, p. 1550.

Fraulini, K. E., and Borchardt, K. C.: Guide to solving postanesthesia problems. Nursing 88, May, 1988, p. 66.

Gallagher, M. T., and Kahn, C.: Lasers: Scalpels of light. RN, May, 1990, p. 46.

Grennan, A. J.: Helping your patient get his strength back . . . first few days at home. RN, March, 1987, p. 70.

Gruendenemann, F. J., and Meeker, M. H.: Alexander's Care of the Patient in Surgery. St. Louis, C. V. Mosby, 1987.

Jackson, M. F.: High risk surgical patients. J. Gerotol. Nurs., Feb., 1988, p. 8.

Leckrone, L.: Preparing your patient for surgery. Nursing 91, July, 1991, p. 46.

Litwack, K.: What you need to know about administering preoperative medications. Nursing 91, Aug., p. 44.

Mangieri, D.: Looking at the tube . . . and we don't mean TV. Nursing 83, April, 1983, p. 47.

McConnell, E. A.: After surgery: How you can avoid the obvious—and not so obvious—hazards. Nursing 83, Feb., 1983, p. 74.

Norheim, C.: Spinal anesthesia: As bad as it sounds? Nursing 86, April, 1986, p. 42.

Rowland, M. A.: Myths and facts about postop discomfort. Am. J. Nurs., May, 1990, p. 60.

Schaefer, A., et al.: Are they ready? Discharge planning for older surgical patients. J. Gerontol. Nurs., Oct., 1990, p. 16.

Spearing, C., and Cornell, D. J.: Incentive spirometry: Inspiring your patients to breathe deeply. Nursing 88, 1988, p. 50.

Strange, J.: An expert's guide to tubes and drains. RN, April, 1983, p. 34.

Unkle, D. W.: Postoperative care after the patient's had a spinal. RN, Sept., 1990, p. 93.

STUDENT STUDY AIDS

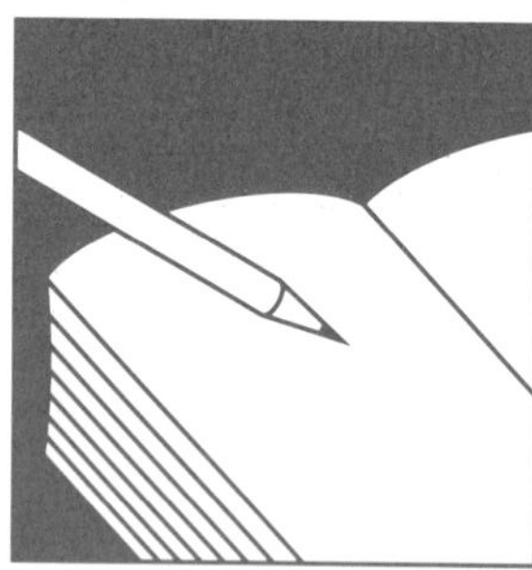

CLINICAL CASE PROBLEMS

Read each clinical case problem and discuss the questions with your classmates.

1. Mrs. Smith, aged 43, is admitted to the surgical unit of the hospital with a diagnosis of acute cholecystitis and obesity. She is the mother of five children and a widow. Mrs. Smith works in a sewing plant to support her family. Her oldest son, aged 19, also works to provide an income for the family.

This patient has never been hospitalized before, except for the birth of her last three children. She is extremely apprehensive about her illness and is worried about her children and the financial status of the family now that she cannot work.

Several days after her admission to the hospital, the acute inflammation responds to treatment sufficiently to permit surgical removal of the gallbladder. The patient gives her consent to the surgery, but she is very frightened and seems to feel that she will never be well again.

- What problems can you see in this situation?
- How can you help reassure Mrs. Smith before surgery?
- What preoperative instructions might you give?
- In what ways might you help Mrs. Smith with her problem of obesity?

  Mrs. Smith returns from surgery with an IV, a "T" tube for bile drainage, an NG tube to low suction, and a Foley catheter.
- What are the points of care for each of these tubes?
- What would need to be documented concerning these tubes?

---

2. You are assigned to care for a 37-year-old male who just had a surgical repair of a ventral hernia with spinal anesthesia.

- How does the care of this patient differ from that of a patient who had inhalation anesthesia?
- If this patient has difficulty voiding after surgery, how could you assist him?

- If he develops a spinal headache, what measures could be taken to decrease his discomfort?

---

3. This is your first day on a surgical unit. You are assigned a patient who is scheduled for surgery at 10:00 A.M. He has preoperative medication ordered: "Demerol 50 mg, Phenergan 35 mg, and atropine 0.04 mg IM on call". You also are assigned two other patients who are ambulatory.

- List what you would check in the surgery patient's chart as part of his preoperative preparation.
- Describe the steps you would take to complete the preoperative checklist and charting for this surgical patient in your assigned hospital.
- What steps are necessary in preparing and administering the preoperative medication?

STUDY OUTLINE

I. Preoperative period

A. Assessment.
  1. Determine patient's readiness for surgery and identify those most at risk.
  2. Chest radiograph; EKG, if patient over 40.
  3. Laboratory data: blood profile, urinalysis.
  4. Nursing assessment.
     a. Vital signs to establish baseline, report abnormalities.
     b. Allergies and drug idiosyncrasies.
     c. Body weight; obesity increases risk: anesthesia, respiratory function, fluid balance, wound healing.
     d. State of nutrition; malnutrition carries greater risk for slow healing.
  5. Nursing history.
     a. Smoking: harmful effect on wound healing, clot formation, and pulmonary function.
     b. Diabetes mellitus: risk for variations in blood glucose level, delayed healing, and infection.
     c. Liver disease: jeopardy for excessive bleeding, poor wound healing, and poor detoxification of drugs.
     d. Respiratory disease: patient at greater risk for atelectasis, hypoxemia, and pneumonia.
  6. Psychologic assessment:
     a. Different expectations for outcome of surgery.
     b. Determine cause of fear and anxiety if possible.
  7. Spiritual assessment: Determine whether patient needs and wants support. Ask usual ways of expressing spirituality and finding comfort.
  8. Assessment of learning needs: What patient and family want to know about? What need to know to reduce anxiety?

B. Intervention—preoperative period
  1. General information: preparation for surgery, preoperative routine, recovery room routine, postoperative routine.
  2. Assess learning needs and do preoperative teaching for patient and family.
     a. Deep breathing, coughing, and incentive spirometry techniques.
     b. Leg exercises, how to turn and get in and out of bed.
     c. Measures for pain control.
     d. Diet restrictions and progression postoperatively.
  3. Reinforce teaching with available hospital audiovisual materials.
  4. Complete preoperative checklist.

5. Preparation for surgery.
   a. Signed consent form.
   b. Diagnostic tests.
   c. NPO 8 to 12 hours before surgery.
   d. Cleansing of intestinal tract; use of nasogastric tube and suction.
   e. Sedation night before surgery.
   f. Indwelling urinary catheter.
   g. Intravenous infusion started.
6. Preoperative routine.
   a. Preoperative medication and purpose.
      (1) Reduce anxiety and promote rest.
      (2) Decrease secretions.
      (3) Prevent nausea and vomiting.
      (4) Enhance anesthesia effect.

II. Anesthesia: loss of sensory perception

A. Given to relieve pain, achieve muscular relaxation, and allay anxiety.
B. Types include inhalants, intravenous anesthetics, regional and topical anesthetics, and hypothermia (see Table 11–2).

III. Hypothermia: reduction of body temperature

A. Used in some types of surgery to lower metabolism and decrease oxygen needs.
B. Methods:
   1. External hypothermia: ice packs or other forms of external cold.
   2. Extracorporeal hypothermia: rerouting the blood outside the body, through a cooling unit, and back into the body.

IV. Postoperative period

A. Recovery room:
   1. Assessed q 15 min until stable.
   2. Maintain airway and respiration.
   3. Discharged to floor after arousal from anesthesia.
B. Observe for shock with circulatory collapse.
   1. Signs and symptoms: drop in BP, rapid thready pulse; cold, clammy skin.
   2. Treatment: fluids, positioning, medication.
C. Postoperative care
   1. Vital signs and dressing check q 30 min × 2h, then q 1 h for 4 h or until stable
   2. Dressing check done with vital signs assessment.
   3. Closely monitor IV fluids.
   4. Monitor for shock, circulatory collapse: drop in blood pressure; rapid, thready pulse; cold, clammy skin.
   5. Treatment: oxygen, IV fluids and medications, appropriate positioning.
   6. Tubes and drains; purpose:
      a. Prevent accumulations of fluids.
      b. Avoid dead air space.
      c. Protect suture line.
      d. Remove specific kinds of fluids (e.g., bile).
   7. Tubes and drains; care:
      a. Location and type; patency.
      b. Suction device; maintain suction.
      c. Amount and characteristics of drainage.
      d. Skin care around drain.
      e. Dressing; all care with aseptic technique.
   8. Wound care
      a. Observe for bleeding and signs of infection: swelling, redness, pain, pulling of sutures, purulent drainage; document findings.

b. Frequent hand washing and aseptic technique for wound care to prevent infection.
c. Dressing checked with each set of vital signs first 24 h.
d. Dressing reinforced as needed until changed by surgeon; then changed at least q 24 h or q 4 h as needed.
e. Dehiscence and evisceration: 5th to 12th day
   (1) Patients at risk: obese, malnourished, wound infected, abdominal distention, multiple trauma, strenuous coughing.
   (2) Signs and symptoms: increased serosanguinous drainage; feel it "give way."
   (3) Cover with sterile towel; if viscera is protruding, moisten towel with sterile saline.

9. Respiratory function assessment:
   a. Auscultate lungs q 4 h × 24 h, then q 8 h; assess for shortness of breath, pain on inspiration, extreme fatigue.
   b. Encourage turning, coughing, deep breathing and leg exercises q 2 h; supervise incentive spirometry.
   c. Splint wound before coughing.
10. Intestinal function assessment: potential ileus.
   a. Auscultate bowel sounds q 8 h; assess for distention.
   b. Signs of ileus: abdominal pain and tenderness, nausea and vomiting, increasing girth, absence of bowel sounds, no passage of flatus rectally.
   c. Treatment: nasogastric tube with suction.
   d. Return of normal bowel function marked by passage rectally of flatus.
11. Urinary function.
   a. Should void within 8 to 10 hours.
   b. Palpate bladder for distention.
   c. Institute measures to assist voiding.
   d. Obtain order to catheterize if needed.
   e. Indwelling catheter: assess patency frequently; observe for signs of infection.
12. Pain relief:
   a. Check for cause before medicating.
   b. Use adjunctive comfort measures.
   c. Administer pain medication before pain is severe for better control.
13. Concerns for the elderly:
   a. Prone to fluid and electrolyte imbalances.
   b. Mild to moderate confusion postoperatively as a result of fluid and electrolyte shifts is not uncommon.
14. Discharge planning
   a. Specific instructions given regarding:
      (1) level of activity.
      (2) care of wound or incision.
      (3) diet.
      (4) signs and symptoms of complications to report.
      (5) medications, schedule, possible side effects.
      (6) when to see physician next.
   b. Answer any questions.
   c. Send patient home with immediate supplies for dressing changes.

CHAPTER 12

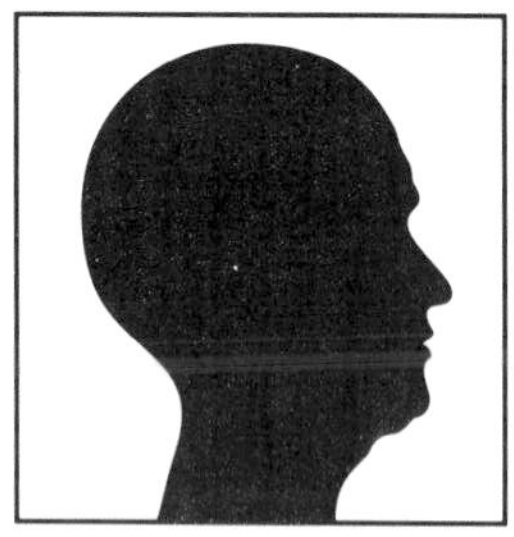

Care of Older Patients

VOCABULARY

conductive hearing loss
disorientation
dyscrasia (blood)
emollient
flatulence
geriatrics
gerontology
motility
parathyroid gland
presbyopia
psyche
reminisce
tactile

Upon completion of this chapter the student should be able to:

1. Describe general attitudes toward elderly persons in our society and how these attitudes can affect their physical and mental health.
2. Identify at least seven physiologic changes that occur with aging and state specific nursing interventions to mitigate the effects of these changes.
3. Identify specific kinds of sensory losses that frequently occur with aging and list nursing interventions appropriate for each.
4. Discuss ways in which mental confusion and disorientation in hospitalized elderly patients can be managed or minimized.
5. Identify nursing interventions to help avoid adverse drug reactions in older adults.
6. List at least five strategies for teaching older adults to care for themselves, including self-administration of drugs.
7. List three kinds of support needed by elderly persons after discharge from an acute-care facility.
8. List at least four developmental tasks of elderly couples and individuals.
9. Cite nursing interventions that can maximize the strengths of elderly persons.
10. Devise innovative ways to care for the elderly persons in our society.

Older adults (over age 65) comprise the fastest growing segment of society in the United States. Population projections estimate that by the end of this century there will be about 29 million Americans who are 65 years of age or older. Stated in another way, persons over the age of 65 currently account for 11% of the total population in this country; by the year 2000 they will account for 15% to 25% of the total. Two major factors that contribute to this change in the makeup of the general population are (1) advances in medical technology and health care that prolong life and (2) lower fertility rates. Extension of the life span and declining numbers of newborn infants inevitably lead to a change in the ratio of older persons to young.

Care of the elderly has always been a responsibility of nursing, but not one of the top priorities of every nurse. In the past, when there were fewer older persons and many of them were ill and disabled, they frequently were moved to the back wards of acute-care facilities or "warehoused" in long-term-care facilities where they sat and waited for the release of death.

Today many nurses recognize the need for more humane and diligent care of the elderly. Increases in the number of older persons needing nursing care have contributed to the development of a specialty called *gerontologic nursing*. Nursing gerontology is the scientific study of the nursing care of older adults, that is, persons over the age of 65. The major goal of gerontologic nursing is to identify the strengths of older adults and help them to use those strengths to maximize independence in the activities of daily living.

Geriatrics deals with the medical treatment of the diseases commonly associated with aging and the later stages of life. Gerontologic nursing focuses on the promotion of health in older adults, preservation of functional capacity, and care of those who cannot recover their health and will need special nursing care for as long as they live.

The knowledge and skills needed by the gerontologic nurse specialist cannot be covered in one brief chapter of a text such as this. However, there are some basic principles and interventions that serve as a foundation for continued study and practice in the care of the elderly. Specific areas of concern in the nursing care of older persons include the following: (1) cultural values associated with aging and social attitudes toward the older adult; (2) physiologic and mental changes that occur during the aging process; (3) the many losses suffered by older persons and the grief work necessary in accepting these losses; (4) the atypical response of the aged to disease and its treatment (e.g., drug therapy); (5) the disabling effects of multiple chronic illness and the degenerative processes associated with aging.

CULTURAL VALUES AND ATTITUDES TOWARD THE AGED

In our society there has been a pervasive negative bias toward aging and the aged, but there also is evidence that more and more people are becoming concerned about our society's failure to recognize the value and rights of older persons.

Gerontologic nursing is not for everyone. It takes a special kind of person to have empathy for and sensitivity to the needs of older persons. However, the profession of nursing has a responsibility to this segment of our population. The elderly are especially in need of the kind of support, caring, patience, and satisfaction with small rewards that nurses can provide. Older persons typically have multiple illnesses, many of which cannot be cured. Their nursing care needs are long term, and most of their illnesses must be managed as long as they live. The gerontologic nurse must have staying power and be willing to stick with the patient through the good and bad times, even when there is no hope for recovery of full health, or even for a return to his former state of health by a patient who has learned to live with a chronic illness but is hospitalized for another health problem.

An important first step toward more effective care of older persons is an examination of one's personal views of aging and the aged. It may help to seek out positive experiences with older persons and systematically look for favorable characteristics of these persons and their lives. Some measure of wisdom, courage, acceptance of one's lot in life, and the virtues of faith, hope, and charity usually can be found if one is willing to take the time to be with and listen to older persons.

Younger people who have had limited exposure to and experience in dealing with older persons usually think of a vigorous person in his 70s or 80s as extremely unusual and not at all typical of a person his age. Many of us cling to the false notion that to be old is to be poor, sick, and lonely. We persist in these negative attitudes and beliefs about what it means to become old in spite of an abundance of evidence to the contrary.

While concern about the truly disadvantaged elderly is praiseworthy, it is important that we recognize the progress that has been made in the health and welfare of older citizens in this country. Surveys of older Americans show that fewer than one in five considers himself or herself to be in poor health. The number of elderly officially counted as "poor" has decreased from 33% in 1959 to 6% in the 1980s. Reasons for these improvements include additional noncash benefits for which the elderly are now eligible, improved housing, and better and more innovative health care.

Older Americans are not typically abandoned and left to fend for themselves or depend on care from governmental agencies. More than 80% have children or other relatives living nearby with whom they are in almost daily contact. About the same percentage own their own homes and live a life of relative independence. Later we will discuss some innovative kinds of care for the elderly that permit those who are able to carry out most of the normal activities of daily living to live in their own homes and maintain contact with the outside world.

Another way to develop positive attitudes toward elderly persons is to become more knowledgeable about the expected physiologic and mental changes that accompany aging, and to realize that with appropriate intervention individuals can be helped to stay as young as possible while growing older.

GENERAL EFFECTS OF AGING

Aging is a very individualized process. All people do not age at the same rate or in precisely the same ways. Some people, because of genetic makeup, temperament, living habits, and external environment, age less rapidly than others. Moreover, although there are several theories about the process of aging, its causes, and ways to impede its progress, there remains a lot that is not known about growing older and being old.

We do know, however, that with age there is a gradual slowing down of all physiologic processes. The cells and tissues become less elastic, and response time increases. Inflexibility and resistance to change are some of the hallmarks of increasing age. Diminished ability to adapt to change is evidenced on all levels—physical, psychological, and social.

In the care of their older patients, nurses must keep in mind that coordination and balance are usually impaired in the elderly, and they are slower to respond physically and mentally. These conditions require a corresponding decrease in the speed at which care is provided for them. A good rule to remember is, "In all care for aged persons, the cardinal principle is that they need time to respond. Their bodies need time to respond to the changes in the temperature of the room, their psyches need time to respond to a new nurse or a new room. They need time to answer questions and to get out of bed."

It is also important to remember that the physiologic changes and deterioration that accompany aging still leave large numbers of functioning cells. This means that rehabilitation is possible and that efforts to improve the functional capacity of older patients are not "wasted" or "useless."

GENERAL PHYSIOLOGIC CHANGES

The external changes associated with aging are obvious to any observer and begin to become evident in middle age. Less obvious are the internal changes that affect all systems of the body and cause problems with nutrition, fluid balance, resistance to infection, skeletal integrity, slower reaction times, decreased mental agility, and dry, fragile skin.

Gastrointestinal System

Aging changes include decreased saliva production, deterioration of teeth, decrease in number of taste buds, loss of strength in muscles of mastication, decreased hydrochloric acid (HCL) in stomach, slower peristalsis and gastric emptying, reduced digestive enzyme secretion, formation of intestinal diverticula, and thinning of mucous membranes with possible decrease in absorption of nutrients.

Assessment factors include state of the mouth, complaints of anorexia and food having little taste, ability to feed self, bloating, indigestion, constipation, flatulence, diarrhea, abdominal pain, diminished bowel sounds, weakened gag reflex, and signs of pernicious anemia and other nutritional deficits.

Possible nursing diagnoses for problems of the gastrointestinal system include:

- Constipation.
- Alteration in nutrition, less than body requirements.
- Potential for injury related to aspiration from impaired mastication and swallowing.
- Pain related to compression of spinal vertebrae as a result of osteoporosis and deterioration.
- Alteration in tissue perfusion related to nutritional anemia.
- Alteration of oral mucous membranes.

Nursing interventions for problems of the gastrointestinal system include increasing bulk and fluids in the diet; obtaining an order for digestive enzymes and artificial saliva; teaching swallowing with the chin down to help prevent aspiration; providing small, frequent, well-balanced meals; obtaining assistance in preparation of meals and a more social atmosphere for eating; increasing calcium intake; encouraging exercise; increasing iron- and vitamin-rich foods in diet; and giving vitamin B_{12} for pernicious anemia.

Musculoskeletal System

Changes include joint stiffness, gout, arthritis, osteoporosis, bunions and other foot deformities, a decrease in muscle strength with a loss of stamina, and loss of bone mass.

Assessment factors include range of motion of all joints, signs of joint inflammation and pain, decrease in height, back pain, foot pain, degree of muscle strength, amount of physical activity, weight gain from inactivity, fatigue, history of bone and joint injuries and falls, history of hormone therapy and calcium supplementation, and family history of gout, arthritis, and osteoporosis (Fig. 12–1).

Possible nursing diagnoses for problems of aging of the musculoskeletal system include:

- Pain.
- Activity intolerance.
- Self-care deficit.
- Alteration in nutrition, more than body requirements, related to inactivity relative to food intake.
- Potential for injury related to falls and "brittle" bones.
- Impaired home maintenance management.
- Disturbance in self-concept related to decreased strength, endurance, and muscle atrophy.

Nursing interventions for problems of aging of the musculoskeletal system include encouraging gentle exercise, particularly walking and stair climbing to help maintain bone and muscle mass. Teaching regarding arthritis medications and exercise programs is helpful. The use of assistive devices for walking and preventing falls, both at home and out, can prevent serious injury. Periods of rest and activity throughout the day can reduce fatigue. Encouraging verbalization of changes in body image can assist with acceptable integration of a new image. Obtaining social support and home help for tasks that the patient can no longer perform is appropriate. Alternative methods of coping with chronic pain (e.g., heat and cold, imagery, relaxation, and diversion) help provide a better quality of life for patients with this problem. A minimal amount of antidepressant medication can sometimes greatly alter the patient's perception of chronic pain.

Cardiovascular System

Degeneration and sclerosis of the heart's conduction system may cause arrythmias. Atherosclerosis and arteriosclerosis, a natural part of aging, may cause vessel and heart changes and resultant problems. Vascular elasticity is considerably diminished, preventing rapid adjustment to changes in position and flow.

Assessment factors include auscultation of heart sounds for murmurs, extra sounds, and

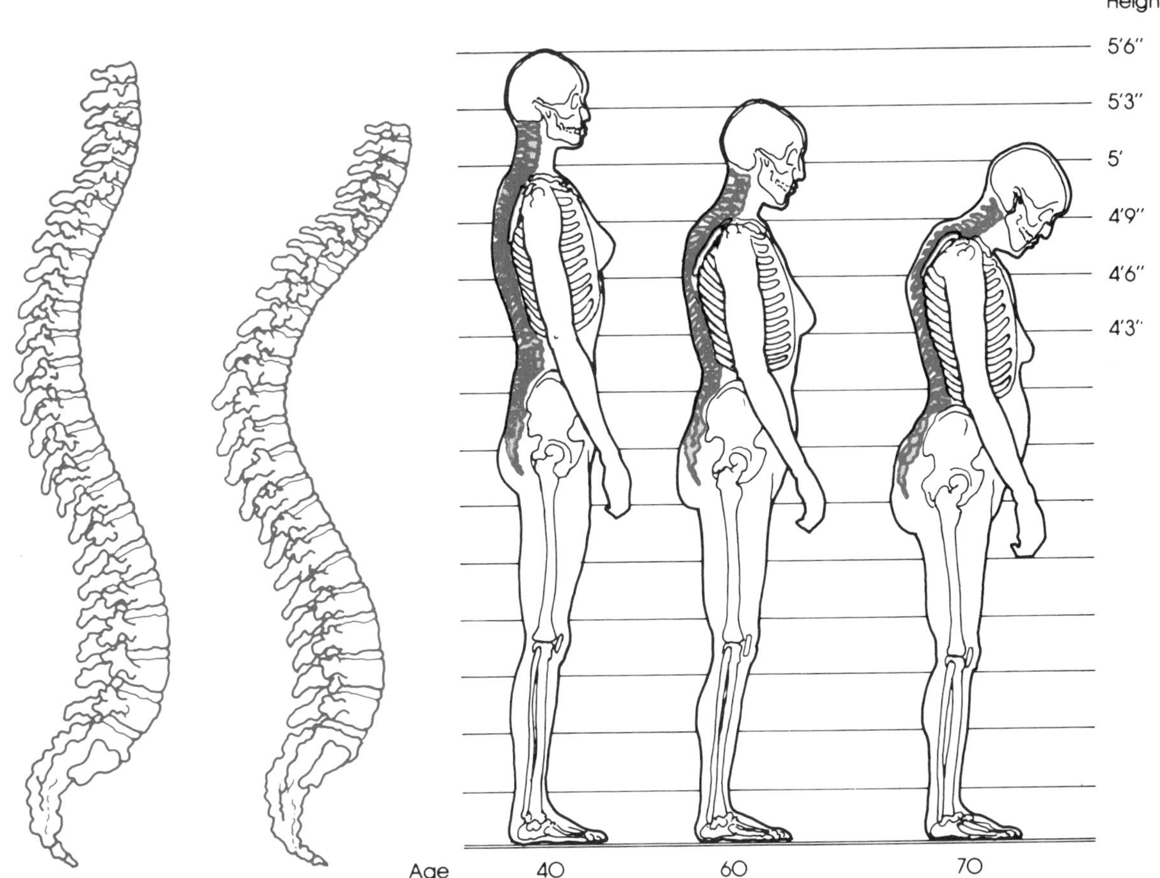

Figure 12–1 Loss of bone mass as a result of osteoporosis produces characteristic changes in the curvature of the spine. At far left are normal curvatures compared with those typical of osteoporosis. Figures to the right show the normal spine at age 40 and osteoporotic changes at 60 and 70 years of age. As shown, these changes bring about a loss of as much as 6 to 9 inches in height, and the so-called dowager's hump in the upper thoracic vertebrae.

irregularity of beat and complaints of fatigue; syncope; dizziness; palpitations, chest pain, and dyspnea on exertion. A history of previous heart problems and current medications is essential. A family history of heart problems is pertinent.

Possible nursing diagnoses common to problems of aging of the cardiovascular system include:

- Alteration in tissue perfusion.
- Pain.
- Anxiety related to cardiac rhythm irregularities.
- Potential for injury related to syncope.
- Fatigue.
- Decreased cardiac output.

Nursing Intervention

On-going assessment of cardiovascular status is very important in the elderly patient. It is particularly important to pay special attention to signs of congestive heart failure, arrhythmias, and evidence of decreased peripheral circulation. Monitoring daily weight and trends in intake and output are essential in the ill, hospitalized patient with cardiovascular problems, as illness can quickly tip the scales, throwing the patient into congestive heart failure.

Monitoring the total picture of all medications the patient is taking is also important, as many times drugs are prescribed for several chronic problems and can interact with each other. Reinforcement of teaching regarding dosage schedule and side effects of cardiovascular medications and self-care measures should be on-going nursing interventions.

Other interventions relate to assisting with activities of daily living (ADL) to conserve the cardiac patient's energy and to provide care to promote safety in the event of syncope.

Genitourinary System

In the female, aging problems of this system result from estrogen deficiency and decreased muscle tone. Stress incontinence is often a problem but is not normal. It is often directly related to cystocele, rectocele, uterine prolapse, and decreased bladder tone. Problems with painful intercourse and vaginal infection are related to the thinning of the vaginal mucosa and decreased secretions, with a consequent change in pH that predisposes the patient to infection.

The male experiences enlargement of the prostate gland and a decrease in bladder capacity with an increase in bladder neck tone. This often leads to problems of urination, backup of urine, and urinary tract infection. Incontinence also occurs but is not normal. The penis and testes decrease in size as a result of sclerosis of the vessels, and a decrease in sexual response time with a greater refractory period after ejaculation is usual. This can be interpreted as impotence by the partner, causing an anxiety reaction on the part of the male.

Both males and females have diminished renal reserve and may begin to exhibit signs and symptoms of early renal failure: elevated blood urea nitrogen (BUN) and creatinine levels, grayish-yellow skin color, fatigue, anemia, and fluid retention.

Assessment factors include patterns of urination (change in the urinary stream, difficulty in starting urination, dribbling), presence of incontinence, history of repeated urinary tract infections, signs of vaginal infection, degree of sexual activity, discomfort on intercourse, difficulty with sexual arousal, current medications that could be causing problems with elimination, especially in the male; and results of urinalysis, BUN, creatinine, and electrolyte tests, complete blood cell (CBC) counts, and Pap smears. Breasts should be checked for lumps, abnormal skin areas, and nipple discharge, and regular mammogram screening should be encouraged.

Possible nursing diagnoses common to problems of aging of the genitourinary system include:

- Urinary retention.
- Alteration in urinary elimination.
- Sexual dysfunction.
- Disturbance in self-esteem related to decrease in sexual interest or ability.
- Potential for infection, either urinary or vaginal.

Nursing interventions for problems of aging of the genitourinary system include encouraging increased intake of fluids to keep urine dilute, teaching pelvic exercises to help prevent stress incontinence, encouraging the patient to seek medical assistance for persistent incontinence, regular prostate examinations, gynecologic consultation for vaginal problems or discomfort with intercourse, health assessment for problems of sexual function, and if diabetes or vascular disease has caused impotence, informing the patient that penile implants are a possible solution for a normal sexual life for the male. Breast self-examination should be taught and stressed for those in this age group.

Integumentary System

The skin becomes dry, loses elasticity (thereby causing wrinkles), pigments unevenly, and develops a variety of lesions with normal aging. Aging skin is more sensitive to sunlight. Sebaceous glands decrease their secretion, and scalp hair becomes thinner and loses color. Facial hair increases in women. The nails become yellowed and thicker, and develop longitudinal ridging. Senile purpura and ecchymoses (bruises) occur after minimal trauma.

Assessment factors for aging of the integumentary system include thorough inspection of the skin for lesions and degree of dryness. The nails should be inspected for signs of fungal infection.

Possible nursing diagnoses for problems of aging of the integumentary system include:

- Potential impaired skin integrity.
- Impaired skin integrity.
- Potential for infection.

Nursing interventions for problems of aging of the integumentary system include teaching the patient to use lubricating lotion immediately after the bath or shower to trap in moisture and decrease skin dryness. Encouraging regular inspection of the skin for lesions and consultation with a dermatologist for suspicious skin lesions is a must for every patient. Protective clothing and an adequate sun screen should be suggested for use any time the patient is outdoors.

Respiratory System

Changes related to aging of the respiratory system include stiffening of the chest wall; a decline in respiratory muscle strength; impaired cough mechanism; decreased ciliary action; and a decrease in alveolar macrophages, phagocytic cells, and immunoglobulin A (IgA), which is responsible for neutralizing nasal and respiratory viruses. All of these factors cause a decrease in respiratory efficiency and increased susceptibility to respiratory infection. There is a greater incidence of chronic obstructive pulmonary disease and of pneumonia in the sixth, seventh, and eighth decades.

Assessment factors include breath sounds, shape of chest, history of smoking and exposure to respiratory irritants, history of lung infection, results of chest radiograph, and spirometry studies.

Possible nursing diagnoses for aging problems of the respiratory system include:

- Impaired gas exchange.
- Activity intolerance.
- Potential for infection.
- Ineffective breathing patterns.

Nursing interventions for respiratory problems include recommending flu and pneumonia immunizations, counseling the elderly to refrain from mingling in large public crowds during the cold and flu season, and encouraging prompt attention for respiratory congestion that lasts longer than a few days.

SENSORY LOSS

The senses of vision, hearing, taste, touch, and smell provide us with information about the world we live in and give us much pleasure and confidence. Impairment or loss of acuity of the senses is an expected characteristic of the process of growing older. When an older person is removed from a familiar environment and moved to a hospital, taken to a health care clinic, or admitted to a long-term-care facility, he needs time to adjust to unfamiliar surroundings. Sensory deficits in the elderly place them at great risk for injury, often weaken self-confidence and change self-concept, and can affect nutrition and other aspects of health.

Visual Loss

The frequency with which visual loss affects persons over 60 years of age is reflected in statistics compiled by the National Center for Health Statistics. Eyeglasses or contact lenses are worn by 92% of all persons over the age of 65. Almost 65% of all known cases of legal blindness are found in persons over the age of 65. Cataracts, glaucoma, and presbyopia are common eye disorders in elderly persons. These and other natural changes in pupil size, clarity of the lens, and decreased reaction of the pupil to changes in light create such problems as decreased sensitivity to light, increased sensitivity to glare, diminished adaptation to changes in light, and altered color vision.

Assessment factors for visual problems of aging include cloudy appearance of the lens, a history of dryness of the eyes with irritation, a family history of glaucoma, use of artificial lenses, previous eye surgery, blurred vision, appearance of "floaters," squinting, difficulty with glare from lights, seeing halos around lights, frequent bumping into objects, difficulty in seeing printed matter, difficulty with night vision, and date of last eye examination.

Nursing diagnoses common to aging problems with vision include:

- Visual sensory perceptual alteration.
- Potential for injury.
- Disturbance in self-esteem.
- Impaired home maintenance management.

Nursing interventions for visual problems include recommending artificial tears for dry eyes, referral to an ophthalmologist, and referral to community resources for assistance in dealing with visual loss and home maintenance. At home or in the hospital, objects in the patient's environment should not be moved once he is oriented to his room or house. Always speak to the patient before touching him.

Hearing Loss

The two most common problems related to impaired hearing in older persons are inability to determine how loud a sound is and difficulty hearing high-frequency sounds. Hearing loss in older persons frequently is caused by changes in the cochlea, the auditory nerve fibers, or the brain cells receiving sound impulses. Accumulations of wax in the outer ear canal also can produce a conductive type of hearing loss. The loss of hearing may not involve both ears, and so it is important to determine which ear is affected and where to position a source of sound so that the patient can hear and understand what he is hearing.

Assessment factors include a history of hearing loss, exposure to loud environmental noise, repeated ear infections, Meniere's disease, and use of a hearing aid. Is there difficulty communicating, blank looks, inappropriate responses to questions and statements, speaking in a loud voice, irritability, confusion, withdrawal, and self-imposed isolation? The ears should be inspected for impacted cerumen (ear wax).

Possible nursing diagnoses for hearing problems in this age group include:

- Auditory sensory perceptual impairment.
- Potential social isolation.
- Disturbance in self-esteem related to the necessity for a hearing aid.

Nursing interventions for problems of hearing include counseling to seek evaluation for problems that can be helped by a hearing aid, learning to lip-read, sharing information about the hearing deficit with significant others, and counseling the patient to avoid environments where there is lots of competing noise. The nurse must provide careful communication and obtain feedback that what she is trying to communicate has been understood by the patient.

Taste Loss

Most noticeable changes in the sense of taste do not appear until after the age of 70. However, by the time a person reaches the age of 60 he has probably lost about half of his taste buds. The first taste buds to be affected are those that allow a person to taste sweet and salty foods. Unfortunately the bitter and sour taste buds remain relatively normal throughout old age.

Assessment factors include complaints that food tastes bitter, increased consumption of sweet and salty foods, changes in appetite (either an increase or a decrease), condition of oral mucosa, and degree of oral hygiene.

Possible nursing diagnoses for problems of taste include:

- Gustatory alteration in sensory perception.
- Alteration in nutrition—more or less than body requirements.

Nursing interventions include preparing and presenting a variety of foods attractively, assisting patients who need to be fed, and feeding one food at a time. Oral hygiene should be scheduled and given regularly. The use of salt and sugar substitutes should be encouraged. Observe for the consumption of excessive amounts of sweets. Family members should be encouraged to bring foods from home that are not restricted by special diet.

Impaired Sense of Smell

The ability to smell is closely associated with the appetite and the sense of taste and therefore affects the enjoyment of food. The ability to smell also is a protective mechanism that warns one of dangerous gases, fumes, and smoke in the immediate environment. In addition, we depend on our sense of smell to warn us of offensive body odors that indicate poor personal hygiene. A decrease in sense of smell has been found to be a sign of Alzheimer's disease in some people.

Assessment factors for problems of smell include strong body and mouth odors that the patient is unaware of, a lack of reaction to strong environmental smells, and a loss of appetite.

The nursing diagnosis appropriate for patients with problems of smell is olfactory sensory perceptual alteration.

Nursing interventions for problems of smell are limited. Teaching good body hygiene and the use of mouthwash and deodorant is helpful.

Chronic Disease in the Elderly

There are many other chronic diseases and conditions that affect the health and well-being of the elderly. Pathologic cardiovascular disease, parkinsonism, rheumatoid arthritis, cancer, cerebrovascular accident (strokes), all of which affect various body systems, and many less common ailments plague the well-being of the aging population.

The nurse needs to make a holistic assessment of the patient and consider all factors that impact the physical and mental health of the patient before devising a care plan for him. Too often focus is placed only on the current problem without considering the ramifications of underlying chronic disorders.

Because the chances of cancer greatly increase with age, every nurse should do a general cancer assessment on each patient. Questions regarding blood in stool or urine, tarry stools, skin changes, bowel habit changes, weight loss, skin and mucous membrane lesions, difficulty swallowing, hoarseness, sores that won't heal, appearance of moles, and breast self-examination should all be asked. Early detection of malignancy provides the best chance of cure.

MENTAL CHANGES IN THE ELDERLY

There are many misconceptions about the mental function of the elderly, primarily because of negative attitudes toward growing old. Moreover, many people assume that mental confusion, forgetfulness, and strange behavior are typical results of the aging process and deterioration of brain cells. Although organic brain disease can occur in older adults, not every person of advanced years is mentally incompetent. The commonly held belief that old people cannot learn and that intelligence typically diminishes with age is simply not true. Although there is a decrease in reaction time as one grows older, there is no loss of intelligence in the normal brain. In fact, the ability to think and reason can actually improve with age and experience.

Lack of knowledge about aging and the fatalistic view that mental confusion and disorientation are typical signs of old age can lead to a misdiagnosis of psychiatric illness instead of a treatable physiologic disorder. Diminishing mental acuity is one of the most common presenting symptoms of a number of organic diseases. For example, stroke, heart attacks, and congestive heart failure can be preceded by mental confusion before other, more apparent, symptoms occur. Additionally, practically all metabolic disorders, as well as blood dyscrasias, can produce altered mental states. It is well known that physical trauma such as a broken hip can bring about mental confusion and loss of memory because of associated shock to the psyche and electrolyte imbalances from disturbed homeostasis.

The nurse who realizes that disorientation and other mental symptoms can have a physiologic basis in the elderly can help avoid the tragedy of a misdiagnosis and resultant lack of proper treatment and recovery. Studies have shown that because of an overlap of physiologic and psychological symptoms, patients are often incorrectly assigned to psychiatric wards, or their symptoms are simply ignored. In some cases failure to administer adequate treatment for a medical disorder has been fatal to patients thought to be hopelessly mentally ill.

In one study of elderly patients, careful medical examinations were done on 116 patients over the age of 65 who had been to the psychiatric division of a large medical center. Of the 116 patients, 71 were found to have medical diseases that accounted for their bizarre and apparently psychotic behavior. Most had been diagnosed as having cerebral atherosclerosis (obstruction to the flow of blood to the brain), which can require admission to a psychiatric facility for long-term custodial care. In reality, many of these patients had treatable disorders such as infections, alcoholism, fractures, and strokes. A large number recovered from their memory loss and disorientation when the underlying physical ailment was corrected.

It is extremely important, then, that an accurate and detailed medical history and physical examination be obtained before judgment is made about the cause of altered mental state in an elderly person. The nurse who is with a patient after admission and has frequent contact with him and his close associates can help avoid misdiagnosis of the patient's problems. She should observe her elderly and confused patients carefully, question them and their associates about events immediately preceding admission, and report the information accurately and promptly.

Because of the frequency with which physical problems of the hospitalized elderly who exhibit altered mental states are either misdiagnosed or ignored, hospitals are beginning to employ gerontologic nurse specialists who act as consultants and patient advocates. The nurse-consultant's task is to look objectively for a cause of mental symptoms and failure to heal and respond to treatment. Descriptions of the cases typically seen by gerontologic nurse-consultants emphasize the need for all nurses to reexamine their attitudes toward the elderly and to heighten their awareness of the importance of a thorough and objective assessment.

One 77-year-old patient, hospitalized for a fractured hip, was still unable to go home after 3 months of intensive physical therapy aimed at getting her to walk again. Her surgical wound did not heal as expected, she was confused and unmotivated, and she did not eat well. After thorough testing and assessment of her health status, she was found to have a tumor of the parathyroid gland, a not uncommon condition. Her parathyroid tumor was treated by surgery, and she improved remarkably and was able to return home and take care of herself within weeks after surgery.

Management of Confusion and Disorientation

There are various techniques and therapies the nurse can use to help the patient regain his sense of who he is, where he is, and what is happening to and around him. These therapies, when properly used, also can help improve an elderly patient's self-esteem. It is important, however, that once a technique is begun, it is used consistently and by everyone in contact with the patient. To do otherwise can only add to the patient's confusion.

Reality orientation involves both the environment and persons who interact with the patient and should be employed 24 hours a day. The environment is structured so that the patient has concrete and continual reminders of the year, day, and time of day. Environmental aids include a readable, up-to-date calendar; a clock; and the daily newspaper or local television or radio news. Consistency in mealtimes, scheduled treatments, and daily personal care also can be helpful. Older patients usually prefer to be called by title (Mr., Mrs., Miss) and surname. Each patient's preference should be known and respected.

Nicknames such as "Granny," "Pops," or "Uncle" are not only demeaning, but can also add to a patient's confusion and disorientation.

Interaction with staff and family members also can give the patient helpful clues. Sometimes people who do not understand the nature of confusion and disorientation in the elderly think it is a kindness to go along with a confused elderly person. They do not gently correct or remind the patient who confuses her daughter with her sister or the nurse with her daughter, nor do they remind the patient where he is when he indicates that he thinks he is at home, rather than at the hospital. A more positive and helpful approach is to continuously respond to the patient's confusion with honest and real information.

Nocturnal confusion is not uncommon in elderly persons who are hospitalized and placed in an unfamiliar and fast-paced environment. Sensory deficits such as impaired sight and hearing add to the patient's confusion and anxiety at night when he is in a strange and darkened environment. Ordinary shapes and sounds can become terrifying, and siderails can be perceived as bars on a jail or cage. Nursing intervention requires creative adaptations of the environment to mitigate the fears of the patient. A night light that gives illumination without shining in the patient's eyes, placing the call bell within reach, frequent visits to calm and reassure the patient, moving the patient closer to the nurses' station, touching, and other signs of caring are all ways in which the nurse can intervene to minimize nocturnal confusion. Restraints, which are often justified on the basis that they protect the patient from falling out of bed, are always a last resort. Their effectiveness in keeping the patient "safe" is questionable, and they usually only add to the patient's anxiety and restlessness.

When older patients do have organic brain disease, Alzheimer's disease, senility, or some other physiologic brain disorder, they require consistent long-term care. An excellent example of the kind of nursing care plan that can be developed for a patient with Alzheimer's disease can be found in an article by Marilyn Pajk in the February 1984 issue of the *American Journal of Nursing* (Pajk, 1984).

DRUGS AND THE ELDERLY PERSON

Chronic illnesses typically affect persons in the later stages of their life, and thus daily medication is a way of life for most older adults. However, drugs present a very real hazard to the elderly. Ninety percent of older people experience adverse reactions to drugs, and 20% of these reactions require hospitalization to treat the drug-induced illness. It is estimated that about 30,000 people die each year as a result of adverse drug reactions.

Many times drug interactions cause problems for the elderly patient. Often various specialists have prescribed medication for the patient, not knowing that he is taking a variety of other medications. The nurse can greatly assist the patient by obtaining a detailed medication history, formulating a list of his medications for him, and encouraging him to always present his list of current medications when he sees a physician or is admitted to the hospital.

Drugs are absorbed, metabolized, and excreted more slowly and less completely in the elderly. Impaired circulation can delay the transport of injected drugs to the tissues they affect. Drugs also can be deposited in fat cells, which have a greater attraction for the drug chemicals than do active cells. Because elderly persons have a higher proportion of fat cells to active cells than do younger persons, they are especially vulnerable to a cumulative effect. Additionally, decreases in kidney and liver function and changes in the chemical binding of proteins in the older person's body fluids alter his ability to detoxify and eliminate harmful drug chemicals and utilize those that are helpful. All of these factors contribute to the accumulation and extended duration of action of drugs taken by an elderly person.

All medications are potentially hazardous, but the medications most dangerous to an elderly patient are tranquilizers, sedatives, and other drugs that alter the mind and change perception. Diuretics and cardiac drugs such as digitalis also pose special dangers and must be given with caution and careful monitoring of the patient's response. Symptoms of toxic reactions and adverse side effects of drugs include diminished level of mental function, increased fatigue, restlessness, irritability, depression, weakness, dizziness, headache, and disorientation. It is important to recognize that these symptoms may be caused by drugs and should not simply be dismissed as "typical" of elderly persons.

Elderly persons must be taught how to take prescription medications and the dangers of taking nonprescription drugs. Failure of the elderly to follow their medication regimens can be caused by a number of personal and environmental factors. The cost of the drug, difficulty in getting it from a pharmacy, poor memory and motivation to take it regularly, depression, and feelings of being overwhelmed by the responsibility of self-medication can all contribute to noncompliance. In some cases arthritis or other disabling physical disease may make getting up and struggling with bottle caps too much of a chore.

Nursing intervention to ensure safe administration of drugs to the elderly at home will depend on the cause of the patient's noncompliance. Sometimes a family member or neighbor can assist the patient and remind him or administer the medication to him. There are many devices for proper administration of timed medication doses that can be most helpful to the forgetful or anxious older person. These are small cabinets or pill boxes with compartments for the daily dose of each drug labeled with the day of the week and the proper time. Some of these devices even have a timer that will ring or buzz when a medication dose is due. In any case, the patient or family member will need instruction in the purpose of the drug and its expected effect, side effects and adverse reactions that should be reported, the dangers of altering the dose or discontinuing the drug without notifying the nurse or physician, and the possibility of drug-drug reactions when nonprescription drugs are mixed with prescription drugs.

The nurse would do well to keep in mind that because liver and kidney function is decreased in the elderly patient, he doesn't metabolize medication as quickly as the younger person and is much more susceptible to side effects and toxicity with normal adult dosages. Monitoring of laboratory values for kidney and liver function should be done routinely, and vigilant assessment for side effects and signs of toxicity is vitally important. If a problem is found, it should be discussed with the physician immediately.

Even with detailed written instructions, elderly patients may not be able to comply with their prescribed regimen for medications. Frequent home visits by a community health nurse or some other health care provider are often necessary to give continued support and instruction and develop creative ways to help the patient take his medications as prescribed. If these efforts fail, other alternatives to self-medication must be considered. For example, a relative or friend may have to administer the medications to a patient who is unable to medicate himself safely.

In acute-care and long-term-care facilities the nurse must follow the basic principles of safe administration of medications and be aware of the vulnerability of elderly persons to adverse side effects and toxic reactions to the drugs she administers.

PSYCHOSOCIAL NEEDS

Persons in the later stages of their lives frequently suffer a series of personal losses that may include a spouse, friends, relatives, job, and social status. The multiple chronic illnesses that are not uncommon in the very old may require a change of lifestyle and lead to a loss of body parts and functions. Sensory losses such as those previously described can mean a loss or diminishing of the simple pleasures of life.

Older persons also are likely to experience some loss of control over their lives. They may become less able to control their home environment and cook, clean, and otherwise maintain a separate household for themselves. They may lose the ability to continue managing their own finances, keep their home in good repair, and drive a car or obtain some other means of transportation to conduct their business. They may also lose control over some body functions, including elimination of urine and feces, and become less able to perform various self-care activities such as bathing, grooming, and feeding themselves.

The losses and grieving experienced by older persons pose complex psychosocial problems. Assistance in meeting the needs of individual patients often requires the services of many members of the health care team and their agencies. Nursing interventions to help elderly persons adjust to and accept their losses are developed only after completion of a thorough assessment of each patient's psychosocial needs. Because each patient is an individual with unique problems, the patient and those close to him must participate in planning for his future care.

Many elderly persons who are lonely, have decreased self-esteem, feel unproductive, and are socially isolated begin drinking more alcohol. Alcoholism is a fairly common problem in the over-60 population. The nurse would be wise to assess for signs of this problem in elderly patients who exhibit the above characteristics. Many times the nurse can be very instrumental in redirecting the person to a life of sobriety and renewed meaning.

When an elderly person is discharged from an acute-care facility, it is important that his future psychosocial needs be considered. Shine suggests the following supports that are needed by elderly persons after they are discharged from the hospital: (1) a supportive environment in which the person can live as active and satisfying a life as possible, including socialization with others, creative and recreational activities, and useful daily activities; (2) a mutually caring relationship with one or more persons; and (3) a mutually caring relationship with one or more health care providers.

Health care providers must be available to the elderly person for consultation and help in dealing with old and new health-related problems and treatment and utilization of community resources. Because of the bureaucracy surrounding governmental agencies designed to help the elderly, an individual may need assistance in dealing with and obtaining services from the resources that are available to him. Because they also must work through their grief over the losses they suffer in the later years of their life, older adults also need knowledgeable support and guidance in the grief process. Grief and acceptance of death and dying are discussed in more detail in Chapter 14.

One of the major goals of nursing care of older persons is to help them maintain reasonable health for as long as possible. Older people need contact with others of all ages to keep themselves mentally alert, bolster their self-esteem, and maintain a healthy outlook on life. Most older adults respond favorably to younger people and are interested in what they are doing in today's world. They also enjoy sharing their memories with younger people. A form of therapy called *reminiscing* provides structured opportunities for the elderly to recall past events and experiences and to write or talk about their memories. This form of therapy has been used to dispel depression, provide social interaction, and improve the self-esteem of the elderly.

Older persons who are still physically active need more than just "something to do" to keep them busy and active. Some have embarked on second and even third careers as they have grown older. Some volunteer their services to those in their community who are less fortunate or to such volunteer agencies as the Cancer Society and the American Heart Association. There are many opportunities for older persons to remain active, have fun, and enjoy the company of others. The socialization of older persons cannot take place, however, if they are not given support, encouragement, and assurance that they are wanted and valued by society.

The nurse can be very instrumental in thinking of creative ways in which an elderly person can contribute something to the community or to others. Even the person who is housebound can be part of a telephone network to provide socialization for other shut-in people. The telephone can also place the person in a network of support people for latchkey children when they come home to an empty house after school. Even those who have no financial resources but are mobile can be useful to various community agencies, which will often provide transportation for a willing volunteer.

DEVELOPMENTAL TASKS

Many of the developmental tasks of the aging person require assistance from nurses and other health care providers. The specific kinds of help an individual needs at any given time will depend on his personal resources and the outside help available to him. When helping older persons complete their developmental tasks, it is extremely important to ensure that they take an active part in any decision making and to encourage them to do as much for themselves as they can. Self-care activities help the older person maintain self-esteem and provide him with a sense of having some control over events in his life. A major developmental task for older adults is to maintain as high a level of health as possible. When teaching older adults to care for themselves and actively take part in the management of their chronic illnesses, the nurse must be aware of potential obstacles to learning. Teaching strategies to facilitate learning in elderly persons are shown in Table 12–1.

Other developmental tasks to be achieved by aging couples or by an aging person alone are to:

- Decide where and how they want to live their remaining years.
- Continue a supportive, close, warm relationship with spouse, relatives, and friends.
- Establish a safe and comfortable home or living arrangement that is compatible with their health and economic status.
- Adjust living standards to retirement income and supplement this income if possible with a salaried job.
- Maintain a maximum level of health by caring for themselves physically and emotionally, having regular health examinations and necessary medical and dental care, eating sensibly and maintaining normal body weight, and maintaining personal hygiene through cleanliness and exercise.
- Maintain interest in people outside the family; accept social and civic responsibility.
- Pursue new interests and add variety to life.
- Work out a significant philosophy of life, finding comfort in religious or philosophic beliefs.
- Adjust to the death of spouse, friends, and loved ones, and prepare for one's own death.

Suggested nursing interventions to help older adults maximize their strengths to accomplish their developmental tasks and achieve fuller self-actualization are listed in Table 12–2.

INNOVATIONS IN HEALTH CARE FOR THE ELDERLY

In recent years, senior citizens have joined together in organizations such as the Gray Panthers and the American Association of Retired Persons (AARP) in order to publicize the cause of elderly Americans and speak up for their rights. They are concerned with mandatory retirement and other regulations imposed on them by a society that often regards "old" as synonymous with "ugly, useless, and troublesome."

Within the past decade, those concerned with gerontology and the plight of the elderly have sought new ways to resolve the problems of the

TABLE 12-1 STRATEGIES FOR TEACHING ELDERLY PATIENTS

1. Take the time necessary to assess learning needs adequately; determine what the patient already knows.
2. Find out how the patient feels he learns best: dialogue, written materials, auditory materials, television presentation, demonstration, etc.
3. Devise an appropriate teaching plan to be utilized when the patient is not preoccupied with other concerns (e.g., illness, grieving, finances, need for a nap).
4. Select visual materials that are geared toward degrees of sensory loss: large print, bright colors, simple design.
5. Select a location for teaching where there are few outside distractions.
6. Position the patient comfortably and with glasses and hearing aid on, if needed.
7. Allow the patient to have some control over the pace of the lesson; be patient and go slow; time is necessary for assimilation. Verify that a point is clear before continuing on to a new one.
8. Try to relate the new items being taught to past experiences or knowledge of the patient.
9. If a sentence needs to be repeated, use the same words initially. Sometimes when processing is slower, the end of the sentence simply isn't heard.
10. Seek feedback and recall of what has been taught, preferably the next day, but at least within a week.

aged. The Department of Health and Human Services has recognized the need for home health care programs that allow the elderly to stay at home rather than enter nursing homes and old-age facilities. The government is providing funds for nursing care in the home and federal grants to hospitals and schools to support the development of special study programs in gerontology.

Day-care centers for senior citizens who need care while their families are away at work are gaining popularity. Such centers are less costly and more beneficial to senior citizens than long-term institutionalization.

Many elderly people do not receive adequate health care, because they cannot afford it or simply do not have the stamina to get themselves to a clinic, wait in long lines, fill out forms, and cope with many different people in the bureaucracy.

An example of how these problems can be resolved is a program instituted by St. Anthony Hospital in cooperation with the Chicago Housing Authority. Two medical centers were set up by the hospital in a newly built housing project that is nearby. The centers are staffed during the day by nurses from the hospital. St. Anthony also provides a bus to transport patients who need backup services to and from the hospital. All

TABLE 12-2 INTERVENTIONS TO MAXIMIZE STRENGTHS OF THE OLDER ADULT

1. Nutrition counseling to ensure adequate dietary intake of nutrients, maintenance of normal body weight; Meals-on-Wheels for those who are unable to prepare their own meals; day-care facilities and residences for the elderly that provide one nutritious meal per day.
2. Enrollment in special exercise programs for the older adult. Teach range-of-motion exercises to patient or family member to preserve mobility during illness and its aftereffects.
3. Encourage use of hearing aid, magnifying glass, contact lenses, and other aids to mitigate sensory loss.
4. Assess level of function; encourage patient to focus on what he is able to do and enjoy.
5. Help older persons keep socially active through volunteer programs for senior citizens (e.g., foster grandparents, continuing education).
6. Encourage consideration of second or third career.
7. Utilize community resources such as Council on Aging, homemaker services, day-care center, visiting nurse and community health nurse agencies, and self-help groups that give support during loss and grieving process.
8. Discourage constant napping during the day.
9. Encourage maintaining a sense of humor and optimistic outlook.

persons 65 years of age or older living in the project and in the surrounding community are eligible for the free health services provided at the centers.

Another new concept in the care of the elderly is that of foster homes for those with no immediate family to care for them. The Arizona Adult Foster Home Registry, founded by Muriel Sieh, a social worker, is an example of this kind of service designed to meet the needs of the elderly.

BIBLIOGRAPHY

American Association of Retired Persons (AARP) and Administration on Aging: A Profile of Older Americans. Washington, DC, U.S. Department of Health and Human Services, 1987.

Anderson, G. P.: Would you know what caused these geriatric emergencies? RN, Aug., 1989, p. 27.

Ashervath, J., and Kizakipunner, K.: Achieving continence in the confused elderly. Adv. Clin. Care, July/Aug., 1990, p. 37.

Campbell, E. B., et al.: After the fall—confusion. Am. J. Nurs., Feb., 1986, p. 151.

Cerrato, P.: Nutritional support—Your elderly patient needs special attention. RN, Sept., 1990, p. 77.

Chenitz, W. C., et al.: Clinical Gerontological Nursing: A Guide to Advanced Practice. Philadelphia, W. B. Saunders, 1991.

Clevenger, F. F.: Interviewing the elderly client. Adv. Clin. Care, Nov./Dec., 1990, p. 26.

Eliopoulos, C.: Health Assessment of the Older Adult, 2nd ed. Redwood City, CA, Addison-Wesley Nursing, 1990.

Harrington, A. M.: 8 steps for evaluating a new long-term care patient. Nursing 89, May, 1989, p. 74.

Heckheimer, E. F.: Health Promotion of the Elderly in the Community. Philadelphia, W. B. Saunders, 1989.

Hogstel, M. O.: Nursing Care of the Older Adult, 2nd ed. New York, John Wiley & Sons, 1988.

Johnson, A. P.: The elderly and COPD. J. Gerontol. Nurs., Dec., 1988, p. 20.

Johnson, E. A., and Jackson, J. E.: Teaching the home care client. Nurs. Clin. North Am., Sept., 1989, p. 681.

Kick, E.: Patient teaching for elders. Nurs. Clin. North Am., Sept., 1989, p. 681.

Lasker, M. N.: Aging alcoholics need nursing help. J. Gerontol. Nurs., Jan., 1986, p. 16.

Lewis, S., et al.: Manual of Psychosocial Nursing Interventions: Promoting Mental Health in Medical-Surgical Settings. Philadelphia, W. B. Saunders, 1989.

Matteson, M. A., and McConnell, E. S.: Gerontological Nursing: Concepts and Practice. Philadelphia, W. B. Saunders, 1988.

Paiva, Z.: Sundown syndrome: Calming the agitated patient. RN, July, 1990, p. 46.

Pajk, M.: Alzheimer's disease: Inpatient care. Am. J. Nurs., Feb., 1984, p. 216.

Phillips, L. R.: Elder-family caregiver relationships: Determining appropriate nursing interventions. Nurs. Clin. North Am., Sept., 1989, p. 795.

Rempusheski, V. F.: The role of ethnicity in elder care. Nurs. Clin. North Am., Sept., 1989, p. 717.

Resnick, B. M.: Rehabilitation is for elderly too! Adv. Clin. Care, May/June, 1991, p. 43.

Wisenbaker, S., and McGill, J.: Caring for the Elderly. Adv. Clin. Care, Jan./Feb., 1990, p. 42.

Whall, A. L.: Self-esteem and mental health of older adults. J. Gerontol. Nurs., April, 1987, p. 41.

Zarle, N. C.: Continuity of care: Balancing care of elders between health care settings. Nurs. Clin. North Am., Sept., 1989, p. 697.

STUDENT STUDY AIDS

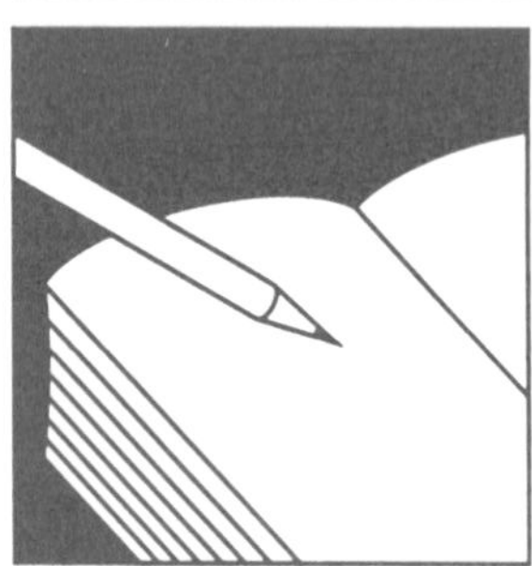

CLINICAL CASE PROBLEM

Read the clinical situation and discuss the questions with your classmates.

1. Mrs. Johnson, age 78, lives in a housing project with her husband, who is 89 years old. Mrs. Johnson has congestive heart failure, chronic obstructive lung disease, and glaucoma. She is 5 feet, 3 inches tall and weighs 200 pounds. She smokes two packs of cigarettes a day. Her husband has arthritis and congestive heart failure and wears a hearing aid for impaired hearing. Neither of them is able to help the other in activities of daily living or health care. Mr. Johnson rarely leaves the apartment and gets little or no exercise each day. Mrs. Johnson occasionally goes out to buy groceries but has no other social contacts.

Digoxin, 0.125 mg, one capsule four times a day, was prescribed for Mrs. Johnson the last time she was hospitalized for her heart condition. Her husband also has had digoxin prescribed for his chronic congestive heart failure. His prescribed dosage is 0.25 mg four times a day. Mrs. Johnson also is supposed to take furosemide, one 20-mg tablet daily. Both of them take nonprescription drugs freely, including aspirin and other analgesics, laxatives, and antacids. Both patients are supposed to limit their sodium intake.

When these elderly persons were visited by the community nurse, she found that they were not taking their prescription drugs as prescribed and often used one another's drugs when they did not have enough of their own or when they thought more medication would make them feel better.

The visiting nurse reviewed the labels on the prescribed drugs and encircled the name and dosage of each so Mrs. Johnson could distinguish her drugs from her husband's. When she returned 2 weeks later, she counted the remaining capsules in each container and found more than there should have been if the drugs had been taken as prescribed. Mrs. Johnson said she could not see the labels well enough to tell one from the other and she was confused about how many capsules to take and when she was to take her medication.

- How would you go about assessing each of these patients' compliance with their prescribed drug therapy and their need for instruction?
- What nursing interventions would you suggest to help improve their ability to take their prescribed drugs safely?
- What nursing interventions might be used to help avoid drug-drug interactions between prescription and nonprescription drugs?
- What other kinds of information do you think these elderly persons might need to help improve their health status?
- What community agencies might be helpful to this couple?

STUDY OUTLINE

I. Introduction

A. Older adults comprise the fastest growing segment of society in the United States.

B. Care of the elderly will become an increasing responsibility of nursing.

C. Nursing gerontology: the scientific study of the nursing care of older adults.

D. Major goal of gerontologic nursing is to identify the strengths of older adults and help them use those strengths to maximize independence in activities of daily living.

E. Specific concerns are:

1. Cultural values associated with aging and social attitudes toward the older adult.
2. Physical and mental changes that occur during aging process.
3. The many losses suffered by older persons.
4. Atypical response of aged to disease and its treatment.
5. Disabling effects of multiple chronic illness and degenerative processes associated with aging.

II. Cultural values and attitudes toward the aged

A. In our youth-oriented society, there has been a pervasive negative bias against the elderly.

B. Gerontologic nursing requires special knowledge, skills, and attitudes. It is not for everyone.

1. Every nurse needs to examine her feelings about aging and the aged.
2. Look for positive experiences with and characteristics of elderly persons.
3. To be old is not the same as being sick, poor, or neglected.
4. Older Americans do not typically think of themselves as unhealthy. Most own their own homes, live near and have contact with relatives, and have an adequate income.

C. With appropriate nursing intervention older persons can be helped to stay as young as possible while growing older.

III. General effects of aging

A. People do not all age at the same rate or in the same ways.

B. With age there is a gradual slowing down of all physiologic processes.

C. Rigidity and resistance to change on all levels are typical of increasing age.

D. Nurses need to slow down their own pace of care and give older patients time.
E. In spite of deterioration of cells and tissues due to aging, there remain many functioning cells. Efforts to improve functional capacity in the elderly are not useless.
F. General physiologic changes:
   1. External changes more obvious. Affect the skin, hair, muscles.
   2. Internal changes affect digestion and nutrition, mobility, circulation, metabolism.
   3. Specific physical changes and activities within the phases of the nursing process are summarized in the text.
   4. Sensory loss occurs gradually in the aged. Assessment and nursing interventions for sensory impairment are summarized in text.
   5. Many chronic diseases impact the health of the elderly.
G. Mental changes in the elderly:
   1. Mental deterioration, forgetfulness, and loss of intelligence are not typical of aging.
   2. Misconceptions about mental changes and fatalistic attitude toward the mental state of the elderly can cause misdiagnosis of physiologic disorders and inadequate or improper treatment.
      a. Important that older patients have an accurate and detailed medical history and examination and thorough nursing assessment when admitted to an acute-care facility.
   3. Management of confusion and disorientation:
      a. Reality therapy involves changes in environment, as well as interaction with staff to help patient remain oriented to reality.
      b. Nocturnal confusion not uncommon in older patients when they are moved from a familiar to a strange environment.
         (1) Provide a night light; visit patient frequently; move patient closer to nurses' station. Restraints can contribute to fear and confusion—used only as a last resort.

IV. Drugs and the elderly person

A. Because older adults often have one or more chronic illnesses, they frequently take medication regularly.
B. Drugs can accumulate more readily and have an extended duration in older persons because:
   1. They are often deposited in the fat cells, which are in higher proportion to active cells in the elderly.
   2. Kidney and liver function can be decreased.
   3. Changes in chemical binding of proteins alter ability to detoxify and eliminate harmful drug chemicals.
   4. High-risk drugs for the elderly include tranquilizers, sedatives, and other mind-altering drugs; diuretics; and digitalis.
   5. Symptoms of toxicity or adverse reaction include those that often are mistaken for "typical behaviors" of the aged.
   6. Older persons need special instructional aids to help them learn about the drugs they are to take on their own.
   7. Nurse should be alert for drug interactions.

V. Psychosocial needs

A. Patients in older age group typically suffer losses and need assistance through the grieving process.
B. Discharge planning before release from an acute-care facility should consider whether patient has:
   1. A supportive environment in which he can live as active and satisfying life as possible.
   2. A mutually caring relationship with one or more persons.

3. A mutually caring relationship with one or more health-care providers.

C. Psychosocial needs are best met by meaningful and loving interaction with others.
D. Alcoholism can be a problem in the lonely elderly person.
E. Developmental tasks are related to where the older person will live, maintaining warm and caring relationships with family and others, having financial security, maintaining health and interest in living, and coping with stresses associated with losses.
F. Strategies for teaching the elderly are listed in Table 12–1.
G. Interventions to help maximize the strengths of the older adult are listed in Table 12–2.

VI. Innovations in health care for the elderly

A. Home health care and homemaker services.
B. Day-care centers
C. Educational programs for senior citizens
D. Neighborhood clinics and health care centers
E. Foster homes for the elderly

CHAPTER 13

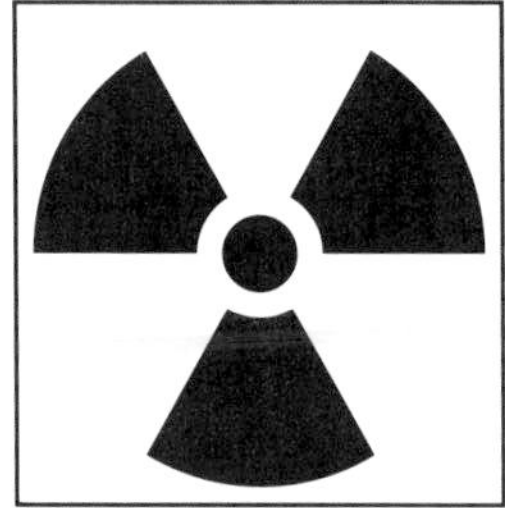

Care of Patients With Cancer

VOCABULARY

adjuvant
benign
biopsy
carcinogen
cytology
cytotoxic
isotope
metastasis
mitosis
mucositis
neoplasm
oncology
precancerous
prognosis
protocol
radiation
replication

Upon completion of this chapter the student should be able to:

1. Give statistical data that justify an optimistic outlook for management of cancer.
2. Briefly describe the tumor classification system.
3. Differentiate localized, regional, and advanced malignancy.
4. Identify at least five factors that contribute to the development of a malignancy.
5. State at least four practices that can contribute to prevention and early detection of cancers.
6. Describe the recommendation of the American Cancer Society for routine checkups for detection of cancers.
7. Debate pros and cons of telling a patient the truth about his diagnosis of cancer.
8. State the major problems and appropriate nursing interventions for a patient coping with expected side effects of radiation.
9. Cite specific nursing interventions necessary to provide safe and effective nursing care for patients receiving internal radiation.
10. Devise a general plan of nursing care for the patient receiving chemotherapy.
11. List three approaches in immunotherapy and the purpose of each.
12. Utilize the standards of care published by the Oncology Nursing Society when evaluating effectiveness of planned nursing care of patients with cancer.
13. Utilize community and regional resources for cancer patients and their families.

THE IMPACT OF CANCER

Few medical terms are as poorly understood as the word *cancer*. Among the more prevalent misconceptions are that cancer is a single disease, that it cannot be cured, and that prolonged suffering and death are its inevitable outcomes. In reality, cancer cannot be defined as a single disease entity. It is a large group of diseases that often have very little in common.

It is probably unfortunate that cancer is called a malignancy because this denotes something terribly evil, destructive, and uncontrollable. Although it is true that cancer cells are characterized by uncontrolled growth and spread, because that is the nature of malignant cells, this does not mean that the progress of a malignant disease cannot be controlled or that all diseases classified as malignant are hopeless and incurable.

For statistical and other purposes, many different kinds and degrees of unwellness are included in the general term *cancer*. As a group, malignancies are the second leading cause of death in the United States (cardiovascular diseases are the first). However, we can be optimistic about the survival of people who develop a malignant disease. In the early 1900s, there was little hope for survival once cancer was detected. By the 1930s, less than one of five people lived more than 5 years after treatment of their malignant disease was begun. In the 1950s, the statistic was one of four, and in the 1970s, one of three. Three out of eight persons who developed cancer in 1986 will be alive 5 years after diagnosis.

Because of the nature of neoplastic diseases, it is considered more realistic to speak in terms of survival rather than cure. Although some malignant growths can be eliminated and the patient considered cured after 1 year, the generally accepted period of time is 5 years. If, after that period, the patient who had been diagnosed as having cancer is still living and shows no signs of the malignancy at its original location or elsewhere in the body, then he is considered as one who has been saved. The primary concern is whether the patient has survived the malignancy.

More lives can be saved if malignancies are treated in their earliest stages. In fact, the American Cancer Society estimates that early detection and prompt treatment could save the lives of half the people who each year are diagnosed as having a malignancy. Figure 13–1 shows the decline in deaths caused by cancer of the stomach, uterus, colon, and rectum. (There is a dramatic increase in deaths from lung cancer.)

In this chapter, we discuss the prevention and control of cancer, current diagnostic and screening techniques that help detect cancer in its earliest stages, therapeutic procedures that are greatly improving a cancer victim's chances for survival, and the role of the nurse in the control and treatment of malignant diseases.

CHARACTERISTICS OF NEOPLASTIC GROWTHS

COMPARISON OF BENIGN AND MALIGNANT GROWTHS

The human body is continuously producing new cells to replace those that are worn out and to repair damage done by illness and injury. An abnormal replication of cells results in a *neoplasm* or new growth of tissue that is not beneficial and often is harmful to the body.

The word* benign *indicates a neoplasm that is usually harmless. Benign growths are almost always encapsulated, which means they are surrounded by a fibrous capsule that prevents the release of cells and their spread to other parts of the body.

These growths can, however, create problems if they obstruct the passage of fluid and air, or if they grow to such a size that they press against and interfere with the normal structure and function of nearby organs.

The cells of malignant growths are quite different from normal cells. Cancer cells are the result of a transformation of normal body cells, probably because of some alteration in the normal cells' deoxyribonucleic acid (DNA). The change in the DNA, which contains the genetic makeup of all future generations of the cell, alters the structure and function of the cancer cell and its progeny. Hence cancer cells do not look like normal cells or behave like them.

The nucleus of a malignant cell is large and irregular. As the cell divides and duplicates itself, it fails to follow the rules that regulate reproduction of normal cells. Malignant cells do not seem to "know" when to stop multiplying. Their offspring proliferate in great numbers and grow more and more disorganized and uncontrollable. Some take on new characteristics so that they do not in any way resemble the cells of the tissues from which they originated.

Because malignant cell growth is not regulated as it is in normal cells, the malignant cells multiply and form tumorous masses, invade neighboring tissues, and travel to other parts of the body, where they establish another colony of malignant cells. Their demand for nourishment depletes the supply of nutrients available for normal cells. This spread of tumor cells is called *metastasis*, a process that is described later in this chapter. *Not all malignant cells metastasize, but the great majority of them do.* This is true because malignant cells are easily broken off from their origi-

TRENDS IN SURVIVAL BY SITE OF CANCER, BY RACE
Cases Diagnosed in 1960-63, 1970-73, 1974-76, 1977-80, 1981-86

SITE	WHITE					BLACK				
	RELATIVE 5-YEAR SURVIVAL					RELATIVE 5-YEAR SURVIVAL				
	1960-63[1]	1970-73[1]	1974-76[2]	1977-80[2]	1981-86[2]	1960-63[1]	1970-73[1]	1974-76[2]	1977-80[2]	1981-86[2]
All Sites	39%	43%	50%	50%	52%*	27%	31%	39%	39%	38%
Oral Cavity & Pharynx	45	43	55	54	53	–	–	35	34	31
Esophagus	4	4	5	6	9*	1	4	4	4	6
Stomach	11	13	14	16	16*	8	13	16	16	18
Colon	43	49	50	53	57*	34	37	46	48	48
Rectum	38	45	49	51	54*	27	30	41	37	41
Liver	2	3	4	3	5	–	–	1	3	4
Pancreas	1	2	3	2	3*	1	2	2	5	4
Larynx	53	62	66	67	69*	–	–	59	58	52
Lung & Bronchus	8	10	12	13	13*	5	7	11	12	11
Melanoma of Skin	60	68	80	81	81*	–	–	69†	49‡	65
Breast (female)	63	68	75	75	78*	46	51	63	63	64
Cervix Uteri	58	64	69	68	67	47	61	63	62	57*
Corpus Uteri	73	81	89	86	84*	31	44	62	56	55
Ovary	32	36	36	37	39*	32	32	41	39	38
Prostate Gland	50	63	67	72	75*	35	55	58	62	62*
Testis	63	72	78	88	92*	–	–	77†	73†	92
Urinary Bladder	53	61	73	76	79*	24	36	47	54	59*
Kidney & Renal Pelvis	37	46	52	51	53	38	44	49	56	51
Brain & Nervous System	18	20	22	24	24*	19	19	28	28	32
Thyroid Gland	83	86	92	92	94	–	–	87	92	96
Hodgkin's Disease	40	67	71	73	76*	–	–	68	73	74
Non-Hodgkin's Lymphoma	31	41	47	49	51*	–	–	48	49	45
Multiple Myeloma	12	19	24	25	26*	–	–	28	32	28
Leukemia	14	22	34	36	36	–	–	30	29	29

Source: Cancer Statistics Branch, National Cancer Institute.

[1] Rates are based on End Results Group data from a series of hospital registries and one population-based registry.

[2] Rates are from the SEER Program. They are based on data from population-based registries in Connecticut, New Mexico, Utah, Iowa, Hawaii, Atlanta, Detroit, Seattle-Puget Sound and San Francisco-Oakland. Rates are based on follow-up of patients through 1986.

* The difference in rates between 1974-76 and 1981-86 is statistically significant ($p < 0.05$).

† The standard error of the survival rate is greater than 10 percentage points.

‡ The standard error of the survival rate is between 5 and 10 percentage points.

– Valid survival rate could not be calculated.

Figure 13–1 Survival rates for various kinds of cancer. Note the poor survival rate for cancer of the lung compared with the improved survival and decline in deaths from cancer of the uterus and the testis.
(From Cancer Facts and Figures 1991. Atlanta, American Cancer Society.)

nal mass of tissue and are able to survive on their own until they reach their new home.

CLASSIFICATION OF TUMORS

Tumors often are classified according to the organs or tissues from which they first began to grow or the substances of which they are formed. The suffix *-oma* means tumor and is used in the names of various kinds of malignancies. However, one should bear in mind that this suffix simply means tumor, which can be any swelling, including one in which there is a collection of fluids, as well as one containing malignant cells. Hematoma, for example, is a combination of *hema-*, meaning blood, and *-oma*, meaning a swelling or collection of fluid or cells.

The prefixes used in classifying neoplasms indicate the kind of tissue where they originated. For example, a "tumor" arising from fatty tissue is called a *lipoma*. A *fibroma* is a tumor composed of fibrous tissue. A *leiomyofibroma* contains both smooth muscle tissue and fibrous connective tissue. Lipoma, fibroma, and leiomyoma are the most frequently occurring types of benign growths.

Malignant growths are divided into four main types. *Sarcomas* arise from mesenchymal tissues, that is, bone, muscles, and other connective tissues. *Carcinomas* originate in epithelial tissues (skin and mucous membranes). These kinds of cancers make up the majority of glandular cancers of the stomach, uterus, lung, skin, and tongue. Cancers of the blood-forming system comprise the *leukemias* and *lymphomas*. Malignancies of the pigment cells of the skin are called *melanomas*.

These are the main groups of cancers. More precise identification can be made by adding modifying prefixes. For example, osteosarcomas arise from bone, and adenocarcinomas arise from glandular structures.

METASTASIS

The word *metastasis* refers to the movement of cells from one part of the body to another. Bacterial cells metastasize and so do malignant cells. Malignant growths can invade normal body tissue by penetrating adjacent tissues, thereby destroying normal cells and taking their place. Malignant cells may also separate from the original tissue mass and travel to distant parts of the body. *Metastasis refers to the moving of these cells to another site.* You will recall that bacterial cells can metastasize by traveling in the blood and lymph. Malignant cells metastasize in much the same way. It is also possible for free malignant cells to be directly transplanted from one organ to another during surgery, when gloves and instruments that have these cells on them serve as vehicles for their transportation. Another way in which malignant cells can "contaminate" normal tissues and organs is by entering a body cavity and coming in contact with a healthy organ. For example, malignant cells may break off from a diseased organ, enter the peritoneal cavity, and attach themselves to an ovary.

The prognosis for a patient with a malignancy depends largely on the extent to which the malignant cells have invaded body tissues. A *localized* growth is one that remains at the original site *(in situ)* and has not yet released its cells even though the growth may have invaded underlying tissues. As long as all of the cells are in the area in which the new growth started, the cancer is said to be localized. At this stage the disease is much more easily eradicated.

A *regional* malignancy is one in which cells from the original mass of malignant growth have broken off and traveled through the lymphatic and blood vessels.

Their journey has been shortened, however, by the body's protective mechanisms, which trap the foreign cells in the lymph nodes. These cells may continue to grow and multiply, and if the regional cancer is not successfully treated, they will eventually break away and spread throughout the body, producing an *advanced* cancer that is inevitably fatal.

One system in which cancers are classified according to the extent to which the malignancy has spread is the *TNM staging system*. The three basic components of the system are *T* for primary tumor, *N* for regional nodes, and *M* for metastasis. The number written beside each letter indicates the extent to which the malignancy has spread and involves other tissues (Table 13–1). For example, T1, N0, M0 means that the tumor is small and localized (no involvement of regional lymph nodes and no metastasis). A designation of T1, N2, M0 indicates a small (T1) tumor with moderate regional involvement (N2) but no metastasis to distant sites (M0).

TABLE 13–1 TNM STAGING SYSTEM FOR CANCER

Tumor	
T0	No evidence of primary tumor.
TIS	Carcinoma in situ.
T1 T2 T3 T4	Progressive increase in tumor size and involvement.
TX	Tumor cannot be assessed.
Nodes	
N0	Regional lymph nodes not demonstrably abnormal.
N1 N2 N3	Increasing degrees of demonstrable abnormality of regional lymph nodes. (For many primary sites, the subscript "a," e.g., $N1_a$, may be used to indicate that metastasis to the node is not suspected; and the subscript "b," e.g., $N1_b$, may be used to indicate that metastasis to the node is suspected or proved.)
NX	Regional lymph nodes cannot be assessed clinically.
Metastasis	
M0	No evidence of distant metastasis.
M1 M2 M3	Ascending degrees of distant metastasis, including metastasis to distant lymph nodes.
M4	Multiple organ involvement.

CAUSATIVE FACTORS

There is no specific cause of cancer. Many harmful agents exist in the external environment that are known to be carcinogenic, that is, cancer causing, and others that are strongly suspect. One can scarcely listen to news broadcasts or read the daily paper without being warned of the possibility of yet another carcinogen in our environment. *Among these harmful agents are certain chemicals, sources of radiation, and viruses* (Fig. 13-2).

In addition to these external causative factors, there are some internal factors that influence an individual's ability to cope with malignant cells. Hormones play an undetermined role in the development and progress of cancer, and although there is no evidence that malignancy follows any pattern of heredity, there is a familial tendency toward the occurrence of cancer in certain organs. This is shown in certain high-risk groups, which are described later in this chapter.

Another factor that enters into the development of a malignancy is age. Although cancer can strike at any age, older people are more susceptible—perhaps because their powers of adaptability are weakened and they have been exposed to carcinogens over a longer period than have younger people.

Immunocompetence, or the capability of one's immune system to deal with foreign cells—bacterial, viral, or malignant—is an important factor in the development of cancers.

CHEMICAL CARCINOGENS

Almost 200 years ago, Sir Percival Pott linked the occurrence of cancer to a substance in the environment when he observed that cancer of the scrotum was common among the chimney sweeps of London. He attributed this high incidence of cancer to repeated accumulations of soot on the skin of these young men, whose occupation required continuous contact with the coal soot in the chimneys they cleaned. Since that time, almost 500 different chemical carcinogens have been identified.

Many of the cancer-producing substances in man's environment are related to occupations that involve repeated exposure to certain substances that are handled or inhaled. For example, cancer of the skin is often related to the handling of pitch, asphalt, crude paraffins, and petroleum products. Lung cancer is linked to irritating sub-

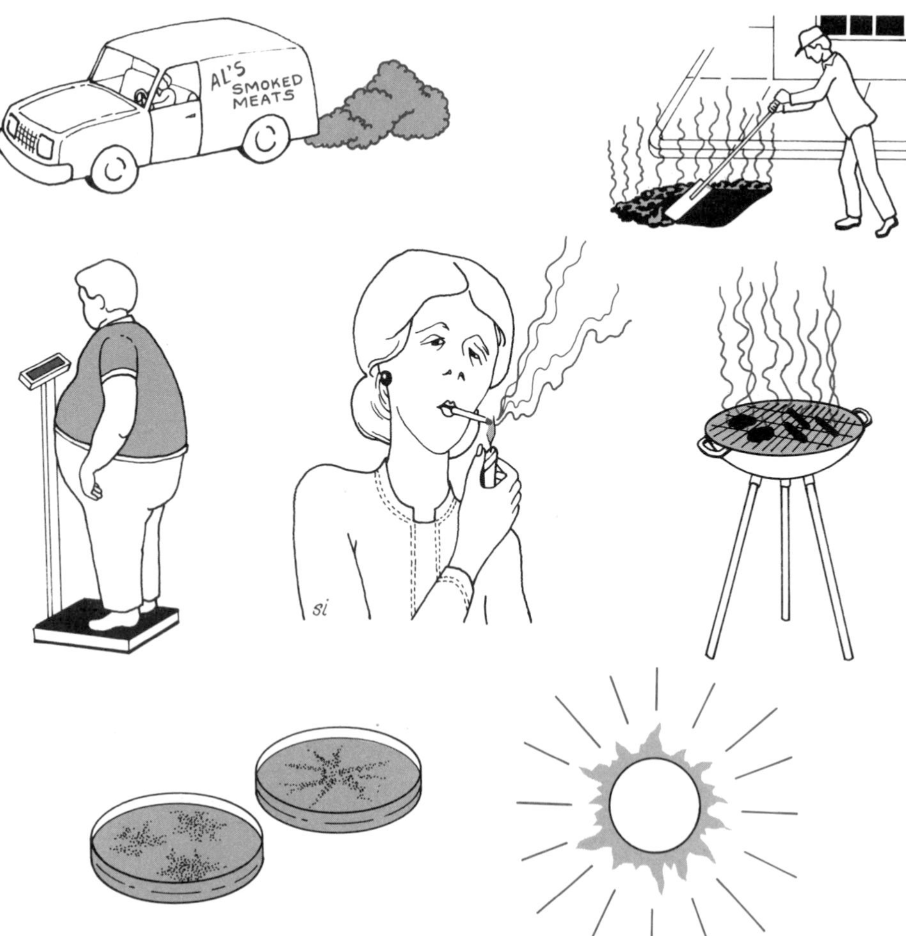

Figure 13-2 Some sources of carcinogens.

stances in the air such as tobacco smoke and chemical wastes from industry and automobiles. Cancer of the bladder is associated with certain substances in aniline dyes, which are present in the environment of workers in that industry. These are but a few of the chemical agents that can contribute to the development of cancer in humans.

DIET AND CANCER

It is only recently that the American Cancer Society has issued nutritional recommendations that are believed to reduce the risk for certain cancers. These recommendations, summarized in Table 13–2, are from a report by a special committee on nutrition and cancer and are based on studies conducted for more than 20 years by the American Cancer Society's Research Program. Although no direct cause-and-effect relationship between diet and cancer has been demonstrated, there is ample evidence that avoidance of obesity and modification of the diet can help prevent some types of cancers.

Obesity is considered to be a risk factor in cancers of the uterus, gallbladder, kidney, stomach, colon, and breast. This was demonstrated by the extensive Cancer Prevention Study conducted by the American Cancer Society between 1960 and 1972. In this study it was noted that men and women who were overweight by 40% or more have a 33% and 55% greater risk, respectively, for developing cancer than do persons with normal weight.

Excessive intake of both saturated and unsaturated fats increases the chance of malignancy of the breast, colon, and prostate. Studies of various populations throughout the world have shown that bowel cancer is more prevalent among groups of people who eat large amounts of fat and very little food fiber. Although there is no universal agreement as to the role of fiber in the prevention of malignancy, high-fiber foods such as fruits, vegetables, and cereals are recommended as a wholesome substitute for fatty foods.

The roles of vitamins A and C and betacarotene and in the prevention of cancer also are not clear. However, human population studies indicate that persons who eat foods high in betacarotene and vitamin A are less likely to develop cancer of the esophagus, larynx, and lung. Those who eat foods with a high content of vitamin C also reduce their chances of developing cancer, particularly of the stomach and esophagus. The exact action of the vitamin is not known, and it may be that other constituents of the vitamin C–rich foods exert a protective effect in the upper gastrointestinal tract.

Moderation in the drinking of alcohol is recommended, because drinking often is accompanied by cigarette smoking. It also can lead to liver damage and possibly to cancer of that organ.

Because the tars in smoke used to prepare smoked and salt-cured meats are carcinogenic, the American Cancer Society recommends limited dietary intake of foods of this kind. There also is evidence that nitrate used in nitrite-cured foods can enhance the formation of nitrosamines, which are potent carcinogens in animals and possibly in humans. Meat processors in the United States have already significantly decreased the amount of nitrite in prepared meats in response to the research findings.

Research has indicated that if foods containing nitrites are eaten in combination with foods containing vitamin C, the formation of nitrosamines is blocked. This means, for example, that if orange juice is consumed along with a meal containing bacon, there is less chance of carcinogenic nitrosamines damaging the body.

Another dietary recommendation is to reduce the amount of charcoal-broiled meat in the diet. The charred portion of the meat is thought to be carcinogenic. This recommendation is undergoing further study at the present time.

TABLE 13–2 RECOMMENDATIONS FOR DIETARY MODIFICATIONS TO MINIMIZE RISK FOR CERTAIN CANCERS

Avoid obesity.
Cut down on total fat intake.
Eat more high-fiber foods (cereals, fresh fruits, and vegetables).
Include foods rich in vitamins A and C in your daily diet.
Include cruciferous vegetables and those containing betacarotene in your diet; e.g., cabbage, broccoli, Brussels sprouts, kohlrabi, cauliflower, and carrots.
Eat minimally of salt-cured, smoked, charcoal-broiled, and nitrite-cured foods.
Keep alcohol consumption moderate, if you do drink.

PHYSICAL CARCINOGENS

The two main types of physical agents capable of causing cancer are radiation and chronic irritation.

Radiation

Radiation may originate from x-ray machines and radioactive elements or from the ultraviolet rays of the sun. These rays are capable of penetrating certain body tissues and causing the development of malignant cells in the affected area. The relationship of intense and prolonged exposure to these rays and the production of cancer cells was first discovered when it was noted that there was a high incidence of cancer, particularly leukemia, among people who pioneered studies of x-rays, radium, and uranium. Later it was found that survivors of atomic blasts at Hiroshima and Nagasaki at the end of the Second World War also suffered an unusually high incidence of leukemia.

Environmentalists continue to be concerned about the dangers that excessive radiation presents, especially the long-term effects that are not immediately apparent but may eventually prove to be related to malignancy. In addition to leukemia, cancers of the skin, bone marrow, and thyroid are believed to be closely linked to exposure to radiation.

The ultraviolet rays of the sun can produce skin cancer if exposure is prolonged and excessive. The deterioration of the earth's ozone layer is causing more ultraviolet rays to reach the earth than in the past, which compounds the problem. The susceptibility of the individual also is a factor. People with fair complexions have less protective pigment and therefore are more likely to develop skin cancer from ultraviolet radiation than are people with darker skin.

Chronic Irritation

In one of the earliest theories about the causes of cancer, a malignancy of the skin and mucous membranes was attributed to long-term chronic irritation of the skin and mucous membranes. Although this condition may be a *contributing cause* of cancer, chronic irritation alone usually does not lead to malignancy. There must be other factors present, particularly a mole and exposure to a chemical carcinogen.

Viruses

In recent years, there has been intensive research directed toward establishing a link between viruses and malignancy. Experiments involving animals have demonstrated that a number of cancers can be produced in animals by injecting them with a filtrate from virus-infected malignant growths. However, there is still no irrefutable evidence that cancers in humans are directly caused by viruses.

After the transformation of a normal cell into a precancerous state, the malignant cell probably requires many conditions favorable to its multiplication and growth into a cancerous tumor. Hence, it is doubtful that viruses can be implicated as the lone causative agents of cancer. However, viruses are capable of introducing new genetic material into a normal cell and transforming it into a malignant one. Furthermore, cell reproduction can be altered when viruses interact with carcinogens. At present it is not known precisely what role viruses play in cancer and whether the process of transforming a normal cell into a malignant one requires many agents acting simultaneously or in some kind of sequence.

Age, sex, and race are considered "predisposing factors" for certain types of cancers. This simply means that statistically, certain types of cancer strike particular age, sex, or racial groups more frequently than others. For example, prostate cancer is far more common in black males than in white males. The incidence of cervical cancer is higher in black women than in white women. Breast cancer is more prevalent in white women than in Oriental women.

Herpes simplex virus 2 and some of the human papillomaviruses that are transmitted sexually are known to predispose to cervical cancer. Better hygiene, reduction of the number of sexual partners, and use of barrier techniques for sexual intercourse can decrease the risk of contracting these viruses.

Research is also revealing that there is probably a genetic predisposition to various types of cancer. It has been known for many years that breast cancer is more likely to occur in women who have a close female relative with breast cancer. In the next decade, genetic markers, or oncogenes, may be found for many forms of cancer. Such markers could identify high-risk individuals, who then could undergo more vigorous, regular diagnostic testing to detect any malignancy in the very earliest stages. Such early discovery would greatly increase survival rates.

Another factor that seems to play an influencing role in the development of cancer is stress. Considerable stress over long periods of time has an adverse effect on the immune system, making it less effective in ridding the body of invading organisms and decreasing the body's ability to destroy abnormal cells. Stress is one more added factor that can perhaps tip the scales in favor of growth of malignant cells.

SCOPE OF CANCER NURSING

Earlier in this chapter it was pointed out that cancer is not a single disease. Nurses are challenged to provide care to cancer patients in a variety of settings. They must assess the status of each patient, any one of whom might be in any stage of the disease process ranging from prediagnosis to terminal illness. Although there are many facilities that treat only those persons who have a malignancy of some kind, almost 85% of all cancer patients receive treatment in the community hospital setting.

In addition, many cancer patients manage their illness at home. Hence they and their families require continued support and guidance while trying to control their symptoms and cope with the biologic, social, emotional, and spiritual needs that the diagnosis of cancer can create.

Anderson and Brown have developed a classification system to help nurses identify specific needs of their cancer patients and organize their thinking in relation to assessment, planning, and implementing nursing care. Their classification is as follows:

1 Patients who are undergoing testing to confirm or exclude a malignant diagnosis and who are trying to deal with the fear of the possible meaning of the symptoms.
2 Patients in whom the diagnosis has been newly established and who are thrust into a position of having to cope with the impact of diagnosis and the resulting interruptions in their lives.
3 Patients who are experiencing the effects and side effects of treatment.
4 Patients who are experiencing an exacerbation of the illness and who are facing the possibility or actuality of recurrence.
5 Patients who, after treatment, have no known evidence of the disease.
6 Patients in advanced (terminal) stages of illness (Anderson, 1980).

In general, patients in all six of these categories will require education to prepare them for management of their problems to the extent that they are capable of self-care. Many of them will also require professional nursing care to meet their needs when they are unable to do so, and to assist them in finding the necessary resources for continued support throughout their illness.

Assessment of the cancer patient can seem overwhelming to even the most experienced nurse. However, it is helpful to keep in mind the reasons why assessment is done and the kinds of information the nurse must have to systematically plan nursing care. Assessment begins with gathering some baseline data so that the nurse can detect changes that might occur. She obtains a nursing history to determine the patient's status in regard to the above classification system. She might find that his most pressing need is for more information about the nature of his illness and the treatment that has been planned. The patient suffering from the side effects of therapy might need relief from his distressing symptoms and prevention of further damage to normal cells.

During her assessment the nurse should seek specific information as to the patient's usual level of functioning and how well he has been able to adapt to changes brought on by his illness. If, for example, the patient has experienced toxic side effects from chemotherapy and has been able to cope with them effectively in the past, the nurse needs to know what measures have been used and how she can incorporate them into the nursing care plan.

Finally, she should try to ascertain how she can assist the patient to make the most of the personal resources and abilities that he currently possesses. This could mean helping him adjust to the emotional impact of only recently learning that he has cancer, or it could require helping him to deal with the pain and discomfort of advanced malignancy and to prepare for a peaceful death.

In the following pages some of the more common nursing activities associated with cancer nursing will be discussed. The information is specific only to the extent that it deals with various forms of therapy and the side effects that can occur with each. Care of the patient with a terminal illness is discussed in Chapter 14.

PREVENTION AND EARLY DETECTION OF CANCER

Although cancers are* not *considered to be infectious diseases, there are some similarities between the two groups of diseases: (1) the body does have protective mechanisms that help ward off bacterial and malignant cells, (2) both kinds of cells can spread to other parts of the body, and (3) the outcome depends on early detection and prompt treatment to minimize their harmful effects.

Screening techniques to identify susceptible and high-risk individuals are essential for reducing the incidence of both infectious and malignant diseases. It is believed by many authorities that a vaccine to provide immunity against certain kinds of cancer will be available in the not-too-distant future. Until it is possible to immunize against malignant diseases, the best defense we have is a concerted effort on the part of the public and health care professionals alike to (1) avoid contact with known carcinogens, (2) identify high-risk people, and (3) utilize scheduled screening techniques to detect precancerous lesions and malignancies in their earliest stages.

AVOIDING AND LIMITING EXPOSURE TO CARCINOGENS

In spite of the fact that there are about 500 known cancer-producing agents in our environment and perhaps many more that are unknown, it is still possible to avoid or at least minimize exposure to them.

The first step toward cancer prevention is knowing which factors are likely to produce a malignancy. (Carcinogenic agents were discussed earlier in this chapter.) The second step is to inform the public and to encourage people to limit their exposure to these substances as much as possible. The incidence of two types of cancer (skin and lung) can be greatly reduced if people can be convinced of the dangers of cigarette smoking and habitual excessive and prolonged exposure to the sun or tanning lights. Other cancers are less easily prevented, but in recent years the occurrence of many occupational malignancies has been dramatically reduced because of safety measures designed to decrease exposure of employees to known chemical carcinogens.

In an effort to instruct the general public in the ways in which it can participate in prevention and early detection of cancer, the American Cancer Society has prepared a list of seven safeguards against cancer (shown on page 275).

IDENTIFYING HIGH-RISK PEOPLE

Studies of individuals who have developed cancer—their medical history, lifestyle, and family history—have shown that some people are more likely to develop certain kinds of cancer than others. Table 13–3 shows information on high-risk groups published by the American Cancer Society in order to develop an awareness of the need for frequent and thorough examinations to detect cancer early in those who are susceptible to the development of a malignancy.

SEVEN SAFEGUARDS AGAINST CANCER

- *Breast:* Regular monthly self-examination of breasts for lumps, nodules, or changes in contour; yearly check by physician.
- *Lung:* Reduction and ultimate elimination of cigarette smoking; avoidance of smoke-filled environments.
- *Colon-rectum:* Rectal examination as routine in annual checkup for those over 40; proctosigmoidoscopy or barium enema colon radiographs at age 50 and each 3 to 5 years thereafter.
- *Uterus:* Pap test for all adult women and high-risk adolescent women.
- *Skin:* Avoidance of excessive exposure to sun or tanning lights.
- *Oral:* Wider practice of early detection measures; regular dental examinations.
- *Basic:* Regular physical examination for all adults.

SCREENING FOR CANCER

The purpose of screening large segments of a population is to identify as many susceptible people as possible. Screening clinics often identify individuals who already have developed malignancies but have no symptoms and are not aware that they are suffering from cancer.

One widely used and useful technique in screening for cancer is the examination of cells under a microscope to determine if they are malignant or premalignant. This technique is called *cytology*, and the most widely used cytologic test is the Papanicolaou smear. Another method of screening for cancer involves teaching women to perform monthly self-examinations of their breasts and teaching men to do monthly testicular examinations. A third method is instructing the public in the seven warning signals for cancer, listed on page 275.

A *cytologic examination* can be done by obtaining a sample of secretions in which there are cells that have been released from adjacent tissue. The technique involves either scraping or brushing a sample of cells from the area or collecting body secretions that contain cells. These secretions may be cervical discharges, sputum, gastric washings, pleural fluid, or urinary washings. The specimen is placed on a slide and sent to a laboratory, where a specially trained technologist or pathologist examines the cells microscopically. If "suspicious" cells are found, the patient is referred to a physician for more extensive diagnostic tests. The "Pap smear," named after Dr. George Papanicolaou, who first developed the procedure, is used in screening for cancer of the uterine cervix. As previously mentioned, the Pap smear is the cytologic technique most often used in screening for cancer.

Self-examination of the breast has been widely publicized in an effort to encourage women to look for a lump or a thickening in the breasts each month, a few days after the onset of the menstrual period. Women who have passed the menopause also are advised to plan a monthly self-examination.

Self-examination for testicular cancer in men also is encouraged, particularly in those who are in the age group most at risk: between 15 and 34 years of age. Malignancy of the breasts, testes, and other reproductive organs is discussed in Chapter 30.

Another screening technique is used for colorectal cancer. This is a simple test for *occult*, or hidden, blood in the stool. The person simply collects one or more stool specimens, depending on the particular test being used, applies a thin smear on the container provided, and returns the slides to the physician or clinical laboratory. Directions for withholding meat and other foods, vitamins, and drugs from the diet for several days before the test must be clear to the patient. Otherwise, a false-positive or false-negative reading might be obtained. Occult blood in the stool

TABLE 13-3 **MAJOR RISK FACTORS FOR CANCER**

Lung	Heavy smoker over age 50 Smoked a pack a day for 20 years Cigarette cough Started smoking at age 15 or before
Breast	Lump or nipple discharge History of breast cancer Close relatives with history of breast cancer Over 35; especially over 50 Never had children; first child after age 30
Colon-rectum	History of rectal polyps Rectal polyps run in family History of ulcerative colitis Blood in stool Over age 40
Uterine-cervical	Unusual bleeding or discharge Frequent sex in early teens or with many partners Low-income background Poor care during or following pregnancy Age 40 to 49
Uterine-endometrial	Unusual bleeding or discharge Late menopause (after age 55) Diabetes, high blood pressure, and obesity Age 50 to 64
Skin	Excessive exposure to sun Fair complexion Work with coal tar, pitch, or creosote
Oral	Heavy smoker and drinker Use of smokeless tobacco Poor oral hygiene
Ovary	History of ovarian cancer among close relatives Age 50 to 59
Prostate	Over age 65 Difficulty in urinating
Stomach	History of stomach cancer among close relatives Diet heavy in smoked, pickled, or salted foods Some link with blood group A

is not always an indication of cancer of the bowel or rectum. Other conditions also can produce this symptom.

Screening techniques such as those just described are needed to detect cancer in its earliest stages, because cancer often does not present symptoms at first. It can cause considerable damage, spreading to other parts of the body before its victim is aware he has been attacked. Because the disease is so insidious, no one can afford to ignore early warning signs of cancer. It is unwise to put off seeking expert advice when there is the slightest suspicion that cancer is present.

Cancer is sometimes called the "great masquerader" because it is capable of causing symptoms similar to those of a variety of diseases. Cancer is, after all, a *group* of diseases. It can strike any organ of the body, affecting different organs with different functions, and therefore can present an untold number of symptoms as it progresses. In order for the nurse to be able to identify the symptoms of cancer in its earliest stages, it is important that she be aware of its warning signals.

SEVEN WARNING SIGNALS OF CANCER

- Change in bowel or bladder habits
- A sore that does not heal
- Unusual bleeding or discharge
- Thickening or lump in breast or elsewhere
- Indigestion or difficulty in swallowing
- Obvious change in wart or mole
- Nagging cough or hoarseness

Recommendations of the American Cancer Society for routine checkups and early detection of cancer are shown in Table 13-4.

TABLE 13-4 ROUTINE CHECKUPS RECOMMENDED BY THE AMERICAN CANCER SOCIETY

Annual cancer-related checkups for men and women past the age of 40.

Checkups every 3 years for those between the ages of 20 and 40.

Colon and rectum: Digital rectal examination at age 40 and annually thereafter. Proctoscopic examinations at 3- to 5-year intervals after age 50, *provided negative results* have been recorded for 2 consecutive years. Guaiac test for occult blood in the stool should be done annually for all persons.

Cervix: Annual Papanicolaou test for all women over the age of 20 and for sexually active women under the age of 20. Test to be done every 3 years *provided* there have been two negative reports 1 year apart.

Breast: Examination by doctor at least every 3 years for women 20 to 30 years of age and annually thereafter. One baseline radiograph recommended for women between the ages of 35 and 39. Women aged 40 to 49 should have mammography every 1–2 years, depending on physical and mammographic findings. After age 50, breast radiograph should be done every year.

Lung: Emphasis on advantages of not smoking. Annual chest radiographs and sputum cytology have not reduced mortality.

High-risk exceptions: More frequent and thorough examinations recommended for: (1) women with personal family histories of breast cancer; (2) women who began having sexual intercourse at an early age or those with many partners; (3) women who have a history of obesity, infertility, failure of ovulation, abnormal uterine bleeding, or estrogen therapy; (4) men and women who have a personal family history of cancer of the rectum, familial polyposis, Gardner's syndrome, ulcerative colitis, or a history of polyps.

Each person also is encouraged to confer with a physician and determine whether these recommendations are adequate in light of his or her personal history and risk factors.

DIAGNOSIS OF CANCER

In addition to the medical history and thorough physical examination that are essential components of any health status evaluation, the physician also conducts certain tests to determine whether a malignancy is present.

Biopsy of a tumor and examination of the cells so obtained is the most certain technique for establishing a diagnosis of malignancy in most neoplasms. Malignancies involving blood cells, as in leukemia, are diagnosed by examination of these cells. Other procedures used to identify lesions that are possibly malignant include radiologic studies, endoscopy, and clinical laboratory testing of enzymes and other substances in the blood.

BIOPSY

A *biopsy* is the removal of living cells for the purpose of examining them microscopically. The cells may be removed by surgical excision of a small part of a tumor, by the aspiration of cells through a needle introduced into the growth, or by brush biopsy. If the tumor is small, the entire growth may be removed. The specimen obtained is examined under the microscope.

Ordinarily, the specimen is prepared in the laboratory by placing it in paraffin and waiting 24 hours before examining it. If, however, the sample is taken in the operating room and the surgeon is waiting for the results in order to determine the extent of surgery needed to remove all the malignant cells, the tissues may be frozen for quick examination. This technique is called *preparing a frozen section.*

RADIOLOGIC STUDIES

X-ray films are particularly helpful in diagnosing tumors affecting the bones and hollow organs. The respiratory, digestive, and urinary tracts can be visualized by x-ray if a radiopaque (not penetrated by the x-rays) substance is used. The substance passes through the hollow organ and, since it is radiopaque, the inner structure of the organ is clearly demonstrated on the x-ray film. A radiopaque substance commonly used is barium, which may be swallowed by the patient or given in an enema. *Mammography* is a radiologic examination of the breast that is useful in diagnosing cancer.

Another radiologic technique involves the use of a radioactive substance *(radionuclide)* that is given to the patient prior to the x-ray filming. The radionuclide is a "tumor-seeking" chemical that searches for the tumor and may or may not concentrate around it. A special scanning apparatus moves back and forth over the subject's body; as it moves, it records information about the concentration of the radionuclide in the area being examined. If the substance is concentrated in the tumor, the growth shows up as a "hot spot" on the screen of the scanning apparatus. If the tumor does not accept the radionuclide, the normal tissue around the tumor concentrates the radionuclide, and the tumor shows up as a "cold spot." This technique is commonly used in the investigation of thyroid tumors.

A commonly used radiologic scanning technique is *computed tomography* (CT scanning). This method is noninvasive and involves relatively small amounts of radiation exposure for the subject. The term *noninvasive* means that no surgical procedures or injections of radiopaque materials are needed to reveal the size, shape, contour, and density of an organ. The procedure is not uncomfortable for the patient and requires minimal preparation.

In CT scanning, the x-ray source moves past the subject in one direction while the film moves in another. In this way, three-dimensional cross sections or "slices" of tissue can be obtained. The scanner rotates an entire 180 degrees (half circle) around the area being examined, filming as it rotates 1 degree at a time. Information received by the scanner is relayed to a computer, which presents an image of the tissues one slice at a time. The "picture" presented by the computer is an interpretation of the varying densities of tissues, fluids, and bones. Tumors, as well as other abnormal structures within the body tissues, can be seen in this way.

ENDOSCOPY

An endoscope is an instrument used for direct visualization of internal body parts. It is designed so that it can be inserted and passed along the interior of hollow organs and cavities. The endoscope has a flexible fiberoptic tube fitted with a lens system so the examiner can view tissues in more than one direction. It has a light to illuminate the area being examined.

Other types of endoscopes include the colonoscope for viewing the colon, the colposcope for examining the vagina and uterine cervix, the bronchoscope for viewing the trachea and bronchi, and the cystoscope for viewing the interior of the bladder. During an endoscopy, the physician may take a sample of cells from a suspicious area so they can be examined more precisely under a microscope (biopsy).

LABORATORY TESTS

Although no one blood test can establish a definite diagnosis of cancer, certain tests are used to ascertain specific information. A complete blood count is helpful in diagnosing leukemia. Levels of the enzyme *acid phosphatase* in the blood can give information about the extent of cancer of the prostate. The enzyme *alkaline phosphatase* is elevated in many patients with metastatic bone cancer and in some who have liver metastasis.

Specialized tests for tumor markers have been developed in the past few years. These detect biochemical substances synthesized and released into the blood stream by tumor cells. However, these are not 100% accurate for diagnosing tumors, because many of these substances are also produced by normal or embryonic cells and are also found in benign conditions. Therefore tumor markers are mainly used to confirm a diagnosis or the response to therapy or to detect a relapse.

A test based on DNA is currently undergoing closer scrutiny to see if it is truly accurate in detecting malignancy of any sort within the body.

INFORMING THE PATIENT OF A DIAGNOSIS OF CANCER

At one time the majority of physicians felt it was best not to tell a patient that his diagnosis was a malignancy. In 1977 a study of physicians' attitudes and practices in regard to telling patients they have cancer revealed that there was a reversal of the trend to withhold the truth from patients. Ninety-eight percent of the physicians surveyed said that their policy was to tell the patient the truth. All agreed that they would want to be told if they had cancer and that the patient has the right to know his diagnosis. Cancer patients who have been told of their diagnosis also agree that they would rather know than be kept in ignorance about what is wrong with them.

Factors that influence the *manner* in which a patient is told of his diagnosis include what the patient has already been told about his illness; any misconceptions he might have; available support from his family or friends; and his age, intelligence, relatives' wishes, and emotional stability.

Any nurse who has close contact with a cancer patient must know whether the patient has been informed of his diagnosis. Some patients may suspect they have cancer but do not want to discuss it. Even those who have been informed may choose not to talk about it or ask any questions about their treatment. The fact that a patient cannot discuss his illness and seek help in dealing with the problems it presents should indicate how very frightened he is and how much he needs help and understanding.

Those patients who know about and accept their illness and strive to learn to live with it might sometimes be less demanding of the doctors' and nurses' time. This does not mean, however, that they require any less information, reassurance, and support than those who cannot adjust to the emotional shock when they learn they have cancer.

TREATMENT OF CANCER AND NURSING IMPLICATIONS

There are three traditional modes of therapy for malignancies: *surgery, radiation,* and *chemotherapy.* A fourth method of treatment, *immunotherapy,* encourages the immune system to destroy and control the growth of malignant cells as it does all foreign cells.

Each of the modes of treatment may be used singly or in combination with one or more of the other methods available. For example, chemotherapy may be used as an *adjuvant* (assisting treatment) after surgical removal of a tumor. No one method is necessarily better or more effective than another except in regard to the location of the malignancy, its type and extent of spread, and the reaction of the tumor itself and the individual patient. The methods of treatment are chosen after due consideration of many factors and are prescribed with the best interest of the patient in mind.

SURGERY

Surgical removal of a malignant growth is the oldest method of treatment. It works very well for tumors that are easily accessible and located in areas where adjacent tissues, such as muscles and lymph vessels, may also be excised. Cutting away apparently normal tissues may seem unnecessarily drastic and mutilating to the person who does not understand the metastasis of cancer cells, but it has been proved that excision of the malignant tumor alone often will not prevent the spread and recurrence of the growth in other tissues of the body.

In recent years, improved surgical techniques and utilization of radiation after, and sometimes during and before, surgery have significantly reduced the need for extensive surgical removal of suspected tissues and decreased the incidence of recurrence.

Newer surgical procedures and techniques have significantly reduced the need for extensive surgical removal of adjacent tissues and structures. Radical mastectomy, for example, involves removal of the entire breast along with underlying pectoral muscle tissues and lymph nodes under the arm on the affected side. This procedure has been replaced almost completely by a modified radical mastectomy, or lumpectomy, combined with radiation and/or chemotherapy, which is far less traumatic and mutilating. If there is no evidence of metastasis, some patients are good candidates for simple removal of the tumor (lumpectomy).

The carbon dioxide laser, which was developed in 1967, is an alternative to hysterectomy or conization for the treatment of preinvasive cancer of the cervix. The laser beam vaporizes the water of malignant cells and thus destroys them. The beam provides pinpoint precision for removal of diseased tissue, thus saving healthy cells from damage. It is accompanied by minimal bleeding because the laser beam coagulates blood vessels and lymphatics. There also is the advantage of greatly reduced risk for infection, since there is no danger of introducing infectious organisms into the operative site and any bacteria or viruses that might be present are destroyed by the beam.

Surgery of the breast and uterus is discussed in more detail in Chapter 30.

Nursing care for patients who have surgical procedures as treatment for malignant growths is discussed throughout this text.

RADIATION THERAPY

The source for radiation therapy is either a high-voltage x-ray machine, electron beam, or a radioactive element. The purpose of radiation is the destruction of malignant cells (which are more sensitive to radiation than are normal cells) without permanent damage to adjacent body tissues.

Ionizing radiation can have both an immediate and a delayed effect on malignant cells. It can damage the cell membrane immediately, causing lysis or decomposition of the cell, or it can cause a break in both strands of the DNA in the cell's nucleus. When a cell is damaged in this way, it will not die until it attempts to divide and replicate itself. The rate at which a particular kind of cell undergoes mitosis determines whether the effects of radiation will occur in a matter of days, months, or years. This is the reason for the delayed effects and side effects of radiation that might not be evident at the time of treatment but appear later.

Radiation therapy may be *external,* in which the source of radiation is outside the patient, or *internal,* in which the source of radiation is a radioactive element that has been implanted or injected into the body.

Because of improvements in tumor localization, beam direction, planning and prescribing the field to be irradiated, and determining the precise dosage needed, radiation therapy is more beneficial and less harmful than it was when this form of treatment was first being pioneered.

The dosage to be administered and the specific areas of the body at which the beam of rays is to be directed are determined by the radiologist, who usually is an oncologist specializing in radiation therapy for malignancies. The *rad*, or *radiation absorbed dose*, is the unit used for measuring dosages of radiation.

The damage to normal tissue can be kept at a minimum in radiation therapy by keeping the dosage or degree of penetration accurate and by aiming the rays from several different angles. The latter technique increases the concentration of the rays in the area of the tumor with a minimum of damage to overlying tissues.

External Radiation Therapy

The *x-ray* machine used for external radiation therapy produces a voltage that is at least a thousand times greater than machines used for diagnostic purposes. It delivers a beam of radiant energy that bombards the malignant cells and destroys them. Because malignant cells are dividing at an abnormally high rate, they are more susceptible to destruction than are normal cells.

Radiation from *radioactive elements* has the same ionizing effect as that from megavoltage x-ray machines; the only difference is the source of radiation. An element that is radioactive is unstable; that is, the nuclei of its atoms decompose naturally and in the process they emit radiant energy. Some elements—for example, radium and uranium—are naturally unstable and therefore radioactive. Other elements such as cobalt and iodine can be made unstable by bombarding them with high-energy particles in a nuclear reactor.

External radiation therapy using a radioactive element is a form of treatment in which the element is housed in a shielded unit located some distance from the patient (Fig. 13-3). The beam of radiation is controlled and directed by collimators and special shielding that localize the area of radiation. It is possible to aim the radioactive beam from any direction; however, the angles most commonly used are similar to those for a chest radiograph—that is, anteroposterior (AP) and right and left lateral.

Modern radiation therapy has improved immensely during the past decade. The use of computers in planning accurate radiation dosage and projectory distributions has decreased the side effects considerably. The use of stereotaxic surgery with the gamma knife is effective for small brain tumors, and research is in progress for other applications. Gamma knife treatment is essentially noninvasive radiosurgery in which the tumor is destroyed by radiation.

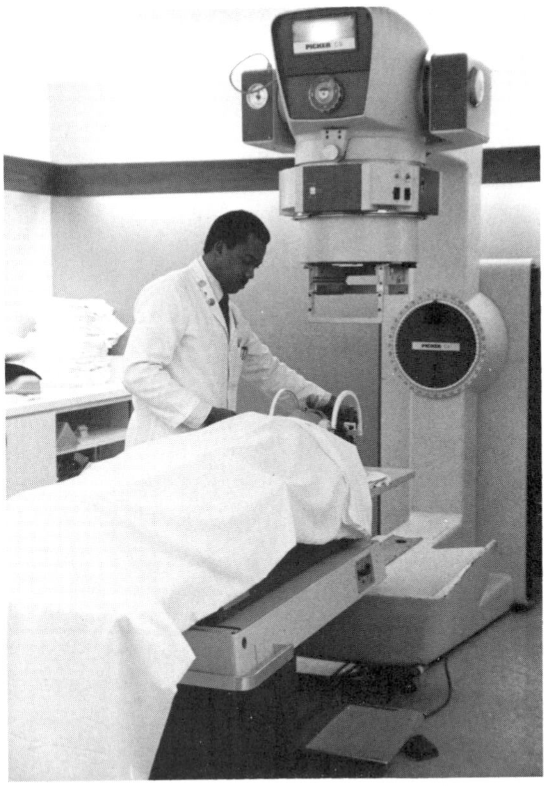

Figure 13-3 Patient being prepared for treatment with a unit containing cobalt 60. The large dial on the machine indicates the degree of angulation at which the patient is to be treated.
(Courtesy of the Department of Radiation Therapy, Athens General Hospital, Athens, GA.)

Nursing Care of Patients Undergoing External Radiation Therapy

Nursing care goals related to radiation therapy for cancer include (1) helping the patient and family or significant others cope with the diagnosis of cancer and its treatment with radiation therapy, (2) minimizing trauma to the skin at the site of entry and exit of radiation, and (3) teaching the patient and significant others how to recognize and manage the expected side effects of radiation.

Helping Patients Cope With Radiation Therapy for Cancer. Most people have a rather limited knowledge of radiation and how it affects cells, normal or otherwise. A lack of knowledge about the side effects of radiation and how to cope with them can greatly add to the anxiety and stress that the patient feels. It is not unusual for a layperson to have some misconceptions about how radiation works, whether a patient can present a hazard to others while undergoing treatment, when he will begin to experience its effects, and how long it will be before he begins to recover from them.

Before the first treatment the patient is told what therapeutic effects are anticipated, what it is like to have a treatment, and what is expected of him during the course of therapy. Because the patient will probably be treated on an outpatient basis, he should be encouraged to keep his scheduled appointments and notify the clinic if he is unable to come when expected. He should also be assured that the source of radiation is in the machine only, and that he cannot "contaminate" others with radioactivity. He should be encouraged to have someone accompany him for each treatment, preferably a family member or a close and trusted friend. Whatever questions he and the person with him wish to ask must be respected and answered to their satisfaction. It is essential that time be set aside for the nurse to establish a trusting relationship with the patient and to communicate with him throughout his course of treatment.

Teaching the patient and significant others how to recognize expected side effects and take an active part in their management is particularly important when the patient is not hospitalized. He will feel less helpless and more in control when he is able to participate in assessing his condition and planning and implementing his care at home. It is unfair to expect either the patient or his significant others to remember everything they are told about his care. Therefore it is essential that they have some written information to refer to once they leave the clinic. They also should be encouraged to write down any questions they might have before the next visit or any points on which they feel they need more information.

In general, most side effects will not begin before a week to 10 days after the first treatment. This will allow the patient time to assimilate the information given to him and to adjust to whatever changes he might experience. The side effects usually continue throughout the course of therapy and begin to subside about 14 days after treatments end.

Minimizing Trauma to Skin. Although the reaction of the skin to therapeutic radiation is similar to a sunburn, it is unwise to use the term *burn* when speaking of irritation of the skin and mucous membranes that sometimes accompanies radiation therapy. The patient should understand that such a side effect is expected and is usually only temporary.

In preparation for radiation therapy the physician will outline the area to be exposed to radiation by marking it with indelible ink or by protecting surrounding areas with a plaster cast or mold or a lead shield. The exposed area may be very fragile and tender and will need special care. Most clinics and hospitals have written procedures and precautions to be used to avoid unnecessary trauma to the exposed areas of skin.

In general, the area is not washed any more than absolutely necessary throughout the course of treatments. When the area is cleansed, a mild unscented soap and tepid water are used. Alcohol, lotions, and salves must not be used, as they either dry out the skin or magnify the radiation damage. If the radiologist will allow a softening agent such as lanolin, pure aloe vera gel, Natural Care gel, desoximetasone (Topicort) ointment, or A and D ointment to be used, he will indicate this in writing.

The patient should be instructed to avoid lying on the area as much as possible and to avoid wearing tight clothing over it. He also should avoid exposing it to sunlight and extremes of cold as well as heat. Areas of damaged skin that are weeping should be cleansed with plain lukewarm water or saline, and a polyethylene film or Vigilon dressing should be applied. Such dressings are removed before the next radiation treatment and then reapplied.

The degree of reaction of the skin to radiation should be assessed daily, either by the patient himself or some other knowledgeable person. There usually is a reddened area resembling a sunburn about 1 week after the first treatment. Later, the skin may appear tanned and might begin to peel. A more severe reaction is blistering and loss of epithelium. The degree of reaction determines what, if anything, should be done. Most of the time all that is necessary is to protect the skin from further injury and allow it to heal once the course of radiation is completed.

Recognizing and Managing Expected Side Effects. Because of the nature of the treatment, side effects from radiation therapy are common. Many patients receiving some form of radiation for control of cancer will experience some degree of skin reaction at the sites of entrance and exit of the radiation. In addition, they will have some loss of appetite and fatigue.

Anorexia often is associated with inflammation of the mouth and tongue and changes in the sense of taste, which can cause the patient great difficulty in eating and drinking. The loss of appetite can quickly lead to deficiencies of protein and calories. The patient with anorexia can experience a significant weight loss (2 or more pounds per week) and suffer from severe malnutrition. A thorough routine for mouth care to minimize damage and anorexia should be started several days before the beginning of radiation therapy.

Weight loss can also occur in cancer patients because of disturbances in their metabolism in which the body metabolizes its own proteins for energy instead of utilizing carbohydrates available in the diet or in body fat.

Initially, the patient's current weight should be noted and recorded and compared with the ideal weight for him. His protein intake should be increased to compensate for the fact that cancer patients often metabolize their own tissues for energy even though glucose may be readily available in the blood. Small, frequent feedings, attention to his preference for foods, and a pleasant and restful environment during meals are often helpful. Supplemental feedings to provide additional protein and calories can help avoid excessive weight loss and protein deficiency. Table 13–5 shows some commonly used supplemental feedings.

An essential part of nursing intervention for anorexia in cancer patients is assessment of the mucosa of the mouth and tongue. The special mouth care needed by some patients receiving radiation therapy is discussed below.

The problem of fatigue may alter the patient's lifestyle slightly or to a great extent. After assessing the extent to which fatigue interferes with the patient's being able to do what he wants to do, the nurse plans with him some realistic goals for periods of rest. Together they can devise ways to conserve his energy and to balance rest with the activities he enjoys.

Coping With Specific Side Effects of Radiation. The specific side effects that can occur will depend on the areas of the body to which the radiation has been administered. It is essential, then, that the nurse assess each patient's status and the location and degree of reaction to radiation and teach the patient how to recognize and deal with these site-specific reactions.

Radiation to the scalp can cause alopecia (loss of hair). The total dose of radiation determines whether the hair loss will be minimal or excessive, temporary or permanent. When less than 3,000 rads are administered, the hair loss can be minimized by gently washing, brushing, and combing the hair. If the dose is larger and the patient has a great loss of hair, wigs, scarfs, and hairpieces can be used to help the patient cope with the psychological impact of sudden baldness. Irritation of the scalp may occur, causing dryness and scaling. K-Y jelly or Natural Care gel will help this condition; both are water soluble. The condition should begin to improve 10 to 14 days after treatment has ended.

Radiation to the head or neck will produce some inflammatory changes in the mouth and often also in the pharynx and esophagus. Measures to combat this expected reaction include frequent oral intake of liquids that are not irritating chemically or otherwise—for example, very hot or highly seasoned liquids; the use of artificial saliva; and frequent and consistent mouth care.

Patients are encouraged to drink water as often as they can to help alleviate the discomfort of

TABLE 13–5 NUTRITIONAL FORMULAS AND PREPARATIONS FOR SUPPLEMENTAL FEEDING

Product Name/ Company	Serving Size	Approx. Content Per Serving: *Cals.*	Approx. Content Per Serving: *Gms Protein*	Special Characteristics
Ensure/Ross	8 oz	250	8.8	Lactose- and milk-free, contains soy protein
Isocal/Mead Johnson	8 oz	250	8.1	Lactose-free, contains soy product
Isomil/Ross	10 oz	200	6.0	Lactose-free, contains soy product
Meritene/Doyle	8 oz	250	14.5	Contains milk
Neo-Mull-Soy/ Syntex	10 oz	200	5.0	Milk- and lactose-free, contains soy protein
Prosobee/Mead Johnson	10 oz	200	7.5	Lactose-free, contains soy protein
Sustacal/Mead Johnson	12 oz	360	21.7	Lactose-free, contains soy protein
Instant Breakfast/ Carnation	1 packet	290	16	Contains milk and soy protein, high lactose
Citrotein/Doyle	1.14 oz	127	7.67	Egg albumin base, lactose-free
Sustacal Liquid/ Mead Johnson	1 packet	360	21.7	Contains milk, high lactose
Sustacal Pudding/Mead Johnson	5 oz	240	6.8	Contains milk

Data from Eating hints: Recipes and tips for better eating during cancer treatment. Bethesda, MD, U.S. Department of Health and Human Services, National Institutes of Health, 1982.

dryness of the mouth and tongue. Extra water also helps the body eliminate the debris from destroyed cells. However, drinking water will not completely resolve the problem. Artificial salivas combat mouth dryness in a different way and help keep the mucous membranes soft and moist. They also help buffer the acidity in the mouth and thus reduce irritation of the oral mucosa. They are available in the form of a spray and can be used by the patient as often as he desires. If artificial salivas cannot be found at a local pharmacy, they can be obtained from any one of the following pharmaceutical companies: Kingswood Laboratories, Inc., Westport Pharmaceutical, Inc., and First Texas Pharmaceuticals, Inc.

A major goal of mouth care, other than protection of the mucosa, is preservation of the teeth and prevention of infections of the gums. To accomplish this, the patient should be encouraged to accept as much responsibility as he can for frequent and consistent oral hygiene. He probably will need to be taught how to brush his teeth using a soft brush and gentle strokes. He also should be taught how to irrigate his mouth to remove debris and counteract acidity. The solutions most often used for this are normal saline, mild solutions of peroxide (1 tbsp. in an 8-oz glass of water), or a bicarbonate of soda solution (½ tsp of baking soda in an 8-oz glass of water). Commercial mouthwashes are not necessary and can be chemically irritating and drying. Fluid intake must be increased to 3,000 mL per day. Viscous lidocaine (Xylocaine) can be used as a mouth swish before meals to decrease discomfort.

Radiation to the chest or upper back can cause inflammation of the esophagus with accompanying nausea and indigestion. Esophageal inflammation is managed as just described in regard to radiation of the head and neck. Management of nausea and vomiting is discussed in Chapter 8. Inflammation of the lung, however, presents a real threat to the patient because of the danger of infection and inadequate aeration of the lungs. Humidifying the air, maintaining an adequate fluid intake, and carrying out coughing and deep breathing exercises daily can help minimize the effects of pneumonitis. Prevention of infection is especially important, and thus the patient must try to avoid contact with persons who have colds and other viral and bacterial infections of the respiratory tract.

Nausea and vomiting and diarrhea are common reactions to *radiation of the abdomen and lower back*. They occur as a result of irritation of the mucous membranes lining the digestive tract. Care of the patient with nausea and vomiting and the patient with diarrhea is discussed in Chapter 8. Another common reaction to radiation of the pelvic area and lower back is cystitis. Measures that can help minimize or alleviate urinary cystitis include increasing fluid intake, promptly emptying the bladder when there is the urge to void, and avoiding foods and beverages that are known to irritate the bladder. Further information on cystitis can be found in Chapter 22.

Internal Radiation Therapy

As previously explained, internal radiation therapy involves introducing a radioactive element into the body. The material may be administered in different ways: (1) it can be placed in a *sealed* container and inserted into a body cavity at the site of the tumor or directly into the tumor or (2) it may be administered in an *unsealed* form and taken orally or injected by syringe.

Cesium is a radioactive element frequently used to treat malignancies of the mouth, tongue, vagina, and uterine cervix. Figure 13–4 shows some of the applicators used for insertion of radium into the vagina and cervix. The illustration also shows capsules in which the cesium is sealed and ready for insertion into the cervix.

Examples of unsealed sources include iodine 131, which is in a solution and is swallowed by the patient, and gold 198, which is administered by injection. Radioactive iodine is useful in the treatment of thyroid malignancies because that gland readily takes up iodine. Thus the radioactive element is delivered to the site of the tumor, where it can be more effective.

During internal radiation therapy, the patient is a source of radiation, because the radioactive element is in his body.

Not all elements that have been made radioactive by artificial means stay radioactive for very long periods. As soon as an element becomes radioactive, it begins to lose its characteristic of radioactivity. The rate at which it becomes less radioactive is called its *half-life*, which is the

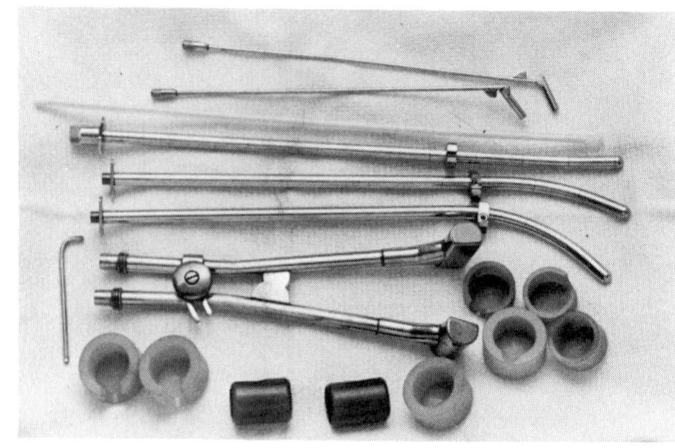

Figure 13–4 Commonly used applicators for gynecologic sealed-source radiation therapy.
(Photo by Ken Kasper.)

amount of time it takes for half of its radioactivity to dissipate.

The half-life of radium is about 1,600 years, whereas the half-life of iodine is only about 8 days. It is important that the nurse caring for a patient receiving sealed or unsealed sources of radiation know the element used, its half-life, and the ways in which it might be eliminated from the body.

Nursing Care of Patients Receiving Internal Radiation

Patients who are treated by internal sources of radiation can be a source of radioactivity. Those who are in close contact with them must therefore take special precautions to protect themselves against unnecessary radiation. Radioactivity is a frightening phenomenon to most people, because they do not fully understand it and are misinformed about how it affects the body.

The effects of radiation may be divided into *short-term* and *long-term effects.* Short-term effects result from relatively large doses received over a short period. These include localized skin burns, fever, hemorrhage due to destruction of bone marrow, diarrhea, fluid loss, and central nervous system dysfunction. The long-term effects may appear years after exposure and usually occur in individuals who have received small doses over an extended period. These include shortened life span, predisposition to leukemia and other malignancies, and development of cataracts. When radiation is directed toward the gonads, genetic mutations may arise. Fetuses cannot tolerate as much exposure as can adults; therefore pregnant women should avoid caring for patients receiving radiation therapy.

When considering the hazards and effects of radiation therapy, one should avoid complacency on the one hand and total panic or paralyzing fright on the other. After all, humans have always been exposed to radiation in their environment. We are continuously bombarded with radiation from the sun's rays, and there are naturally occurring radioactive materials in the earth and therefore in the foods we eat and the water we drink. This does not mean that we should be content with haphazard efforts toward protection or complacent about the dangers of excessive radiation. Nurses simply must put these dangers in their proper perspective; for example, although we know that oxygen supports combustion and creates a fire hazard when it is administered to a patient, we still administer it, taking the necessary precautions during oxygen therapy so that the patient may enjoy its benefits.

It is also important that the nurse know whether the radioactive element is sealed and inserted into the body to remain for a certain time, or if it is an unsealed source that may be eliminated through body secretions and excreta. Unsealed sources usually have a very short half-life, which means they are not radioactive for as long as sealed sources are.

Principles of Radiation Protection

In general, the amount of radiation a nurse might receive while caring for a patient being treated with radioactive elements depends on three factors: (1) the distance between the nurse and the patient, (2) the amount of time spent in actual proximity to the patient, and (3) the degree of shielding provided.

Distance is an important factor in reducing exposure to radiation. By doubling one's distance from a radioactive element or x-ray beam, the exposure is reduced to one fourth, and tripling the distance reduces it to one ninth (Fig. 13–5).

Time spent near the source of radiation can be controlled by the nurse who plans her nursing care carefully so that she can spend less time with the patient without sacrificing the quality of care given (Fig. 13–6). The occasions for application of this principle will most often be those in which the patient is hospitalized for implantation of a radioactive element.

Shielding from radiation exposure must take into account the type of rays being emitted. The more dense the shielding material, the less the possibility of penetration by the rays and the better the protection. A lead shield that is 1 cm thick offers the same amount of protection as 5 cm of concrete or 30 cm of wood. Portable lead shields can be used to provide some protection for the nurse caring for a patient who is confined to bed for implantation therapy (Fig. 13–7). Lead aprons give protection from diagnostic x-rays but do not provide adequate shielding from the *gamma rays* emitted by radium, cesium 137, and cobalt 60. Anyone coming into contact with or proximity to a source of radiation should wear a radiation dosimeter badge. This badge measures the exposure to radiation the individual has received.

Precautions for Sealed Sources. Hospitals where sealed sources of radiation are implanted into the body tissues to treat malignancies usually have written policies and procedures to guide personnel who are responsible for patient care. The precautionary measures listed below cover general areas of concern.

- Place a sign on the patient's door indicating that the patient is receiving internal radiation therapy.
- Observe principles of time and distance. Limit time spent in the room. Work as quickly and

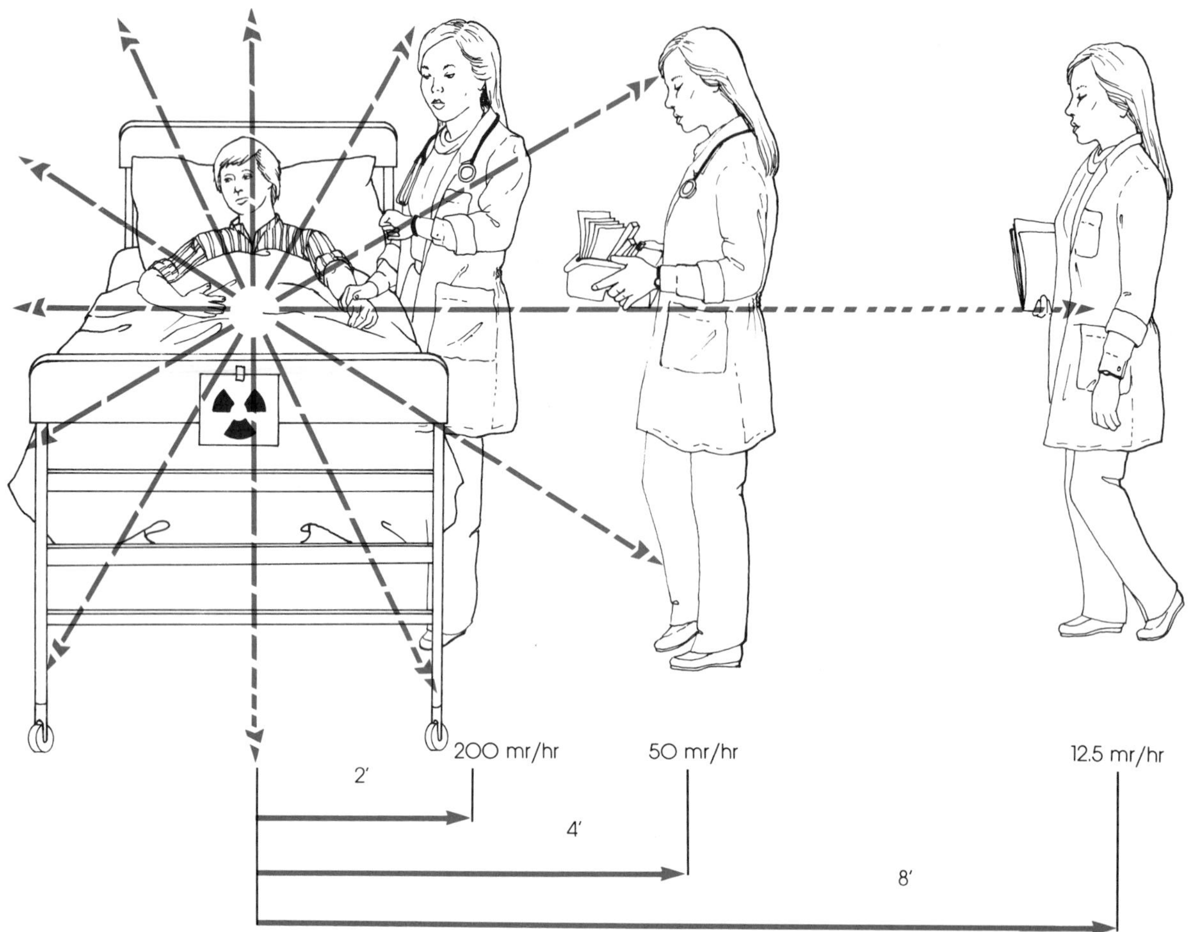

Figure 13-5 The nurse nearest the source of radioactivity (the patient) is more exposed; at two feet, exposure is more than 15 times that at eight feet.

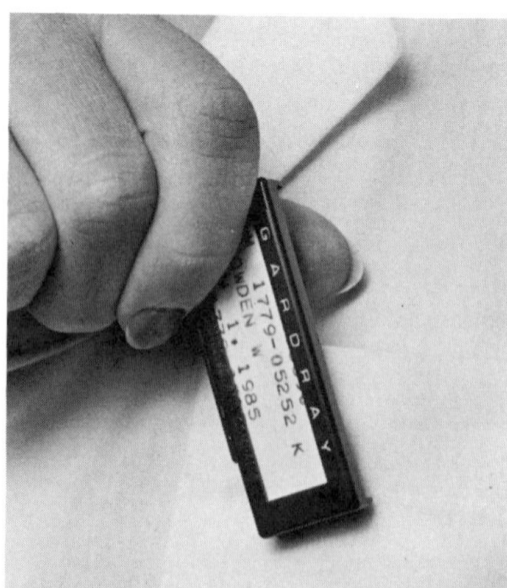

Figure 13-6 Badge worn by personnel who might be exposed to radiation. The badge records a cumulative dose of radiation and is used to monitor exposure over a period of time (for example, 1 month).
(Photo by Ken Kasper.)

as efficiently as you can. Avoid standing near the part of the patient's body where the radioactive element is located.

- Check all linens, bedpans, and emesis basins routinely to see if the sealed source has been accidentally lost from the tissue.
- If a sealed source is dislodged, but has not fallen out of the patient's body, notify the physician at once. If the source has fallen out, *do not pick it up with your bare hands.* Use forceps and place it in a lead container.
- Most patients are placed on bed rest and instructed to remain in certain positions so that emanations from the element will reach the correct area.
- Visitors will be limited in the amount of time they can stay in the room.

After the physician removes the source, the patient is no longer in need of special precautionary care. Special observations are necessary, however, in the event a systemic reaction develops. In addition to the anorexia, nausea and vomiting, diarrhea, and urinary frequency that were mentioned previously, the patient also may

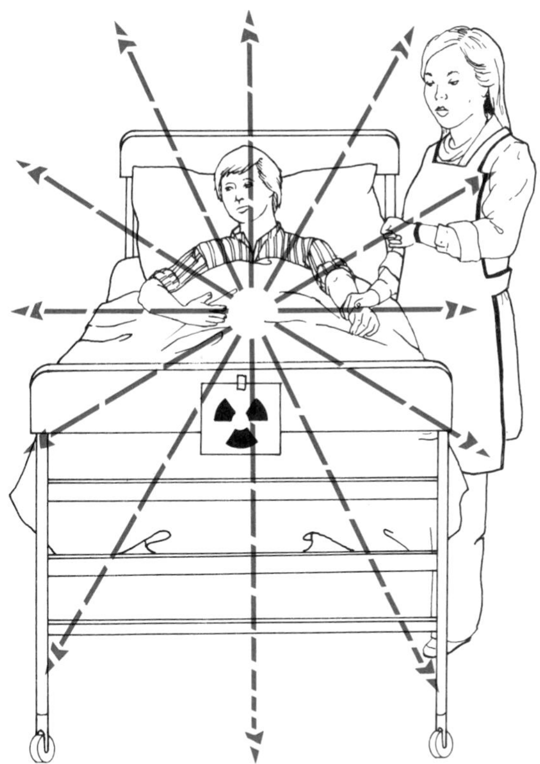

Figure 13-7 Wearing a lead apron will reduce the nurse's exposure to radiation.

develop an elevated temperature. Should any of these symptoms appear, the physician should be notified. Patients receiving radiation therapy are easily dehydrated, and thus a record should be kept of their intake and output and their hydration status.

Precautions for Unsealed Sources. The most commonly prescribed unsealed sources of radiation are iodine 131, phosphorus 32, and gold 198. The radioactive element is in a solution; it is not sealed in a container. The solution may be taken orally or injected into a vein or a body cavity. It is eliminated through body secretions such as sweat, sputum, vomitus, urine, and feces. The major hazard from radioactive iodine is in the patient's urine; therefore special precautions must be taken according to hospital policy. Again it is stressed that hospital policies and procedures must be followed when caring for a patient receiving an unsealed source of radiation.

Some special precautions that should be observed when caring for a patient receiving internal radiation therapy from an unsealed source are listed below.

- Observe the principles of time, distance, and shielding for radiation protection.
- Wear gloves when handling bedpans, bed linens, and patient's clothes.
- Dispose of urine, feces, and vomitus according to policy.
- Handle dressings with forceps and dispose of them according to policy.
- Follow hospital procedure for disposal of patient's bed linens and clothing.

CHEMOTHERAPY

The oncologist has a wide variety of drugs from which to choose when planning a course of treatment for a patient with cancer. He may choose to give a particular drug alone or in combination with other drugs. Chemotherapy also is used with other forms of therapy—for example, following surgery and before, during, or after radiation treatments and immunotherapy.

Among the drugs used to treat malignancies are the *antineoplastic* agents. The overall effect of antineoplastic drugs is to decrease the number of malignant cells in a generalized malignancy, such as leukemia, or to reduce the size of a localized tumor and thereby lessen the severity of symptoms. Antineoplastic drugs are *cytotoxic* (poisonous to cells), and their damaging effects are not limited to malignant cells. However, normal cells do not reproduce in exactly the same way as malignant cells and are able to repair themselves more rapidly and effectively.

Chemotherapy is the preferred treatment for various kinds of leukemias, some lymphomas, multiple myeloma, and many types of tumors resulting from metastasis.

The specific aim of many antineoplastic agents is to attack malignant cells in one of the four major phases of their reproductive cycle. These are called *cell-cycle-specific* drugs, and include mitotic inhibitors (vinblastine and vincristine), and antibiotics such as bleomycin and mithramycin. Some cell-cycle-specific drugs affect metabolic activities of the cell; these are called *antimetabolites*. Examples of antimetabolites include folic acid antagonists such as methotrexate sodium (MTX), purine antagonists such as 6-mercaptopurine (6-MP), and pyrimidine antagonists such as cytosine arabinoside.

Cell-cycle-nonspecific drugs can destroy cells in all phases of the cell cycle, resting or proliferating. Examples of cell-cycle-nonspecific drugs include the alkylating agents, nitrosuoureas, cisplatin, and dacarbazine. Other drugs used for the treatment of cancers include the hormones such as estrogens, progestins, androgens, and corticosteroids.

Newer techniques of administration of antineoplastic agents include intraarterial, intraperitoneal, intraventricular, and intrathecal infusion. Cancers of the liver, ovary, and brain have sometimes shown better remission with infusion treatment. Another advance in chemotherapy is the use of lower doses of multiple drugs to treat various types of malignancies. Because side effects are lessened when lower doses of a drug are used, several drugs can be used in combination to hit all phases of the cell cycle, destroying more malignant cells.

Nursing Care of Patients Receiving Chemotherapy

Nursing management of the patient receiving chemotherapy requires special knowledge and skills beyond those of basic nursing. The nurse oncologist is a specialist who is able to give comprehensive nursing care because of years of study and experience. A full discussion of care of the patient receiving chemotherapy is therefore beyond the scope of this text. There are, however, some general principles that can be helpful to the nurse who encounters a patient receiving a course of chemotherapy for cancer or experiencing some of the toxic side effects of antineoplastic drugs.

Not all neoplastic drugs produce every toxic side effect, and the oncologist plans therapy so that destruction of malignant cells is maximized and toxicity is kept at a minimum. The toxicity associated with chemotherapy is most evident in the cells of the body that have a short life span and must continuously reproduce to provide the body with the normal cells it needs. These include the blood cells, hair follicles, and epithelial cells of the mucous membranes lining the digestive tract.

The more common toxic side effects of chemotherapy and their implications for nursing are summarized in Table 13–6. Some of the toxic side effects of chemotherapy are similar to the expected effects of radiation. Although the causes of the problems are different, assessment of the patient and symptomatic relief measures are the same.

Nursing interventions for selected problems in a patient receiving chemotherapy for cancer are summarized in Nursing Care Plan 13–1.

THERAPY USING BIOLOGIC RESPONSE MODIFIERS

Biologic response modifiers (BRMs) are agents that manipulate the immune system in hopes of controlling or curing a malignancy, with little or no toxic effect on normal cells. These agents either stimulate or suppress immune activity. There are basically three groups of such agents. The first group includes interferons, interleukins, the bacille Calmette-Guérin (BCG) vaccine and *Corynebacterium parvum*, and tumor antigens, which work to restore, modulate, or augment immune activity in the body. The second group includes monoclonal antibodies and tumor necrosis factor, both of which have direct antitumor effects. Genetic engineering techniques can produce the monoclonal antibodies, and thus this form of therapy holds much promise for the future.

The third group contains miscellaneous agents that have different functions. Some stimulate undifferentiated cells into maturing so that they can be more easily killed; others prevent metastasis.

All the biologic response modifiers are still undergoing clinical trials to determine effectiveness on various types of malignancies. They are not without side effects, but the most common side effects are fatigue and flulike symptoms such as fever, chills, muscle aches, and headache, which are much less life-threatening than some of the side effects of chemotherapy.

PHOTODYNAMIC THERAPY

Photodynamic therapy is currently used for bladder cancer. A photosensitizing substance is given intravenously. This agent concentrates in the tumor tissue, and then a laser beam is used to destroy the cells. The tumor cells are much more sensitive to this light source than normal tissue and therefore can be sought out and destroyed. Clinical trials are in progress for treatment of other types of tumor cells by this method.

NURSING DIAGNOSES

Nursing diagnoses that may be appropriate for the patient with cancer include:

- Alteration in nutrition (less than body needs), related to increased metabolic demand and nausea, vomiting, diarrhea, or mucositis.
- Potential for infection related to bone marrow depression from therapy.
- Impaired skin integrity related to surgical or radiation therapy.
- Disturbance in body image related to weight loss or hair loss.
- Potential for injury to patient, staff, and visitors related to exposure to radioactive implant.
- Impaired physical mobility related to restricted activity because of radioactive implant.
- Diarrhea related to effects of cancer treatment.
- Constipation related to effects of chemotherapy.
- Activity intolerance related to fatigue.
- Knowledge deficit related to drugs and side effects.
- Self-care deficit related to weakness and fatigue.
- Fear related to possibility of dying.

TABLE 13-6 **TOXIC SIDE EFFECTS OF CHEMOTHERAPY, ASSESSMENT, AND NURSING INTERVENTIONS**

Toxic Effect	Nursing Assessment	Nursing Intervention
Lowered resistance to infection due to leukopenia.	Monitor lab data for WBC count less than 3,000 and granulocyte count of less than 2,000. Notify physician if temp. reaches 101°F, especially if accompanied by chills. Observe for early signs of infection.	Teach patient good personal hygiene, mouth care, and proper care of nails. Help patient avoid contact with infectious agents: reverse isolation may be indicated.
Impaired clotting due to thrombocytopenia.	Monitor lab data for platelet count of less than 100,000. Observe for hematuria, bruising, bleeding into joints.	Keep trauma at a minimum. Give stool softener to prevent straining at stool and episodes of bleeding during Valsalva maneuver. Modify diet to avoid irritating foods. Avoid IM injections whenever possible. If IM injection is necessary, apply pressure to site after puncture. Do not take temperature rectally.
Alopecia due to chemical damage to hair follicles.	Obtain history of onset; determine what he has done to minimize hair loss, how he has coped with balding up to now.	Teach patient to avoid further trauma from hair dryers, curlers, permanent wave solutions, dyes, and bleaches. Instruct patient to comb and brush hair gently. Apply head tourniquet, hypothermia cap to inhibit blood flow and access of chemicals to hair follicle cells during chemotherapy. Encourage patient to use scarf, wig, or hairpiece during transient period of hair loss. Remind patient that alopecia is temporary in most cases.
Potential for injury due to nerve damage by chemicals	Observe for poor coordination, unsteady gait, constipation, hoarseness, ptosis. Obtain data about loss of sensation, changes in pattern of bowel elimination, clumsiness, needing help to climb stairs, get into and out of car.	Protect from falls. Assist patient when walking. Use fecal softeners to combat decreased peristalsis. Give diet high in fiber. Teach patient to avoid strain on vocal cords by limiting speech and speaking softly.

- Ineffective individual coping related to denial of significance of cancer.
- Ineffective family coping related to inability to function as a result of anxiety over patient's prognosis.

EVALUATING THE EFFECTIVENESS OF MEDICAL TREATMENT AND NURSING INTERVENTION

MEDICAL TREATMENT

The oncologist conducts an ongoing evaluation of each patient's status to determine how effective the prescribed treatment has been and to plan for a future course of therapy should it be needed. He is particularly interested in knowing whether there has been a reduction in the size of the tumor and an abatement of the patient's symptoms.

A newer test for monitoring the effectiveness of treatment is a measurement of carcinoembryonic antigen (CEA) levels. This particular antigen is a glycoprotein that is produced during fetal life but is not normally present after birth. Its production may resume again, however, and CEA levels can be increased by some kinds of liver disease, heavy cigarette smoking, and benign and malignant tumors. Because of the many and diverse conditions that can elevate CEA levels, the test cannot be used to diagnose cancer. However, it can be used to evaluate the effectiveness of treatment, because CEA levels usually fall to

.. the normal range about 1 month after successful treatment of cancer. If the serum CEA level is higher than normal prior to treatment and remains elevated after treatment, this suggests that there are malignant cells remaining in the body.

NURSING INTERVENTION

The relief and remission of symptoms and the patient's ability to cope with his diagnosis of cancer and the problems it may bring about are of primary concern to the nurse. The Oncology

NURSING CARE PLAN 13–1

Selected nursing diagnoses, goals/outcome criteria, nursing interventions, and evaluations for a patient receiving chemotherapy for cancer

Situation: Harold Pole is receiving chemotherapy for leukemia. This is his third round of weekly intravenous treatments. His platelet count is down to 185,000; he has had difficulty eating as a result of mucositis and anorexia. He states that he is mildly nauseated most of the time. He is 15 pounds underweight.

Nursing Diagnosis	Goals/Outcome Criteria	Nursing Intervention	Evaluation
Potential for infection related to bone marrow suppression. SUPPORTING DATA Receiving chemotherapy drugs that suppress bone marrow.	Patient will remain free of infection.	Monitor WBCs (more susceptible to infection when <3,000 and granulocyte count is <2,000. Assess for signs of infection every shift. Teach good hygiene, mouth care, hand washing before meals and after using bathroom. Restrict visitors; allow no one to visit who has an infection. Use protective isolation techniques if needed. Encourage good nutrition and hydration.	WBCs, 3,200; temp. 98.8°F; no signs of infection; visitors monitored; taking sufficient food and fluid; continue plan.
Potential for injury related to impaired blood clotting ability. SUPPORTING DATA Chemotherapy treatment lowers platelets and causes extended bleeding time.	Patient will not experience hemorrhage.	Monitor blood count; assess for bruising and bleeding into joints q shift. Observe for signs of bleeding: hematuria, melena, etc. Give stool softener as ordered to prevent straining at stool and bleeding. Refrain from needle sticks as much as possible. Do not take temperature rectally.	No signs of bleeding; platelet count 180,000; stool softener administered; BM soft.
Alteration of nutrition (less than body requirements), related to nausea, vomiting, and mucositis.	Patient will verbalize relief from nausea. Patient will be able to eat with minimal discomfort. Patient will maintain present weight.	Keep room odor free; give mouth care before meals. Give ordered antiemetic before and during chemotherapy. Use distraction, meditation, relaxation techniques. Give small, frequent feedings. Assess mouth and mucous membranes q shift. Give meticulous mouth care every 2 hours. Give antiemetics on a regular schedule during chemotherapy treatment times. Encourage added calories in meals and food supplements between meals.	Mouth care: 7, 9, 11, 1, and 3 o'clock; antiemetic 45 min before meals; mucous membranes reddened, but intact; enriched shake between meals taken; has not vomited this shift; continue plan.

NURSING CARE PLAN 13-1, *Continued*

Nursing Diagnosis	Goals/Outcome Criteria	Nursing Interventions	Evaluation
Body image disturbance related to alopecia and weight loss. SUPPORTING DATA "I look awful; I don't want any visitors to see me."	Patient will adjust to new body image within 3 weeks as evidenced by verbalization.	Encourage him to maintain sense of humor. Use wig, scarfs, eyebrow pencil, and false eyelashes as needed; assure him that hair will eventually grow back. Encourage verbalization of feelings; focus on strengths. Establish and maintain trusting relationship. Assess spiritual needs; help patient achieve spiritual consolation. Encourage him to obtain clothing that fits.	Has not yet lost hair; checking on purchase of wig; family is bringing in head scarfs; talking more about feelings regarding weight loss and appearance; continue plan.
Fear related to diagnosis of cancer. SUPPORTING DATA "Do you really think the treatment will cure my cancer?" "I'm afraid that I'll go through all this and it will just come back in a few months."	Patient will verbalize fears and develop coping mechanisms to decrease fear.	Encourage verbalization and identification of specific fears. Help him to explore ways to cope with fears. Assess spiritual needs; contact chaplain or other as patient desires. Offer support by active listening, offering hope in some form, and being there for patient. Encourage expression of fears to significant others.	Is verbalizing fears; encouraged to do same with family; used to meditate; encouraged to do so; began teaching imagery techniques; continue plan.

Nursing Society has developed a set of standards for the practice of cancer nursing and prepared outcome criteria and rationales for each standard. The complete set of standards, outcome criteria, and rationales can be obtained from the American Nurses' Association, 2420 Pershing Road, Kansas City, MO 64108.

Patient care that is systematically planned and coordinated is certainly the goal of all nursing care. Although nurses who specialize in oncology nursing are expected to have a greater depth of knowledge and to function as leaders in the care of cancer patients, all nurses should have an understanding of the standards of practice and the long-term goals of cancer nursing. The 11 standards proposed by the Oncology Nursing Society are presented in Table 13–7 so that the reader can make a meaningful contribution to the achievement of the stated goals and will be better able to evaluate the effectiveness of her own efforts to meet the published standards.

SOURCES OF HELP FOR THE CANCER PATIENT AND FAMILY

Through the efforts of professional health care providers, laypersons, and governmental and voluntary associations, there is an abundance of resources for the cancer patient and his family. In view of the standards of care listed in Table 13–7, it is apparent that there is a need for utilizing some of the resources to help the patient and family learn about his illness and get the support they need while trying to cope with his diagnosis and treatment.

Family, friends, individuals, and community groups are among the sources of support and encouragement that the cancer patient might need to care for himself and attain some level of independence and peace of mind. Two excellent references for help in locating existing support

TABLE 13–7 **STANDARDS OF ONCOLOGY NURSING PRACTICE**

Professional Practice Standards

I. Theory
The oncology nurse applies theoretical concepts as a basis for decisions in practice.

II. Data Collection
The oncology nurse systematically and continually collects data regarding the health status of the client. The data are recorded, accessible, and communicated to appropriate members of the multidisciplinary team.

III. Nursing Diagnoses
The oncology nurse analyzes assessment data to formulate nursing diagnoses.

IV. Planning
The oncology nurse develops an outcome-oriented care plan that is individualized and holistic. This plan is based on nursing diagnoses and incorporates preventive, therapeutic, rehabilitative, palliative, and comforting nursing actions.

V. Intervention
The oncology nurse implements the nursing care plan to achieve the identified outcomes for the client.

VI. Evaluation
The oncology nurse regularly and systematically evaluates the client's responses to interventions in order to determine progress toward achievement of outcomes and to revise the data base, nursing diagnoses, and the plan of care.

VII. Professional Development
The oncology nurse assumes responsibility for professional development and continuing education and contributes to the professional growth of others.

VIII. Multidisciplinary Collaboration
The oncology nurse collaborates with the multidisciplinary team in assessing, planning, implementing, and evaluating care.

IX. Quality Assurance
The oncology nurse participates in peer review and interdisciplinary program evaluation to assure that high-quality nursing care is provided to clients.

X. Ethics
The oncology nurse uses the *Code for Nurses** and *A Patient's Bill of Rights*† as guides for ethical decision making in practice.

XI. Research
The oncology nurse contributes to the scientific base of nursing practice and the field of oncology through the review and application of research.

* American Nurses Association: Code for Nurses with Interpretive Statements. Kansas City, MO, 1985.
† American Hospital Association: A Patient's Bill of Rights. Chicago, 1972.
From American Nurses Association and Oncology Nursing Society, 1987: Standards of Oncology Nursing Practice. Kansas City, MO, American Nurses Association. Reprinted with permission.

groups in a community are (1) Blumberg, B. D., and Flaherty, M.: Services available to persons with cancer. JAMA, *244*(15):1715, 1980; and (2) Hartman, J. B.: *Taking Time: Support for People with Cancer and the People Who Care for Them.* Bethesda, MD, U.S. Department of Health and Human Services, 1987 (NIH Publication No. 88-2059).

Local chapters of the American Cancer Society and American Lung Association have a wide variety of services available to professionals and laypersons interested in care of the cancer patient. These include an annotated bibliography of public, patient, and professional information and education materials, pamphlets and booklets, and audiovisual programs. To obtain materials from the American Cancer Society, one can write or call the nearest ACS division. The national office number is 1-800-877-1710. In addition, there are more than 3,000 local ACS unit offices in the United States and Puerto Rico. The local telephone directory carries a list of local unit offices in the area. There also may be a regional Cancer Information Service that provides information about local resources for specific problems, such as pain control. For information, one can call 1-800-4-CANCER.

If there is a local hospice program, the services provided might include professional volunteers who visit the patient in his home and provide care the family is not able to give, and lay volunteers who help meet the emotional, social, and spiritual needs of the terminally ill patient and his family. Additionally, some hospitals and proprietary health care agencies provide home health care as an extension of hospital care after discharge.

Table 13–8 lists some of the organizations that can provide assistance and the kind of aid and services available.

TABLE 13-8 **COMMUNITY RESOURCES**

Organization	Financial Aid	Equipment	Miscellaneous
American Cancer Society	$25 per month, up to $200 per year for medication for relief of pain Reimbursement of 6 cents per mile (if patient can arrange own transportation) Reimbursement of $25 per month for 3 months of colostomy expenses	Hospital beds and equipment Dressings Prostheses Miscellaneous supplies	Recruitment of volunteers to take clients to health care facility Free educational information on any cancer Rehabilitation programs Reach to Recovery Nu-Voice Club Ostomy Association I Can Cope
Cancer Information Center			Provides educational materials for the lay and professional person
Hospice Programs			Provide care to the terminally ill
Leukemia Society	Limited funds for monetary assistance Reimbursement up to $600 per year for chemotherapy		Transportation assistance to health care facilities
Miriam Foundation	Monetary aid for cosmetic items (wigs, prostheses)		
Peregrine Society	Reimbursement up to $100 per month for cancer-related medications	Supply Sustagen and Ensure (nutritional aids) Dressings Beds, wheelchairs Catheters Colostomy and postoperative appliances	Transportation to clinics for treatments

From Dwyer, J. E., and Held, D. M.: Home management of the adult patient with leukemia. Nurs. Clin. North Am., Dec., 1982, p. 671.

BIBLIOGRAPHY

Amenta, M. O., and Bohnet, N. L.: Nursing Care of the Terminally Ill. Boston, Little, Brown, 1986.

American Cancer Society: Cancer Facts and Figures—1991. Atlanta, 1991.

American Nurses' Association and Oncology Nursing Society: Standards of Oncology Nursing Practice. Kansas City, 1987.

Anderson, J. L., and Brown, M. L.: The cancer patient in the community: A nursing challenge. Nurs. Clin. North Am., June, 1980, p. 373.

Beare, P. G., and Myers, J. L.: Principles and Practice of Adult Health Nursing. St. Louis, C. V. Mosby, 1990.

Blank, J. J., et al.: Perceived home care needs of cancer patients and their caregivers. Cancer Nurs., April, 1989, p. 78.

Camp-Sorrell, D.: Controlling adverse effects of chemotherapy. Nursing 91, April, 1991, p. 34.

Cawley, M. M.: Recent advances in chemotherapy: Administration and nursing implications. Nurs. Clin. North Am., June, 1990, p. 377.

Collins, P. M.: Tumor markers and screening tools in cancer detection. Nurs. Clin. North Am., June, 1990, p. 283.

D'Agostino, N. S.: Managing nutrition problems in advanced cancer. Am. J. Nurs., Jan., 1989, p. 50.

Gullatte, M. M.: Nursing management of external central venous catheters. Adv. Clin. Care, July/Aug., 1990, p. 12.

Hogan, C. M.: Advances in the management of nausea and vomiting. Nurs. Clin. North Am., June, 1990, p. 475.

Hydzik, C. A.: Late effects of chemotherapy: Implications of patient management and rehabilitation. Nurs. Clin. North Am., June, 1990, p. 423.

Ignatavicius, D. D., and Bayne, M. J.: Medical-Surgical Nursing. Philadelphia, W. B. Saunders, 1991.

Malloy, J.: Administering intraperitoneal chemotherapy: A new approach. Nursing 91, Jan., 1991, p. 58.

Mayer, D. K.: Biotherapy: Recent advances and nursing implications. Nurs. Clin. North Am., June, 1990, p. 291.

McGown, K. L.: Radiation therapy: Saving your patient's skin. RN, June, 1989, p. 24.

Muller, R. A., and Pelczynski, L.: You can control cancer pain with drugs but the proper way may surprise you. C. E. Test Handbook, Vol. 3, 1987–1988. Springhouse, PA, Springhouse Corp., p. 43.

National Cancer Institute: Eating hints: Recipes and tips for better nutrition during cancer treatment. Publication no. 87-20079. Bethesda, MD, 1987.

Oncology Nursing Society: Standards of Oncology Nursing Education. Pittsburgh, 1989.

Schlesselman, S.: Understanding oncologic emergencies. Adv. Clin. Care, July/Aug., 1990, p. 21.

Spindler, J.: Seeing through the mask of cancer. Nursing 91, May, 1991, p. 37.

Strohl, R. A.: Radiation therapy: Recent advances and nursing implications. Nurs. Clin. North Am., June, 1990, p. 309.

Tenenbaum, L.: Cancer Chemotherapy: A Reference Guide. Philadelphia, W. B. Saunders, 1989.

Valente, S. M., and Saunders, J. M.: Dealing with serious depression in cancer patients. Nursing 89, Feb., 1989, p. 44.

Weisman, A. D.: Coping With Cancer. New York, McGraw-Hill, 1979.

Ziegfeld, C. R., ed.: Core Curriculum for Oncology Nursing. Philadelphia, W. B. Saunders, 1987.

STUDENT STUDY AIDS

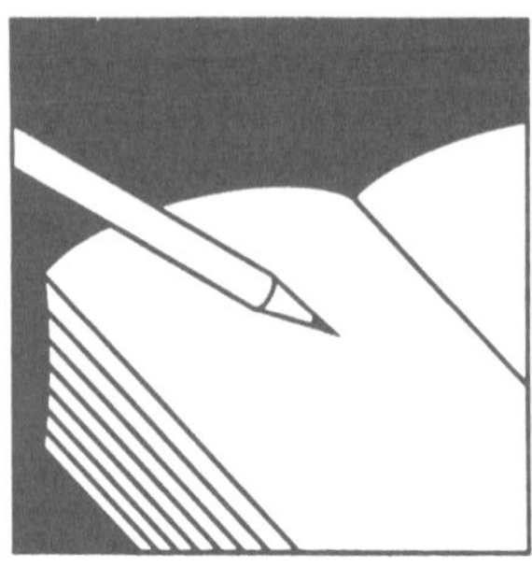

CLINICAL CASE PROBLEMS

Read each clinical situation and discuss the questions with your classmates.

1. An acquaintance tells you that she has had a mole on her back for several years and it appears to be getting larger and darker. She admits that it could be malignant, but she argues that there is no point in going to a physician, because there is nothing to be done for cancer, and she does not want to burden her family with doctor bills and hospital bills that will not accomplish anything.

- What is your obligation as a nurse in regard to encouraging this person to see a physician at once?
- What is your own attitude toward cancer and the treatment of the disease?

---

2. Mrs. Allgood went to her physician for a regular physical checkup and was told that she had malignant cells in the cervical secretions obtained for a Papanicolaou smear. She had a biopsy of the cervix, and this, too, proved to contain malignant cells. She was admitted to the hospital, cesium was implanted in the cervix, and Mrs. Allgood was kept isolated during the treatment.

- If you were assigned to give A.M. care to this patient, what special precautions would you take to protect yourself from excessive radiation?
- What would be some signs and symptoms that you would watch for to determine whether Mrs. Allgood is having either a local or a systemic reaction to radiation?

---

3. Mary is a 19-year-old college student receiving chemotherapy for bone cancer. Identify *specific* problems you would expect Mary to have, and state the measures you would suggest to help her deal with them.

---

4. Mr. Hopkins, age 66, has metastatic lung cancer. He is to undergo radiation therapy.

- What would you tell Mr. Hopkins the treatments will be like?
- What instructions would he need regarding the inked target lines and skin care?
- What precautions should Mr. Hopkins take regarding use of deodorants, type of clothing, and exposure to the sun?
- What type of side effects might Mr. Hopkins experience with radiation therapy to the chest?
- What nursing interventions would be appropriate for the above side effects?

STUDY OUTLINE

I. The impact of cancer

A. Cancer is not a single disease; it is a large group of over 100 diseases that have very little in common.

B. Malignancies are the second leading cause of death in the United States.

C. Three out of every eight persons who developed cancer in 1986 will be alive 5 years after diagnosis.

D. More lives could be saved by early detection and prompt treatment.

II. Characteristics of neoplastic growths

A. Comparison of benign and malignant growths.

1. Benign growths are almost always encapsulated.
2. Benign growths can create problems by pressing against and interfering with functions of adjacent organs, but do not metastasize.
3. Malignant cells are the result of transformation of normal cells, probably because of change in the cells' DNA.
4. Growth of malignant cells is not regulated; they and their offspring are disorganized and uncontrollable by normal mechanisms.
5. Most but not all malignant cells metastasize.

B. Classification of tumors.
   1. Typed according to the kinds of tissue from which they arise.
   2. Suffix *-oma* simply means tumor. Lipoma is a tumor arising from fatty tissue.
   3. Sarcomas arise from mesenchymal tissues; carcinomas from epithelial tissue.
   4. Leukemias and lymphomas are cancers of blood-forming organs.
   5. Malignancies of pigment cells of skin are melanomas.
   6. More precise identification made by adding modifying prefixes; for example, osteo- (bone) sarcoma.

C. Metastasis: movement of cells to a distant site.
   1. Extent to which malignant cells have spread influences prognosis.
      a. Localized ("in situ") at original site.
      b. Regional—extended to lymph nodes.
      c. Advanced—spread throughout the body.
   2. Staging system: (T) primary tumor, (N) regional nodes, (M) metastasis.

III. Causative factors

A. There is no one specific cause of cancer. It is not one disease but many kinds of malignancies.

B. Susceptibility influenced by age, familial tendency, exposure to carcinogens, and immunocompetence.

C. There is a relationship between dietary intake and the occurrence of some kinds of cancers.

D. Carcinogens include chemicals, radiation, and physical irritation. Viruses also play a role in cancer development, probably by introducing new genetic material into a normal cell and transforming it into a malignant cell.

E. Predisposing factors for the development of cancer:
   1. Genetic predisposition is evident in breast and some types of colon cancer.
   2. Age, sex, and race are predisposing factors for certain types of cancer: black men have more prostate cancer; cervical cancer is higher in black women; breast cancer is more prevalent in white than in Oriental women.
   3. Herpes simplex virus 2 and some forms of the human papillomavirus that are transmitted sexually are linked to cervical cancer.
   4. Stress decreases efficiency of the immune system and seems to make certain people more susceptible to cancer.

IV. Scope of cancer nursing

A. Classification system can help nurses assess and identify each patient's needs. Categories range from those who are being tested to confirm or exclude a malignant diagnosis to those in the terminal stages of advanced cancer.

B. Assessment of a cancer patient can be overwhelming. Nurse keeps in mind the purpose of her assessment and the specific kinds of information she needs to give individualized nursing care.
C. Many nursing diagnoses may be appropriate, but they must be individualized to the patient (see Nursing Care Plan 13–1).

V. Prevention and early detection

A. Avoiding and limiting exposure to carcinogens.
B. Identifying high-risk persons.
C. Screening large segments of a population to identify malignancy in its early stages.
D. Encouraging self-examination of the breasts and testes.
E. Increasing general public's awareness of the seven safeguards against cancer.
F. Encourage routine checkups as recommended by the American Cancer Society.

VI. Diagnosis of cancer

A. Biopsy—microscopic examination of living cells. Can give a definitive diagnosis of malignancy. Other test results suggest cancer.
B. Radiologic studies:
   1. Radiographs.
   2. CT scanning.
   3. Radionuclide studies.
   4. Mammography.
C. Endoscopy: direct visualization.
D. Laboratory tests: blood analysis, acid and alkaline phosphatase levels, tumor markers.
E. Informing the patient of a diagnosis of cancer.
   1. Ninety-eight percent of physicians surveyed have policy of telling the patient the truth.
   2. Cancer patients interviewed also say they would rather know their diagnosis.
   3. Manner in which patient is told is important.
   4. Any nurse in close contact with a cancer patient should know whether patient has been informed of his diagnosis.

VII. Treatment of cancer and nursing implications

A. Surgery—removal of malignant growth and adjacent tissue. Newer techniques less traumatic and mutilating.
B. External radiation. Sources—high-voltage x-ray machine, radioactive element such as cobalt 60 housed in a shielded unit, linear accelerator; Gamma knife.
   1. Nursing care of patients undergoing external radiation therapy:
      a. Helping patient cope with side effects of radiation.
         (1) Instruct patient and significant others in purpose and goals of radiation therapy.
         (2) Assure patient he cannot be a source of radiation for others.
         (3) Important that patient keep to scheduled treatments.
         (4) Teach patient and significant others how to recognize and take an active part in managing expected side effects.
         (5) Most side effects begin a week to 10 days after first treatment and usually continue for several weeks after last treatment.
      b. Minimizing trauma to skin.
         (1) Avoid friction, sunlight, and application of alcohol, lotions, or salves to exposed areas.
         (2) Teach patient to assess degree of reaction daily.

c. Recognizing and managing expected side effects.
   (1) Anorexia: a common side effect. Caused by irritation of mucous membranes of mouth and gastrointestinal tract and changes in taste perception, dryness of mouth, sore tongue.
      (a) Note current weight, compare with ideal weight.
      (b) Daily weight to recognize significant (2 or more pounds per week) weight loss.
      (c) Assess condition of oral mucosa; start oral care program before treatment begins.
      (d) Give small, frequent feedings; attend to preferences for food; provide restful and pleasant environment.
      (e) Give supplemental feedings as necessary to maintain adequate protein intake.
   (2) Fatigue.
      (a) Can alter patient's lifestyle.
      (b) Help patient plan realistic goals for periods of rest balanced with activities.

d. Coping with specific side effects of radiation.
   (1) Radiation to scalp—produces alopecia, usually temporary.
      (a) Teach patient to avoid harsh treatment of hair and scalp.
      (b) Encourage use of wigs, scarfs, hairpieces to maintain self-image until hair grows back.
   (2) Radiation to head and neck—inflammation of oral mucosa, pharyngitis, and esophagitis.
      (a) Encourage fluid intake.
      (b) Use artificial saliva.
      (c) Good oral hygiene, gentle tooth brushing.
      (d) Use saline, peroxide, or bicarbonate of soda solution to counteract acidity and cleanse the mouth. Avoid full-strength commercial mouthwashes.
   (3) Radiation to chest and upper back—nausea and indigestion, inflammation of lung tissue.
      (a) Humidify inhaled air.
      (b) Maintain adequate fluid intake.
      (c) Coughing and deep breathing exercises.
      (d) Avoid respiratory infections.
   (4) Radiation to abdomen and lower back—nausea and vomiting, diarrhea, cystitis.
      (a) Increase fluid intake.
      (b) Empty bladder promptly.
      (c) Avoid irritating foods and beverages.

C. Internal radiation. Source of radioactivity is in the patient's body. Source is either sealed in container or unsealed, as in liquid that is ingested or instilled.
   1. Nursing care of patients receiving internal radiation:
      a. Nurse should know effects of radiation, source being used, and where it is in the patient.
      b. Principles of radiation protection (time, distance, shielding) must be observed.
      c. Special precautions and policies and procedures of institution must be followed.
      d. If source is unsealed, for example, radioactive iodine, nurse needs to know how it is excreted and its half-life.

D. Chemotherapy. Use of drugs either alone or in combination with other drugs or other forms of therapy.

1. Overall effect of antineoplastic drugs is to reduce size of tumor and lessen symptoms.
2. Preferred treatment for leukemias, some lymphomas, multiple myeloma, and metastatic cancer.
3. Cell-cycle-specific drugs attack malignant cells at one phase of cell's reproductive cycle.
4. Cell-cycle-nonspecific drugs can destroy cells in all phases.
5. Nursing care of patients receiving chemotherapy:
   a. Not all neoplastic drugs are cytotoxic.
   b. Toxicity most damaging to cells that have a short life span, such as those in the hair follicles.
   c. More common toxic effects and nursing care are summarized in Table 13–6.

E. Biologic response modifiers.
1. Purpose of BRM therapy is to stimulate, suppress, or assist immune system to combat malignant cells.
2. Three approaches:
   a. Active nonspecific immunization: BCG vaccine, *Corynebacterium parvum*, interferons and interleukins, tumor antigens.
   b. Second group: monoclonal antibodies and tumor necrosis factor, both of which have direct antitumor effects.
   c. Third group: miscellaneous agents that have different functions; some stimulate undifferentiated cells to mature, others prevent metastasis.

F. Photodynamic therapy: photosensitizing agent given intravenously that is taken up by tumor cells; laser light is then used to destroy tumor cells.

VIII. Evaluating effectiveness of treatment and nursing care

A. Reduction in size of tumor, abatement of symptoms.
B. CEA levels.
C. Nursing intervention. Standards of oncologic nursing provided by Oncology Nursing Society.

IX. Sources of help for the cancer patient and family

A. American Cancer Society.
B. Cancer Information Service.
C. American Lung Association.
D. See Table 13–8.

CHAPTER 14

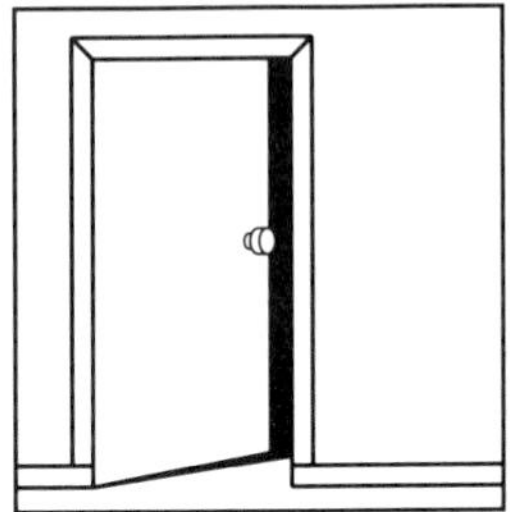

Care of Terminally Ill and Dying Patients

VOCABULARY

cephalic
ethical
euthanasia, active and passive
hypostasis
moral
rationalization
role model
reprisal
resolution
unresponsiveness

Upon completion of this chapter the student should be able to:

1. Describe the essential task of the dying patient and that of those who care for him.
2. Describe the five stages proposed in Kübler-Ross's stage theory of dying.
3. Identify nursing interventions appropriate for allaying the fears commonly experienced by the dying.
4. List five desirable attitudes and attributes of the nurse caring for a dying patient.
5. Debate the issue of a patient's right to know or his desire not to know his prognosis.
6. Describe the special physiologic needs of terminally ill patients.
7. Utilize standards of care for terminally ill patients, their families, and caregivers.
8. Define the nurse's responsibility for participating in decision making regarding issues related to death and dying.

From the beginning of human history the meaning of life and death has fascinated and perplexed philosophers, theologians, scientists, artists and writers, and ordinary people in all walks of life. Contemplation of one's own death or the death of a loved one can cause anxiety, fear, and a tentative denial of its existence, even though it is as much a part of life as birth, growth, and maturity. In a youth- and beauty-oriented society, coming to terms with human mortality is not a top priority, yet it is in the study of death that one can come to a better understanding of the meaning of life. Helping others confront and deal with death and dying and related issues can provide the helper with opportunities for personal growth and maturity.

Not too many years ago, health professionals were poorly prepared to identify and meet the needs of dying patients. There were few guidelines and even fewer role models for effectively assisting the dying. Because death was not openly and honestly discussed, most health care givers were not taught even the barest essentials of care of the terminally ill and dying. Until the 1960s it was common practice to relegate "hopelessly ill" and dying patients to back wards and other less visible places. Since it was believed that there was nothing more that medical science could do for these patients, they were essentially abandoned and left to be tended by ministers or family members or sometimes by no one at all.

Today, death and the special needs of the dying are no longer denied or ignored. Death and the process of dying have become subjects of scientific research, popular literature, and open discussion among laypersons and professionals.

In this chapter we will be talking about the clinical care of those patients for whom death is imminent. We also will consider the bereaved, those who grieve over their loss of a family member, friend, or patient.

The task of the dying patient is to work his way through psychological responses ranging from total disbelief and rejection to whatever resolution is characteristic of him. The task of the nurse and other health professionals is to help the dying person live his life as fully as possible, or as much on his own terms as possible, until he dies.

STAGES OF DYING

In 1965 Dr. Elisabeth Kübler-Ross, a renowned psychiatrist, was approached by four students of the Chicago Theological Seminary for assistance with a research project on death as a major event in human life. The subsequent interviews with patients and the conclusions drawn from the data thus obtained led Kübler-Ross to write *On Death and Dying*, which was published in 1969.

When the researchers first began their study of the phenomenon of death and its psychological impact on the dying person and those in contact with him, they often met denial, rationalization, and even open hostility on the part of the hospital staff. Under the illusion of kindness to dying patients, nurses and doctors refused to admit that there were any such patients under their care. Kübler-Ross reported that there seemed to be a thinly disguised conspiracy to protect dying patients from anyone who showed interest in openly talking with them about their approaching death.

Kübler-Ross wrote that she was hopelessly naive when she entered the wards seeking interviews with terminally ill patients. Her purpose and that of the students under her direction was to question the patients about how they felt, how they were being treated, and how they would like to be treated so that their final days could be more meaningful and less frightening.

An outcome of the studies conducted by Kübler-Ross was a stage theory of dying. These so-called stages represent the adaptive strategies of a dying person who is trying to come to grips with the finality of his terminal illness. It should be emphasized that the concept of persons going through a sequence of psychological responses to personal death does not mean that all dying persons proceed through these stages in accordance with the proposed sequence. Many patients alternate from one stage to another. Sometimes a patient will appear to have moved toward acceptance, and then some event will trigger feelings and behaviors that indicate regression toward denial.

Unfortunately, when it was first proposed, the stage theory was accepted without question and misapplied by well-intentioned persons who were desperately looking for some way to assist and provide appropriate care for the terminally ill. Death, like life, is unique to the individual. No two people share the same life experiences or have the same inner resources to deal with life's difficulties. However, knowing that there are some commonalities shared by people who confront death can be of benefit to those who care for them.

In general, the psychological responses to one's impending death begin with denial and progress through anger, bargaining, and depression to an idealized final stage of acceptance.

Acceptance may or may not be achieved no matter how good the care, nor how sensitive the support. These reactional stages are not limited to adaptation to dying. They are familiar to many of us because we experience them to some degree whenever we are faced with any important change. Every change involves some loss, the end of something familiar and the beginning of something new. If we are unhappy about the change and attendant loss, our first reaction might be to deny it and behave as if it never happened. If we adapt to the change in a healthy manner, we accept it and get on with the task of adjusting to it.

Study of the effect of death on survivors also has shed some light on the stages of grief felt by those whom the dying person leaves behind. In 1964, Dr. George Engel proposed that grief over the loss of a loved one brings about psychological responses not too different from those exhibited by patients who are themselves dying. Moreover, several authors have noted that severely handicapped and disabled persons who must abruptly change their lifestyle might also go through a process in which they move from denial, anger, and depression toward acceptance of a new way of life. The manner in which these persons adjust to the "death" of their former selves and the emergence of a new self often bears some resemblance to the adaptive stages of the dying person.

DENIAL AND DISBELIEF

The initial response to the knowledge that one is dying is shock and disbelief. The person does not seem to be able to believe that death is imminent or inevitable. Most patients initially reject the idea; the typical response to the news that they have a terminal illness is "No, not me. It's not possible." This denial of one's death is usually temporary, a kind of holding action until progression to the next stage is possible. A small percentage of patients, however, continue to deny that they are dying to the very end. *Denial can be useful if the period is used to find a way to deal with death.*

If the patient feels that family, friends, and hospital staff expect or need him to continue his denial, that they are not willing to discuss death with him, and that they prefer to ignore the issue, he will be much less likely to proceed toward acceptance. The result is that the patient is not provided the comfort of talking about his feelings and expressing his fears and anxieties about his death. He is also cheated of the opportunity to take care of unfinished business or financial matters. He is not given a chance to communicate to his loved ones certain feelings that he might have about them and his life with them, and finally, he loses some control over what happens to him in the final days of his life.

It is inevitable that nurses, who are devoted to the preservation and improvement of the quality of life, will often have difficulty finding the appropriate words and attitudes needed to help a patient through the first stage of the coping process. The nurse might have a strong desire to encourage the patient in his denial, telling him that he is going to be all right and agreeing with him that he is not dying. She probably considers such actions helpful in making it easier for the patient to pass through the final days of his life. Although it might seem a kindness to support the patient in his denial, such support is in reality a serious obstacle to his progress toward a peaceful and realistic resolution of his conflicts with the reality of death. This is not to suggest that the nurse, or anyone else, should force on the patient an acceptance of his condition or engage in arguments with him when he denies the fact that he is dying, but she should recognize denial as only the first step in a progression toward acceptance.

In all instances, the patient should be assisted through the stages of his coping process and helped to face issues as honestly as he can. The nurse need only let the patient know that she is available to talk about whatever he or she wishes to discuss. She does not force the subject on the patient.

ANGER

A second common and important response to the knowledge that one's life is ending is that of frustration and anger. The patient no longer denies the fact that he is dying. Instead, he asks, "Why me?" It seems unfair to him and he retaliates by becoming belligerent, uncooperative, and critical of those around him. Visiting relatives and friends may irritate him; they may visit too often, not enough, or at the wrong time. The physician is not prescribing the right medicines and treatments and might, in fact, be seen by the patient as the one who is responsible for his impending death. Nurses, too, become objects of abuse and criticism. Efforts to comfort the patient, such as a back rub or straightening the bed linen, might be met with an angry outburst or a surly "Get out of here and leave me alone." One is tempted, of course, to take the patient at his word and leave him isolated in his room, left to his own devices. Sometimes, one might feel that the only sensible response is one of reciprocal anger toward the patient, giving him exactly what he asked for. Neither of these responses to his anger will be of much help. He does not intend his remarks to be taken personally. The anger he feels is not directed toward any one person but toward circumstances and events over which he has no control and against which he feels helpless. When a dying patient wants to express his anger and rage it is best to let him do just that—say whatever he feels, cry, curse, scream, or do whatever he needs to do to release his pent-up feelings.

It should be noted that sometimes the very things nurses do or say in an effort to be helpful can be the most annoying to the patient who is terminally ill. For some patients, the efficient, smiling, healthy nurse who bustles cheerfully about the room serves as a source of irritation simply because she *is* healthy and full of life. Through no fault of her own she represents the things he is losing. The patient might see her as a reminder that he is unattractive and no longer free to escape the restrictions his illness has imposed upon him.

The dying patient has a need for self-esteem, as do all human beings. Basic to this feeling are his needs for some degree of physical comfort, for acceptance of him and his condition as they are, to be able to express angry feelings, and to speak out about whatever is causing those feelings.

Many people *never* get past the anger stage. Anger is certainly the most characteristic and long-lasting response to the certain knowledge of one's own imminent death. The nurse should always keep this in mind. Many dying people remain angry while they have the energy and then go into a withdrawal as they become weaker when death approaches.

BARGAINING

The bargaining stage, if it occurs, may follow the anger phase closely. The patient says, "Yes, me, but. . . " and then begins to make some kind of arrangement whereby he gives something in order to gain more days of life. Kübler-Ross observes that most bargaining is done with God and that it often is a promise in exchange for prolongation of life. For example, the patient might vow to change his way of life, to become more generous, or to give up something valuable as payment for a few more months or years.

The classic example of bargaining given by Kübler-Ross is the terminally ill patient who suffered severe pain, requiring medication around the clock. One day she asked if it would be possible for her to leave the hospital to attend her son's wedding. Permission for the day's leave of absence was granted, and the patient went to the wedding, remained free of pain during the entire day, and returned that evening. As soon as the patient saw Kübler-Ross she said, "Don't forget, Dr. Kübler-Ross, I have another son." Kübler-Ross cited this as the briefest, quickest example of the bargaining stage that she could give.

DEPRESSION

In another stage, the patient drops the "but" and recognizes that the facts cannot be escaped. "Yes, me . . . " he says, and by that he means that he knows he is approaching the end of his life. He may become depressed and begin to grieve for all that he knows he will soon lose. When he admits this and can face the reality of his loss, he may be able to grieve and mourn his loss.

Many patients become silent in this stage. They sit quietly, tears rolling down their faces, or sob uncontrollably when they are alone. Many do prefer to be alone in their grief, asking that visitors not come because they do not want to talk with anyone. The patient who is silently grieving may be more difficult to cope with than the one who is venting his anger. There seems to be so little one can say to console him and so little one can do to comfort him. All one can do is listen, to "be there." The nurse can provide companionship and allow him to express his grief in his own way without fear of reprimand or ridicule. She strives to maintain communication with the patient, letting him know by her presence that she is aware of his suffering and that she is concerned for him. She gives him permission to withdraw, accepting his efforts to cope with the problem on his own for a while as a natural process.

ACCEPTANCE

In some cases the patient may consciously and openly accept his imminent death and find some degree of peace within himself. Kübler-Ross describes acceptance as different from resignation or resentful giving-in to the inevitable forces of "fate." In acceptance the patient is not what we commonly understand as happy but appears to have come to terms with his struggle with fear and grief. He seems to be indicating that he knows that death is near and that it is all right. He is willing to stop resisting death and to rest quietly. The "acceptance" described by Kübler-Ross is seldom seen in practice.

In the last days or hours of life, the patient might choose only one person with whom he wishes to spend his remaining time. He wants only the comfort of being with a loved one or someone he trusts. He appreciates having a time of togetherness that does not necessarily involve extensive conversations or expressions of his feelings. Although his depression might appear profound, it is a natural state and should not be cause for alarm or indication of a need for psychiatric help.

It must be remembered that the stages of the Kübler-Ross coping mechanism are not clearly defined in every patient who is dying. The limits of time have little relevance to these stages; some patients might not have sufficient time to progress to acceptance. Others might rapidly progress through all the stages within a very short period, sometimes within hours. Some others might seem calmly accepting and after a symptom-free day go back to denial.

Recent research studies indicate that all terminally ill patients exhibit some withdrawal or depression shortly before dying. Two explanations are suggested:

- The depression is the result of an increase in the severity of symptoms or the loss of a body part.
- The physical decline of the patient results in energy depletion and decreased ability to make sense of and cope with environmental stimuli.

It is likely that both factors are responsible.

FEARS EXPERIENCED BY THE DYING PERSON

Dying persons typically experience some specific fears about what is happening to them and how they will be treated by others during their final days and hours.

Williams (1978) has identified three common fears of persons who know they are dying: fear of pain, fear of abandonment, and fear of meaninglessness.

FEAR OF PAIN

Pain and death are almost synonymous in the minds of many people. Perhaps they have been influenced by literary references to "the throes of death," the "last agony," and other phrases melodramatically describing the final moments of human existence. Whatever the source of fear of the pain of death, there is no basis for the assumption that physiologic pain necessarily accompanies death. There is the psychological pain of separation, anxiety, and depression associated with the dying process, but physical agony and mental torment are not inevitable companions of death.

The patient who is terminally ill and does have physical pain must be assured that medication is available to him when he needs it. This assurance is followed up with prompt response to his reports of pain and discomfort. The medication for pain need not cloud the patient's mind and deprive him of meaningful interaction with others. Allowing the patient to take part in deciding the frequency and strength of dosage helps diminish the fear that when the pain returns, relief will not be available. Pain medication regimens are individualized for each patient.

Noninvasive techniques of pain control can be utilized to prevent or alleviate the pain of the terminally ill and can be combined with administration of pain medication. Relaxation techniques, meditation, imagery, therapeutic touch, massage, and other methods can be very effective in helping to control pain in a majority of patients.

Whatever medications and noninvasive techniques are used to either prevent or alleviate the pain of the terminally ill, they must be administered with compassion and understanding of the complexity of the phenomenon of pain. In general, the goal should be to prevent the pain, rather than wait for it to occur and then attempt to relieve it.

Addiction, which is sometimes a concern of nurses who administer frequent doses of a narcotic, is not a valid concern when there is no hope for recovery from an illness and death is inevitable. The nurse should always try to mentally put herself in the patient's shoes when considering pain control issues.

Relatives and friends of the dying patient often are relieved to know that everything possible is being done so that the patient will not suffer. They also need assurance that the final moments of a person's life are more likely to be tranquil than turbulent, and he is more likely to be unconscious or semiconscious than fully aware of what is happening.

Table 14–1 gives the dying person's bill of rights.

FEAR OF LONELINESS AND ABANDONMENT

In their study of the dying, thanatologists have found that those who are approaching death usually do not want to be left alone. Many are afraid of being abandoned, because they sense that others cannot bear the spectacle of their death or are not equipped to deal with a dying person or one who is sick, incontinent, and emaciated. They seem to be afraid that no one will witness their departure from this life, that no notice will be taken of their going. It is especially comforting to the patient if there is someone he knows and trusts sitting calmly and lovingly at his side. Nothing need be said or done unless the patient specifically requests it. He may ask for and be comforted by prayers, or he may want to share his own thoughts. He may ask to be remembered or to have a message given to someone who cannot be with him at the moment. There may also be hours and days when he wants no communication at all—maybe just a pat now, a sip of water then, or the bedclothes straightened. Whatever is done while staying with a person who is dying, the purpose of providing human presence and companionship is to give him a sense of security and peace.

FEAR OF MEANINGLESSNESS

This third fear of the dying has to do with being afraid that one's life really had no meaning. There is regret that so many good intentions

TABLE 14–1 A DYING PERSON'S BILL OF RIGHTS

The person who is dying has the right to
- be treated as a person until death.
- caring human contact.
- have pain controlled.
- cleanliness and comfort.
- maintain a sense of hope whatever its focus.
- participate in his care or the planning of it.
- respectful, caring medical and nursing attention.
- continuity of care and caregivers.
- information about his condition and impending death.
- honest answers to questions.
- explore and change religious beliefs.
- maintain individuality and express emotions freely without being judged.
- make amends with others if desired and settle personal business.
- terminate with family members and significant others in private.
- assistance for significant others with the grief process.
- withdraw from social contact if desired.
- die at home in familiar surroundings.
- die with dignity.
- respectful treatment of the body after death.

were never acted on, so many noble thoughts were never expressed, and so many golden opportunities to make a difference in this world were missed. Each of us could say the same about our own lives, but then we expect to have another chance. We can look forward to tomorrow and perhaps to future opportunities to do the things we think give meaning and purpose to our lives.

The dying person needs to know that he has done some things right in his life. Even the most desolate and self-deprecating of patients respond to mention of the positive aspects of their lives. Relatives and friends can be asked to jog their memories and reminisce with the patient about the happy times spent together and the good deeds done by the patient. This can assure him that he will be missed and that others will remember him kindly.

The nurse herself can point out something favorable about the patient that she has noticed while caring for him. Perhaps he has retained his sense of humor, talked about his great love for a son or daughter, exhibited great patience during tedious procedures, or shown concern for and kindness toward other patients on the unit.

Religious practices and rituals can have great significance for some patients, though others might not share these beliefs and are not consoled by them. Whatever the patient's religious and philosophic orientation, the prayers, thoughts, and feelings that give comfort to him and help him find purpose and meaning in his suffering should be identified and made available to him. The nurse remains nonjudgmental, respecting the beliefs of her dying patient regardless of whether they conflict with or are in accord with her own beliefs and personal convictions.

HOPE AND DESPAIR IN THE DYING PATIENT

The dying patient typically experiences a high level of tension between hope and despair, the will to live and the desire to die. Hope looks to the future and provides comfort in the conviction that whatever is wished for will be attained. Absence of hope can lead to despair and loss of the will to live. The dying patient is particularly vulnerable to feelings of despair, even though hope persists to some degree regardless of what it is that the patient looks forward to.

Clinicians who have studied the emotions and attitudes of the terminally ill tell us that these patients rarely give up all hope of recovery. Even those who have apparently accepted the reality of their impending death seldom deny the possibility of a last-minute reprieve through a newly discovered drug or treatment.

The hopes expressed by these patients lift their spirits during difficult times and can give meaning to the suffering they endure. At first, the patient might want to think that his illness is not really serious or that a wrong diagnosis was made. Later he might hope that a treatment can be found that will cure his illness or at least prolong his life. Finally, he might find assurance in believing that he will continue to exist and have life after death. Not every person can accept the concept of an immortal soul that enters into another form of life after this one. For many people the words *everlasting life* have little meaning until they are confronted with the reality of their own death, and even then they might question whether immortality of the soul has any relevance to their own situation. Another patient might believe in reincarnation or a totally different spiritual framework. The nurse must respect the patient's beliefs and not try to impose her own religious beliefs on him.

Whatever the patient chooses to believe and rely on as his source of confidence, he has the right to and a need for the hope of something better than what he is presently experiencing. The nurse can listen to and perhaps share in the patient's experience of optimism, but she must be honest and cannot give him false expectations for recovery or cure when realistically there are none. What she can do is give him hope for a better day tomorrow, hope of a good laugh about something that happens, hope of obtaining a favorite food or seeing a favorite person, or even hope of seeing an especially beautiful sunrise or sunset. There are so many small things that are pleasurable that can happen in one day of life. Even hope of a few small pleasant things can sometimes lift the patient's spirits. The creative, thoughtful nurse can find some way to bring a little pleasure and hope to a terminally ill patient's day.

Death itself can be a welcome relief and actively sought by a patient. However, the nurse must be careful not to give the patient the impression that she agrees that his death would be desirable and therefore is willing to "give up" on him. In some situations the patient may put his desire into action and ask the nurse to make it easier for him to end his life (commit suicide), or to end it for him (active euthanasia). Feigenberg writes that an appeal for a quick end to life, either by suicide or an act of euthanasia, is not really a request for death but a cry for help. It is an indication that the support the patient needs to get him through the dying process is not available to him.

COMMUNICATION WITH THE DYING PATIENT

Not every patient who is dying wants to talk about himself and what is happening to him, and there are times when even the most outspoken of patients would rather remain silent and aloof. It is important, however, that the patient have opportunities for companionship, conversation, and ventilation of his feelings. He should be allowed to choose the time, the topic, and the person with whom he wishes to communicate.

Nonverbal communications can be as meaningful as verbal ones, if not more meaningful. A gentle touch, a willingness to spend time with the patient, and an attitude of patience and acceptance can convey compassion and concern. Terminal illnesses often are accompanied by deterioration of body tissues, unpleasant sights and smells, and messy lesions and discharges. If the patient sees that the nurse is not repulsed by these problems and is willing to make an effort to keep him clean and presentable, he is assured by her actions that she has not chosen to abandon him.

In her dealings with the dying patient it helps both the nurse and the patient if she can maintain a sense of humor in spite of the gravity of the situation. Everyone appreciates occasional comic relief from unrelenting grief and tragedy. Humor and laughter should be natural and healthful parts of everyone's life. The patient who is dying is still living. He still can enjoy whatever contributes to the fullness of his life in his final days, laughing or crying, being creative or appreciating creation, giving love or receiving it.

Nurses who have had extensive experience working with the dying agree that the best way to develop skill in clinical thanatology is through reading actual case histories and first-hand experience meeting the challenges and rewards of caring for patients who are approaching death. Some brief case situations and a suggested reading list are presented at the end of the chapter. Desirable attitudes and personal attributes of nurses and others who care for the dying are summarized in Table 14–2.

A touching and informative plea of a young student nurse longing for communication with and companionship from her fellow nurses is presented below. It is typical of the kinds of reading that can help the inexperienced nurse know and appreciate the psychological needs of the dying. The article was published anonymously in the February 1970 issue of the *American Journal of Nursing* and has been reprinted many times.

> I am a student nurse. I am dying. I write this to you who are, and will become, nurses in the hope that by sharing my feelings with you, you may someday be better able to help those who share my experience.
>
> You slip in and out of my room, give me medications and check my blood pressure. Is it because I am a student nurse, myself, or just a human being, that I sense your fright? And your fears enhance mine. Why are you afraid? I am the one who is dying!
>
> I know you feel insecure, don't know what to say, don't know what to do. But please believe me, if you care, you can't go wrong. Just admit that you care. That is really for what we search. We may ask for why's and wherefore's, but we really don't expect answers. Don't run away—wait—all I want to know is that there will be someone to hold my hand when I need it. I am afraid. Death may be routine to you, but it is new to me. You may not see me as unique, but I've never died before. To me, once is pretty unique!
>
> If only we could be honest, both admit our fears, touch one another. If you really care, would you lose so much of your professionalism if you even cried with me? Just person to person? Then, it might not be so hard to die—in a hospital—with friends close by.

THE PATIENT'S RIGHT TO KNOW

A terminally ill patient's right to know his diagnosis and prognosis is directly related to his ability to give informed consent to whatever medical and surgical treatments are being contemplated by health professionals. There seems to be no question that the patient who asks about

TABLE 14–2 DESIRABLE ATTITUDES AND ATTRIBUTES OF NURSES AND OTHERS WHO CARE FOR THE DYING

1. High sense of purpose in life; comfort with personal philosophy of life, religious beliefs, or value system.
2. Consciously aware of own feelings about death and able to remain nonjudgmental when talking with patients who have different value systems; comfortable dealing with death.
3. Listen actively and encourage patient's expressions of his feelings; comfortable with silence.
4. Remain calm when patients exhibit agitated or angry behavior; accepting of such behavior.
5. Comfortable with own body image and sexuality; demonstrate forthrightness.
6. Highly flexible and creative; can function independently.
7. Good sense of humor, which is used appropriately.
8. Acceptance without show of distaste of manifestations of physical deterioration; willing to touch and minister to the dying body with compassion.
9. Assess the physiologic needs of dying patients, alter nursing care as appropriate, and obtain assistance from other disciplines as needed.
10. Comfortable with own limitations.

his condition has a right to know. It is generally agreed that if the patient is informed about the nature of his illness and the treatments prescribed for it, he will be better able to take care of himself and actively participate in planning his medical and nursing care. Problems arise, however, when members of the health care team do not agree on what or when the patient should be told, do not know what he has been told, or are not aware of or do not care about the patient's wishes in the matter.

Some patients do not want to know the seriousness of their condition.

Every patient has a right to know the expected outcome of his illness, if that is what he wants, but he has a corresponding right to not want to know.

Most patients who are dying already know that they are dying, but not every patient wants to talk about or be completely informed about his condition. If it is apparent that the patient does not want to openly admit and talk about his impending death, his wish must be respected. This does not mean, however, that he might not change his mind and ask for information later on. Lines of communication are always kept open so that the patient is always free to ask questions and express his thoughts and feelings.

Some dying patients do want to be fully informed. They want to know approximately how long they have to live and what is likely to happen during the final stages of their illness. Knowing his true status gives the patient an opportunity to maintain some control over his life, plan for his survivors, make peace with his family and his God, if applicable, and settle his business and financial affairs while he is still able to do so.

Everyone in close contact with the patient should be informed as to whether the patient knows his diagnosis and prognosis. If he says he wants to know "the truth" but senses that some people are not being entirely honest with him and are evading his questions, his trust in them will be badly damaged, if not destroyed. Any therapeutic relationship with a patient, dying or otherwise, must be based on mutual trust and respect.

PHYSIOLOGIC DEATH AND THE DYING PROCESS

Thanatologists make a distinction between death and the process of dying. In his discussion of what death means, Kastenbaum (1977) points out that death might be described as an event, a state, or an analogy. It does not have the same meaning for everyone, nor does it have precisely the same emotional impact. *Dying is a completely subjective and private experience.* For some it is a separation from all hope of companionship; for others it is an opportunity to rejoin those who have gone before them and to be with their God and Father in heaven. Cultural and religious differences can cause us to misunderstand the death-related behavior of others. Those who care for the dying patient must be aware that in order to understand what death means to another person one must listen and observe attentively and nonjudgmentally.

Dying is not, like death, a static event that occurs at a specific moment in time. It is, rather, a physiologic and psychosocial process that can take place in a matter of minutes, hours, or months. Dying is actually a stage of life. Thinking philosophically about dying, one might say that we begin the process of dying from the moment we are born. From the medical point of view, the process of dying begins when a person has a disease that is untreatable and inevitably ends in death or is in the final stages of a disease that is fatal.

If it is evident that a patient's disease is untreatable and he is considered to be in the terminal stages of disease, it is the responsibility of the nurse to speak to the physician about the possibility of a "do not resuscitate" (DNR) order. If no such order is written in the chart, all medical personnel are legally responsible for making every effort to resuscitate the patient in the event of a cardiac or respiratory arrest. The physician should be the one to speak to the patient and family about whether a DNR order should be written. For a terminally ill patient who wishes to be released from his body, going through the process of CPR, which is both painful and frightening, seems an insult to his dignity and only prolongs his low-quality existence.

Signs that death has actually occurred are the result of the disintegration of cell structures. There is a loss of body heat, stagnation of the blood, and rigidity (rigor mortis). Because of the medicolegal and ethical problems associated with continuing life-support systems and obtaining viable organs for transplantation, it has become necessary to establish some criteria by which to judge whether brain death or irreversible coma is present.

The most widely accepted of these criteria were developed during several medical conferences held in the late 1960s at Harvard Medical School. They are as follows:

- Coma with cerebral unresponsiveness unrelated to drug depression or hypothermia.
- Cessation of movement and breathing, including no spontaneous breathing for 3 minutes after artificial ventilation is discontinued.
- Dilated and fixed pupils.
- Absence of cephalic responses and brain stem reflexes.

Repetition of testing is customary, and the electroencephalogram is recommended for confirmation of brain death. If there is a flat encephalogram reading at the time of presumed death and a second flat reading 24 hours later, the person can be declared dead.

NURSING ASSESSMENT AND INTERVENTION

When a person is terminally ill, all the body systems gradually become less able to maintain their specific functions of protection and adaptation. The patient becomes progressively weaker, more prone to infection and injury, and more likely to suffer some degree of discomfort.

Assessment of a dying patient's physiologic status and diagnosis of his specific nursing care needs is essentially the same as for any patient with a pathologic condition. In the early stages of the process the patient may be able to do many things for himself and should be encouraged and helped to do so. As he becomes more debilitated and more dependent, he will need increased support so that he is more comfortable physically and psychologically.

The following nursing interventions are presented according to body systems for purposes of convenience. Not every dying patient will have the same needs for nursing intervention.

THE SKIN AND MUSCULOSKELETAL SYSTEM

As the terminally ill patient's physical condition declines, he loses protective fat, his skin becomes more fragile, and he is therefore more subject to pressure sores. As his muscles weaken he is less able to move himself about in bed in order to relieve pressure and assume a more comfortable position. Nursing interventions for the prevention of pressure sores and positioning the patient for comfort have been covered in Chapter 9. Whatever is done for the patient should be done with extreme gentleness and care to avoid further damage to the skin.

We all move about in bed to get comfortable, even when we are asleep. The terminally ill patient may lack the strength and energy to change his position and must rely on the nurse to do this for him. Although the process of moving him might cause some discomfort, most patients are more relaxed and better able to rest and sleep when their positions are changed often. The frequency with which a patient should be turned depends on his general condition and capacity for turning himself without assistance. All nursing measures to provide comfort, protection, and good personal hygiene should be scheduled as far as possible according to a patient's individual needs, rather than the routine times allotted for bathing, turning, feeding, and other aspects of personal care. Seek the help of family members or volunteers to help with personal care. Many times family members feel more comfortable around the patient if they can be doing things for him, rather than just sitting and wondering what to say. Both family members and volunteers can be extremely helpful in augmenting the care the staff nurses have time to give to the patient.

Pillows, blanket rolls, towels, and padded footboards are used to support the body and limbs in good alignment. It might be necessary to pad the siderails so as to prevent bruises and injury to the skin.

Muscular weakness also can lead to urinary and fecal incontinence, and there usually is diaphoresis. All these situations necessitate frequent sponging, partial baths, and changes of linen to keep the patient dry and free of offensive odors. Common sense dictates that sponging and bathing for the sake of cleanliness do not take priority over the patient's need to rest undisturbed.

Dressings should be changed as often as necessary to minimize unpleasant sights and smells. Room deodorizers are helpful, but using one odor to cover up another should never be considered the primary method of dealing with odors. All soiled dressings and linens must be removed from the patient's room or bathroom promptly. It is important to the patient's self-esteem that he not view himself as repulsive to others.

The profuse sweating that often occurs in the final days or hours of life is the result of diminishing blood flow. The perspiration cools the body surface, no matter how hot or cold the environment might be. Body temperature will begin to rise, and the patient is likely to feel hot even though his skin is cold. He may kick away covers and toss or attempt to remove bed clothing that is too hot. Lighter clothes, fresh circulating air, and only a light cover can help make him more comfortable. The top cover should not be tucked tightly over the lower extremities, as this can restrict movement and cause discomfort.

It is difficult for relatives and others less familiar with the dying process to understand that even though the patient's skin feels cold, he may feel uncomfortably hot. A simple explanation for the light, loosely fitting covers and clothing usually is all that is necessary to calm any fears they might have that the patient does not feel comfortably warm.

If the patient is able to respond to questions, he can indicate whether he wants more or less warmth. If he is not able to respond, the nurse should look for clues in his bodily movements, such as pulling at covers to remove them or drawing himself up and huddling his body to preserve warmth.

GASTROINTESTINAL SYSTEM

As muscle tone diminishes, the involuntary muscles of the gastrointestinal tract become more sluggish, causing accumulations of flatus and feces and possibly nausea and vomiting. An antiemetic medication might be given to help relieve the nausea. Other measures include taking sips of water or ginger ale, eating ice chips, and frequent mouth care. Care of the patient with nausea and vomiting is discussed in Chapter 8.

Bowel and bladder elimination should be monitored carefully in order to detect early signs of such problems as abdominal distention, retention of feces in the rectum, fecal impaction, and retention of urine in the bladder.

RESPIRATORY SYSTEM

Because of decreased movement of the muscles involved in respiration, the air passages can become congested with accumulations of mucus, causing or aggravating shortness of breath and producing coughing and general discomfort. Placing the patient in the semi-Fowler's position might help relieve the dyspnea. Low doses of oxygen by nasal prongs also could be helpful. Infrequently, secretions that cannot be coughed up by the patient may have to be removed by suctioning and inhalation therapy.

As the patient's condition continues to decline, his breathing may become more difficult and his breath sounds louder. Accumulations of the mucus in the air passages produce a gurgling sound (sometimes called the "death rattle") that can be particularly distressing to family members who are present.

CENTRAL NERVOUS SYSTEM

The dying patient's senses are often diminished or distorted as death approaches. Although the sensation of touch may be depressed, the dying person can sense pressure. If the patient has exhibited a desire to be touched and derives comfort from being touched by another, simply holding his hand, placing a hand on his arm, or gently stroking him can let him know that he is not alone. However, touch is a very personal thing, and some people who have never been demonstrative do not want or appreciate being touched.

Dying persons are not always comatose or totally unconscious. One who appears comatose or partially conscious should be spoken to in exactly the same way as if he were fully conscious and responsive. He should be told what is going to be done before it is done to him. He deserves an explanation of noises and other unfamiliar sensory stimuli that he could be aware of.

Hearing is thought to be the last sense that is lost when a patient either lapses into deep coma or is close to death. It is imperative that conversations held by others within hearing of the patient be conducted as if he were able to hear and respond. Whispering is never acceptable; it is rude, and it can increase the patient's anxiety and cause him to distrust those who care for him.

Nurses who specialize in the care of the dying report that the dying person almost invariably turns his head toward the light. This is probably because as sight and hearing fail the patient strives to see the objects and people near him. Indirect lighting can help avoid unnecessary stimulation. The person sitting with him should be at the head of the bed, near the patient so that the patient can see and hear him more easily. There is a tendency for well-meaning family members to lower the blinds or shades in the room, so that the dying person is in semidarkness. This does the patient a disservice and can increase his discomfort and anxiety. Again, he might feel that he is being hidden or that others are hiding from him because they do not want to confront him and help him deal with his dying.

In the study of clinical thanatology the best teachers are the patients. Each person reacts differently during the dying process, and each has needs that are not always shared by every other dying person.

If there are any "experts" in the care of the dying, they are the patients themselves.

Nursing Care Plan 14-1 presents nursing interventions for a terminally ill patient.

PSYCHOSOCIAL CARE

Patience, empathy, honesty, and an understanding of the grief process can provide the nurse with the necessary tools to be of help to the terminally ill patient. A variety of interventions have proved helpful to the psychosocial well-being of the patient and the family. Helping the patient to live each day to the fullest and focusing on the best quality of life that can presently be obtained can do much to diminish the fear of death.

The nurse must carefully assess the patient's mood and needs before undertaking the following psychosocial interventions. Caution is to be exercised in encouraging the terminal patient to share feelings and deal with issues of death. This should not be done before he is ready. A patient's defenses should never be taken away from him.

Allow the patient to make as many decisions as possible, even if it is over something small, such as which arm he would like to have washed first. This is especially important as he loses control over bodily functions such as defecating and urinating. Seek his input on how and when he wishes to receive visitors and how many he wishes to see. As death approaches, he may prefer to see only one or two close family members or a significant other. At that time a "No Visitors" sign on the door is advisable.

Help the patient to maintain his dignity by always providing privacy and showing concern for him during procedures that are embarrassing to him. When the patient expresses feelings of dependency, loss, anxiety, or despair, help him to explore and express those feelings rather than discounting them with a quick reassurance. Let him live his past or present regrets. Assist the patient to go through a "life review" with a special person or with you. Chronologically reviewing one's life and sharing experiences has proven to be very beneficial to the peace of mind of the dying individual. Be available to listen and encourage family members to share good memories of past events of which the patient was a part.

One of the most difficult parts of dying is losing relationships. It is appropriate to mourn and grieve over relationships that are to be lost at death. Remembering the positives of those relationships and sharing the memories can be pleasurable. Encourage the patient to give or leave special messages to the people who are most meaningful to him.

Sustaining hope when the end is in sight is important, but the focus shifts to hope for relief from pain, for a time of complete rest, for a visit from a special person, or to complete some task before death.

At an appropriate time, talk with the patient and the family about their wishes regarding organ transplants and artificial means of life support.

There is as much work to be done with the family as with the patient as death nears. The family needs to understand that withdrawal emotionally by the patient is a natural occurrence as death approaches. Each family member may be in a different stage of grief.

At the time of death, it is best to ask if the patient and/or family wishes you to remain with them. After death has occurred, many times the only honest thing that can be said is "I'm sorry this has happened," or just "I'm so sorry." It is okay to cry with the family, if the nurse can control her reaction and appropriately stop crying. She must remember that she is there to support the family, not have them support her.

STANDARDS OF CARE FOR THE TERMINALLY ILL

In 1974 the first international conference of specialists in dying and death was held to discuss the problems and needs of the terminally ill. Those who attended the conference were representative of almost all of the disciplines responsible for direct care of terminally ill persons. At this meeting of practitioners and researchers in clinical thanatology, a task force was formed to identify explicit standards of care for the terminally ill. It was felt by the group that the practices of care typically provided in medical facilities were developed and carried out to meet the needs of the staff and the institution, rather than those of the dying patient and his family. The goal of the conference was to develop patient and family-oriented standards of care. Additionally, it was felt that attention should be paid to the needs of staff members who provide care for terminally ill patients and their families, so staff-oriented standards were added as a third category. The standards developed by the task force are shown in Table 14-3.

THE GRIEVING PROCESS

Grieving, like any loss, is a process through which one works ideally toward the ultimate stage of acceptance. In the case of the bereaved, grief is over the loss of a spouse, parent, child, friend, or other loved one who has died. In the grieving process, the task of the bereaved person is to accept the finality of his loss. The manner in which he does this varies greatly, as does the length of time it takes to work through the grieving process. In general, persons who have a positive self-image, are able to relate to others easily, have a sound religious faith or value system, and are willing to take the initiative find

NURSING CARE PLAN 14–1

Selected nursing diagnoses, goals/outcome criteria, nursing interventions, and evaluations for a terminally ill patient with end-stage renal disease

Situation: Mrs. Cox, age 60, has been ill with renal disease for the past 10 years. In spite of biweekly hemodialysis treatments, her condition has worsened, and she has but a few months to live. She is a widow with three children: two married sons who live nearby and one daughter who lives at home.

When she learned of her prognosis during hospitalization, Mrs. Cox asked to be allowed to go home for her final days. She seems to have resolved her feelings of denial and anger and is moving toward accepting her impending death as inevitable. She is in no great physical distress but does have congestive heart failure, anemia, fatigue, drowsiness, and decreased attention span.

Nursing Diagnosis	Goals/Outcome Criteria	Nursing Intervention	Evaluation
Impaired gas exchange related to fluid in lungs SUPPORTING DATA Bilateral rales, dyspnea, color ashen.	Patient will state that anxiety over difficulty in breathing is lessened.	Maintain in semi-Fowler's or Fowler's position. Administer oxygen via nasal cannula at 3 to 5 L per minute. Auscultate lung fields q shift; suction as needed. Administer morphine as ordered to ease breathing and lessen anxiety.	Oxygen at 3 L/min per nasal cannula continuous; suctioned × 3 this shift; morphine at 8, 11, 2; breathing easier; continue plan.
Anxiety related to feeling of having "unfinished business." SUPPORTING DATA "I'm not ready to die; I have too many things to attend to."	Patient will express sense of having taken care of business and disposal of personal items.	Help patient identify things she wants to take care of and ways in which she can accomplish these tasks. Encourage family members to assist patient and participate in decision making when she requests them to do so.	Made list of tasks to be completed—will, finances, etc.; will meet with attorney tomorrow; daughter included in meeting; continue plan.
Anticipatory grieving related to impending death. SUPPORTING DATA Crying a lot; states she is very sad and is not ready to say goodbye to family and friends. "It hurts so bad to think of leaving everyone."	Patient will express sense of peace in regard to impending death.	Provide opportunities for verbalization of grief. Support and encourage her to communicate her thoughts and feelings with family members and share love and memories with them. Help patient feel free to cry and express her sense of loss. Establish trusting relationship with patient and family members. Reply honestly to her questions; respect confidentiality of information she divulges. Assess spiritual needs. Help patient identify resources for spiritual solace. Comply with request to call minister, rabbi, or whomever; obtain reading material, and if requested to do so, pray with her. Respect patient's beliefs, values, and philosophic outlook.	Discussed feelings for 15 min; is talking with family members and saying goodbye; crying lessened; minister visiting each A.M.; continue plan.

NURSING CARE PLAN 14–1, *Continued*

Nursing Diagnosis	Goals/Outcome Criteria	Nursing Intervention	Evaluation
Ineffective family coping, compromised, related to daughter's denial of impending death of mother. SUPPORTING DATA Daughter states: "She's looking much better now." Heard to tell someone on the phone that she feels her mother may be able to go to a relative's wedding 2 months from now.	Daughter participates in physical care and psychological support of mother while dying. Mother expresses deepening bond and sense of unity with daughter and feels more at ease with her.	Help daughter identify personal strengths that make accepting and dealing with her mother's chronic illness less difficult. Allow daughter to express her grief and sense of loss. Encourage her to reminisce with her mother, remember happy times together. Reinforce mother's right to refuse intensive treatment and to choose the place and manner in which she wants to spend her final days.	Daughter assisting with care; talked with her alone for 15 min this P.M.; is beginning to realize her mother is terminal; continue plan.

it easier to complete the process and go on with their lives after suffering the loss of someone very dear to them.

In Western culture, people often are embarrassed by signs of grief. We do not seem to recognize that grief serves a very useful purpose in helping people who have suffered the loss of a loved one adjust to new ways of living and eventually resolve their grief. As a reminder to those of us who wish to ignore, neglect, or hasten the grief process, Barckley wrote:

> All grief must not be thought of as dreary and destructive. The world would be worse without it. If no man's life were significant enough to cause weeping, if birth and death were unmarked, if the measure of our years on earth were nothing, we might better be houseflies rather than human beings made in God's image. Profound grief is preceded by deep love, which gives life meaning. In the deepest sense, our days would be empty and futile if we never grieved, or if dying never left an emotional chaos behind us.

PHASES OF GRIEVING

Therapists whose goal is to provide support and guidance during the grieving process admit that they still have much to learn. However, thanatologists from many different disciplines have noted that there seem to be rather roughly defined stages in the grieving process as in the dying process. Although the number and names of the stages described may vary from one author to another, there is a general consensus that there are three major phases of grieving.

The process begins when the person has been told or is otherwise aware that death has occurred. This first *impact* or *awareness* phase is followed by a *recoil* phase, in which the bereaved responds with feelings of anger, depression, or hostility toward the self and others. Finally, there is a *recovery* or *adjustment* phase, during which strong emotional ties with the past are gradually broken and the bereaved person becomes reinvested in the present and future.

Awareness Phase

The person who is suffering from acute grief is in a state of shock caused by the news of actual or impending death. The physiologic signs commonly seen at this time are fainting, a feeling of tightness in the throat, shortness of breath and a need to sigh, waves of nausea or sensations of somatic distress lasting from 20 minutes to more than an hour, a feeling of emptiness in the abdomen, and a strong sensation of tension or pain. Other signs that a person is suffering from acute grief include inability to sleep, forgetfulness and absentmindedness, and a tendency to repeat the same behavior over and over again. The person may cry uncontrollably or sit withdrawn and unresponsive.

Recoil Phase

After the first wave of shock and grief, the bereaved person usually moves into the second phase, in which he experiences powerful emotions that he has difficulty controlling. His atti-

TABLE 14–3 STANDARDS OF CARE FOR THE TERMINALLY ILL, HIS FAMILY, AND CAREGIVERS

Patient-oriented standards

1. The terminally ill person's own preferences and lifestyle must be taken into account. Each person's personality and needs are considered when criteria for his care are developed. Routine care, rigid rules, and institutional regulations should not be applied indiscriminately.
2. Symptomatic relief is a goal of treatment. Regardless of the length of time before his death, efforts must be made to maintain functional capacity and relieve discomfort.
3. Control of pain is a goal of treatment. This standard is implied in the above standard, but it is considered of such importance that it is given the status of a separate standard.
4. The "living will" or a similar document will be considered appropriate information clearly stating the patient's preferences and intentions. Such information is taken into account along with the rights and responsibilities of family members and staff and current state and federal laws.
5. The patient should feel that he is safe and secure in the care of his caregivers and that they will perform their functions and communicate with him in an appropriate manner.
6. The patient will have opportunities for leave-taking and saying his goodbyes to people who are important to him.
7. The patient will have the opportunity to experience his final moments in a way that is meaningful to him. He will be able to be with whomever he chooses, and with or without physical contact, depending on his preference.

Family-oriented standards

1. Family members should have opportunities to discuss dying, death, and related emotional needs with staff. Expressions of the need to share their feelings should be honored by the staff, and time should be taken to allow for this.
2. The family should have the opportunity for privacy with the dying person while he is still living and immediately after death. Some families may have special customs they wish to follow, such as dressing the corpse or having someone in constant attendance, even accompanying the body to the funeral home. Others may simply need some time alone with the newly dead person. Viewing the body can help them realize the finality of the death and facilitate the beginning of the grief process.

Staff-oriented standards

1. The caregivers should be given adequate time to form and maintain personal relationships with the patient.
2. A mutual support network should exist among the staff, who frequently are among the bereaved. There should be some place for the individual staff member to turn for support and comfort.

Data from Kastenbaum, R. J.: Death, Society, and Human Experience, 3rd ed. New York, Macmillan, 1986, p. 218. Reprinted with permission of Merrill, an imprint of Macmillan Publishing Company.

tude is indicative of an attempt to run away or hide from a situation he finds completely repugnant. He may be so angry that he is compelled to withdraw from others, and he will probably try to find someone or something to blame for the catastrophe that has befallen him. He might blame God or some other authority figure such as the physician or nurse. It is even possible that the bereaved will feel anger against the person who has died or is dying and leaving him, or he might feel terrible guilt, wondering what he might have done to prevent the death.

Destructive feelings such as anger and guilt need to be admitted to the conscious mind and dealt with by the bereaved. This is necessary so that he can resolve his grief and resume his life without the loved one.

Resolution and Acceptance

If he is to work through his grief and move forward to resolution, the grieving person must accept the finality of his loss with mind *(cognitive resolution)*, feelings *(affective resolution)*, and behavior *(conative [action] resolution)*.

During cognitive resolution the person is beginning to realize that the loved one is indeed dead and will not return, but his loss is not yet fully believed. The person may exhibit searching behavior in which he continues to look for and expects to see and be with the deceased person. He may continue to speak of the person as if he were still alive but simply away for a while. The bereaved will be sad and disconsolate, but he still clings to the hope that by some miracle or clearing up of a misunderstanding he will awaken from a nightmare and find that nothing has really changed. Eventually he *knows* in his mind that the death is a reality and he is able to speak of the person as dead or "gone."

Affective resolution is initially manifested by the disappearance of hope and the emergence of despair. At this point the person may exhibit apathy and an inability to maintain relations with others. There is overwhelming sadness, but as he progresses through the grief process there is a gradual emotional detachment and letting go.

Conative resolution is sometimes called the *reorganization* phase. The bereaved person begins to reorganize his life and do certain things in order to get on with living. Activities that are typical during this phase of resolution include cleaning out closets and drawers in the loved one's room, and giving away his clothes, books, and tools; changing the listing in the telephone directory; removing wedding rings; redecorating the home; getting a job; and going out to be with others in church, social, and civic gatherings.

GRIEF AND TIME

Persons who are learning to work with the bereaved often ask how long it takes for a person to work through the process to final acceptance and resolution. Sometimes well-meaning friends will tell a grieving person that time heals all things. However, how much time is needed for resolution and healing depends on the individual, the circumstances of the loss of a loved one, and social and cultural customs. In many cases reorganization behavior begins 3 to 4 months after bereavement and becomes more evident 6 months to a year later. This is not necessarily a goal or something to be forced on the bereaved. It is simply the average length of time required before resolution can be expected.

The action-oriented person usually begins reorganization behavior earlier than the passive and nonassertive person. It is not so much a matter of how much time it takes to recover from the death of a loved one as what is done with the time the bereaved person has. Arnaldo Pangrazzi, a Roman Catholic priest who serves as a hospital chaplain, has coordinated numerous support groups for the bereaved, and has conducted seminars on grief, suggests ten ways in which a grieving person can use time to recover from the loss of a loved one. The ten suggestions and a brief explanation of each are presented in Table 14–4.

SUPPORT FOR THE NURSE OF THE TERMINALLY ILL

A great many books and articles have been published since Kübler-Ross pioneered the field of thanatology in this country. However, until recently, little has been offered in the way of help to the nurse who works with the terminally ill and their families. Nurses see themselves as healers and often are uncomfortable in the role of helping someone to die. Most have not had sufficient experience in dealing with death and are not confident that they will be able to say and do the right and humane things that will comfort the patient and his family.

It is emotionally draining to care for someone who is dying. If the nurse is truly involved in working with the patient as he progresses through the stages of dying, she has needs of her own that must be met. If she is to recover from her personal loss of someone she has grown close to, she needs support and understanding in order to sustain her inner strength needed to help other patients.

Someone must be available to listen as she expresses her feelings. Just as the dying patient uses denial to adjust to the news that his life will soon end, the nurse also uses denial as a time to collect herself and gather her strength. She, too, becomes angry and has doubts about her ability and that of her colleagues to provide the kind of care that the patient needs.

The nurse might bargain by asking that she be relieved of some of the duties that bring her into direct contact with the patient. Her feelings of helplessness and inability to cope are understandable. Perhaps she does need relief so that when she returns to the patient, she can be available to him as a caring person.

When the nurse has experienced the loss of a patient, she too should have opportunities to grieve without fear of reprisal or ridicule, a soft shoulder to cry on, an understanding embrace, words of comfort that say, "Of course you're sad. You too have suffered a loss and by acknowledging it you may develop some insight."

Sometimes it might be necessary for the nurse to have a day off in order to replenish herself after having given of herself emotionally and physically. Those nurses who are continuously exposed to terminally ill patients might benefit from a temporary transfer to a less stressful tour of duty. If that is not feasible, they can be assigned to tasks that keep them occupied but do not require prolonged contact with a dying patient.

Nurses are no less in need of self-esteem, security, love, and respect from their peers than any other human beings. Mutual support can help the nurse and her colleagues deal more effectively with death and the natural and expected

TABLE 14-4 TEN SUGGESTIONS FOR OVERCOMING GRIEF

1. *Take time to accept death.* Facing and accepting death is a necessary condition for continuing with one's own life.
2. *Take time to let go.* Life is a series of letting go—sometimes temporarily, sometimes permanently. Letting go occurs when we are able to endure and accept the feelings that accompany death. It occurs when we are able to tolerate the helplessness and insecurity, when we are willing to face the tears, to wait, trust, and hope again.
3. *Take time to make decisions.* Be patient with yourself and learn to make independent decisions. Start with small decisions; write out a schedule for the day and set up tasks to be done. Planning helps you look forward to visits with friends, eating out, vacations. Making decisions about our life helps us gain control over it and increases self-confidence.
4. *Take time to share.* The greatest need of the bereaved is to have someone to share their pain, their memories, their sadness. Bereaved people need others to give them time and space to grieve.
5. *Take time to believe.* At times our grief can shake up our faith. To survive is to find some meaning in suffering because suffering that has meaning to it is endurable. For many people, religion—with its rituals, promise of an afterlife, and its community support—offers a comforting and strengthening base in the lonely encounter with helplessness and hopelessness.
6. *Take time to forgive.* Forgive yourself for the things you did not do, the words you did not say to the loved one. Forgive others for their hurtful comments or actions, insensitivity or avoidance. Forgive the deceased one who has left you bereaved and angry.
7. *Take time to feel good about yourself.* The death of a loved one does not sentence you to a life of sorrow. It does alter our lifestyle and change our self-image, but grief can help us discover new independence and a new outlook. Explore new interests, develop new hobbies, engage in activities that build self-confidence and provide a feeling of newness, satisfaction, and pleasure.
8. *Take time to meet new friends.* Try to find a new sense of belonging. Take steps to move out of safe boundaries and interact with others. Old friends might be there to offer security and comfort; new friends will be there to offer opportunities.
9. *Take time to laugh.* In life there are as many reasons to laugh as there are to cry. Laughter helps us to survive, to reenter life, and to accept our limitations, and develops hope in the present.
10. *Take time to give.* The best way to overcome our loneliness and pain is to be concerned about the loneliness and pain of others. Getting involved with others gives us the feeling that life goes on, and takes us away from self-pity.

From Pangrazzi, A. Overcoming grief: Ten suggestions. *St. Anthony Messenger.* Cincinnati, St. Anthony Messenger Press, June, 1983.

psychological reactions to it. Standards for care of bereaved staff members are included in Table 14-3.

HOSPICE CARE FOR THE DYING AND BEREAVED

Hospice originally meant a medieval guest house or way station for pilgrims and travelers. Many of the hospices of twentieth-century England are free-standing facilities unaffiliated with hospitals and autonomous in terms of professional procedures. These hospices were the predecessors of the hospice movement in the United States. A hospice as currently conceived is not necessarily a specific kind of institution or facility, but a program of care that is specially designed to meet the needs of the terminally ill and their families. The hospice program can be implemented in an institution or in the patient's home.

The National Hospice Organization (NHO) was organized in the United States in 1978. The Hospice Nurses' Association was founded in 1986. (Their current address is P. O. Box 8166, Van Nuys, CA 91409-8166.)

Hospice is a concept or philosophy based on universal humanitarianism; it accepts death as a natural part of the life cycle. The purpose of a hospice program is to serve persons with a terminal illness through grief and death and to serve those supporting them through the death process and bereavement. Through an interdisciplinary approach, skilled medical and nursing care is given to meet medical, social, psychological, and spiritual needs of the patient and significant others.

A hospice program is concerned with symptom management that maximizes client comfort, enhances feelings of self-worth and well-being, and encourages client participation in decisions affecting his living and dying. Such a program lends support to both the patient and significant others as their activities and relationships undergo change. The support continues into the periods of grief and bereavement.

Most hospices have services that are available on a 7-day-per-week, 24-hour-per-day basis and continue uninterrupted, regardless of the patient's ability to pay for that care.

The hospice program has been approved and encouraged by the American Medical Association, the American Nurses' Association, and other professional organizations. Information about hospice programs in the United States and training programs for professional persons interested in this area of practice can be obtained by writing to The National Hospice Organization, 1901 North Vroome Street, Arlington, VA 22209.

ETHICAL AND MORAL ISSUES

Nurses have a right and a responsibility to participate in decisions that are made about the effects of certain treatments on a patient's quality of life and the sustaining of life at all costs, even when the patient's prognosis offers no hope for recovery. Nurses are qualified for involvement in the decision-making process because (1) the focus of nursing care is on the patient's responses to health problems, (2) a nurse's education includes social sciences and the humanities, which can contribute to making informed moral decisions, and (3) it is the nurse who has continuous and intimate contact with the patient and is therefore able to provide important insights and speak on his behalf when he is unable to do so.

Participating in deliberations about ethical questions related to death and dying carries with it the responsibility to clarify one's own values and philosophy of life. This can be done by attending seminars and conferences, by informal discussions, and by reading about various points of view. Professional nursing journals frequently carry articles on bioethical and moral dilemmas confronting those who practice in the health care field.

Among the ethical and moral questions surrounding the topics of death and dying and the continued use of life-support systems are:

- Who should be the decision makers?
- Does hospitalization mean that one is obligated to accept all forms of active treatment?
- Is there an appropriate time to let a patient die?
- How does one measure rationality or a person's mental competence to decide that he wants life-support measures to be discontinued?
- What values should enter into the decision making?
- Does the dying patient or his family have the right to allow him to die?
- Is there a moral responsibility for a physician or other caregiver not to force the patient and his family into a position where active euthanasia is the only alternative?
- Is it always best to act on the side of life?
- Should nurses be dedicated to the inherent value of human life?
- Is it true that human life that is externally valued (that is, its worth measured in terms of economic, social, and personal considerations) is subject to the whimsy of others?

There are no simple answers to such complex questions. One must know what one believes in and then act accordingly. Modern technology has brought many benefits to mankind, but it also has brought the burden of bioethical dilemmas that were unheard of 30 or 40 years ago.

LEGAL ASPECTS OF LIFE AND DEATH ISSUES

In recent years many state legislatures have passed laws that allow an adult to authorize, by means of a written directive, the withholding of life-sustaining measures in the event of his own terminal illness. The so-called living will or similar document is intended to protect a person's right to die. A sample living will is shown in Figure 14–1.

A durable power of attorney is a most useful document, because unlike a regular power of attorney, it is not voided when the principal (person) becomes incapacitated. It is written so that it can be executed at any time but does not take effect until the person desires or until a specific set of criteria are met (e.g., health decline reaching mental disability or the inability to make decisions on one's own). An example of a durable power of attorney is also shown in Figure 14–1.

These legislative actions provide adults with the means to control decisions related to life-support procedures. The main features of such laws are (1) a written document that gives directives regarding withholding or withdrawing life-support measures, (2) a definition of "terminal illness," (3) verification of the patient's prognosis

To My Family, My Physician, My Lawyer And All Others Whom It May Concern

Death is as much a reality as birth, growth, and aging—it is the one certainty of life. In anticipation of decisions that may have to be made about my own dying and as an expression of my right to refuse treatment, I, ____ (print name), being of sound mind, make this statement of my wishes and instructions concerning treatment.

By means of this document, which I intend to be legally binding, I direct my physician and other care providers, my family, and any surrogate designated by me or appointed by a court, to carry out my wishes. If I become unable, by reason of physical or mental incapacity, to make decisions about my medical care, let this document provide the guidance and authority needed to make any and all such decisions.

If I am permanently unconscious or there is no reasonable expectation of my recovery from a seriously incapacitating or lethal illness or condition, I do not wish to be kept alive by artificial means. I request that I be given all care necessary to keep me comfortable and free of pain, even if pain-relieving medications may hasten my death, and I direct that no life-sustaining treatment be provided except as I or my surrogate specifically authorize.

This request may appear to place a heavy responsibility upon you, but by making this decision according to my strong convictions, I intend to ease that burden. I am acting after careful consideration and with understanding of the consequences of your carrying out my wishes. *List optional specific provisions in the space below. (See other side.)*

Durable Power of Attorney for Health Care Decisions (Cross out if you do not wish to use this section)

To effect my wishes, I designate ____________________________, residing at ____________________________ ____, (phone #) ________________________, (or if he or she shall for any reason fail to act, __________________________________, residing at ____ ____, (phone #) __________________________) as my health care surrogate—that is, my attorney-in-fact regarding any and all health care decisions to be made for me, including the decision to refuse life-sustaining treatment—if I am unable to make such decisions myself. This power shall remain effective during and not be affected by my subsequent illness, disability or incapacity. My surrogate shall have authority to interpret my Living Will, and shall make decisions about my health care as specified in my instructions or, when my wishes are not clear, as the surrogate believes to be in my best interests. I release and agree to hold harmless my health care surrogate from any and all claims whatsoever arising from decisions made in good faith in the exercise of this power.

I sign this document knowingly, voluntarily, and after careful deliberation, this ______ day of __________________, 19_____.

____
(signature)

Address _______________________________________
____

I do hereby certify that the within document was executed and acknowledged before me by the principal this ______ day of __________________, 19_____.

____
Notary Public

Witness _______________________________________
Printed Name __________________________________
Address _______________________________________
____

Witness _______________________________________
Printed Name __________________________________
Address _______________________________________
____

Copies of this document have been given to:

This Living Will expresses my personal treatment preferences. The fact that I may have also executed a declaration in the form recommended by state law should not be construed to limit or contradict this Living Will, which is an expression of my common-law and constitutional rights.

(Optional) my Living Will is registered with Concern for Dying (Registry No. ______)

Distributed by Concern for Dying, 250 West 57th Street, New York, NY 10107 (212) 246-6962

----- (Detach here) --

Figure 14–1 Living will and durable power of attorney for health care decisions.
(Reprinted with permission of Concern for Dying, 250 West 57th Street, New York, NY 10107.)

How to Use Your Living Will

The Living Will should clearly state your preferences about life-sustaining treatment. You may wish to add specific statements to the Living Will in the space provided for that purpose. Such statements might concern:

- Cardiopulmonary resuscitation
- Artificial or invasive measures for providing nutrition and hydration
- Kidney dialysis
- Mechanical or artificial respiration
- Blood transfusion
- Surgery (such as amputation)
- Antibiotics

You may also wish to indicate any preferences you may have about such matters as dying at home.

The Durable Power of Attorney for Health Care

This optional feature permits you to name a surrogate decision maker (also known as a proxy, health agent or attorney-in-fact), someone to make health care decisions on your behalf if you lose that ability. As this person should act according to your preferences and in your best interests, you should select this person with care and make certain that he or she knows what your wishes are and about your Living Will.

You should not name someone who is a witness to your Living Will. You may want to name an alternate agent in case the first person you select is unable or unwilling to serve. If you do name a surrogate decision maker, the form must be notarized. (It is a good idea to notarize the document in any case.)

Important Points to Remember

- Sign and date your Living Will.
- Your two witnesses should not be blood relatives, your spouse, potential beneficiaries of your estate or your health care proxy.
- Discuss your Living Will with your doctors; and give them copies of your Living Will for inclusion in your medical file, so they will know whom to contact in the event something happens to you.
- Make photo copies of your Living Will and give them to anyone who may be making decisions for you if you are unable to make them yourself.
- Place the original in a safe, accessible place, so that it can be located if needed—not in a safe deposit box.
- Look over your Living Will periodically (at least every five years), initial and redate it so that it will be clear that your wishes have not changed.

The Living Will Registry

In 1983, Concern for Dying instituted the Living Will Registry, a computerized file system where you may keep an up-to-date copy of your Living Will in our New York office.

What are the benefits of joining the Living Will Registry?

- Concern's staff will ensure that your form is filled out correctly, assign you a Registry number and maintain a copy of your Living Will.
- Concern's staff will be able to refer to *your* personal document, explain procedures and options, and provide you with the latest case law or state legislation should you, your proxy or anyone else acting on your behalf need counselling or legal guidance in implementing your Living Will.
- You will receive a permanent, credit card size plastic mini-will with your Registry number imprinted on it. The mini-will, which contains your address, Concern's address and a short version of the Living Will, indicates that you have already filled out a full-sized witnessed Living Will document.

How do you join the Living Will Registry?

- Review your Living Will, making sure it is up to date and contains any specific provisions that you want added.
- Mail a photo copy of your original, signed and witnessed document along with a check for $25.00 to: Living Will Registry, Concern for Dying, 250 West 57th Street, Room 831, New York, New York 10107.
- The one-time Registry enrollment fee will cover the costs of processing and maintaining your Living Will and of issuing your new plastic mini-will.
- If you live in a state with Living Will legislation, send copies of any required state documents as well.
- If you have any address changes or wish to add or delete special provisions that you have included in your Living Will, please write to the Registry so that we can keep your file up to date.

Figure 14-1 *Continued*

by one or more physicians, and (4) provisions that protect the physician and health care agency against legal action.

Some opponents of the living will argue that it is not necessary, because the patient has an inherent right to die. When a person engages the services of a physician, he retains his right of self-determination. Thus physicians are "servants" rather than "masters" of their patients and must respect their wishes.

Another argument against legislation related to fatal illness is that although it may give a patient self-determination, lack of such a document signed by the patient may have the opposite effect. In other words, in the absence of a written directive, is the physician obligated to use extraordinary means to prolong life? And if he chooses not to use extraordinary means to sustain life, is he likely to be accused of malpractice or even homicide?

A third objection concerns the length of time between the signing of the will and its application to a specific event at some future time in the patient's life. It is difficult to give informed consent when one does not know what procedures, possible cures, and other conditions might exist years after the will was signed. In answer to this objection, some state legislatures have incorporated a time limit such as 7 years for the document to be valid.

Written directives about what should be done in the event of a terminal illness are not the perfect answer to the issue of a person's right to die. They can be a source of conflict among family members and omit some or all of them from the decision-making process. They intrude into the physician-patient relationship and suggest mistrust. However, nurses and other health professionals must ask whether in every instance a person's right to die as he wishes (aside from suicide or active euthanasia) has been honored, and if his rights have been denied, why and how they were denied, and how they could have been protected.

BIBLIOGRAPHY

Amenta, M. O., and Bohnet, N. L.: Nursing Care of the Terminally Ill. Boston, Little, Brown, 1986.

American Nurses' Association: Standards and Scope of Hospice Nursing Practice. Kansas City, 1987.

Barckley, V.: Grief: A part of living. Nurs. Digest, Summer, 1977, p. 75.

Blues, A. G., and Zerwekh, J. V.: Hospice and Palliative Nursing Care. Orlando, FL, Grune & Stratton, 1984.

Clark, C., et al.: Hospice care: A model for caring for the persons with AIDS. Nurs. Clin. North Am., Dec., 1988, p. 851.

Coco, P.: How should I help my grief-stricken clients cope with their loss? Adv. Clin. Care, Sept./Oct., 1990, p. 9.

Coolican, M., et al.: Helping survivors survive. Nursing 89, Aug., 1989, p. 52.

Editors of Nursing 91: Meeting the challenge of a dying patient. Nursing 91, Feb., p. 42.

Feigenberg, L.: Terminal Care. New York, Brunner/Mazel Publishers, 1980.

Gifford, B. J., and Cleary, B. B.: Supporting the bereaved. Am. J. Nurs., Feb., 1990, p. 48.

Kastenbaum, R. J.: Death, Society, and Human Experience. 3rd ed. New York, Macmillan, 1986.

Kübler-Ross, E.: Death: The Final Stage of Growth. Englewood Cliffs, NJ, Prentice-Hall, 1975.

Kübler-Ross, E.: On Death and Dying. New York, Macmillan, 1969.

Lewis, S., et al.: Manual of Psychosocial Nursing Interventions: Promoting Mental Health in Medical-Surgical Settings. Philadelphia, W. B. Saunders, 1989.

Leverett, P., Pickren, J., and Wells, C.: Evelyn had plans and they didn't include dying. Nursing 90, Nov., p. 44.

Martocchio, B. C.: Living While Dying. Bowie, MD, Robert J. Brady, 1982.

McCaffrey, M., and Beche, A.: Giving narcotics for pain: A problem-solver handbook. Nursing 89, Oct., 1989, p. 161.

National Hospice Nurses' Association: Quality Assurance for Hospice Patient Care. Escondido, CA, 1988.

National Hospice Organization: Standards of a Hospice Program of Care. Arlington, VA, 1982.

Omery, A., et al.: Ethical perspectives. Crit. Care Nurs. Clin. North Am., March, 1989, p. 165.

Pangrazzi, A.: Overcoming grief: Ten suggestions. *St. Anthony Messenger*, Jan., 1983.

Parkes, C. M., and Weiss, R. S.: Recovery From Bereavement. New York, Basic Books, 1983.

Perton, L.: Share what you feel. RN, July, 1990, p. 41.

Post, H., et al.: Letting the family in during a code. Nursing 89, March, 1989, p. 43.

Schwartz, E. A.: Your Jewish patient is dying. AD Nurse, Jan.–Feb., 1989, p. 12.

Stephany, R. M., and Benaer, P.: A death in the family. Am. J. Nurs., April, 1990, p. 54.

Ufema, J.: Facing death: Look to the past. Nursing 88, Nov., 1988, p. 93.

Welter, K. M.: Night watch . . . a nurse reflects on how little and how much she can offer a dying patient. Nursing 89, May, 1989, p. 105.

Williams, J. C.: Allaying common fears. *In* Dealing With Death and Dying. Nursing 78 Skillbook Series. Jenkintown, PA, Intermed Communications, 1978, p. 27.

Worden, W.: Grief Counseling and Grief Therapy: A Handbook for the Mental Health Practitioner. New York, Springer, 1982.

SUGGESTED READINGS

Carroll, D.: Living With Dying. New York, McGraw-Hill, 1985.

Craven, M.: I Heard the Owl Call My Name. Garden City, NY, Doubleday and Co., Inc., 1973.

Gunther, J.: Death Be Not Proud. New York, Harper & Row, 1949.

Grollman, E.: Living When a Loved One Has Died. Boston, Beacon Press, 1977.

Parkes, C., and Weiss, P.: Recovery From Bereavement. New York, Basic Books, 1983.

Simos, B.: A Time to Grieve: Loss as a Universal Experience. New York, Family Service Association of America, 1979.

STUDENT STUDY AIDS

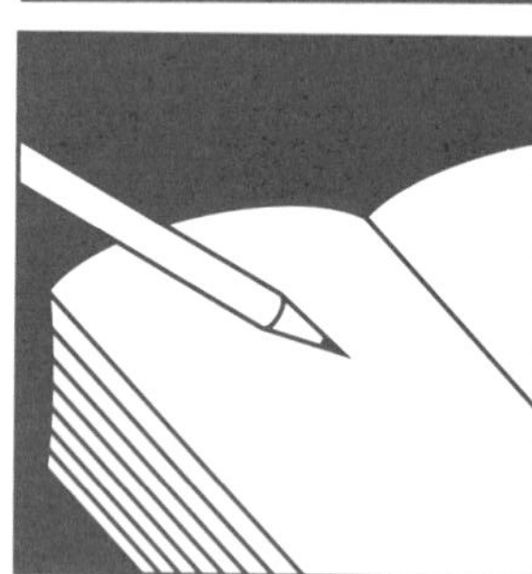

CLINICAL CASE PROBLEMS

Read each clinical case problem and discuss the questions with your classmates.

1. You are assigned to care for Mr. Roberts, age 38, who is terminally ill. He is emaciated, short of breath, and near death. His wife is a nurse who is unable to be with him more than a few hours a day because of her responsibilities at home and at work. Mr. Roberts is very difficult to care for because of his belligerent attitude. He refuses to eat and insists that he does not need A.M. care or any other kind of attention. The other nurses on duty do not go into Mr. Roberts' room except when absolutely necessary because "he has asked to be left alone, we are busy, and, anyway, it is depressing to be around him. He is so young to die."

- What stage of adjustment do you think Mr. Roberts is experiencing?
- How can you help him?
- What personal attributes and attitudes are lacking in the nurses who choose to leave Mr. Roberts alone?
- What kinds of physiologic needs might Mr. Roberts have?

---

2. The husband of a patient with terminal cancer refuses to accept the doctor's diagnosis and insists that she be kept alive at all costs. The patient has accepted her condition and wishes to discuss her feelings about her approaching death. She asks that you contact a minister but that you not tell her husband about the request. She also asks how you feel about using heroic measures to keep someone alive when he or she is hopelessly ill and willing to accept death.

- What would you do about notifying the minister?
- How would you answer her second question?

---

3. Your aunt, age 58, has only recently been widowed. The death of her husband was completely unexpected, and she still has not recovered from the shock. Family members urge you to help her "snap out of it" and get on with her own life. "After all," they say, "he has been dead 6 weeks now."

- How would you respond to your relatives who are anxious for your aunt to finish her grieving and look to the future instead of the past?
- What behavior might you expect to see in your aunt as she works her way through her grief?
- What kinds of support might you give your aunt during her grieving?

---

4. Mrs. Stinson, age 55, has metastatic liver cancer and is in the terminal stages. She and her husband agree that she would rather leave the hospital and enter the hospice program, which will allow her to die at home. They have two grown children in their late 20s and a 15-year-old daughter. The children disagree with this choice and want her to stay in the hospital where constant care is available.

- How would you go about putting her in contact with the hospice program in your area?
- How would you deal with the children and their desire for their mother to stay in the hospital?
- What particular support and counseling would you suggest for the 15-year-old daughter?
- What support network can you provide for the other members of the family?

STUDY OUTLINE

I. Introduction

A. Death is an integral part of life; in a study of death one can find the meaning of life and an opportunity for growth.

B. Health professionals are beginning to develop more positive attitudes toward and competence in dealing with death and dying.

C. Death and the dying process have become subjects of scientific research, popular literature, and discussions among lay persons and professionals.

D. The task of the dying person is to work his way toward acceptance of his death. The task of the nurse is to help him live his life more fully until he dies.

II. Stages of dying

A. Theory first proposed by Dr. Elisabeth Kübler-Ross.

B. Stages represent psychological responses or coping mechanisms used by dying persons to resolve conflicts.

C. Criticisms of stage theory point out that no two persons react to the inevitability of personal death in exactly the same way.

D. The work of Kübler-Ross and other thanatologists has helped caregivers be more sensitive to the needs of the dying person and his family.

E. Death represents change and separation. Stages of dying are similar to responses in other change situations.

1. Denial and disbelief: "No, not me, it's not possible."
2. Anger: "Why me?"
3. Bargaining (usually with God): "Yes, me, but . . ."
4. Depression: "Yes, me."
5. Acceptance: person is not happy but appears to have won his struggle with grief and fear.

III. Fears experienced by the dying person

A. Fear of pain.
   1. Physical pain need not be an inseparable companion to death.
      a. Patient is to be kept comfortable and assured that analgesic medication is readily available.
      b. Combinations of oral and parenteral analgesia or intrathecal analgesia can allow patient to remain lucid and free of pain.
   2. Goal of pain management is to prevent rather than treat it once it occurs.

B. Fear of loneliness and abandonment.
   1. Dying persons often express fear that they will be alone when they die and no notice will be taken of their leaving.
   2. Patient should be free to choose whom he wants for companionship and what he needs from others.
   3. Human companionship and contact can give patient sense of security and calm.
   4. Pain control is possible for many patients.
   5. Pain control is a major nursing function.

C. Fear of meaninglessness.
   1. Patient needs reassurance that his life has been worthwhile and has had some meaning for others.
   2. Family and friends can reminisce and recall good times spent with dying person and good deeds he has done.
   3. Nurse can point out favorable attributes noted while patient goes through the dying process.
   4. Religious practice, prayers, and rituals can be comforting and give meaning and purpose to life and suffering.

D. Dying person's Bill of Rights—see Table 14–1.

IV. Hope and despair in the dying patient

A. There is tension between hope and despair, the will to live and the desire to die.

B. Patients rarely give up all hope. They need a belief in something better to lift their spirits and give them strength to go on. There might be hope for:
   1. A mistaken diagnosis.
   2. Discovery of a cure or some means of postponing death.
   3. Life after death.
   4. Relief from pain.
   5. A better day.
   6. Living for a particular event.
   7. A good laugh.

C. Tension between will to live and desire to die related to hope and despair.
   1. Death can be a welcome relief and source of hope.
   2. Caregivers must not give the impression they have "given up" on the dying person.
   3. Request for active euthanasia or threat of suicide is a plea for help that the patient is not getting.

V. Communication with the dying patient

A. Patient should be free to express his feelings and needs.

B. Important for caregivers to maintain sense of humor.

C. There is need for opportunities to relieve tension, release pent-up emotions, and experience grief.
D. Desirable attitudes and personal attributes of nurses who care for the dying (see Table 14–2).

VI. The patient's right to know

A. Should be told diagnosis and prognosis if he indicates a need to know.
B. Patient has a corresponding right to not want to know.
C. Most dying patients are aware of the seriousness of their condition, but not every one wants to talk about it.
D. Lines of communication always kept open to give patient an opportunity to ask questions and discuss his condition.

VII. Physiologic death and the dying process

A. Death is an event, a state. Does not have the same meaning for everyone.
   1. Dying is a subjective and private experience.
   2. It is a dynamic process; a stage of life.
   3. Cultural and religious differences can create misunderstanding of death-related behaviors.
B. From a medical point of view, dying begins when the person has an untreatable and fatal disease.
   1. When death is inevitable, a "do not resuscitate" order is appropriate.
C. Signs of death are the result of cell destruction: loss of body heat, stagnation of blood, and rigor mortis.
D. Criteria to determine irreversible coma used to make decisions about continuing life-support systems and procuring viable donor organs.
   1. Cerebral unresponsiveness not related to drugs or hypothermia.
   2. Cessation of spontaneous movement and breathing.
   3. Dilated and fixed pupils.
   4. Absence of cephalic responses and brain stem reflexes.
   5. Repetition of testing and encephalography is customary.

VIII. Nursing assessment and intervention

A. Skin and musculoskeletal system:
   1. Protective body fat diminishes, skin more fragile. Measures taken to maintain skin integrity, prevent pressure sores.
   2. Muscle weakness requires repositioning to provide comfort.
   3. Nursing intervention to provide comfort, protection, and good personal hygiene scheduled according to patient's needs.
   4. Muscle weakness can lead to urinary and fecal incontinence.
   5. Patient and environment kept clean and odor free. Dressing changes, bathing, and mouth care scheduled to allow patient sufficient rest.
   6. Profuse sweating, tossing about, and kicking off covers probably indicate that the patient feels hot, even though his skin may be cold to the touch.
B. Gastrointestinal system:
   1. Diminished involuntary muscle function can cause accumulations of feces and flatus.
   2. Nausea and vomiting can occur.
   3. Nursing intervention to help manage these symptoms.
   4. Bowel and bladder elimination monitored to detect early signs of retention and fecal impaction.
C. Respiratory system:
   1. Air passages can become congested. Nursing interventions include positioning to relieve shortness of breath, turning, help

with coughing and deep breathing, and possibly suctioning and inhalation therapy.

D. Central nervous system:
   1. Senses become less acute. Touching may or may not be desired by patient.
   2. Comatose and semiconscious patient must be talked to and told what is being done to and for him even though he cannot respond.
   3. Conversations held within patient's hearing should be held as though patient were fully alert and aware of what is being said.
   4. Room should not be darkened or shades drawn.
   5. Person sitting with dying patient should sit at head of bed where patient is better able to see and hear the person.

E. Psychosocial care
   1. Help patient to live each day to the fullest.
   2. Be cautious; assess mood and needs; defenses should never be taken from patient.
   3. Allow patient to make decisions over anything he can, no matter how small.
   4. Maintain patient's dignity by providing privacy and showing concern for embarrassing procedures.
   5. Help patient express feelings of dependency, loss, anxiety, or despair and explore them, rather than just offering reassurance.
   6. Assist patient to go through a "life review."
   7. Assist patient to mourn relationships that will be lost.
   8. Provide psychosocial support for the family as well.
   9. Ask patient and family their preference as to your presence at time of death and respect their wishes.
   10. It is okay to grieve and cry with the family as long as the nurse's grief can be controlled; nurse is there to support the family.

IX. Standards of care for the terminally ill (see Table 14–3)

X. The grieving process

A. The task of the bereaved is to accept the finality of the loss he has suffered.

B. Grief serves a useful purpose during period of adjustment to new life without loved one.

C. Phases of grieving:
   1. Impact or awareness phase: person may experience physiologic symptoms of shock.
   2. Recoil phase: person reacts with anger, depression, or hostility.
   3. Recovery phase: adjustment period during which strong emotional ties are severed; bereaved become reoriented to present and future.
   4. Moving toward acceptance and resolution:
      a. Cognitive resolution: bereaved is beginning to mentally acknowledge loss, but it is not yet fully believed. Person may exhibit searching and pining behavior.
      b. Affective resolution: disappearance of hope that loved one will return. Strong emotions of anger, etc.
      c. Conative resolution: the reorganization phase. Person begins to reorganize environment and life in order to live without the lost one.

D. Grief and time:
   1. Length of time it takes to work through grief to acceptance is highly individualized.

2. Action-oriented, assertive person more likely to begin reorganization behavior early than one who is passive and withdrawn.
3. Ten suggestions for use of time for grieving listed in Table 14–4.

XI. Support for nurses of the terminally ill

A. Care for terminally ill can create special needs for support and consolation.

B. Caregiver can experience bereavement and grief over loss of patient.

XII. Hospice care

A. A concept or program of care for the terminally ill and his family.

B. Nurse-coordinated program that can be implemented in an institution or the patient's home.

XIII. Ethical issues

A. Nurses have a right and responsibility to participate in moral and ethical decisions about treatments and prolonging life of terminally ill.

B. Some ethical considerations surround reverence for life, the quality of life, and the right to die with dignity and grace.
1. Who should decide?
2. Must one accept all forms of treatment?
3. Is there an appropriate time to let a patient die?
4. Should family and patient be forced into a position where active euthanasia is their only alternative?

C. The optimal time for a family to discuss death is before they must deal with issues of death and dying.

XIV. Legal aspects

A. The "living will" is an attempt to document a person's wishes in regard to sustaining his life.

B. A "durable power of attorney" is effective only when the person becomes incapacitated. See Figure 14–1.

CHAPTER 15

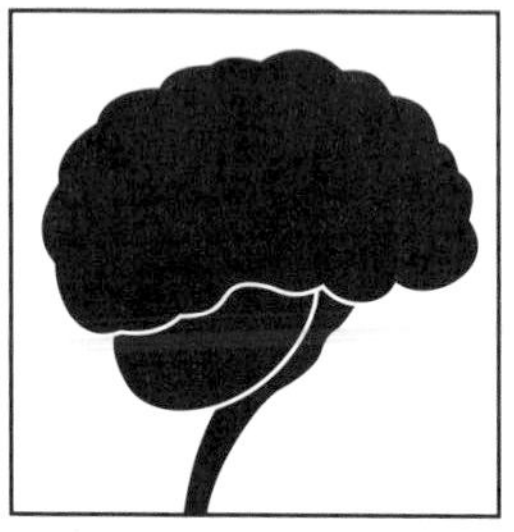

Care of Patients With Neurologic Disorders

VOCABULARY

aura
conjugate
demyelination
hemiparesis
hemiplegia
intention tremor
neuropathy
nuchal rigidity
nystagmus
quadriplegic
sequelae

Upon completion of this chapter the student should be able to:

1. Demonstrate a "neurologic check" and describe the thorough neurologic nursing assessment.
2. State the appropriate preparation and postprocedure care of patients undergoing lumbar puncture (spinal tap), electroencephalogram, and radiologic studies of the brain and cerebral vessels.
3. Write a nursing care plan for the patient who is experiencing increased intracranial pressure.
4. Prepare discharge instructions for the patient leaving the emergency department after sustaining a head injury and concussion.
5. Identify four specific ways in which a nurse can contribute to prevention of cerebrovascular accidents.
6. Develop and implement a comprehensive nursing care plan for a patient who has suffered a cerebrovascular accident.
7. List appropriate nursing diagnoses and interventions for patients who have suffered a spinal cord injury.
8. Compare the pathophysiology, diagnosis, and treatment of parkinsonism, multiple sclerosis, Guillain-Barré syndrome, trigeminal neuralgia, and myasthenia gravis.
9. Describe the nursing actions and observations for a patient experiencing a seizure.
10. Formulate a teaching plan for the patient newly diagnosed with epilepsy.
11. Write nursing care plans for the following nursing diagnoses: impaired physical mobility; self-care deficit; alteration in bowel and urinary elimination related to incontinence; impaired verbal communication related to aphasia; and body image disturbance related to paraplegia.

The nervous system is the communication system of the body. It coordinates all sensory and motor activities by receiving, interpreting, and relaying messages that are vital to the proper performance of all the body's activities. The nervous system is composed of nerve cells and their branches, which interlace with one another to form a dense network of nerve tissue. There are a number of different types of nerve cells, but they all have two physiologic properties in common: excitability and conductivity.

Nerve cells are excited, or spurred into action, by a stimulus. This stimulus sets up an impulse, which is conducted along the nerve pathways until it reaches the tissues of the organ controlled by the nerve cells. If anything happens to impair the ability of certain nerve cells to receive and conduct impulses, the tissues controlled by the nerve cells cease to function normally. An example of this is trauma to the spinal cord. All parts of the body below the point of injury would be paralyzed and have no sensation of heat, cold, pressure, or pain if the spinal cord had been severed and the flow of impulses interrupted.

Unlike almost every other kind of cell in the body, the nerve cell, or neuron, cannot be replaced once it has been destroyed. The central nervous system, composed of the brain and spinal cord (Fig. 15-1), and the peripheral nerves are made up of highly specialized cells and tissues. Respiratory, circulatory, and digestive activities and endocrine functions all depend on an intact and normally functioning autonomic nervous system.

Because the skull is a closed bony structure, it is unable to expand. Any lesion that begins to take up space within the cranial cavity causes an increase in the pressure within the cavity. Therefore any swelling of the brain tissue from injury or surgery, leakage of blood from ruptured cerebral vessels, or tumors, abscesses, or any other lesion within the skull presents the danger of increased intracranial pressure. Nerve cells are particularly sensitive to hypoxia and cannot be replicated once they have been destroyed. Pressure against cerebral veins and arteries interferes with the flow of blood, producing a local ischemia. Pressure against the cells themselves can interfere with their vital functions. If intracranial pressure (ICP) rises very high and remains high for very long, it can cause death.

The supersensitivity of the nervous system to a lack of oxygen supply is evidenced by the speed with which some neurons die when deprived of oxygen. The skeletal muscles build up what is called an "oxygen debt," so that neuromuscular neurons can continue to live for a short while without a fresh supply of oxygen. However, the brain's neurons cannot survive anoxia for more than 4 to 6 minutes. After that time there is permanent damage to the brain cells.

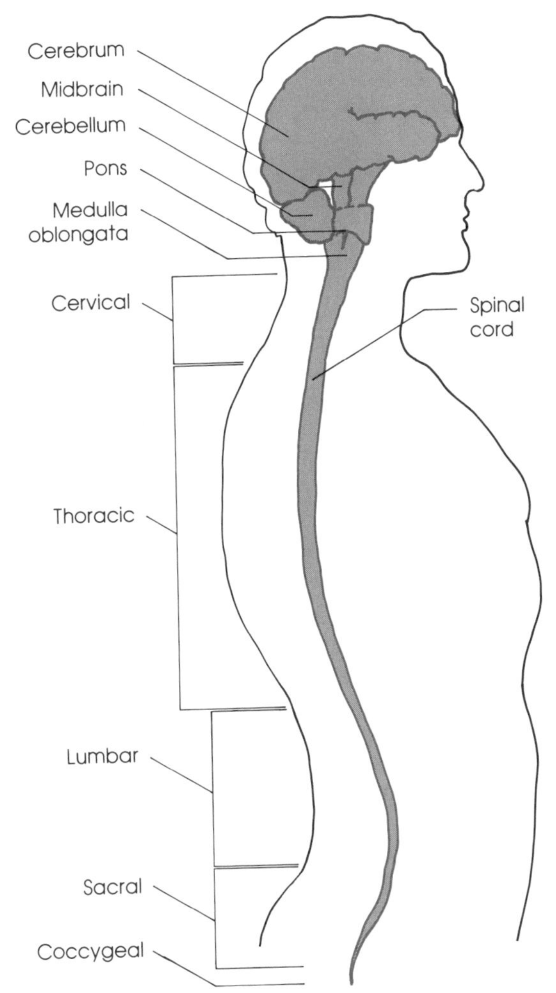

Figure 15-1 Major anatomic divisions of the central nervous system.

CAUSATIVE FACTORS IN NEUROPATHOLOGY

Any one or more of the disease-producing factors mentioned in Unit 2 can affect the nervous system and bring about a neurologic disorder. The major categories of neuropathies are:

- Developmental disorders: genetic and acquired.
- Trauma: chemical and physical.
- Inflammation: infective and allergic.
- Neoplasm: benign and malignant.
- Degeneration: vascular, other.
- Metabolic and endocrine disorders.

TERMS COMMONLY USED IN NEUROLOGIC PATHOLOGIES

As with other medical terms, those used in neurology are combinations of Greek and Latin prefixes and suffixes. The prefixes *a-*, *dys-*, *hypo-*, and *hyper-* are familiar to every student in nursing. Some prefixes and less commonly used suffixes related to disorders of the nervous system may not be so familiar. The following is a list of terms frequently encountered in neurologic nursing:

- *aphasia*—loss of the function of speech.
- *dysphasia*—impairment of or difficult speech.
- *aphonia*—loss of the ability to form vocal sounds.
- *anarthria*—inability to articulate words.
- *dysarthria*—slurring or indistinct articulation.
- *atrophy* or *hypotrophy* of muscle—muscle wasting.
- *hypertrophy* of muscle—enlargement of muscle tissue.
- *ataxia*—unsteadiness or lack of coordination.
- *apraxia* or *dyspraxia*—loss or impairment of acquired motor skills.
- *agnosia*—loss of the ability to recognize and interpret sensory information.
- *hypoesthesia* (sometimes called *hypesthesia*)—reduced sensation.
- *hyperpathia*—increased sensitivity to painful or unpleasant sensory stimuli.
- *hemiparesthesia*—reduced sensation on one side.
- *monoplegia*—weakness of one limb.
- *hemiplegia*—paralysis of arm and leg on one side of the body.
- *paraplegia*—paralysis of the lower limbs.
- *quadriplegia* (sometimes called *tetraplegia*)—paralysis of all four limbs.
- *monoparesis*—weakness of one limb.

EVALUATION OF NEUROLOGIC STATUS

The complete neurologic examination systematically measures the ability of the body to perform its myriad motor and sensory functions. Mental acuity, memory, and emotional stability are also assessed. The physical examination to identify problems of motor and sensory function is a very long procedure and may be performed by the physician in stages over several days. However, gross assessment of the cranial nerves, coordination and balance, muscle strength, and reflexes is standard for every patient with a neurologic complaint.

CRANIAL NERVES

The 12 cranial nerves (designated as CN I through CN XII) control both sensory and motor activities within various parts of the body. The patient may be tested for his sense of smell (CN I), sight (CN II, III), and hearing (CN VIII). The ability to change facial expression (CN V, VII, XII), gag reflex and swallowing (CN IX, X), ability to move his eyes (CN IV, VI), and head and shoulder movement (CN XI) are also evaluated.

COORDINATION AND BALANCE

This portion of the neurologic examination evaluates functions controlled by the higher centers of the brain—the cerebrum and cerebellum. During the examination, the patient is asked to stand with his feet together and close his eyes. If his sense of balance is normal, he will maintain a steady posture and not sway from side to side. He is then asked to walk across the room, and his gait is assessed. Next the examiner stands in front of the patient, holds up a finger, and asks the patient to touch his finger and then his own nose; the examiner moves his own finger to different locations in front of the patient. This tests both the ability to follow directions and coordination.

NEUROMUSCULAR FUNCTION TESTING

Groups of large muscles are tested for strength and coordination. The physician may evaluate the patient's gait while running, the strength of his hand grip, and the strength of his arms and legs as he pushes against resistance. More sophisticated tests include electromyography (Table 15–1).

REFLEXES

A reflex is a reflected action or movement that is built into the nervous system and does not need the intervention of conscious thought to take place. In other words, it is an automatic response. The knee jerk is an example of the simplest type of reflex. When the knee is tapped, the nerve that receives this stimulus sends an impulse to the spinal cord, where it is relayed to a motor nerve. This causes the quadriceps muscle at the front of the thigh to contract and jerk the leg upward. This reflex, or simple reflex arc, involves only two nerves and one synapse. The leg begins to jerk up while the brain is just becoming aware of the tap on the knee.

The knee jerk, or patellar reflex, tests nerve pathways to and from the spinal cord at the level of the second through fourth lumbar nerves. In addition to testing the patellar reflex, a neurologic examination also might include testing the biceps reflex (pathways for the fifth and sixth cervical nerves), triceps reflex (seventh and eighth cervical nerves), brachioradialis reflex (fifth and sixth cervical nerves), and achilles tendon reflex (first and second sacral nerves).

Another reflex action widely used as a diagnostic aid in disorders of the central nervous system (CNS) is the *Babinski reflex*, which is elicited by scraping an object along the sole of the foot. In a normal response to this stimulus the toes will bend downward. In a *positive* Babinski reflex, the great toe bends backward (upward) and the smaller toes fan outward. A positive Babinski reflex indicates an abnormality in the motor control pathways leading from the cerebral cortex (Fig. 15–2).

To test brain stem function, the oculocephalic ("doll's eyes") and oculovestibular reflexes are assessed. For the doll's eyes reflex, the examiner places both hands on the sides of the patient's head, using the thumbs to gently hold open his eyelids; while watching the patient's eyes, the head is rotated briskly from side to side or up and down and eye movement is observed in relation to head movement. If the brain stem pathways are not intact, the eyes appear to move in a direction opposite to that of the head movement. The oculovestibular reflex is assessed by *calorics* testing. With the patient's head elevated at least 30 degrees, 20 to 200 mL of cold or ice water is instilled into the ear with a catheter-tipped syringe. While the external ear canal is irrigated, the patient's eye movements are observed. Normally the eyes will show nystagmus, darting away from the irrigated ear. Absence of eye movement indicates a brain stem lesion.

DIAGNOSTIC TESTS

The major diagnostic tests most commonly used for evaluation of the neurologic system are presented in Table 15–1. Basic physiologic testing is also done to rule out disease in some other system that might be affecting the condition of the patient. A chest radiograph, electrocardiogram (EKG), complete blood cell (CBC) count, urinalysis, and basic tests for electrolytes, liver function, kidney function, nutritional parameters, and lipid metabolism (such as are included on a Sequential Multiple Analyzer [SMA] profile) are performed. A nerve or muscle biopsy may be done to determine pathologic changes in these tissues.

NURSING ASSESSMENT OF NEUROLOGIC STATUS

Neurologic nursing requires special training and experience in observation, critical judgment, and specific skills to help patients cope with a myriad of problems. The nurse not only must be aware of subtle changes in the patient's condition but also must recognize the *significance* of these changes and act promptly when medical attention is needed. In a text such as this we can cover only the most basic of skills and knowledge required in neurologic nursing. It is extremely important that the nurse who is sharing in the responsibility for the care of a patient with a neurologic disorder know her own strengths and weaknesses and seek guidance when she is not sure of her ability to observe and evaluate a patient's status.

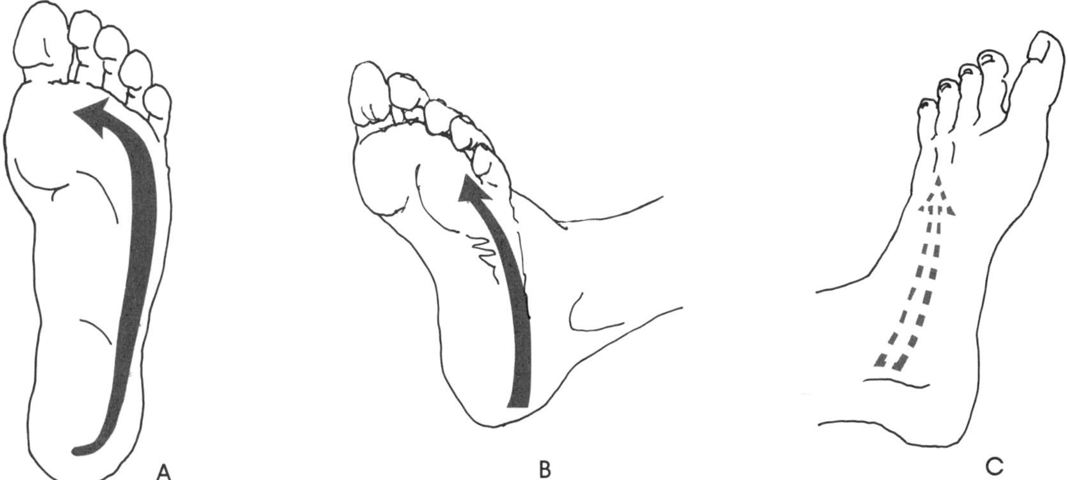

Figure 15–2 Normal and Babinski reflexes. *A*, Line of stimulation: outer sole, heel to little toe. *B*, Plantar (normal) reflex. Toes curl inward. *C*, Positive Babinski reflex (always abnormal). Great toe bends upward; smaller toes fan outward.

TABLE 15-1 **DIAGNOSTIC TESTS FOR NEUROLOGIC PROBLEMS**

Test	Purpose	Description	Nursing Implications
Lumbar puncture (spinal tap)	To determine if CSF pressure is elevated; to determine if there is a blockage to the flow of CSF; to inject medication; to detect the presence of blood from subarachnoid hemorrhage; to obtain fluid for chemical analysis and culture.	Physician performs a sterile puncture into the arachnoid space, using local anesthetic, between L-3 and L-4 or L-4 and L-5 (Fig. 15-3); opening pressure is obtained; fluid is aspirated and placed in sterile test tubes labeled 1, 2, 3. Fluid is analyzed for color, pH, cell count, protein, chloride, and glucose; a culture is usually done.	Obtain signature on consent form. Obtain sterile lumbar puncture tray, local anesthetic, sterile gloves, and tape. Assist patient into position with back bowed, head flexed on chest, and knees drawn up to the abdomen. Patient may be lying or sitting. Assist him to maintain position and to hold still during procedure. Reassure patient and provide emotional support. Appropriately label tubes with patient data afterward and transport them to the laboratory immediately. Keep patient flat in bed to reduce headache for 6 to 8 hours after procedure and encourage fluid intake unless contraindicated.
Electroencephalogram (EEG)	To detect abnormal brain wave patterns that are indicative of specific diseases such as seizure disorder, brain tumor, CVA, head trauma, and infection; to determine cerebral death.	May be performed while asleep, awake, drowsy, or undergoing stimulation such as hyperventilation or rhythmic bright light. Hair should be clean and dry. No sleeping pills or sedatives the night before test; check with physician regarding other drugs to be held; restrict coffee, tea, caffeine, and alcohol for 24 to 48 hours; tracing is taken with patient in reclining chair or lying down (Fig. 15-4). Test takes 45 minutes to 2 hours. A mesh cap containing the electrodes is snugly applied to the head. If a sleep EEG is ordered, patient may need to be kept up most or all of the night prior to the test; do not keep NPO, as hypoglycemia can affect the test.	Explain purpose of test to the patient; assure him he will not receive an electric shock, the test is not painful, and that the machine does not determine intelligence or read his mind. Test may be done at the bedside or in the EEG lab.
Electromyography (EMG)	To measure electrical activity of skeletal muscle at rest and during voluntary activity to determine abnormalities in muscular contraction. Helpful in diagnosing neuromuscular, peripheral nerve, and muscular disorders.	With the patient sitting in a chair or lying on a table, needle electrodes are inserted in selected muscles. Tracings of electrical activity are taken with the muscles at rest and then with various voluntary activities that produce muscle contraction. The test takes 1 to 2 hours depend-	Obtain signed informed consent. Explain the procedure to the patient; tell him that there is a small amount of discomfort when the electrodes are placed. Check with physician regarding medications to be withheld; muscle relaxants, cholinergics, and anticholinergics can influ-

TABLE 15-1 **DIAGNOSTIC TESTS FOR NEUROLOGIC PROBLEMS** *Continued*

Test	Purpose	Description	Nursing Implications
		ing on how many muscles are tested.	ence test result. There is no food or fluid restriction. If serum enzymes are ordered, they should be drawn before the EMG.
Myelogram	To detect spinal lesions: intervertebral disc problems, tumors, or cysts.	Air or a radiopaque substance is injected into the spinal canal (Fig. 15-5), and fluoroscopic examination and radiographs are made. The study is contraindicated if the patient has increased ICP. The patient is placed prone and strapped to the x-ray table for the spinal puncture; as the contrast medium is injected, the table is tilted. After the test, if oil-base medium was used, it is withdrawn. The patient is kept in bed with head of bed elevated 60 degrees or flat depending on the contrast medium used. Procedure takes 1 hour.	Requires a signed consent. Explain what to expect. Patient may feel a warm flush when contrast medium is injected. Bowel evacuation regimen may be ordered the night before. Keep NPO for 4 to 8 hours prior to procedure. Check for medications to be withheld before and for 48 hours posttest. Assess for allergy to iodine or shellfish. Dress in myelogram pajamas; administer preoperative sedative or analgesic. Posttest: monitor VS q 30 min × 2 h, then 1 h × 4 h. Assess pulses and sensation in extremities; monitor urinary output; catheterize if patient cannot void in 8 h as ordered; encourage increased fluid intake. Observe for signs of meningitis.
Computerized Axial Tomography (CAT or CT Scan)	To examine the brain from many different angles, obtaining a series of cross-sectional images that provide views from three dimensions. To identify hematomas, tumors, cysts, hydrocephalus, cerebral atrophy, obstruction to CSF flow, and cerebral edema.	May be done with or without contrast dye enhancement. Patient lies on a narrow table with his head cradled and is moved so that his head is inside the circular opening of the machine. A security strap is wrapped snuggly around him. CT scanner produces a narrow x-ray beam. Various clicking and whirring noises are heard as the machine rotates the scanner for different views. If contrast dye is used, the patient will feel a warm flush and have a metallic taste in his mouth as it is injected. The test takes 45 minutes to 1½ hours. The patient may need to be sedated if he is prone to claustrophobia; the table can be uncomfortable for those with arthritis or back problems. He will be able to communicate with the machine's operator.	A consent form is required. Explain the procedure and what he will see, hear, and feel. Patient should be NPO for 3 to 4 hours prior to test if contrast dye is to be used to prevent vomiting. Assess for allergy to iodine or shellfish. Remove all hairpins, jewelry, and metal from the head and neck.

Table continued on following page

TABLE 15–1 **DIAGNOSTIC TESTS FOR NEUROLOGIC PROBLEMS** *Continued*

Test	Purpose	Description	Nursing Implications
Cerebral angiography	To visualize the structure of the cerebral arteries to determine presence of stricture, tumor, aneurysm, thrombus, or hematoma.	Radiopaque liquid is injected through a catheter inserted into the common carotid artery, and a series of radiographs is taken. Fluoroscopy is used during the procedure. Digital subtraction angiography (DSA) is done by utilizing a computer along with the angiography procedure.	Consent form is required. Assess for allergy to iodine and shellfish. Explain procedure; patient will be supine on x-ray table; local anesthetic will be used to introduce the catheter; an IV will be started in case of need for emergency drugs; patient will feel a flush as the dye is injected; test takes 1 to 2 hours. Should be NPO 8 to 12 hours prior to test; anticoagulants are discontinued beforehand. May be given preprocedure sedative, antihistamine, or steroid to decrease possibility of allergic reaction to dye. Postprocedure: assess for bleeding; perform neurologic checks; monitor vital signs q 15 min × 1 h; q 30 min × 2 h; q 1 h × 4 h or until stable. Assess for dysphagia and respiratory distress that could indicate internal bleeding in the neck. Activities are restricted for 24 hours.
Radionuclide imaging (brain scan)	To detect an intracranial mass: tumor, abcess, hematoma, aneurysm.	A radioisotope is administered IV. Abnormal tissue usually absorbs more of the isotope than normal tissue. After a 1- to 3-hour waiting period for absorption, a scintillation scanner is used to image the brain. The test takes ½ to 1 hour.	Explain the procedure; patient will sit or lie on a table; the scanner makes clicking noises; the amount of radioactivity is very low and is not dangerous to the patient or others. He will need to lie or sit still during the scanning. A drug may be given the night before to block uptake of the radioactive element by the thyroid and salivary glands. There is no food or fluid restriction; no special aftercare.
Magnetic resonance imaging (MRI)	To visualize soft tissue without the use of contrast media or ionizing radiation; provides excellent images of soft tissue, eliminating bone; can visualize lesions undetected by CT scan. To detect white matter areas in nervous system that represent demyelination, as in multiple sclerosis.	An electromagnet is used to detect radio frequency pulses produced by alignment of hydrogen protons in the magnetic field. Computer produces tomographic images with high contrast of area studied. Cannot be used in the presence of metal. Is quite expensive.	Inform patient that the test is painless; no dietary restrictions. Remove all metal objects before test. Patient must be still during test. Explain that body part to be imaged is moved inside large machine; some patients become claustrophobic.
Ultrasound arteriography (Doppler flow studies)	To study flow and determine areas of constriction or obstruction in cerebral ar-	Noninvasive test. Doppler image scanning device is used with computer to vi-	Tell patient that the test is painless. A small Doppler wand is positioned over

TABLE 15-1 **DIAGNOSTIC TESTS FOR NEUROLOGIC PROBLEMS** *Continued*

Test	Purpose	Description	Nursing Implications
	teries. To detect arterial spasm.	sualize anatomy of major cerebral arteries.	particular "window" areas on the skull (temples), and with the computer, sound waves are directed so as to produce an image of the interior arteries and their blood flow. No special preparation or aftercare.
Evoked potential studies	To measure response of the CNS to visual, auditory, or sensory stimulus. Helpful in detecting tumor of CN VIII, blindness in infants, or brain stem lesions. Also useful in diagnosing multiple sclerosis.	May be done in conjunction with EEG. Electrodes are used to pick up and transmit impulses to a computer while a stimulus is delivered to the patient. Signals are displayed on an oscilloscope, and data are stored for later interpretation.	Explain the procedure to the patient. Visual evoked responses: stimulus may be a bright flashing light or checkerboard patterns. Somatosensory evoked potentials require stimulation of a peripheral sensory nerve with a mild electric shock. Auditory brain stem evoked potentials utilize various noises or tone bursts through earphones. Discomfort is minimal. Test takes 30 to 60 minutes.
Cerebrospinal fluid analysis and culture	To detect abnormalities that are indicative of specific neurologic problems and determine which organism is responsible for infection.	CSF is obtained by lumbar puncture. It is analyzed for color, cell count, protein, chloride, and glucose. The fluid is cultured to detect the presence of organisms; if present, an antibiotic sensitivity test is done to determine which drug will best kill the organism. CSF pressure is also measured. Normal CSF values for the adult are: Color: Clear Cell count (WBCs): 0 to 8 cu mm Protein: 15 to 45 mg/dL Chloride: 118 to 132 mEq/L Glucose: 40 to 80 mg/dL Pressure: 75 to 175 mm H_2O	Follow lumbar puncture procedure (above). Label the test tubes #1, 2, 3 and be certain they are filled with at least 3 mL of CSF in this order. Do not refrigerate the tubes; transport to the lab immediately. Maintain universal precautions.

PATIENT HISTORY

Because neurologic disorders can be present in conjunction with or in addition to disorders of other systems of the body, the nurse should always include questions about neurologic status in her initial and ongoing assessments of all her patients. For example, a surgical patient could well have had a previous stroke, a history of seizures, or an existing neuromuscular disease such as multiple sclerosis. Although these may not be the primary reason for his admission to a hospital, they will certainly influence the course of the illness or injury for which he has been admitted.

Most admissions forms used by the nurse in her assessment include questions about the patient's personal or family history of epilepsy or any genetic disorder of the nervous system. In addition, it would be helpful to know if at the present or in the past the patient has or had any change or difficulty in concentrating or remembering, speaking, or expressing his thoughts. Other questions might include changes in muscle strength or coordination, recent or past injury to the head, or infections that could affect the ner-

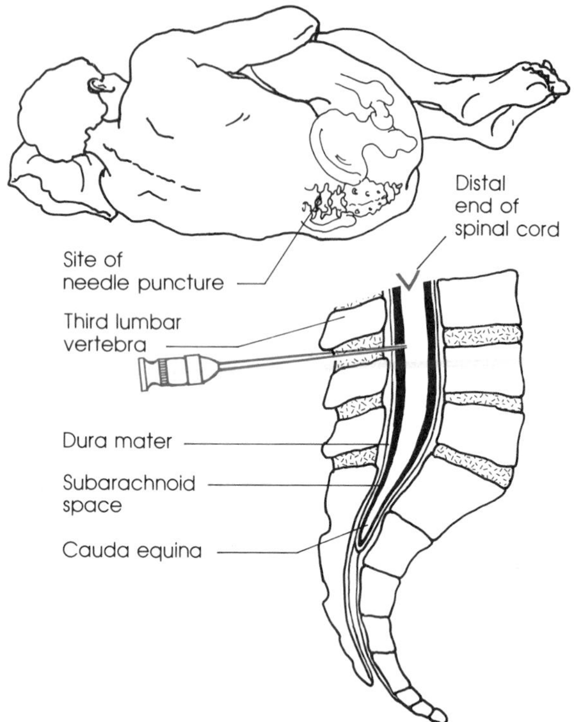

Figure 15-3 Lumbar puncture technique. The needle is inserted between the vertebrae and advanced through the dura mater to the subarachnoid space. Cerebrospinal fluid is thus withdrawn from the spinal cavity during a spinal tap.

vous system. These infections are not limited to meningitis and encephalitis, but also include infections affecting tissues near the brain (for example, sinusitis, middle ear infection, abscessed teeth, and pustules on the skin such as those accompanying severe acne).

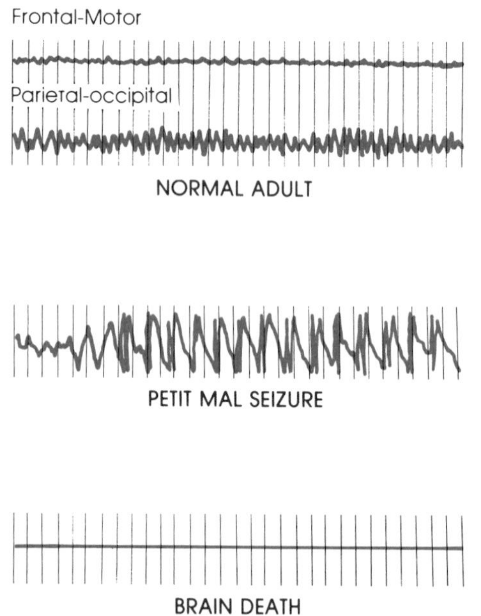

Figure 15-4 Samples of EEG tracings showing normal activity, seizure activity, and brain death.

Symptoms that the patient might have noticed and that are significant in assessing his neurologic status include muscle weakness, tremors, or spasms; fainting, dizziness, or episodes of unconsciousness; ringing in the ears; blurred vision; changes in his sense of taste or smell; numbness or tingling of the extremities; and loss of coordination.

ASSESSMENT OF A PATIENT WITH A DIAGNOSED NEUROLOGIC DISORDER

There are many times when a patient will need frequent, systematic monitoring to determine his neurologic status. For example, monitoring is necessary following a traumatic head injury, after ingestion of an overdose of a drug or other chemical, or any other condition in which the patient has lost or may lose consciousness.

In many institutions a checklist for neurologic assessment ("neuro check") is available for the nursing staff to use as a guide for objective assessment of a patient's status. The neuro check is meant to avoid subjective and vague terms that do not give precise information. Such terms as *comatose, semiconscious,* and *stuporous* do not provide reliable data for drawing valid conclusions and making decisions. The format of the neurologic assessment sheet varies from one place to another, but four major components are usually included.

The four major areas to be assessed in a patient with a problem of altered state of consciousness are (1) level of consciousness (LOC), (2) neuromuscular responses, (3) reactions of the pupils to light, and (4) vital signs.

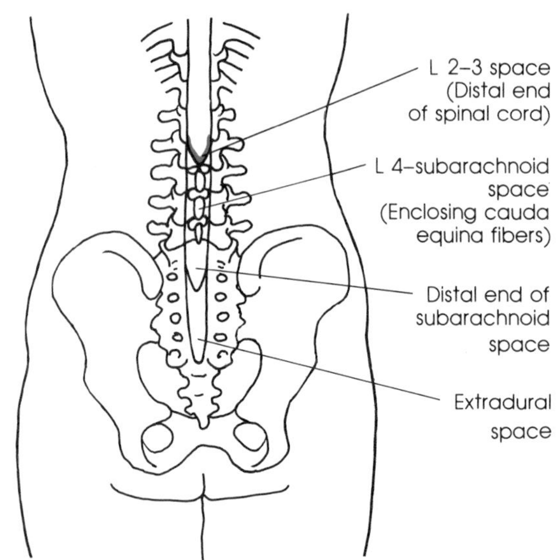

Figure 15-5 Relationship of spinal cord and vertebrae. Note the location of the distal end of the spinal cord.

Level of Consciousness

The ability of the patient to respond appropriately to whatever is going on around him usually is not simply an "on/off" or "yes/no" situation. Patients experience varying levels of awareness and ability to respond. Thus the observation that a patient is unconscious has little meaning in terms of his neurologic status at any given time. It is more accurate to determine where the patient is on a scale of varying degrees of consciousness, the extremes of the scale being alert wakefulness and deep coma (no responsiveness at all).

In observing a patient for level of consciousness, the best assessment is based on established criteria or standards that are understood by the observer as well as by others who will be reading the results of the observations. The Glasgow Coma Scale is a tool that is universally used in one form or another for this purpose (Table 15–2). The nurse gives a rating to the patient in three different categories. The first category is eye opening, the second is best verbal response, and the third is best motor response. A number is assigned for each category depending on what the assessment reveals. Assessment within the first and last category determines whether the patient can respond to voice commands or to pain or doesn't respond at all. Verbal responses are evaluated according to whether the patient is oriented and "making sense," confused, making inappropriate remarks, incomprehensible, or silent. The score in each area is added together, and the sum is compared to a score of 15, indicating a fully alert patient, and a score of 3, indicating a totally comatose patient. Coma level is indicated by a score of 7 or less. Some of the criteria are: Does he awaken easily? Is he oriented as to person (himself as well as others), place, and time? Is he able to follow commands? Does he fail to respond to any stimulus, even painful ones? Is he restless? Combative? Does he respond to pain with abnormal posture?

TABLE 15–2 GLASGOW COMA SCALE

Eye opening	
Spontaneous	4
To sound	3
To pain	2
Never	1
Motor response	
Obeys commands	6
Localizes pain	5
Normal flexion (withdrawal)	4
Abnormal flexion posturing	3
Extension posturing	2
None	1
Verbal response	
Oriented	5
Confused conversation	4
Inappropriate words	3
Incomprehensible sounds	2
None	1

A score of 7 or less indicates coma.
The highest possible score is 15.

Neuromuscular Responses

This aspect of assessment is concerned with the function of the motor pathways. Each of the upper and lower extremities is tested. If the patient is not able to respond to verbal commands to move his arms and legs, another stimulus may be necessary. Gentle pressure over the tendons and joints in the extremities is preferred to pinching, deep pressure, and other painful stimuli. Applying pressure to the nail bed with your own fingernail or an object such as the cap of a pen is also acceptable.

> ***The levels of response are (1)* purposefully *withdrawing from the stimulus or an attempt to push it away; (2)* nonpurposeful *response, in which the patient may frown or move his arm or leg in a random fashion; and (3)* failure to respond *at all.***

Nonpurposeful responses to pain occur in two ways. Flexor (decorticate) posturing, in which there is extension of the legs and internal rotation and adduction of the arms with the elbows bent upward, occurs with damage to the cortex. In extensor (decerebrate) posturing, the arms are stiffly extended and held close to the body, and the wrists are flexed outward. This response means there is damage to the midbrain or brain stem and indicates a very serious injury.

Pupillary Reactions

Changes in pupil size in response to a bright light are frequently used to determine whether the areas of the brain stem that help control consciousness are functioning normally. First, if at all possible, one should know the state of the pupils that is normal for the patient. Although pupils of equal size are considered normal, some people have pupils that are unequal in size. The size of the pupils also may vary from person to person. See Figure 15–6 for a chart showing pupil sizes in millimeters.

The pupils should be checked in a darkened room, in which one would expect the pupils to be dilated. A bright light is then directed into each eye from the side. One should observe whether the pupil into which the light is shone constricts and whether it does so quickly or slowly.

Pupils that remain dilated and fixed in the presence of a bright light are indicative of brain

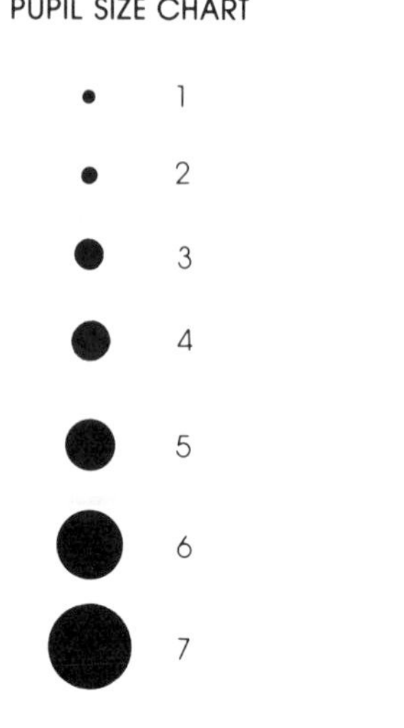

Figure 15-6 Chart showing pupil sizes in millimeters.

damage. One pupil remaining fixed and dilated indicates increased ICP. If both pupils remain constricted, there probably is damage to the pons.

Extraocular muscle movements are also checked. Ask the patient to follow your finger while you make a wide "H" in the air. Note whether both eyes move together (conjugate) or one deviates. If there is deviation, it is important to note in which direction the deviation is. It should be noted if there is any quick back-and-forth oscillation (nystagmus) of the eye at the end points of each direction. Nystagmus can indicate abnormality or can be a side effect of medication such as phenytoin (Dilantin). Warning signs of increasing intracranial pressure and impending cerebral disaster are summarized in Table 15-3.

Although changes in the pupils such as unequal constriction and decreased rate of constriction are indicators of increased ICP, sometimes changes in pupils can be caused by medications. For example, atropine and scopolamine can produce dilated pupils, and the opiates can cause constriction (Table 15-4).

Vital Signs

Assessing and recording temperature, pulse, respirations, and blood pressure are essential parts of a neurologic check. Temperature is important for a number of reasons; an infection may be developing, or there may be damage to the temperature control mechanisms within the brain.

If there has been a decrease in blood supply to the brain and ICP is rising, the heart may begin to beat strongly, elevating the blood pressure. This is, however, only a temporary change. If it is not reported promptly and action is not taken to relieve the increasing ICP, the blood pressure will begin to fall, and the pulse rate will compensatorily increase. Changes in respiratory rate and character also must be reported promptly, because they may indicate impaired function of the parts of the brain that control respiration.

INFECTIOUS DISEASES

MENINGITIS

Meningitis is an inflammation of the membranes covering the brain and spinal cord. The membranes can become infected in a number of ways, because infectious agents can be carried (1) through the blood stream by direct extension from an infected area of the brain, spinal cord, and sinuses; (2) through an opening in the skull in a head injury; and (3) by accidental introduction of infectious agents into the spinal canal during spinal puncture.

Many different strains of bacteria and viruses can cause meningitis, including pneumococcal and influenzal bacilli, but when the disease occurs in epidemic form, the causative agent usually is meningococcal (*Neisseria meningitidis*).

TABLE 15-3 **WARNING SIGNS OF INCREASING INTRACRANIAL PRESSURE AND IMPENDING CEREBRAL DISASTER**

Sign	Nursing Assessment
Change in level of consciousness	Note change in awareness, whether increasing or decreasing; orientation; decreasing response to stimulation.
Change in limb motion	Extreme restlessness; muscle weakness or paralysis.
Change in pupil size	Bilateral or unilateral dilatation.
	Unilateral dilatation may be sign of cerebral hemorrhage with rapid deterioration.
Change in vital signs	Slowing pulse rate; widening pulse pressure; labored, irregular breathing; rising body temperature.

TABLE 15-4 PUPILLARY ABNORMALITIES AND POSSIBLE CAUSES

Assessment Data	Appearance	Possible Causes
Unilateral, fixed, dilated pupil. Unreactive to light. May be accompanied by ptosis and deviation to side and downward.		Damage to oculomotor nerve related to increased intraocular pressure, compression of oculomotor nerve, head trauma with epidural or subdural hematoma.
Bilateral dilated and fixed pupils that do not react to light.		Hypoxia associated with cardiopulmonary arrest. Pressure on midbrain. Severe CNS disorder. Anticholinergic drug overdose.
Bilateral small, fixed pupils that do not react to light. Accompanied by motor deficits, drowsiness, confusion, headache, vomiting, incontinence when due to damage to diencephalon.		Side effect of opiates such as morphine. Miotic eye drops. Hemorrhage into the pons. Damage to the diencephalon.
Unequal pupil size; both pupils react to light unless there is underlying pathology.		Ocular inflammation. Congenital aberration. Adhesion, as of iris to cornea or lens. Disturbance of neural pathways.

Symptoms and Medical Diagnosis

The most outstanding symptom of meningitis is a severe and persistent headache that is greatly aggravated by shaking the head. Other signs of meningeal irritation include pain and stiffness of the neck (nuchal rigidity), exaggerated deep tendon reflexes, irritability, photophobia, and hypersensitivity of the skin. Seizures frequently are present, as are nausea and vomiting and signs of an upper respiratory infection.

When meningitis is suspected, a spinal tap is performed and the cerebrospinal fluid (CSF) examined for the number and type of organisms in it. The CSF pressure is usually elevated. *When meningitis is present, the spinal fluid may appear milky as a result of the increased number of white cells suspended in the fluid.* Other abnormal findings include the presence of protein and decreased amounts of glucose.

Medical Treatment

Successful treatment of meningitis and prevention of permanent disability depend on early recognition and prompt treatment. Once the causative organism has been identified, specific antibiotics to which the organism is sensitive are administered. A combination of two drugs is often utilized. The disease usually responds well to intravenous (IV) antibiotic therapy given for 2 weeks, followed by several days of oral doses. Anticonvulsive drugs are given to control seizures, and aspirin or acetaminophen is given for headache. Narcotics are never used for pain control in patients with neurologic problems, as they cause sedation and prevent accurate neurologic assessment. They can also mask signs of increasing ICP. Prophylactic antibiotics are usually given to those in close contact with the patient to prevent the spread of the infection.

Nursing Assessment

In addition to noting the specific signs and symptoms of meningitis, the nurse must assess the patient for subjective and objective data relevant to each of the patient care problems that might accompany the disease. Examples include convulsive seizures, elevated body temperature, nausea and vomiting, delirium, pain, increased ICP, and fluid and electrolyte imbalances. Each of these problems and assessment of the patient are discussed in the section "Common Neurologic Patient Care Problems."

Nursing Intervention

Ongoing, vigilant neurologic assessment is a high priority. Specific nursing interventions in the care of the patient with meningitis are primarily concerned with measures to conserve the strength of the patient and promote healing. Prevention of the spread of infection will include some precautionary measures. The type of precautions and isolation will depend on the type of meningitis present. Meningococcal meningitis is spread by droplet infection, so the recommended procedure is *respiratory precautions.*

The patient's room should be quiet and dimly lit. Sudden noises or a bright flash of light, such as occurs when an overhead light is switched on, can cause a seizure. It is obvious from outward appearance that the patient with meningitis is acutely ill. He must be turned very gently and positioned to prevent joint stiffness. Range-of-motion exercises must be done regularly. Care and treatments are coordinated to allow as much rest as possible. Meningitis often produces mental confusion and delirium, as well as the possibility of seizures. The nursing care of patients with these problems is discussed later in this chapter.

Herpes simplex (fever blisters) frequently accompanies meningitis. The presence of these sores, plus drying of the lips and mouth as a result of high temperatures and dehydration, requires special mouth care. The lips and mouth should be cleansed and lubricated at least every 2 hours during the acute stage of the disease.

Fluid volume deficit is often a problem; thus the patient's intake and output should be measured. Excessive vomiting or outward signs of early dehydration should be reported promptly so that fluids may be given intravenously when necessary.

A decrease in the peristaltic action of the intestines often occurs in meningitis and can lead to an accumulation of flatus and fecal material with severe abdominal distention. The patient's abdomen should be checked for distention and his bowel sounds noted and recorded. Rectal tubes, suppositories, or *small, low* enemas may be ordered for relief of this condition. Large amounts of fluid should not be given rectally, because they may increase ICP by being absorbed into the body's fluid compartment and causing fluid excess.

The patient will need support and reassurance from the nurse, because the severity of this illness is frightening. If he is confused, he will need frequent orientation. The family will need information and reassurance also.

Once the acute stage of the disease is over, the patient is allowed to gradually resume his former activities. Residual effects of the disease such as paralysis, deafness, and visual defects sometimes occur, but these sequelae of meningitis do not usually occur if the disease is diagnosed and treated in the early stages before permanent damage is done.

ENCEPHALITIS

Encephalitis is an inflammation of the tissues of the brain that causes cerebral edema and diffuse nerve cell destruction. The disease is most often caused by a virus or the toxins produced by the organisms that cause chickenpox, measles, and mumps. Some chemicals such as lead and arsenic also can produce encephalitis.

The severity of the illness may be mild or fatal. Encephalitis is most commonly transmitted by the bite of an infected mosquito or tick.

Symptoms

The onset of encephalitis may be either sudden or insidious and is characterized by headache, high fever, stiff neck or back, muscular weakness, and extreme restlessness or lethargy. CNS signs appear 1 to 4 hours after the other symptoms. Mental confusion, visual disturbances, and disorientation may be present. The lethargy may progress to coma. Diagnosis is confirmed by the presence of the virus in the CSF or blood stream.

Medical Treatment and Nursing Intervention

The treatment of encephalitis is primarily symptomatic, with general supportive measures to maintain the strength of the patient, promote healing, and prevent complications.

Specific nursing measures are essentially the same as for any patient who is subject to seizures, high fever, delirium, and altered levels of consciousness.

GUILLAIN-BARRÉ SYNDROME

Guillain-Barré syndrome is a relatively rare disease that affects the peripheral nervous system, especially the spinal nerves outside the spinal cord. It also can affect the cranial nerves. Pathologic changes include demyelination (loss of the fatty sheath around the nerves), inflammation, edema, and compression of the nerve root. These changes bring about the paresthesia, pain, and progressive, ascending paralysis that are typical of the syndrome.

The cause of Guillain-Barré syndrome is not known, but it usually follows a respiratory infection or gastroenteritis within 10 to 21 days. Because one half to two thirds of patients with the syndrome report a febrile condition before its clinical onset, some authorities believe the disease is related to an autoimmune response.

Diagnosis and Medical Treatment

Objective and subjective symptoms of Guillain-Barré syndrome include mild sensations of numbness and tingling in the feet and hands, followed by muscle pain, tenderness, and aching, especially in the shoulder, pelvis, and thighs. There is progressive muscle weakness, usually starting in the lower extremities and tending to move upward over 24 to 72 hours. However, it can also affect the facial muscles first and move downward. Sensory loss also can occur but is not as common as motor loss.

Diagnosis of Guillain-Barré syndrome is difficult, because its characteristic signs and symptoms are similar to those of several other diseases. Analysis of the CSF is helpful. Typically there is an elevated protein content that tends to rise as the disease progresses, peaking in 4 to 6 weeks. The number of leukocytes remains within normal limits, as does CSF pressure. For the most part, the physician must depend on the clinical picture presented by the patient in order to diagnose Guillain-Barré syndrome.

Medical treatment is mainly supportive. Plasmapheresis, in which the patient's plasma is removed and "washed" to remove antibodies, hastens recovery in some patients.

Nursing Assessment and Intervention

There are three stages of Guillain-Barré syndrome, each demanding different kinds of monitoring and intervention. During the *acute phase*, the goals are to sustain life, prevent complications related to immobility, and promote rest and comfort. Respiratory problems are particularly troublesome and may require suctioning, tracheostomy care, artificial ventilation, and other life-support measures.

Vital signs must be checked frequently. Alterations in the autonomic nervous system can cause drastic changes in blood pressure, particularly hypotension. Cardiac arrhythmias also frequently occur.

The paralysis and loss of control that occur with Guillain-Barré syndrome come on so suddenly and are so overwhelming that the patient becomes very frightened. Because the course of the disease usually extends for months with a very slow recovery, the patient begins to have feelings of hopelessness, despair, and isolation. If the respiratory muscles are affected, the patient will be placed on a ventilator.

The *static* phase is a kind of plateau the patient reaches 1 to 3 weeks after the onset of his illness. During this time the motor loss and paresthesias no longer progress, and the patient's condition becomes somewhat stabilized; he gets no better and no worse. This phase can last from a few days to months.

During the static phase, nursing care is concerned with preventing complications of immobility and helping the patient deal with his feelings of anger, depression, and anxiety. Exercises are usually begun but are limited to passive and gentle range-of-motion and stretching exercises. There must be a balance of rest and exercise and no sudden changes in posture or position, lest blood pressure suddenly drop.

Meticulous skin care is essential. Monitoring for thrombophlebitis is important, as this is a frequent complication. Elastic stockings or alternating compression boots are used along with anticoagulant therapy to try to prevent thrombophlebitis.

The final phase—*rehabilitation*—is one of gradual recovery. The patient may become elated over the change in his condition and must be prevented from overexertion, which can lead to a relapse. As muscle function returns, the level of exercise and activity is slowly increased.

HEAD INJURIES

The brain is safely encased in a rigid skull to protect it from traumatic physical blows, which is consoling, but this structural feature of the head can be harmful when the contents of the skull swell or are otherwise enlarged. For example, tumors composed of either benign or malignant cells and those filled with blood from damaged vessels will occupy space reserved for the tissues of the brain. Swellings within the rigid skull produce an increasing *intracranial pressure*, which compresses the brain and brings about symptoms of sensory and motor damage.

Head injuries are the most frequent cause of death in people between the ages of 1 and 35 years. Those who survive initial head injury require meticulous observation and care so that damage to the brain cells can be kept at a minimum.

TYPES OF INJURIES

A blow to the head may cause *open* injuries, with lacerations of the skin and scalp and fracture of the skull, or *closed* injuries, in which the scalp and skull remain intact, but the underlying brain tissue is damaged.

The term* concussion *is used to describe a closed head injury in which the brain is compressed by a portion of the skull at the time of the blow and temporary ischemia of the brain tissue results. In a* contusion, *the brain tissue is bruised and blood from broken vessels accumulates, causing increased intracranial pressure.

A contrecoup injury, also called an acceleration-deceleration injury, occurs when the head is moving rapidly and hits a stationary object such as a windshield. The contents within the cranium hit the inside of the skull and then bounce back and hit the bony area opposite the site of impact, causing a second injury.

Subdural hematoma is a common result of head injury. A hematoma is a blood-filled swelling. When a blow is delivered to the head, it may rupture the blood vessels that lie between the delicate arachnoid membrane covering the brain and the tough, fibrous dura mater. As the blood leaks under the dura mater (subdural), the hematoma grows in size, pressing against the softer arachnoid and the brain tissue it is covering (Fig. 15–7).

An *epidural hematoma* rarely occurs, but when it does, there is rapid leakage of blood from a relatively large artery, which quickly elevates ICP. This constitutes a medical emergency. A craniotomy is needed to repair the damaged vessel and relieve pressure.

SYMPTOMS AND MEDICAL DIAGNOSIS

The severity of brain damage from a head injury is best judged by the symptoms presented by the patient, neurologic assessment, the history of the type of blow received, and whether the victim lost consciousness and for how long. No head injury should be considered completely harmless. They are all potentially dangerous, because there may be a delayed reaction in which there is hemorrhage into the brain tissues or the formation of a blood clot. These conditions build up over a period of time and result from weakening and rupture of the small blood vessels in the brain. Sometimes the bleeding is so slow that it takes weeks or even months for the symptoms of pressure within the skull to appear.

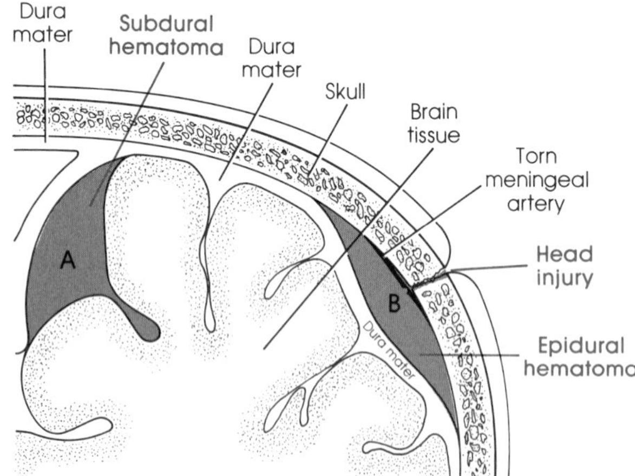

Figure 15–7 Subdural and epidural hematoma. *A*, Subdural hematoma. As a result of trauma to the head, small ruptured blood vessels leak blood into the space under the dura mater. The hematoma forms between the dura mater and the arachnoid membrane. *B*, Epidural hematoma, the result of a head injury that tears a large meningeal artery, causing the collection of a large amount of blood above the dura mater. The large epidural hematoma compresses brain tissue. If not relieved, subdural and epidural hematomas can be fatal.

The outward symptoms of head injury are fairly obvious; these include bruising, swelling, lacerations, and bleeding. However, the symptoms indicating a buildup of pressure within the skull are more subtle and less easily detected. In effect, the nurse observing a patient with a head injury, infectious diseases of the central nervous system, brain tumor, or intracranial surgery is observing for signs of *increased intracranial pressure* as well as other pathologic changes.

Diagnostic tests and examinations commonly used to determine the extent of head injury include a radiograph of the skull, a computed tomographic (CT) scan, cerebral angiography, electroencephalography, and brain scanning.

MEDICAL AND SURGICAL TREATMENT

The patient with a head injury usually is treated conservatively at first, unless a serious emergency such as greatly increased ICP arises, or a compound fracture of the skull demands surgical débridement of the wound and removal of splintered bone from the brain tissues.

Increased Intracranial Pressure

The patient with greatly increased ICP is placed in an intensive care unit. Increased ICP is treated with supportive care to keep the pressure from rising further and with mannitol, an osmotic diuretic, to remove fluid from the body, including the brain. Dosage is determined by body weight, and electrolytes are monitored every 6 hours, as mannitol's action can cause electrolyte imbalances. The patient is kept in a slightly dehydrated state with fluid restriction and a "keep open" IV set at about 50 mL/h. Dexamethasone (Decadron) is given to decrease the inflammatory response and reduce cerebral edema. The patient is positioned with the head of the bed at 15 to 30 degrees to promote venous drainage from the head. The head and neck must be kept in midline so that venous drainage into the body is not restricted. If ICP is dangerously high, an intraventricular catheter can be inserted into the ventricle, through which CSF can be drained in small amounts to relieve the pressure. A pressure-monitoring device is attached to monitor the ICP changes. Cerebral perfusion pressure (CPP) must be kept above 60 mm Hg in order to ensure oxygenation of the brain tissue. (CPP = mean arterial pressure − intracranial

TABLE 15–5 **SOME DO'S AND DONT'S IN CARE OF PATIENTS WITH INCREASED INTRACRANIAL PRESSURE**

Do:

1. Conduct neuro checks at least once every hour unless more frequent monitoring indicated.
2. Report changes immediately.
3. Maintain a patent airway and adequate ventilation to ensure proper oxygen and carbon dioxide exchange.
4. Elevate the head of the bed 15 to 30 degrees to facilitate return of blood from the cerebral veins.
5. Use measures to maintain normal body temperature. Elevations of temperature raise blood pressure and cerebral blood flow. Shivering also can increase ICP.
6. Monitor intake and output. Restrict or encourage fluids according to physician's order.
7. Give passive range-of-motion exercises.

Don't:

1. Allow patient to become constipated or have any reason to perform Valsalva maneuver.
2. Hyperextend, flex, or rotate the patient's head.
3. Flex the patient's hips (as in female catheterization).
4. Place patient in Trendelenburg position for any reason.
5. Allow patient to perform isometric exercises.

pressure.) Table 15–5 provides general guidelines for the care of patients with increased ICP.

Barbiturates are sometimes used along with continuous brain wave monitoring when patients do not respond to the more common therapies for reduction of ICP. In general, the short-acting barbiturates are used (for example, pentobarbital [Nembutal] and thiopental [Pentothal]).

Because carbon dioxide is a vasodilator and can increase blood volume within the cranial cavity, hyperventilation is used to combat the increased ICP. A CO_2 level between 25 and 30 mm Hg will improve oxygenation to the brain, avoid vasodilation of cerebral vessels, reduce blood flow to the brain, and decrease jugular vein pressure.

Subdural hematoma is removed surgically either via burr holes or by craniotomy incision. Epidural hematoma, which almost always is associated with skull fracture, necessitates immediate surgery to stop the bleeding and evacuate the hematoma to prevent death from increased ICP.

NURSING ASSESSMENT AND INTERVENTION

Early recognition of increasing pressure is extremely important in the prevention of permanent damage to the tissues of the brain, the cranial nerves, and the motor and sensory nerve pathways that are within the cranium.

The earliest symptoms of increased ICP include restlessness and irritability, disorientation, and decreasing levels of consciousness as the pressure builds up. The patient may have projectile vomiting without nausea. Deep coma is a sign that serious damage has been done to the cells.

Major aspects of the assessment and care of a patient with a head injury are (1) maintenance of an open airway and adequate aeration of the lungs, (2) frequent "neuro checks" to determine neurologic status and monitor for increasing ICP, (3) observation for leakage of spinal fluid, and (4) proper positioning and care to avoid increasing the ICP.

Maintenance of an open airway and adequate respiration may require suctioning and possibly a tracheostomy with mechanical ventilation. These procedures are necessary if the head injury resulted in damage to the respiratory control centers in the brain. The patient whose consciousness level is decreased and whose gag and swallowing reflexes are impaired is in danger of aspirating blood, vomitus, mucus, and other material into the air passages.

Unless the patient has a tracheostomy or an oral airway in place, he should be positioned on his side or abdomen, not on his back, as the tongue may occlude the airway, and mucus cannot drain naturally.

Careful neurologic assessment with monitoring

of the patient's level of consciousness, pupillary reactions, level of neuromuscular activity, and vital signs is essential to an accurate evaluation of the patient's progress. The following indications that ICP may be rising should be reported immediately:

- Changes in the patient's blood pressure, pulse, or respiration; widening pulse pressure; a slow, bounding pulse.
- Extreme restlessness or excitability following a period of apparent calm.
- Deepening stupor and decreasing levels of consciousness.
- Headache that is unrelenting and increasing in intensity.
- Vomiting, especially persistent, projectile vomiting.
- Unequal size of pupils and other abnormal pupillary reactions.
- Leakage of CSF from the nose and ear. Table 15–2 summarizes four warning signs that indicate increasing ICP.

Leakage of spinal fluid should be watched for in all patients with head trauma, as well as in those who have had brain surgery. To be sure that a drainage is spinal fluid, it may be tested for sugar with a strip of testing tape such as Clinistix. *Spinal fluid will give a positive reaction for sugar; mucus will not.* If blood is mixed in the fluid, the test is not reliable, as blood contains glucose.

Cerebrospinal fluid may leak from the nose, the ear, or both. It appears as a clear yellowish fluid that might be slightly blood-tinged. If the fluid leaks onto the pillowcase or sheet, it often looks like a "halo"; that is, it has a pinkish center surrounded by a ring of a lighter shade. When this is noticed, the piece of linen should be set aside for the physician to see.

If it has been determined that there is indeed leakage of spinal fluid through the nose, ear, or an open wound, special precautions must be taken to prevent infection. These include the following:

- Keep the patient on absolute bed rest with the head of the bed elevated 30 degrees.
- Cover a draining ear with a sterile gauze square, changing it periodically to look for drainage.
- Instruct the patient *not* to blow his nose or pick at it.
- Remind the patient that he is not to change his position in any way unless he has been told it is all right to do so. Specific nursing diagnoses are listed in Nursing Care Plan 15–1.

Observation of a patient treated in an emergency department for head injury and released to go home requires specific techniques. Table 15–6 includes instructions for the patient's family.

CEREBROVASCULAR ACCIDENT (CVA, STROKE)

INCIDENCE AND CAUSES

Stroke is a common disease, more common than many of us realize. Autopsy studies have shown that nearly half the people who die from other causes have had minor strokes without ever having been aware of them or understanding their significance as a warning that a major stroke is impending. In recent years, the incidence of CVAs accidents has decreased despite the lengthening life span for the general population. This decrease in the incidence of stroke can be attributed to successful preventive measures such as those presented below.

A CVA usually is the result of an interruption to the flow of blood to a specific area of the brain (that is, *cerebral ischemia*). The ischemia can be caused by (1) cerebral thrombosis (formation of a blood clot in a cerebral artery), (2) cerebral hemorrhage (the blood vessel ruptures and leaks blood into brain tissue), (3) an embolus (occlusion of a cerebral vessel by a traveling clot, tumor, fat, bacteria, or debris), or (4) pressure on a blood vessel (Fig. 15–8).

The carotid arteries supply a major portion of the blood that goes to the brain (Fig. 15–9). If plaque forms in these arteries as a result of atherosclerosis, the person is at risk for a stroke. Less common causes of stroke are arterial spasms and compression of cerebral vessels by a tumor, local edema, rupture of cerebral aneurysm, and other disorders.

Persons most at risk for a CVA include those with hypertension, atherosclerosis, heart disease, and other cardiovascular disorders. Obese persons, heavy smokers, and those with diabetes mellitus also are at increased risk.

STROKE PREVENTION

Many strokes can be and have been prevented by either surgical procedures or medical management of diseases that predispose a person to a CVA.

Surgical procedures for the prevention of a major stroke involve either the removal of plaque laid down on the inner wall of the carotid artery (carotid endarterectomy) or the rerouting of blood around an obstructed artery. Extracranial-intracranial bypass grafts the superficial middle temporal artery to the middle cerebral artery. About one third of all strokes can be traced to obstruction of any one of the four arteries in the neck that supply blood to the brain. These arteries are readily accessible, so the surgeon can open the artery and remove the obstruction. He then sutures the vessel wall or sews a dacron patch over the incision, leaving the vessel larger than before. If a long section of

NURSING CARE PLAN 15–1

Selected nursing diagnoses, goals/outcome criteria, nursing interventions, and evaluations for a patient with a head injury

Situation: A 16-year-old male who suffered a head injury in an automobile accident is assigned to you. He is groggy but arousable.

Nursing Diagnosis	Goals/Outcome Criteria	Nursing Intervention	Evaluation
Alteration in cerebral tissue perfusion related to increased intracranial pressure from head injury. SUPPORTING DATA Alteration in LOC; confused as to where he is, what day it is; somewhat combative; hit head on dashboard on right side.	No further increase in ICP.	Monitor neurologic status q 2 h using Glasgow Coma Scale; notify physician of any pupil changes or signs of increasing ICP such as widening pulse pressure, change in respiratory pattern, slowing of pulse, increase in temperature, or decrease in LOC. Monitor for seizure activity; institute seizure precautions. Keep head of bed at 30 degrees and body in correct alignment; turn side to side q 2 h. Maintain IV at 50 mL/h; administer dexamethasone as ordered; keep room calm and softly lit; do not disturb more than necessary; talk to patient while giving care; allow rest periods between any invasive procedures; monitor intake and output; reorient frequently.	PEARL; still groggy; no change in BP and pulse; no sign of seizure activity; states name, age; still confused as to place; continue plan.
Self-care deficit related to confusion, grogginess, and increased ICP. SUPPORTING DATA Falls asleep during attempts at bath, etc. Is confused about how to use ordinary objects such as toothbrush.	Adequate hygiene, nutrition, activity will be maintained. Patient will resume own self-care by discharge.	Provide assistance with all ADL's while groggy and confused. Inspect when turning; place foam pad on bed. As LOC improves, encourage self-care activities.	Assistance for all ADL provided; skin intact; turned 8, 10, 12, and 2; voiding quantity sufficient; able to drink liquids; continue plan.
Ineffective family coping related to anxiety about patient's condition. SUPPORTING DATA Mother states she is afraid he will die. She keeps trying to arouse him when she is in the room.	Mother's anxiety will decrease as she gains information about her son's condition and prognosis.	Explain to family that confusion and grogginess is usual after head injury. Explain that the danger is if the ICP keeps increasing; tell what measures are being done to minimize increasing ICP; explain all procedures; explain that calm, rest, and positive talk in the room will help. Encourage family members to share their fears and concerns with each other. Call hospital chaplain or own minister if family desires. Keep family informed of changes in patient's condition.	Discussed condition with mother; states she understands the need for quiet and vigilance; appears less anxious.

the artery is blocked, he may reroute the blood through a dacron tube grafted onto the occluded vessel.

Medical preventive measures are aimed at eliminating or managing some of the conditions that predispose a person to stroke. Control of hypertension and the effective treatment of rheumatic heart disease and atherosclerosis have significantly reduced the incidence of stroke. Efforts to control diabetes mellitus, reduce choles-

TABLE 15-6 INSTRUCTIONS FOR HOME CARE AFTER HEAD INJURY

1. Avoid strenuous physical activities for at least 24 hours after injury.
2. Apply icebag to areas of swelling—continue for at least 24 hours after injury.
3. Light diet for 24 hours after injury.
4. Arouse patient every 2 hours, day and night, for at least 24 hours.

Call doctor immediately or return to emergency department if:

1. Patient becomes confused, irrational, disoriented, "talks out of head," doesn't know where he is.
2. Unable to arouse patient.
3. Patient continues to be nauseated and/or vomits more than once, especially if projectile.
4. Patient has trouble with his balance.
5. Patient complains of double or blurred vision.
6. Headache persists, or becomes more intense 12 hours after the injury.

Courtesy Emergency Department, St. Mary's Hospital, Athens, GA.

terol levels, prevent obesity, and encourage cessation of smoking are examples of measures to prevent stroke in high-risk persons.

Medications that reduce platelet aggregation and decrease the chance of thrombosis are widely used. Low-dose aspirin, dipyridamole (Persantine), or sulfinpyrazone (Anturane) is prescribed for patients who have transient ischemic attacks, or to prevent the recurrence of stroke from thrombosis.

Another factor in prevention of a so-called completed stroke and its devastating neurologic effects is early detection and prompt treatment of early warning signals. Many patients with a narrowing of the lumen of the arteries supplying the brain experience what are called *transient ischemic attacks* (TIAs). Although they usually are not recognized as such, TIAs are often warnings that a more serious neurologic event is likely to occur. During the attack the person may feel a weakness or numbness on one side of the body, slurring of speech or inability to talk, visual disturbances such as blindness or double vision, and staggering or uncoordinated walking. These symptoms last only a few minutes to an hour or so, however, and unless the person has been told about them and their importance, he usually will not seek medical treatment and further investigation. However, about 25% to 35% of those persons who experience TIAs will eventually have a completed stroke.

Cerebral ischemia caused by thrombosis has signs that progress slowly. Lodging of an embolus in a major cerebral vessel causes sudden neuro-

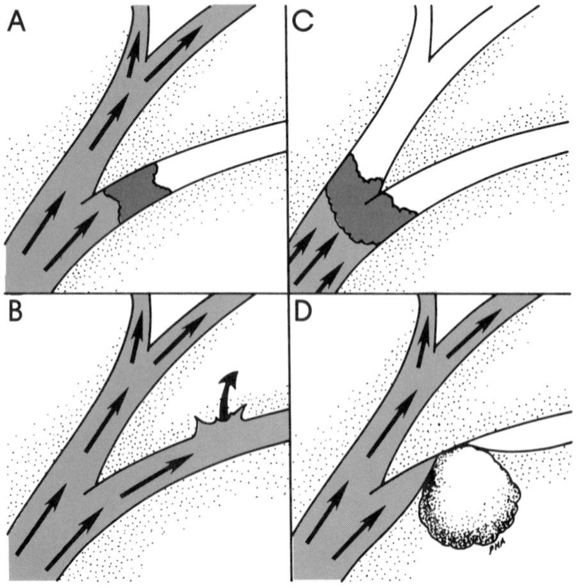

Figure 15-8 Causes of cerebrovascular accident. *A*, Blood clot forms in vessel (cerebral thrombosis). *B*, Wall of blood vessel ruptures (cerebral hemorrhage). *C*, Blood clot or other material from another part of vascular system flows to the brain and obstructs the cerebral vessel (cerebral embolism). *D*, Tumor exerts pressure on a blood vessel.

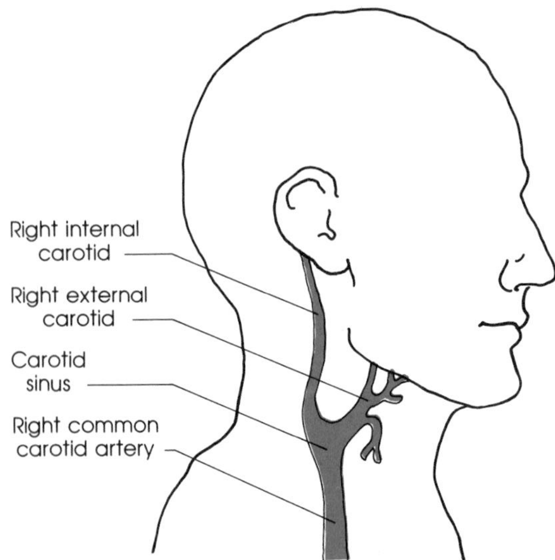

Figure 15-9 The carotid arteries are the principal arteries supplying the head and neck. Surgical bypass to reroute blood flow to the brain and other procedures to remove obstruction in a carotid artery have contributed to prevention of stroke.

logic deficit. Intracerebral bleeding (subarachnoid hemorrhage [SAH]) often causes rapid onset of neurologic deficit and loss of consciousness. A leaking cerebral aneurysm may cause a severe headache. However, some bleeding is slower, producing a more gradual progression of headache, neck stiffness, and other neurologic signs such as blurred vision.

MEDICAL DIAGNOSIS AND TREATMENT

In addition to a complete physical and neurologic examination, the physician may order a CT scan, cerebral angiogram, or magnetic resonance imaging (MRI) scan to determine the specific cause of the stroke. A lumbar puncture may be done to confirm SAH if there are no signs of greatly increased intracranial pressure. If the ICP is high, a lumbar puncture can cause herniation of the brain down onto the brain stem, causing death. Bloody CSF confirms intercerebral bleeding or SAH. An electroencephalogram is then performed, and brain scans or Doppler flow studies may be ordered.

Once the specific cause has been determined, the physician is able to plan a more effective regimen of care. For example, anticoagulant therapy is indicated when cerebral thrombosis is present but is certainly contraindicated if the patient is suffering from cerebral hemorrhage.

EMERGENCY CARE

Immediately after a person is suspected of having suffered a stroke, it is especially important to maintain an open airway. All constricting clothing around his neck should be removed, and he should be turned to one side to prevent aspiration of saliva and obstruction of the air passages. No attempt should be made to move the person until an ambulance has arrived. Reassure the patient regardless of whether he is able to respond. If he is conscious, elevate the head slightly to reduce ICP. *Never* try to stimulate or arouse a person who is unconscious from a stroke.

NURSING ASSESSMENT AND INTERVENTION

The neurologic effects of stroke can range from mild motor disturbances to profound coma. Figure 15–10 shows some control zones of the brain and some motor and sensory functions likely to be affected by a stroke. When the stroke patient is first admitted to the hospital, he is assessed for his general state of health and for the residual effects of his stroke. Care of the hospitalized stroke patient can be divided into three phases: *phase one*, or initial care; *phase two*, which is concerned with rehabilitation efforts while the patient is still in the hospital; and *phase three*, during which plans are made for continuity of care once he returns home. These are not phases in the sense that one begins only after another is finished. There is much overlapping of activities in each phase. Because about 80% of all stroke victims survive the first or initial phase of their illness, rehabilitation and plans for self-care are of the utmost importance.

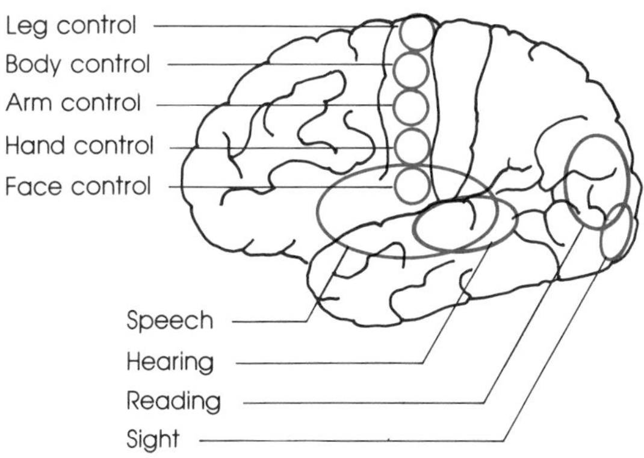

Figure 15–10 Control zones of the brain. When a cerebrovascular accident deprives brain cells of their blood supply, the area of the body controlled by the affected cells becomes unable to function.
(Redrawn from Strokes: A Guide for the Family. Reproduced with permission. © American Heart Association.)

Phase One

Initial care of the stroke patient requires careful assessment to determine the extent to which his neurologic functions have been affected. Complete hemiplegia is a common effect of stroke. Paralysis on the left side indicates focal damage to the right side of the brain, because the motor pathways cross to the opposite side before extending down to the spinal cord. Aphasia often indicates ischemia of the brain cells on the left side and is usually accompanied by right-sided hemiplegia. The nurse's observations of the patient can be very helpful in diagnosing the cause of his cerebrovascular accident.

Nursing diagnoses for the patient who has experienced a CVA commonly include:

- Impaired physical mobility related to weakness or paralysis.
- Altered nutrition that is less than body requirements, related to impaired swallowing and hemiparesis or hemiplegia.
- Self-care deficit related to inability to perform ADL (feeding, bathing, grooming) without assistance.
- Urinary incontinence, related to neurologic deficits.
- Bowel incontinence, related to impaired mobility and neurologic impairment.
- Potential for impaired skin integrity, related to decreased mobility, paresis, or paralysis.
- Impaired verbal communication, related to

inability to clearly verbalize or inability to comprehend communication.

- Alteration in sensory perception: visual, related to loss of vision in parts of visual field; kinesthetic, related to decreased sense of touch on one side of the body.
- Self-esteem disturbance related to alteration in body image and dependence on others.
- Depression related to loss of usual lifestyle, neurologic deficits, and dependence on others.

The amount of activity permitted a stroke patient during the initial acute stage of his illness will depend on the cause of his CVA. If there is danger of continued hemorrhage from a ruptured artery and resultant increase in ICP, his physical activity will necessarily be limited, and the patient care problems he presents will not be the same as for a patient with stroke from another cause. When there is no danger of further damage to his brain, the patient usually is encouraged to become active as soon as his condition has stabilized.

Once the patient is stabilized, assessment is conducted in a systematic way, considering the possibility that any of the above problems could be present. Assessment of and nursing intervention for the patient with problems of immobility, incontinence of urine and feces, aphasia, delirium or confusion, and altered levels of consciousness are discussed in the section "Common Neurologic Patient Care Problems."

Planning for the accomplishment of specific goals for the patient must take into account the individual patient's previous lifestyle, age, general health-illness status, and specific problems of care. The 80-year-old retired person will not have the same goals for rehabilitation and recovery as the 47-year-old mother of three who had been working full time as a schoolteacher before her attack.

Major goals during the first phase are (1) to establish baseline data regarding vital signs, level of consciousness, neuromuscular function, and neurologic status; (2) to preserve joint and muscle function; and (3) to prevent complications that may interfere with rehabilitation.

Phase Two

Both phases one and two are concerned with rehabilitation while the patient is still in the hospital. Plans for rehabilitation should begin the moment the patient is admitted. This means maintenance of an adequate airway and aeration of the lungs, proper positioning, range-of-motion exercises for affected limbs, adequate nutrition and fluid intake and output, prevention of decubitus ulcers, and all other nursing measures directed toward the goal of maintaining normal body functions until the patient is able to maintain them on his own (Nursing Care Plan 15–2).

If dependent disabilities from inactivity are avoided, rehabilitation of the patient has a much better chance of success. During phase two, various members of the health care team begin to work with the patient and his family to help resolve psychosocial as well as physical problems. Among the team members helping the stroke victim may be the physical therapist, speech pathologist, social worker, psychologist, and occupational therapist.

During phase two, the patient is encouraged to strengthen his muscles as well as his resolve to help himself. He will need to exercise his muscles actively and retrain them. *The stroke has not directly affected his muscles, but it has damaged the centers that control muscular activity.*

NURSING CARE PLAN 15–2

Selected nursing diagnoses, goals/outcome criteria, nursing interventions, and evaluations for a patient with a stroke

Situation: A 63-year-old female with a 20-year history of hypertension and severe obesity suffered a right-sided CVA. Before the CVA, she kept house and cooked for her husband, who is retired; she did needlework and was active in church groups.

Nursing Diagnosis	Goals/Outcome Criteria	Nursing Intervention	Evaluation
Impaired mobility related to left-sided hemiplegia. SUPPORTING DATA Right-sided CVA; partial hemiplegia with hemiparesis of left leg and arm; cannot bear weight or functionally use arm.	Patient will maintain full range of motion on left side. Patient will learn to transfer to chair and bed using aids within 6 weeks. Patient will ambulate with assistive devices within 3 months.	Assist her to turn q 2 h when in bed; position extremities in correct alignment; support feet. Perform ROM at least tid. Teach patient and family how to transfer from bed to chair and back. Reinforce physical therapy exercises for muscle strengthening. Prepare for use of walker or cane for ambulation.	Performing own ROM exercises on left and assisting with those on right side; can pull self up on side of bed; teaching transfer to chair; continue plan.

NURSING CARE PLAN 15–2, *Continued*

Nursing Diagnosis	Goals/Outcome Criteria	Nursing Intervention	Evaluation
Alteration in sensory perception: visual and kinesthetic. SUPPORTING DATA Unable to see in left half of visual field; diminished sense of touch on left side.	Patient will learn to turn head to take in left visual field within 3 weeks. Patient will avoid injury to left side by attending to limbs and taking safety precautions. Patient will adjust to diminished vision and be able to resume needlework projects within 4 months.	Place bedside console and frequently used articles on right side of bed; approach from right side. Train her to turn head to see what is on left half of plate; give ruler to use when reading; remind her to turn head to left until cue becomes instinctive. Teach her to protect left extremities when transferring and to check their position frequently. Teach her to check condition of left extremities each day at bath time to prevent infection from breaks in the skin. Encourage attempts to move left extremities and to use grasp with left hand; teach her to do passive ROM exercises on left extremities.	Beginning to turn head more automatically to see left visual field area; using ruler to read; attends to left arm most of time, occasionally forgets when being transferred; working on left hand grasp; continue plan.
Altered nutrition that is more than body requirements. SUPPORTING DATA Is 100 lbs overweight; has not been able to stick to a diet for more than 3 to 4 weeks; eats considerable quantities of sweets and bread.	Patient will express desire to lose weight within a month. Patient will lose 2 lbs per week until normal weight is reached by sticking to 1,500-calorie-per-day diet. Patient will maintain adequate nutrition and weight loss for 5 years.	Explain danger of excessive weight and hindrance to mobility, as well as possibility of further CVA. Take thorough nutritional history of usual food eaten —quantities, snacks, etc. —for normal week at home. Obtain dietary consult to plan 1,500-calorie diet that considers food preferences. Refer her to community support group for assistance with changing eating patterns. Assist her to set own goals for weight loss.	Doesn't have much appetite, as she has difficulty eating; states "I should lose weight this way"; continue plan.
Self-esteem disturbance related to hemiplegia and hemiparesis and inability to perform self-care and participate in usual activities. SUPPORTING DATA Withdrawn and depressed affect; states she hates having others do things for her; worried about how husband will cope; doesn't see how she will be able to walk again or lead a meaningful life.	Patient will verbalize positive aspects of being alive within 3 weeks. Patient will interact with others and participate in all aspects of therapy. Patient will set own small goals for achievement. Patient will verbalize positive outlook within 4 months.	Assist her to focus on pleasures of being alive; interacting with family and friends; watching grandchildren grow, etc. Have other patients who are recovering from CVA and making progress talk with her; enlist person from community support group to offer help. Assist her to set own goals; give considerable encouragement for all attempts at self-care; praise for each accomplishment; encourage patience; continue to stress patient's strengths and contributions.	Achieving small goals; pleased with slight movement in left hand, but easily discouraged; grandchild to visit tomorrow; continue plan.

There are many little things the nurse can do to encourage the patient. Instead of feeding him every item on his tray, she can let him hold bread and other "finger foods," suggesting that he feed himself while she handles the more difficult items. Strange as it may seem, solids and semisolids are easier to ingest than water and juices for the patient who has difficulty swallowing without strangling. Chewing may be very slow at first; the patient should not be hurried, nor should he be allowed to chew to the point of exhaustion. Eating is often difficult and messy, and privacy must be provided.

Combing and brushing the hair is good exercise for the arm and shoulder, as are brushing the teeth and washing the face and hands. The patient may not be able to carry all these procedures through to completion at first, but with encouragement he can gradually improve until he is able to perform much of his own personal care.

The patient who has suffered brain injury becomes fatigued very quickly, and the nurse must keep this in mind when encouraging self-care activities. Encouragement and praise for the smallest accomplishment can help the patient's tattered self-esteem.

The stroke patient is prone to rapid mood swings and spontaneous weeping. The nurse must be patient and accepting, and an explanation to the patient that this is very common after a stroke can ease his embarrassment.

Phase Three

Plans are made for discharge and referral to individuals and agencies outside the hospital who will help the patient and his family adjust to his new way of life. The patient who is retired or for whom a return to employment is not possible will need help in finding recreational activities and other ways to help pass the time. Sometimes retraining for a different occupation is possible through vocational rehabilitation programs within the community. Referral and introduction to a community-sponsored stroke club should be made before discharge. Sharing with other stroke victims in informal gatherings is most beneficial. Such clubs may be sponsored by the local chapter of the American Heart Association, a hospital, public health department, senior citizen group, or others interested in providing emotional support, guidance, and encouragement to stroke victims and their families.

INTRACRANIAL TUMORS

Neoplasms within the confines of the skull are space-occupying lesions and thus create problems of increasing ICP by compressing adjacent tissues. If the tumor arises from cells of the brain, the cranial nerves, or the pituitary gland, the neoplastic cells can infiltrate and destroy these structures. *About 50% of all brain tumors are malignant.*

Intracranial tumors may begin in the substance of the brain itself, or they may begin in the meninges, cranial nerves, or pituitary gland. Primary malignant brain tumors rarely metastasize outside the brain, but an intracranial tumor may be secondary to malignant lesions outside the skull—for example, a malignancy of the breast.

SYMPTOMS AND MEDICAL DIAGNOSIS

There can be as many symptoms of intracranial tumors as there are functions of the structures within the skull. The symptoms are dependent on location and may appear gradually, or if the tumor is a highly malignant, fast-growing type, they may appear suddenly. In a slow-growing type of tumor, the patient may first show personality changes, disturbances in judgment and memory, loss of muscular strength and coordination, or difficulty in speaking clearly. Headache, vomiting, visual problems, and other signs of increased ICP *do not* appear early in the disease.

Diagnostic procedures to identify the site and extent of intracranial tumors include MRI, arteriography, and CT scan.

MEDICAL AND SURGICAL TREATMENT

The four modes of therapy for intracranial tumors are the same as those for neoplastic diseases elsewhere in the body: surgery, radiation therapy, chemotherapy, and immunotherapy. These are discussed more thoroughly in Chapter 13.

Whenever possible, intracranial tumors are removed surgically, and the other modes of treatment are utilized to destroy remaining cells. Sometimes, however, the tumor has infiltrated vital parts of the brain that must not be traumatized by surgical procedures. If the tumor is located in the cerebrum, an operation called a *craniotomy* is done. A flap of scalp and bone is cut and pulled down, the dura is opened, and the tumor is removed. Tumors in or near the *cerebellum* are removed through an incision under the occipital bone. This is called a *suboccipital craniectomy*, in which part of the skull is permanently removed, leaving a defect in the skull. IV mannitol, an osmotic diuretic, and dexamethasone (Decadron), a corticosteroid, are given to reduce inflammation and fluid volume, thereby lowering ICP.

If the tumor is found while it is still very

small, a stereotaxic gamma knife procedure can destroy it. This procedure uses a domed steel head covering with ports through which gamma radiation is directed. Measurements are calculated by a computer to precisely locate the tumor, and the radiation is delivered only to the tumor. This procedure can be used for small recurrent tumor growth also.

If all of the tumor cannot be removed, a portion of the skull (usually in the temporal region) may be removed to relieve compression of the brain against the skull. The tumorous mass then bulges through the opening. This procedure is only a temporary measure to relieve the patient's symptoms.

NURSING CARE OF PATIENTS HAVING INTRACRANIAL SURGERY

Preoperative Care

Unless an emergency exists, the patient who is scheduled for intracranial surgery receives essentially the same care as other surgical patients. The exceptions are physical preparation, neurologic assessment, and intervention for management of such problems as altered levels of consciousness, seizures, and increased ICP. Psychological preparation is also important.

The operative site usually is not shaved until the patient is under anesthesia in the operating room. A shampoo may be ordered the evening before surgery. Any scalp lesions or other unusual conditions that are noted at this time should be reported. Usually the entire head is not shaved, and if the patient has long hair, any hair that is cut off may be saved to be used as a hairpiece until the patient's hair grows back.

Postoperative Period

During the immediate postoperative period, the patient will be in the intensive care unit for continuous monitoring and attention. Essentially, his care will be the same as that for a patient who has had a head injury. Additional specific points in the postoperative care of the patient who has undergone intracranial surgery are as follows:

- Position the patient according to written orders from the attending surgeon. *Make no exceptions.*
- Keep the neck in midline and prevent excessive hip flexion.
- Use nasal suctioning *only* if there is a written order allowing this.
- Watch carefully for signs of leakage of CSF from the nose, ear, and operative site and report evidence of leakage immediately. Use aseptic technique in applying dressings to collect the drainage.
- Provide a quiet, nonstimulating environment.
- Do not restrain the patient unless absolutely necessary and only if there is a written order.
- Administer only those treatments, comfort measures, and medications for which there are specific written orders.
- Report promptly any changes in the neurologic status of the patient.

SPINAL CORD INJURY

A person may suffer from injury to the spinal cord in a number of ways. When we speak of injury, our first thought is a violent, traumatic injury in which the spinal cord is severed or partially severed by a direct blow. Automobile accidents, gunshot wounds, and other forms of violence often do inflict severe damage to the spinal cord, but tumors, degenerative disease, and infections also can impair the functions of the spinal cord and its branches.

Generally speaking, spinal cord injuries are classified according to their anatomic location; that is, cervical, thoracic,* or *lumbosacral.

Whatever the cause of spinal cord injury, the clinical manifestations of the injury are the same. A complete severance of the cord results in a total loss of sensation and control in the parts of the body below the point of injury. If the cord is severed in the cervical region, the paralysis and loss of sensory perception will include both arms and both legs. Severe injury to the cord above the level of the fifth cervical vertebra is often fatal because the *phrenic* nerves have their origin in the third, fourth, and fifth cervical segments. Branches of these nerves play a major role in the control of respiration. Table 15–7 presents activities possible at varying levels of cord injury.

Injury to the spinal cord that does not involve complete severance of the cord may result in a temporary paralysis, which will subside as the spinal cord recovers from the swelling and initial shock of the injury.

MEDICAL AND SURGICAL TREATMENT

There are four main objectives in the treatment and nursing care of the patient with an injury of the spinal cord: (1) to save the victim's life, (2) to prevent further injury to the cord by careful handling of the patient, (3) to repair as much of the damage to the cord as possible, and (4) to establish a routine of care that will improve and maintain the patient's state of health and prevent complications, so that eventual physical, mental, and social rehabilitation is possible.

TABLE 15–7 ACTIVITIES POSSIBLE AT VARYING LEVELS OF SPINAL CORD INJURY

Activities	Spinal Cord Level						
	C-5	*C-6*	*C-7*	*T-1*	*T-6*	*T-12*	*L-4*
Self-care: Eating	–	+/–	+	+	+	+	+
Dressing	–	–	+/–	+	+	+	+
Toileting	–	–	+/–	+	+	+	+
Bed independence	–	+/–	+/–	+	+	+	+
Wheel chair independence	–	+/–	+/–	+	+	+	+
Ambulation: Functional	–	–	–	–	+/–	+	+
Vocation: Homebound	–	–	+	+	+	+	+
Outside	–	–	–	+/–	+/–	+	+

From GraBois, M.: Nursing guidelines for the rehabilitation of the quadriplegic and paraplegic patient. J. Pract. Nurs., April, 1971, p. 22.
+ = capacity to accomplish task.
+/– = questionable capacity to accomplish task.
– = will not be able to accomplish task.

Immediate Care

As soon as a person suffers a sudden injury to the spinal cord, he must be handled with extreme care. Because the nurse or doctor may not be at the scene of the accident to supervise the moving of the victim, laypersons should learn the proper emergency care of such injuries. If the injured person complains of neck pain and cannot move his legs and has no feeling in them, he must be treated as if he has a spinal cord injury.

Transfer of the patient to the hospital should be done only by trained emergency medical technicians or others qualified to administer first aid. A cervical collar is applied if there is any question of neck injury. The victim is moved on a stretcher or board and taken directly to the hospital. His back must be kept straight and be well supported. To avoid flexion of the neck, *no pillow or other kind of support is placed under the head.*

In the emergency department of the hospital, the patient's condition is stabilized and a thorough examination is conducted to establish the extent of his injuries. A large dose of corticosteroid is given as soon as the examination and diagnosis of cord injury is made. Cervical spinal cord injury usually is treated with traction to immobilize the affected vertebrae and maintain them in alignment. Traction can be accomplished by a head halter; skeletal traction using Crutchfield tongs with ropes, pulleys, and weights (Figure 15–11); or a halo ring and fixation pins (Figure 15–12).

Selection of the type of bed to be used for a patient with spinal cord injury depends on many factors. Some physicians and nurses prefer placing the patient in a standard bed, rather than on a canvas and metal frame (called a *wedge turning frame* or *Stryker frame*). Figure 15–13 shows a drawing of a patient in cervical traction with halo fixation that can maintain stability of the cervical vertebrae while the patient is in or out of bed. "Logrolling" the patient must be done with extreme care to avoid twisting the vertebral column and further damaging the spinal cord (Fig. 15–13).

Once the patient is in bed or on the orthopedic frame, the true test of nursing care begins. All the nursing measures designed to prevent the disabilities that may result from immobility, to promote healing, and to avoid complications are utilized to help the patient achieve the goals of rehabilitation. Bladder and bowel training programs, as well as instruction in moving from bed to chair and other aspects of self-care, may be necessary. Realistic goals should be set for the patient and every effort made to achieve them.

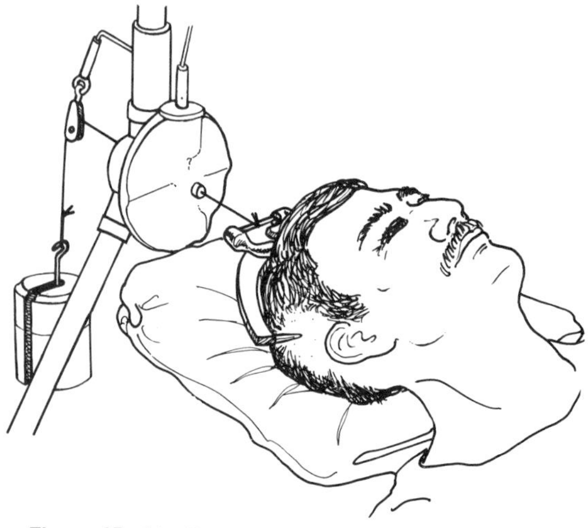

Figure 15–11 Crutchfield tongs for skeletal traction.

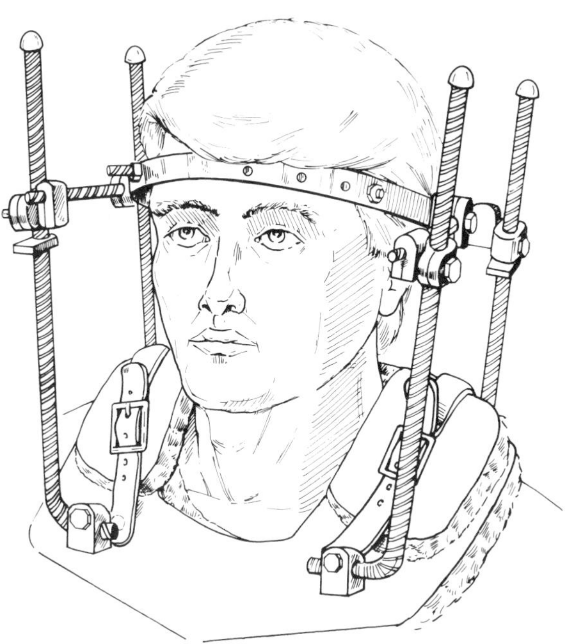

Figure 15-12 Halo ring and apparatus for traction.

MUSCLE SPASMS

Immediately after a cord injury, the patient will usually have a flaccid type of paralysis. Later, as the cord adjusts to the injury, the paralysis will become *spastic*, and there will be strong, involuntary contractions of the skeletal muscles.

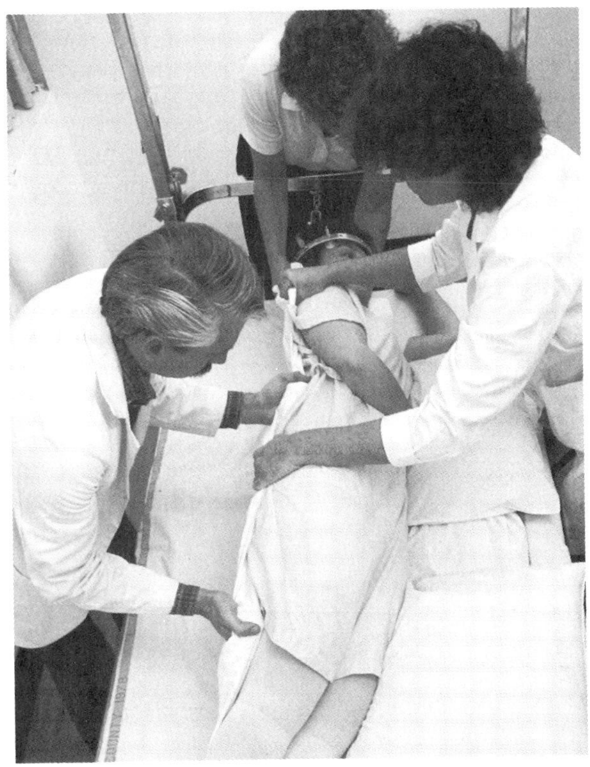

Figure 15-13 Logrolling a patient in cervical traction.
(From Agee, B. L., and Herman, C.: Cervical logrolling on a standard hospital bed. Am. J. Nurs., March, 1984, p. 315.)

These muscle spasms, which may be violent enough to throw the patient from his bed or wheelchair, must be anticipated and the patient secured so that accidents can be avoided. If the patient is on a frame, a protective strap is placed across the thighs. If the upper extremities are involved, he is likely to tip over glasses, water pitchers, or anything within reach of his arms when he is seized with uncontrollable muscle spasms.

The patient and his family may interpret these spasms as a return of voluntary function of the limbs and will thus have false hopes of complete recovery. It is best if the nurse in charge or the physician explains to them that such is not the case.

To avoid stimulating the muscles when moving the patient and thereby precipitating a spasm of the muscles, the nurse should avoid grasping the muscle itself. The palms of the hands are used to support the joints above and below the affected muscles.

AUTONOMIC DYSREFLEXIA (HYPERREFLEXIA)

Autonomic dysreflexia (AD) is an uninhibited and exaggerated reflex response of the autonomic nervous system to some form of stimulation. It is a response that occurs in 85% of all patients who have spinal cord injury at or above the level of the sixth thoracic vertebra (T-6). The response is potentially dangerous to the patient, because it can produce vasoconstriction of the arterioles with an immediate elevation of blood pressure. The sudden hypertension can, in turn, cause a seizure, hemorrhage into the retina of the eye, or a stroke. Less serious effects include severe headache, changes in pulse rate, sweating and flushing above the level of the spinal cord lesion, and pallor and "goose bumps" below the level of injury.

It is important for nurses and others participating in the care of a patient with quadriplegia and other kinds of spinal cord disorders at or above the T-6 level to be aware of the circumstances that can trigger AD, its manifestations, and the correct measures to take if it happens. The problem can occur at any time after a spinal cord injury; in some cases it has first appeared as late as 6 years after the injury.

There are many kinds of stimulation that can precipitate AD. Most are related to the bladder, bowel, and skin of the patient. For example, catheter changes, a distended bladder, the insertion of rectal suppositories, enemas, and sudden changing of position can provide the stimulation that results in AD.

Once the patient exhibits symptoms of AD, an emergency exists. Efforts should be made to lower his blood pressure by placing him in a sitting position or elevating his head to a 45-degree angle. If the cause of the stimulation is known—for example, an impacted bowel or overdistended bladder, or pressure against the skin—the stimulus should be removed as gently and quickly as possible. The physician should be notified immediately so that the appropriate medications can be prescribed and administered.

Patients who experience repeated attacks of AD may require surgery to sever the nerves responsible for the exaggerated response to stimulation.

PSYCHOLOGICAL IMPACT

The short-term and long-term psychological changes brought about by spinal cord injury and paralysis are difficult, if not impossible, to measure. Adjustment to such a drastic change in one's lifestyle is a continuous process that may well last a lifetime.

We are fortunate that today there are many health care professionals other than the physician and the nurse who are prepared to counsel and guide the patient in his efforts at adjustment. Nurses who feel uncomfortable and unknowledgeable about the best way to help a patient deal with emotional and psychosocial problems should feel free to discuss their own feelings with and seek help from other professionals. It is encouraging to know that in recent years the trend has been toward a *team approach to health care*, with each team member giving support to other members as well as to the patient.

One area of concern to the patient and his family members that has formerly been ignored for the most part is that of sexual function and sexuality following spinal cord injury. Discussions of sexual conduct and the larger concept of human sexuality are not easily approached and participated in by many individuals. The issue involves moral values, social taboos, and cultural attitudes, which are not always the same for each of the individuals involved in the discussion. When these values and attitudes differ, there is a temptation to moralize and make judgments about the personal worth of those who think and feel differently about the subject.

The nurse who wishes to help a patient deal with problems of sexuality must first come to terms with her own feelings and attitudes and clarify her own values. She should also try to be uncritical and nonjudgmental in her dealings with her patients. The patient and his partner must be encouraged to verbalize their concerns and questions and should be given guidance in alternative ways to express sexuality and meet sexual needs.

There often is a tendency to treat a physically disabled patient as if he were something less than a "whole" person with the same desires, hopes, and anxieties that all humans share. The nurse can best serve her patients by reacting to and interacting with them in an open and honest manner. When she feels unprepared to handle a certain problem, there is no reason not to readily admit her embarrassment, confusion, or lack of information and seek assistance from other members of the health care team.

RUPTURED INTERVERTEBRAL DISC ("SLIPPED DISC")

The bodies of the vertebrae lie flat on one another like a stack of coins. Between the vertebral bodies there is a disc of fibrous cartilage that acts as a cushion to absorb shocks to the spinal column. This disc may be ruptured by an injury, such as strain caused by lifting a heavy object or wrenching or falling on the back. When the disc ruptures, part of it squeezes out from between the vertebrae and pinches the adjacent nerve root by pressing it against the bone (Fig. 15–14). Thus the person suffers from what is sometimes called a "slipped disc." Another name for this condition is *hernia of the nucleus pulposus* (HNP).

SYMPTOMS AND MEDICAL DIAGNOSIS

About 95% of all ruptured or slipped discs occur in the lower back at the fourth and fifth intervertebral spaces in the lumbar spine. The patient experiences pain in the lower back radiating down the back of the leg to the foot. Walking is extremely painful, and the discomfort is aggravated by coughing, sneezing, or straining. Many times young patients give a history of "feeling something give way" in their backs.

When the ruptured disc is located in the cervical region, the patient complains of pain in the neck, shoulder pain radiating down the arm into the hand, and tingling and numbness of the hand and fingers.

Diagnosis usually is confirmed by myelography or MRI.

MEDICAL AND SURGICAL TREATMENT

In most instances, the physician will treat the condition with conservative measures in the hope that surgical correction will not be necessary.

The patient is placed on a firm cotton mattress with bed boards under it. The bed is kept flat, and the patient is placed on bed rest. When he is turned off his back, he is "logrolled"—that is, he

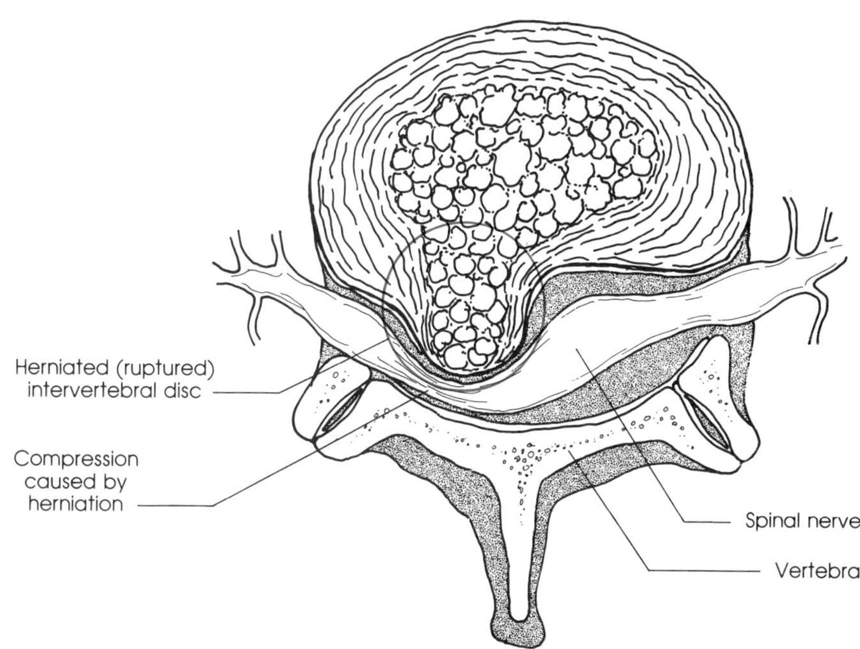

Figure 15-14 Cross section of intervertebral disc with herniation pressing against spinal nerve.

is turned without bending his back. In order to accomplish this, the patient folds his arms over his chest, flexes the knee opposite the side on which he is to turn, and is rolled over, just as a log would be rolled.

Hydrocollator packs (or some other form of local heat) or ice packs are applied to reduce muscle spasm in the back. Pelvic traction may be applied and mild exercises ordered by the physician. These treatments are usually done under the guidance of a physical therapist. Specially designed corsets or back braces are sometimes used to maintain proper alignment of the spine when the patient is allowed out of bed.

Occasionally chemonucleolysis is used as an alternative treatment for some patients. A drug derived from the papaya plant (chymopapain) is injected into the central, jellylike portion of the ruptured disc. The drug is an enzyme, pharmacologically akin to a meat tenderizer, that causes the disc to shrink in size and thereby relieves pressure on the affected nerve root. However, complications of spinal damage and anaphylactic shock have diminished the use of this treatment.

Nursing Assessment and Intervention

Before the procedure the nurse should question the patient about allergies. Anaphylaxis is the most serious complication of chemonucleolysis. Patients who have an allergy to tenderized meat, beers that contain papaya derivatives, or any other source of papaya are disqualified from having the procedure. Other contraindications include any bowel or bladder dysfunction; pregnancy; a sedimentation rate greater than 20 in females (because studies have shown that anaphylactic reactions occur more frequently in women who have high sedimentation rates); and a history of previous treatment with chymopapain, which could increase the possibility of an allergic reaction. If the nurse discovers any of these conditions during her history taking and assessment, she should notify the surgeon immediately.

During the postoperative period the patient is carefully assessed for the development of three major problems: (1) anaphylaxis, (2) alteration in neurologic status, and (3) alteration in comfort related to muscle spasm or pain. Nursing assessment activities and intervention for each of these problems have been discussed previously.

SURGICAL PROCEDURES

For those patients who cannot find relief through conservative measures, surgical removal of the damaged disc may be the only alternative. A diskectomy is often performed. This is a microsurgical technique that utilizes a very small incision through which the herniated intervertebral disc material is dissected and extracted. If the area cannot be handled with microsurgery, a laminectomy, which involves removal of the posterior arch of the vertebra along with the disc, is done. A spinal fusion is necessary in some patients to stabilize the spine. In a spinal fusion, a piece or pieces of bone from another part of the body are grafted onto the vertebrae to strengthen them. This procedure may be done for conditions other than a ruptured disc—for example, for such degenerative diseases of the spine as Pott's disease (tuberculosis of the spine), for fractures of the spine, and for spinal dislocation. Once a laminectomy has healed, the fused vertebrae are immobile.

Nursing Intervention

Preoperatively, a baseline neurologic assessment is performed and documented. Other preoperative care is the same as for other types of general surgery.

The major concern after spinal fusion, laminectomy, or diskectomy is keeping the spinal column in alignment so that healing can take place and no further injury is done to the spinal cord. If the surgeon allows the patient to be turned onto his side, he must be logrolled to avoid twisting the spine. Sometimes the surgeon will allow the patient to be positioned only on his back or abdomen. Whenever the patient's position is changed, there should be ample help to move him.

A small bedpan is used, and the patient's back is firmly supported while he is resting on the pan. His back and legs should be supported so that all of his body is on the same plane. To promote healing, circulation to the back, head, and neck can be stimulated by gentle massage.

When the patient is allowed out of bed, the physician may order a back brace or corset to support the spinal column until complete healing has occurred. The patient is not allowed to sit for any length of time for several weeks. He must stand or lie down.

The diskectomy patient is usually up and about the day after surgery. However, weeks to many months of exercises and physical therapy are necessary before recovery is complete.

SPECIFIC NEUROLOGIC DISORDERS

PARKINSONISM

Parkinsonism, formerly called *Parkinson's disease* after James Parkinson, who first described the syndrome in 1871, is no longer considered a specific disease. It is, rather, a group of symptoms (i.e., a syndrome) that are neurologic in nature and become progressively more incapacitating. It is also called "shaking palsy," because the outstanding manifestation is a tremor or involuntary motion of the muscles.

Parkinsonism is considered a major health problem because of its crippling effects; it is considered by some to be the third most crippling disorder in the United States. It is a progressive disorder, beginning rapidly at first and then advancing more slowly. It affects more men than women and usually occurs between the ages of 45 and 80 years.

Classification of the syndrome may be based on the causative factor. It is a disorder of the part of the brain that controls balance and coordination. The most common type of parkinsonism is *idiopathic*—that is, the primary or specific cause is not known. Other types include atherosclerotic, drug-induced (especially by some tranquilizers), toxic (as in carbon monoxide and mercury poisoning), and traumatic.

Symptoms and Medical Diagnosis

Two groups of symptoms are characteristic of parkinsonism. The first, *tremor*, occurs when the body is at rest, decreases when there is voluntary movement, and is absent when the patient is asleep. If the patient suffers stress and emotional tension, the tremor becomes more pronounced. The second symptom, *rigidity*, affects the skeletal muscles and produces poor body balance, a characteristic gait, loss of motion, and body restlessness.

There may be slowness in the initiation and execution of movements. The cause of parkinsonism is uncertain but is thought to occur from dopamine deficiency in the brain. The characteristic symptoms of the disease are used to diagnose parkinsonism. Laboratory tests usually reveal findings within normal ranges.

Medical Treatment

Treatment of parkinsonism usually includes drug therapy, physical therapy, and considerable emotional support. Amantadine hydrochloride (Symmetrel) is tried first, is effective in two thirds of patients, and sometimes can be used alone in early cases. If it is ineffective, L-dioxyphenylalanine (L-dopa or levodopa) or a combination of levodopa and carbidopa (Sinemet) is given. L-Dopa is given in increasing doses until there is control of the symptoms. It is not without side effects, but these are relatively minor. Other drugs used, either along with L-dopa or sometimes alone to treat early stages of parkinsonism or to minimize the side effects of L-dopa, include antispasmodic and anticholinergic drugs. Bromocriptine mesylate (Parlodel) is also prescribed for some parkinsonism patients; it activates postsynaptic dopamine receptors.

Stereotaxic neurosurgery may be done if drug therapy fails. In this procedure the area in the thalamus that is causing the involuntary movements is destroyed. The surgery only relieves the symptoms; it is not a cure.

Depression is frequent in parkinsonism patients, and most people respond well to a tricyclic antidepressant.

Recent research has shown some success in relieving parkinsonian symptoms by transplanting tissue from the adrenal medulla into the brain or by implanting cells that produce dopamine from tissue cultures or fetal sources (Andreoli et al., 1990). This may some day be an accepted treatment.

MULTIPLE SCLEROSIS

Multiple sclerosis (MS) is a neuromuscular disorder that affects primarily the central nervous system. It usually, but not always, tends to be progressive. Its cause is not known, and there is no cure. Symptoms most often appear in young adults in their teens and 20s. MS is usually diagnosed when these individuals are between 20 and 40 years old. The neuromuscular dysfunctions characteristic of MS are unique to each person and can vary greatly from time to time in the same person.

Clinical manifestations of MS reflect the pathologic changes that occur as a result of inflammation and subsequent scarring of myelin covering the nerves. This protective sheath around the axons that transmit electrical impulses from one neuron to the next acts as a thick, protective insulator. When myelin is eroded by inflammation and replaced by scar tissue (demyelinization), nerve impulses cannot travel along the damaged neurons. Thus the muscles served by the affected nerves do not receive the impulses they need to perform in a well-coordinated and useful manner.

Symptoms and Medical Diagnosis

There is no laboratory test that will definitively establish a diagnosis of MS, although most patients have elevated gamma immunoglobulin (IgG) levels in their spinal fluid with the presence of oligoclonal bands. MRI usually shows characteristic white-matter lesions scattered through the spinal cord and brain, which confirms the diagnosis of MS. However, the clinical signs and symptoms presented by a patient usually are sufficiently characteristic of the disorder to allow the neurologist to make a diagnosis that the patient possibly or probably has MS. The clinical manifestations of the disease reflect the extent to which inflammation and scarring of the myelin have occurred.

The disorder typically follows a course of unpredictable flare-ups that unaccountably are followed by periods of partial or complete remission. The very nature of the disease affects a patient's life in terms of ability to make a living, maintain satisfying interpersonal relationships with family and friends, and maintain a positive self-image.

The more common manifestations of MS are as follows:

- *Motor dysfunction* can include weakness or paralysis of limbs, trunk, and head; diplopia caused by oculomotor weakness; and spasticity of the muscles.
- *Sensory dysfunction* might include numbness, tingling, burning, and painful sensations; patchy or total blindness or blurring of vision in one or both eyes; dizziness; ringing in the ears and hearing loss; and Lhermitte's sign (a sensation like an electric shock down the spine when the neck is flexed).
- *Problems of coordination* include ataxia, intention tremor of limbs and eyes, slurring speech, and dysphagia.
- *Mental changes* usually are limited to depression and possibly inappropriate euphoria. Intellectual function is *not* adversely affected.
- *Fatigue* is a characteristic of MS and is worsened by heat; for example, a hot bath or hot weather.
- Other problems that occur late in the disease are related to urinary and bowel incontinence and disordered sexuality—for example, loss of male and female self-esteem, physical impotence in the male, and diminished sensation.

Medical Treatment

Because there is no specific preventive treatment or cure for MS, most therapeutic efforts are centered on supportive measures to maintain resistance to infection, reduce muscle spasticity, and manage specific symptoms such as diplopia, speech disorders, muscle weakness, and others listed above.

In addition, the patient should be provided the support and physical and psychological means necessary to develop a positive and hopeful outlook. A positive and affirming mental attitude can have beneficial physiologic and biologic effects on the MS patient. There is an understandable tendency to become depressed and pessimistic about one's future when confronted with the realities of muscle weakness, incontinence, sexual impotence, and any combination of disabilities likely to be experienced during the course of MS.

Nursing Assessment and Intervention

Appropriate care for the patient with MS depends on the severity of the disease and the symptoms. Care is individualized for each patient. During the diagnostic phase the patient and family will need a great deal of emotional support, as most patients know that there is no cure.

Ongoing care is focused on safety, prevention of complications, assistance with physical therapy, and emotional support. The patient should not be exposed to excessive heat or hot baths, as this causes his weakness to become much worse. Care of the particular common problems of the neurologic patient is covered later in this chapter. The importance of proper nutrition with adequate fluids and roughage in the diet should be stressed to maintain proper bowel function and decrease the likelihood of urinary tract infections.

The nurse helps the patient and family to establish a consistent daily routine that will promote optimum level of functioning for the patient. The routine should include daily physical exercise balanced by rest periods to prevent fatigue.

Patient teaching involves (1) education about the unpredictability of the disease and the need to avoid stress, infections, and fatigue in order to maintain independence as long as possible and (2) referral to the National Multiple Sclerosis Society and local support groups.

Additional information and local sources of help for the patient with MS and his family can be obtained by writing to the National Multiple Sclerosis Society, 205 East 42nd St., New York, NY 10010.

AMYOTROPHIC LATERAL SCLEROSIS

Amyotrophic lateral sclerosis (ALS), also called *Lou Gehrig's disease,* is a progressive neuromuscular disease characterized by degeneration of the gray matter in the anterior horns of the spinal cord and the lower cranial nerves. It is a relatively common disease that has an estimated incidence of 2 to 7 per 100,000 people. It most often occurs in persons between the ages of 40 and 70 years and affects males two to four times more often than females. Although some persons with ALS can survive for many years, the disease usually progresses rapidly, producing a prognosis of death within about 3 years of the onset of symptoms.

There is no known cause of ALS and no satisfactory treatment for control or cure. Eventually the muscle paralysis renders the patient totally dependent because of inability to move, swallow, speak, and, ultimately, breathe.

Symptoms and Medical Diagnosis

One of the first clinical manifestations of ALS is weakness of the voluntary muscles, especially of the distal muscles of the extremities. Some patients may notice difficulty swallowing and speaking clearly because of oropharyngeal weakness. As the disease progresses there is atrophy of the muscles. Until atrophy is complete, however, there may be spontaneous contractions or spasticity of the muscles and abnormal sensations (paresthesias) such as tingling or prickling. The patient also may report pain, which is probably caused by undue strain on weakened muscles.

Only the motor neurons are affected in ALS; therefore the patient remains mentally alert and has no sensory impairment. Mental depression is relatively common as a result of the unrelenting progression of muscle weakness and atrophy.

There is no laboratory test to confirm a diagnosis of ALS. Other neuromuscular disorders such as multiple sclerosis, myasthenia gravis, and progressive muscular dystrophy must be ruled out.

Nursing Assessment and Intervention

During her first contact with the patient with ALS, the nurse conducts a thorough assessment of his neurologic status. As the disease progresses, periodic assessments can identify the specific needs of each patient. Nursing diagnoses likely to be associated with ALS include:

- Ineffective airway clearance related to paralysis of oropharyngeal and respiratory muscles.
- Constipation related to immobility.
- Altered nutrition that is less than body requirements, related to dysphagia.
- Self-care deficit, related to muscle weakness.
- Potential for impairment of skin integrity, related to immobility.
- Impaired verbal communication, related to oropharyngeal muscle weakness.
- Self-esteem disturbance, related to dependence on others.
- Individual ineffective coping, related to changes in lifestyle and prognosis of disease.
- Pain, related to muscle cramps.

In the latter stages of ALS the patient and his family will probably need more assistance and guidance to maintain some level of independence and comfort for the patient. Rehabilitation efforts include obtaining equipment and devices such as a walker, wheelchair, hospital bed, suction machine, and nasogastric or gastrostomy tube feeding supplies.

Because of the nature of the disease, problems related to terminal illness, death, and the grieving process are likely to be present (see Chapter 14). The services of a visiting nurse or a hospice program can provide appropriate instruction and physical and emotional support.

TRIGEMINAL NEURALGIA (TIC DOULOUREUX)

This disorder involves one or more branches of the fifth cranial (trigeminal) nerve. The three branches of this nerve are the ophthalmic, the mandibular, and the maxillary (Fig. 15-15). In most cases of trigeminal neuralgia the ophthalmic nerve is not involved. The motor and sensory functions affected by trigeminal neuralgia include chewing and facial movements and sen-

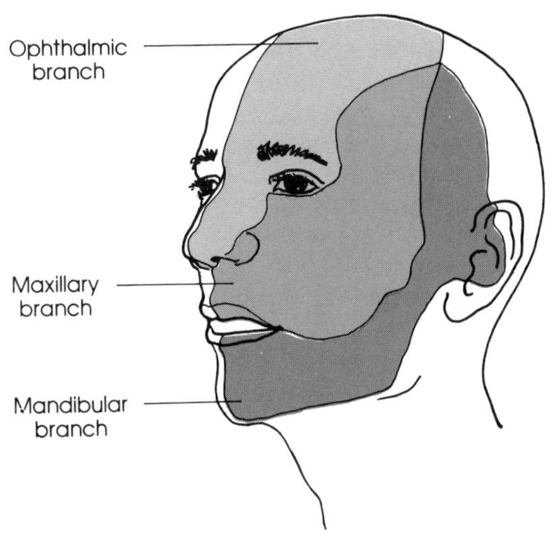

Figure 15-15 Areas of innervation by each of the three branches of the trigeminal nerve.

sations of the face, scalp, teeth, nasal cavities, and ear drum.

The cause of trigeminal neuralgia is not known, though it can be related to pressure on the nerve root by a tumor or to a lesion of the blood vessels. Sometimes the disorder is associated with herpes zoster and multiple sclerosis. In most cases, however, the cause cannot be found.

Symptoms and Medical Diagnosis

The most notable symptom of trigeminal neuralgia is severe pain, which is described as sharp and intense, lasting for 1 to 2 minutes, and located along the pathway of one of the branches of the trigeminal nerve. The pain is localized on one side of the face, rarely affecting both sides. It can extend from the midline of the face across the cheek and jaw to the ear.

Attacks are usually triggered by exposure to cold drafts or drinking cold or very hot liquids, chewing, brushing the hair, shaving, or washing the face. Between acute flare-ups the patient may experience no pain, or he may report a dull ache. The pain during the acute phase is so severe that many patients live in constant fear they will do something to provoke an attack.

Diagnosis is based on the patient's history and chief complaint. There is no test to confirm the diagnosis, and there are no observable pathologic changes.

Medical and Surgical Treatment

Medical management usually is preferred to surgical intervention, because the latter involves dissection of nerve rootlets with resultant loss of motor and sensory function. Microsurgical techniques have improved the precision with which nerve tissue can be destroyed without affecting large segments of tissue served by the nerves.

The drugs most frequently prescribed to prevent or relieve spasmodic pain are phenytoin, an anticonvulsant, carbamazepine (Tegretol), and baclofen (Lioresal). Relief of severe pain during an acute attack usually can be obtained by injection of either alcohol or glycerol into the terminal branch of the trigeminal nerve.

Nursing Assessment and Intervention

Observation of the patient between acute attacks can help identify clues to affirm the presence of trigeminal neuralgia. The patient may not wash his face or shave, and he will guard his face or hold it immobile to avoid an attack. He is very sensitive to any contact with his face and will indicate the area of pain by pointing to but never touching it.

The universal nursing diagnosis for patients with trigeminal neuralgia is, of course, pain. Because chewing can provoke an attack of pain, the patient may be susceptible to nutritional deficit. Small, frequent feedings consisting of food that is moderately warm can help provide adequate nutrition and at the same time avoid precipitating an acute attack.

Nursing intervention for the patient who is being treated medically includes instruction about the expected actions and adverse side effects of the drug he is taking. Phenytoin can produce ataxia, skin eruptions, overgrowth of the gums, and nystagmus. Carbamazepine can damage the bone marrow and produce such hematologic reactions as leukopenia, aplastic anemia, and decreased platelet count. Skin eruptions also can occur as a reaction to carbamazepine or baclofen. The patient's blood count and liver function must be closely monitored to detect early signs of drug toxicity. Baclofen may cause transient drowsiness, nausea, weakness, or fatigue.

Surgical treatment of trigeminal neuralgia brings about problems related to potential for damage to the cornea when the ophthalmic branch is dissected. The patient must be taught to avoid rubbing his eyes or exposing them to foreign objects, because the normal protective corneal reflex is no longer functional. He should get into the habit of wearing protective goggles when there is the possibility of getting dust and debris in his eyes and to try to blink his eyes often to cleanse their surface.

Dissection of the second or third branches of the trigeminal nerve produces problems of potential damage to the oral mucosa and teeth. The patient cannot feel hot liquids and foods and could be burned, he could bite the inside of his mouth without realizing it, or he may have dental caries that will not cause pain. Good oral hygiene and periodic dental examinations are particularly important when the body's natural warning system is not operative.

MYASTHENIA GRAVIS

The words *myasthenia gravis* literally mean *grave muscle weakness*. The disease is a chronic disorder manifested by fatigue and exhaustion that are aggravated by activity and relieved by rest. The muscular weakness can be so mild that it causes a minor inconvenience, or so severe that it is life-threatening because of its effect on breathing and swallowing.

Myasthenia gravis is believed to be an autoimmune disease in which circulating autoantibody is directed against the postsynaptic acetylcholine receptors at the neuromuscular junction (the point at which nerve impulses are transmitted to muscle tissue). The antibody reduces the number of functional receptor sites and thereby interferes with total neural stimulation of the muscle, which in turn produces muscle weakness.

Symptoms and Medical Diagnosis

Symptoms of myasthenia gravis include ptosis (drooping eyelid), diplopia (double vision), and difficulty in chewing and swallowing. Severe muscle weakness is the outstanding symptom of the disorder. Any of the skeletal muscles might be involved; muscles of the intestine, bladder, and heart are not affected.

The onset is gradual, and muscle weakness often is first noted when the patient tries to walk upstairs, get up from a sitting position, raise his arms over his head, or lift a heavy object. The fatigue is relieved by rest but soon returns and is more severe than expected from the amount of exertion put forth.

Diagnosis is established by administering an injection of edrophonium (Tensilon); a marked increase in muscular strength is noted within 1 minute of injection if the patient has myasthenia gravis.

Medical Treatment

There are two main modes of therapy, the choice depending on the severity of the symptoms. In milder cases the physician may manage the disease by dealing with the specific symptoms, rather than trying to induce a remission of the disease. In more severe cases efforts are made to manage the underlying cause of the symptoms.

Because 80% to 90% of myasthenia gravis patients have autoantibodies against acetylcholine receptors, plasmapheresis can be an effective treatment. The purpose of the plasma exchange is to remove the circulating autoantibodies from the patient's blood. This mode of therapy may bring clinical improvement in some patients, but it is not a cure for myasthenia gravis.

Anticholinesterase therapy is the earliest form of treatment for myasthenia gravis. Anticholinesterase agents inactivate acetylcholinesterase, a substance that prevents accumulations of acetylcholine at the neuromuscular junction. Acetylcholine must be present at the point where nerve impulses are transmitted to muscle in order for there to be sustained repetitive muscle contraction. Anticholinesterase agents temporarily increase muscle strength by inhibiting the enzyme acetylcholinesterase and allowing the acetylcholine to work, but they do not cure the problem. Two drugs commonly used as anticholinesterase agents are neostigmine (Prostigmin) and pyridostigmine (Mestinon). Pyridostigmine is more commonly used, because it can be taken orally.

The dosage of anticholinesterase drugs is precisely calculated for each patient, the aim being to achieve a delicate balance between too much and too little acetylcholine at the neuromuscular junction. Stress can quickly alter a patient's need for acetylcholine; hence overmedication or undermedication can occur rather suddenly. Unfortunately, the symptoms of too much medication are quite similar to those of too little medication, so it is often difficult to adjust the dosage correctly.

Another method of treatment is removal of the thymus gland, which decreases the antibody production. Immunosuppression also is a form of therapy for myasthenia gravis, inasmuch as it is believed to be an autoimmune disorder. The patient may, therefore, be given corticotropin (also known as adrenocorticotropic hormone [ACTH]), prednisone, azathioprine, or cyclophosphamide (Cytoxan).

Nursing Intervention

As with other neurologic disorders, nursing care of patients with myasthenia gravis will be based on the specific nursing diagnoses presented. When a person with this disorder is admitted to the hospital, special care and precautions must be taken, regardless of whether he was admitted for a condition related to his myasthenia gravis.

Infection, surgery, and other physical and emotional stresses can precipitate a myasthenic crisis. During the crisis frequent monitoring is essential. The patient's ability to swallow and breathe on his own can be seriously compromised. Suctioning, tracheostomy, and artificial ventilation may be necessary to maintain life until the crisis is over.

Education of the patient and his family must include instruction about the nature of the illness and the adverse effects of emotional upsets, respiratory infections, and similar stresses. Rehabilitation goals include instruction and support for the patient and family so that the patient remains as independent as possible.

Because he can become critically ill and in immediate need of medical attention at any time, the patient with myasthenia gravis should at all times wear a Medic-Alert emblem that identifies him as having the disease.

The patient, as well as members of his family and the nurses who care for him in the hospital or at home, should know the symptoms of improper dosage of anticholinesterase agents. These include dyspnea; poor tongue control, which produces difficulty in chewing, swallowing, and speaking; generalized muscle weakness; and neurologic symptoms such as restlessness, anxiety, and irritability. If any of these symptoms occur, the physician should be notified immediately.

In addition to problems arising from the anticholinesterase drugs, the myasthenic patient can also suffer from exaggerated and bizarre effects from a variety of drugs. These include the steroids and thyroid compounds; sedatives and respiratory depressants, such as morphine; tranquilizers, such as the phenothiazines; the mycin antibiotics; and some cardiac drugs, such as quinine and quinidine. Because so many drugs are potentially dangerous to a patient with myasthenia gravis, it is imperative that the nurse check with the physician ordering a medication to be sure he is aware that the patient has myasthenia gravis and that she give the prescribed drugs with great caution.

The Myasthenia Gravis Foundation, whose headquarters are at 61 Gramercy Park North, New York, NY 10010, promotes research for discovery of the cause and cure for the disease, and distributes information through its local chapters.

SEIZURE DISORDERS AND EPILEPSY

A seizure or convulsion is an attack of uncontrollable muscular contractions that may affect all (*generalized seizure*) or part (*partial* or *focal seizure*) of the body. With *tonic* convulsions, there is continued contraction of all muscles and the body becomes rigid. *Clonic* convulsions are characterized by alternate contraction and relaxation of the muscles, which give the affected part a rhythmic, jerking motion. A combination *tonic-clonic* convulsion is typical of the grand mal seizure of epilepsy.

There are several ways to classify epilepsy. The International Classification of Epileptic Seizures defines four groups: partial seizures, generalized seizures, unclassified seizures (because of insufficient data), and status epilepticus. The first group, partial seizures, is further divided into three subgroups: simple partial seizures, in which consciousness is not impaired but there are other motor, sensory, autonomic, or psychological symptoms; complex partial seizures, in which there is some impairment of consciousness with or without automatisms (repetitive, automatic actions such as lip smacking); and partial seizures that become generalized as the seizure continues.

Generalized seizures have symptoms or activity that is bilaterally symmetric and include absence, myoclonic, clonic, tonic, tonic-clonic, atonic, and infantile spasms (usually caused by fever). Absence seizures are also called *petit mal* and tonic-clonic seizures are called *grand mal*.

The third major group, unclassified seizures, simply means that not enough data have been obtained to determine which type of seizure the patient is experiencing.

The fourth designation, status epilepticus, indicates prolonged partial or generalized seizure without recovery between attacks.

Seizures can be symptomatic of a large number of disorders. Brain injury, infectious diseases with high fever, end-stage renal disease with uremia, toxicity (such as that occurring in eclampsia during pregnancy or in drug poisoning), epilepsy, and tetanus are but a few examples of seizure-producing disorders. Seizures can also occur any time the brain is deprived of oxygen.

Epilepsy is a chronic disturbance of the nervous system characterized by recurrent seizures that are the result of abnormal electrical activity of the brain. In epilepsy there is an excessive firing of brain cells, but this abnormal discharge occurs only occasionally; at other times the firing is normal.

Partial seizures with elementary symptomatology are also called *simple* or *focal* seizures and result from an abnormal localized cortical discharge. Partial seizures with complex symptomatology, also called *psychomotor* or *temporal lobe seizures*, usually, but not always, originate in the temporal lobe of the brain.

Generalized seizures are bilaterally symmetrical (affecting both sides of the body equally) and *do not* have a local onset; that is, they do not typically begin in one part of the body. Partial seizures can be unilateral, with involvement on only one side of the brain and activity only on one side of the body.

In classifying epileptic seizures on the basis of origin, the seizures are grouped as either idiopathic or symptomatic. *Idiopathic* epilepsy has no known cause. *Symptomatic* epilepsy has a known physical cause (e.g., brain tumor, injury to the head at birth, a wound or blow to the head, or an endocrine disorder).

Symptoms and Medical Diagnosis

The manifestations of epilepsy depend on the area of the brain where the abnormal firing occurs. *Absence* or *petit mal* seizures last only a few seconds. The onset is sudden, with no aura or warning and no postictal (after-seizure activity) symptoms. Seizures of this type usually affect children between 5 and 12 years of age and disappear during puberty. There usually is a twitching about the eyes and mouth. The person remains standing or sitting and appears to have had no more than a lapse of attention or a moment of absent-mindedness.

Grand mal or *tonic-clonic* seizures usually begin with bilateral jerks of the extremities or focal seizure activity. There is loss of consciousness and both tonic and clonic convulsions. The patient may be incontinent during the attack, and there is danger of biting the tongue. In the postictal phase the person is confused and drowsy.

Atonic or *akinetic* seizures are characterized by loss of body tone that results in nodding of the head, weakness of the knees, or total collapse and falling. The person usually remains conscious during the attack.

Status epilepticus is a grave condition in which there is a rapid, unrelenting series of convulsive seizures without intervening periods of consciousness. Irreversible brain damage can occur if the seizures are not controlled. Treatment of status epilepticus depends on its cause. Many times patients who are known to have epilepsy arrive in the emergency department with status epilepticus because, for one reason or the other, they stopped taking their medication for control of their seizures. Treatment in this instance would involve administration of diazepam, phenytoin, or phenobarbital in a dose sufficient to stop the seizures.

Uncontrolled seizures secondary to hypoglycemia (as in uncontrolled diabetes mellitus) can be relieved by intravenous administration of 50% dextrose. If the unrelenting seizures are caused by chronic alcoholism or withdrawal, treatment consists of intravenous administration of thiamin. Although these kinds of seizures are known as status epilepticus, they should not be confused with chronic epileptic seizures.

A diagnosis of epilepsy is confirmed by electroencephalogram and MRI. These tests help locate the site, or *locus*, and possibly the cause of the seizures. Skull radiographs are also part of the diagnostic workup when epilepsy is suspected.

Medical and Surgical Treatment

When the cause of seizures is known, as in cases of high fever or drug toxicity, medical treatment is aimed at controlling or eliminating whatever is responsible for the seizures. However, when there are recurrent seizures, as in epilepsy, the condition usually is managed with anticonvulsant drug therapy.

The major antiepileptic drugs are phenytoin (Dilantin), phenobarbital, primidone (Mysoline), and carbamazepine (Tegretol) for complex partial tonic-clonic seizures and valproic acid (Depakene), ethosuximide (Zarontin), and clonazepam (Klonopin) for absence epileptic seizures. Anticonvulsants are capable of interacting with other drugs and decreasing or enhancing their specific action. Among the drugs that interact with anticonvulsants are warfarin, digoxin, aspirin, certain antibiotics, antacids, folic acid, and narcotics.

All of the anticonvulsant drugs can produce some unpleasant side effects such as fever and leukopenia and, in the case of phenytoin, gingival hyperplasia and rash. Physical dependence can become a problem for patients taking either phenobarbital or primidone, which is largely converted to phenobarbital in the blood stream. Toxic side effects such as ataxia, drowsiness, nausea, sedation, and dizziness are not uncommon. Because of these and other toxicities associated with anticonvulsant therapy, patients taking these drugs regularly must have periodic laboratory tests performed and must remain under close supervision.

Patient education is extremely important, because the patient will need to report any untoward effects to the physician or nurse clinician so the dosage can be adjusted or the drug changed.

Through the efforts of the Epilepsy Association of America, located at 815 15th Street NW, Suite 528, Washington, DC 20005, the general public has become increasingly aware of the true nature of epilepsy. Research continues in an effort to find the cause and cure for this disease. In the meantime, we all have a responsibility to help those afflicted with epilepsy gain steady employment and lead useful, active lives. Most individuals who suffer from epileptic seizures are perfectly normal between seizures; they are not mentally retarded and are quite capable of becoming contributing members of our society if only they are given the chance to prove their worth.

Surgical treatment of epilepsy is an alternative for about 5% of all persons who have the disorder. The procedure involves removal of the portion of brain tissue that is the source of the seizures. Surgery of this kind is not without danger and is reserved for those patients whose seizures cannot be managed by medical treatment and in whom the focus of the seizures is accessible.

Nursing Assessment and Intervention

Patients with a known seizure problem usually are treated on an outpatient basis. However, these patients also are seen in hospitals or long-term care facilities and must be assessed carefully in order to provide optimal safety and care.

Significant information that should be obtained from these patients includes the kind of seizures they experience, whether they have any sensation (aura) just before the appearance of clinically observable signs, what medications they are taking, and what measures are known to be helpful either to prevent a seizure or while they are having a seizure and afterward.

When caring for a patient who is likely to experience a seizure during an acute illness, the nurse should periodically observe the patient for tremors, unexplained sensory or motor changes, mental changes that indicate confusion or disorientation, and restless or agitated behavior. In many cases, a change in the neurologic status of a patient can signal the possibility that a seizure might occur.

Nursing care of patients with epileptic seizures is concerned with immediate care during and after a seizure and long-term management and control of seizures and their psychosocial implications.

Assessment should include any factors that could have triggered the seizure (e.g., hyperventilation, bright lights [photosensitivity], alcohol and other drugs, fluid and electrolyte imbalances, lack of sleep, and emotional stress).

A major concern of those caring for a patient subject to seizures is protecting him from injury. Although witnessing a seizure for the first time can be a frightening experience, the movements the person is making are just exaggerations of normal body movements.

The nurse's first responsibility is to stay calm, remain with the patient, and send for assistance.

The environment of a patient at risk for seizure should be made as safe as possible. If the patient is very likely to have seizures, the siderails and headboard of the bed are padded. If the nurse can observe a patient in the preictal (before seizure) stage, she can slip a folded washcloth or padded tongue blade into the mouth to protect the tongue from chewing movements. It is not usual to be able to do this before the jaws are clenched, however, and the nurse should never try to pry open the mouth or insert something into it once the jaws are clenched and the seizure motor activity has begun.

If a seizure comes on without warning, the patient should be left wherever he is lying. If he is on a hard surface, his head should be protected from injury by placing a pillow or a rolled blanket or coat under it. The head should be turned to the side, if possible, to prevent aspiration. Do not attempt to restrain the patient's movements or to move him to a bed or chair during the seizure. If supplemental oxygen is near, it should be administered. When the seizure is over, turn the patient to the side.

Observations during a patient's seizure should include as much of the following as possible:

- The time the seizure began, whether the patient experienced an aura, and the length of time the seizure lasted.
- What the patient was doing just before the seizure.
- Where in the body the seizure began and what parts of the body were involved.
- The character of the movements (tonic or clonic) and whether they changed during the seizure.
- Whether the head or eyes turned to one side and, if so, which side.
- Whether there was incontinence of urine or stool, vomiting, bleeding, or foaming or frothing at the mouth.
- If the eyes are open, in which direction they were positioned.
- The effects of the seizure on the patient's vital signs.
- Changes in skin color or profuse perspiration.

Postictal (after seizure) assessment should include information about the presence of lethargy, confusion, headache, speech impairment, and muscle soreness.

The long-term management of epileptic seizures is primarily focused on providing the patient with the information and support he needs to care for himself and avoid recurring and debilitating seizures.

Patient Teaching

Self-care for the person with epilepsy requires that he understand the nature of his disorder, the purpose of his prescribed medications, their side effects, and the signs of toxicity that should be reported to the physician. He must understand the necessity for compliance with the prescribed regimen in order to avoid recurrent seizures. He will need assistance in developing coping mechanisms to deal with the psychosocial impact of having epilepsy.

The teaching plan should also include information about possible seizure-triggering mechanisms and the importance of avoiding them whenever possible. Alcohol is especially contraindicated for the patient with seizures, as it interferes with the effectiveness of the medications, causes excessive sedation, and may trigger seizures. Fatigue can also make the patient more prone to seizure activity. He must be helped to plan for adequate rest each day.

The patient is taught not to swim or participate alone in activities that could have dangerous effects if he had a seizure and was alone. Women need to know that menstruation puts additional stress on the body, and they are more prone to seizures during this period each month.

Persons with epilepsy should wear a Medic-

Alert bracelet or necklace and carry a list of the medications they are taking and names and phone numbers of their physician and others to be notified in an emergency.

Psychosocial support is necessary in encouraging the patient to talk about his fears and concerns. Lifestyle changes will have to be made if he is not permitted to drive. Most states allow resumption of driving when a patient has been seizure free for 1 year. A referral to the local epilepsy society for connection with a support group can be very helpful for both the patient and family.

Nursing interventions for selected problems in a patient subject to seizures are summarized in Nursing Care Plan 15–3.

NURSING CARE PLAN 15–3

Selected nursing diagnoses, goals/outcome criteria, nursing interventions, and evaluations for a patient subject to seizures

Situation: A 27-year-old male is admitted to your unit after suffering a generalized seizure at work. He has a history of epilepsy but had not had a seizure in 6 months and had decided to quit taking his phenytoin (Dilantin). He did not return to his physician, because he did not like the side effects of the medicine and didn't want to take anything.

Nursing Diagnosis	Goals/Outcome Criteria	Nursing Intervention	Evaluation
Potential for injury related to seizure activity. SUPPORTING DATA Known history of epilepsy; had grand mal seizure at work; has not taken anticonvulsant medication for past 10 days.	Patient will not sustain injury during a seizure.	Administer anticonvulsant as ordered; monitor neurologic status; ask him to ring for nurse if he experiences any warning (aura) of a seizure about to occur. Pad headboard and siderails. Keep room softly lit and avoid turning on overhead lights to prevent triggering a seizure. Immediately obtain oxygen and suction apparatus in room as ordered; utilize if patient has seizure. If he has seizure, do not force anything into his mouth; protect head; turn to side when motor activity is over and establish airway; allow him to recover from postictal state; reorient and reassure him. If seizure activity continues for more than 15 minutes, establish an airway and call physician.	Anticonvulsant administered per schedule; no sign of seizure activity.
Noncompliance related to stopping medication and not obtaining follow-up care. SUPPORTING DATA Stopped taking anticonvulsant; did not consult physician.	Patient will adhere to treatment regimen.	Discuss dangers of not taking anticonvulsant medication. Explain advantages of continued medical care on a regular basis; explain that when one medication is not satisfactory, another can be tried.	Discussed need for continued medication on regular schedule; states he doesn't want to have another seizure, but the side effects of the medication were getting to him; states he won't stop his medicine again.
Knowledge deficit related to disease and treatment (medications). SUPPORTING DATA Unaware of things that can trigger seizures; did not know that medications other than phenytoin (Dilantin) can be effective.	Patient will verbalize dangers of continued seizures by time of discharge. Patient can describe treatment options and advantages of controlling his epilepsy by time of discharge.	Teach him about oxygen deprivation to the brain during seizure activity. Teach him about factors that can trigger seizures and how to avoid them. Teach him about anticonvulsant medications: side effects, monitoring levels, proper dosage schedule; explain need to take them even when there is no seizure activity.	States he understands now that seizures can cause brain damage if uncontrolled; identifies proper rest and nutrition, decreased stress, and avoidance of alcohol as measures he can take to help prevent seizures; continue plan.

NURSING CARE PLAN 15–3, *Continued*

Nursing Diagnosis	Goals/Outcome Criteria	Nursing Intervention	Evaluation
Anxiety related to fear of losing job and friends because he has epilepsy. SUPPORTING DATA States that he feels shame when he thinks about his coworkers seeing him have the seizure. Does not think his boss will let him keep his job as a shipping clerk.	Patient will talk to boss about his job status before discharge. Patient will begin to discuss his epilepsy with his closest friends by time of discharge.	Encourage verbalization of fears and concerns; listen actively. Encourage him to seek information about his job as an alternative to "fearing the unknown"; assure him that physician or nurses will educate his boss about the disorder and likelihood of control of seizure activity with medication. Encourage him to be "up front" with friends and to seek their support; have him assess what disabilities people that he knows have and whether that has interfered with his friendship for them. Encourage contact with the local chapter of the Epilepsy Society and a support group.	Seems interested in an epilepsy support group; talked at length about being "different" from his friends; does have some friends with diabetes and one with cystic fibrosis; is thinking about how to approach his boss; discussed pathophysiology of seizures; focused on how well controlled he had been when taking his medication; reviewed other aspects of self-care.
Self-esteem disturbance related to occurrence of seizure and diagnosis of epilepsy. SUPPORTING DATA States he thinks people will see him as a "freak."	Patient will express confidence that seizures can be controlled. Patient will verbalize that he can still hold a job, maintain friendships, and be productive.	Project a calm and matter-of-fact attitude about his epilepsy; focus on fact that seizures can be controlled. Emphasize how good self-care can prevent triggering seizures. Assist him to look at positive strengths he has to offer job and friends. Have someone of similar age who has well-controlled epilepsy talk with him.	States he understands that he most likely can control his seizures if he takes his medication and follows instructions regarding self-care; made list of strengths he has for his job to discuss with boss.

CEREBRAL PALSY

Cerebral palsy includes a group of paralytic disorders in which muscle coordination is lost as a result of cerebral damage that is generally thought to occur at or near the time of birth. The exact cause is not known, but the condition is believed to be associated with oxygen lack.

Symptoms

Although cerebral palsy can cause a wide variety of muscular disorders and some disturbances of sensory perception, it can be categorized into three general types: (1) *spastic paralysis*, in which there are exaggerated reflexes, increased deep tendon reflexes, and muscle spasms; (2) *athetoid type*, in which there are random and purposeless movements and a high degree of muscle tension; and (3) *ataxic type*, in which there is a disturbance of coordination with poor balance and a staggering gait. The patient also may suffer from defects of hearing, vision, or speech. The impairment may be severe or minimal.

Treatment

There is no cure for cerebral palsy, but early muscle training and special exercises can be of benefit if they are started before a child develops faulty habits of movement and incorrect muscle patterns. In some cases, orthopedic surgery and devices such as braces and casts can be used to correct orthopedic deformities and disabilities. Treatment is lifelong and individualized, attempting to prevent complications and to help individuals lead the fullest life possible, limited only by the imposed muscular and sensory disturbances.

Attitudes Toward Cerebral Palsy Victims

Most victims of cerebral palsy, be they men, women, or children, long to be treated as normal, sane individuals. For some reason, many people assume that the speech difficulties and uncoordinated movements characteristic of cerebral palsy indicate mental retardation or total disability. Although the cerebral palsy victim may be somewhat slow and clumsy in accomplishing relatively simple tasks or difficult to understand when he is talking, he can be fairly independent if one is patient with him and willing to make the effort to communicate with him. Patients who have entered hospitals for an unrelated illness and are sufferers of cerebral palsy often are treated in a humiliating and degrading manner by personnel who assume that because the patient is uncoordinated in his movements and cannot speak clearly he is also mentally retarded, unable to comprehend what is happening to him, and unaware of the fact that he is not thought of or treated as a rational, thinking human person. A young patient wrote the following after being admitted to a hospital for an appendectomy: "There were many depressing moments during my hospital stay. Some could not have been avoided; others might have been if personnel had known that what I needed most was to be treated as any patient would be—as the 19-year-old adult I am."

ALZHEIMER'S DISEASE

Alzheimer's disease is a form of dementia that occurs from pathologic changes in the brain tissue of the patient. Unfortunately the changes can be detected only at autopsy. The cause of Alzheimer's disease is unknown, and considerable research is in progress to better define this disease. It can occur during middle age or during the later decades of life and causes devastation to the patient and family. The disease has a slow onset, progresses at varying rates of speed through several stages, and is eventually fatal.

Early signs and symptoms are those of beginning mental deterioration: forgetfulness, recent memory loss, difficulty learning and remembering, inability to concentrate, and a decline in personal hygiene, appearance, and inhibitions. Later the patient becomes quite confused and unable to make judgments, has difficulty communicating, suffers losses in motor function, and becomes dependent on others.

There is no cure or specific treatment for Alzheimer's disease. Care is supportive and is directed at assisting the patient to maintain as much ability to perform activities of daily living for himself as possible. Preservation of dignity is another goal for these patients.

COMMON NEUROLOGIC PATIENT CARE PROBLEMS

Disorders affecting the central nervous system are many and varied, but they all share some common problems related to impaired control or loss of sensory and motor functions. Patients may have incontinence because of a stroke, multiple sclerosis, or a spinal cord injury, but regardless of the cause, each can be helped to some degree by a bladder or bowel training program. Several types of neurologic disorders cause problems with mobility, and there is much the nurse can do to help the patient achieve greater independence. Specific nursing actions for these and other common problems of neurologically impaired patients follow.

IMPAIRED MOBILITY

The nurse, the physical therapist, and the patient work together to help the patient cope with his muscle weakness or paralysis. Activities such as proper positioning and range-of-motion exercises are started immediately in order to preserve proper alignment of joints and limbs and prevent contractures and muscle atrophy. Assistive devices such as splints and slings may be utilized. The patient who suffers paralysis and loss of sensation in an extremity is taught to become aware of where that arm or leg is when he turns, transfers to a chair, etc., in order to avoid injury to the extremity.

The hemiplegic patient is taught how to transfer from the bed to a chair and back and how to best utilize assistance from others, if needed, for these activities. He is taught how to protect his skin in areas of decreased sensation.

The patient who has hemiparesis (one-sided weakness) is taught how to strengthen his muscles and use assistive devices such as walkers, crutches, or canes to walk. He is taught the best ways to get out of bed and into and out of a chair.

The quadriplegic patient (i.e., with all four limbs paralyzed) is helped to learn to cope with this drastic alteration in his life and how he might direct his energies at different, but attainable, goals.

All patients who have suffered an impairment in mobility need assistance with the grieving process, help in establishing healthy and effective coping patterns, and assistance with depression.

Attention to the relief of pain and muscle spasm is necessary in order for the patient to achieve the highest level of rehabilitation of which he is capable. Paralyzed extremities are subject to the formation of edema and should be elevated when the patient is at rest in order to decrease this problem. The patient needs to be turned frequently to prevent problems from pressure and sluggish circulation.

Chapter 9 studies the effects of immobility on each of the body's systems in detail, along with the nursing activities necessary to avoid disabilities resulting from inactivity. The principles and practices presented in that chapter are relevant to the nursing care of a patient with a neurologic disorder that produces some type of paresis or paralysis.

INCONTINENCE (ALTERATION IN BOWEL AND URINARY ELIMINATION)

There are few problems more exasperating to the patient and more challenging to the nursing staff than those presented by the loss of control over urination and defecation. In recent years, some very positive steps have been taken to establish successful bladder and bowel training programs and to improve the effectiveness of collection devices and protective undergarments when complete control is not a realistic goal.

Perhaps the first step in planning and implementing either a bladder or a bowel training program is to convince the nursing staff and the patient and his family that *something can be done* to improve, if not completely relieve, the situation. A negative attitude and lack of persistence can doom a program to failure before it is started. One must be content with small successes at first, setting short-term goals that will eventually lead to a satisfactory resolution of the problem.

Bladder Training Program

This is a program designed to help a person with some degree of loss of normal bladder function and a resulting disturbance of voiding and bladder control. Loss of control can occur in a variety of neurologic disorders, including stroke, spinal cord injury, and tumors and lesions of the spinal cord.

The purposes of a bladder reconditioning program are to prevent urinary complications such as infection and calculi (stones) and to allow the patient freedom from fear of embarrassment and loss of self-esteem.

Assessment of bladder function is conducted to determine the optimal neural and muscular control that can realistically be expected in view of the physiologic cause of loss of control and the patient's mental and emotional ability to cooperate and take an active part in carrying out the program.

The cause of urinary incontinence must be known, and the specific symptoms manifested by the patient must be clearly defined. Significant data would include information about (1) difficulty in initiating voiding, (2) any methods the patient may use to initiate voiding (for example, pressure on the bladder), (3) degree of awareness of the need to void, (4) ability to empty the bladder completely and amount of residual urine, (5) signs of bladder distention and dribbling or overflow, (6) night incontinence, (7) stress incontinence, and (8) usual times for voiding.

Spinal cord injuries and lesions produce what is known as a *cord bladder* or *neurogenic bladder*. Patients with disorders of this type are not aware of the need to void and must be trained in techniques to initiate voiding and empty the bladder.

The second step in a bladder training program is to keep an accurate record of actual voiding times for a 2- to 3-day period. Some problems of incontinence can be corrected by a simple scheduling of voiding times. Offering a bedpan or getting the patient up to the bathroom one-half hour before times he is usually incontinent may remedy the problem.

A bladder retraining program usually begins with a 2-hour schedule for toileting. The patient should attempt to drink 2,000 to 3,000 mL of fluid between waking up and 6 P.M. Coffee, tea, alcoholic beverages, and soda with caffeine should be avoided near bedtime, because they have a diuretic effect. The patient is toileted before retiring for the night. The maintenance of an accurate retraining record is essential. A trial of 6 weeks is necessary before determining whether the retraining is successful.

Various drugs that affect the voiding process may be helpful for certain types of patients. The nurse must assess whether the medication is beneficial.

Patients who have nerve damage and paralysis are trained in specific techniques to empty the bladder. The Crede technique, in which the open hand is pressed over the bladder and directed toward the suprapubic area, can facilitate emptying a flaccid bladder. Self-catheterization is taught to paralyzed patients so that they are not dependent on an indwelling catheter or on other people for their urinary elimination.

Some patients are candidates for the implantation of an artificial sphincter to control bladder release of urine. More and more types of successful devices are developed each year, but these are primarily for the patient who has no neurologic control over the bladder.

Every patient undertaking a bladder retraining program needs a great deal of understanding and encouragement and a positive attitude in order to be successful. Praise for each small achievement should be given. Accidents should be expected and not looked on as "failures." Achieving total continence takes considerable time and effort, but for many patients it is possible.

Bowel Training Program

Bowel training for the neurologic patient is done to correct incontinence or prevent constipation and impaction. The bowel training program begins with assessment of the specific patterns of elimination. It also helps to know the patient's former bowel pattern before illness or injury: Has he regularly relied on the use of enemas or laxatives? Has he been prone to constipation in the past? Next, the nurse needs to establish whether the patient is aware of the urge to defecate or has any warning that his bowels are about to move.

A bowel training program for either constipation or incontinence should incorporate an exercise program that is within the patient's ability, a high-fiber diet, and adequate liquid intake during the day. An accurate recording of bowel movements correlated with times of oral intake over a 2- to 3-day period will help establish the most opportune times to try to stimulate evacuation and thus establish a habit. If incontinence has occurred at specific times after eating, toileting 30 minutes sooner and using a rectal suppository to stimulate the urge to defecate may alter the pattern. Gradually the use of the suppository is discontinued.

For the patient who is prone to constipation and then incontinence, increasing liquid intake and adding a stool softener to the above suggestions can be effective. Otherwise, a planned regimen of suppository or enema use may be necessary to assist with evacuation at a desired time, thus preventing incontinence.

All patients need to be comfortable when attempting to evacuate the bowel. A raised, padded toilet seat, handrails, and perhaps a footstool can provide enough comfort to allow the patient to relax so that evacuation can occur naturally. Privacy is essential.

Most of all, a positive attitude on the part of staff members that the problem can be overcome is needed. If the nurse and the patient are optimistic and patient, success can be achieved a great deal of the time.

APHASIA

Aphasia is a defect or loss of the power of expression by speech, writing, or signs or of comprehension of spoken or written language. It is caused by disease or injury of the brain centers controlling language comprehension and expression.

Aphasia may be *receptive, expressive,* or *global.* The person with receptive aphasia has difficulty interpreting communications to him in either spoken or written form. In expressive aphasia, the person has difficulty expressing himself in speech or writing. Global aphasia is where the person has a combination of receptive and expressive aphasia. Aphasias vary in degree and in type of deficit. For example, a person may be able to write a message but cannot form the words to say it.

Assessment

A comprehensive assessment of the patient who has some type of aphasia usually is a team effort carried out under the leadership of a specially trained speech therapist. Nurses and others responsible for the care of the aphasic patient can assist by noting specific abilities or inabilities of the patient to communicate with them. Some important questions the nurse might ask herself while observing and assessing the status of a patient who has difficulty communicating because of a neurologic disorder include the following:

- Can he understand yes/no questions?
- Can he point or look toward objects you have named that are in his line of vision?
- Can he name the objects?
- Is he able to follow simple directions (e.g., "Turn your head")?
- Can he repeat simple words? Complex words?
- Can he repeat sentences?
- Can he follow simple written requests?
- Can he write answers to questions?
- Can he write requests?
- Can he read questions or directions?

Nursing Intervention

The patient who suddenly has a problem speaking or understanding words or signs is likely to suffer from isolation and experience extreme frustration unless an effort is made to establish some means of communicating with him as quickly as possible. Once the patient's specific problem is identified (and it could be relatively simple or extremely complex), measures are taken to help the patient communicate as fully as his condition will allow.

Goals for the care of the aphasic patient are focused on stimulating communication without undue frustration and gradually guiding him to appropriate responses and requests. Reaching these goals may take weeks or months, but there are helpful principles and techniques that can be used by all members of the health team and by family members and friends.

Perhaps the most important rule of all is to *avoid talking to the aphasic person as if he were mentally incompetent.* His inability to communicate does not mean a lack of intelligence. He should be spoken *to,* not spoken *about* as if he cannot hear and understand what others are saying in his presence.

Do not shout at the aphasic person. Speak slowly and distinctly as you are facing him. Use body language and sign language to communicate if they seem to be helpful to the patient. Your facial expressions, posture, and gestures can often say more than the words you are saying.

Give the aphasic patient time to respond to questions. Do not ask more than one question at a time. It takes longer for an aphasic person to process what is being said to him. If you need to repeat a statement or question, use exactly the same words. He may have comprehended only half of the sentence the first time. Only one person in the room should speak at a time. Be certain to establish eye contact with the patient before speaking.

It is especially important that the aphasic patient be in an orderly and relaxed environment that is relatively free from distractions that make it difficult to concentrate on communicating.

The speech therapist will plan the patient's therapy program and will share with the nurse the details of how best to work with each individual patient. Some general guidelines include: (1) give praise for attempts at communication and for each correctly expressed word or sentence; (2) do not correct the patient's pronunciation, as he is liable to become too frustrated and give up speaking; and (3) be very patient.

Problems with aphasia sometimes resolve spontaneously in 3 or 4 months after a CVA. Total speech rehabilitation can take many months and may never reach the prestroke level.

Among the techniques used to stimulate communication and help the patient deal with his problem of aphasia are self-talk, parallel talk, expansion, and modeling. *Self-talk* helps the aphasic person associate activities with specific words and phrases. The nurse or other person talks about what she is doing while performing a task (for example, making the bed). Self-talk is done in the presence of the patient so he can make connection between what is being said and what he sees being done.

Parallel talk describes for the patient what he is doing while he is performing some activity. In *expansion*, the person communicating with the patient completes the patient's sentences when he is able to verbalize but cannot yet speak in complete sentences. No new information is added during expansion. In *modeling*, the patient's sentences are completed, and new information is added.

All of the above techniques are helpful in improving communication. They are forms of therapy, however, and are used only in a planned program that has been designed to meet a patient's individual needs. Whatever techniques are chosen and used, they should not be used in a condescending manner, nor should the patient be treated as a child.

The plan of care for the aphasic patient should not neglect the physical condition of his mouth and tongue. Good oral hygiene is needed to keep the oral mucosa clean and moist and in optimal condition so that it is easier for the patient to form words.

CONFUSION

Confusion may be acute and short term, or it may be a permanent state. Confusion may also be mild or severe and may be accompanied by anxiety, agitation, and refusal to cooperate. The person is in a state of disorientation, and until the symptoms subside, he cannot behave rationally. He must be supported and protected, or he may injure himself.

In states of severe confusion, once called *delirium*, the patient may experience hallucinations, delusions, and severe agitation. This is usually an acute, short-term state caused by fever or metabolic imbalance.

Patients who experience confusion after a head injury often become combative as their intracranial pressure rises. It is not advisable to restrain these patients, and the nurse must be very careful to stay out of range of flailing arms.

Assessment

The nurse should be alert to signs of confusion in any patient with a CNS problem. Subjective and objective assessment data include (1) loss of orientation to person, place, or time; (2) inability to cooperate fully with simple tasks and requests such as eating and bathing; (3) inappropriate statements or answers to questions; (4) restlessness and agitation; (5) hostility and anxiety; (6) hallucinations or delusions; and (7) other signs of inability to maintain control over thought processes and behavior.

Nursing Intervention

The patient who is confused needs above all else a stable and calm environment. His thought processes are, in a sense, "fractured" and somewhat beyond his control. Stimuli entering his brain are frightening and threatening to him, and he simply cannot make sense out of most of what is going on around him. A calm, consistent, and orderly approach combined with a set daily routine is most helpful.

After assessing her patient and determining as precisely as possible what kind of altered consciousness the patient is experiencing, the nurse plans intervention to minimize his confusion and help him regain control. A care plan for a delirious or confused patient should include the following nursing interventions:

- Be sure the patient is using whatever sensory aids he usually needs to see and hear; for example, eyeglasses, contact lenses, and hearing aid.
- Turn off the television and radio when communicating with patient.
- Utilize methods of reality therapy to help orient him to who he is, where he is, and what has happened and is happening to him. Do not "go along" with his disorientation. Calmly reorient him, but without arguing or attempting to refute or elaborate on his delusional thinking. If the patient persists in talking about his delusions, gently change the subject, saying something like, "I would rather talk about something else."

- Communicate with him face-to-face and only with simple, direct, and descriptive statements. Do not bombard him with unnecessary explanations and questions.
- Provide the *proper* level of stimulation, giving the patient the information he needs to recognize what is going on, but without making him feel threatened or overwhelmed with information.
- Provide safety measures for the patient who is hallucinating, extremely agitated, confused, or paranoid. Use physical restraints only when necessary to prevent injury and to allow for treatments such as IV fluids or indwelling catheters and tubes. Constant attendance may be necessary until the confusion subsides.
- Maintain a calm, tolerant, and uncritical manner. Do not laugh at the patient or treat him in a condescending way. Accept his behavior as one way in which some people cope with what is to them a world they cannot understand.
- Administer antipsychotic and antianxiety drugs as prescribed.
- Help the patient to perform activities of self-care; do for him only what he is unable to do.

PROBLEMS OF SELF-CARE

Disturbances in motor function and inability to carry out the most basic of self-care activities can erode a person's sense of independence and self-esteem. Although we are dependent on one another for satisfaction of our basic human needs, each of us wants and needs some degree of autonomy and independence. The ability to feed and clothe ourselves and take care of functions of elimination is an important part of that independence. Regaining some level of self-care in these areas is of particular concern to the adult who, because of neurologic dysfunction, may have to relearn ways to perform the simplest of daily activities.

Assessment

Nursing assessment of the patient with a neurologic disorder must consider what the patient and his significant others know about his disability and its limitations on his ability to care for himself. The ability of significant others to learn how to care for the patient and their willingness to do so is an important part of assessing and planning for rehabilitation. Other assessment data include the patient's current status in regard to bowel and bladder control programs that have been initiated to help him achieve control and his motivation and level of adaptability to disability. An assessment of the patient's ability to perform self-care activities such as bathing, feeding, dressing, and grooming must be completed.

Long-term goals for a patient with impaired mobility must take into account the prognosis for recovery of sensory and motor function. Often the patient with a neurologic disorder has some permanent disability that requires careful assessment of his potential for self-care and the support he is likely to receive from family and friends once he is discharged. Goals for rehabilitation must be realistic and mutually agreed on by the patient, his family, and the nurse.

There are many assistive devices available to help patients with neurologic deficits to feed and dress themselves. Occupational therapists can help the patient relearn how to perform elementary tasks necessary to daily living. Patients are retaught how to feed themselves, how to get in and out of bed or a chair, how to select and put on clothes and fasten them, and how to bathe, brush teeth, and comb their hair.

The nurse provides assistance when the patient cannot do a task completely, and most of all, she provides encouragement and praise for efforts made. When pursuing self-help rehabilitation, the nurse needs to remember that the patient tires easily, and tasks must be spaced apart so that energy is available for achievement. Pushing the patient to try yet another task when he is too tired only sets him up for failure and frustration.

Psychosocial Concerns

In addition to physical rehabilitation, attention must be paid to restoring the patient's self-esteem. He will need time and assistance in adapting to an altered body image. Counseling is often needed in order to restore or maintain an optimal level of sexual health.

Vocational rehabilitation may be needed so that the patient can remain a productive member of society and can contribute to the welfare of his family.

Reentry into the community and a normal social life is another area for intervention. Often the patient has been out of touch with his normal social circles for many months during his illness and recovery process. Plans should be made before discharge for social contact to be reinstated.

The social worker is a valuable part of the health care team and can direct the patient and family to the appropriate agencies for assistance with social rehabilitation. In addition, the American Heart Association and the other agencies for specific diseases mentioned in this chapter have considerable literature and advice available to patients and families.

Concerns for the Elderly

Although there is loss of neurons in the nervous system with aging and brain weight may drop considerably after age 70, these factors do not correlate with a decrease in intellectual function. People with gross brain atrophy found at autopsy were reported to be "sharp as a tack" before death. Others with relatively little evidence of brain atrophy showed signs of considerable impairment of intellectual function while alive.

Simple reaction time is decreased with age, largely as a result of vision impairments that occur with age and a decrease in the dendrites that conduct nerve impulses. It has been shown that the elderly often make up for a decrease in psychomotor speed by an increase in accuracy and are therefore able to do things just as well as the younger person when there is no time pressure involved. In some patients the loss of dendrites may be responsible for the decreased intellectual responsiveness and abstract reasoning ability, impaired perception and integration of sensory input, failing short-term memory, and decreased learning ability. Changes in the production and metabolism of the neurotransmitters in the CNS may also account for these changes.

Loss of neurons and slower nerve conduction cause a decrease in efficiency of the autonomic nervous system in old age. Body homeostasis is more difficult to maintain or regain. For this reason, the elderly are subject to death from hypothermia (prolonged, profound cold) or from hyperthermia (excessive heat). Adaptation to physiologic stress takes much longer, and recovery is often incomplete.

The nurse who works with the elderly needs to remember that the elderly do not adapt to stress as readily as younger people. Teaching the patient about the dangers of becoming cold or hot is necessary. Physical exertion must be countered with sufficient rest.

As they reach their later years, more patients have diseases that affect the nervous system. Arthritis, osteoporosis, parkinsonism, diabetic peripheral neuropathy, deafness, and cataracts are just a few of the disorders that can affect posture, balance, and movement.

By performing a total assessment of the patient and considering his problems holistically, the nurse can provide high-quality, individualized care that can maximize the patient's potential for living an independent, satisfying life.

BIBLIOGRAPHY

Andreoli, T. E., et al.: Cecil Essentials of Medicine, 2nd ed. Philadelphia, W. B. Saunders, 1990.

Aumick, J. E.: Head trauma: Guidelines for care. RN, April, 1991, p. 3.

Barker, E.: Brain tumor: Frightening diagnosis, nursing challenge. RN, Sept., 1990, p. 46.

Barker, E., and Higgins, R.: Managing a suspected spinal cord injury. Nursing 89, April, 1989, p. 52.

Beck, C., and Heacock, P.: Nursing interventions for patients with Alzheimer's dementia. Nurs. Clin. North Am., March, 1988, p. 95.

Burns, E. M., and Buckwalter, K. C.: Pathophysiology and etiology of Alzheimer's disease. Nurs. Clin. North Am., March, 1988, p. 11.

Chadwick, A. T., and Oesting, H. H.: Caring for patients with spinal cord injuries. Nursing 89, Nov., 1989, p. 53.

Coderre, C. B.: Meningitis: Dangers when the diagnosis is viral. RN, Aug., 1989, p. 50.

Delgago, J., and Billo, J.: Care of the patient with Parkinson's disease: Surgical and nursing interventions. J. Neurosci. Nurs., June, 1988, p. 142.

Dudas, S.: Nursing diagnoses and interventions for the rehabilitation of the stroke patient. Nurs. Clin. North Am., June, 1986, p. 345.

Eliopoulos, C.: Health Assessment of the Older Adult, 2nd ed. Redwood City, CA, Addison-Wesley, 1990.

Ferguson, J. M.: Helping an MS patient live a better life. RN, Dec., 1987, p. 22.

Fode, N. C.: Subarachnoid hemorrhage from ruptured intracranial aneurysm. Am. J. Nurs., May, 1988, p. 673.

Gardner, D.: Acute management of the head injured adult. Nurs. Clin. North Am., Dec., 1986, p. 555.

Gilliam, E. E.: Intracranial hypertension—advances in intracranial pressure monitoring. Crit. Care Nurs. Clin. North Am., March, 1990, p. 21.

Goetter, W.: Nursing diagnoses and interventions with the acute stroke patient. Nurs. Clin. North Am., June, 1986, p. 309.

Gray-Vickery, V. P.: Evaluating Alzheimer's patients—the importance of being thorough. Nursing 89, Dec., 1989, p. 39.

Hall, G.: Care of the Alzheimer's patient living at home. Nurs. Clin. North Am., March, 1988, p. 31.

Harper, J.: Use of steroids in cerebral edema: Therapeutic implications. Heart Lung, Jan., 1988, p. 70.

Hart, G.: Strokes causing left vs. right hemiplegia: Different effects and nursing implications. Ger. Nurs., March/April, 1990, p. 67.

Hickey, J.: The Clinical Practice of Neurological and Neurosurgical Nursing. Philadelphia, J. B. Lippincott, 1985.

Hughes, M. C.: Critical care nursing for the patient with a spinal cord injury. Crit. Care Nurs. Clin. North Am., March, 1990, p. 33.

Ignatavicius, D. D., and Bayne, M. J.: Medical-Surgical Nursing. Philadelphia, W. B. Saunders, 1991.

Jeter, K., et al.: Nursing for Continence. Philadelphia, W. B. Saunders, 1990.

Kaufman, J.: Nurse's guide to assessing the 12 cranial nerves. Nursing 90, June, 1990, p. 56.

Lewis, S., et al.: Manual of Psychosocial Nursing Interventions: Promoting Mental Health in Medical-Surgical Settings. Philadelphia, W. B. Saunders, 1989.

Luchka, S.: Working with ICP monitors. RN, April, 1991, p. 34.

Matteson, M. A., and McConnell, E. S.: Gerontological Nursing: Concepts and Practice. Philadelphia, W. B. Saunders, 1990.

O'Brien, K.: Managing the seizure patient. Nursing 91, Jan., 1991, p. 63.

Rakel, R. E., ed.: Conn's Current Therapy 1990. Philadelphia, W. B. Saunders, 1990.

Rhynsburger, J.: How to fight MS fatigue. Am. J. Nurs., March, 1989, p. 337.

Scheinberg, L., and Holland, N.: Multiple Sclerosis: A Guide for Patients and Families, 2nd ed. New York: Raven Press, 1987.

Sherman, D. W.: Managing an acute head injury. Nursing 90, April, 1990, p. 47.

Springhouse Corp.: Illustrated Manual of Nursing Practice. Springhouse, PA, 1990.
Walleck, C. W.: Controversies in the management of the head injured patient. Crit. Care Nurs. Clin. North Am., Jan., 1989, p. 67.
Weber-Jones, J. E.: Patient-teaching guide: Performing clean, intermittent self-catheterization. Nursing 91, Aug., 1991, p. 56.

STUDENT STUDY AIDS

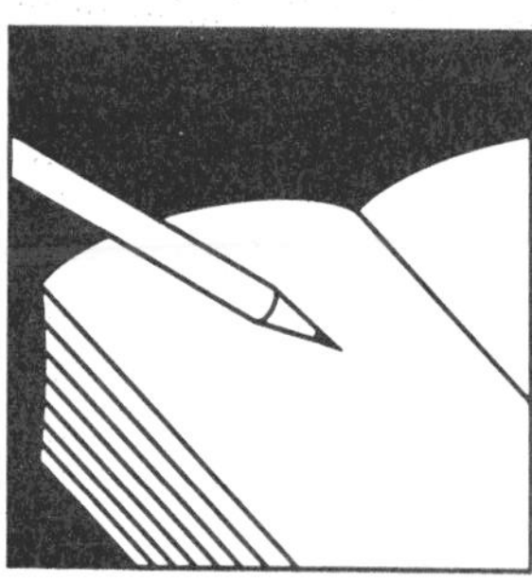

CLINICAL CASE PROBLEMS

Read each of the following clinical situations and discuss the questions with your classmates.

1. Mr. Long is to have several diagnostic tests done to determine the cause of his neurologic symptoms, which include headache, visual disturbance, muscular weakness, and personality change.

- How would you explain an EEG to Mr. Long? A lumbar puncture? CT scan? MRI?

---

2. Martha is a 22-year-old college student who has suffered a head injury in an automobile accident. She had no illnesses prior to her accident. She was stabilized in the emergency department and admitted to the neurologic intensive care unit. She is confused and groggy and has leakage of spinal fluid from one ear and irregular respirations.

- What assessments would you do on Martha?
- What specific nursing measures would you include in your care plan concerning the leaking CSF?
- What measures would you take to provide appropriate respiratory care?

---

3. Mr. Foster is a 77-year-old retired teacher who complained of a severe headache during dinner and then slumped over the table, unconscious. He was rushed to the hospital, and a tentative diagnosis of CVA was made.

- What diagnostic tests might be appropriate for Mr. Foster?
- What emergency care could you have given Mr. Foster if you had been present at dinner?

  Mr. Foster's diagnostic tests indicate a SAH from a ruptured aneurysm. He is comatose; his pupils are equal and reactive to light; and he responds to pain with flexor posturing, opens his eyes at random, and seems to be paralyzed on the right side.

- Write a nursing care plan for Mr. Foster, including appropriate nursing actions for each nursing diagnosis.

---

4. George Black is a 40-year-old truck driver who received a severe spinal injury when he was shot in the back by a hitchhiker. The bullet severed the spinal cord at the sixth thoracic vertebra.

- What kinds of activities should Mr. Black eventually be able to perform?
- How would you plan his care during the acute stage of his illness so that efforts at rehabilitation might be successful?
- What other members of the health care team might participate in his care and rehabilitation?

STUDY OUTLINE

I. Introduction

A. Nervous system coordinates all sensory and motor activities by receiving, interpreting, and relaying messages.

B. When something happens to impair the ability of the nerves to send or receive impulses, the tissues controlled by those nerves cannot function normally.
C. Neurons cannot be replaced when destroyed.
D. The skull is a closed bony cavity, and increases in its contents of tissue, cerebrospinal fluid, and blood cause intracranial pressure to rise.
E. Greatly increased intracranial pressure can cause death.
F. Neurons are very sensitive to hypoxia and lack of nutrients and will die if deprived of them for very long.
G. Neurologic terminology combines prefixes and suffixes often used in medical terminology.

II. Evaluation of neurologic status is done by history, physical assessment, and diagnostic testing.

A. Mental acuity, memory, and emotional stability are also assessed.
B. The 12 cranial nerves are tested for normal function.
C. Specific tests for coordination and balance are done to determine if problems exist in the cerebellum.
D. Neuromuscular tests assess muscle strength and coordination.
E. Diagnostic tests are listed in Table 15–1.
F. Reflexes: A reflex is an action or movement built into the nervous system; it does not require conscious thought to respond to stimulus.
   1. Knee jerk reflex tests innervation of spinal cord at second, third, and fourth lumbar levels.
   2. Biceps reflex and brachioradialis reflex test innervation at fifth and sixth cervical levels.
   3. Triceps reflex tests innervation at seventh and eighth cervical levels.
   4. Achilles tendon reflex tests innervation at first and second sacral levels.
   5. Babinski reflex indicates abnormality of motor control pathways.
   6. Oculocephalic ("doll's eyes") and oculovestibular reflex assess brain stem function.

III. Nursing assessment of neurologic status

A. Objectivity important in observing and recording findings; vague terms should be avoided.
B. History-taking:
   1. Past and current neurologic disorders.
   2. Symptoms noticed by patient.
   3. Observations of nurse.
C. Assessment of patient with diagnosed neurologic disorder:
   1. Four major components of "neuro check":
      a. Level of consciousness (LOC).
      b. Neuromuscular responses: ability to move limbs in response to stimulus.
      c. Pupillary reactions to light, equality in size.
      d. Vital signs.
   2. Glasgow Coma Scale (Table 15–2) used to determine level of consciousness (LOC).
   3. Earliest signs of increasing intracranial pressure are subtle and include restlessness and change in LOC.
   4. Classic signs of increasing intracranial pressure are decreasing LOC, widening pulse pressure, and slow, bounding pulse, but these occur very late.
   5. Pupils that are unequal in size, sluggish to react, or dilated and

will not constrict signal an emergency, and the physician should be notified immediately.

IV. **Infectious diseases**
   A. Meningitis: inflammation of coverings of the brain.
      1. Causative organisms: bacteria and viruses.
      2. Symptoms and medical diagnosis:
         a. Headache, stiffness of neck, irritability, photophobia.
         b. Spinal tap and analysis of spinal fluid for definitive diagnosis.
      3. Medical treatment: symptomatic; antibiotics and anticonvulsants.
      4. Nursing assessment directed toward accompanying problems such as increased intracranial pressure, seizures, fever, nausea and vomiting, delirium, pain, electrolyte imbalance.
      5. Nursing interventions directed at decreasing intracranial pressure and supportive measures to prevent complications and promote healing.
   B. Encephalitis: inflammation of brain tissue.
      1. Causative organism usually viral; lead, arsenic, and other heavy metals can also cause encephalitis.
      2. Symptoms: headache, fever, extreme restlessness, lethargy, confusion, visual disturbances, delirium.
      3. Treatment is symptomatic.
   C. Guillain-Barré syndrome: inflammatory disease affecting myelin, with edema and compression of the nerve root.
      1. Symptoms: paresthesia, pain, and progressive paralysis.
      2. Diagnosis difficult, because it mimics many other disorders.
      3. Spinal fluid shows elevated protein levels, but leukocyte count is normal.
      4. Nursing assessment and intervention:
         a. During acute phase, goals are to sustain life, prevent complications of immobility, and promote rest and comfort.
         b. Vital signs monitored frequently.
         c. Avoid stimulation and Valsalva maneuver; otherwise extreme changes in blood pressure can be triggered.
         d. Static phase: patient gets no worse and no better; provide a balance of rest and activity (passive exercise and range of motion).
         e. Rehabilitation phase: gradual recovery.

V. **Head injuries**
   A. Brain is encased in rigid skull, with very little room for expansion.
   B. Types: open fracture and closed injuries.
      1. Closed types include concussion, contusion, and hematoma.
      2. Symptoms and medical diagnosis:
         a. Outward signs: evidence of fracture, bleeding, scalp laceration, etc.
         b. Increased intracranial pressure.
         c. Skull radiograph, angiogram, electroencephalogram, and brain scan.
      3. Medical and surgical treatment:
         a. Treated conservatively at first. Surgery may be necessary to relieve intracranial pressure, débride wound.
      4. Nursing assessment and intervention:
         a. Maintain open airway and adequate ventilation.
         b. Head of bed at 30 degrees, proper positioning.
         c. Frequent assessment per Glasgow Coma Scale, neuro check, and vital signs.
         d. Observe for leakage of CSF.

e. Instruction of patient and family when head injury has been treated and patient released from emergency department.
f. See Nursing Care Plan 15–1.

C. Treatment for increased intracranial pressure:
1. IV mannitol to promote fluid excretion.
2. Fluid restriction.
3. Mechanical ventilation with hyperventilation to decrease levels of CO_2 and promote vasoconstriction.
4. Insertion of intracranial pressure monitor.
5. Intraventricular catheter to drain small amounts of CSF.
6. Surgical removal of hematoma by burr holes or craniotomy.

VI. Cerebral vascular accident (CVA, stroke)

A. Cerebral ischemia caused by thrombosis, hemorrhage, or occlusion of cerebral blood vessel by embolus.
B. Persons most at risk: those with hypertension, atherosclerosis, heart disease, obesity.
C. Stroke prevention:
1. Incidence of stroke has decreased as a result of better control of hypertension, better management of heart disease, early recognition of impending stroke.
2. Surgical procedures include removal of plaque and rerouting of blood around obstructed carotid artery.

D. TIA causes temporary symptoms; provides warning that stroke may occur.
E. Medical diagnosis: CT scan, angiogram, EEG, MRI scan, lumbar puncture.
F. Emergency treatment: loosen constricting clothing, turn head to side, elevate head slightly, monitor pulse and respirations.
G. Stabilize vital signs, promote adequate respiration, decrease intracranial pressure.
H. Heparin is given for thrombosis.
I. Aneurysm repair if needed.
J. IV dexamethasone (Decadron) to decrease inflammation and ICP.
K. IV mannitol to decrease ICP.
L. Nursing assessment and intervention:
1. Closely monitor neurologic status.
2. Prevent complications; decrease ICP.
3. Assist with rehabilitation.
4. See Nursing Care Plan 15–2 for care of stroke patient.

VII. Intracranial tumors

A. Symptoms: headache, vomiting without nausea, visual problems, personality changes, and disturbances in judgment, memory, coordination, and speech.
B. Medical treatment: surgical removal, chemotherapy, radiation, gamma knife procedure.
C. Nursing care: preoperative psychological preparation and thorough baseline neurologic assessment.
D. Postoperative care: position only per orders, watch for CSF leak, monitor for increasing ICP.

VIII. Spinal cord injury

A. Degree of motor function depends on level of injury.
B. Immediate care: move victim only after neck and back have been splinted.
C. Traction may be applied to stabilize spinal column; Gardner-Wells tongs, Crutchfield tongs, halo.
D. Patient may be placed on special bed (Rotorest; Stryker frame) to facilitate care.

E. Muscle spasms and autonomic dysreflexia require skilled nursing assessment and intervention.

F. Goals of medical and surgical treatment:
1. Stabilize vital signs.
2. Prevent further cord damage by splinting and traction, and give large doses of corticosteroid to decrease inflammatory response and swelling.
3. Repair damage to spine and cord as much as possible.
4. Prevent complications and maintain as much function as possible.
5. Promote rehabilitation.

G. Efforts of health care team members necessary to help patient and family deal with psychosocial impact of paralysis.

IX. Ruptured intervertebral disc ("slipped disc")

A. Fibrous cushion between vertebrae slips out of place (herniates) and pinches adjacent nerve.

B. Symptoms and medical diagnosis:
1. Pain in lower back radiating down leg; history of feeling something "give way."
2. Cervical ruptured disc: pain in neck and shoulder, radiating down arm.
3. Diagnosis confirmed by myelography, MRI.

C. Medical and surgical treatment:
1. Bed rest on firm mattress with bed board; heat, cold, pelvic or head traction, mild exercises, back brace.
2. Muscle relaxants, antiinflammatory agents, and analgesics for muscle spasm and pain.
3. Surgical procedures: microdiskectomy or laminectomy; may do spinal fusion.
   a. Must be "logrolled" for turning; back must be kept straight; physical therapy exercises.

X. Specific neurologic disorders

A. Parkinsonism: group of symptoms, including tremor, poor coordination, rigidity of muscles.
1. Most often idiopathic.
2. Treatment: medications (L-dopa) and physical therapy.

B. Multiple sclerosis: a neuromuscular disorder affecting primarily the central nervous system. Most often affects those between 20 and 40 years of age.
1. Symptoms and diagnosis:
   a. Clinical manifestations reflect inflammatory changes and demyelinization of the spinal cord nerves and neurons in the brain.
   b. Clinical manifestations indicate diagnosis.
   c. Symptoms include motor dysfunction, sensory changes, problem of coordination, mental changes (depression and inappropriate euphoria), and fatigue worsened by heat.
2. Medical treatment: There is no cure. Supportive measures taken to prevent infection, reduce muscle spasticity, and manage specific symptoms.
3. Nursing assessment and intervention:
   a. Identification of specific problems related to immobility, incontinence, diplopia and other visual problems, speech disorders, sexual impotence, muscle spasticity, and other manifestations of disorder.
   b. Intervention requires well-coordinated planning with patient, family, and appropriate members of health team.

C. Amyotrophic lateral sclerosis (Lou Gehrig's disease).
   1. Progressive degeneration of gray matter in the anterior horn cells and lower cranial nerves.
   2. No known cause and no satisfactory treatment for control or cure.
   3. Symptoms: Voluntary muscle weakness, usually beginning in hands. Difficulty speaking and swallowing. Eventually patient is unable to move, speak, swallow, and finally breathe. There is some pain; patient remains mentally alert and continues to have sensation.
   4. Nursing assessment to determine patient's level of optimal physical activity and specific problems related to muscle paralysis.
   5. Nursing intervention aimed at providing physical comfort, emotional support to patient and family, and full utilization of resources for maximum independence of patient within limitation of his disability.

D. Trigeminal neuralgia (tic douloureux).
   1. Pain along pathways of one or more branches of the trigeminal nerve.
   2. Sometimes caused by tumor or vascular disease, but most often cause is not known.
   3. Symptoms: acute attacks of severe, sharp pain localized on one side of the face and extending from the midline of the face across the cheek and jaw to the ear.
      a. Acute attack often triggered by exposure to heat or cold, chewing, brushing the teeth, or washing or shaving the face.
   4. Medical treatment: administration of anticonvulsant such as phenytoin (Dilantin), carbamazepine (Tegretol), or baclofen (Lioresal).
   5. Surgical treatment: dissection of trigeminal nerve branch rootlets.
   6. Nursing intervention:
      a. Help patient avoid triggering attack. Instruct about side effects of prescribed medication.
      b. Following surgery, patient may need instruction to avoid damage to cornea, inside of mouth, and teeth, depending on branch of nerve removed.

E. Myasthenia gravis: Chronic disorder manifested by fatigue and exhaustion that are aggravated by activity and relieved by rest. Believed to be an autoimmune disease with circulating antibodies acting against neuromuscular receptor sites.
   1. Symptoms and medical diagnosis:
      a. Severe muscle weakness is the principal symptom; also ptosis, diplopia, and difficulty in chewing and swallowing.
      b. Diagnosis established by injection of edrophonium (Tensilon) followed by marked increase in muscle strength.
   2. Medical treatment:
      a. Anticholinesterase therapy.
      b. Plasmapheresis to mechanically remove autoantibodies.
   3. Nursing intervention:
      a. Monitor hospitalized patient frequently for signs of myasthenic crisis.
      b. Education of patient and family about the disease.

F. Epilepsy: chronic disturbance of electrical activity of the brain.
   1. Idiopathic: no known cause.
   2. Symptomatic: related to brain tumor, injury, endocrine disorder, etc. which cause the seizures.

3. Seizures classified under four major groups—partial, generalized, unclassified, and status epilepticus—with various subgroups under each.
4. Symptoms and medical diagnosis:
   a. Absence or petit mal: usually only slight twitching around mouth or eyes, no loss of consciousness.
   b. Grand mal or tonic-clonic: bilateral jerks of the limbs; loss of consciousness, incontinence.
      (1) Tonic convulsions: continued muscle contraction.
      (2) Clonic convulsions: alternate contraction and relaxation of muscles.
   c. Atonic or akinetic seizures: loss of body tone, weakness of knees, or total collapse and falling; usually no loss of consciousness.
   d. Status epilepticus: unrelenting series of convulsions. An emergency treated with anticonvulsants and diazepam. If seizures are caused by hypoglycemia or alcohol withdrawal, treatment may consist of IV 50% dextrose or IV thiamin.
   e. Diagnosis confirmed by EEG, CT scan.
5. Medical and surgical treatment:
   a. Antiepileptic drugs.
   b. Surgical removal of abnormal brain tissue.
6. Nursing assessment and intervention:
   a. Two major areas: assessment and care of patient during seizure and long-term support for management of seizures and coping with psychosocial effects of epilepsy.
      (1) Education of patient about nature of illness, importance of compliance, side effects and symptoms of toxicity of medications.
      (2) Avoidance of factors that trigger seizures.
      (3) Information about community resources for social interaction and information.

G. Cerebral palsy: a type of paralysis accompanied by poor muscle coordination.
1. Caused by cerebral damage possibly stemming from lack of oxygen at birth, traumatic birth, premature delivery, or infection.
   a. Symptoms: exaggerated reflexes, poor coordination of voluntary muscles, high muscle tension, and sometimes defect of speech, hearing, or sight.
   b. Treatment: early muscle training and special exercises; orthopedic surgery, braces, or casts can correct some deformities and disabilities.
   c. Patient instructed in self-care.

H. Alzheimer's disease: pathologic changes that cause a dementia.
1. Slow onset; progresses through stages at varying speeds; eventually fatal.
2. Symptoms progress from forgetfulness and memory loss to decline in personal hygiene and inhibitions; later, severe confusion, helplessness, and difficulty communicating, until totally dependent.
3. Goals: promote ability to perform ADL as long as possible; protect from injury; preserve dignity.

XI. Common neurologic patient care problems

A. Impaired mobility: help patient cope with muscle weakness or paralysis.

1. Prevent contractures and muscle atrophy.
2. Teach use of assistive devices and techniques to promote mobility.
3. Assist with grieving process; treat for depression.
4. Review problems of mobility and nursing care from Chapter 9.

B. Incontinence.
1. Bladder training program:
   a. Assess bladder function and patterns of incontinence; determine optimal neural and muscular function that can be expected.
   b. Design program according to patient's needs; try different techniques until successful.
2. Bowel training program:
   a. Assess former and present bowel patterns.
   b. Determine expected neural and muscular capability for bowel elimination.
   c. Set objectives with patient.
   d. Increase fiber and fluids in diet; employ rectal suppositories for retraining if needed.
   e. Keep accurate record of BMs.

C. Aphasia.
1. Assessment: Note specific abilities and disabilities of patient in area of communication.
2. Nursing intervention:
   a. Goals focused on stimulating communication without undue frustration for patient.
   b. Helpful principles and techniques to be used by nurses, family, and all others who deal with patient.
   c. Good oral hygiene helps patient form words more easily.

D. Disorientation and confusion.
1. Cause may be organic or temporary, secondary to illness or toxicity.
2. Assess degree of problem; may fluctuate from day to day.
3. Use principles of reality orientation.
4. Provide calm, stable environment; help patient focus on what he is able to do; give instructions one step at a time.

E. Problems of self-care.
1. Goal is for patient to assume as much responsibility for his care as he can.
2. Assessment of patient's capabilities and of family's ability and willingness to assist him.
3. Combined efforts of nurses, physical therapist, and occupational therapist for optimal function.
4. Goals must be realistic and agreed on by patient and family.
5. Encouragement and attention to psychosocial concerns is essential.

F. Psychosocial concerns.
1. Assist with mental adjustment; treat depression.
2. Build self-esteem and help to integrate new body image.
3. Provide emotional support and encouragement.
4. Obtain counseling for sexual problems or concerns.
5. Refer for vocational rehabilitation if appropriate.
6. Plan with patient for renewed social life.

XII. Concerns for the elderly

A. Decrease in brain weight not correlated with decrease in mental ability.

B. Reaction time slower; visual acuity decreased.
C. Elderly cannot adapt to physiologic stress as well as younger people and are subject to hypothermia and hyperthermia.
D. Older patients often have other diseases and conditions that affect the neurologic system: arthritis, hearing loss, visual loss, diabetic neuropathy, etc.

CHAPTER 16

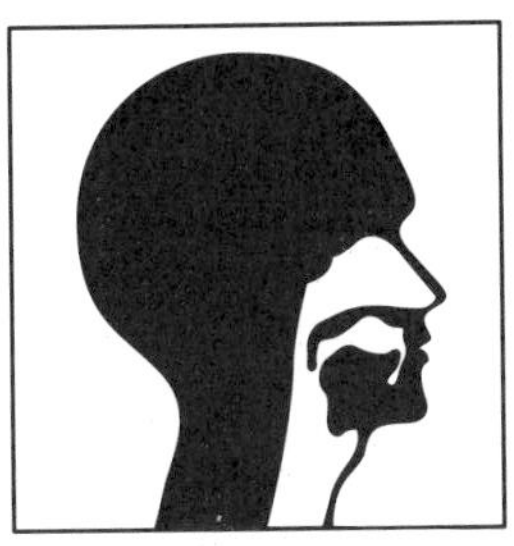

Care of Patients With Disorders of the Nose and Throat

VOCABULARY

expectorate
lozenge
stoma
tracheostomy

Upon completion of this chapter the student should be able to:

1. Describe assessment of patients with disorders of the sinuses, pharynx, and larynx.
2. Describe the pre- and postoperative care for the patient undergoing a tonsillectomy.
3. List the risk factors and warning signs of cancer of the larynx or throat.
4. Devise a nursing care plan for the patient who has had a laryngectomy.
5. Describe safety factors to be considered when caring for the patient with a tracheostomy.

Air flows into the nasal cavity through the nostrils (nares), which are separated by the nasal septum. The nasal cavity warms, filters, and humidifies air as it is drawn into the body. The respiratory mucosa lines the nasal cavity along with nasal hairs located just inside the nares. The mucosa secretes mucus, which forms a layer that traps dust particles. The action of cilia then propels them toward the larynx, where they are swallowed or expectorated (spit out). The multitude of blood vessels in the cavity, along with the mucus, provides warmth and water for humidification of the air. The olfactory cells are in the roof of the nose and the floor of the anterior cranial fossa.

The paranasal sinuses include the maxillary, frontal, sphenoid, and ethmoid sinuses. These are air-filled cavities lined with mucous membrane and situated among the facial bones around the nasal cavity. The exact function of the sinuses is not known, but they, too, secrete mucus, which drains via the turbinates into the nasal cavity.

The throat has been described as the "crossroads of the human body." It has openings leading from the nose and ears and also serves as a passageway for food and air (Fig. 16–1). It is little wonder, therefore, that inflammation of the throat (pharyngitis) is such a common condition. Considering the exposure of the throat to the hordes of bacteria present in our environment, it is remarkable that more infections do not occur there.

The most common disorders of the larynx are inflammation and tumors. Laryngitis usually accompanies infections of the lower respiratory tract (for example, laryngotracheobronchitis involving the larynx, trachea, and bronchi). Tumors of the larynx are less common than neoplasms in other parts of the body and, like other tumors, can be either benign or malignant.

DIAGNOSTIC TESTS AND EXAMINATIONS

VISUAL EXAMINATION OF THE NOSE, MOUTH, AND THROAT

The interior of the nose, mouth, pharynx, and the tonsils can be inspected by an examiner using a tongue blade and a good source of light. The nose is inspected for redness, swelling, and lumps. With the head tilted upward, the inside of the nares are inspected for pallor, redness, swelling, and polyps and for mucus color, consistency, odor, and amount. The examiner obtains a better view if a nasal speculum is used. The hard and soft palates are inspected, and the mobility of the soft palate is evaluated by asking the patient to say "ah." The pharynx can be brought into view by asking the patient to say "ee." The examiner is looking for signs of inflammation, lesions, plaques, exudates, or a gray membrane. The paranasal sinuses are assessed by observing for purulent discharge in the nares and by palpating over the sinus areas for tenderness. Sometimes sinus radiographs will be ordered.

LARYNGOSCOPY

Inspection of the larynx is done in one of two ways: by *indirect laryngoscopy* or *direct laryngoscopy*. Indirect laryngoscopy is a relatively simple office procedure that does not require

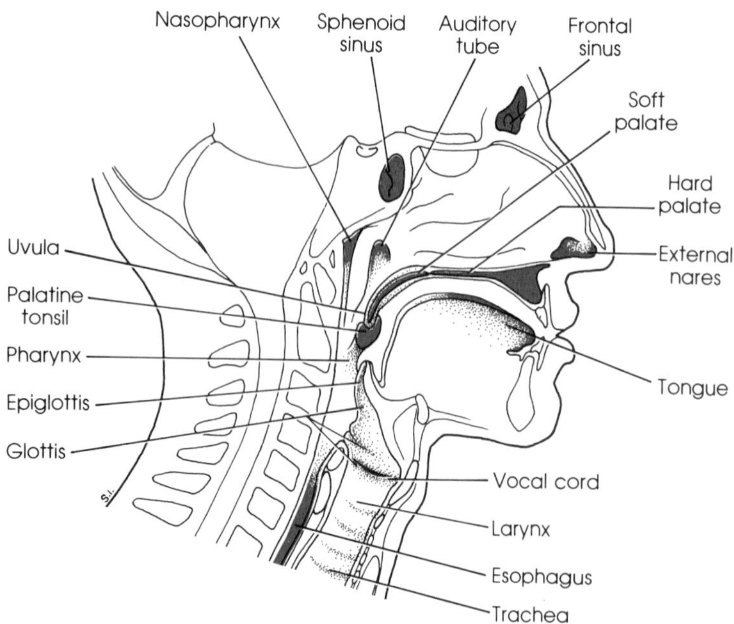

Figure 16–1 Upper respiratory tract.

local anesthesia unless the patient has a very sensitive gag reflex. The patient is placed in a sitting position directly in front of the examiner. A warm laryngeal mirror is placed at the back of the throat, and the soft palate is gently lifted up. The examiner wears a head mirror, which reflects light from a source near the patient's head. While the throat is at rest the examiner can see only the upper part of the epiglottis, the base of the tongue, and the back of the pharynx. The larynx is brought into view by asking the patient to make an "ee" sound. During indirect laryngoscopy the examiner is looking for inflammation, ulceration, mucosal irregularity, and tumors and polyps. Polyps can be removed easily at the time of indirect laryngoscopy.

Direct laryngoscopy requires the use of a fiberoptic endoscope (laryngoscope) that is introduced through the mouth and past the pharynx to the larynx. It may be performed as an outpatient procedure. Direct laryngoscopy permits visualization of areas that cannot be seen by indirect laryngoscopy. During the procedure, specimens of exudate or tissue can be obtained or foreign bodies removed.

Direct laryngoscopy may be done to obtain a biopsy or to locate benign lesions, malignant tumors, or strictures that interfere with breathing.

Direct laryngoscopy requires local or general anesthesia. The patient is prepared by withholding food and drink for 6 to 8 hours before the test. The procedure and its purpose should be explained to the patient. A mild sedative usually is administered, along with atropine to reduce secretions. The patient should know that the procedure will be performed in a darkened room. The laryngoscope is passed through the mouth, but it will not obstruct breathing.

After the procedure, nursing intervention is similar to that for a patient having a bronchoscopy. The patient's vital signs are monitored and he is watched carefully for signs of adverse reaction to the anesthetic and medications administered before and during the test. Laryngeal edema and discomfort are reduced by applying an ice collar. Any signs of airway obstruction from edema, epiglottitis, or laryngospasms must be reported immediately.

Foods and fluids are restricted for 4 to 8 hours or until the gag reflex has returned. The patient should be given an emesis basin and instructed to expectorate saliva rather than swallow it. Saliva and other secretions from the mouth are observed for blood, which should not be present in more than very small amounts. The patient also is instructed not to cough or clear his throat, especially when a biopsy has been done. To do so may initiate fresh bleeding from the biopsy site.

Loss of the voice (aphonia), hoarseness, and a mild sore throat are expected after laryngoscopy, but these discomforts should not last more than a day. Warm saline gargles and throat lozenges (medication that dissolves when sucked on) can be soothing but are not allowed until the gag reflex has returned.

THROAT CULTURE

The most common reason for culturing pharyngeal secretions is to establish a definitive diagnosis of infection with *Streptococcus pyogenes*. A culture permits prompt and appropriate treatment of a potentially dangerous infection that can have such sequelae as rheumatic heart disease and glomerulonephritis. Rheumatic fever has increased alarmingly since 1985. A throat culture also is sometimes done to identify carriers of various organisms or to establish a diagnosis of diphtheria, meningitis, or whooping cough. These diseases can be particularly harmful to elderly, debilitated, or very young patients and therefore require prompt diagnosis and treatment.

NURSING ASSESSMENT

HISTORY TAKING

Infections and inflammations of the throat and larynx frequently are treated on an outpatient basis. The patient often will have a history of exposure to a specific person with a respiratory infection or to a large group of people at school or work where there are likely to be frequent occasions for contact with infected persons.

The patient's personal history also might include recurrent respiratory infections and sore throats, known allergies, or chronic sinusitis.

SUBJECTIVE AND OBJECTIVE DATA

Patients with sinus problems complain of headache, malaise, a bad taste in the mouth, nasal congestion or obstruction, and purulent drainage from the nose. Those with pharyngitis usually report a sore or "scratchy" throat, malaise, headache, and sometimes a cough. There may be facial puffiness over the affected sinus. Dysphagia also might be a problem for patients with pharyngitis, because swallowing involves pushing the food back against the inflamed oropharynx. Hoarseness and loss of the voice are common symptoms of laryngitis. However, if either dysphagia or hoarseness persist for more than 4 to 6 weeks and there are no other signs of infection or inflammation, a tumor should be suspected.

Objective data include fever and other signs of infection, productive or nonproductive cough, and hoarseness. Palpation of the neck may reveal enlarged lymph nodes.

SINUSITIS

Sinusitis is an inflammation of the mucosal lining of the sinuses. Causes include infection that has spread from the nasal passages to the sinuses and blockage of normal sinus drainage routes. Sinusitis often occurs after colds or other respiratory infections. People with a deviated nasal septum or allergy problems tend to have recurrent sinusitis.

Treatment of sinusitis is directed at relieving pain, promoting sinus drainage, controlling infection, and preventing recurrence. Hot, moist packs over the sinus area can be helpful. Inhaling moist steam and increasing fluid intake helps promote drainage. Medications are prescribed to promote vasoconstriction, reduce swelling, and promote drainage. Decongestants may also be used. Infection is treated with an antibiotic or antiinfective agent. Rest, reduced stress, a balanced diet, and control of allergies can help prevent recurrence. Analgesics are given for pain.

Acute or chronic sinus infection should not be ignored, as the infection can cause a variety of complications, including septicemia, meningitis, or brain abcess.

EPISTAXIS

Epistaxis (nosebleed) is a common occurrence. Nosebleeds may occur for many reasons. Decreased humidity, excessive nose blowing, allergy with inflammation, and nose picking are some causes. Nosebleeds can also result from trauma, hypertension, and blood dyscrasias such as leukemia.

When epistaxis occurs, the patient should sit forward and apply direct pressure to the nose for 3 to 5 minutes. Cold compresses or ice, which will constrict the blood vessels, may be applied to the nose or face. The patient is warned not to blow the nose for 4 to 8 hours after the nosebleed has stopped. If needed, the nose may be loosely packed with gauze along with the application of pressure. The gauze should be left in place for several hours and then very gently removed and pressure applied again for several minutes. If a nosebleed cannot be stopped in this manner, the patient should go to the emergency department, where a physician will cauterize the bleeding vessels or solidly pack the nose to stop the bleeding. Otherwise the patient will continue to slowly hemorrhage.

PHARYNGITIS

Inflammation of the pharynx, usually called a *sore throat,* is such a common occurrence that almost everyone has experienced it at one time or another. The symptoms familiar to us all include a dry, "scratchy" feeling in the back of the throat, mild fever, headache, and malaise. Dysphagia also is present, with greater discomfort when swallowing one's own saliva than when swallowing food. Unfortunately, pharyngitis also is accompanied by a constant urge to swallow. The usual course for uncomplicated pharyngitis is 3 to 10 days. All patients should be assessed for the warning signs of cancer of the larynx and throat: hoarseness or sore throat that lasts more than 2 weeks, pain on swallowing, dysphagia, hemoptysis, or enlarged cervical neck nodes.

The diagnosis of pharyngitis is confirmed by clinical manifestations such as the previously mentioned symptoms and a red and inflamed throat. A throat culture is sometimes done to confirm or rule out streptococcal and other bacterial infections.

MEDICAL TREATMENT AND NURSING INTERVENTION

Uncomplicated viral pharyngitis usually responds to such conservative measures as rest, warm saline or aspirin gargles (one aspirin tablet and one-half teaspoon of baking soda dissolved in a glass of warm water), throat lozenges, plenty of fluids, and a mild analgesic for aches and pains.

Bacterial pharyngitis requires antibiotic therapy, particularly if the infecting organism is *Streptococcus.* Chronic pharyngitis may require diagnostic procedures to determine the underlying cause (for example, an infection elsewhere in the respiratory tract) and therapeutic measures such as humidification and filtering of environmental air.

TONSILLITIS

An inflammation of the tonsils is usually caused by streptococci or staphylococci and is completely different from pharyngitis, even though the symptoms may be somewhat alike. Acute tonsillitis may occur repeatedly, especially in those who have a low resistance to infection. Chronic tonsillitis usually produces enlargement of tonsillar tissue and adjacent adenoidal tissue as well.

SYMPTOMS

Acute tonsillitis occurs most often in young children. There is an elevation of temperature, sore throat, general malaise, and chills. Inspection of the throat reveals redness and swelling of the tonsils and surrounding tissues.

Chronic infection of the tonsils produces symptoms that may not be as dramatic as those of acute tonsillitis but most certainly are capable of making the person uncomfortable. The child with chronic tonsillitis and enlarged adenoids has frequent colds and appears to be in poor health. He gives the impression of being dull or mentally retarded, because he constantly holds his mouth open to breathe and often has difficulty in hearing. These children also are mouth breathers when they sleep and are very likely to snore.

TREATMENT AND NURSING INTERVENTION

A throat culture is done before treatment is begun to check for the presence of *Streptococcus*, which can cause rheumatic fever or glomerulonephritis if not treated promptly. Acute tonsillitis is treated with hot saline throat gargles and the administration of specific antibiotics for the destruction of the causative organism. Bed rest, nursing measures to reduce the fever, and a liquid diet to minimize trauma to the tonsils are also included.

Surgery is used to treat tonsillitis when it is recurrent or when enlargement of the tonsils and adenoids obstructs airways. The physician's rule of thumb is usually to consider surgery if the patient has more than five episodes of tonsillitis per year. Surgery is performed after the acute infection has cleared.

NURSING CARE OF THE PATIENT UNDERGOING A TONSILLECTOMY AND ADENOIDECTOMY

Preoperative Care

Physical preparation of the patient having a tonsillectomy involves administration of preoperative medications as ordered and restriction of the patient's diet for 6 to 8 hours prior to surgery. It is especially important that the child be observed for signs of fever. An elevation of temperature or any signs of an upper respiratory infection should be reported. Surgery is usually postponed if these signs are present.

Tonsillectomy and adenoidectomy may be done as outpatient or inpatient procedures. When tonsillectomy is performed using a laser, there is very little swelling and little bleeding. The patient also has an easier time swallowing postoperatively.

Postoperative Care

Following tonsillectomy or adenoidectomy, the nurse's chief concern is observation for hemorrhage.

Although tonsillectomy and adenoidectomy patients usually recover from surgery rapidly and rarely suffer any complications, nurses should be vigilant, because hemorrhage is a real danger. Vital signs are checked frequently, and the patient is observed for frequent swallowing, which may indicate bleeding in the throat. Restlessness can be another clue to excessive bleeding. An ice collar may be placed around the neck to reduce swelling and prevent the oozing of blood from the operative site.

Although it is difficult to keep a child in one position for very long, he should be kept on his side or abdomen as long as there is drainage from the surgical wound. If the child is thrashing about in the bed when recovering from the anesthesia, it is best to collect secretions from the mouth in a large towel rather than use a metal emesis basin, which may injure him. Older children may sit up in a semi-Fowler's position after they have recovered from the anesthesia and are often more comfortable this way. A younger child usually can be kept calm and quiet if someone holds him and rocks him. He needs to keep as quiet as possible to prevent hemorrhage from the operative site, and he also needs love and affection to reassure him at a time when he is frightened and uncomfortable.

The postoperative diet usually consists of ice cold liquids, popsicles, and gelatin, progressing to ice cream, custards, and other semisolid foods for the first 24 hours. Citrus fruits, hot fluids, and rough foods should be avoided until the throat has completely healed.

CANCER OF THE LARYNX

Cancer of the larynx occurs most often in men in their 50s to 70s, but it can strike anyone, especially those over the age of 18. It is one of the most easily cured of all malignancies because of its location and adjacent tissues, and about 90% of all patients treated by early radiation and/or surgery are cured. The cause of cancer of the larynx is not known, but there is some evidence that predisposing factors are cigarette smoking, alcohol use, chronic laryngitis, abuse of the vocal cords, and a familial tendency toward cancer. Exposure over long periods to environmental pollutants such as asbestos, diethyl sulfate, mustard gas, or wood dust is also considered a risk factor.

MEDICAL SYMPTOMS AND DIAGNOSIS

Because the larynx, sometimes called the voice box, is directly involved with production of vocal sounds, a tumor of the larynx will quickly produce persistent hoarseness that does not respond to usual methods of treatment. After the cancer has spread beyond the vocal cords (and is much more difficult to treat), the symptoms may include difficulty in swallowing or breathing, a sensation of having a lump in the throat, cough, enlarged lymph nodes in the neck, and pain in the region of the Adam's apple.

Diagnosis is established by visualization of the larynx via a laryngoscope, CT scan of the larynx and throat, MRI scan, and microscopic examination of a sample of tissues taken from the tumor.

SURGICAL TREATMENT

There are several types of surgical procedures that may be performed for treatment of laryngeal malignant disease. If the tumor is restricted to the vocal cords, the surgeon may perform a *partial laryngectomy* in which the thyroid cartilage is split, and only the tumor and involved portion of the vocal cords are removed. A partial laryngectomy does not permanently eliminate voice sounds. A tracheostomy may be done for temporary facilitation of breathing, but the opening made by the stoma operation eventually is closed, and the patient may resume talking after the affected area is healed completely.

Microlaryngoscopy combined with laser is now the choice for removal of vocal cord polyps and carcinoma in situ. Cure rates for malignancy of the true vocal cords treated by laser are equal to those for combined traditional surgery and radiation therapy. Other advantages include the absence of mechanical trauma and swelling when laser is used, which means that the patient returns to normal activities within about 3 days. There is also no need for extended voice rest; 2 days is usually sufficient.

A total laryngectomy is done if the tumor has progressed to the point of paralyzing the vocal cords. The surgeon excises the entire larynx, epiglottis, thyroid cartilage, hyoid bone, cricoid cartilage, and 2 or more rings of the trachea.

If the tumor has extended to the lymph nodes, a radical neck dissection is also performed on the side of the lesion. All the muscle, lymph nodes, and soft tissue from the lower edge of the mandible to the clavicle and from the top of the trapezius muscle to the midline is removed. A tracheostomy is performed at the same time. The trachea is diverted to a surgically constructed opening (stoma) in the neck. The patient then has a permanent tracheostomy with no connec-

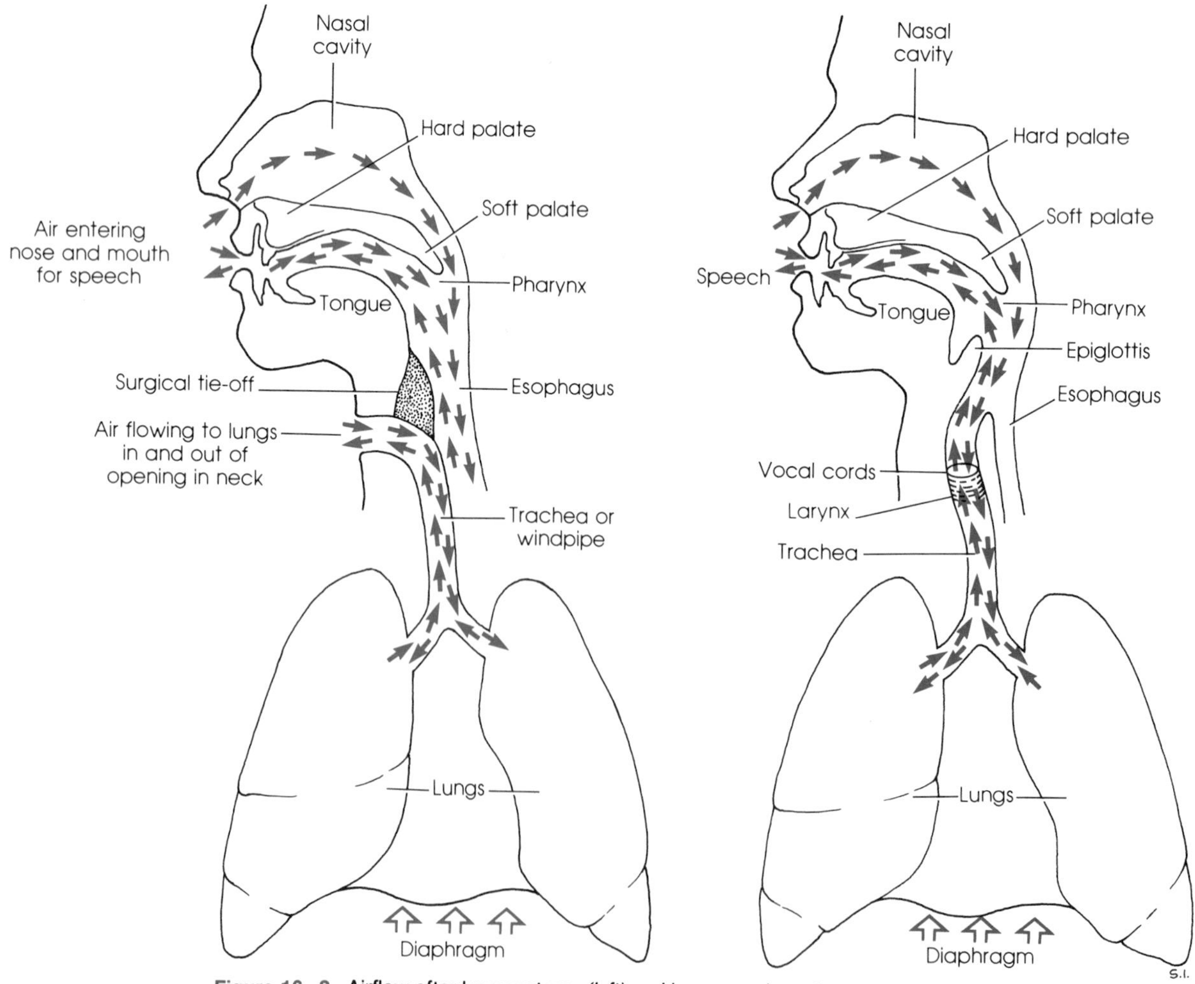

Figure 16-2 Airflow after laryngectomy *(left)* and in a normal respiratory tract *(right)*.

tion between the nose and mouth and the lower respiratory system; he must depend on the stoma for breathing (Fig. 16–2). A laryngectomy tube, which is shorter and wider than a tracheostomy tube, is put into place before discharge. After the stoma is completely healed and matured, about 6 weeks after surgery, the tube can be left out as long as there is no compromise of the airway.

A thin feeding tube is placed during surgery for postoperative use for about 10 to 14 days. The patient has only IV fluids initially but then progresses to regular tube feedings. When healing is far enough along that the danger of contamination of the operative site is not a concern, training in eating and swallowing is begun. If the patient has been discharged from the hospital earlier than 2 weeks, a visiting nurse or clinic nurse will work with the patient on eating skills. Some patients have to rely on a feeding tube, as they cannot master the swallowing procedure without aspiration. The indwelling tube is then replaced with a tube that the patient can insert and then remove after feedings himself.

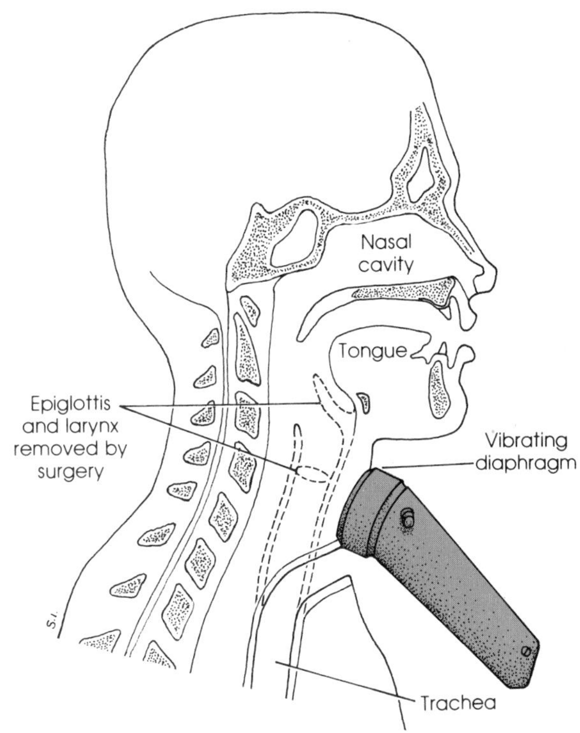

Figure 16–3 External larynx. The vibrating cap of the electronic artificial larynx is held against the throat with sufficient pressure to maintain firm contact. Sound vibrations are transmitted into the lower portion of the pharynx and transformed into speech by the normal movements of the tongue, lips, and teeth.

NURSING INTERVENTION

The patient who has had a laryngectomy will require adequate instruction in the care of his stoma and laryngectomy tube. He will need help and guidance in facing a future in which he will not be able to speak until he learns esophageal speech or uses an artificial "voice box" (Fig. 16–3). He also may have difficulty eating and swallowing until he gets accustomed to the sensations of choking and gagging that frequently occur with a laryngectomy.

Immediate postoperative care focuses on maintenance of a patent airway and observing for hemorrhage. If the patient has a tracheostomy, it will need to be suctioned very frequently during the first 24 to 48 hours. His air exchange is dependent on the nurse maintaining a patent airway for him. *Totally aseptic technique* must be used when suctioning in order to prevent lung infection. Special care must be taken when the ties that hold the tracheostomy tube in place are changed; otherwise the tube may be dislodged by coughing, which movement of the tube tends to cause (see Chapter 17 for tracheostomy care). Good aseptic technique is a must when caring for the tracheostomy and the neck incisions in order to prevent infection of the incision areas.

The patient will go through a grief process over losing his natural voice if a total laryngectomy has been done. A radical neck dissection creates further problems with alteration of body image, as the procedure is somewhat disfiguring. Depression is a common problem initially, but contact with others who have had the surgery and are leading full productive lives may help the patient focus on the benefits of the surgery in saving his own life.

Protection of the tracheal opening from dust and lint can be accomplished through the use of a simple gauze covering or high-necked clothing. The patient also should be told to avoid swimming and to use care when taking a shower or tub bath so that water is not aspirated through the opening. In order to protect the patient from inhalation of extremely cold air (he no longer breathes through his nose and mouth, which normally warm the inspired air) the patient may wear a small scarf over the opening during the winter.

Proper rehabilitation of the patient plays a very important part in his acceptance of surgery and its consequences. Nursing Care Plan 16–1 lists some problems and nursing interventions for the laryngectomy patient. Many people are able to learn esophageal speech in which they first master the art of swallowing air and then moving it forcibly back up through the esophagus. They then learn to coordinate lip and tongue movements with the sound produced by the air passing over vibrating folds of the esophagus. The sounds may be somewhat hoarse, but they can be understood as speech and are more natural than the sounds produced by an artificial larynx. For patients who cannot master esophageal

NURSING CARE PLAN 16–1

Selected nursing diagnoses, goals/outcome criteria, nursing interventions, and evaluations for a patient with a laryngectomy

Situation: Mr. Cato had a supraglottic laryngectomy 5 days ago. He is withdrawn and having difficulty adjusting to his tracheostomy and states, with pencil and paper, that he doesn't feel he can learn to speak again.

Nursing Diagnosis	Goals/Outcome Criteria	Nursing Intervention	Evaluation
Ineffective airway clearance related to discomfort and secretions resulting from surgery and tracheostomy. **SUPPORTING DATA** Unable to cough secretions out of tracheostomy tube; becomes anxious when secretions build up, decreasing air flow.	Tracheostomy will be cleared by suctioning as needed. Patient will learn to suction own tracheostomy effectively by discharge. Patient will learn to clear tracheostomy by coughing effectively.	Suction as needed, at least q 4 h. Encourage patient to assist with procedure: hold water for moistening catheter, turn on suction. Teach to attach catheter to suction tubing; teach to suction self using mirror. Praise for all attempts. Point out advantages of not being dependent on others for care of airway. Medicate for discomfort and encourage him to cough to remove secretions without suctioning.	Suctioned approximately q 2 h; assisting with equipment; first teaching session on suctioning complete; will cough on command.
Impaired skin integrity related to surgical incisions. **SUPPORTING DATA** Supraglottic laryngectomy and tracheostomy.	No infection at incision sites as evidenced by no redness, swelling, or purulent discharge. Skin integrity is intact within 6 weeks.	Clean incision lines with H_2O_2; apply antibiotic ointment as ordered q shift. Clean around tracheostomy with acetic acid and change gauze pad as needed. Change tracheostomy ties q 24 h, being very careful not to dislodge tracheostomy tube. Observe for signs of infection.	Incision cleaned with H_2O_2; antibiotic ointment applied; trach cleaned and dressed; stoma reddened, without signs of pus or excessive swelling; continue plan.
Impaired verbal communication related to loss of larynx. **SUPPORTING DATA** Laryngectomy and tracheostomy.	Patient will show interest in learning new style of speech within 6 weeks.	Assist him to use Magic Slate or paper and pencil for communication; show patience. Obtain order for visit from rehabilitated laryngectomy patient who has mastered some form of speech. Encourage affiliation with community support group for laryngectomy patients.	Using Magic Slate for communication; becomes frustated with time it takes to communicate; spoke to physician about referral to Lost Cord group.
Anxiety regarding aspiration when tries to swallow; doesn't feel he'll be able to eat by mouth again. **SUPPORTING DATA** Chokes when tries to swallow saliva; tends to aspirate.	Lungs will remain clear. Patient will learn to swallow without aspirating within 6 weeks.	Teach patient to hold his breath and perform the Valsalva maneuver while swallowing; teach him to keep his neck relaxed forward when swallowing and forcibly exhale after swallowing.	Still very anxious when tries to swallow; still coughing a lot with each attempt; get consult with speech therapist for swallowing exercises; continue plan.

speech in this manner, a tracheoesophageal prosthesis can be implanted. A fistula is created by connecting the esophagus and the trachea. A silicone prosthesis is inserted after healing has taken place. The patient can cover the opening of the prosthesis with a finger or close it with a special valve that diverts air from the lungs up through the trachea into the esophagus and out of the mouth. Speech is formed by the lip and tongue movement as the air is expelled.

A mechanical vibrator device known as an electronic artificial larynx can be used externally when applied to the skin of the esophagus to simulate speech. These are battery powered; they do not produce voicelike speech, but they do provide understandable sounds and make it possible for the patient to communicate.

In various parts of the United States, there are several groups organized for laryngectomy patients who wish to get together for social and rehabilitation purposes. These clubs have names like Lost Cord, New Speech, New Voice, and Esophageal Speech. Information regarding these clubs and other aspects of postlaryngectomy rehabilitation can be obtained by writing to the American Speech-Language-Hearing Association, 10801 Rockville Pike, Rockville, MD 20852. Local chapters of the American Cancer Society also are good sources of information and assistance for the laryngectomy patient and his family. Further information regarding care of the laryngectomy patient who has cancer can be found in the chapter on care of the cancer patient.

Concerns for the Elderly

Patients older than 75 sometimes have decreased strength in the muscles that are responsible for swallowing. For this reason they are more at risk for aspiration and aspiration pneumonia. Many patients in this age range also have suffered a stroke that has resulted in dysphagia.

In elderly men who have a long history of smoking and of heavy alcohol use, more incidence of throat cancer is seen. A good history for these risk factors should be sought by the nurse.

BIBLIOGRAPHY

Biggs, C. B.: The cancer that cost a patient his voice. RN, May, 1987, pp. 44–51.

Feinstein, D.: What to teach the patient who's had a total laryngectomy. RN, April, 1987, pp. 53–57.

Ignatavicius, D. D., and Bayne, M. J.: Medical-Surgical Nursing. Philadelphia, W. B. Saunders, 1991.

Kersten, L. D.: Comprehensive Respiratory Nursing: A Decision Making Approach. Philadelphia, W. B. Saunders, 1989.

Lockhart, J. S., and Griffin, C.: Action STAT! epistaxis. Nursing 86, 1986, p. 33.

Sigler, B. A.: Nursing care of the head and neck cancer patient. Oncology, Dec., 1988, pp. 49–53.

Smalley, P. J.: Lasers in otolaryngology. Nurs. Clin. North Am., Sept. 1990, pp. 645–656.

Ulrich, S. P., et al.: Nursing Care Planning Guides: A Nursing Diagnosis Approach, 2nd ed. Philadelphia, W. B. Saunders, 1990.

STUDENT STUDY AIDS

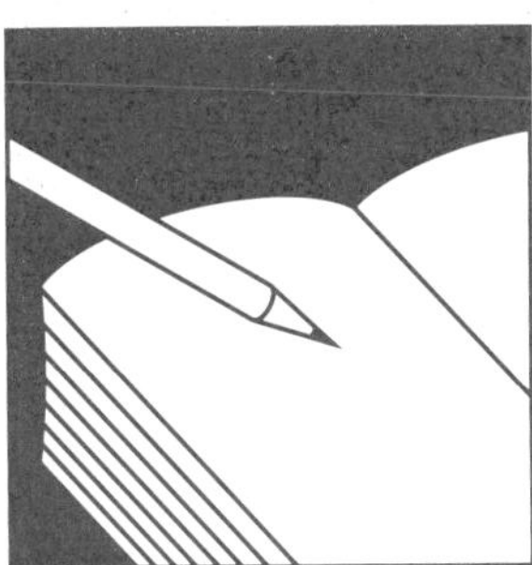

CLINICAL CASE PROBLEM

Read the following clinical situation and discuss the questions with your classmates.

1. Mr. King has undergone diagnostic procedures to confirm suspected cancer of the larynx. He has been admitted to the hospital for a hemilaryngectomy.

- Describe the teaching plan that would be used for a patient undergoing a direct laryngoscopy.
- What diagnostic tests would have been done on Mr. King?
- Devise a postoperative nursing care plan for Mr. King, including interventions for psychosocial problems.
- What resources in the community could be suggested to help Mr. King adjust to his laryngectomy?

STUDY OUTLINE

I. Introduction

A. Nasal cavities and mucosal lining warm, humidify, and clean the air as it passes through to the lungs.

B. Function of sinuses is unknown; they do secrete mucus, which flows into the nasal cavities.

C. Throat serves as passageway for food and air and plays role in production of sound.
D. Disorders of the larynx usually are inflammations and tumors.

II. Diagnostic tests and examinations

A. Nasal passages are inspected with nasal speculum and light.
B. Visual examination of mouth and throat.
  1. Requires only a tongue blade and good light.
C. Laryngoscopy: visualization of larynx.
  1. Indirect laryngoscopy: relatively simple office procedure.
    a. Examiner uses a warm laryngeal mirror, head mirror, and light source.
    b. No anesthetic required unless patient has strong gag reflex.
  2. Direct laryngoscopy: endoscopic examination of larynx.
    a. Local or general anesthetic required.
    b. Patient fasts 6 to 8 hours prior to examination.
    c. Postexamination care similar to that for bronchoscopy.
    d. Resuscitative equipment must be close at hand in case of laryngeal edema, epiglottitis, or laryngeal spasm.
    e. Hoarseness, aphonia, and mild sore throat expected.
D. CT and MRI scans performed to locate tumors and other pathologic abnormalities of the larynx and esophagus.
E. Throat culture: usually to establish or rule out streptococcal infection.

III. Nursing assessment

A. History taking—recent exposure to infectious agents, known allergies, chronic sinusitis. (Many cases of pharyngitis and other throat infections treated on outpatient basis.)
  1. Complaints of headache, malaise, bad taste in the mouth, nasal congestion, purulent drainage from nose indicate possible sinus infection.
B. Subjective and objective data—sore throat, malaise, fever, dysphagia, hoarseness, aphonia, cough, enlarged lymph glands.
  1. Persistent hoarseness and dysphagia should be further investigated for possible malignancy.

IV. Pharyngitis: inflammation of the pharynx

A. Diagnosis by history, symptoms, and throat examination and culture.
B. Uncomplicated viral infections respond to conservative measures.
C. Bacterial infections treated with antibiotics.

V. Sinusitis: inflammation and infection of the sinuses

A. Symptoms: headache, fever, tenderness over sinuses, purulent drainage from nose, malaise.
B. Uncontrolled sinus infection can lead to meningitis or brain abscess.
C. Treated with 10 to 14 days of antibiotics; control of allergies.
D. Surgery is sometimes necessary to open drainage tract and clear purulent material.

VI. Epistaxis: nosebleed; caused by many factors: irritation from nose blowing, hypertension, trauma, blood dyscrasias, decreased humidity, and nose picking

A. Apply direct pressure to nose to stop bleeding.
B. Cold compresses or ice are helpful.
C. If bleeding doesn't stop, a physician's attention is necessary to prevent slow hemorrhage.

VII. Tonsillitis: inflammation of the tonsils; usually streptococcal or staphylococcal infection

A. Symptoms: fever, sore throat, chills, malaise.

B. Chronic infection can lead to enlargement of tonsils and adenoids.
C. Treatment and nursing intervention—warm saline gargles, throat lozenges, rest, antibiotics. Surgery indicated in few cases.
D. Nursing care of patient undergoing tonsillectomy and adenoidectomy:
  1. Preoperative care routine. Monitor for elevated temperature.
  2. Postoperative care: vital signs checked frequently, patient kept on side or abdomen as long as there is drainage from the throat; diet limited to soft, nonirritating foods until throat is no longer sensitive.

VIII. Cancer of the larynx

A. Most easily treated of all malignant diseases.
B. Predisposing factors: smoking, alcohol use, chronic laryngitis, abuse of vocal cords.
C. Symptoms: persistent hoarseness at first; later, pain in throat, dysphagia, lump in throat, pain in region of Adam's apple.
D. Surgical treatment: laser tumor treatment, partial or total laryngectomy, radical neck dissection.
  1. Patient who has had partial laryngectomy retains function of speech.
  2. Total laryngectomy patient has permanent opening in trachea and must learn new speech pattern.
E. Nursing intervention: special care problems (see Nursing Care Plan 16–1).

IX. Concerns for the elderly

A. Weakened muscles predispose to aspiration.
B. Many patients in this age group have suffered strokes and have dysphagia.
C. Elderly men with a long history of smoking and heavy alcohol use most likely to develop throat cancer.

CHAPTER 17

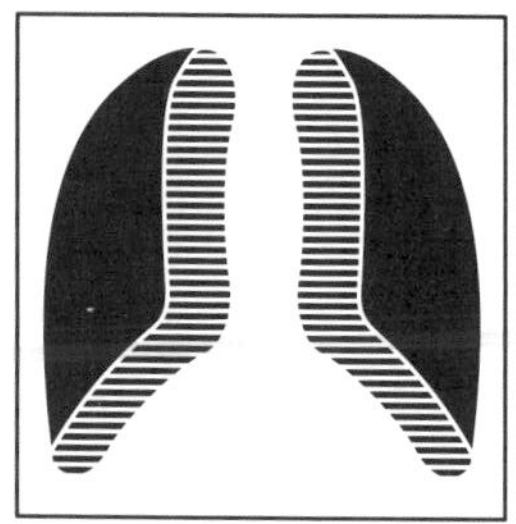

Care of Patients With Respiratory Disorders

VOCABULARY

atelectasis
compliance
COPD
emphysema
excursion
hypoxemia
hypoxia
kyphosis
mucolytic
orthopnea
perfusion
pneumothorax
respiration
scoliosis
shunting
ventilation

Upon completion of this chapter the student should be able to:

1. Identify three measures people can take to prevent respiratory disorders.
2. Describe the pre- and posttest care for the patient undergoing the following: chest radiograph, bronchoscopy, pulmonary function testing.
3. Describe the procedure for nursing assessment of the respiratory system.
4. Compare and contrast commonalities and differences in nursing care for patients with bronchitis, influenza, pneumonia, pleurisy, and empyema.
5. Complete a nursing care plan, including home care, for the patient with chronic obstructive pulmonary disease (COPD).
6. List four ways a nurse can contribute to prevention and prompt treatment of tuberculosis.
7. Describe the specifics of nursing care for the patient who has had thoracic surgery and has chest tubes in place.
8. List at least three nursing interventions appropriate for care of patients experiencing the following: persistent cough, increased secretions in the respiratory tract, dyspnea, alteration in nutrition and hydration related to respiratory disorder, and fatigue related to hypoxia.
9. Devise a nursing care plan for the tracheostomy patient on oxygen therapy and a mechanical ventilator.

PHYSIOLOGY

The respiratory tract is composed of a system of hollow tubes through which we breathe. These tubes are constructed so that they resemble a tree; therefore the term *bronchial tree* is frequently used to describe the respiratory tract. The trunk of the tree is the trachea, the branches are the bronchi, and the twigs, or smaller branches, are the bronchioles. As a breath of air travels down the bronchial tree, it eventually ends its journey in tiny air sacs called *alveoli*. These minute sacs constitute most of the tissues of the lungs. It is in the alveoli that the exchange of carbon dioxide and oxygen takes place (Fig. 17-1).

Each lung is covered with a membranous sac called the *pleura*. There are two layers of the pleura, and between these layers there is a fluid that acts as a lubricant to prevent friction when the lung expands and deflates. The pleural sac, which encloses each lung, is an airtight compartment. The pressure within the pleural cavity is less than that of the outside atmosphere. Thus if the pleural layers are penetrated from the outside, air will rush in and collapse the lung.

Whereas the outer surface of the lungs and bronchial tree are normally protected from contamination by outside sources, the inner lining of the respiratory tract is constantly exposed to dust, germs, and other foreign materials in the air. For defense against these substances, the mucous membranes contain tiny hairlike projections called *cilia*. These tiny projections trap and help to remove small foreign particles that are inhaled. The membrane also secretes a mucoid substance that helps prevent infection by cleansing foreign substances from the respiratory tract.

Within the alveoli are macrophages, which contribute to defense of the lung by quickly phagocytizing inhaled bacteria and other foreign particles. Such particles are then moved up the smaller airways. The cough reflex works to expel unwanted substances from the airways. *Surfactant* is a substance secreted by cells in the alveoli that reduces surface tension so that the alveoli do not collapse during exhalation.

In order to maintain constant levels of oxygen and carbon dioxide in the arterial blood, the body has a complex respiratory control system. It manages to keep concentrations of these gases within a very narrow range, even though oxygen demand can fluctuate widely during the course of a day's activities. When a person is engaged in very strenuous exercise, he can consume 20 times the amount of oxygen used while asleep.

The regulatory mechanisms that control breathing patterns do so in response to metabolic demands and increased cardiac output. The central nervous system controls both involuntary and voluntary respiration. The vagus nerve supplies the pharynx, larynx, respiratory airways, and lungs. The muscles of respiration are dependent on nerve impulses from the spinal cord. Involuntary breathing is regulated by the medulla and pons in the brain stem, whereas voluntary respi-

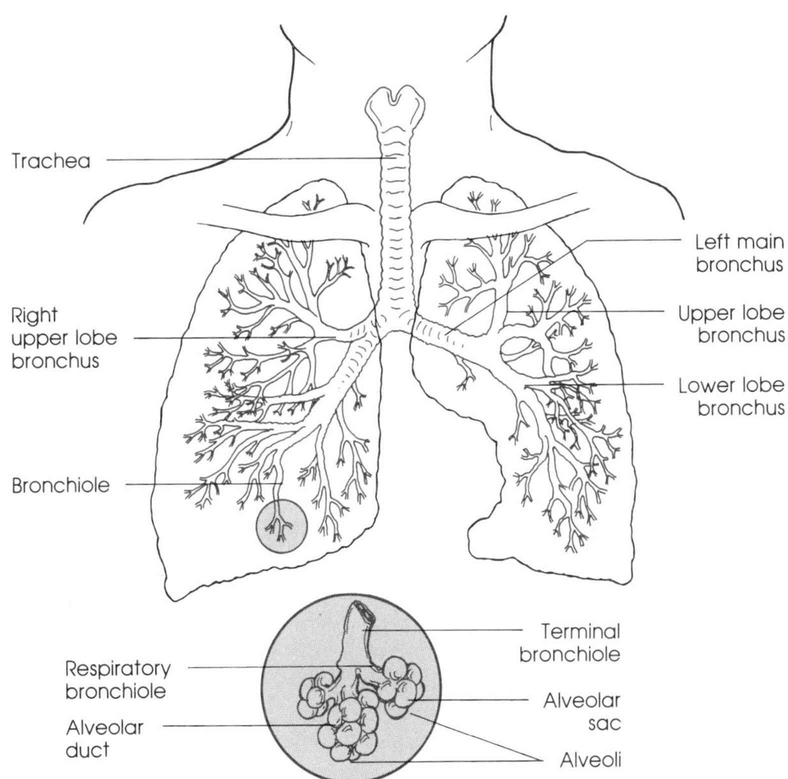

Figure 17-1 Respiratory tract. *Inset*, alveoli.

ration is controlled by the cerebral cortex. CO_2 and hydrogen ions in the cerebrospinal fluid stimulate the central chemoreceptors, causing an increase in the rate and depth of breathing; thus excess CO_2 is blown off, lowering the acidity of the blood. Low oxygen content in the blood stimulates the peripheral chemoreceptors in the carotid arteries and the aorta, and messages are sent from the respiratory center for the respiratory muscles to work harder to raise the oxygen level. These muscles include the diaphragm and the intercostals and other accessory muscles used for respiration.

PATHOLOGIC FACTORS

The respiratory system is particularly susceptible to harmful substances in the external environment. Inhalation of bacteria and other organisms can quickly produce an infection in either the upper or lower respiratory tract. Tobacco smoke, allergens, poisonous gases, and other toxic substances cause irritation and inflammation of the air passages and can eventually lead to chronic inflammation, obstructive diseases, and tumors.

Furthermore, adequate exchange of oxygen and carbon dioxide depends on sufficient blood supply to lung tissues. Hence cardiac disease, emboli, and other disorders of the heart and pulmonary blood vessels will eventually produce problems in the respiratory system.

Aside from infection of the respiratory tract, there are two major types of ventilatory diseases: *restrictive* and *obstructive*. Each group has different causative factors and pathophysiologic effects.

Restrictive diseases are a group of disorders characterized by decreased lung capacity. They are not necessarily primarily lung disorders, but their eventual effect is to limit expansion of the lung and chest wall, and they can include a large variety of illnesses. Examples include scoliosis and kyphosis, both of which decrease the size of the chest cavity; arthritis, which increases stiffness of the chest wall; pneumothorax (collapsed lung), which diminishes lung space; neuromuscular disorders that weaken the strength of the muscles of respiration (e.g., myasthenia gravis); and disorders of the lung that increase stiffness and decrease lung volume (e.g., pneumonia and atelectasis).

Obstructive pulmonary diseases are characterized by problems moving air into and out of the lungs. Narrowing of the openings in the tracheobronchial tree increases resistance to the flow of air, making it difficult for oxygen to enter and contributing to air trapping, as exhalation is also difficult. Asthma, emphysema, and chronic bronchitis are examples of obstructive lung diseases.

PREVENTION OF RESPIRATORY DISEASES

Elimination of such widespread respiratory diseases as the common cold and influenza is hardly possible, considering the many daily contacts a person has with viruses and other infectious organisms. There are, however, certain common sense measures that can reduce one's chances of catching an upper respiratory infection. These include adequate rest and good nutrition, especially during the time of year when respiratory infections are most prevalent. In addition, it is important to practice good personal hygiene, including frequent hand washing and avoiding as much as possible direct contact with people who have a respiratory infection. Following respiratory precautions while caring for patients whose condition indicates such precautions can help protect the nurse from unnecessary exposure.

For some persons, particularly the elderly and the chronically ill, vaccination against influenza is an effective means of reducing the incidence of respiratory disease. The U.S. Public Health Service Advisory Committee on Immunization recommends annual vaccination for high-risk persons. Immunization against pneumococcal infection that occurs secondary to viral infection is also recommended on a one-time basis to high-risk persons. Those considered at high risk are people over 65 years of age, those confined to long-term-care facilities, and persons with (1) chronic respiratory disorders, (2) congenital or chronic cardiovascular disorders, (3) chronic renal disease, (4) diabetes mellitus and other chronic metabolic disorders, and (5) conditions compromising the immune response.

Physicians, nurses, and others involved in providing health care, and therefore often exposed to influenza viruses, also should be immunized.

Although there is some danger in taking the vaccine, the benefits far outweigh the risks. Among the more serious reactions to influenza vaccine are allergic reactions, fever, malaise, muscle soreness, and possibly the development of Guillain-Barré syndrome. This latter reaction occurs in only about 1 in 100,000.

Vaccination against influenza is not recommended for children under the age of 8 years. Persons who are allergic to eggs, chicken protein, or feathers also should not be given the vaccine, because it is prepared from chick embryos.

Other actions that can be taken to avoid serious respiratory disease include prompt treatment of upper respiratory infections, especially in children. An acute respiratory infection that is not completely eliminated can develop into a chronic disorder and cause problems throughout the person's life.

Perhaps one of the most important preventive measures is avoiding prolonged and repeated inhalation of irritating substances. Such substances include tobacco smoke, industrial gases, coal dust, soot and other carbons, and air polluted by automobile exhaust.

TERMS COMMONLY USED IN RESPIRATORY CARE

As with other specialties in health care, there are some terms that are used almost exclusively in respiratory care. A selection of these terms and their definitions follow:

- *diffusion*—the movement of oxygen and carbon dioxide across the alveolar-capillary membrane. It takes place between the gas in the alveolar spaces and the blood in the pulmonary capillaries.
- *elastance*—the extent to which the lungs are able to return to their original position after being barely stretched or distended.
- *lung compliance*—the ability of the lungs to distend in response to changes in volume and pressure of inhaled air. Lung compliance first increases and then decreases with age as the lungs become stiffer and the chest wall more rigid.
- *hypoxia*—a broad term meaning diminished availability of oxygen to the body tissues.
- *hypoxemia*—deficient oxygenation of the blood.
- *resistance*—the force working against the passage of air. The major determinant is the radius of the airway.
- *respiratory failure*—an abnormality of gas exchange with either an excess of carbon dioxide or a deficit of oxygen, or both.
- *perfusion*—the passage of a fluid through the vessels of a specific organ. Perfusion of blood through the pulmonary vessels is an essential function of respiration. The other two essential functions are ventilation and diffusion of gases.
- *shunting*—turning aside or diverting. Intrapulmonary shunting is the diverting of blood so that it does not take part in the exchange of gas at the alveolar sites. When intrapulmonary shunting occurs, blood enters the left side of the heart without being oxygenated. It is, therefore, a possible cause of hypoxemia.
- *surfactant*—a complex lipoprotein produced by cells lining the alveoli and essential to ventilatory function. Its primary purpose is to lower surface tension within the alveoli. It prevents collapse of the lung by stabilizing the alveoli and decreasing capillary pressures.
- *ventilation*—the movement of air from the external environment to the gas exchange units of the lung. It can be spontaneous or done by a mechanical ventilator.

DIAGNOSTIC TESTS AND PROCEDURES AND NURSING IMPLICATIONS

A complete blood cell (CBC) count with hemoglobin and hematocrit determinations is done to detect any deficiency in oxygen-carrying capacity of the blood. Pulmonary function tests are useful in screening for gross abnormalities in the respiratory system. Table 17–1 lists the specific tests for respiratory problems.

Figure 17–3 shows two spirograms, one depicting the tracings made by a healthy young person, the other those of a patient with emphysema. The *forced vital capacity* (FVC) is affected by diseases that restrict lung motion. *Forced expiratory volume in 1 second (FEV_1)* gives some estimate of the amount of *obstruction* to the patient's airflow. FEV_1 is reduced in obstructive pulmonary diseases such as emphysema and chronic bronchitis.

The results of spirometry tests often are recorded in the following terms:

- *total lung capacity* (TLC)—the volume of gas the lung can hold at the end of a maximal inspiration.
- *vital capacity* (VC)—the volume (amount of gas that a person can exhale after inhaling as much air as he can [maximal inspiration]).
- *tidal volume* (TV)—the volume of gas either inspired or exhaled during each breath.
- *functional residual capacity* (FRC)—the volume of gas remaining in the lungs when the lungs and chest wall are at resting end-expiratory position (that is, at rest at the end of a normal expiration).
- *residual volume* (RV)—the volume of gas remaining in the lungs after a person has exhaled as much air as he can (maximal expiration).

Figure 17–4 shows the various subdivisions of total lung capacity.

Magnetic resonance imaging (MRI) is sometimes used to better define the extent of a lesion found by other diagnostic tests.

NURSING ASSESSMENT OF RESPIRATORY STATUS

HISTORY TAKING

Information about the patient's past and current respiratory status is used to plan systematic and goal-oriented nursing care. If the patient

Text continued on page 392

TABLE 17–1 **DIAGNOSTIC TESTS FOR RESPIRATORY PROBLEMS**

Test	Purpose	Description	Nursing Implications
Chest radiograph	To determine pathologic conditions in the lungs such as pneumonia, lung abscess, tuberculosis, atelectasis, pneumothorax, and tumor. Also gives indication of heart size.	Front, back, and lateral views are taken; fluoroscopy may be used to visualize lung and diaphragm movement. Tomograms, which give enhanced pictures of "slices" of lung tissue, may be done; tomograms better define location and size of known lesions in the lung. More sophisticated tomograms can be obtained by CT.	Tell patient he will need to remove his clothes down to the waist and put on an x-ray gown so that it ties in the back. Will be asked to take a deep breath and hold it while the radiograph is taken. Radiographs take 15 to 45 minutes.
Bronchogram	Visual anatomy of the bronchial tree; evaluate presence and severity of bronchiectasis.	Chest radiographs are taken after bronchial instillation of a radiopaque dye. A topical anesthetic is used. The patient is placed in various positions to coat the bronchial tree with the dye.	Requires a consent form. NPO for 6 to 8 h before test. Assess for iodine allergy. Provide good oral hygiene before test to decrease bacteria. A sedative and atropine are administered 1 h beforehand. Pharynx and trachea will be sprayed with topical anesthetic. Catheter is introduced via the nose into the trachea, and contrast dye is administered. Postprocedure nebulization treatment may be given, followed by postural drainage to drain the dye. Check gag reflex before giving anything by mouth.
Lung ventilation and perfusion scan	To assess lung ventilation and lung perfusion; to locate pulmonary embolism and diagnose tumor, emphysema, bronchiectasis, or fibrosis.	*Perfusion scan:* An IV injection of radioactive dye is given. Decreased blood flow to any part of the lung is shown by decreased radioactivity in that area. *Ventilation scan:* Radioactive gas is inhaled and, when scanned, presents a pattern of ventilation in the lungs.	Assess for allergy to iodine. Ask patient to remove all metal jewelry from around the neck. Assure him that amount of radioactivity used is very small and is not harmful. Either iodine- or technetium-based dye is used. An IV access will be inserted. Patient will be asked to hold breath for a short period for the ventilation scan. Images are viewed by use of a scintillation scanner.
Pulmonary angiography	To visualize pulmonary vasculature; to locate pulmonary embolus or other abnormality.	Radiopaque dye is injected via a catheter into the right side of the heart or the pulmonary artery. Radiographs are taken; fluoroscopy is used.	Check consent form. Assess for allergy to dye. Explain that patient may feel warm flush as dye is injected. Posttest: monitor vital signs and check pressure dressing for signs of hemorrhage.
Bronchoscopy	To inspect bronchi; to remove foreign objects or mucus plugs; to biopsy lesions.	Preoperative sedation (diazepam) is usually given. Throat is sprayed with local anesthetic. With neck hyperextended, a	NPO for 6 h prior to test. Check consent form; administer preoperative sedative. Give mouth care just before test. Posttest:

TABLE 17-1 **DIAGNOSTIC TESTS FOR RESPIRATORY PROBLEMS** *Continued*

Test	Purpose	Description	Nursing Implications
		flexible fiberoptic bronchoscope is guided into bronchi; biopsies are taken if needed. Oxygen is administered; a patent IV line is necessary in case emergency drugs are needed.	monitor vital signs and for bleeding, dyspnea, and swelling of face and neck; sputum will be slightly blood-tinged at first. Position patient on side until gag reflex has returned. Check for return of gag reflex by having patient take small sips of water. When gag reflex has returned, throat lozenges may be used for sore throat.
Pulmonary function tests	To determine integrity of mechanical function and gas exchange function of the lungs: volume of air lung can hold, rate of flow of air in and out of the lung, and the elasticity, or compliance, of the lung.	Patient breathes in as much air as possible and then breathes out as much air as possible into a spirometer indicating the forced vital capacity (FVC); Forced expiratory volume in 1 second (FEV_1) is measured. Other measurements include total lung capacity (TLC), vital capacity (VC), tidal volume (TV), functional residual capacity (FRC), and residual volume (RV).	Should not be done within 1 to 2 h of eating; explain procedure to patient. Posttest: monitor vital signs and allow patient to rest, as test can be fatiguing.
Arterial blood gas analysis	To determine if there is adequate exchange of carbon dioxide and oxygen across the alveolar membrane; to determine acid-base balance within the body; to determine hypoxemia.	Useful in care of patients with respiratory disorders, problems of circulation and the distribution of blood, body fluid imbalances, and acid-base imbalances. Arterial blood sample is drawn and tested for pH, $Pa{O_2}$, $Pa{CO_2}$, and HCO_3. (See Chapter 8 for detailed discussion.)	Explain procedure to patient; arterial puncture is briefly painful. Apply firm pressure for 5 to 10 min after specimen is drawn. Compare lab results to normals: pH: 7.35–7.45 $Pa{O_2}$: 80–100 mm Hg $Pa{CO_2}$: 35–45 mm Hg HCO_3: 22–26 mm Hg
Sputum analysis	To examine sputum from lower respiratory tract for bacteria, bacilli, or malignant cells; to determine color, consistency, and sensitivity of bacteria to specific antibiotics.	Sputum specimen is examined and cultured for bacteria; acid-fast stain and Gram stains are done for tuberculosis bacillus; cytologic studies are done to search for malignant cells. If bacteria are present, sensitivity studies to antibiotics are performed.	Explain that specimen is desired from lower areas of lungs; may require respiratory therapy in order to obtain proper specimen or coaching in proper coughing technique. Best specimen is obtained in A.M. before eating or mouth care. Provide mouth care after obtaining specimen. Specimen is expectorated into sterile container.
Oximetry	To noninvasively monitor arterial oxygen saturation ($Sa{O_2}$). To allow comparison of oxygenated hemoglobin to total hemoglobin.	Device attaches to earlobe, pinna of ear, tip of nose, or fingertip. Sensor warms skin, increasing capillary blood flow. Light beam is used to obtain reading, which is displayed by number on oximeter monitor.	Explain equipment to the patient. Keep sensor intact on patient. Monitor $Sa{O_2}$ readings and record. Report readings persistently below 95% to physician.

Table continued on following page

TABLE 17–1 **DIAGNOSTIC TESTS FOR RESPIRATORY PROBLEMS** *Continued*

Test	Purpose	Description	Nursing Implications
Thoracentesis	To remove pleural fluid, instill medication, or obtain fluid for diagnostic studies.	With local anesthetic, a large-bore needle is inserted through the chest wall into the pleural space, and fluid is withdrawn with a large-bore syringe. Aseptic technique must be used. Specimens are obtained for culture, microscopic examination, and stains. Medication may be instilled. Usually done at the bedside (Fig. 17–2).	Explain procedure to patient. Take baseline vital signs. Position patient sitting, facing side of bed, and leaning over the overbed table with arms crossed on it; pillows or the back of a chair can also be used. Monitor respirations and skin color during procedure. Assist patient to remain still. Chest radiograph may be ordered after procedure. Monitor vital signs q 15 min for 1 h or until stable, then routinely. Auscultate breath sounds frequently. Rapid breathing, cyanosis, changes in breath sounds, and tachycardia should be reported immediately. Chart amount and appearance of fluid and condition of patient.

is in obvious respiratory distress, only a few questions about his present illness and chief complaint are asked. Later, during a formal admission interview and informal discussions with the patient and his family, more information can be obtained to plan individualized nursing care.

Some of the more pertinent areas to be covered in a thorough respiratory disease history are listed in Table 17–2. The table also includes implications for planning patient care on the basis of data obtained.

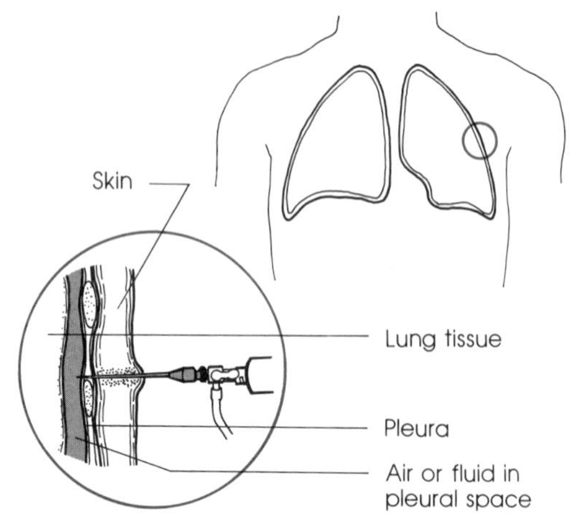

Figure 17–2 Technique of thoracentesis. The needle is advanced only as far as the pleural space.

OBSERVATION

Assessment of respiratory status demands careful and frequent observation of the patient. The nurse notices the posture of the patient, the amount of effort he must exert to breathe, the way he uses abdominal muscles and other accessory muscles of respiration, the number of words he can say between breaths, and, of course, the rate and depth of ventilation. These specific ob-

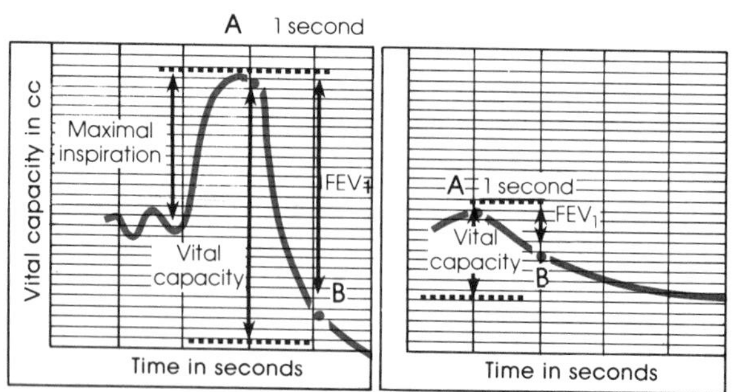

Figure 17–3 A normal spirogram made by a healthy young person would look like that in the illustration at the left. The forced vital capacity (FVC) is large, and the forced expiratory volume (FEV_1) shows the patient can expire about 85% of his inspired air in 1 second. Contrast this with a typical curve of a disease state, which has a more gradual slope. The spirogram at the right was made by an elderly person suffering from emphysema. His inspiration is impeded, his vital capacity is considerably reduced, and his FEV_1 shows he can expire only about half of his lung volume in 1 second because of obstructive lung disease.

(Redrawn from Spirometry: How it helps detect impaired pulmonary function. Nursing Update, March, 1974, p. 14. Reprinted with permission.

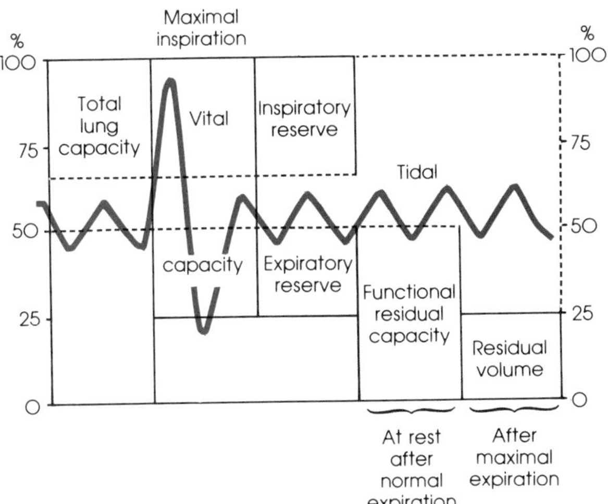

Figure 17–4 Subdivisions of total lung capacity. Note the rise and fall of tidal volume, peaks and valleys with maximal inspiration, and residuals after maximal expiration.

(Adapted from Goddard, R. F., and Luft, U. C.: Pulmonary function tests for infants and children. Albuquerque, Lovelace Foundation for Medical Research and Education, 1980).

servations are more helpful than simply saying that a patient has dyspnea.

A patient with chronic obstructive pulmonary disease usually leans forward in a sitting position and uses his abdominal muscles to force air out of his lungs. Other significant movements during ventilation are elevating the shoulders and ribs, tensing the neck and shoulder muscles, and flaring the nostrils. A retraction of the spaces below and around the sternum also might be observed in a patient in respiratory distress.

TABLE 17–2 **RESPIRATORY ASSESSMENT**

Area	Specifics
Present illness: chief complaint	When started; exposure to infection; history of respiratory infections? Description of symptoms.
Precipitating factors	Any allergies? Sinusitis? Asthma? Emphysema? Chronic bronchitis? Exposure to dust or other irritants?
Risk factors	Smoke? Number of packs per day for how many years? Exposure to occupational air pollutants? Exposure to tuberculosis?
Cough	Type of cough? When occurs? Productive? Quantity and color of sputum? Odor and taste?
Dyspnea	Any shortness of breath? On exertion? Any wheezing? Use of accessory muscles?
Measures for symptom relief	Humidifier? Over-the-counter medicines? Antihistamines? Decongestants? Cough medicines? Bronchodilators? Other medications?

The nurse might also notice that the patient uses two pillows to prop himself up or asks to have the head of his bed raised to facilitate breathing. Other indications of respiratory difficulty are extreme restlessness and agitation.

Skin color can be significant in a respiratory assessment, but cyanosis of the skin is not a reliable indicator of hypoxemia.

Cyanosis occurs late in the process of oxygen depletion and, as previously explained, could indicate problems of circulation or hemoglobin deficiency. The skin of a person with emphysema can have a pinkish color in spite of the fact that he does not have adequate oxygenation of his blood.

Observation of the shape of the patient's chest can give a clue that an obstructive disease is present. Obstructive disorders can cause enlargement of the front-to-back measurement of the chest wall, giving a barrel-like appearance to the chest. This is due to the presence of trapped air in the lungs and inadequate recoil. These forces prevent the chest from returning to its original position at the end of each expiration. Over a period of time there is a gradual elevation of the resting level of the chest, which produces an increase in the size of the chest wall.

Other deformities of the thoracic cage might include kyphosis or scoliosis, either of which can cause restrictive pulmonary disorders.

Clubbing of the fingers is frequently seen in patients with chronic respiratory disease (Fig. 17–5). The fingers are wider than normal at the distal end, similar in shape to a baseball bat or club. There also is marked curvature of the fingernails. These physical changes result from inflammatory changes in the bones of the fingers. However, the primary cause of the pathologic bone changes is not known.

INEFFECTIVE BREATHING PATTERNS

Hyperventilation and hypoventilation were discussed in Chapter 8, as was the effect of either of these abnormal breathing patterns on the acid-base balance of body fluids. *Hypercapnia* (also called *hypercarbia*) is the retention of excessive amounts of carbon dioxide. It is the result of hypoventilation, during which the usual amount of carbon dioxide is not eliminated by exhalation.

Carbon dioxide is a respiratory stimulant; hence the body responds to excessive levels of carbon dioxide by increasing the rate of respirations in an effort to "blow off" larger quantities of the gas. If, however, the respiratory centers in the brain are exposed to higher than normal levels of carbon dioxide over a long period of

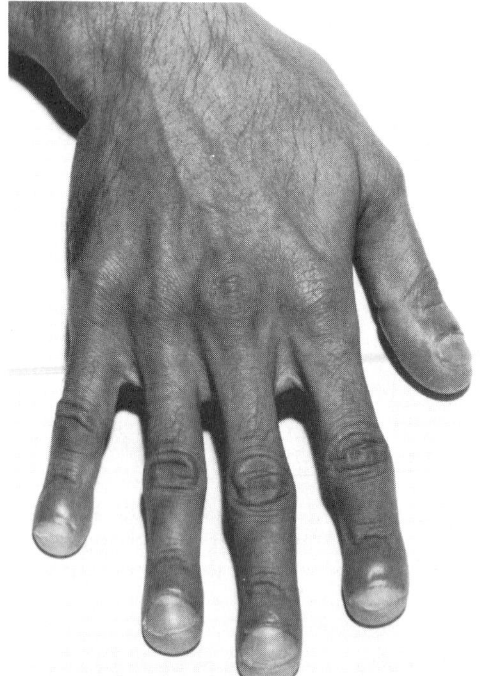

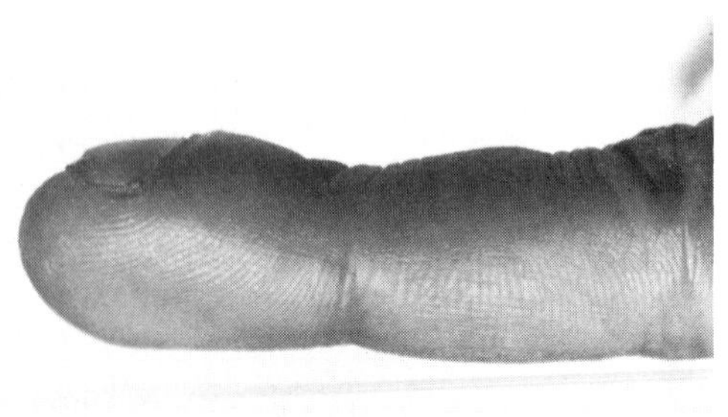

Figure 17-5 Clubbed fingers of patient with diffuse interstitial lung disease. Top view of right hand and side view of index finger.
(From Hinshaw, H. C., and Murray, J. F.: Diseases of the Chest, 4th ed. Philadelphia, W. B. Saunders, 1980.)

time, they cease to react and a drop in the respiratory rate occurs. The patient then becomes mentally confused, his senses become less acute, and eventually he may fall into a coma. The heart rate increases in an attempt to meet the tissues' need for more oxygen. Mental confusion and an increase in pulse and heart rate are, therefore, indicators of inadequate oxygenation of the blood and tissues. If the slowing down of respiration is not corrected, the accumulation of carbon dioxide continues, and a vicious cycle begins. The final outcome can be cardiac arrest from respiratory acidosis.

Blood gas analysis is the best way to determine whether respiratory acidosis is either threatening or already present. Results of the analysis will show a high level of $Paco_2$, high carbonate (HCO_3) level, and a low pH (acidosis) if the condition has been present for several days.

Hypocapnia, which is a deficit of carbon dioxide, occurs as a result of hyperventilation and eventually produces respiratory alkalosis. Conditions associated with hypercapnia include (1) those in which there is an increased metabolic rate, such as thyrotoxicosis, persistent fever, and hysteria; (2) salicylate overdosage; and (3) improper use of mechanical ventilation.

Clinical signs of respiratory alkalosis include hyperactive neuromuscular reflexes, tetany, vertigo, blurred vision, and diaphoresis. Blood gas analysis will show a low $Paco_2$ and a high pH (alkalinity).

Other abnormal respiratory patterns are as follows:

- *Biot's respiration*—respiration that is characterized by irregular periods of apnea alternating with periods in which four or five breaths of identical depth are taken. A respiratory pattern of this kind is seen in patients with increased intracranial pressure.
- *Cheyne-Stokes respiration*—breathing characterized by rhythmic waxing and waning of the depth of respiration, with regularly recurring periods of apnea. This kind of respiration is often seen in patients in coma resulting from a disorder affecting the central nervous system.
- *Kussmaul's respirations* (also called *air hunger*)—respiration characterized by a distressing difficulty in breathing that occurs spasmodically at irregular intervals. This abnormal breathing pattern is often seen in patients with diabetic acidosis and coma.
- *apneustic respiration*—prolonged gasping inhalation, followed by short, ineffective exhalation. The pattern is indicative of damage to the respiratory centers in the brain.

ADVENTITIOUS BREATH SOUNDS

Auscultation of lung sounds using a stethoscope, once a procedure carried out exclusively by physicians, is rapidly becoming a nursing activity during assessment. Learning to use a stethoscope to listen to lung sounds and interpret what all the various sounds mean is not within the scope of this text. The best way to learn to do this is not by reading about it but by listening to tapes and to actual breath sounds and gaining experience in distinguishing one sound from another.

There are, however, some breath sounds the nurse can learn to distinguish when using a stethoscope. With experience she can become very adept at noting adventitious (abnormal) breath sounds and what each might indicate.

The lungs should be auscultated with the patient in a sitting position. Ask him to breathe deeply through the mouth while you listen with the diaphragm of the stethoscope. Listen to the front, back, and lateral areas of the chest in a systematic, symmetric manner. Move from one side of the midline of the chest to the equivalent location on the other side of the midline, comparing one side's sounds with the other. Begin above the clavicles and progress downward in the intercostal spaces to above the sixth rib. On the back, start above the scapula and progress along the sides of the spine, inside the scapular area, on down and then toward the lateral areas above the tenth thoracic vertebra. Laterally, listen in the midaxillary line in three descending locations to just above the diaphragm. (See Figure 17-6).

Wheezing is probably familiar to everyone who has been around a person suffering from asthma. It is a whistling, musical, high-pitched sound produced by air being forced through a narrowed airway.

Rhonchi, which sometimes can be heard without a stethoscope, are coarse, low-pitched, sonorous, rattling sounds caused by secretions in the larger air passages. Crackles, which nearly always require a stethoscope to hear, are produced by air passing through moisture in the smaller airways. Crackles are either fine or coarse. Fine crackles are high in pitch and can be heard in patients who have atelectasis, fibrosis, pneumonia, or early congestive heart failure. Coarse crackles are louder and low in pitch and are heard in patients with bronchitis, pulmonary edema, and resolving pneumonia.

"Croaking" sounds (also called *stridor*) can be heard when there is partial obstruction of the upper air passages. They are typically heard in children with croup but can also occur in adults with some kind of obstruction. The inflammation that is producing the obstruction often also affects the larynx, producing hoarseness.

Another adventitious sound is that of a *pleural friction rub*, which is a grating or scratchy sound similar to creaking shoe leather or an opening door that occurs when irritated visceral and parietal pleura rub against each other.

COUGH

Because there are different kinds of coughs, each giving some clue as to the kind of ventilation problem presented by the patient, information noted by the nurse can help establish a medical diagnosis and identify problems amenable to nursing care.

Nursing observations of a patient with a cough include (1) whether the cough is productive or nonproductive of sputum; (2) whether it is dry and hacking or deep and moist-sounding; (3) events or circumstances that occurred immediately before the attack of coughing and seemed to trigger it; (4) time of day when the cough is most noticeable; (5) measures (if any) that help relieve coughing; and (6) other symptoms that occur simultaneously with the cough—for example, a change in vital signs, pain, breathlessness or dyspnea, and fatigue.

A *productive* cough is moist and deep, often accompanied by bronchial crackles or wheezing, and ends in production of fairly large amounts of sputum. The amount and character of the spu-

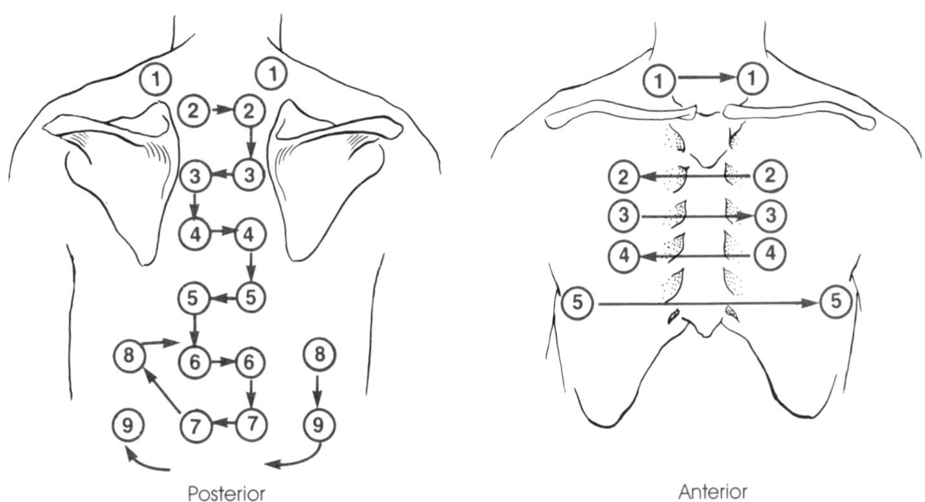

Figure 17-6 Sites for auscultation of the lungs.

tum is significant in assessment of the patient and will be discussed later.

A *nonproductive* cough is dry and harsh; the patient is unable to bring up any mucus from the bronchial tree. Patients who have a generalized obstruction of the airways may cough frequently, but the cough is ineffective in bringing up sputum and may cause only exhaustion and pain.

The manner in which a patient coughs can indicate a need for instruction in more effective and less tiring coughing techniques.

SPUTUM

It is important to remember that *sputum* refers to the material brought up from the bronchi and bronchioles and *not* to nasal secretions, mucus and other debris that has drained from the sinuses, or saliva from the mouth. Table 17–3 shows various characteristics of sputum and what each might indicate.

In addition to the character of sputum, assessment should include the amount expectorated after coughing.

ACUTE RESPIRATORY DISEASE

THE COMMON COLD

The common cold is an inflammation of the upper respiratory tract caused by a virus. It is the most prevalent infectious disease among people of all ages. There are so many different strains of viruses that can produce the symptoms of a common cold that immunity is difficult, if not impossible, to establish. Avoiding exposure to those who have a cold and maintaining a state of good health are the only ways one can avoid catching a cold.

TABLE 17–3 CHARACTERISTICS OF SPUTUM AND POSSIBLE CAUSES*

Characteristic	Possible Cause
Thick, tenacious, and "ropy"; difficult to cough up	Chronic bronchitis, emphysema
Scant, sticky, rust-colored	Pneumococcal pneumonia
Frothy, pinkish or blood-tinged	Pulmonary edema
Yellow, yellow-green, or grayish-yellow, with foul odor or taste	Pulmonary infection
Blood-tinged, bloody, or blood-streaked	Tuberculosis, or ulcerated pulmonary vessel, or bronchogenic carcinoma
Large amounts	Pneumonia or bronchitis
Scanty	Asthma
Very thick and viscous	Inadequate hydration

* Note: Normal sputum is white and slightly viscous and has no odor or taste.

Symptoms

The common cold usually starts with a mild sore throat or a hot, dry, prickly sensation in the nose and back of the throat. Within hours after the onset of a cold, the nose becomes congested with increased secretions, the eyes begin to water, and sneezing and an irritating, nonproductive cough appear. There is usually no elevation of temperature; if a fever does develop, it is low-grade.

Medical Treatment and Nursing Intervention

There is no cure for the common cold. The thousands of nonprescription cold remedies bought each year by Americans may relieve the symptoms of a cold, but they do not prevent, cure, or shorten the course of the infection.

A major goal in the care of a common cold is prevention of a secondary bacterial infection. For their own sake as well as that of people around them, persons with a cold should avoid contact with others so as to avoid picking up a bacterial infection or giving their viral infection to someone else. A person with a cold is contagious for about 3 days after his symptoms first appear.

Colds can, of course, be spread by droplet infection, and most people realize that coughing and sneezing can send literally millions of viruses into the air. Some are also aware of the danger of spreading a cold by sharing drinking glasses and cups with others. They might not know, however, that a cold can be transmitted by hand. Coughing and sneezing into tissues does limit the viruses' travel by air, but they are also very likely to be on the person's hands, where they can be transferred to anything he touches. Hand washing, then, is an important part of teaching patients about preventing the spread of his cold to others.

The patient should be instructed to stay indoors, preferably in bed or resting during the first few days of his illness. His fluid intake should be increased. Fruit juices are recommended, especially citrus juices, because of their vitamin C content.

Aspirin or some other mild nonprescription analgesic can help relieve the muscle aches and headache of a cold. Nose drops or sprays for the relief of nasal congestion can have a rebound effect, leaving the nose "stuffier" than before. Antibiotics do not cure a common cold, which is a viral infection.

If a "cold" persists for more than a week to 10 days, or if the patient begins to feel worse, has a temperature of 102°F (38.9°C), and develops chest pains or coughs up purulent sputum, he is showing signs of a bacterial infection that should be treated medically, probably with an antibiotic.

ACUTE BRONCHITIS

Acute bronchitis frequently is an extension of an upper respiratory infection involving the trachea (tracheobronchitis) and is usually viral in origin. Causes other than infectious agents are physical and chemical agents that are inhaled in air polluted by dust, automobile exhaust, industrial fumes, and tobacco smoke.

Acute bronchitis is most often encountered in small children and the elderly and debilitated. It is particularly dangerous in the very young, because their bronchi are smaller and more easily obstructed.

Symptoms and Medical Diagnosis

Early symptoms of acute bronchitis are similar to those of the common cold. In acute bronchitis the symptoms progress to chest pain, fever, and a dry, hacking, and irritating cough. Later the cough becomes more productive of mucopurulent to purulent sputum. The fever may be moderate with accompanying chills, muscle soreness, and headache. There is no specific test that will give a definitive diagnosis of bronchitis. In most instances the physician relies on clinical manifestations to make his diagnosis.

Medical Treatment and Nursing Intervention

Acute bronchitis is treated conservatively; antibiotics are used only as indicated by sputum that contains specific organisms. Symptomatic treatment includes the use of humidification using either warm or cool moist air, cough mixtures and aerosols to reduce coughing and soothe the irritated tracheal and bronchial mucosa, and bed rest to promote healing. Nutritional and fluid balance should be maintained. A period of convalescence is recommended to avoid progression of an acute condition to a chronic one.

INFLUENZA

Influenza is an acute, highly infectious disease of the respiratory tract, and is caused by any of three major types (A, B, and C) and numerous subtypes of viruses. It occurs as isolated cases, or in epidemics and pandemics. The most virulent form is type A, which usually affects young adults first and then spreads to the very young and very old in the community.

Influenza is spread by direct and indirect contact with infected persons by coughing and sneezing and by sharing items such as drinking and eating utensils or towels.

Symptoms and Medical Diagnosis

The first symptoms of influenza appear 2 to 3 days after exposure. They come on rather suddenly and include dry, hacking cough, headache, fever, chills, muscle aches, sore throat, fever blisters, and red and watery eyes.

Chest radiograph and auscultation usually show no abnormality. The white cell count is normal or slightly below normal. Diagnosis is based on clinical findings, as there is no specific laboratory test for influenza.

Medical Treatment and Nursing Intervention

Uncomplicated influenza usually is managed more effectively by nursing intervention than by drugs or other forms of medical treatment. Antibiotics are given only if there is evidence of bacterial infection secondary to the viral infection.

If a person is known to be at high risk for influenza and has been exposed to type A influenza, the physician may choose to provide prophylaxis with an antiviral agent such as amantadine hydrochloride (Symmetrel).

Prevention of influenza was discussed earlier under "Prevention of Respiratory Diseases."

Nursing diagnoses commonly associated with influenza include sleep pattern disturbance related to cough and fatigue; activity intolerance; fluid volume deficit related to fever; pain; and alteration in oral mucous membrane related to mouth breathing.

Nursing interventions for patients with these kinds of problems might include the following:

- Administer suppressant cough medicine at bedtime and during the night as prescribed.
- Mouth care at least every 4 hours, before each meal, and more frequently if patient reports bad taste in mouth or has halitosis from sputum.
- Cater to patient's food and drink preferences within limits of dietary restrictions.
- Schedule procedures and medications to allow periods of uninterrupted rest.
- Perform sponge bath and other temperature-reducing measures to reduce fever.
- Increase oral intake to at least 3,000 mL per 24 hours.
- Humidify inhaled air.
- Splint chest and abdomen with pillow during coughing attacks.
- Administer cough medicine and analgesics promptly.
- Encourage patient to ask for analgesics when discomfort first appears.
- Emollient to lips and nares as needed.
- Clear nostrils as much as possible to prevent mouth breathing.

PNEUMONIA

Pneumonia is an extensive inflammation of the lung with consolidation of the lung tissue as it fills with exudate. It can affect one or both lungs or only one lobe of a lung (lobar pneumonia). There are two general types of *infectious* pneumonia: typical, or bacterial, pneumonia and *atypical* pneumonia, which can be viral or due to *Mycoplasma pneumoniae*. The most common causative organism is *Streptococcus pneumoniae*, which is also called *pneumococcus*. However, some pathogenic microorganisms are always present in the upper respiratory tract. They usually cause no harm unless resistance is lowered by some other factor, such as chronic disease, alcoholism, physical inactivity, or extremes in age (very young or very old). Those patients who are in a weakened condition are particularly susceptible to pneumonia.

Pneumonia also can result from inhalation of poisonous gases *(chemical pneumonia)*, accidental aspiration of foods or liquids *(aspiration pneumonia)*, or a blow or injury to the chest that interferes with normal respiration *(traumatic pneumonia)*. *Hypostatic pneumonia*, which is due to lying in bed for extended periods of time, is always a threat to those with impaired mobility. Lack of physical exercise and inadequate aeration of the lungs are major factors in the development of hypostatic pneumonia.

Prevention

Elderly, weak and debilitated, and immobilized persons are all prime candidates for pneumonia, as are those who have some kind of chronic pulmonary disease.

A variety of nursing interventions can help prevent pneumonia. These include (1) using nursing intervention to strengthen the patient's natural defenses and avoid infection; (2) frequent turning, coughing, and deep breathing by postoperative patients or those who are otherwise unable to ventilate their lungs adequately; (3) carefully watching and properly positioning those vomiting patients who are in decreased states of consciousness, such as the patient recovering from anesthesia; (4) elevating the head of the bed when administering tube feedings and when assisting a patient to eat; (5) avoiding giving liquids to patients who are prone to aspiration; (6) faithfully following principles of cleanliness and asepsis when caring for debilitated patients and those most susceptible to infection; and (7) administering pneumonia vaccine when prescribed for those most at risk for developing the disease.

Symptoms and Medical Diagnosis

Symptoms of pneumonia vary according to type. In typical, infectious pneumonia there usually is a high fever accompanied by chills, a cough that is productive of rusty or blood-flecked sputum, chest pain that is made worse by respiratory movements, and a general feeling of malaise and aching muscles. Diagnosis is confirmed by chest radiograph, which reveals densities in the affected lung.

The diagnosis of atypical pneumonia might be missed because of a lack of symptoms usually indicative of pneumonia. Body temperature can be normal or subnormal, breath sounds can be good with perhaps only occasional rales and wheezing, no pleural involvement and therefore no pain, a dry cough, and feeling of extreme fatigue. Chest radiograph reveals diffuse, patchy areas of density.

Cytomegalovirus has become a cause of pneumonia in immunocompromised patients, particularly those with AIDS or transplant patients on immunosuppressive drugs.

Medical Treatment

Typical pneumonia is treated with antibiotic agents such as penicillin, erythromycin, cephalosporins, aminoglycosides, or ciprofloxicin (Cipro), depending on the type of bacteria responsible and the degree of sensitivity to various antibiotics. Atypical pneumonia caused by *Mycoplasma* is usually treated with either erythromycin or tetracycline. Viral, atypical pneumonia requires no antiinfective therapy. *Pneumocystis carinii* pneumonia associated with AIDS is treated with pentamidine.

Nursing Intervention

The nursing care plan for a patient with pneumonia should include interventions to promote oxygenation, control elevated temperature, maintain fluid and electrolyte balance, promote adequate nutrition, provide adequate rest, monitor vital signs and respiratory status, relieve pain and discomfort, provide good oral hygiene and care for "fever blisters" (herpes), prevent irritation of the lungs by smoke and other irritants, and avoid secondary bacterial infections. It is important that the nurse assess for signs of increasing impairment of gas exchange. Because abdominal distention, nausea, and vomiting may also accompany pneumonia, nursing intervention to deal with these problems may be indicated. Other problems that could be presented by the patient include altered states of consciousness (delirium and confusion) and the development of such complications as empyema (see below) and congestive heart failure.

PLEURISY

Pleurisy is an inflammation of the pleural membranes surrounding the lungs. In *pleurisy with effusion*, there is also an increase in the amount of serous fluid within the pleural cavity.

The most outstanding symptom of pleurisy is a sharp, stabbing pain in the chest. The pain is aggravated by taking a deep breath. Pleurisy may occur alone or in conjunction with another disease of the respiratory system.

Medical Treatment

The patient with pleurisy is placed on bed rest and observed carefully for signs of development of an infection in the respiratory tract. Nonsteroidal antiinflammatory drugs are used to decrease inflammation and control pain. This offers some relief.

When pleurisy is accompanied by effusion of serous fluid, the physician may perform a thoracentesis (removal of fluid from the pleural cavity) for diagnostic tests or relief of symptoms. It is not uncommon for as much as 500 mL to be removed at one time during a thoracentesis (see Table 17–1 for further information on this procedure).

EMPYEMA

When the fluid within the pleural cavity becomes infected, the exudate becomes thick and purulent, and the patient is said to have *empyema*. The organisms causing the infection may be staphylococci or streptococci.

Medical Treatment

Empyema is treated by eliminating the infection through the use of specific antibiotics and the removal of the excess fluid from the pleural cavity by insertion of an empyema tube. A specimen of the fluid is sent to the laboratory for a culture and sensitivity study. This test determines the exact antibiotic that will most effectively destroy the organism causing the infection.

FUNGAL INFECTIONS

Pneumocystis carinii pneumonia has a high incidence in AIDS patients. *P. carinii* is either a protozoon or a fungus. It is only found in immunocompromised patients and is highly lethal.

Histoplasmosis and coccidioidomycosis are fungal lung infections caused by the inhalation of spores. Both can cause pneumonia. They are diagnosed by history, signs and symptoms, and skin test reaction to the fungus. Treatment is IV amphotericin B.

SARCOIDOSIS

Sarcoidosis is a group of interstitial lung diseases characterized by granulomas. These diseases cause fibrotic changes in the lung tissue over a period of time. They affect other tissues in the body as well as the lungs. A cellular immune response seems to be responsible for the tissue changes. Sarcoidosis is 10 times more common in blacks than in whites, and most cases occur in those between ages 20 and 40. The fibrotic changes cause a reduction in functioning lung tissue.

CHRONIC OBSTRUCTIVE PULMONARY DISEASE

The term *chronic obstructive pulmonary disease* (COPD) is used to describe a condition that is common to three diseases: *pulmonary emphysema*, *chronic bronchitis*, and *bronchial asthma*. Although the clinical history, manifestations of the specific illness present, treatment, and course of each of the diseases may vary, the term *COPD* describes one condition that is common to all three. This condition is *obstruction of the small airways*. Because the obstruction is located in the bronchioles and alveoli, the condition is sometimes called *chronic obstructive lung disease* (COLD) and *chronic airway obstruction* (CAO).

COPD ranks fifth among the major causes of death in the United States, and the number of its victims is increasing.

Since 1950, the death rate from COPD and related disorders has risen steadily. COPD accounts for billions of dollars in economic loss as a result of inability to work and the expense of repeated visits to the physician and hospitalizations. The American Lung Association estimates that about 14 million Americans suffer from COPD.

The dramatic increase in the rate of morbidity and mortality due to COPD is attributed to increases in habitual cigarette smoking and rising levels of air pollution. A third factor is genetic susceptibility to the destruction of lung tissue. A serum protein, *alpha$_1$-antitrypsin* (AAT) is deficient in certain people, and the deficiency runs in families. This protein inhibits the activity of the enzyme *elastase*, which tends to break down lung tissue. In the absence of AAT, lung tissue is more easily destroyed by the enzyme.

MECHANICS OF COPD

Pulmonary Emphysema

Emphysema is characterized by a permanent distention of the bronchioles and destruction of the walls of the alveoli (Fig. 17–7). It is essentially a disease of the *terminal* respiratory units. Air that is inhaled becomes trapped, causing the victim to work harder to *exhale* air than to inhale it. One patient who has had emphysema for more than 26 years suggests that a healthy person can get some idea of the effects of emphysema by doing the following: Take a deep

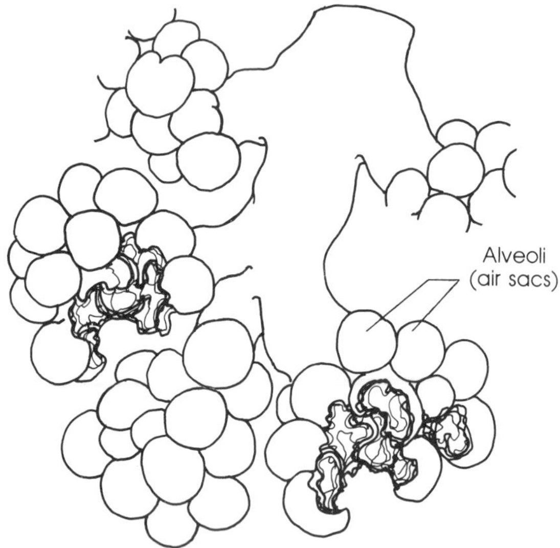

Figure 17-7 Emphysematous alveoli. Irreversible breakdown of walls of individual air sacs creates large air spaces. Small air tubes collapse, trapping air and making exhalation difficult.

breath and then exhale only about one third of the air you have breathed in. Now continue trying to breathe while retaining two thirds of the air you breathed in.

As pulmonary emphysema progresses, the patient suffers further loss of lung elasticity. The diaphragm becomes permanently flattened by overdistention of the lungs, the muscles of the rib cage become rigid, and the ribs flare outward. This produces the "barrel chest" that is typical of patients with COPD.

In order to compensate for the loss of the muscular action that normally aids respiration, the patient begins to use other muscles, mainly those of the neck and shoulders. He holds his shoulders high in an attempt to enlarge the space in which his lungs can expand. His facial expression conveys the anxiety and tension that result from his struggle to get enough air into his lungs.

The patient with almost pure emphysema—that is, no asthma and very little bronchitis—has only a small amount of mucus. His skin is a pinkish color, even though he may be hypoxic. He usually does not retain carbon dioxide and therefore is not likely to suffer acid-base imbalances.

Chronic Bronchitis

Inflammation of the bronchi is considered chronic when the recurrent cough is present for at least 3 months of each year for at least 2 years. Chronic bronchitis can range from a mildly irritating "cigarette" cough in the morning with production of small amounts of sputum to a severe disabling condition. The latter extreme is characterized by increased resistance to airflow, hypoxia, and frequently hypercapnia and *cor pulmonale.* Cor pulmonale is a heart condition characterized by pulmonary hypertension and an enlarged right ventricle, both of which are secondary to chronic lung disease. Cor pulmonale places the patient at risk for right-sided heart failure.

The primary clinical characteristics of chronic bronchitis include a productive cough due to hyperplasia of the bronchial glands and increased secretion of mucus, and the breathing difficulties typical of obstructive lung disease. Pulmonary function testing reveals an increased residual volume due to premature closure of the narrowed airways during exhalation. The patient has a marked increase in his $Paco_2$ levels and a marked decrease in his Pao_2 levels. The retention of carbon dioxide and deficiency of oxygen give his skin a reddish-blue color. The reddish color is also due to an increase in his red blood cell count *(polycythemia).* Laboratory tests also will show elevated hemoglobin and hematocrit levels. The increase in production of red blood cells is an attempt by the body to compensate for the chronic hypoxia.

Asthma

The person with asthma has a hypersensitivity of the trachea and bronchi to various kinds of stimuli (Fig. 17-8). It is likely that no single cause is responsible for the group of symptoms known as asthma, but that a combination of two or more factors is responsible. Among the factors implicated in the development of asthma are allergens, infectious agents, occupational and environmental toxins, and psychological disturbances.

The symptoms of asthma are due to construction of the bronchi, inflammatory changes in the mucosa, accumulations of secretions in the lumen of the bronchi, and changes in the elastic recoil of the lungs.

Some asthmatics are without symptoms between attacks, but pulmonary function tests may occasionally reveal some abnormalities even though there is no wheezing, coughing, or other outward signs. Cough is a common symptom of asthma in adults and usually indicates obstruction of the larger airways. Dyspnea, another common symptom, is indicative of edema or mucus in the smaller airways.

Recognizing the specific symptoms of a patient suffering from asthma can be helpful not only in establishing a diagnosis, but also in deciding the most effective medical treatment and nursing intervention.

Because asthma is a chronic disease, the patient should know the intended effect of his medications. Ideally, he will eventually be able

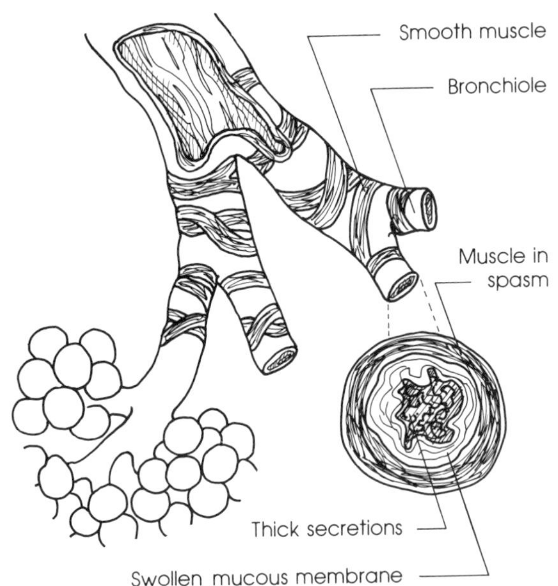

Figure 17-8 Bronchial asthma. The bronchiole is obstructed during expiration by muscle spasms, swollen mucous membranes, and thick mucous secretions within air tubes and sacs.

to adjust dosage and therapy as his condition changes, using guidelines provided by the physician or nurse. As with any chronic disease, the patient with asthma periodically consults the physician for continued management of his illness.

MEDICAL TREATMENT

Because emphysema, chronic bronchitis, and asthma are often seen in combination in patients with COPD, the first step in designing therapy is to determine which aspects of these diseases the patient displays. Treatment is aimed at management of the underlying symptoms.

The goals of medical treatment are to (1) minimize irritation of the air passages and relieve obstruction by secretions, edema, or bronchospasm; (2) prevent or control infection and allergy; (3) increase the patient's tolerance for activity; and (4) determine the best drug combination in the least amounts that will control symptoms.

Drugs that may be prescribed to achieve these goals include antibiotics, which are used to treat infection or are given prophylactically to prevent an overwhelming infection from occurring if the patient experiences a viral respiratory illness.

Bronchodilators in the form of beta-adrenergic agonists, theophyllines, or anticholinergic agents such as ipratropium bromide (Atrovent) are used as the main form of therapy. Beta-adrenergic agonists in inhalant form are now the primary drug of choice for asthma. These drugs cause bronchodilation and inhibit mast cell release; examples include albuterol (Proventil, Ventolin), metaproterenol sulfate (Alupent, Metaprel), and terbutaline (Brethine, Brethaire). Addition of other drugs for maintenance therapy depends on whether the disease is chronic or intermittent. Theophylline in oral form is added for patients with chronic asthma. In children, cromolyn sodium (Intal) in inhalant form is often substituted for theophylline. Corticosteroids are used orally for 1- to 2-week periods in patients uncontrolled by other drugs alone. If needed on a long-term basis, they are given in inhalant form, as this seems to cut down on the many serious side effects these drugs cause. Elimination of allergens in the immediate environment and desensitization for those asthma patients with known allergies are other very important aspects of therapy.

Bronchodilators promote bronchial drainage by relaxing the smooth muscle surrounding the bronchi and thereby enlarging the lumen of the tubes. They also promote better ventilation. Mucolytic agents are administered as necessary to help break down and separate mucous strands from airway walls and thus aid in their removal by coughing. Examples include wetting agents such as tyloxapol (Alevaire) and acetylcysteine (Mucomyst), which actually are detergents that affect the surface tension of mucus. Other medications include cromolyn sodium and corticosteroids.

Oxygen is prescribed for moderate and severe hypoxemia. For acute episodes of COPD with hypoxemia, oxygen is given to raise the PaO_2 to 60 mm Hg. Oxygen is used in patients with chronic COPD who have consistent PaO_2 levels less than 55 to 59 mm Hg. Oxygen is always used cautiously in patients with COPD, as they have adjusted to high levels of CO_2, which normally provides the drive to breathe, and are dependent on low oxygen levels to stimulate breathing. If too much oxygen is given, the patient may cease to breathe and require mechanical ventilation.

Oxygen is also prescribed for moderate and severe cases of dyspnea. Patients who continue to experience exertional dyspnea after discharge may be taught to administer their own oxygen at home. A portable oxygen tank can be used to allow the patient to increase his level of activity without triggering severe and frightening episodes of dyspnea.

NURSING INTERVENTION

Rehabilitation and education of the patient and family are the chief long-term goals of nursing intervention.

With proper home care the patient with COPD can live longer and have a higher quality of life, reduce the number of hospitalizations and visits to his physician, and have fewer psychosocial problems related to inactivity and a feeling of hopelessness.

It is very important that the family, as well as the patient, be educated so that there will be an understanding of the need for appropriate exercise and activity and of the desire for independence. Families often tend to become very overprotective of the patient because of their fear of episodes of dyspnea. Rehabilitation needs to be a joint effort by the patient and family to help the patient attain as high a quality of life as possible while avoiding the complications of COPD.

The major problem of chronic, diffuse, and irreversible obstruction of the airways must be dealt with in a systematic way. This means working with the patient to identify the specific difficulties he is experiencing, assessing his current ability to cope with them, and devising plans to accomplish specific goals for improvement. In general, no matter what the primary cause of the disorder, patients with COPD will require some nursing interventions to help them (1) maintain optimal health status, (2) achieve a balance of maximal exercise and adequate rest, (3) utilize techniques to facilitate breathing (for example, breathing through pursed lips and diaphragmatic breathing), and (4) cough effectively to remove secretions. In order to prevent frequent hospitalizations for acute flareups of his disease, the patient will need to be taught how to avoid bronchial irritation and infection and prevent such complications as right-sided heart failure (cor pulmonale). Tables 17–4 and 17–5 show some helpful tips and techniques for the patient with COPD.

Encouragement to quit smoking is of major importance for those with COPD who still smoke. Continued smoking will seriously compromise the extent and quality of life for this patient. The American Lung Association has both literature and community programs directed to assist COPD patients with this problem.

Psychosocial concerns are another area for nursing intervention. The patient often needs help with adjustment to alterations in roles and lifestyle. He may have problems with self-esteem, body image, and sexuality that stem from his chronic disease. A trusting relationship between nurse and patient opens the way for discussion of the most personal concerns and provides a means to explore possible solutions or adaptations for problems in these areas. Referral to community support groups can also be beneficial, as the patient then has an opportunity to see and hear how others in his situation have learned to cope and adapt.

The teaching plan for the COPD patient is extensive and includes (1) management of medications and side effects, (2) use of respiratory therapy measures and care of equipment, (3) management of dyspnea, (4) control of the immediate environment and avoidance of allergens, (5) maintenance of nutrition, (6) balancing exercise and adequate rest, (7) signs of complications, and (8) the need for close medical supervision.

Education of the patient and family can be overwhelming if it is not planned carefully, allowing enough time for them to gain confidence in one aspect of care before introducing more information.

Detailed information on nursing intervention and the specifics of teaching follow in the section "Common Respiratory Patient Care Problems." A sample plan for a patient with COPD is shown in Nursing Care Plan 17–1.

Most patients with COPD have difficulty getting sufficient rest and sleep because of their dyspnea, anxiety, and decreased mobility. Sedatives and tranquilizers are contraindicated, because they tend to depress respiration. Tension

TABLE 17–4 TIPS FOR THE PATIENT WITH COPD

1. To make mucus more liquid and easier to cough up, drink at least 2 and preferably 3 quarts of liquid every day.
2. When you exert yourself, as in lifting something or getting up from your chair, *exhale* slowly through pursed lips rather than holding your breath. You should do the same thing when you are walking for exercise. It is natural for all of us to hold our breath when we exert ourselves, so you may need practice to get into the habit of exhaling on exertion.
3. Eat three or four small, balanced meals rather than one or two large ones each day.
4. Practice your breathing exercises every day without fail.
5. Try to avoid crowds during the flu and cold seasons.
6. Do not take over-the-counter drugs. They can interact with your prescribed drugs and some may be harmful because of their effects on your breathing. Antihistamines can dry out the mucus even more and make it more difficult for you to clear your air passages.
7. Don't smoke or inhale the tobacco smoke of others.

Note: Normal sputum is white and slightly viscous and has no odor or taste.

TABLE 17-5 TECHNIQUES TO IMPROVE BREATHING

Technique	Instructions
Pursed-lip breathing	1. Purse your lips as if you were going to whistle or blow out a candle. 2. Inhale slowly through your nose. 3. *Slowly* exhale through your pursed lips; control the flow of exhaled air as you would if you wanted to cause a candle flame to flicker but not go out. 4. Do not force exhaling. It should last about twice as long as inhaling or as long as is comfortable for you.
Abdominal ("belly") or diaphragmatic breathing	1. You can do this in bed, resting against a partially raised backrest. Later, when you have mastered the technique, you can do this while standing or performing exercises. 2. Inhale through your nose, with your abdomen relaxed. Your diaphragm should move slightly downward. 3. Exhale through pursed lips while the nurse or someone else gently pushes inward and upward, helping the diaphragm move up in the chest. As you exhale, tighten your abdominal muscles. This should help your respiratory muscles force air out of your lungs. 4. Exhalation time should be about two to three times longer than inhalation, but don't worry if you cannot exhale for that long a period of time. As you improve, your exhalation time will get longer. 5. You can use diaphragmatic breathing as a controlled breathing pattern while you are doing something else, such as walking or exercising.
Positioning while sitting	1. Sit in a chair and spread your feet so they are shoulder-width apart. 2. Lean forward with your elbows on your knees and your arms and hands completely relaxed. This should help you breathe easier and become less tense.
Positioning while standing	1. Stand with your back and hips against a wall. 2. Spread your feet apart to shoulder width and about a foot from the wall. 3. Relax and bend your shoulders slightly forward. You should be able to breathe easier in this position.

Data from Rifas, E. M.: How you and your patient can manage dyspnea. Nursing 80, June, 1980, p. 34. Reprinted with permission from the June issue of Nursing 80.

and anxiety often can be relieved if the patient is taught some relaxation techniques. It should be emphasized that these techniques must be *taught to the patient.* Simply telling him to relax or to stop worrying will not be helpful; he is using almost every muscle in his body to struggle for breath or is extremely tense in anticipation of an attack of breathlessness.

The exact ways in which a patient learns to relax can vary, but the purpose of using a relaxation technique is always to "let go" of his muscles. First he is told to assume a comfortable position either sitting in a chair or lying in bed. His head, upper chest, shoulders, and arms should be well supported. Next he is told to "talk to" individual muscle groups in his body. Starting with the muscles in his face and head he tells them to "let go" each time he exhales. His exhalation should be slow and "sighing." He then tells his shoulder and arm on one side to let go, then his shoulder and arm on the other side, and so on moving down the body until all muscles are totally relaxed.

BRONCHIECTASIS

Bronchiectasis is a chronic respiratory disorder in which one or more bronchi are permanently dilated. It is thought to occur as a result of frequent respiratory infections in childhood. It is often classified with COPD, and its management is similar.

Cystic fibrosis is a major cause of bronchiectasis. It is a genetic disease in which there is excessive mucus production because of exocrine gland dysfunction. The lungs, intestines, sinuses, reproductive tract, sweat glands, and pancreas are all affected. It is diagnosed by history, physical examination, and a positive sweat test.

Lung damage occurs in cystic fibrosis patients

NURSING CARE PLAN 17–1

Selected nursing diagnoses, goals/outcome criteria, nursing interventions, and evaluations for a patient with COPD

Situation: Vince Thompson, age 72, lives with his wife in a small apartment in the center of the city. He has been hospitalized repeatedly during the past 6 years with respiratory infections, severe dyspnea, and anxiety. He has chronic bronchitis and emphysema. He smoked 1½ packs cigarettes for 46 years and quit 5 years ago. He worked as a cabinet maker and likes to fish and garden but can't do much any more. His physician has enrolled him in the community ambulatory clinic for further patient teaching to try to decrease his episodes of infection.

Nursing Diagnosis	Goals/Outcome Criteria	Nursing Intervention	Evaluation
Impaired gas exchange related to decreased airflow and respiratory muscle fatigue. SUPPORTING DATA "I can't take 10 steps without becoming breathless." Pao_2, 62; Pco_2, 49; HCO_3, 30. Very thick sputum.	Patient will utilize modified breathing techniques to facilitate ventilation. Patient will display increased ability to tolerate nonstrenuous activity by walking short distances without breathlessness.	Reinstruct him in techniques of pursed-lip, diaphragmatic breathing, deep breathing, and coughing; teach relaxation techniques. Review medication dosages and schedule with patient; assess effectiveness and compliance. Begin stepped exercise program to improve muscle function and promote efficient oxygen use by muscles. Help him to formulate plan for pacing activities of daily living. Assess sputum and obtain culture for infection if indicated. Assess diet and nutritional status; assist him to choose foods high in calories but easy to chew and swallow; suggest small, frequent meals.	Practicing pursed-lip breathing; walking to door and back without breathlessness; continue plan.
Ineffective airway clearance related to viscous sputum. SUPPORTING DATA Thick, tenacious sputum that is hard to cough up. Fluid intake of only 1,000 mL/day.	Thinner mucus that is easier to cough up. Fluid intake will increase to at least 2,000 mL/day. Patient will demonstrate proper use of nebulizer.	Explain effect of inadequate fluid intake on liquidity of mucus; assess what fluids patient likes; advise him to drink 8 oz of fluid every hour while awake; suggest use of room humidifier at home; review technique for using nebulizer and mucolytic agents.	Intake 3,400 mL; mucus is thinner than yesterday; using nebulizer properly; effective.
Potential for respiratory infection related to compromised respiratory system and decreased resistance. SUPPORTING DATA History of frequent respiratory infections, chronic emphysema, and bronchitis. Difficulty clearing mucus from lungs.	Patient will have no more than one respiratory infection per year.	Review ways to decrease contact with respiratory infectious organisms: avoiding those with colds, flu, and other infections; frequent hand washing. Teach him to avoid respiratory irritants; stay in house when air pollution index is high; avoid smoke, dust, and cold air. Observe sputum for changes in color, consistency, odor, and amount; call clinic promptly if signs of infection occur. Give influenza and Pneumovax vaccines. Encourage him to maintain adequate nutrition.	Reviewed guidelines for prevention of respiratory infection; states that he understands; continue plan.
Disturbance in self-concept related to inability to do much of anything.	Patient will express improvement in self-concept within 3 months. Patient will be able to fish	Allow him to verbalize concerns; assist him to focus on activities he can still do; explore ways of continuing	Verbalizing dismay at not being able to do the things he used to do; discussed how he might at least fish some; continue plan.

NURSING CARE PLAN 17–1, *Continued*

Nursing Diagnosis	Goals/Outcome Criteria	Nursing Intervention	Evaluation
SUPPORTING DATA "I have to sit down and rest even when I'm just showering and dressing in the morning; I can't really garden or fish anymore."	or garden for short periods within 3 months.	favorite activities using modification (i.e., fishing in afternoon when air is warmer; picking spots that do not require much walking to reach; gardening in a small area rather than keeping up the whole yard). Give encouragement and praise for efforts in stepped exercise program.	

as a result of excessive secretion of abnormally thick mucus, impairment of ciliary action in the lungs, airway obstruction, and repeated infections, which cause scarring. Cystic fibrosis eventually results in COPD. It was once solely a pediatric disease, because children with cystic fibrosis died before reaching adulthood. Today 20% of cystic fibrosis patients are adults. Some cystic fibrosis patients live into their 30s and 40s because of aggressive respiratory treatment and antibiotics.

Research has finally identified the gene responsible for cystic fibrosis, and work is continuing on ways to isolate and replace the missing gene in order to prevent or cure the disease.

TUBERCULOSIS

PULMONARY TUBERCULOSIS

Pulmonary tuberculosis is an infectious disease of the lung characterized by lesions within the lung tissue. The lesions may continue to degenerate and become necrotic, or they may heal by fibrosis and calcification. The causative organism is the true tubercle bacillus, *Mycobacterium tuberculosis.*

Contrary to popular beliefs, tuberculosis is *not* highly contagious. Infection most often occurs after prolonged exposure to the tubercle bacillus, but not everyone contracts the disease, even after close and extensive contact with infected persons.

Tuberculosis is still a major health problem in many countries throughout the world, and unfortunately its incidence is rising again in the United States. Poor living conditions, especially in urban areas, malnutrition, and immune incompetence all increase susceptibility to the tubercle bacillus. Homeless individuals in the cities, users of recreational drugs, and AIDS patients are the main groups in which the increase in tuberculosis is seen.

Diagnosis

Early detection of tuberculosis is of great importance because (1) the antituberculotic drugs are more effective in the early stages of the disease, (2) the period of disability is much shorter, and (3) the complications are fewer.

To aid in the identification and prompt treatment of potential and active cases of tuberculosis, the National Lung Association has determined five basic classifications of tuberculosis and suspected tuberculosis in children and adults (Table 17–6).

Skin Testing

Skin testing for tuberculosis may be done by either the *Mantoux* or the *tine* method. Of these, the Mantoux test is considered more accurate. In this test, 0.1 mL of purified protein derivative (PPD) tuberculin containing 5 tuberculin units is injected intradermally. The test is *positive* when the swelling at the site of injection is more than 10 mm in diameter 48 to 72 hours after injection.

A positive tuberculin test indicates that the person has been infected with the tubercle bacillus. It does not ***indicate whether the disease is active or inactive at that time, only that the body tissues are sensitive to tuberculin. A positive reaction indicates a need for further evaluation.***

Radiographs

An x-ray examination of the chest may or may not reveal tubercular lesions in the lung, but calcified and healed lesions as well as active lesions usually can be seen on radiographs. A *diagnosis of active tuberculosis is established when the tubercle bacillus has been found in the sputum.* Because people are quite likely to swallow sputum rather than expectorate it, a sample

TABLE 17–6 CLASSIFICATION OF TUBERCULOSIS

0. NO TUBERCULOSIS EXPOSURE, NOT INFECTED (no history of exposure, reaction to tuberculin skin test not significant).
1. TUBERCULOSIS EXPOSURE, NO EVIDENCE OF INFECTION (history of exposure, negative reaction to tuberculin skin test).
2. TUBERCULOUS INFECTION, NO DISEASE (positive reaction to tuberculin skin test, negative bacteriologic studies [if done], no clinical and/or radiographic evidence of tuberculosis).

    CHEMOTHERAPY STATUS (preventive)
    - None
    - Receiving chemotherapy since (date)
    - Chemotherapy terminated (date)
        - Complete (prescribed course of therapy)
        - Incomplete
3. TUBERCULOSIS: Clinically active (*M. tuberculosis* cultured [if done], otherwise, *both* a positive reaction to tuberculin skin test *and* clinical and/or radiographic evidence of current disease).

    LOCATION OF DISEASE
    - Pulmonary
    - Pleural
    - Lymphatic
    - Bone and/or joint
    - Genitourinary
    - Disseminated (miliary)
    - Meningeal
    - Peritoneal
    - Other

    The predominant site should be listed. Other sites may also be listed. Anatomic sites may be specified more precisely.

    BACTERIOLOGIC STATUS
    - Positive by
        - Microscopy only (date)
        - Culture only (date)
        - Microscopy and culture (date)
    - Negative (date)
    - Not done

    CHEMOTHERAPY STATUS
    - Receiving chemotherapy since (date)
    - Chemotherapy terminated, incomplete (date)

    The following data are necessary in certain circumstances:

    RADIOGRAPH FINDINGS
    - Normal
    - Abnormal
        - Cavitary or noncavitary
        - Stable or worsening or improving

    TUBERCULIN SKIN TEST REACTION
    - Positive
    - Negative
4. TUBERCULOSIS: Not clinically active (history of previous episode(s) of tuberculosis, or abnormal stable radiographic findings in a person with a positive reaction to tuberculin skin test, negative bacteriologic studies [if done], no clinical and/or radiographic evidence of current disease).

    CHEMOTHERAPY STATUS
    - None
    - On chemotherapy since (date)
    - Chemotherapy terminated (date)
        - Complete
        - Incomplete
5. TUBERCULOSIS SUSPECT (diagnosis pending)

    CHEMOTHERAPY STATUS
    - None
    - Receiving chemotherapy since (date)

From American Lung Association: Diagnostic Standards and Classification of Tuberculosis, 1990.

of stomach contents may be examined (gastric analysis).

Symptoms

The onset of tuberculosis is gradual; a patient may have an active and progressing lesion before symptoms appear. Typical symptoms are cough, low-grade fever in the afternoon, anorexia, loss of weight, fatigue, night sweats, and sometimes hemoptysis.

Medical Treatment

Before the advent of antituberculotic drugs, patients with pulmonary tuberculosis were treated in sanatoria, where they were isolated in order to avoid spreading the disease. Since the 1960s, the trend has been toward treating patients with active tuberculosis in general hospitals for a short time and then sending them home on medication.

If the patient is able to carry out his regimen of care at home, he may be allowed to return home after one negative sputum smear and go back to work after three consecutive negative smears. Smears are usually negative after 2 to 3 months of drug therapy. Many patients can be treated on an outpatient basis in this way. Effective cure can be obtained in about 9 months for all but 2% of the patients with pulmonary tuberculosis.

Tuberculosis was once greatly feared, because it was considered to be highly contagious, and the treatment and confinement to an institution could last for years. Now, however, it is considered far less threatening. This change in attitude has come about because of the chemotherapeutic agents that quickly render the patient noninfectious. A second factor is the knowledge that tuberculosis is essentially an air-borne infectious disease requiring respiratory precautions rather than strict isolation of the patient. Information about drugs commonly used in the treatment of tuberculosis is summarized in Table 17–7. The drugs are prescribed in combinations of two or three antituberculotic agents (for example, the primary drug INH and a secondary drug such as RMP).

Chemotherapy is the preferred method of treatment for most patients with tuberculosis, but some may require surgery if the disease has progressed to an advanced stage, or if drug-resistant infection has developed. Surgical treatment involves removal of the affected lung tissue.

Nursing Intervention

Because tuberculosis is an infectious disease, nursing goals are similar to those for other diseases of this type. Nursing objectives concerned with prevention and control of infectious diseases are (1) to control the spread of the infectious agent, (2) to promote immunity to infectious diseases, and (3) to support and strengthen the capacity for recovery in a patient who has an infectious disease.

Control of Infection

Pulmonary tuberculosis is transmitted principally by way of the respiratory tract. Acid-fast bacillus precautions are recommended for the hospitalized patient who has an active case of tuberculosis and is just beginning drug therapy.

Another aspect of infection control is identification and prompt treatment of potential and active cases of tuberculosis. The nurse should be thoroughly familiar with the five basic classifications of tuberculosis described earlier in this chapter.

Promotion of Immunity

A vaccine is available that is made from live, attenuated bacilli. It is called BCG (bacille Calmette-Guérin) and is capable of offering some protection from tuberculosis but cannot be depended on to provide complete immunity. The BCG vaccine has the disadvantage of causing a positive reaction to the tuberculin test (this interferes somewhat with the usefulness of tuberculin testing programs). Public health officials in this country advise the administration of BCG vaccine only to those who live in communities that have a very high rate of tuberculosis.

In countries where there are high rates of tuberculosis, the World Health Organization strongly recommends the widespread use of BCG, which is credited with having a favorable impact in reducing the morbidity of tuberculosis.

Fortunately, tuberculosis is one of the most easily avoided of all serious respiratory illnesses. The body's innate immune system cannot work well, however, when a person is malnourished, physically debilitated, and subject to extreme physical and emotional stress. Improvement of living conditions and carrying out sound health practices are essential to maintaining a natural resistance to tuberculosis.

Preventive therapy with isoniazid (INH) has been particularly successful in reducing the transmission of tuberculosis. It is estimated that the drug is 85% effective in reducing the chances of contracting tuberculosis by persons who are most exposed. The drug is given prophylactically once daily for a full year. Those for whom a course of INH therapy is recommended include (1) those living in the house with or closely associated with a person who is newly diagnosed as having tuberculosis; (2) people who have positive skin reactions but normal chest radiographs; (3) positive skin reactors who suffer from a

TABLE 17-7 **DRUGS COMMONLY USED IN THE TREATMENT OF TUBERCULOSIS**

	Dosage		Most Common Side Effects	Test for Side Effects	Remarks
	Daily	*Twice Weekly*			
Primary					
Isoniazid (INH)	5–10 mg/kg up to 300 mg PO or IM	15 mg/kg PO or IM	Peripheral neuritis, hepatitis, hypersensitivity, jaundice	AST/ALT (not as a routine)	Bactericidal. Pyridoxine 10 mg as prophylaxis for neuritis; 50–100 mg as treatment
Secondary					
Ethambutol	15–25 mg/kg PO	50 mg/kg PO	Optic neuritis (reversible with discontinuation of drug; very rare at 15 mg/kg), skin rash	Red-green color discrimination and visual acuity	Use with caution with renal disease or when eye testing is not feasible
Rifampin (RMP)	10–20 mg/kg up to 600 mg PO	Not recommended	Hepatitis, febrile reaction, purpura (rare)	AST/ALT (not as a routine)	Bactericidal. Orange secretion color. Affects action of other drugs
Streptomycin	15–20 mg/kg up to 1 gm IM	25–30 mg/kg IM	VIIIth cranial nerve damage, nephrotoxicity; hypersensitivity	Vestibular function, audiograms; BUN and creatinine	Use with caution in older patients or those with renal disease
Pyrazinamide	15–30 mg/kg up to 2 g PO	Not recommended	Hyperuricemia, hepatotoxicity	Uric acid, AST/ALT	Under study as first-line drug in short-course regimens
Tertiary Drugs					
Kanamycin	15–30 mg/kg up to 1 gm IM	Tertiary drugs are not recommended for twice-weekly dosage.	Similar to streptomycin	BUN, creatinine	Increase hydration; evaluate hearing before therapy starts
Capreomycin	15–30 mg/kg up to 1 gm IM		Similar to streptomycin	BUN, creatinine	Periodic hearing evaluation needed
Cycloserine	10–20 mg/kg up to 1 gm PO		Depression, psychosis, hypersensitivity	Neurologic exam	Warn to avoid alcohol; monitor serum blood levels of drug
Ethionamide	15–30 mg/kg up to 1 gm PO		Peripheral neuritis, GI distress, dermatitis	AST/ALT	Pyridoxine used for neuropathy Give with meals; avoid alcohol
Para-amino salicylic acid	150 μg/kg up to 12 gm PO		GI distress, hepatotoxicity, hypersensitivity	AST/ALT	Give with meals; monitor for hepatotoxicity

ALT = Alanine aminotransferase; AST = aspartate aminotransferase; BUN = blood urea nitrogen.
Adapted from Farer, L. S.: Tuberculosis: What the physician should know. American Lung Association, 1982.

chronic disease (for example, diabetes mellitus), are taking steroids, or have had a gastrectomy; and (4) those who have recently shown a positive skin reaction in spite of a history of negative reactions.

Support

Even though studies of the effectiveness of INH and RMP consistently show a very high success rate (98%) in the control of tuberculosis, many people still have a dread of the disease. When a person first learns that he has tuberculosis, he will need reassurance and continued support in sorting out his feelings and overcoming any fears and misinformation he might have.

Additionally, it is important that the patient name all close contacts so that they can be reached and started on preventive therapy. Giving the names of contacts may be very difficult for the patient because of the social stigma that is still attached to tuberculosis in certain cultural groups.

The vast majority of newly diagnosed tuberculosis patients are treated on an outpatient basis. Only those who are very debilitated or suffering from another chronic illness are hospitalized. Because much of the responsibility for his care probably will rest on the patient himself and possibly on family members, health education is a major intervention in the management of tuberculosis.

Education of the patient, his family, and close contacts should include information about how the disease is transmitted, how it affects the lungs, the importance of taking prescribed medications continuously and without fail, and the risks involved in failing to take both therapeutic doses and preventive doses of medication.

Instruction in personal hygiene and nutrition is included in the program of health care teaching if the patient needs this information. Specifically, the patient and family are taught measures to cope with a cough, handle secretions properly, and observe sputum and report any change in its characteristics. A balance of rest and physical activity also should be stressed if it appears that the patient is overexerting himself either by working or by indulging in a debilitating social life.

EXTRAPULMONARY TUBERCULOSIS

It is possible for the tubercle bacillus to attack and damage parts of the body other than the lungs. This is called *extrapulmonary tuberculosis.* The areas most frequently affected are the bones, meninges, urinary tract, and reproductive system.

Tuberculous meningitis involves infection of the meninges, which line the brain and spinal cord. This disease can be fatal unless it is promptly treated with antituberculotic drugs. The symptoms of this disorder are essentially the same as those in other types of meningitis.

Tuberculous infection of the bone is less common than it formerly was because of better methods of detecting pulmonary tuberculosis and the elimination of contaminated milk as a source of infection. Because of extensive bone destruction in a tubercular infection, there can be serious orthopedic deformities in this disease. Tuberculosis of the spine, called *Pott's disease,* is now quite rare in the United States. The deformity most commonly seen in Pott's disease is *kyphosis,* or "hunchback."

CANCER OF THE LUNG

In 1930, the death rate from lung cancer for males was 3.6 per 100,000 population; in 1986 the rate had increased to approximately 73.8 per 100,000. Today, whereas death rates from other forms of cancer are decreasing or remaining stable, lung cancer has become a leading cause of death in males, and the death rate for females is rapidly increasing. Factors that contribute to this include increasing air pollution, more cigarette smoking by young people, and the growing numbers of older people in the population. Lung cancer is found most often in men 40 years of age or older. About 12.5% of patients diagnosed with lung cancer survive more than 5 years (American Cancer Society, 1990).

SYMPTOMS

Most lung tumors begin in the epithelial lining of the bronchi. There are few symptoms at first, usually only a cough and some wheezing. As the tumor grows larger, the patient may have some pain or discomfort in the chest, exertional dyspnea, and expectoration of blood-streaked sputum. More specific symptoms depend on the location and size of the malignant tumor and the areas to which it has metastasized. If, for example, the malignancy has involved the esophagus, there will be ulceration, bleeding, and dysphagia. Tumors pressing against the trachea can produce hoarseness and paralysis of the vocal cords.

The oncologist may choose from a variety of diagnostic tests and procedures to establish a definite diagnosis of lung cancer. These include chest radiograph and cytology, which is examination of cells obtained by mediastinoscopy, bronchoscopy, thoracentesis, and needle biopsy of the tumor. Lung scans also are used in the diagnosis of lung cancer.

TREATMENT

It may be possible to remove the affected area of the lung by surgery if the malignancy is in its earliest stages and is localized. Radiation may be used after surgery; however, there are some types of lung cancers that are radioresistant. Small cell tumors respond dramatically to chemotherapy, but the malignancy tends to recur. As with other forms of cancer, the oncologist chooses specific therapies on the basis of the type of malignancy affecting the lung and its stage of development.

CHEST INJURIES

Injury to the chest wall and underlying structures can range from minor bruises to major trauma to the pulmonary and cardiovascular systems. Thoracic trauma is a major cause of accidental death, exceeding head and facial injuries. Whenever there is evidence of chest injury, a very real state of emergency exists, because the condition of the victim can rapidly deteriorate to death.

The major complications of chest trauma involve either the lungs and air passages or the heart and major blood vessels, or both. Pneumothorax and hemothorax frequently occur as a result of a blunt (nonpenetrating) or penetrating injury to the chest wall. These conditions can cause partial or total collapse of one or both lungs. There also can be contusion of the myocardium, rupture of the aorta, and tracheobronchial or tracheoabdominal injuries. The procedure for correction of pneumothorax or hemothorax is insertion of a thoracostomy tube (chest tube) (Fig. 17–9).

Major concerns in the care of patients with chest injuries are (1) maintenance of an airway, (2) assurance of adequate ventilation, and (3) treatment of circulatory problems to ensure circulation of oxygenated blood.

The emergency care of patients with such chest injuries as open "sucking wounds" and flail chest is discussed in Chapter 36.

PNEUMOTHORAX AND HEMOTHORAX

The space within the pleural membranes is an airtight compartment. Pressure within this compartment is less than that of the atmosphere and therefore is called a *negative pressure*. This negative pressure is necessary to allow sufficient space for normal breathing in which the tidal movement of air in and out of the lungs inflates and deflates them. If, however, there is a break in the airtight compartment, either along the surface of the lung or from outside the pleural sac, air rushes in and collapses the lung. The presence of air or gas within the pleural cavity is called *pneumothorax* (Fig. 17–10).

Pneumothorax is always a threat in chest injury, as well as in the period following chest surgery. However, the condition also can occur spontaneously when there is a pathologic opening on the surface of the lung that allows a leakage of air from the bronchi into the pleural cavity. This condition is called a *spontaneous pneumothorax*.

Treatment for spontaneous pneumothorax may require nothing more than rest and the administration of oxygen to relieve discomfort. Thoracentesis may be performed to remove excess air

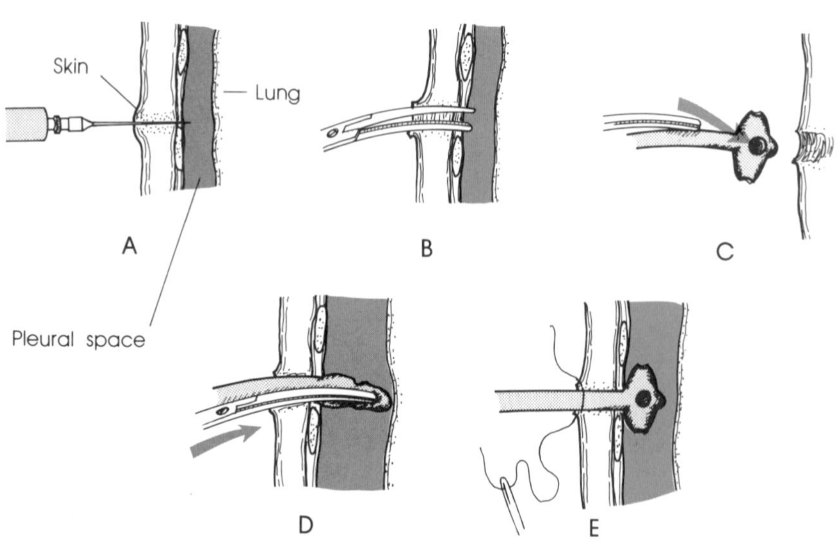

Figure 17–9 Procedure for thoracostomy. If the procedure is done in an emergency, a local anesthetic is injected at the site of insertion of the thoracostomy tube *(A)*. The intercostal space is infiltrated with anesthetic, and the incision is made through the skin and underlying tissues only as far as the pleural space. Care is taken not to puncture the lung. (If a general anesthetic is used, step *A* is not necessary.) The incision is widened *(B)*, and the tube inserted *(C* and *D)*. To avoid accidental removal, it may be sutured in place *(E)*. The free end of the tube is connected to a closed drainage system.

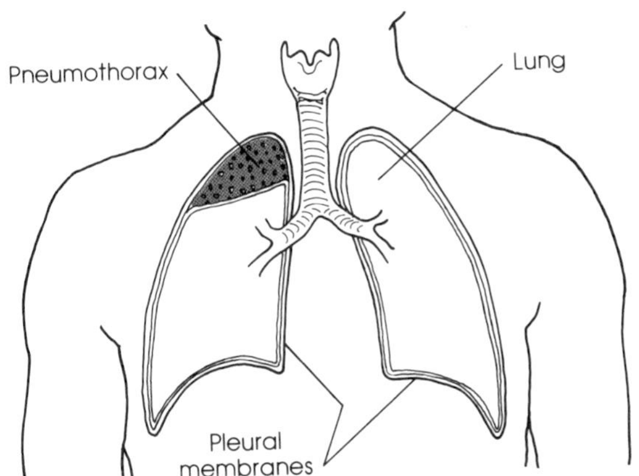

Figure 17-10 Pneumothorax. Air within the pleural cavity has entered some of the space normally occupied by the lung, thus preventing its expansion and causing partial collapse. Note the location, which usually is in the upper segment; hence a thoracic tube for the drainage of air would be located in the upper chest.

and allow for gradual reexpansion of the lung. If air continues to leak into the pleural space, the physician may insert chest tubes to remove the air.

Tension pneumothorax develops when air enters the pleural space on inspiration but remains trapped there rather than being expelled on expiration. It can occur from trauma, mechanical ventilation, or rib fracture during CPR. The air in the pleural space increases with each breath, and the pressure within the chest builds, which gradually collapses the lung. If unrelieved, this increasing pressure will cause a *mediastinal shift*, resulting in a decrease in cardiac output and blood pressure. Mediastinal shift means that the structures in the mediastinum—the heart, great vessels, trachea, and esophagus—are all shifted to the unaffected side of the chest. In this case, emergency thoracentesis is necessary to remove the air from the pleural cavity. The insertion of chest tubes may be necessary to provide a means of removing air from the chest cavity.

Hemothorax is the presence of blood within the pleural cavity. It can occur as a result of laceration of the lung, heart, and blood vessels within the thorax. The accumulation of blood in the pleural cavity can have the same effect as accumulations of gas or air—that is, it fills up space and causes partial or total collapse of the lung. There also is the possibility of mediastinal shift in hemothorax and the likelihood of impaired venous return in the pulmonary blood vessels.

Assessment of a patient for pneumothorax, hemothorax, or a combination of the two (hemopneumothorax, Fig. 17-11), includes awareness of the patient's history in regard to acute or chronic respiratory disease, accidental injury to the chest, or chest surgery. The condition is suspected when the patient complains of sudden chest pain or a feeling of tightness in the chest. There will be an increase in both pulse rate and rate of respirations, a drop in blood pressure, and the absence of normal chest movements on the affected side when the patient breathes.

FLAIL CHEST

When a patient experiences severe chest trauma in an automobile accident or fall, several ribs are often broken. When three or more ribs are broken in two or more places, the chest wall becomes unstable. This condition is called *flail chest*. When the patient breathes in, the fractured portion of the chest is drawn inward instead of expanding outward as the rest of the chest does; when he exhales, the flail portion expands outward as the rest of the chest collapses normally. This interferes with oxygenation, as the lungs cannot expand normally.

Flail chest is treated by intubating the patient and placing him on mechanical ventilation while the ribs heal. This causes considerable pain, and the patient usually has to be given a skeletal muscle-paralyzing agent (pancuronium bromide [Pavulon]) to prevent him from fighting the action of the ventilator. He is given IV morphine or meperidine for pain control and sedation along with the paralyzing agent to decrease his anxiety over being totally paralyzed.

PULMONARY EMBOLISM

Pulmonary embolism occurs when a pulmonary vessel is plugged with a mass or clot. Emboli can occur in solid, liquid, or gas forms and can occur from fracture of a long bone (fat embolus), from amniotic fluid during childbirth, from

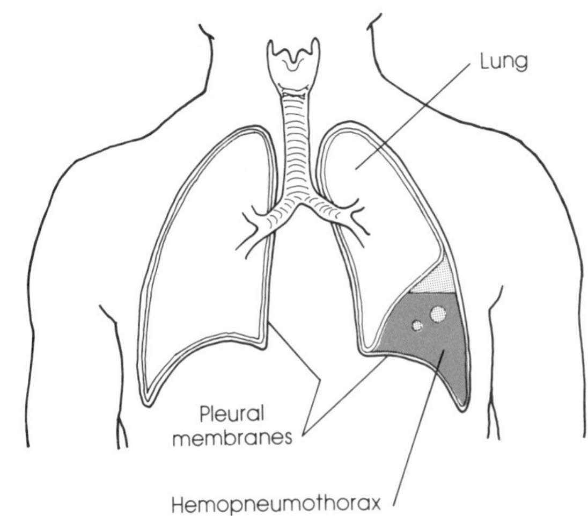

Figure 17-11 Hemopneumothorax. A collection of air and blood in the pleural space causes inadequate lung expansion. Note its location, which is typically in the lower segment of the chest; thus a thoracic tube for the drainage of blood would be located in the lower chest.

air introduced through a central line, and from clots formed elsewhere in the body, such as from a deep vein thrombosis or thrombi that form in the heart when the patient has arrhythmias. Regardless of the origin of the embolus, the result is the same: interference with blood flow in the lung distal to the point where the embolus lodges.

Symptoms depend on the size and location of the clot and whether there is one clot or multiple small clots. The general symptoms are respiratory distress with dyspnea, chest pain, cough, hemoptysis, and anxiety. Consequences of pulmonary embolism can be minor or life threatening.

Treatment depends on the size and location of the embolus. The nurse should stay with the patient, begin low-flow oxygen therapy if there is oxygen in the room, assess vital signs, notify the physician of the patient's symptoms, and administer heparin when it is ordered.

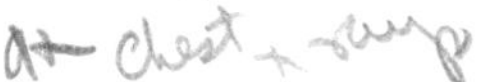

CARE OF THE PATIENT HAVING INTRATHORACIC SURGERY

Many kinds of surgical procedures require opening the chest wall and entering the pleural cavity. For example, in addition to resection of lung tissue and other pulmonary structures, intrathoracic surgery also is necessary for repair of the heart and great vessels, and the correction of defects of the esophagus.

PREOPERATIVE CARE

Assessment of the patient's respiratory status prior to chest surgery will depend on whether the surgery is elective or in response to accidental trauma. If there is time, history taking and obtaining subjective and objective assessment data will be essentially the same as described earlier in the section, "Nursing Assessment of Respiratory Status."

In general, the preoperative period for the patient scheduled for chest surgery is somewhat longer than for other kinds of surgery. During this time efforts are made to improve the respiratory status of the patient as much as possible. Special exercises may be prescribed to strengthen chest and shoulder muscles and accessory muscles of respiration and to remove accumulated secretions from the air passages.

Arm and leg exercises also are taught preoperatively to avoid thrombophlebitis in the lower extremities and problems with movement of the arm on the operative side. Movement of the arm may be very painful, because of either the position in which the patient was placed during surgery or the surgical severing of muscles that control the arm. If the arm is not moved in spite of discomfort, it is possible that the patient will develop a "frozen" (immobile) shoulder.

Preoperative patient education also should include teaching the patient any techniques he will be expected to use after surgery to improve ventilation to his lungs. He will need to know about chest tubes, suctioning, mechanical ventilation, and any other procedures that are anticipated as a part of his care postoperatively.

POSTOPERATIVE CARE

During the immediate postoperative period, nursing assessment and intervention are focused on special observations (in addition to routine postoperative ones), positioning, routine turning, coughing and deep breathing, and attention to chest tubes and the closed drainage system. In spite of the tubes and machines used postoperatively, the patient with chest surgery usually must ambulate early.

Observations

Special observations include watching for signs of pneumothorax, hemothorax, or both; symptoms of respiratory distress; and auscultation and palpation of the upper chest and neck for swelling caused by *subcutaneous emphysema*, which is an accumulation of air or gas under the skin. It usually occurs after thoracic surgery when air leaks into the tissues around chest tubes. It could be a sign of malfunctioning of the drainage system and should be reported. Assessment for signs of infection, both respiratory and incisional, is very important.

Gastric distention and paralytic ileus also are possible complications of thoracic surgery. Distention of the stomach and intestines is particularly hazardous for the postthoracotomy patient, as it can cause these organs to push up on the diaphragm and impair ventilation, which is already severely compromised by the surgery.

Positioning

Positioning for comfort, optimal ventilation, and adequate drainage of the operative site is an important aspect of postthoracotomy care. In most cases the patient is allowed to lie on his back and operative side. Many surgeons do not permit lying on the unaffected side, because this position diminishes expansion of the good lung. There also is danger of infection of the good lung by drainage from the side of the affected lung if the patient lies with the operative side uppermost. When the patient has a tube inserted for drainage from the operative site, lying on the operative side facilitates the flow of drainage. Care must be taken when positioning the patient to prevent kinking the chest tubes.

A pneumonectomy patient is *never turned onto his unoperated side.* There are two reasons for this. First, tension pneumothorax and mediastinal shift could occur. Second, the bronchial stump where the lung was removed could burst, and the patient could drown in accumulated fluids.

When in doubt about positioning a patient who has had chest surgery, it is always best to check the physician's orders before turning the patient or raising the head of the bed.

Chest Tubes and Closed Drainage

Of all the special procedures and techniques used in the care of a patient who has had chest surgery, the use of tubes and a drainage system to allow reexpansion of the lung is probably the most anxiety-producing for many nurses (Fig. 17–12).

Tubes and drainage systems need not be so threatening if one understands the anatomy and physiology of the bronchi, lungs, and pleura and the basic laws of physics.

Care of Patients With Chest Tubes and Closed Drainage

Chest tubes inserted during surgery may be attached to any of a variety of drainage systems. Among these are *water-sealed drainage bottles,* which may be one, two, or three in number. Disposable, self-contained systems include Pleur-evac and the Argyle Double-Seal. Whatever system is used, its purposes are (1) to provide for drainage of air and blood from within the pleural cavity and (2) to allow for gradual reexpansion of the lung. Figure 17–13 shows one-bottle, two-bottle, and three-bottle closed drainage systems. Note that the water serves as a seal to avoid the return of air to the chest cavity. Figure 17–14 shows a Pleur-evac apparatus, which is more commonly used. This is a disposable unit that contains all three chambers in one. The collection chamber is calibrated for more accurate measurement of drainage from the chest. It also contains float valves, which prevent the entry of air or fluid back up into the chest.

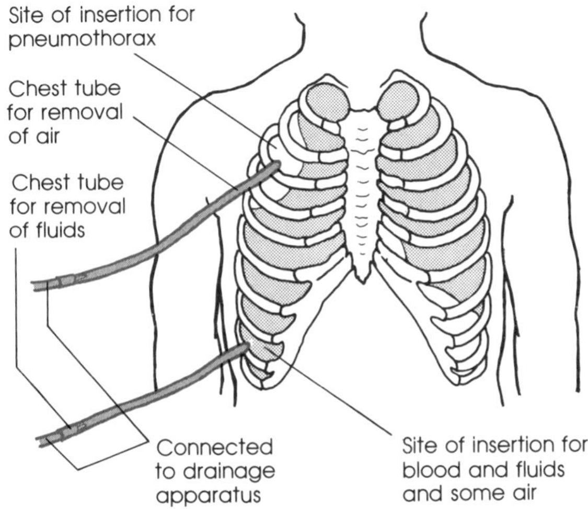

Figure 17–12 Location of sites for insertion of chest tubes for drainage of air and fluids. The tube in the upper chest is for removal of air. The lower tube is for removal of blood, fluids, and some air.

A flutter valve may be substituted in closed chest drainage systems. This valve permits the flow of air and fluid from the pleural space into a collection area but prevents the return flow of air or fluid and is inserted between the chest tube and the drainage collection apparatus.

CARING FOR A CLOSED DRAINAGE SYSTEM

- Remember that the pleural cavity is an airtight compartment. The apparatus and all connections must remain airtight at all times.
- Do not raise the drainage bottle from a thoracotomy tube above the level of the surgical incision. To do so may cause air and possibly drainage fluid to reenter the thoracic cavity.
- Do not allow the tubing to become kinked or obstructed by the weight of the patient.
- Never pin the tubing to the bed clothes.
- Do not empty thoracotomy drainage bottles. If the bottle becomes full, replace the bottle according to hospital procedure.
- Dressings may be reinforced but are not changed except by order of the surgeon.

Special Aspects of Patient Care. Regular and frequent monitoring of the patient with a chest tube is an essential part of his nursing care. There are three major areas of assessment: the respiratory status of the patient, the site at which the tube is inserted into the chest, and the drainage tubing attached to the chest tube.

The patient is assessed for ease of breathing, pain or discomfort, level of consciousness and orientation, and anxiety and restlessness. The rate and character of respirations are noted, as are breath sounds.

The entry site is assessed for unusual drainage, integrity of sutures, and the presence of subcutaneous emphysema.

The drainage tubing must be patent at all times, unless clamped off by the surgeon or momentarily in an emergency when there is leakage of air. It cannot be occluded by kinks, compression, or dependent loops; otherwise gas, air, and fluid have no way of escaping from the pleural cavity. It must be airtight; otherwise air will enter the pleural cavity and collapse the lung. All connections should be taped.

In addition to respiratory distress in the pa-

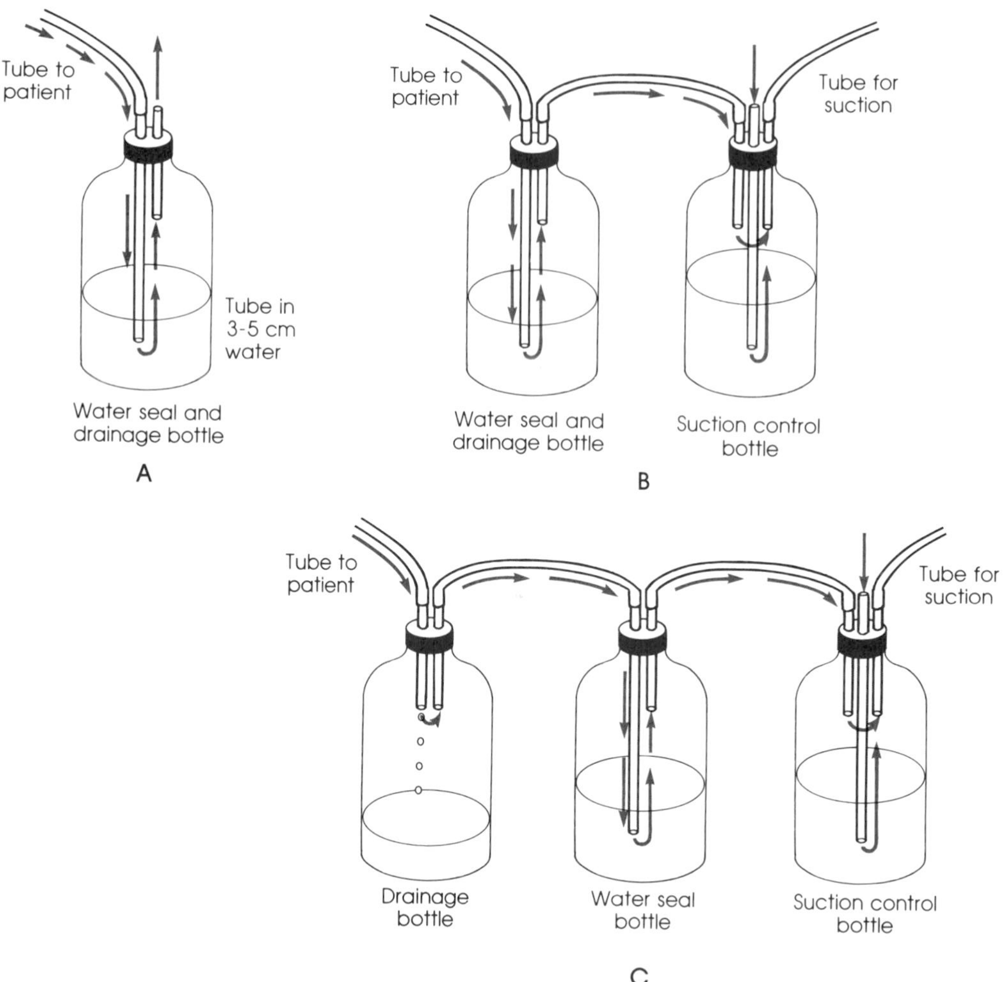

Figure 17-13 One-, two-, and three-bottle methods for providing a closed drainage system. *A*, In the one-bottle system the drainage via the chest tube enters the bottle through the glass tube that has one end submerged under water to form a seal. This provides a one-way valve that prevents a backflow of air into the pleural cavity, which could collapse the lung. As fluid and air from the pleural cavity enter the drainage bottle, the air that is displaced in the bottle is vented through the short tube above water level. *B*, The second bottle in the two-bottle system acts as a trap to control and decrease the amount of suction within the chest tube. Otherwise, the suction might be too forceful and damage the pleural membrane. No drainage enters this bottle. Its only purpose is to control the force of suction applied. *C*, The third bottle in the three-bottle system also is used to regulate the amount of suction. This can be done by adjusting the length of the glass tube that is under water.

tient, conditions that require immediate attention are:

- Persistent bubbling in the underwater seal. Fluid in the tube *should* fluctuate as the patient breathes air in and out.
- Fluid drainage through the chest tube accumulating at a rate of more than 100 mL per hour.
- A "puffed-up" appearance caused by leakage of air (subcutaneous emphysema) into the subcutaneous tissues in the upper chest and neck.
- Leakage of air around the junctions in the chest tube and drainage tube and bottles or Pleur-evac or Argyle Double-Seal.

When the surgeon removes the chest tubes, he probably will cover the incision with a dressing containing sterile petroleum jelly to close off the opening so that air does not enter the pleural space. Eventually the incision will seal itself.

A sample plan for care of a patient having thoracic surgery is shown in Nursing Care Plan 17-2.

COMMON RESPIRATORY PATIENT CARE PROBLEMS

INEFFECTIVE AIRWAY CLEARANCE

When a person coughs, he suddenly and noisily expels air from the pulmonary alveoli. A cough usually is a reflex triggered by a foreign substance or some other irritant in the respiratory tract. Sometimes, when coughing is needed to bring up secretions from the lower respiratory

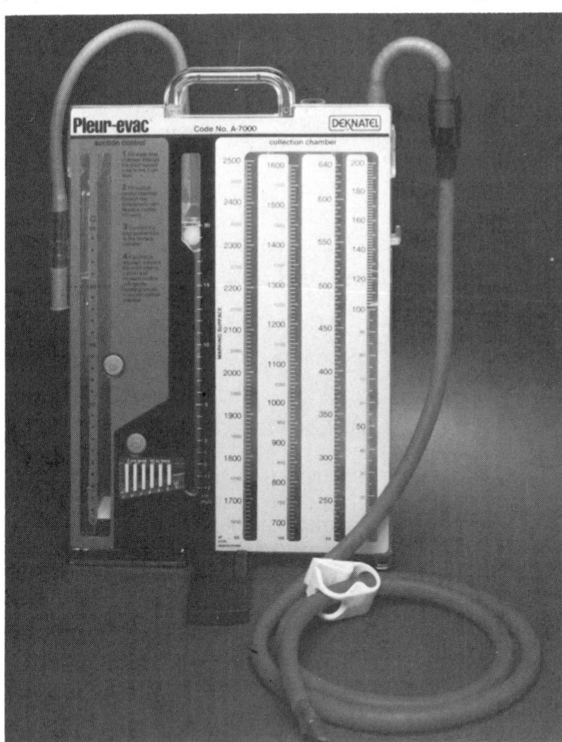

Figure 17–14 Pleur-evac.
(Courtesy of Deknatel, Floral Park, N.Y.)

tract, the patient is instructed to cough voluntarily.

Coughing can be beneficial if it is effective in clearing the air passages and removing accumulations of stagnant mucus. It can be harmful if done excessively, because it can exhaust the patient and traumatize the respiratory tissues and thoracic structures. A chronic cough can greatly limit one's activities, even eating, because the person hesitates to do anything that might trigger a bout of severe coughing.

Prolonged coughing in patients with cardiac problems can be very serious. The Valsalva maneuver can, as previously explained, increase the workload of the heart and increase intracranial pressure. Effective coughing techniques usually must be taught to the patient. *He should be told that it is better to avoid unnecessary and ineffective coughing as much as possible.* Sometimes, if he will voluntarily suppress a cough for a moment or two, when he does cough he will be better able to remove secretions.

The nurse should explain that deep breathing and coughing maneuvers are the most effective ways to remove sputum.

When administering medications prescribed for a cough, the nurse should know the expected action of the medication and the correct procedure for giving cough mixtures. Not all cough medicines have the same effect and not all are given to suppress coughing.

Antitussive agents inhibit the cough reflex in the cough center in the brain. Many sedative cough mixtures contain codeine or other drugs that decrease the desire to cough. *Expectorant cough medicines* aid in the raising of mucus from the bronchial tree so that they are more easily expectorated. The liquefying agents and diluents discussed later in this chapter are examples of expectorants.

Cough syrups are given to soothe the nerve endings in the respiratory mucosa. These medications are given in small doses to coat and protect the throat. *Water should not be taken immediately after a cough syrup.*

SECRETIONS

Many acute upper respiratory infections are transmitted by droplet infection; that is, the causative organisms are expelled along with the liquid secretions released during coughing and sneezing. Cores of the droplets expelled from the nose or mouth continue to float in the air after the liquid evaporates. These cores are called *droplet nuclei,* and they are teeming with bacteria or viruses when an infection is present.

In order to avoid the transmission of infectious agents from the respiratory tract, the nurse should carefully avoid contaminating herself and should instruct the patient in the proper ways of handling and disposing of secretions. She should stand to the side of a patient who is coughing and sneezing. After each contact with the patient or with articles contaminated by secretions, the hands should be washed thoroughly.

Most patients are not offended by tactfully being told to place a folded tissue over the nose and mouth while sneezing and to turn the head away from the nurse whenever close contact is necessary, as in a bed bath or other nursing procedures.

Care must be used in handling all nasal secretions and sputum. Disposable tissues are used and discarded in a small plastic or paper bag within reach of the patient. A used tissue should never be put in the pocket of one's clothing. If a patient has such a copious amount of sputum that tissues are not practical, he should be given a waxed sputum cup with a cover and instructed in its use.

In bacterial infections and chronic respiratory diseases, the sputum often is foul smelling, leaving a bad taste in the mouth and offensive breath odor. Frequent oral hygiene is important for patients with this problem. Mouth care is especially needed before meals, when the taste or odor of the sputum may adversely affect the appetite. *Frequent mouth care also helps remove pathogenic microorganisms from the oral cavity and thereby diminishes the possibility that they will be aspirated deep into the air passages.*

Mechanical suctioning of excessive amounts of secretions in the respiratory passages is indicated when the patient cannot clear his airway. Removal of secretions from the nose, mouth, and throat (nasopharyngeal suctioning) is a relatively safe and simple procedure. Deep tracheal suctioning, whether through the nose, mouth, or tracheal tube, however, should only be per-

NURSING CARE PLAN 17–2

Selected nursing diagnoses, goals/outcome criteria, nursing interventions, and evaluations for a patient having thoracic surgery

Situation: A 58-year-old male smoker with a diagnosis of early lung cancer is scheduled for a right thoracotomy and lobectomy. He has no other medical problems except mild arthritis, for which he occasionally takes aspirin.

Nursing Diagnosis	Goals/Outcome Criteria	Nursing Intervention	Evaluation
Knowledge deficit related to postoperative care for thoracotomy. SUPPORTING DATA "I've never had surgery before."	Patient will demonstrate leg and arm exercises. Patient will verbalize understanding of postoperative routine of frequent monitoring of vital signs, chest tube care, and respiratory treatments	Teach deep breathing, coughing, arm and leg exercises; obtain return demonstration. Explain kind and purpose of tubes, drainage apparatus, and oxygen equipment. Explain need for early ambulation. Describe methods of pain control.	Returned demonstration of turning, coughing, exercises, and deep breathing; states tubes he will have postoperatively; verbalizes understanding of pain control method with PCA pump.
Postoperative period: Potential impaired gas exchange related to surgical removal of portion of lung and possible complications. SUPPORTING DATA Thoracotomy and lobectomy.	Patient will display normal respiratory rate and normal blood gas exchange within 36 hours.	Position patient on back or operative side; turn, cough, and deep breathe q 2 h; splint incision with small pillow to minimize pain. Administer humidified oxygen as ordered. Monitor vital signs q 4 h and respirations frequently; auscultate lung fields q shift; monitor blood gas levels. Medicate adequately for pain control to promote better cooperation with respiratory therapy, coughing, and deep breathing, but avoid oversedation and respiratory depression. Maintain intact, functioning closed chest drainage system. Observe for signs of subcutaneous emphysema; assess for signs of pulmonary embolism. Monitor abdomen for signs of distention or ileus, which could cause pressure on diaphragm.	TCDB, 8, 10, 12, and 2; splinting with pillow; oxygen per nasal cannula on continuously; lung fields clear to auscultation; using PCA appropriately; chest tube system intact, fluid fluctuating properly; blood gases: Po_2, 76; Pco_2, 46; HCO_3, 26. resp., 26 min; continue plan.
Potential for infection related to surgical incisions and chest tubes. SUPPORTING DATA Thoracotomy and lobectomy; chest tube in place.	No signs of infection as evidenced by clean incision, temperature in normal range, normal WBC count, and clear breath sounds.	Use aseptic technique for dressing changes and care of chest tube. Assess temperature trends q 24 h; monitor WBCs. Auscultate lungs q shift. Observe wound for signs of infection. Protect from people with infections; maintain adequate nutrition and fluid intake.	Incision clean and dry; temp., 100°F; WBC, 10,000; breath sounds clear bilaterally; continue plan.

NURSING CARE PLAN 17–2, *Continued*

Nursing Diagnosis	Goals/Outcome Criteria	Nursing Intervention	Evaluation
Anxiety related to diagnosis of cancer of the lung, treatment, and prognosis. SUPPORTING DATA "I'm scared. I don't want to die of cancer. Will I have to have chemotherapy? Will there be a lot of pain?"	Patient will cope positively with diagnosis of cancer by determined attitude to do whatever he can to fight the cancer by discharge.	Establish trusting relationship; use active listening. Encourage verbalization of fears and concerns; answer questions honestly. Establish hope; discuss what patient can do to optimize chances of survival: quit smoking, exercise program, diet, relaxation techniques, stress reduction. Advise that oncologist will discuss modes of treatment after full pathology report is back. Focus on positives of his life now and for each day in the future; assure him that pain control is possible.	Asking questions about radiation therapy; has quit smoking; wants to learn relaxation techniques; continue plan.

formed using strict aseptic technique by someone experienced in the correct procedure.

The need for suctioning should be determined on an individual basis. Some patients may require suctioning only once or twice daily to remove deeply situated pools and plugs of mucus that cannot be brought up by coughing. Others require suctioning every 10 to 15 minutes to clear their air passages. It should be remembered that the purpose of suctioning is to facilitate breathing and allow for an adequate exchange of carbon dioxide and oxygen in the lungs. Even though the procedure may be necessary, the suctioning process removes oxygen, which is the very substance the patient needs to relieve his distress.

There are some basic guidelines that should be helpful to the nurse in avoiding the serious consequences of oxygen removal by suctioning.

1. ***Preoxygenate the patient before suctioning by (a) using an Ambu bag attached to 100% oxygen for 2 minutes or (b) using the sigh mechanism on the ventilator 2 to 3 times over a few minutes. Repeat this procedure after suctioning and between repeated sessions of suctioning.***
2. ***Suction no longer than 10 to 15 seconds; holding your own breath while suction is applied is one way to avoid suctioning too long.***
3. ***Suction gauge pressure should be between 80 and 100 mm Hg when the tubing is unoccluded; no higher pressure should be used.***
4. ***If tachycardia or other cardiac arrhythmia develops during suctioning, stop and hyperoxygenate unless the airway is badly occluded by secretions.***

The reader is cautioned that these are only *basic guidelines*. Anyone attempting to suction the bronchi and trachea of a patient in respiratory distress should have additional instruction in the technique and adequate supervision until he or she becomes proficient at it.

DYSPNEA OR BREATHLESSNESS

We have all experienced at some time in our lives the near panic one feels when breathing is obstructed. It is understandable how the patient who must struggle for breath or feels that he is smothering is suffering from mental anxiety as well as physical stress. Unfortunately, the mental anxiety can only aggravate the situation and increase the distress.

Nursing actions that can help relieve dyspnea and its consequences include proper positioning so that the respiratory passages are able to function as best they can, administering oxygen as prescribed by the physician, and assuring the patient that everything possible is being done to bring relief.

The position that best facilitates breathing is the semi-Fowler's or high Fowler's position. The shoulders and back should be supported with a pillow to allow for full expansion of the lungs

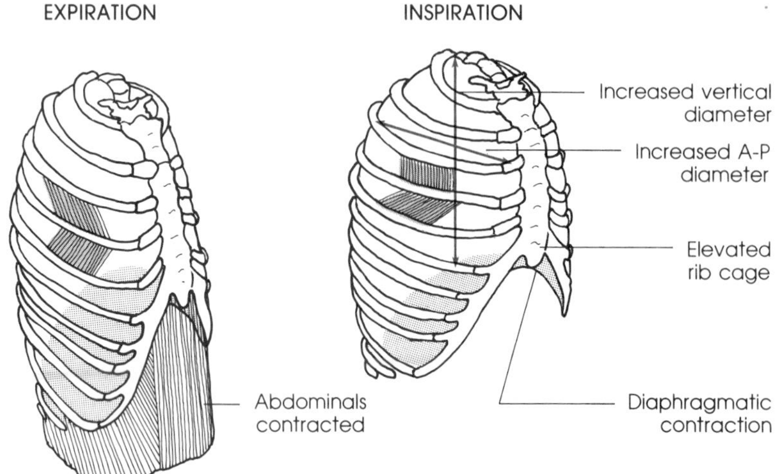

Figure 17-15 Expansion and contraction of the thoracic cage during inspiration and expiration, illustrating especially diaphragmatic contraction, elevation of the rib cage, and function of the intercostals.

(Redrawn and adapted from Guyton, A. C.: Human Physiology and Mechanisms of Disease, 4th ed. Philadelphia, W. B. Saunders, 1987.)

and to keep the chin off the chest. The diaphragm and the intercostal muscles are responsible for the mechanical expansion of the thoracic cavity, which allows the lungs to inflate with air. Downward movement of the diaphragm during inspiration lengthens the chest cavity; upward movement has the opposite effect. During inspiration the intercostals elevate the ribs and increase the diameter of the chest (Fig. 17-15). Proper positioning and support of the body parts will allow these muscles to function at their maximum efficiency.

For severe dyspnea, the orthopneic position is most effective. The term *orthopnea* means the ability to breathe only in the upright position (Fig. 17-16). The patient should sit upright, lean over the overbed table, which is padded with pillows, and elevate and round the shoulders to allow maximum expansion of the lungs.

Another factor to be considered in caring for the dyspneic patient is that of pressure from organs below or near the lungs and diaphragm. A full stomach can contribute to dyspnea by limiting the amount of space available for expansion of the lungs. For this reason, small, frequent feedings are preferred to three large meals a day. Abdominal distention due to a collection of flatus and fecal material also can make breathing more difficult.

ALTERATIONS IN NUTRITION AND HYDRATION

Anorexia and inadequate nutrition are not uncommon in patients with respiratory disorders, particularly when the disorder is chronic in nature.

Reasons for this are (1) the senses of taste and smell may be impaired by nasal congestion, (2) the patient might be afraid that chewing and swallowing will bring on an attack of coughing, (3) purulent sputum leaves a bad taste in the mouth and can cause nausea, and (4) fatigue can deprive the patient of the will to expend the energy needed to feed himself.

Nursing intervention to help overcome the problem of loss of appetite and poor nutrition should start with the environment in which the patient eats his meals. His hospital room should be kept clean, uncluttered, and orderly. Used tissues are disposed of promptly, and sputum cups are kept covered and out of sight.

Good oral hygiene and frequent mouth care can help diminish mouth odor and nausea. Smaller, more frequent feedings of nutritious liquids and foods are preferable to three large, heavy meals.

Because there is an increased energy expenditure when breathing is difficult, many patients

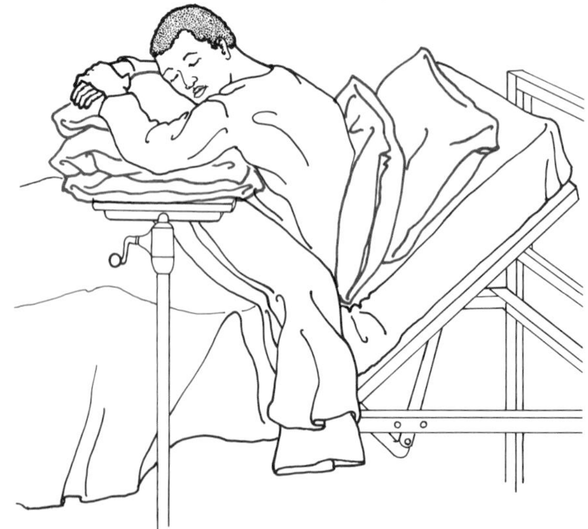

Figure 17-16 Orthopneic position, used when the patient has difficulty breathing and is more comfortable in a sitting position. Pillows are used to support the back. Other pillows are placed on an overbed table to support the weight of the arms, shoulders, and head.

have difficulty maintaining weight even when they do take in normal amounts of calories. Supplements are now available that have increased fat content and provide more calories in smaller quantities than can be accomplished with carbohydrate substances. Pulmocare is one such supplement. When a patient is receiving mechanical ventilation his caloric needs rise considerably. Sometimes total parenteral nutrition (TPN) or lipid infusions are necessary in order to prevent malnutrition in a patient with severe COPD.

A fluid deficit is likely in patients with respiratory disorders because there is an increased loss of fluid in repiratory secretions. The patient usually breathes through his mouth and exhales large amounts of moisture from his body. Without adequate replacement of these fluids, he can become dehydrated very quickly. Unless contraindicated the patient is encouraged to drink at least 3,000 mL of liquid each day. These should include low-sodium bouillon, fruit juices, and other liquids in addition to water.

Humidifying the air breathed by the patient is an effective way to minimize dehydration and liquefy secretions in the air pasages. It is especially important to the patient whose secretions are thick and tenacious and difficult to cough up. Humidification of inhaled air is covered below under "Common Therapeutic Measures."

FATIGUE

Hypoxia, which is an oxygen deficit in the tissues, produces a loss of energy because it causes a disturbance in cellular metabolism. Patients with respiratory disorders often have hypoxia and, to make matters worse, must use the little energy they have to struggle for breath and cough up secretions.

Patients with respiratory disorders, whether acute or chronic, have some degree of intolerance to physical activity and therefore need periods of rest throughout the day. Treatments and medications should be scheduled so that the patient can rest without interruption. As with any inflammation, repair of damaged tissue is facilitated by rest of the affected part. In order to rest the lungs, the patient should lie down for short periods. Long naps during the day are not recommended, because they interfere with a restful sleep at night.

Although rest is needed, we also cannot ignore the dangers of physical inactivity and the disabilities that can result. The goal of nursing care, therefore, should be to achieve a satisfactory balance of rest and activity.

Deep breathing exercises and coughing techniques should be planned whenever the patient is able to do these on his own or with some assistance. These activities should be followed by good mouth care and a short period of uninterrupted rest. A schedule of *purposeful* activity and adequate rest can be most beneficial to the patient in helping him avoid additional disabilities.

The problem of fatigue and nursing intervention for the patient with chronic lung disease were covered earlier in this chapter.

COMMON THERAPEUTIC MEASURES

MEDICATIONS

A wide variety of drugs are used to treat respiratory disorders. Patients often are taking several drugs simultaneously, and it is vitally important that the nurse monitor for side effects and drug interactions. Theophylline preparations are tolerated better if they are taken after meals so that there is less stomach upset. The pulse should be assessed before and after the patient takes this medication. If the pulse increases more than 20 to 30 beats, the physician should be notified. Patients taking theophylline derivatives should have serum drug levels assessed periodically; therapeutic range is 8 to 20 gm/mL. Patients receiving IV aminophylline must be monitored for hypotension.

When corticosteroids are part of the patient's drug therapy, he must be closely watched for infection, as steroids mask the signs and symptoms. He must be cautioned never to abruptly stop taking a steroid drug; it is to be slowly tapered over several days to prevent the serious problems of abrupt steroid withdrawal. Potassium loss must be replaced and monitoring for elevated blood glucose performed.

Antihistamines are used to treat respiratory manifestations of an allergic disorder. They reduce secretions of the nasal and bronchial mucosa. *Decongestants* are prescribed for symptoms of the common cold and sinusitis.

Metered dose inhalers are used to deliver a variety of drugs to the respiratory patient. The patient should be taught to exhale completely, insert the mouthpiece of the inhaler into his mouth, and depress the cylinder while inhaling deeply. The breath is then held for a few seconds before exhaling. It is important to have the patient demonstrate his use of an inhaler in order to determine if his technique is correct.

Bronchodilators are drugs that act directly on the smooth muscle of the bronchi to relax them and thereby relieve bronchospasms. Among the bronchodilators are *aminophylline*, *epinephrine hydrochloride* (adrenalin and Vaponefrin), *isoproterenol hydrochloride* (Isuprel), *ephedrine sulfate*, and adrenergic drugs such as *metaproterenol* (Alupent) and *terbutaline* (Brethine).

Liquefying agents and *diluents* help to thin the

bronchial secretions, making them more liquid and less tenacious. Preparations of this type include *acetylcysteine* (Mucomyst), distilled water, and *tyloxapol* (Alevaire).

Antiinfectives are helpful in controlling infectious agents in the respiratory tract. These include the tetracyclines, penicillin, cephalosporin antibiotics (cephalothin, Keflin), ciprofloxacin (Cipro), streptomycin, and the sulfa drugs.

Bronchodilators, liquefying agents, and some anti-infectives may be adminstered directly onto the mucous membranes of the respiratory tract by means of nebulizers and mechanical ventilators.

HUMIDIFICATION

The respiratory passageways are constructed so that air passing through the nose and on through the airways is warm and moist when it reaches the lower structures. A respiratory infection can interfere with this normal process of *humidification* of inhaled air. In order to provide the humidity needed, *aerosols* are sometimes used.

Aerosols are fine suspensions of very small particles of a liquid or solid that constitute a gas. Water is the most important of all aerosols in respiratory therapy. Without adequate humidity, mucous secretions become extremely thick and tenacious, and the mucous membranes become dry, crusted, and irritated. They are then more susceptible to invasion by pathogenic microorganisms. Aerosols other than water include the aforementioned drugs.

The four general purposes of aerosol and humidity therapy are (1) relief of edema and spasms of the bronchi, (2) liquefaction of bronchial secretions, (3) delivery of medication, and (4) humidification of the respiratory mucosa.

Instruments used to produce aerosols are called *nebulizers* and *humidifiers*. Nebulizers are designed to deliver a maximum number of particles of drugs or water to the respiratory tract. They produce an aerosol by forcing air or oxygen through a solution. There are simple hand nebulizers as well as more complex ones, such as those attached to oxygen systems and mechanical ventilators.

When a hand-held nebulizer is used, the patient should sit upright with the chin pointed slightly upward. The nebulizer cartridge should be shaken before beginning the treatment. The patient fully exhales, begins inhaling, and depresses the cartridge fully, continuing to inhale slowly and as deeply as possible. He should hold his breath for a few seconds and then slowly exhale. Equipment should be cleaned after each treatment to minimize the risk of infection.

Humidifiers are designed to deliver a maximum amount of water vapor into the air the patient breathes. They actually humidify the air in a room. They are most helpful in diseases of the upper respiratory tract, because they do not break the water into particles small enough to be inhaled deep into the bronchioles.

Patients should be instructed in the purposes of humidification; otherwise they may resist the treatment. When humidification is first started, it may temporarily increase the difficulty in breathing, because the water further obstructs the passage of air. However, as the secretions are liquefied and more easily coughed up, the air passages become less obstructed, and breathing becomes easier. The patient will, of course, need to know how to cough effectively so that maximum benefit of the treatment can be achieved.

PULMONARY HYGIENE

Patients with chronic pulmonary disease can benefit from a program of pulmonary hygiene that is designed to (1) remove secretions for more efficient exchange of oxygen and carbon dioxide and (2) help them control their breathing so that it is more effective in moving air in and out of the lungs.

Pulmonary hygiene programs are achieved by the administration of prescribed drugs, humidification of the air inhaled, intermittent positive pressure breathing (IPPB) therapy, nebulizer and metered dose inhaler therapy, chest physiotherapy, and breathing exercises.

Medications and humidification have been discussed; IPPB therapy is covered later in this chapter.

Chest physiotherapy includes postural drainage when possible, and percussion and vibration. *Postural drainage* involves positioning the patient so that the forces of gravity can help in the removal of secretions deep in the bronchi and lungs. The nurse who assists a patient with postural drainage should obtain specific directions from the physician or physical therapist so that she can position the patient properly. She also may need to use certain tapping, clapping, and vibrating techniques during postural drainage. These measures are carried out for the purpose of dislodging mucus plugs so that they can be coughed up more easily. They must be done with precision and only by someone who has received adequate instruction in the proper technique. Improper clapping and vibrating can cause much discomfort to the patient and accomplish little more than upsetting him to the point that he refuses the treatment. Family members can be taught the procedures if they are to be continued after the patient goes home.

Because there is likely to be some gagging during coughing episodes that take place during postural drainage, it is best to carry out the procedure before meals, when the stomach is relatively empty and vomiting is less likely.

If the patient is to have postural drainage only once a day, it should be done in the morning when he awakens. At this time, secretions that have accumulated during the night can be removed. After postural drainage is completed, good mouth care, including tooth brushing and a refreshing mouth wash, should be done.

The most important aspects of breathing exercises include blowing through pursed lips, exhaling slowly, and *not* forcing the air out of the lungs (this can bring about collapse of the airway structures). Breathing through pursed lips is described in Table 17–5.

The mechanics of respiration can become less efficient as chronic respiratory disease progresses. The patient suffers a loss of lung elasticity, a flattened diaphragm, and fixation of the rib cage as he becomes more and more dependent on the muscles of his upper chest and neck for breathing. The purpose of breathing exercises is to help correct this situation by strengthening the abdominal muscles so that they can push upward against the diaphragm and assist in the expiration of air from the lungs. These exercises also help overcome rigidity of the thorax so that the lungs can inflate and deflate more easily.

Patients who follow the exercises prescribed for them often find that they can lead more active and useful lives than formerly possible, because their exertional dyspnea is less severe. This means that they can make better use of all the muscles of their body and are less likely to develop complications that accompany immobility. They also are better able to cough up secretions that would otherwise remain in the lower bronchi and serve as a growth medium for bacteria or as a cause of atelectasis. The psychological value of being able to indulge in ordinary activities that once left the patient breathless cannot be overestimated. Abdominal and diaphragmatic breathing are also described in Table 17–5.

OXYGEN THERAPY

The air we breathe contains about 20% oxygen. Under normal circumstances, this percentage is adequate for maintaining a balance between supply and cellular demand for oxygen. Tissues vary in their oxygen requirements. The cerebral cells, for example, receive 20% of the body's oxygen supply and can live for only a few minutes if their oxygen supply is cut off. Other cells, such as those of the myocardium, can survive as long as 30 to 40 minutes without a fresh supply of oxygen. We can see why it has been said that hypoxia not only stops the machine, it also wrecks the machinery.

Dosage

Because oxygen acts as a drug, it must be prescribed and administered in specific doses in order to avoid oxygen toxicity. The dosage of oxygen is stated in terms of *concentration* and *rate of flow*.

High concentrations above 50% may be prescribed to treat acute conditions in which the patient can benefit from prompt treatment of hypoxia, as in cardiovascular failure and pulmonary edema. The rate of flow may be as high as 12 liters per minute.

Moderate concentrations of oxygen usually are prescribed when increased metabolic rate raises the consumption of oxygen, or when there is poor distribution of oxygen because of either congestive heart failure or pulmonary embolism. The concentrations of oxygen given in a moderate dosage are about 23% at a rate of flow of 4 to 7 liters per minute.

Low concentrations of oxygen of about 23% delivered at a rate of 1 to 4 liters per minute are indicated when the patient needs oxygen over an extended period. Patients with chronic respiratory insufficiency who can utilize only a minimum amount of oxygen in a given period of time usually are given low doses of oxygen.

The above percentages and rates of flow are approximate amounts. The exact dosage depends on the method of administration and the patient's individual need for additional oxygen supply.

Short-term oxygen therapy, which is the administration of oxygen to treat hypoxemia, is indicated when (1) there is an inadequate intake of oxygen because of obstruction or restriction of the flow of air through the air passages, (2) oxygen is not distributed throughout the body because of circulatory failure, (3) there is an inadequate supply of hemoglobin to transport the oxygen, and (4) carbon dioxide or other gases displace the oxygen in the blood. Objective criteria for oxygen needs include $Pa{O_2}$ less than 60 mm Hg or $Sa{O_2}$ less than 90%.

Outward signs of hypoxia vary in patients and therefore cannot be completely relied on as indications that additional oxygen is needed. The most reliable indicators are the results obtained from blood gas analysis and determination of the blood pH. Not all patients with hypoxia can benefit from oxygen therapy.

Long-term oxygen therapy for patients with COPD is used (1) to relieve hypoxemia; (2) to reverse tissue hypoxia and its signs and symptoms; and (3) to allow the patient to function better mentally and physically, thereby allowing greater self-reliance. Home oxygen units and portable units are available for patients who require long-term therapy.

The patient with COPD may suffer adversely from inappropriate dosages of oxygen. Over a long period of time, these patients can gradually adapt to a diminished supply of oxygen. The brain normally responds to oxygen deficiency by increasing the respiratory rate; however, after repeated warnings that more oxygen is needed, the brain no longer responds in this way. Thus the respiratory control center of a patient with COPD does not react to hypoxia, and his respiratory rate is not increased.

Because the reaction of the respiratory center to the presence of oxygen causes a decrease in respiratory movements, oxygen is said to be a *respiratory depressant.* If it is given in high concentrations and at a rapid rate to a patient with a chronic respiratory ailment that has caused him to hypoventilate habitually, the oxygen only serves to further depress the respirations and slow down the intake of oxygen. The result is a buildup of carbon dioxide in the blood and eventual respiratory acidosis.

Oxygen Toxicity

Even though oxygen is essential to life, excessive amounts can have serious adverse effects on the tissues of the body. High concentrations of inhaled oxygen can bring about collapse of the alveoli, because the oxygen displaces some of the nitrogen there. Another effect of high oxygen concentration is an interruption in the production of *pulmonary surfactant.* This is a substance that stabilizes the alveoli and prevents atelectasis.

In certain situations, the eyes and the central nervous system can be irreparably damaged by high levels of oxygen. The eyes of premature babies who are exposed to excess oxygen can be permanently injured. The condition is called *retinopathy of prematurity* and can produce permanent blindness because of pathologic changes in the structures behind the lens of the eye.

Modes of Administration

The manner in which additional oxygen is supplied to a patient depends on his particular need for oxygen and his physical condition.

Oxygen by Nasal Cannula

This is the simplest, most convenient, and most commonly used means of administering oxygen (Fig. 17–17). The two-pronged nasal cannula is inserted one-fourth to one-half inch into each nostril. *This method does not provide sufficient oxygen concentration for a patient with severe hypoxemia.*

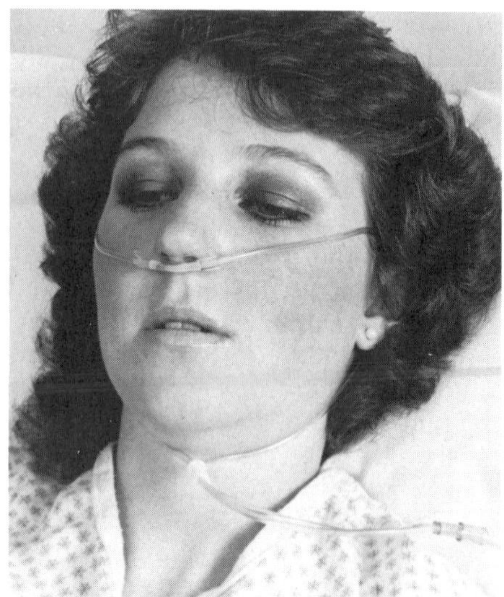

Figure 17–17 Oxygen by nasal cannula. (Photo by Ken Kasper.)

Oxygen by Mask

If oxygen is administered by mask, care must be taken to ensure that the mask fits snugly and follows the contour of the face (Fig. 17–18). It is comforting to the patient to have the mask removed periodically so that his face can be washed to prevent irritation of the skin. Obviously this procedure is carried out quickly, so that the patient does not suffer from a loss of oxygen therapy while the mask is removed.

The patient inhales from the mask, which is connected to 30% to 60% oxygen at a flow rate of

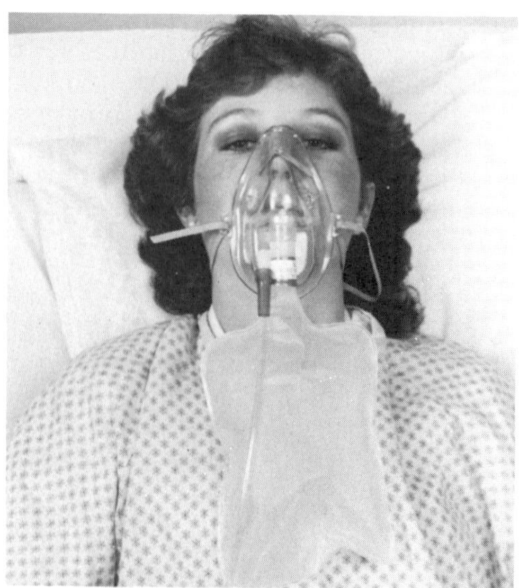

Figure 17–18 Oxygen by mask. (Photo by Ken Kasper.)

5 to 10 liters per minute. The mask is used for short-term therapy.

Oxygen by Partial Rebreathing Mask. The partial rebreathing mask is similar to the face mask but has a reservoir bag attached to it. Oxygen-rich air plus some room air from the exhalation ports in the mask is inhaled from the reservoir bag. About one-third of the exhaled air goes back into the reservoir bag. It provides 40% to 60% oxygen at 6 to 10 liters per minute and is used for acutely ill patients. The bag should not deflate completely.

Oxygen by Nonrebreathing Mask. This device has a one-way valve between the mask and the reservoir bag that prevents exhaled air from entering the bag. There are also flaps or valves on the sides of the mask to allow air to be exhaled out into the room, but no air from the room can be inhaled through these openings. The patient breathes pure oxygen from the reservoir bag. This mask provides 90% to 100% oxygen. The patient should be kept on this mask for as brief a time as possible to restore adequate PaO_2, as oxygen in this concentration can cause toxicity.

Oxygen by Venturi Mask. This mask can deliver the most precise dose of oxygen. It has a circle of holes on the sides and a flexible tube attached to the bottom of it. A concentration of 24% to 50% oxygen is mixed with room air in the flexible tubing. The amount of room air is controlled by an orifice whose opening can be adjusted. The exhaled air exits through the side exhalation ports. This mask can be used for both short- and long-term therapy.

Special Considerations

Regardless of the mode of administration, humidification of the oxygen is necessary to avoid drying out of the respiratory tract mucosa and thickening of secretions any time the liter flow is greater than 3 to 4 liters per minute. Humidity may be provided by passing the oxygen through water as it is administered to the patient or by aerosolizing the water and adding it to the oxygen.

Oxygen is *not* explosive. However, it does support combustion, which means that a spark or flame can cause a major fire in a very short time. The special precautions necessary for the prevention of such a catastrophe should be clearly stated in every hospital policy book or procedure manual. They must be followed without exception.

Other precautions include paying attention to conditions that can interfere with the flow of oxygen from the source to the patient. These may include kinks in the tubing, loose connections, and faulty humidifying apparatus. If there is some question about whether the oxygen is flowing properly, listen for the hissing sound of air passing into the catheter, mask, or tent. To determine whether the tubing is open and oxygen is passing through it, hold your finger over the end of the tube momentarily and then release it. You should hear a "pftt" sound as the oxygen escapes through the end of the tube. Remember that it is not unusual to find that a patient who is supposedly receiving oxygen therapy is actually getting less oxygen than he would under normal circumstances. The physician decides when the patient is to receive oxygen and by what method and in what concentration, but it is the nurse or respiratory therapist who must see to it that the oxygen is administered as prescribed.

Infection control is especially important so that cross-infection does not take place by way of the equipment that is used to administer oxygen. Humidifiers and nebulizers, being warm and moist, serve as excellent "hothouses" for the growth of pathogenic microorganisms. Although the use of disposable equipment reduces the possibility of contamination of the patient, it does not relieve nursing personnel and others who are concerned with patient care from the responsibility of observing basic principles of cleanliness and asepsis.

When oxygen therapy is discontinued, it is done so gradually. The patient is "weaned" from dependence on oxygen by reducing the dosage and then alternating periods of breathing room air with periods of breathing low concentrations of oxygen.

MECHANICAL VENTILATION

Mechanical ventilation is needed when the patient cannot maintain adequate ventilation because of respiratory, neurologic, or neuromuscular problems or trauma. There are two major types of basic ventilators used to give support to patients with ventilatory problems: negative-pressure and positive-pressure ventilators. Negative-pressure ventilators are mainly used for patients with normal vital capacities who have neuromuscular disease, CNS disorders (e.g., spinal cord damage), and COPD. Negative-pressure ventilators include the iron lung, cuirass, poncho, and body wrap ventilators.

Positive-pressure ventilators are seen far more frequently. There are several types of positive-pressure ventilators: (1) pressure-cycled, (2) time-cycled, (3) volume-cycled, and (4) high-frequency ventilation machines. These work by delivering a positive driving pressure to the patient's airway. The pressure delivered is greater than that within the airway and alveoli; therefore gas flows into the lungs and either assists or controls inhalation. When the pressure is released, exhalation takes place without effort on the part of the machine or the patient.

Pressure-cycled ventilators are those in which cycling is primarily dependent on a buildup of pressure within the patient's lungs. Gas continues to flow into the lungs until a preset airway pressure is reached. When the desired amount of pressure has been exerted, the flow of gas stops, and exhalation takes place spontaneously. This type of ventilator is used for short-term therapy, primarily for giving intermittent positive-pressure breathing (IPPB) treatments and to deliver medication to the bronchial tree such as bronchodilators and liquefying agents.

Time-cycled ventilators deliver air into the lungs for a preset length of time. The volume of gas delivered may vary. The Babybird and the Siemens Servo are examples of this type. These are mainly used for infants and children.

Volume-cycled ventilators deliver a preset volume of gas to the bronchi and lungs. Pressure limits are also set. If the ventilator meets with too much pressure to deliver the selected volume of gas, an alarm sounds to tell the nurse that the patient is not receiving the correct tidal volume. Most commonly this occurs because there is a buildup of secretions in the lungs and the patient needs to be suctioned. Ventilators of this type are most often used in a critical care setting in which severe chest disease or surgery has severely compromised normal respiratory function. This type of ventilator will deliver adequate tidal volume even when airway resistance is great (for example, in patients suffering from severe obstructive lung disease). Examples of volume-cycled ventilators include the MA-1 and the Bear-2.

Microprocessor-controlled ventilators are becoming more common as high-tech features are integrated into the various types of ventilators. They are mainly used for patients with adult respiratory distress syndrome, major burns, or multisystem failure.

High-frequency jet ventilation is used to supplement volume ventilation. It provides good ventilation of the patient with the use of relatively small tidal volumes at very high respiratory rates. The oxygenation and ventilation are accomplished by gas diffusion and convection rather than high flow of gas. Because the intrathoracic pressures needed for this type of ventilation are much lower, there are fewer of the complications (e.g., barotrauma, hypotension, and pneumothorax) associated with other types of ventilation.

There are several modes used for positive-pressure ventilation. In *controlled-mode* ventilation, the machine is set to deliver a fixed number of breaths per minute, no matter how the patient tries to breathe. This is used during periods of central nervous system depression such as during anesthesia and drug overdose.

In *assist mode*, the frequency of ventilation is determined by the patient. When he does take a breath, the machine is triggered to deliver a set tidal volume. This mode is not used alone in the clinical setting but is combined with the control function to provide an *assist-control mode*. If the patient's respiratory rate falls, the machine will deliver a set number of breaths per minute; if the patient is breathing within the set rate, the machine only assists by delivering the set tidal volume. This mode is mostly used in the clinical setting. It considerably decreases the work of breathing for the patient.

Intermittent mandatory ventilation (IMV) and *synchronized intermittent mandatory ventilation* (SIMV) are the most common modes of ventilation found in critical care settings. These modes allow the patient to breathe spontaneously and yet provide a preset number of ventilator breaths at a preset tidal volume to ensure adequate ventilation without respiratory muscle fatigue.

IMV can "stack" breaths when the machine delivers a breath at the end of normal inspiration on the part of the patient. SIMV is activated by the patient's own breath and is therefore synchronized with his breathing pattern. One of the main advantages of these modes is that the respiratory muscles do not become as weak during mechanical ventilation from lack of use, and it is then easier to wean the patient from the ventilator by steadily decreasing the number of mandatory breaths per minute.

Positive end-expiratory pressure (PEEP) can be delivered by most ventilators also. When using PEEP, the pressure in the airways never falls below a certain level (usually between 5 and 15 cm H_2O). This has the effect of holding the smaller air passages open and thus limiting atelectasis. It also holds alveoli in expansion so that there is more time for gas to diffuse across the alveolar membrane and hopefully correct hypoxemia. It is used for adult respiratory distress syndrome and respiratory failure where there is PaO_2 of less than 50 and a PCO_2 of greater than 50.

Continuous positive airway pressure (CPAP) can be used for patients who are breathing spontaneously but are showing signs of hypoxemia. It is used for infants with mild respiratory distress syndrome and for adults in the early stages of respiratory failure. The patient does not have to be intubated for CPAP to be used. It can be given with nasal prongs.

Nursing Intervention

Nursing responsibilities for patients on mechanical ventilation include checking the physician's order each shift and then the ventilator for the proper settings: mode, FIO_2, respiratory rate, tidal volume, peak inspiratory pressure, and PEEP. Alarms are checked to see that they are turned on. Alarms should not be turned off when disconnecting the patient to suction. Tubing should be kept clear of pooled water.

The patient is observed for signs of complications, such as gastric distention, pneumothorax, and impaired cardiac output from decreased venous return, and the need for increasingly higher pressures to deliver the set tidal volume, which can indicate stiffening of the lungs (decreased compliance). The nurse auscultates the lung fields to be certain that both lungs are being ventilated. Arterial blood gas levels are monitored to determine the effectiveness of ventilation treatment.

For ventilation to be effective, the lungs must be kept clear of secretions. Many patients can cough up secretions and do not need to be suctioned; others may need suctioning as frequently as every 15 minutes. Endotracheal and tracheal suctioning must be done with strict aseptic technique. Mechanical ventilation places the patient at considerably greater risk of respiratory infection because of its invasive nature.

The intubated patient on the ventilator cannot talk and must be given an alternative means of communication such as a Magic Slate or paper and pencil. Being hooked up to a ventilator is very frightening for most patients, and it is important that the nurse assure the alert patient that he will not be left alone.

Any time a patient is turned or repositioned, the endotracheal or tracheal tube must be checked to be certain that the ventilator tubes are not pulling on it too much.

Attention must be paid to adequate nutrition, as the patient cannot eat by mouth when he is connected to a ventilator. Additional calories are needed just to maintain weight when a ventilator is used. Continuous enteral feeding is the method most often used to prevent malnutrition in these patients; but whatever method is used, the nurse should keep an eye on nutritional parameters to assess whether nutrition is adequate.

If a ventilator alarm sounds and the problem cannot be located quickly, the patient should be disconnected from the machine and ventilated with an Ambu bag and oxygen until the problem is solved. Table 17–8 summarizes the dangers of mechanical ventilation.

Care for a patient who is being ventilated artificially by a ventilating machine is extremely complex. No one should care for such a patient without extensive training and supervised practice. The patient will require protection from infection, continuous monitoring of the vital signs, observations for hypoventilation and hyperventilation, measurement of intake and output, and prevention of the disabilities of inactivity.

Intermittent Positive-Pressure Breathing Therapy

Intermittent positive-pressure breathing treatments are used to expand the lungs more than is usual with spontaneous deep breathing. It is helpful in preventing atelectasis and pneumonia in bedridden patients.

IPPB therapy helps overcome bronchial resistance to the inward flow of air, allows for more uniform distribution of oxygen to the alveoli, aids in the removal of carbon dioxide, and makes coughing more effective in the removal of secretions that have accumulated in the lower respiratory tract.

TABLE 17–8 **DANGERS OF MECHANICAL VENTILATION**

Danger	Manifestations
Barotrauma	Sudden increase in peak inspiratory pressure; absent breath sounds over one area or lung; pneumomediastinum; pneumothorax; subcutaneous emphysema; high-pressure alarm goes off frequently.
Oxygen toxicity	Parenchymal damage and absorption atelectasis; alveolar membrane damage; nonproductive cough; decreasing vital capacity; decreased compliance; increased peak inspiratory pressure.
Impaired cardiac output	Decreased BP; poor peripheral perfusion; decreased level of consciousness.
Infection	Change in sputum color, quantity, and consistency; crackles and rhonchi; increased WBC count; fever; infiltrate on chest radiograph.
Fluid retention	Increasing body weight; fluid intake more than output; peripheral edema; crackles in lungs or diminished breath sounds.
Gastric distention	Increasing abdominal girth; complaint of distention; tender to palpation.
GI bleeding	Positive stool guaiac; "coffee grounds" aspirate from gastric suction; dropping hemoglobin; black or bloody stool.

For many years IPPB was the main method of delivering aerosol medications for liquefaction of secretions and the promotion of effective coughing in patients with COPD. Treatments are given at a clinic or outpatient department, or at home. Many patients own or rent their home machine.

The humidified gas is inhaled under positive pressure through the mouth and exhaled passively. Treatments are usually 15 to 20 minutes in length. Medication is added via a nebulizer device.

Nursing responsibilities for the patient receiving IPPB treatments include monitoring vital signs before and after treatment, giving encouragement, and seeing that the patient utilizes the equipment properly if the respiratory therapist is not on hand. The patient should be allowed a rest period after the treatment. IPPB treatments may be followed by chest physiotherapy or postural drainage treatment.

Aerosol Therapy by Jet Nebulization

Aerosol therapy is used to deliver medication or large amounts of liquid to help liquefy respiratory secretions so that they can be mobilized. *Aerosol* means liquid or solid particles suspended in a gas. Aerosols are delivered by a *nebulizer.* There are several types of nebulizers: (1) a metered-dose device (inhaler), (2) a hand-held nebulizer, and (3) an IPPB device. Aerosol is delivered by face mask, face tent, or tracheostomy collar. Most aerosols are produced in a jet nebulizer in which a high-velocity gas shatters the liquid into small aerosol particles. Many COPD patients have been switched from IPPB nebulization treatments to hand-held nebulizers for delivery of their aerosol medications. In the hospital the nebulizer is attached to oxygen so that hypoxemia can be treated as medication is being administered. There are a variety of home nebulizer units in use such as the Puritan nebulizer or the Ohio Deluxe nebulizer. Nebulizer treatments are usually 20 to 30 minutes in length and are given two, three, or four times a day.

The patient is taught to breathe through the mouth during the treatment. He should sit in a comfortable chair. Halfway through the treatment and after the treatment, deep breathing and coughing are performed to raise loose mucus. Equipment is cleaned and dried before storing.

ENDOTRACHEAL INTUBATION AND TRACHEOSTOMY

Endotracheal intubation means that an endotracheal tube is inserted into the trachea via the nose or the mouth. An endotracheal tube is placed for airway protection against aspiration when there is upper airway obstruction and when mechanical ventilation is necessary. Endotracheal tubes are used for short-term respiratory support such as during anesthesia or for a few days postoperatively.

A *tracheostomy* is a surgical incision into the trachea for the purpose of inserting a tube through which the patient can breathe.

Tracheostomy is done for the following reasons: (1) to assist or control ventilation by mechanical means over a prolonged period of time; (2) to facilitate suctioning of secretions in the air passages of patients unable to cough; (3) to prevent aspiration of oral and gastric secretions (as in unconscious or paralyzed patients); and (4) to bypass a constricted or obstructed upper airway (as results, for example, from edema of the larynx, presence of a foreign body or tumor, surgical procedures involving the neck, severe burns, facial trauma, or chest trauma.

Tracheostomy may be an emergency procedure or an elective operation. When the passage of an endotracheal tube through the nose or mouth is impossible or extremely difficult, a tracheostomy may be done to provide an airway. Some patients, because of changes in the structure of the throat, will need a tracheostomy tube for the rest of their lives. In general, an endotracheal tube is used when the patient is expected to be able to breathe normally within a few days or weeks; for example, after surgery. A tracheostomy tube is inserted when the patient is expected to need an artificial airway for an extended period (Fig. 17–19).

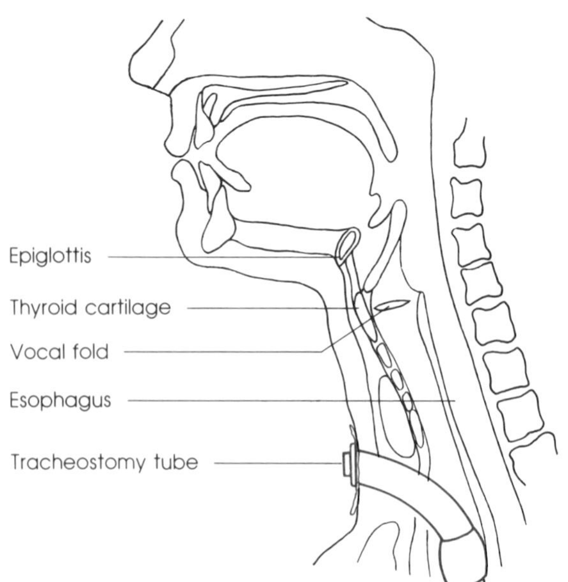

Figure 17–19 Tracheostomy, with tube in place.

Types of Tracheostomy Tubes

Tracheostomy tubes are available in a variety of materials and styles. Most of the newer models are made of plastic or rubber. Tubes made of metal alloys are used chiefly for patients who need a tracheostomy for an extended period of time. The three styles of tracheostomy tubes are single cannula, double cannula, and fenestrated.

Single-cannula tubes are made of pliable materials that conform to the shape of the trachea more easily than do double-cannula tubes. In a *double-cannula* tracheostomy tube, the outer cannula acts as a sleeve for the inner cannula, which can be removed for cleaning (Fig. 17–20). The obturator is used during insertion as a guide (the olive tip extends beyond the end of the tube) and for protection against scraping the sides of the trachea with the sharp edge of the tube.

Fenestrated tubes have a small opening in the outer cannula that allows for the escape of some air through the larynx. This helps prepare the patient for the time when the tracheostomy tube will be removed and he breathes normally again.

A one-way tracheostomy valve box can be fitted into the tube opening. It allows air to be inhaled through the tracheostomy opening, but the valve closes when the patient exhales. This diverts the exhaled air through the larynx and enables the patient to speak. Other types of speaking tracheostomy tubes are now available for the patient who must have the tracheostomy for the rest of his life.

The *cuffed tracheostomy tube* has a small balloon encircling its tracheal end (Fig. 17–21). It is sometimes called a *balloon tracheostomy tube.* When the ballon is inflated, it fills the space between the outside of the tracheostomy tube and the trachea, thereby providing a seal and preventing the escape of air around the tube. When positive-pressure artificial ventilation is administered, the air passes through the tracheostomy tube *only,* thus providing sufficient pressure to inflate the lungs. The cuffed tracheostomy tube also reduces the chance of aspiration of mucus and fluids by those patients whose protective reflexes in the larynx and trachea are impaired.

Foam-cuffed tracheostomy tubes have the cuff bonded to the tube and, of course, do not need to be inflated and deflated. They are disposable and cause minimal tissue necrosis.

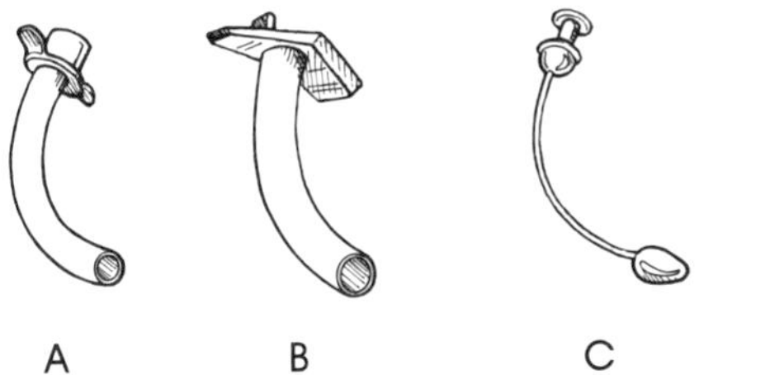

Figure 17–20 Parts of the tracheostomy tube. *A*, Inner cannula. *B*, Outer cannula. *C*, Obturator.

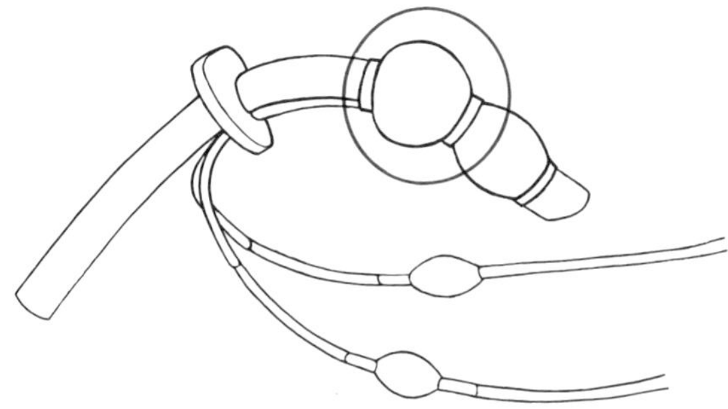

Figure 17–21 Two-cuff tracheostomy tube. The advantage of the two-cuff tube is that during prolonged artificial respiration, the cuffs may be inflated alternately to prevent pressure necrosis. The circle indicates the portion of the tube inflated after insertion in patients.

Because the lumen of the tube is the only source of air for the patient, he must be watched closely for signs of obstruction of the tube. If the lumen is not suctioned frequently and kept open, the patient will suffocate. To avoid depression of the surface blood vessels in the tracheal wall and resultant necrosis, the cuff must be inflated just enough to seal the trachea without causing extreme pressure against the tracheal wall. Cuff pressure is checked each shift and each time the cuff is reinflated.

Nursing Intervention

A patient with a new tracheostomy requires very specialized nursing care, especially if he is receiving artificial ventilation through the tube.

During the first 24 hours, the patient is monitored continuously for signs of respiratory distress. If the patient is unable to cough to remove mucus and drainage, tracheal suctioning is necessary. However, adequate humidification of the inhaled air helps reduce the need for such frequent suctioning.

The tracheostomy tube is an artificial airway, the *only* passageway for the inhalation and exhalation of air if the tube is cuffed. It is essential to keep the tube open and clear of secretions. The lungs should be auscultated (1) before suctioning to assess the need and (2) afterward to verify that the procedure has successfully cleared the airways. Suctioning is done with a sterile suction catheter, sterile normal saline or water to lubricate the catheter, sterile gloves, and a hookup to suction with a drainage container. Sterile technique is important, as the patient with a tracheostomy is very susceptible to respiratory infection. Suction pressure should never exceed 80 to 100 mm Hg when the tubing is unoccluded. The catheter should not remain in the trachea with suction on for more than 10 to 15 seconds. Either intermittent suction or a twisting motion should be used to reduce possible damage to the respiratory mucosa. The patient should be allowed to rest and should be reoxygenated between suctionings.

Prevention of infection is another nursing responsibility. The incision is an open wound with minimal dressings, is frequently exposed to sputum that is coughed up, and is an ideal entryway for infectious organisms. Tracheostomy care is a sterile procedure until the stoma (opening) is well healed.

If the patient is to go home with a tracheostomy, he or a family member must be taught the techniques for suctioning and providing the necessary tracheostomy care.

The stoma wound is usually cleaned with acetic acid solution, removing all secretions. The slit gauze pad is replaced as frequently as needed, and the twill tape ties that hold the tube in place are replaced whenever they become soiled. It is best to have two people help change the ties, as movement of the tube can easily cause the patient to cough and expel the tube from the stoma. The tube must be securely held in place while the ties are loose. The nurse will quickly learn that it is best to stand to the side of the patient, as he frequently will cough and expel mucus during the cleaning procedures.

No nurse should suction a patient without sufficient supervised practice in this technique. Considerable skill is necessary to maintain sterile technique while suctioning, yet perform the maneuver quickly and efficiently.

Psychological support of the tracheostomy patient and his family is an essential component of nursing care. The patient is having to learn to breathe in a totally different way, and he cannot speak or call out for help. He will need continued reassurance both verbally and by actions that show that the nurse is aware of his apprehension and readily available should he need help. Some means of communicating with him must be devised until he is able to speak again. He should be told what is being done and the reason it is necessary, so that if he needs to care for his tracheostomy later he will have learned from his nurses the correct way to go about it.

Concerns for the Elderly

Adults age 70 and older have some degree of alteration of connective tissue that affects lung function and ventilation. Total body water decreases to 50% after age 70, which means that the mucous and respiratory membranes are not as moist as in younger individuals. Mucus becomes much thicker. There is some degree of impairment of the ciliary action in the airways, which makes it more difficult to remove mucus, and retained mucus provides a breeding ground for bacterial infection.

There is a loss of normal elastic recoil of the lung during expiration, and the patient must use muscle action to complete expiration.

Connective tissue changes and loss of elastic tissue in the alveoli cause the alveolar membranes to become thickened, decreasing the ease with which gases can diffuse across the membranes. Oxygen saturation decreases, with PaO_2 dropping to 75 to 80 mm Hg from the usual 80 to 100 mm Hg. Essentially these changes mean that the elderly patient has less respiratory reserve. He cannot meet demands made on the body for increased oxygenation.

The decreased ability of the immune system to ward off infection makes the elderly patient more susceptible to respiratory infections. Elderly patients should be protected from exposure to colds and other respiratory ailments whenever possible. Patients in long-term-care facilities and those at home need to be closely monitored for beginning respiratory problems at all times.

BIBLIOGRAPHY

American Cancer Society: Cancer Statistics 1990. Atlanta, 1990.

American Lung Association: Facts in brief about lung disease. New York, 1990.

Anderson, S.: Six easy steps to interpreting blood gases. Am. J. Nurs., Aug., 1990, p. 45.

Andreoli, T. E., et al.: Cecil's Essentials of Medicine, 2nd ed. Philadelphia, W. B. Saunders, 1990.

Bolgiano, C. S., et al.: Administering oxygen therapy: What you need to know. Nursing 90, June, 1990, p. 47.

Carrol, P. F.: Good nursing gets COPD patients out of hospitals. RN, July, 1989, p. 24.

Caruthers, D. D.: Infectious pneumonia in the elderly. Am. J. Nurs., Feb., 1990, p. 56.

Cuzzell, J. B., et al.: How to use a bag-valve-mask device for artificial ventilation. Am. J. Nurs., July, 1989, p. 932.

Dickinson, S. P., and Bury, G. M.: Pulmonary embolism: Anatomy of a crisis. Nursing 89, April, 1989, p. 41.

Erickson, R. S.: Mastering the ins and outs of chest drainage, part 1. Nursing 89, May, 1989, p. 43.

Erickson, R. S.: Mastering the ins and outs of chest drainage, part 2. Nursing 89, June, 1989, p. 36.

Fareer, L. S., et al.: TB today: Don't count it out. Patient Care, Nov., 1987, p. 141.

Ferland, P. A.: Are you ready for ventilator patients? Nursing 91, Jan., 1991, p. 42.

George, M. R.: CF: not just a pediatric problem anymore. RN, Sept., 1990, p. 64.

Grandstrom, D., et al.: A better way to deliver long-term oxygen therapy. RN, Sept., 1989, p. 58.

Guyton, A. C.: Textbook of Medical Physiology, 8th ed. Philadelphia, W. B. Saunders, 1991.

Hefti, D.: Chest trauma. RN, May, 1991, p. 28.

Ignatavicius, D. D., and Bayne, M. J.: Medical-Surgical Nursing. Philadelphia, W. B. Saunders, 1991.

Johnson, A. P.: The elderly and COPD. J. Gerontol. Nurs., Dec., 1988, p. 35.

Kersten, L. D.: Comprehensive Respiratory Nursing: A Decision Making Approach. Philadelphia, W. B. Saunders, 1989.

Mapp, C.: Trach care: Are you aware of all the dangers? Nursing 88, July, 1988, p. 34.

Matteson, M. A., and McConnell, E. S.: Gerontological Nursing: Concepts and Practice. Philadelphia, W. B. Saunders, 1987.
Mims, B. S.: Interpreting ABGS. RN, March, 1991, p. 42.
Openbriar, D. R., et al.: What patients on home oxygen therapy want to know. Am. J. Nurs., Feb., 1988, p. 198.
Orsi, A. J.: Asthma—the danger is real. RN, April, 1991, p. 58.
Rakel, R. E., ed.: Conn's Current Therapy 1990. Philadelphia, W. B. Saunders, 1990.
Sonnesso, G.: Are you ready to use pulse oximetry? Nursing 91, Aug., 1991, p. 60.
Spector, N.: Nutritional support of the ventilator-dependent patient. Nurs. Clin. North Am., June, 1989, p. 407.
Spyr, J., and Preach, M. A.: Pulse oximetry: Understanding the concept, knowing the limits. RN, May, 1990, p. 38.
Ulrich, S. P., et al.: Nursing Care Planning Guides: A Nursing Diagnosis Approach, 2nd ed. Philadelphia, W. B. Saunders, 1990.
Wilson, E. B., et al.: Discharge planning for the patient with a new tracheostomy. Crit. Care Nurse, Jul./Aug., 1990, p. 73.
Ziegfeld, C. R., ed.: Core Curriculum for Oncology Nursing. Philadelphia, W. B. Saunders, 1987.

STUDENT STUDY AIDS

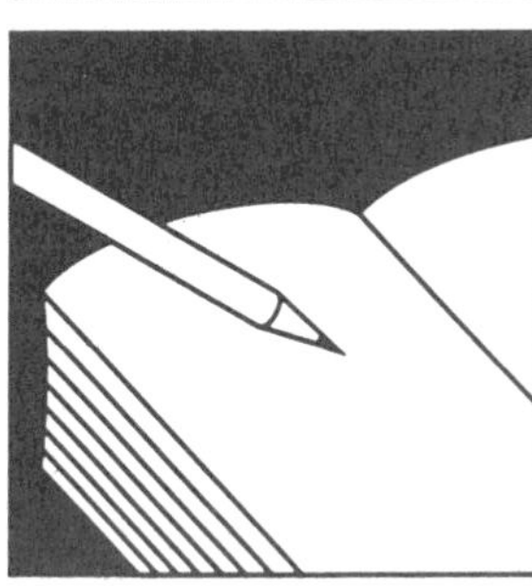

CLINICAL CASE PROBLEMS

Read each clinical situation and discuss the questions with your classmates.

1. You are assigned to take care of Lisa Gibson, a 16-year-old who has pneumococcal pneumonia. She is receiving oxygen by nasal cannula at 5 L/min. She is on bed rest with BRP. She is receiving nebulization, chest physiotherapy, and postural drainage treatments from respiratory therapy. She is very weak and runs a temperature of 104.6°F in the afternoons and evenings, which sometimes seems to cause delirium.

- What would be an appropriate plan of care for Lisa?
- How would you evaluate the effectiveness of the nursing interventions listed on the plan of care?
- What psychosocial problems might Lisa have? How would you help her with these?

2. Mrs. Williams is 62 years of age. She has suffered from emphysema for several years but has not sought help in coping with the problems it presents. While in the hospital with an acute respiratory infection, she becomes very depressed and says she will never be able to take care of herself again because of her breathlessness. She is not willing to give up smoking and has not been taught any techniques for pulmonary hygiene.

- What do you think might be the attitude of some health care professionals in regard to Mrs. Williams' problems?
- Devise a teaching plan to help her with her problem of fatigue and breathlessness.
- List interventions that would be appropriate in helping with her nutritional and hydration needs.

3. Mr. Cook is admitted to the hospital for pneumonectomy. His diagnosis is cancer of the lung. He is 56 years old and has worked in a cotton mill since he was 16. He is slightly underweight but is physically strong and has an optimistic outlook about his surgery and chances for recovery.

- What special preoperative instruction would you expect Mr. Cook to need?
- What nursing interventions would you expect to be on his nursing care plan postoperatively?
- How would you help Mr. Cook deal with the diagnosis of cancer, treatment, and prognosis?

STUDY OUTLINE

I. Physiology

A. Bronchial "tree" made up of trachea (trunk), bronchi, bronchioles, and alveoli, which are the terminal units of ventilation.

B. Lung defense system: macrophages, cilia, mucus, cough reflex; surfactant helps keep alveoli open.
C. CNS controls respiration: vagus nerve, medulla, and pons regulate involuntary breathing; cortex regulates voluntary breathing.
D. Increased CO_2 and hydrogen ion concentration in CSF stimulate chemoreceptors, causing increased rate and depth of respiration.
E. Decreased oxygen content in blood stimulates chemoreceptors in carotid arteries and aorta, causing increased action of respiratory muscles, which increases respiration.

II. Pathologic factors

A. Inhalation of infectious organisms and chemical irritants.
B. Cardiac disease and other conditions that interfere with perfusion and distribution of gases.
C. Two major types of ventilatory diseases: restrictive (decreased lung volume) and obstructive (narrowed air passages).

III. Prevention of respiratory disease

A. Good health practices: rest, nutrition, personal hygiene.
B. Vaccination against influenza and pneumococcal pneumonia.
C. Prompt treatment of respiratory infections.
D. Avoidance of irritants such as tobacco smoke, industrial pollutants.

IV. Terms commonly used in respiratory disease nursing (see page 389)

V. Diagnostic tests and procedures and nursing implications (Table 17–1)

A. General health screening.
B. Pulmonary function tests: spirometry.

VI. Nursing assessment of respiratory status

A. History taking (see Table 17–2).
B. Observation:
   1. Posture, amount of effort to breathe, use of abdominal muscles and other accessory muscles of respiration, rate, depth, and character of respirations.
   2. Skin color: cyanosis appears late in oxygen depletion.
   3. Shape of chest: barrel-shaped? kyphosis? scoliosis?
   4. Clubbing of fingers.
C. Ineffective breathing patterns:
   1. Hyperventilation.
   2. Hypoventilation.
   3. Biot's respirations; Cheyne-Stokes respiration; Kussmaul's respirations; apneustic respiration.
D. Adventitious breath sounds:
   1. Auscultation of lungs in systematic manner.
   2. Wheezing, "croaking" or stridor, hoarseness.
   3. Rhonchi: coarse, rattling sounds due to secretions in the air passages.
   4. Crackles: produced by air passing through moisture. Dry crackles produced by thick secretions.
E. Ineffective airway clearance
   1. Productive or nonproductive of sputum.
   2. Events that trigger cough; time of day; measures that help relieve; other symptoms occurring simultaneously, e.g., fatigue, dyspnea, change in vital signs.
F. Sputum (see Table 17–3).

VII. Acute respiratory disease

A. Common cold: caused by many different viruses.
   1. Rest, fluids, mild analgesic for aches and soreness.

2. If cold persists and high fever develops, patient should have medical attention.

B. Acute bronchitis: frequently an extension of an upper respiratory infection.
   1. Treated conservatively with humidification, cough suppressant, bed rest, nutritious meals.

C. Influenza: caused by any of three major types of virus (A, B, and C) and numerous subtypes.
   1. Spread by direct and indirect contact.
   2. Symptoms come on rather suddenly: fever, chills, headache, sore throat, and dry, hacking cough.
   3. Common nursing diagnoses include activity intolerance, sleep pattern disturbance, ineffective airway clearance, pain, potential for nutrition deficit, potential for fluid deficit.

D. Pneumonia: extensive inflammation of lung tissue with consolidation. Various causes, ranging from infectious agents and chemicals to atelectasis.
   1. Prevention: nursing intervention to avoid hypostatic and aspiration pneumonia.
   2. Diagnosis by radiograph.
   3. Typical pneumonia responds to antibiotic therapy.
   4. Atypical pneumonia caused by *Mycoplasma* treated with erythromycin or tetracycline. Viral atypical pneumonia requires no antiinfective therapy.
   5. *Pneumocystis carinii* pneumonia associated with AIDS; treated with pentamidine.
   6. Nursing care plan should include measures to control fever, maintain fluid and electrolyte balance, meet needs for nutrition, rest, comfort; avoid irritating substances and secondary infections. Abdominal distention, nausea and vomiting, and altered states of consciousness are frequent problems.

E. Pleurisy: inflammation of pleural membranes.
   1. Pleurisy with effusion: an increase in serous fluid in pleural cavity.
   2. Symptoms: sharp, stabbing pain in chest.
   3. Treatment includes bed rest and prevention of infection. Thoracentesis may be needed to remove excess fluid.

F. Empyema: thick and purulent fluid within pleural cavity.
   1. Treated by antibiotics and thoracentesis: empyema tube.

G. *Pneumocystis carinii*: high incidence in AIDS patients; histoplasmosis and coccidioidomycosis caused by fungus.

H. Sarcoidosis: interstitial lung disease characterized by granulomas.

VIII. Chronic obstructive pulmonary disease (COPD)

A. Ranks fifth among major causes of death in the U.S.

B. Increased incidence from tobacco smoke and air pollution.

C. Mechanics of COPD:
   1. Pulmonary emphysema is essentially a disease of the terminal respiratory units. Walls of the alveoli are damaged, bronchioles permanently distended.
      a. Patient has more difficulty exhaling because of loss of lung elastance.
   2. Chronic bronchitis: increased residual volume due to premature closure of the airways during exhalation.
   3. Asthma: hypersensitivity of trachea and bronchi to various stimuli. Bronchospasm usually reversible with drug therapy.

4. Bronchiectasis: bronchi become dilated; caused by frequent respiratory infections, and cystic fibrosis.
5. Adult cystic fibrosis patients have form of COPD.

D. Medical treatment goals:
1. Minimize irritation of air passages and their obstruction by secretions, edema, etc.
2. Prevent or control infection.
3. Increase tolerance for physical activity.

E. Nursing intervention:
1. Rehabilitation and education of patient for self-care are major goals.
2. Techniques and tips for patient with COPD listed in Tables 17–4 and 17–5.

IX. Tuberculosis

A. Pulmonary tuberculosis.
1. Infectious disease caused by tubercle bacillus. *Not* highly contagious; opportunistic and therefore have increased incidence in AIDS patients.
2. Categories can help identify those needing treatment or preventive therapy.
3. Symptoms: cough, low-grade fever in the afternoon, weight loss, night sweats, hemoptysis.
4. Diagnostic tests: tuberculin skin tests, chest radiographs, examination of sputum and gastric contents for causative organism.
5. Treatment, rest, good nutrition, proper handling of secretions, control of coughing.
6. Specific antituberculotic drugs: isoniazid (INH), rifampin (RMP), and streptomycin. Drugs selected according to sensitivity of organisms in sputum.
7. Preventive therapy for selected groups. INH is 85% effective in preventing tuberculosis in high-risk persons.
8. Nursing intervention primarily concerned with education of patient and family to assure control and prevent transmission.

B. Extrapulmonary tuberculosis: bacillus affects organs other than the lungs.

X. Cancer of the lung

A. A leading cause of cancer deaths in males and females; major factor is smoking.
B. Tumors usually begin in epithelial lining of bronchi.
C. Symptoms appear late in disease.
D. Treatment includes surgery, chemotherapy, and radiotherapy.

XI. Chest injuries

A. Can be life-threatening because of possible damage to respiratory and cardiovascular systems.
B. Major concerns are:
1. Maintenance of airway.
2. Ensurance of adequate ventilation.
3. Control of circulatory problems.

C. Pneumothorax and hemothorax two major complications. Unrelieved tension pneumothorax can lead to mediastinal shift and can be fatal.
D. Flail chest may require intubation and mechanical ventilation.
E. Pulmonary embolism: mass or clot occludes pulmonary vessel; can be a mild problem or fatal.
1. Many types of emboli: blood thrombus, fat, amniotic fluid, air.

2. Symptoms depend on site and location of embolus; dyspnea, chest pain, cough, hemoptysis, and anxiety.
3. Treatment: oxygen, anticoagulation, clot removal.

XII. Care of patients having intrathoracic surgery

A. Preoperative care: assessment of patient's respiratory status; arm and leg exercises; explanation of chest tubes, closed drainage system, suctioning, any other procedure anticipated.

B. Postoperative care: special observations, positioning, and chest tubes.

C. Care of patients with chest tubes and closed drainage.
1. Apparatus can be one-, two-, or three-bottle system for closed drainage or disposable self-contained unit.
2. Purpose is to allow for gradual reexpansion of lung and prevention of hemothorax and pneumothorax.
3. System must be airtight at all times; tape connections.
4. Note conditions that require immediate attention:
   a. Persistent bubbling in underwater seal.
   b. More than 100 mL drainage per hour.
   c. "Puffed up" appearance in chest and neck.
   d. Leakage of air around connection.
5. See Nursing Care Plan *17–2*.

XIII. Common respiratory patient care problems

A. Ineffective airway clearance
1. Report observations accurately.
2. Teach patient effective breathing and coughing maneuvers.
3. Help patient avoid prolonged coughing.
4. Not all cough medicines have the same effect.

B. Secretions:
1. Respiratory precautions to avoid spreading infection.
2. Teach patient proper handling and disposal of secretions.
3. Frequent oral hygiene.
4. Observe amount and characteristics of sputum.
5. Mechanical suctioning procedure and hazards.

C. Dyspnea or breathlessness:
1. Position patient properly.
2. Relieve abdominal distention.
3. Avoid overfilling stomach.

D. Alterations in nutrition and hydration:
1. Anorexia common problem; increased work causes increased calorie need.
2. Nursing intervention: clean, odor-free environment; good oral hygiene; small, frequent feedings; supplements (Pulmocare).
3. Fluid deficit not uncommon because of increased secretions and abnormal breathing patterns.
4. Patient should drink at least 3,000 mL per day.
5. Humidification of air can help prevent fluid deficit.

E. Fatigue:
1. Caused by hypoxia.
2. Provide periods of uninterrupted rest.
3. Balance rest with purposeful physical activity (i.e., deep breathing and coughing exercises).

XIV. Common therapeutic measures

A. Medications: antihistamines, bronchodilators, liquefying agents and diluents, antiinfectives; cromolyn sodium, corticosteroids.

B. Humidification: aerosol and humidity therapy; nebulizers.

1. Relief of bronchial edema and spasms.
2. Liquefaction of secretions.
3. Delivery of drugs.
4. Moisten mucous membranes.

C. Pulmonary hygiene: purposes are (1) removal of secretions in the air passages and (2) breathing control.
   1. Intermittent positive-pressure breathing.
   2. Chest physiotherapy includes postural drainage, percussion, and vibration.
   3. Breathing exercises and effective coughing.

D. Oxygen therapy:
   1. Indicated when there is either inadequate intake or poor distribution of oxygen.
   2. Oxygen toxicity: damage to cells from excess O_2 in their environment.
      a. Dosage must be specific in regard to concentration and rate of flow.
   3. Administration by nasal cannula, mask, and tent.
   4. Special considerations to avoid fire hazards; measures to control infection.
   5. Patient is "weaned" from oxygen dependence.

E. Mechanical ventilation:
   1. Two types of ventilators: positive-pressure and negative-pressure.
   2. Positive-pressure ventilators: pressure-cycled, time-cycled, volume-cycled, high-frequency.
   3. Modes of delivery:
      a. Controlled artificial ventilation for patient who cannot breathe on his own.
      b. Assisted ventilation helps patient breathe more deeply.
      c. IMV allows patient to breathe spontaneously between controlled breaths.
      d. PEEP delivers pressure at the end of expiration; for patients who have been intubated and require assisted ventilation.
      e. CPAP delivered continuously to patients who are breathing spontaneously.
      f. All ventilators provide humidification of inspired air and measurement of expired volumes.
   4. Nursing intervention:
      a. Check physician's orders and compare with settings on ventilator.
      b. Ventilator settings: mode, FIO_2, respiratory rate, tidal volume, peak inspiratory pressure, PEEP.
      c. Keep alarms turned on.
      d. Keep tubing cleared of water.
      e. Assess patient for signs of complications: pneumothorax, gastric distention, impaired cardiac output, decreased compliance.
      f. Auscultate lung fields frequently.
      g. Monitor arterial blood gas levels.
      h. Suction with aseptic technique.
      i. Provide means of communication.
      j. Assess nutritional adequacy.

F. IPPB therapy helps overcome resistance to inspired air and allows for more uniform distribution of oxygen to alveoli.
   1. Nursing responsibilities:
      a. Assess condition before and after treatment.

b. Supervise use of machine if respiratory therapist is not on hand.

G. Aerosol therapy by jet nebulization for humidification and medication.

H. Endotracheal intubation and tracheostomy: an artificial airway.
1. Types of tubes: single-cannula, double-cannula, fenestrated.
2. Cuffed tracheostomy tube allows for passage of air through the tube only.
3. Patient care requires specific instruction and supervised practice. Major concerns are:
   a. Maintaining open airway.
   b. Preventing infection.
   c. Maintaining integrity of skin around stoma and mucous membranes of respiratory tract.
   d. Psychological support of patient and family.

XV. Concerns for the elderly

A. Connective tissue changes and decreased elasticity.
B. Thickened mucus as a result of decreased water content of body.
C. Thickened alveolar membrane causes drop in PaO_2 to 75 to 80 mm Hg.
D. Less efficient immune system: more susceptible to respiratory infection.

CHAPTER 18

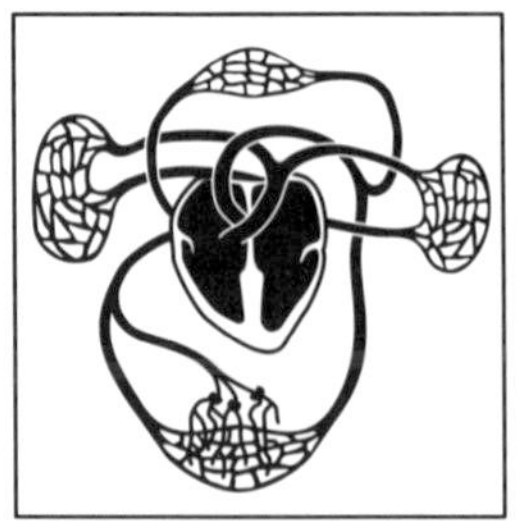

Care of Patients With Disorders of the Blood, Blood-Forming Organs, and Lymphatic System

VOCABULARY

aplastic
dactylitis
dyscrasia
ecchymosis
erythropoiesis
hemarthrosis
hemolysis
hypovolemia
iatrogenic
infarction
leukocytosis
lymphadenopathy
petechiae
polycythemia
splenomegaly
thrombosis
viscous

Upon completion of this chapter the student should be able to:

1. State the major functions for each of the formed elements in the blood.
2. Describe the functions of the three plasma proteins.
3. Identify the nurse's role in the prevention of blood dyscrasias.
4. List at least five different kinds of information that can be obtained from a complete blood cell count.
5. Describe the factors considered when performing nursing assessment of hematologic status.
6. List at least four nursing diagnoses related to blood disorders, with appropriate nursing interventions for each.
7. Describe the pathology and clinical manifestations of sickle cell disease, leukemia, and hemophilia.
8. List the major nursing interventions for each of the above disorders.
9. List appropriate nursing interventions to help patients with problems associated with lymphedema.

The life of each cell in the body is dependent on a system of transportation to bring nutrients to its immediate environment and carry away its wastes. The cardiovascular system is such a transportation system. It is composed of a fluid medium for vital substances (the blood), a pump to move the blood throughout the body (the heart), and an interconnecting network of tubes through which the blood flows (veins, arteries, and capillaries). Any disorder that affects one or more of these components of the cardiovascular system threatens the health and life of the entire body. In this chapter, disorders that affect the blood and its formed elements, the organs that produce the various blood cells, and the lymphatic system, which drains the fluid from the spaces around each cell and eventually empties into the circulatory system, will be discussed.

Plasma is a clear yellow fluid in which the blood cells and other solutes are carried. Plasma proteins, consisting of albumin, globulins, and fibrinogen, are the main substances other than the blood cells in the plasma. When the plasma proteins and other solutes are separated out of the plasma fluid, only serum remains.

The blood has many important functions in the body. It provides transportation to and from the cells for nutrients, hormones, enzymes, and waste products. It takes part in regulating fluid volume, electrolyte distribution, and body temperature and in protecting the body against harmful agents.

PATHOPHYSIOLOGY

The blood is actually a tissue. Slightly more than half of it is plasma, whereas the remainder (about 45%) is made up of several different kinds of cells or formed elements.

The formed elements of blood are the erythrocytes (red blood cells, or RBCs), leukocytes (white blood cells), and thrombocytes (platelets) (Fig. 18–1).

ERYTHROCYTES

The RBCs are by far the most numerous of the blood's formed elements, outnumbering the white blood cells about 1,000 to 1. RBCs contain

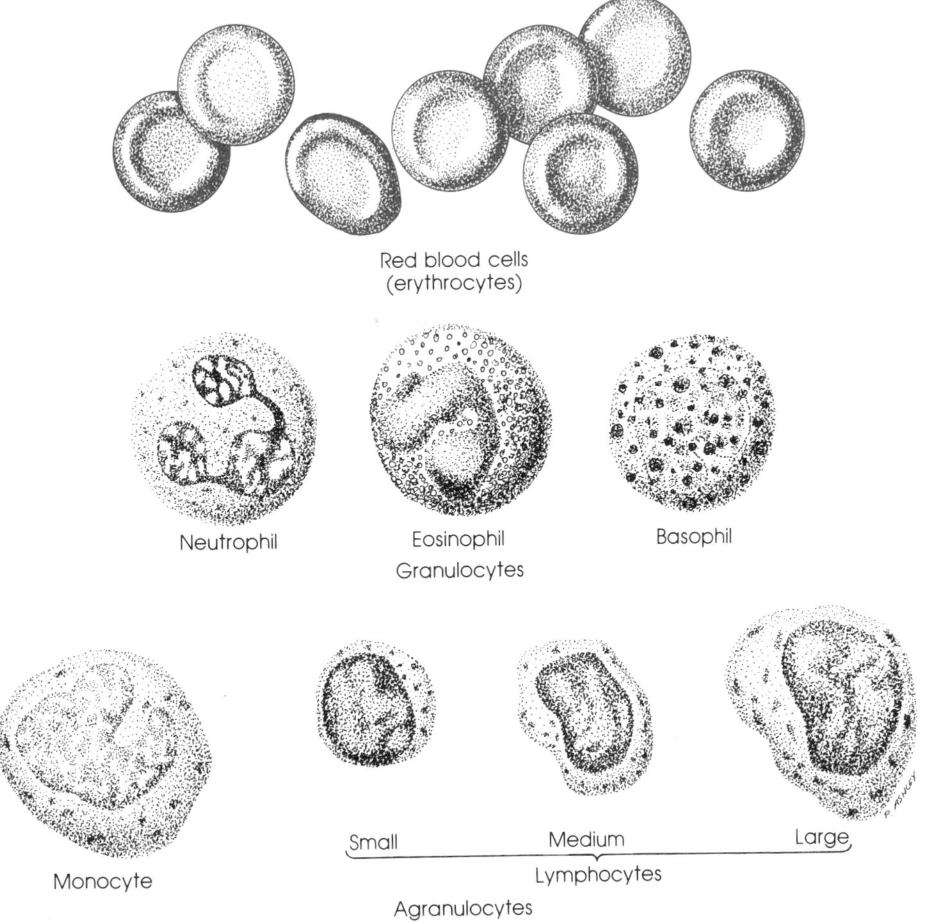

Figure 18–1 Red and white blood cells.

hemoglobin, which gives the cells their red color and provides the cell with the ability to carry oxygen and carbon dioxide.

Erythrocytes are formed in the red bone marrow by a process called *erythropoiesis.* The average life span of a red blood cell is only about 2 to 3 months, so erythropoiesis must continue throughout a person's life in order to meet the oxygen requirements of the tissues. This process requires iron; vitamins B_{12}, C, and E; folic acid; and amino acids and protein.

Pathologic conditions related to erythrocytes range from a deficit in supply (resulting in various types of anemia) to an excessive amount of RBCs, which is called *polycythemia.* An abnormality in the shape of erythrocytes also can cause difficulties, as we shall see later when we discuss sickle cell disease.

LEUKOCYTES

White blood cells (WBCs) are primarily involved in protection of the body against invasion and infection by harmful agents, including bacteria, viruses, and other antigens. Even though leukocytes are among the formed elements of blood, their primary functions are outside the blood—that is, in the tissues. The circulatory system provides transportation for the various kinds of leukocytes to get them where they need to go to do their specific jobs.

Leukocytes are divided into granulocytes and agranulocytes, meaning *with* and *without granules* in the cell nucleus. There are five main types of leukocytes: *Granulocytes* provide the first line of defense against microbial invasion. *Neutrophils* are the most numerous of the granulocytes, making up 50% to 70% of the total white count. They engulf and destroy bacteria by a process called *phagocytosis.* An infection in the body stimulates increased production of neutrophils, resulting in a higher than normal leukocyte count, or *leukocytosis.*

Eosinophils make up 1% to 5% of the total number of white blood cells. They help to detoxify foreign proteins. Eosinophils increase in number during allergic reactions and in response to parasitic infections.

Basophils constitute only 0% to 1% of the total white cell count. They function to prevent clotting in the small blood vessels and release histamine in response to allergens.

Agranulocytes consist of both lymphocytes and monocytes. *Monocytes* change into macrophages when they move out into the tissue and play an aggressive role in phagocytosis. *Lymphocytes* are divided into B lymphocytes and T lymphocytes and are active in the immune responses of the body. T lymphocytes produce antigen-reactive cells, and B lymphocytes can change into plasma cells that produce the immunoglobulins that are responsible for the humoral immune response.

A differential blood cell count, which gives information about the numbers of the different types of leukocytes present in the blood, yields information about the type of inflammatory process that is occurring in the body and is an important diagnostic tool.

Among the pathologic conditions affecting the leukocytes are the leukemias, which are a group of neoplastic disorders involving the peripheral blood leukocytes and their precursors.

PLATELETS

Thrombocytes provide the first line of protection to prevent bleeding when the wall of a blood vessel has been damaged. They are able to stick to foreign surfaces and to bunch together in large masses to begin the formation of a clot. Platelets also release several factors necessary for the clotting of blood.

Platelets are actually fragments of a very large cell *(megakaryocyte)*, and their life span is only about 10 days. A reduced platelet count can result from either inadequate production or excessive destruction. For example, diseases of the bone marrow, infection, and cytotoxic drugs can interfere with the production of platelets, and infections, alcohol, and mechanical injury can result in their excessive destruction. Although the body can withstand a substantial drop in the number of platelets, when the platelet count is low there is risk of spontaneous bleeding into the skin, kidney, brain, and other internal organs.

PLASMA

The liquid noncellular portion of blood, called *plasma*, is part of the extracellular fluid. It is almost exactly the same as the fluid in the tissue spaces, except that plasma contains a higher percentage of protein. The three major plasma proteins are albumin, the globulins, and fibrinogen. The major function of albumin is to cause osmotic pressure at the capillary membrane, which prevents fluid in the plasma from leaking out of the capillaries and into the tissue spaces. The alpha and beta globulins are involved in transporting other substances such as drugs and lipids that combine with them. The gamma globulins are chiefly the antibodies that do battle with foreign agents entering the body. Fibrinogen is essential to the function of the body's clotting mechanism.

LYMPHATIC SYSTEM

The lymphatic system is made up of small vessels (or channels), ducts, and nodes. It is an accessory system by which fluids can flow from the tissue spaces into the blood. The lymphatic fluid that returns to the circulatory system is extremely important, because it contains large particles such as proteins that cannot easily pass through the pores of the venous capillaries.

Lymph nodes, sometimes mistakenly called *lymph glands,* are small collections of lymphatic tissue scattered along the course of the lymphatic vessels. They produce lymphocytes and release them into the blood to fight infection and provide immunity. The lymph nodes also "police" the extravascular fluids, filtering out leukocytes and cell debris from inflammations and infections. In severe infections the lymph also may contain bacterial or chemical agents, and thus the lymph nodes themselves can be secondarily infected or inflamed *(lymphadenitis).*

The lymph nodes are rarely the site of primary disease except in lymphomas, which include Hodgkin's disease as well as other proliferative disorders. The infections that cause lymphadenitis are many and varied and usually do not result in major problems unless there is an overwhelming infection. When this happens the inflammatory reaction can spread to adjacent nodes and then to more distant ones along the chain of pathways. If the lymphatic system cannot contain the infection, the infectious agents (bacterial or viral) enter the blood stream and produce a septicemia. The same is true of malignant cells, which can metastasize from the original tumor and involve the lymph nodes along the way.

SPLEEN

The spleen is the largest unit of the monocyte-macrophage system. This system is a loosely organized network of organs, tissues, and cells that have a wide variety of functions including the immune response, phagocytosis, filtration of blood and tissue fluids, and the production of blood elements. The spleen stores and releases blood and removes old blood cells from circulation. Not all of the functions of the spleen are yet known.

Aside from trauma and rupture of the spleen, the most frequently occurring abnormality is enlargement *(splenomegaly).* The organ is rarely the primary site of disease but enlarges in response to systemic infections, congenital and acquired hemolytic anemias, and congestive states related to hypertension of the portal circulation. Enlargement of the spleen can be an important clue in the diagnosis of a primary disease that secondarily affects the spleen.

CAUSES OF BLOOD DYSCRASIAS

Many disorders involving the blood and lymphatics are not easily prevented, because they are either inherited or secondary to a primary disease that is itself difficult to treat. Genetic counseling is a part of the overall management of such inherited conditions as hemophilia and sickle cell disease.

There are, however, some blood disorders that are *iatrogenic;* that is, they are brought on by medical treatment. For example, blood dyscrasias or other pathologic conditions of the blood can be induced by drugs through at least three kinds of actions: (1) bone marrow suppression, which interferes with the production of blood elements; (2) inhibition of normal cell function; and (3) destruction of the blood cells by cytotoxic drugs.

Some antineoplastic drugs, for instance, act to depress the bone marrow, which inevitably causes reduced supply of blood elements. Other drugs, such as phenytoin (Dilantin), primidone (Mysoline), barbital derivatives, and oral contraceptives can produce anemia by interfering with the absorption and utilization of folic acid, a substance needed for the production of red blood cells.

Diuretics such as furosemide (Lasix) and hydrochlorothiazide (Hydrodiuril) can cause decreased numbers of white cells *(leukopenia),* aplastic anemia, and abnormally low counts of platelets and granulocytes. Procainamide hydrochloride (Pronestyl) and quinidine, which are used to correct arrhythmias of the heart, also can cause thrombocytopenia, agranulocytosis, and aplastic anemia. In fact, it is well to remember that most drugs are powerful chemicals that are capable of producing undesirable side effects, even though they can be of help in managing a patient's primary disease.

Although bone marrow suppression is an expected action of some antineoplastic agents, the same effect can be caused by an idiosyncrasy or hypersensitivity to other kinds of drugs. The dilemma facing the physician who prescribes drugs that adversely affect blood cells is not easily resolved. The nurse can help him decide when to alter dosage or substitute another drug by carefully noting and documenting patients' reactions to the medications they are taking. She should be aware of the possible side effects of drugs that she administers and be especially alert for them when observing patients' individual reactions to them.

Incompatibility of blood types also can contribute to blood disorders by causing hemolysis (destruction of blood cells) and can in many cases be prevented by careful administration of blood and blood products that contain RBCs. The nurse is obligated to follow the procedure to the letter when checking labels for donor and recipient blood. She also must monitor every patient receiving a transfusion and promptly report any indications that the patient is having a reaction. Transfusion reaction is discussed in detail in Chapter 8.

DIAGNOSTIC TESTS AND PROCEDURES

A surprising amount of information can be obtained from a stained blood film using only a 5-mL sample of uncoagulated blood. Each of the formed elements can be studied for shape, maturity, and number. Other kinds of studies include those done on the plasma to measure the rate at which RBCs settle out from plasma (called the *sedimentation rate*) and to separate and classify various kinds of proteins, including antibodies, in the plasma.

The nurse's responsibility in relation to tests on the blood is to explain the venipuncture procedure and the purpose of the test to the patient. Many patients have a great fear of needles. Others are concerned about having what seems like a lot of blood withdrawn. A few words of assurance and explanation can do much to relieve anxiety about a needle stick and promote cooperation. If the nurse is to perform the venipuncture, she must follow aseptic technique and use the correct tubes for each sample. Rubber gloves should be worn by the nurse any time a venipuncture is performed, and equipment must be disposed of according to universal precautions.

Leukocytes may be studied for total number of white cells per millimeter (WBC count) and for a differential count. A differential white cell count determines the numbers of various kinds of leukocytes present in the sample of blood (Table 18-1). A distinction should be made in the reading of reports of differential WBC counts. If the count is reported as *absolute*, it is the *exact* number of the specific type of leukocytes present in the sampling of blood. A *relative* count indicates the *percentage* of the specific type of leukocyte when compared with all other types present in the specimen. For example, the absolute count of lymphocytes may be 2,100/mm^3; the relative count, 25%.

TABLE 18-1 DIFFERENTIAL LEUKOCYTE COUNT

Cell Type	Range	Percentage
Total WBC	4,500–11,000	
PMN neutrophils	4,100–6,500	36–66
Band neutrophils	100–2,100	<5 or 0–5
Esosinophils	0–700	1–3
Basophils	0–150	0–1
Lymphocytes	1,500–4,000	24–44
Monocytes	200–950	2–8

From Bennington, J. L., ed.: Saunders Dictionary and Encyclopedia of Laboratory Medicine and Technology. Philadelphia, W. B. Saunders, 1984.

Platelets, also called *thrombocytes*, are minute particles suspended in the blood. As their name implies (*thrombo*—clot, *cyte*—cell), they are essential to the clotting of blood. Information about the number and different types of platelets is valuable in diagnosing a variety of diseases affecting or affected by the clotting of blood.

Hemoglobin studies include determination of the amount of hemoglobin per 100 mL of whole blood. The normal range for hemoglobin is 14.5 to 16 gm per 100 mL of blood in males and 13.0 to 15.5 gm per 100 mL of blood in females.

A study also may be made of the concentration of hemoglobin in erythrocytes. The *mean corpuscular hemoglobin concentration (MCHC)* is the average hemoglobin content per 100 mL of packed red blood cells. The MCHC value indicates the amount of hemoglobin in a 100-mL sample of blood from which the plasma and other cellular components have been removed, leaving only the red blood cells. The normal value is 33% to 38% or 33 to 38 grams per 100 mL.

There are at least 12 different types of hemoglobin in human blood. The types are designated by letters—for example, hemoglobin A is normal adult hemoglobin, hemoglobin F is normal fetal hemoglobin, and hemoglobin S is found in sickle cell disease.

A *hematocrit* is a test that measures the volume of blood cells in relation to the volume of plasma. When there has been a loss of body fluids but no loss of cells, as in dehydration, the cell volume is high in proportion to the amount of liquid (plasma) in the blood stream. On the other hand, when either hemorrhage or anemia has depleted the supply of cells, the blood is "thinned" and the cell volume is low. The normal range for the hematocrit is 45 to 50 mL per 100 mL of whole blood in males and 40 to 50 mL per 100 mL of whole blood in females.

BONE MARROW BIOPSY

Examination of cells taken from the bone marrow is a common procedure for diagnosis of blood dyscrasias. The cells usually are withdrawn by needle from the sternum, in which case the procedure is called a *sternal puncture*. Sometimes, other accessible bones such as the crest of the ilium are used.

The cells that are withdrawn from the bone marrow are examined in the laboratory under a microscope. In this way, erythrocytes, platelets, and leukocytes can be examined in the various stages of development, and their size, number, and shape can be determined. This information is helpful in identifying certain types of anemia, leukemia, and platelet deficiency (*thrombocytopenia*).

Nursing Responsibilities

A bone marrow biopsy is usually done at the bedside. If the patient is extremely apprehensive, it is best to administer an analgesic an hour before the procedure. After the skin is prepped with iodophor solution, a local anesthetic is injected, and the physician inserts a biopsy needle into the bone marrow of the chosen site and aspirates a marrow specimen. The patient must hold absolutely still during the procedure. A sharp, brief pain occurs with aspiration. Afterward, pressure should be applied to the site to prevent hematoma formation.

A test should not have to be repeated because the patient was not prepared properly. This may sound obvious, but numbers of tests are repeated in hospitals for just this reason.

Instructions for care of the patient before and during a bone marrow aspiration usually can be found in the hospital or clinic nursing procedure book. After the procedure is done the site of needle insertion should be checked routinely. There usually will be some bleeding that should respond to firm pressure on the site and the application of ice packs. If these measures are not taken, a painful hematoma could form. Continued tenderness at the site and the appearance of redness and swelling should be reported, as they could indicate development of an infection.

SCHILLING TEST

The Schilling test determines the patient's ability to absorb vitamin B_{12} and is used to diagnose pernicious anemia. Vitamin B_{12} is necessary for the formation of RBCs. Radioactive B_{12} is given orally, along with an IM injection of B_{12}, and then a 24-hour urine specimen is collected. Subnormal levels of B_{12} in the urine indicate a problem with secretion of intrinsic factor, which facilitates absorption of vitamin B_{12}.

SICKLE CELL TEST

The sickling test (Sickledex) is a blood screening test for the presence of hemoglobin S (Hgb S) in people suspected of having sickle cell anemia or sickle cell trait. The normal adult has no Hgb S. Individuals in whom 50% or less of their hemoglobin consists of Hgb S are *carriers* of the sickle cell trait. Those who have 90% or more of Hgb S have sickle cell anemia. If the sickling test is positive, hemoglobin electrophoresis is done to determine the amount of Hgb S present.

NURSING ASSESSMENT OF HEMATOLOGIC STATUS

HISTORY TAKING

Some blood dyscrasias are more common in certain racial and geographic groups, particular age groups, and sexes. For example, sickle cell disease is predominant in members of the black race, some hemophilias affect only males, and pernicious anemia occurs more frequently in Northern Europeans. It is important, therefore, that the race, ethnic background, age, and sex of the patient be noted in a patient's biographic data. Most of this information is readily available in other areas of the patient's chart. The point is that during her assessment the nurse should be aware of the significance of these particular kinds of data when a blood dyscrasia is suspected.

Other significant data include a history of abnormal bleeding; feelings of weakness and fatigue; pain in the joints; neurologic symptoms such as dizziness, irritability, drowsiness, numbness, and tingling in the extremities, and pounding headache; cardiovascular symptoms such as tachycardia and dyspnea; and indications of gastrointestinal involvement such as flatulence, vomiting, diarrhea, and soreness of the mouth and tongue.

Internal bleeding in either the urinary or gastrointestinal tract can occur in blood dyscrasias, especially those affecting the platelets. It would be helpful, therefore, to question the patient about the color of stools, whether they have been very dark or tarry, and the color of urine, whether it has been smoky, hazy, or brown.

Inability to tolerate cold also is significant in patients with anemia. The nurse might ask whether the patient uses extra blankets, is comfortable in cold weather, or typically wears sweaters, thick socks, and other warm clothes when others are dressed more lightly.

A history of repeated infections or frequent bouts of fever could indicate either a deficiency in number or abnormal function of white blood cells. Swollen lymph nodes in the armpit, groin, neck, or elsewhere are typically found in patients with a pathologic condition of the lymphatic system or with a systemic infection and elevated production of leukocytes.

ASSESSMENT

Certain specific objective and subjective signs and symptoms are related to hematologic disorders. In addition to the usual initial and ongoing assessment conducted by the nurse caring for a patient, some special observations are relevant to assessment of patients with blood disorders.

Skin

Although pallor is a sign of anemia, it is not the most reliable. Many other factors can affect a person's complexion and skin color, including thickness of the skin, amount of skin pigment, and number and distribution of blood vessels near the surface of the skin. When pallor of the skin, nail beds, and conjunctiva is noticed, it should be documented, but being pale or ashen or having a sallow complexion does not in itself indicate anemia.

Jaundice, or a yellowing discoloration of the skin and sclera of the eyes, can occur as a result of excessive destruction of red blood cells (*hemolysis*). When red blood cells are ruptured, bilirubin is released. The pigment eventually finds its way into the blood stream, where it causes jaundice. It is interesting to note that although eating large amounts of carrots and other yellow vegetables can cause a yellowish cast to the skin, it will not cause a change in the color of the sclera and mucous membranes.

Bruises and small red patches (*petechiae*) are typical of purpura, a hemorrhagic disease sometimes associated with a decrease in the number of circulating platelets. Bleeding under the skin and formation of bruises in response to the slightest trauma frequently occur in anemias, leukemias, and diseases affecting the bone marrow and spleen.

A very ruddy complexion of red, florid appearance (*plethora*) is typical of excessive numbers of red blood cells (*polycythemia*). Enlargment of the spleen, which also accompanies polycythemia and several other blood disorders, might be described by the patient as a feeling of fullness on the left side of the upper abdomen. Cyanosis, or a bluish tint, can indicate hypoxia resulting from inadequate numbers of circulating erythrocytes.

Mucous Membranes

Nutritional deficiences and hypoxia resulting from inadequate blood supply can contribute to sore and painful gums and tongue. For example, the nurse might notice that the patient does not eat all the food served to him and, on questioning him, might learn that "it hurts too much to chew," or when assisting the patient with mouth care, she may notice swollen and bleeding gums.

Stools and Urine

Stools are observed for signs of fresh blood or old blood (tarry or coffee-ground stools). The urine also is observed for signs of internal bleeding. Bright red blood rarely goes unnoticed, but the smoky, brownish color caused by old blood in the urine may not be recognized as important unless one is aware of its significance.

Swollen and Painful Joints

Bleeding into the joints (*hemarthrosis*) is not uncommon in certain kinds of anemia, especially sickle cell disease. The nurse might notice the swelling and some redness in the area of the joints, or she might observe the patient moving more slowly and with obvious discomfort. When questioned, the patient might give subjective evidence of his painful joints and identify those that are involved.

Lymph Node Involvement

Enlarged lymph nodes are significant in a number of different blood disorders as well as in infections and immune disorders. The nodes most often inspected and palpated are those under the arm, in the neck, and in the inguinal region. Lymph node enlargement often can be found while bathing a patient and helping him with activities of daily living.

Nodes covered by red streaks in the skin or with streaks leading to and from the node are indicative of lymphadenitis. There usually is a local site of infection nearby.

Mental State

Irritability and mental depression are often found in patients with blood disorders. Irritability, dizziness, and difficulty in concentrating could be caused by a decreased supply of blood to the brain. Depression is certainly understandable when one considers the chronic lack of energy, difficulty in eating and enjoying food, and the many other problems patients with blood dyscrasias often suffer. Lack of energy can prevent them from doing the things they want to do and may interfere with social activities. The patient simply may not want to expend the energy it takes to participate in social interaction and so is denied the enjoyment of being with other people.

Activity Intolerance

Physical activity increases the demand for oxygen, but if there are not enough circulating RBCs to provide the necessary oxygen, the patient becomes physically weak and unable to engage in physical activity without severe fatigue. When helping a patient with his activities of daily living, the nurse can note whether he is able to do things for himself or needs help to complete specific tasks. The nurse might ask him how much he is able to do at home in regard to such activities as bathing and dressing and whether he needs assistance. To get more specific data she could ask how far he can walk without feeling tired, how he feels after walking up a flight of stairs, and how much work he can do at home without stopping to rest.

Common nursing diagnoses and appropriate interventions for patients experiencing blood dyscrasias are listed in Table 18–2.

ANEMIA

The term *anemia* is actually a misnomer, because it means, in the strictest sense, an absence of blood. In reality, anemia is an *abnormality in*

TABLE 18–2 COMMON NURSING DIAGNOSES AND INTERVENTIONS FOR PATIENTS WITH BLOOD DISORDERS

Nursing Diagnosis	Intervention
Alteration in nutrition, less than body requirements, related to:	Instruct in foods that meet required needs. Obtain dietary consult as needed.
Iron deficiency from inadequate intake or blood loss	Administer iron preparation; if liquid, give through straw. Give with vitamin C–containing juice or food. Warn that stool may be greenish-black.
Vitamin B_{12} deficiency	Administer vitamin B_{12} as ordered; advise that lifetime therapy is needed.
Stomatitis	Give gentle mouth care before meals and q 2 h. Provide bland, easily chewed foods. Monitor CBC count for evidence of increase in RBCs and Hgb.
Activity intolerance related to decreased RBCs or Hgb A	Administer oxygen by nasal cannula at 3–6 L/min as ordered for patient with sickle cell crisis. Space activities, allowing rest periods for patient with fatigue. Assist with ADL to prevent fatigue. Maintain skin integrity. Turn frequently. If dizzy, caution to change position slowly; call for assistance with ambulation.
Pain related to ischemia and swollen joints	Elevate swollen joints and apply hot or cold packs. Encourage high fluid intake. Monitor IV fluid therapy. Teach to avoid strenuous exercise. Use bed cradle to support bed covers. Administer analgesics as ordered prn.
Potential for injury, related to low platelet count	Assess for signs of internal bleeding: bruises, urine, stool. Minimize trauma; handle gently. Apply ice packs and gentle pressure if hematoma seems to be forming. Monitor administration of platelets prn. Use small-gauge needle for injections; rotate sites.
Potential for infection, related to decreased leukocytes	Observe for early signs of infection and report. Use strict aseptic technique for wound care and invasive procedures. Reverse isolation as indicated. Teach patient good personal hygiene. Maintain integrity of skin and mucosa. Administer antiinfectives precisely as ordered.
Knowledge deficit, related to substances that damage bone marrow	Assess for exposure to substances that could have damaged the bone marrow. Teach about drugs and chemicals that are harmful to bone marrow and how to prevent damage. Seek feedback to validate understanding of content taught.
Anxiety related to unknown outcome of diagnostic tests and knowledge of disease, treatment, and prognosis	Provide teaching regarding each diagnostic test. Encourage verbalization of fears. Offer emotional support to patient and family.
Self-esteem disturbance, related to inability to perform usual activities	Assist to cope with limitations of the illness. Help to plan ways to maintain appropriate activity. Help him focus on the things he can still do. Obtain counseling referral if psychological disturbance indicates need.
Potential ineffective family coping, related to expense of treatment and possible death of patient	Refer leukemia patients to community resources such as the American Cancer Society for assistance. Assist family and patient to understand the disease, treatment modalities, and their implications. Encourage attendance for all family members in a support group. Obtain referral to social worker for further assistance. Encourage open communication within family.

the number and characteristics of red blood cells circulating in the blood. In a healthy person, there is a balance maintained between production of new cells and the disposal of old, "worn out" cells. When something happens to upset this balance or interfere with maturation of cells, anemia results.

The functional definition of anemia refers to transport of oxygen to tissues; that is, anemia is a state in which there are insufficient numbers of functioning red blood cells to meet the demands of the tissues for oxygen.

CLASSIFICATION

There are three major classifications of anemia according to cause: (1) anemia resulting from blood loss, (2) anemia resulting from a failure in blood cell production, and (3) anemia associated with an excessive destruction of red cells.

A blood loss that leads to anemia may result from severe trauma to the blood vessels and massive hemorrhage or may be more gradual, as in a small, bleeding peptic ulcer.

Anemia caused by a failure in cell production is the result of either a deficiency of certain substances necessary for the formation of red blood cells or abnormal function of bone marrow. Examples of this type of anemia are (1) nutritional anemia, in which there is an inadequate intake of foods containing proteins and iron, and (2) pernicious anemia, in which there is faulty absorption of specific nutrients such as vitamin B_{12} and iron.

Anemias associated with excessive destruction of red blood cells are exceedingly rare. They are known as *hemolytic anemias* (*hemolysis* means the destruction of red blood cells). Some of the hemolytic anemias are inherited, whereas others are caused by exposure of the erythrocytes to poisonous agents such as chemicals or certain bacterial toxins.

Another way in which anemias are classified is according to the *morphologic characteristics* of erythrocytes—that is, their various sizes and shapes. This classification is based on objective laboratory findings.

The kind of data used to classify anemias morphologically includes (1) the mean corpuscular volume (MCV), which is a measure of the volume of the average erythrocyte in cubic microns; (2) the mean corpuscular hemoglobin (MCH), which indicates the amount (by weight) of hemoglobin in the erythrocytes in the blood sample; and (3) the mean corpuscular hemoglobin concentration (MCHC), which represents the concentration of hemoglobin in the average erythrocyte.

The term *mean* indicates a mathematical average. Therefore, the data obtained through the tests are purely objective and not as susceptible to error as is information about the causes of anemia. Morphologic classification provides a very accurate description of the exact type of anemia present.

The microscopic appearance of the red cells on a film of blood that has been spread over a slide gives information about abnormalities in size, shape, and color of erythrocytes circulating in the patient's blood stream.

The prefix *normo* refers to normal, the suffix *cyte* refers to cell, and the suffix *chrom* refers to color. Thus a normocytic, normochromic anemia is characterized by cells that are normal in size and color but have a deficiency in the number of RBCs and in the hematocrit. This type of anemia usually occurs as a result of sudden blood loss.

A hypochromic, microcytic anemia is characterized by decreased levels of hemoglobin (not enough color) and small (micro) cells. This type of anemia is typical of an iron deficiency anemia.

SIGNS, SYMPTOMS, AND MEDICAL TREATMENT

Rapid, severe bleeding leads to hypovolemia (decreased volume of circulating blood) and shock. The bleeding may be external or it may be internal and therefore more difficult to detect. The classical signs and symptoms of hypovolemia are falling blood pressure; rapid, weak pulse; cool, damp skin; thirst; decreased urine output; and restlessness progressing to decreased consciousness. The best treatment is restoration of blood volume with fluids and blood by transfusion.

Signs and symptoms of anemia from other causes are essentially the same and include pallor, fatigue, headache, and dizziness or faintness. These all relate directly to the decreased ability of the blood to transport sufficient oxygen to the tissues.

Anemia from chronic, slow blood loss is treated by correcting the underlying problem and then building replacement blood cells with good nutrition and iron intake. Anemia caused by inadequate iron or protein intake is managed with oral iron supplements and diet adjustment.

Pernicious anemia is treated by regular injections of vitamin B_{12}, as the deficiency of intrinsic factor prevents adequate absorption of this vitamin from food.

For hemolytic anemia, the underlying cause is found and corrected if possible, and then the blood volume is rebuilt with added iron and appropriate diet. If the anemia is severe, blood transfusion may be indicated.

NURSING INTERVENTION

Intervention begins with an understanding of the particular kind of anemia affecting the patient. Anemia from blood loss presents problems quite different from those related to chronic, and possibly incurable, anemia.

Actions are directed toward preventing complications for patients with anemias that interfere with clotting and tend to cause bleeding episodes. Assistance with activities of daily living is essential for any patient with anemia severe enough to cause fatigue. Planned rest periods must be provided for these patients.

Administration of blood, iron, B_{12}, and folic acid and monitoring for desired effect is a nursing function. Patient teaching regarding needed dietary adjustments is also done. Analgesia for headache or joint pain is given as ordered, and the patient is monitored for adverse side effects. Table 18–2 identifies nursing diagnoses commonly used for patients with anemia and lists appropriate interventions.

POLYCYTHEMIA VERA

Excessive production of red blood cells results in polycythemia vera. White cell numbers also increase. The cause of this disorder is unknown. The blood becomes more viscous (thick) from the increased numbers of cells, and there is a tendency to develop blood clots. Signs and symptoms include a reddish face with deep red-purple lips, fatigue, weakness, dizziness, headache, and enlarged spleen (splenomegaly). Minor injury may result in excessive bleeding.

Treatment is aimed at reducing the number of blood cells. Antineoplastic agents, radiation therapy, and phlebotomy are all used. In phlebotomy, a blood vessel is pierced, and blood is drawn off. As much as 500 mL at a time may be withdrawn. Increased fluid intake is essential to decrease blood viscosity, and aspirin is used to decrease platelet clumping and clot formation.

IDIOPATHIC THROMBOCYTOPENIA PURPURA

Idiopathic thrombocytopenia purpura is a disorder in which the platelets are decreased in number either from decreased manufacture or from increased destruction of platelets by the spleen. *Idiopathic* means without known cause. Signs and symptoms include purpura (small areas of hemorrhage in the skin and mucous membranes) or large bruised areas called *ecchymoses*. Bleeding can occur in any part of the body.

Some patients recover spontaneously. Otherwise, transfusion of platelets is used to control hemorrhage. Splenectomy is done if the patient does not respond to other therapy with the hope that this will remove the cause of platelet destruction.

Nursing care is focused on prevention of bleeding by careful handling of the patient, close observation for signs of spontaneous bleeding, and quick intervention.

SICKLE CELL DISEASE

Sickle cell disease is a genetic disorder in which the gene is inherited from both parents (homozygous). It is characterized by erythrocytes that contain more hemoglobin S than hemoglobin A.

In the United States, the most common disorders related to the presence of this specific type of hemoglobin are *homozygous sickle cell anemia, sickle cell thalassemia,* and *sickle cell hemoglobin C disease.* Of these, homozygous S, or sickle cell anemia, is by far the most common. *Sickle cell trait,* in which only about 50% of an individual's total hemoglobin is affected, is present in about 1 of every 10 to 12 blacks in this country.

Sickle cell disease is found mostly in African-Americans, but also affects some people whose ancestors were from the Mediterranean region, the Middle East, and India.

Nearly 10% of the black population of the United States have the trait, are therefore carriers, and can transmit the gene to their children. Therefore genetic counseling and adequate screening for early detection of the disease are considered extremely important in the control of sickle cell anemia. Figure 18–2 illustrates the statistical probabilities of transmission.

When the patient with sickle cell disease experiences lower oxygenation than normal, the defective hemoglobin forms clumps in the red cells, causing them to assume a sickle shape (Fig. 18–3). The deformed cells cannot move along in the blood stream as easily as normal cells, and they have difficulty passing through the smaller blood vessels. They tend to break apart and pile against one another. This obstruction to the flow of blood deprives the hemoglobin of the oxygen it needs, and thus a vicious cycle of oxygen deprivation and cell malformation is begun. Thrombosis (clotting) in the vessels leads to infarction (tissue death) in areas not receiving blood. Infarction can occur in the brain, lungs, bone marrow, or spleen (Fig. 18–4). Lower oxygenation occurs at high altitudes or with strenuous exercise, severe illness, or sometimes anesthesia. Sickling can also occur with acidosis or dehydration.

Infants are not usually affected until about 6 months of age, when sufficient fetal hemoglobin has been replaced with hemoglobin S. In young

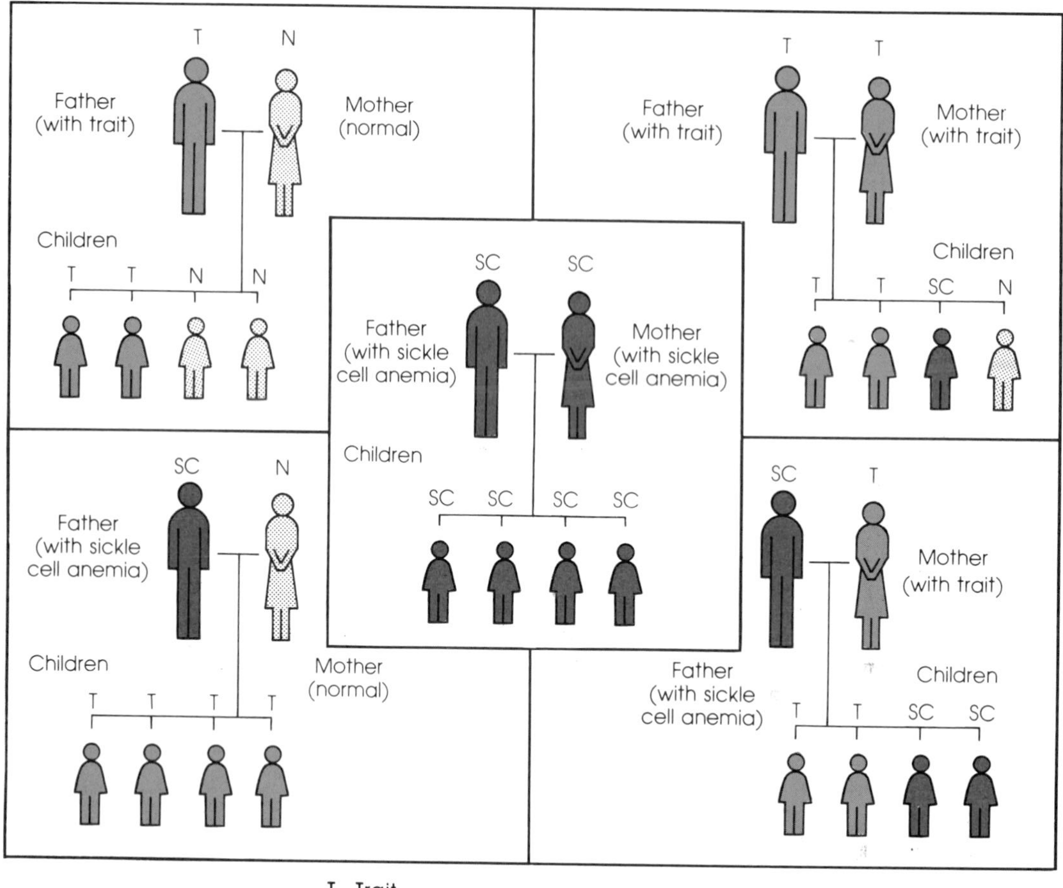

Figure 18-2 Statistical probabilities of inheriting sickle cell anemia.

children, painful and swollen fingers and toes (dactylitis) and enlargement of the liver and spleen may be the earliest signs.

Sickle cell trait occurs in people who have only one gene, rather than a pair of genes, for sickle cell anemia. They usually do not have problems with sickling unless they experience severe deprivation of oxygenation (Fig. 18-2).

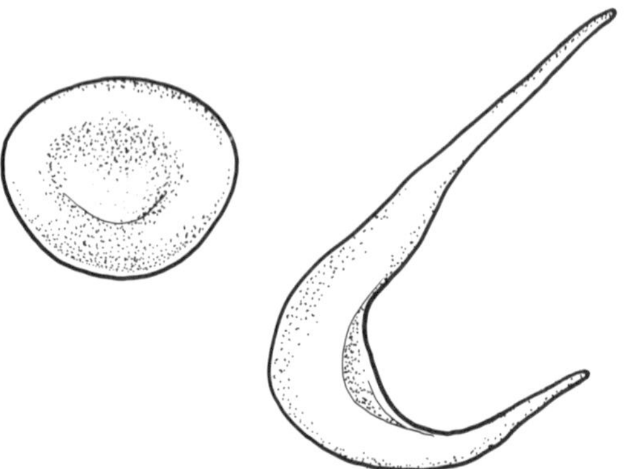

Figure 18-3 Normal and sickled red blood cell.

SIGNS AND SYMPTOMS

Pallor and lethargy may indicate that a "sickle cell crisis" is about to occur. Swelling and limitation of movement of joints may occur next. When sickling causes thrombosis, signs resulting from decreased blood supply to organs and tissues occur. There may be pain from ischemia and swollen joints, decreased urine output from decreased blood flow through the kidneys, or signs of neurologic damage if infarction occurs in the brain. The signs and symptoms depend on which organs and tissues are affected. Leg ulcers can develop from thrombosis in the microcirculation, especially around the ankles.

Signs typical of anemia also occur after sickle cell crisis, as the abnormally shaped cells are very fragile and break easily. The RBC and hemoglobin count can drop very quickly during a crisis.

MEDICAL TREATMENT

There is no cure for sickle cell anemia; treatment is primarily symptomatic and preventive.

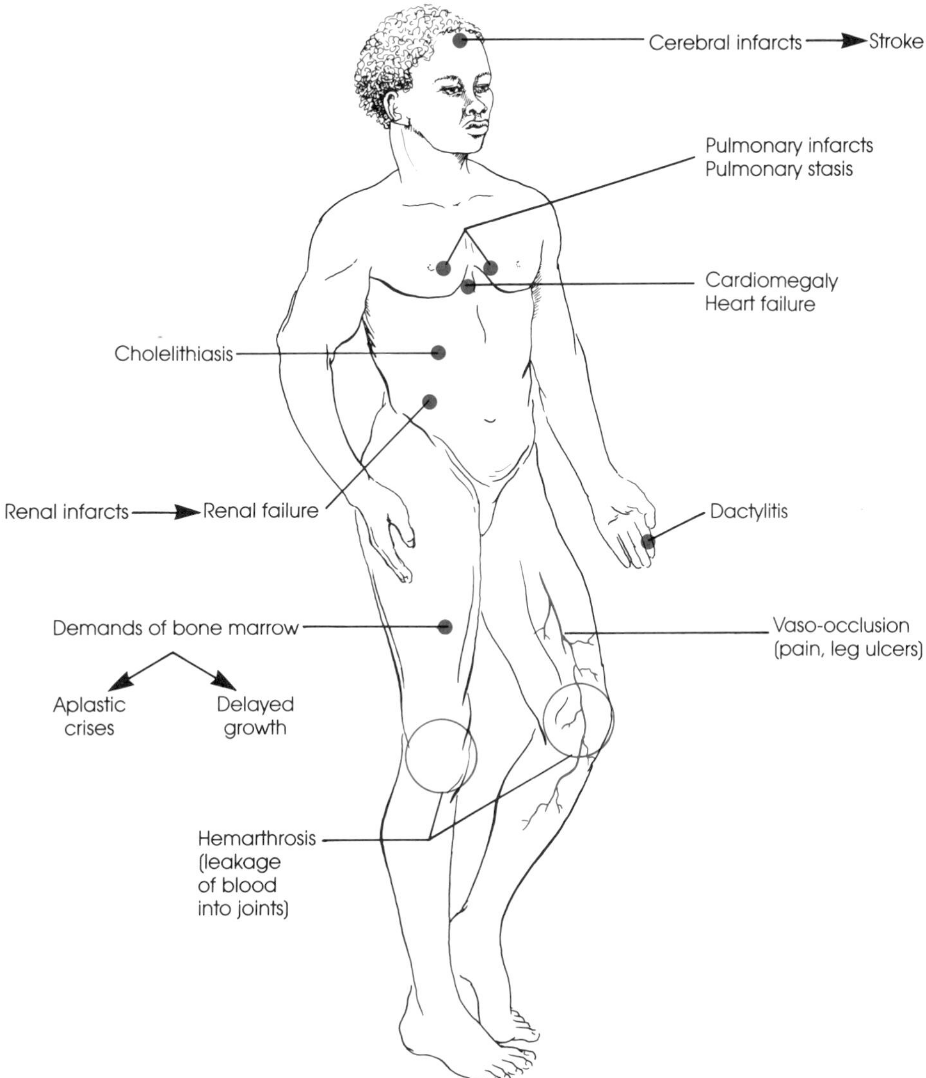

Figure 18-4 Potential effects of episodes of sickling. The fragility of the abnormal red blood cells results in their destruction, the formation of emboli and infarcts, and leakage of blood into the joints. Virtually every system of the body can be adversely affected.

The patient is usually treated at home with bed rest, adequate fluids, and analgesics. If his hemoglobin drops considerably or his condition suddenly deteriorates, he is hospitalized, given oxygen, and transfused with packed red cells. IV fluids are given, and narcotic analgesics may be needed to control pain. An attempt is made to mobilize the sickled cells and prevent infarction of major organs. Infection is treated with appropriate antibiotics.

NURSING INTERVENTION

Prevention of complications is a major goal in the nursing management of sickle cell anemia. Education of the patient and his family and the general public about differences between sickle cell trait and sickle cell anemia can do much to allay unnecessary anxiety and worry. When the diagnosis is sickle cell anemia, the nurse must have a thorough understanding of the disease and its potential harm to virtually every organ in the body.

Adequate nutrition, increased fluid intake, avoidance of infections, and regular visits to the clinic or physician are essential for prevention and early detection of adverse responses to the illness. See Table 18-2 for specific nursing intervention.

Sickle cell disease is an inherited disorder and therefore can affect decisions about whether to have children when one or both parents either have the disease or are carriers of the trait. Genetic counseling should be encouraged. Nursing care of the patient experiencing a sickle cell crisis is presented in Nursing Care Plan 18-1.

At the present time there are several sources of help for improving understanding of the disease

NURSING CARE PLAN 18–1

Selected nursing diagnoses, goals/outcome criteria, nursing interventions, and evaluations for a patient experiencing a sickle cell crisis

Situation: John Talbert, a 28-year-old black male, has sickle cell disease. He had the flu last week and now is in sickle cell crisis. He is experiencing severe pain, joint swelling, and splenomegaly. He is hospitalized for pain relief and treatment.

Nursing Diagnosis	Goals/Outcome Criteria	Nursing Intervention	Evaluation
Alteration in tissue perfusion related to sickling of red blood cells. SUPPORTING DATA Known sickle cell disease; experiencing sickling episode with pain, joint swelling, pallor, and lethargy.	Organ damage from infarction will be prevented; sickling will be halted within 3 days.	Oxygen at 5 L/min continuous by cannula or mask as ordered. Monitor cardiac rate and rhythm q 4 h or more often if he experiences further chest pain. Auscultate lungs q 4 h; assess peripheral pulses and circulation q 4 h. Observe urine for signs of blood indicating impairment of kidney function. Maintain on bed rest with bathroom privileges if allowed. Maintain IV and oral hydration to promote blood circulation.	Continuous oxygen given; IV flow rate maintained; joint swelling slightly decreased; urine negative for blood; no sign of cardiac, kidney, or other organ infarction; continue plan.
Pain related to sickling interference with microcirculation and joint inflammation. SUPPORTING DATA Sickle cell crisis; knees, ankles, and elbows all swollen; grimacing and guarding against movement; states pain is severe.	Pain will be controlled with analgesia within 12 h. Pain will be absent at discharge.	Medicate with IV narcotic as ordered; assess effect of medication; utilize oral analgesics between narcotic doses as ordered. Encourage relaxation techniques and imagery to decrease pain. Utilize distraction activities. Apply warm packs to swollen joints to ease pain and promote blood circulation. Keep well hydrated to promote better blood circulation.	Demerol and aspirin are controlling pain; warm packs applied, swelling reduced; hydration status good; continue plan.
Infection related to influenza virus and superimposed sinusitis. SUPPORTING DATA Had influenza last week; temperature 100.8°F; purulent drainage from nose; cough; sinus headaches; boggy turbinates and some pus evident.	No infection at discharge, as evidenced by lack of colored nasal secretions, normal temperature, no productive cough.	Administer ordered antibiotics on schedule; monitor for side effects. Monitor temperature and WBCs for signs that infection is resolving. Keep well hydrated. Keep oxygen flow well humidified. Instruct him to contact physician at first sign of infection in order to get early treatment and prevent sickle cell crisis.	Antibiotics administered on schedule; less sinus congestion; secretions still yellow; drinking lots of fluid; teaching regarding infection reinforced; continue plan.
Activity intolerance related to pain and joint swelling of sickle cell crisis. SUPPORTING DATA Ankle, knee, and elbow joints all swollen and reddened; experiencing severe pain on movement; bed rest ordered.	Patient will not develop leg ulcer as result of this sickle cell crisis. Patient will maintain bed rest until crisis is resolved, as evidenced by decreased pain and swelling and lab data indicating lack of sickling.	Maintain bed rest as ordered. Assist to reposition q 1 to 2 h; pad joint areas and inspect pressure points and legs each time position is changed. Encourage rest to help resolve crisis. Assist with all ADL to conserve energy and avert pain.	Maintaining bed rest; pressure points without skin breakdown; repositioned at 8, 10, 12, and 2; assisted with all ADL; rested for 1 h both A.M. and P.M.; continue plan.

and for helping families cope with the multitude of problems it can cause. There are Comprehensive Sickle Cell Centers scattered throughout the country that can provide educational material and support. Other sources for educational materials include:

- National Association for Sickle Cell Disease, Inc.
  4221 Wilshire Blvd.
  Suite 360
  Los Angeles, CA 90010
- Sickle Cell Center
  Howard University College of Medicine
  2121 Georgia Ave., N.W.
  Washington, DC 20059
- National Sickle Cell Program
  Division of Blood Diseases and Resources
  National Heart, Lung, Blood Institute
  National Institutes of Health
  Sickle Cell Disease Branch
  Room 4 A-27, Building 31
  Bethesda, MD 20014

APLASTIC ANEMIA

Aplastic anemia may develop after a viral infection, as a reaction to a drug, or as a result of an inherited tendency for it. The disease is characterized by bone marrow depression. Red cells, white cells, and platelets are decreased. Toxic effects of certain substances such as benzene, insecticides, or drugs such as chloramphenicol (Chloromycetin), phenylbutazone (Butazolidin), or antineoplastic agents such as nitrogen mustard can be responsible for aplastic anemia. Many other drugs can potentially cause aplastic anemia, but this adverse effect is rare. Radiation exposure is another factor in the development of the disorder.

Signs and symptoms are the same as those of iron deficiency anemia but also include ecchymosis, petechiae, and hemorrhage from thrombocytopenia (too few thrombocytes). Infection without inflammation also occurs because of the very low leukocyte count.

Diagnosis is by blood count with differential, by bone marrow biopsy, and by ruling out other disorders. Treatment must eliminate any identifiable underlying cause. Packed red cells and platelets are administered. Reverse isolation is necessary to prevent infection in those with low leukocyte counts. Antibiotics are given for identified infection; oxygen is administered to those patients with low erythrocyte counts. Bone marrow transplant is the treatment of choice for those with severe bone marrow depression.

NURSING INTERVENTION

Prevention of hemorrhage and infection are top priorities. Psychological support of the patient and family is important when they are faced with this life-threatening condition. Nursing diagnoses and interventions are listed in Table 18–2.

Another responsibility of the nurse is to monitor blood studies carefully for all patients who are receiving any drug that is potentially damaging to the bone marrow. All nurses should promote public education about the dangers of toxic agents. It is vitally important that people read and follow the label instructions on all cleaning agents, insecticides, and chemical compounds.

LEUKEMIA

The word *leukemia,* when translated literally, means *white blood.* Actually, the white blood cells would have to number 1,000,000/mm³ before the blood would have a milky white appearance, and though leukemia is characterized by an increase in the number of leukocytes, they rarely rise above 500,000/mm³. In addition to the increase in number, however, the leukocytes of the patient with leukemia are abnormal cells that do not function as normal white cells do. Malignant proliferation of WBCs causes the disease.

An *acute* leukemia is one in which there are a lot of primitive cells, called *blasts.* In *chronic* leukemia, the predominant cells are more mature. Leukemias are also classified by the origin of the abnormal cells. *Myeloid leukemia* arises from the bone marrow, whereas *lymphoid leukemia* has its origin in the lymphatic system. There are four types of leukemia: acute myelogenous leukemia (AML), chronic myelogenous leukemia (CML), acute lymphocytic leukemia (ALL), and chronic lymphocytic leukemia (CLL).

Acute leukemia is the most common form of cancer in children, although it also occurs in adults. About 13,900 people develop this disorder annually (American Cancer Society, 1990). In acute leukemia there is a sudden, rapid proliferation of immature blast or stem cells, rapid progression of the disease, and a short survival time if the disease is not treated.

Chronic forms of leukemia have a more gradual onset, slower disease progression, and a relatively longer survival time. Chronic lymphocytic leukemia is common in men over age 50 and accounts for one third of the new cases of leukemia annually. Chronic myelogenous leukemia is most common in young and middle-aged adults. Over time it progresses to the acute form, and eventual death is inevitable.

CAUSATIVE FACTORS AND EFFECTS

As with other types of cancers, the exact cause of leukemia is not known. There are, however, some factors that are considered to be closely linked with the development of leukemia. Exposure to *ionizing radiation* in relatively large doses is one such factor. Another is exposure to certain *chemicals*, such as benzene, that are toxic to bone marrow. The third factor, one that has been the subject of much research in the past few years, is the theory that *tumor viruses* are in some way linked to the development of leukemia. No one has yet been able to isolate a virus that can be identified as the specific cause of leukemia. There has been a chromosomal link found for chronic myelogenous leukemia. About 90% of patients with CML have the Philadelphia chromosome.

There are three major effects of leukemia: (1) increased numbers of abnormal, immature leukocytes, (2) accumulations of these cells within the lymph nodes, spleen, and other organs, and (3) eventual infiltration of the malignant cells throughout the body.

The symptoms produced by these pathologic changes are presented in Table 18–3.

DIAGNOSIS AND MEDICAL TREATMENT

Treatment is aimed at (1) slowing down the growth of the malignant blood cells; (2) maintaining a normal level of red cells, hemoglobin, and platelets; and (3) management of the symptoms and meeting the special needs of each patient.

The patient with leukemia usually complains of fatigue and malaise and may complain of frequent infections. Diagnosis is made by physical examination, complete blood cell count with differential, and bone marrow studies to rule out other disorders.

Acute leukemia treatment consists primarily of chemotherapy with a combination of antineoplastic agents that are targeted at different phases of the cell cycle. Radiation therapy is sometimes used supplementally. Cure is sometimes possible, as has been evidenced in children with ALL. Results in adults have not been as good. Bone marrow transplantation is being investigated as a treatment for patients under age 30 who have had an initial remission with chemotherapy. Eventually it is hoped that monoclonal antibody treatment can be combined with bone marrow transplant to provide lasting remission.

Chronic lymphocytic leukemia is not treated until the patient experiences symptoms. At that time alkylating agents such as chlorambucil and prednisone are used.

Chronic myelogenous leukemia is managed with oral alkylating agents or hydroxyurea. Research with recombinant human alpha interferon to induce remission for CML is ongoing. Leukopheresis (extraction of WBCs) may be done to reduce the massive number of circulating leukocytes that clog organs and cause infarction.

Transfusions of blood components are prescribed to maintain a near-normal blood picture. Antibiotics are given immediately to control infections, because the body's defense mechanisms are seriously compromised.

TABLE 18–3 BASES FOR CLINICAL MANIFESTATIONS OF LEUKEMIA

Manifestations	Bases
Severe infections	Immature and abnormally functioning leukocytes, even though there is an increased number of them.
Symptoms of anemia	Rapidly proliferating white cells apparently "crowd out" developing red cells and platelets.
Enlarged spleen, liver, lymph nodes	Excess white cells accumulate within organs, causing distention of tissues.
Weakness, pallor, and weight loss due to elevated metabolic rate	Increased production of white cells requires large amounts of amino acids and vitamins. Increased destruction of cells leads to more metabolic wastes that must be disposed of by the body.
Renal pain, urinary stones and obstruction to flow of urine, and infection	Large amounts of uric acid are released when white cells are destroyed by antileukemic drugs.
Headache, disorientation, and other CNS symptoms	Abnormal white cells infiltrate the central nervous system.

NURSING INTERVENTION

Among the problems presented by a patient with leukemia are potential for infection, abnormal bleeding, anemia, nutritional alteration with severe cancerous cachexia, altered urine elimination related to increased levels of uric acid in the urine and blood, and psychosocial problems related to the effects of the disease as well as the prescribed treatment.

Infection is a threat to the patient with leukemia either because of abnormal function of bone marrow that is characteristic of the disease or because of suppression of bone marrow function as a result of therapy. Infections from bacteria, viruses, and fungi are the most common cause of death in persons with leukemia. Nursing measures such as those described in Chapter 6 are essential to prevention of this very serious complication of leukemia.

Abnormal bleeding as a result of a very low platelet count is the second most common and dangerous complication of leukemia. Observation of the patient, awareness of his current platelet count, and prevention of trauma to body tissues and blood vessels are primary concerns in the nursing management of leukemia.

Anemia and its attendant problems of fatigue, hypoxia, gastrointestinal upsets, and cardiovascular complications such as circulatory overload is always a threat and in many cases a reality in patients with leukemia. The anemia can result from the disease itself, from excessive bleeding, or from the therapy administered. Nursing measures previously described for the patient with anemia are appropriate to the care of the patient with leukemia.

Nutritional problems arise from any of a number of conditions. Extreme weight loss and emaciation are nearly always seen in patients with cancer. Failure to eat sufficient amounts of nutritious foods is not the only reason this is so. As was explained in Chapter 13, metabolic changes that occur with the proliferation of malignant cells in the body also are responsible for weight loss and emaciation. If nursing measures to alleviate or minimize stomatitis, nausea, and vomiting are not effective, parenteral nutrition may be necessary.

Intensive chemotherapy and the rapid destruction of cells can bring about an increase of uric acid in the urine and blood. If the uric acid crystals settle out in the kidney structures, the patient can experience impaired renal function. Maintenance of adequate hydration and administration of drugs to decrease production of uric acid are important nursing measures, as is close observation of fluid intake and urinary output.

The emotional impact of a diagnosis of cancer and the psychosocial needs of the cancer patient and his family were discussed in Chapter 13.

HEMOPHILIA

Hemophilia is an inherited disorder in which there is a deficiency of specific clotting factors. Classic hemophilia, also known as *hemophilia A* and *factor VIII deficiency*, affects more than 80% of all hemophiliacs. It is characterized by a delayed blood coagulation time that produces a prolonged period of bleeding after injury or surgery. This type of hemophilia almost always occurs in males and is transmitted through the female. Although the female does not have the disease herself, she and all her female descendants can transmit classic hemophilia to their offspring.

There are other types of hemophilia, similar to classic hemophilia, that can affect both men and women.

In all types of hemophilia, there is a decrease in the amount of activity of one of the 11 different clotting factors normally present in blood and essential to the formation of clots.

Hemophilia A results from a *deficiency* of factor VIII. Hemophilia B, or Christmas disease, is the result of a deficiency of factor IX. In von Willebrand's disease, there is a decrease in the *activity* of factor VIII, even though the factor is present in normal amounts in the plasma. The blood of a hemophiliac forms a clot immediately after injury, but the clot is unstable and does not effectively impede bleeding.

There are varying degrees of severity in the types of hemophilia, depending on the amount of the factor present and the role of the factor in clot formation. For the patients with mild cases, who have 25% to 50% of the deficient factor present in the serum, symptoms may not appear at all until a severe injury or surgery is followed by prolonged bleeding and the hemophilia is thus discovered. In very severe cases, in which less than 1% of the factor is present, the affected individuals may bleed spontaneously without injury, and severe hemorrhage can develop very quickly whenever an injury does occur.

SYMPTOMS

The most obvious symptom of hemophilia is, of course, bleeding. However, it is not surface bleeding that causes the most serious complications of hemophilia. Bleeding most often occurs internally, with leakage of blood into the joints, the intestinal wall or peritoneal cavity, and the deeper tissues of the body. Hemarthrosis, or bleeding into the joints, produces swelling, pain, warmth, and limitation of movement similar to that suffered by the patient with rheumatoid arthritis. If the bleeding occurs in the intracranial spaces and thereby increases intracranial pressure, the patient may experience convulsions and brain damage that can be fatal. Other serious complications from internal bleeding in the hemophiliac include obstruction of the airway as a result of hemorrhage into the neck or pharynx and intestinal obstruction resulting from bleeding into the intestinal wall or peritoneum.

MEDICAL TREATMENT

Plasma concentrates are used to replace the missing factors in the more common types of hemophilia. These factor replacements include those needed to treat von Willebrand's disease, factor VIII deficiency (classic hemophilia), and factor IX deficiency (Christmas disease). The availability of these replacement factors has greatly improved the outlook for those with hemophilia and helped the hemophiliac person live a more normal life.

Many patients with hemophilia have been receiving blood products for a number of years. Unfortunately some patients have been infected with the human immunodeficiency virus (HIV) from contaminated plasma concentrates. Before the invention of an HIV-specific blood test just a few years ago, there was no way to tell whether blood donors carried the virus. This problem has created additional psychological stress for the patient with hemophilia. There is considerable fear of AIDS and people infected with the HIV virus, and those who have developed AIDS are frequently shunned.

Hemophilia is a complex disease requiring individual treatment and nursing care based on the needs of each patient. The hemophiliac should be encouraged to lead an active life insofar as he is able to avoid situations that predispose him to injury and illness. The parents of a child with hemophilia should avoid overprotecting him, because treating him as an invalid and sheltering him from normal childhood activities deny him the opportunity to develop into a healthy, well-adjusted person.

NURSING INTERVENTION

In addition to administering the necessary clotting factors, interventions include elevating the injured body part, applying cold packs, controlling pain, observing for further bleeding, and providing psychological support for the patient and family. The nurse should also encourage genetic counseling for family members if this has not been done previously.

DISORDERS OF THE LYMPHATIC SYSTEM

Unlike the circulatory system, the lymphatic system has no central pump. The movement of lymph along the extensive network of channels, capillaries, vessels, and nodes depends on massage by the skeletal muscles and arteries, intestinal peristalsis, respiratory movements, and response to gravitational pull.

The lymph itself is the fluid that is drained from the tissue spaces (interstitial fluid) and emptied into the lymphatic vessels. In the abdominal lymphatic system, a steady flow of digested fatty food elements (called *chyle*) is transported from the intestinal mucosa to the thoracic duct, where it enters the blood circulation.

Disorders of the lymphatic system include malignant lymphomas and other proliferative blood disorders; inflammation of the lymph nodes (*lymphadenitis*) and lymph vessels (*lymphangitis*); and obstruction to the flow of lymph, which results in swelling of the tissues served by the obstructed lymph vessels (*lymphedema*).

DIAGNOSTIC TESTS

Physical examination of the lymph nodes can reveal redness, swelling, hardness, tenderness, and other signs of inflammation and infection of the lymph nodes.

Radiologic examination of the lymphatic vessels (*lymphangiography*) requires injection of a radiopaque medium directly into the lymphatic vessels in the hands and feet. The procedure aids in the diagnosis of metastatic involvement of lymph nodes by malignant cells and bacterial and viral cells. The presence and extent of involvement in the lymph nodes at the time of the lymphangiography can be determined. Moreover, because the contrast medium is retained in the lymphatic system for 4 to 6 weeks after injection, reductions in malignant growth as a result of treatment can be observed.

LYMPHANGITIS

Inflammation of the lymph vessels is usually diagnosed when red streaks and tenderness are noted along a part of the body near a site of infection. These red streaks follow the course of the infected and inflamed lymph vessel and extend from the site of infection to the nearest lymph nodes.

Treatment of lymphangitis is aimed at relieving the infection at the primary site. If these efforts fail, the infection spreads to the circulatory system, resulting in septicemia (called "blood poisoning" by many laypersons).

LYMPHEDEMA

Swelling of the tissues drained by the lymphatic system occurs as a result of obstruction to the flow of lymph along the vessels. It is especially common in the lower extremities and other dependent organs. The obstruction may be the result of a *congenital* condition in which there is hypoplasia of the lymphatic system of a lower extremity. This condition chiefly affects females and most often becomes apparent during the middle teens to early 20s.

Acquired lymphedema is the result of an obstruction caused by trauma to the lymph vessels and nodes, as following surgical resection of the nodes, for example in mastectomy. Other causes of obstruction include extensive soft tissue injury and scar formation and, in tropical countries, parasites that enter and occlude lymph channels.

NURSING INTERVENTION

Lymphedema that involves an extremity often can be treated conservatively using simple nursing measures. Prevention and treatment of lymphedema of the arm and hand following mastectomy is covered in Chapter 13. In general, any lymphedema of an extremity responds to the following measures.

- Elevate the extremity to the level of the heart. This reduces hydrostatic pressure within the veins.
- Active exercise of the skeletal muscles. This promotes massage of the lymph vessels and the movement of lymph.
- Application of elasticized stockings or gloves. This increases pressure on interstitial fluid and encourages venous return.

LYMPHOMAS

Lymphomas are malignant neoplasms that affect the lymphoid tissue and lymph nodes. The two main types of lymphoma are Hodgkin's disease and non-Hodgkin's lymphoma. The most common sign of both is one or more enlarged lymph nodes.

Hodgkin's Disease

Hodgkin's disease primarily affects young adults. The disorder is often discovered when lymphadenopathy is found on a routine examination or an employment physical examination. Some patients experience fever, night sweats, or weight loss. Diagnosis is made by the presence of Reed-Sternberg cells in the blood. Lymphangiography is used to help determine progression of the disease and appropriate therapy. Treatment depends on how far the disease has progressed. Remission and cure are often achieved with the use of radiation, chemotherapy, or both. Stage IA and IIA disease patients have a greater than 90% 5-year survival rate, which will probably translate to a cure.

Non-Hodgkin's Lymphoma

Several similar neoplasms are classified as non-Hodgkin's lymphoma. The cause of lymphoma is unknown, but viruses, immunosuppression, and radiation are all thought to be possible contributors to the disorder. This type of lymphoma tends to have more widespread involvement of lymphoid tissue than found in Hodgkin's disease. Treatment is with chemotherapy or radiation, depending on the stage of disease, and offers relief of symptoms but often does not alter survival. However, aggressive chemotherapy with a combination of drugs has been effective for some patients with advanced disease.

Nursing Intervention

Nursing care is directed toward supporting the patient through the diagnostic process and observing for and treating side effects of radiation and chemotherapy. Chapter 13 contains information on specific nursing diagnoses and interventions for the patient with cancer.

THE SPLEEN

Although all kinds of disorders can have an adverse effect on the spleen, the organ itself is rarely the original site of disease. Because of the nature of its many functions, the spleen is involved in all systemic inflammations, in blood disorders, and in many metabolic disturbances.

The most common disorders are (1) rupture of the spleen as a result of a crushing injury or blow and (2) splenomegaly (enlarged spleen). An enlarged spleen usually is palpable below the rib cage. Radioactive scanning can show the organ's size and shape, and any infarcts and abnormal masses. The radioactive substance is injected intravenously and consists of radiolabeled red cells, platelets, or colloids, which are readily taken up by the reticuloendothelial system.

SPLENECTOMY

Indications for surgical removal of the spleen include (1) severe trauma to and rupture of the spleen; (2) splenomegaly, in which the destructive functions of the organ are greatly accelerated; and (3) certain blood disorders.

Although the known functions of the spleen are important and other functions have not yet been identified, the spleen is not an indispensable organ. The other organs of the monocyte-macrophage system take over many of its chores once it has been removed. However, those persons who no longer have a functioning spleen, whether as a result of disease or surgical removal, are at a very high risk for the development of life-threatening infections, especially those caused by pneumococci. It is recommended that these persons receive vaccination against 14 strains of pneumococcal bacteria and that they be sure to consult a physician and take preventive antibiotics as prescribed when they experience a supposedly trivial respiratory infection.

The patient with a ruptured or torn spleen is in immediate danger of hemorrhage and shock. Whenever an accidental blow, stab wound, or gunshot wound occurs in the vicinity of the spleen, the patient must be watched closely for signs of internal bleeding.

After surgery, the patient is observed for early signs of infection, abdominal distention, and other more general complications of abdominal surgery.

THERAPIES FREQUENTLY USED IN THE MANAGEMENT OF BLOOD DISORDERS

TRANSFUSIONS

A blood transfusion is the administration of whole blood or one or more of its components. In order to minimize the risks of circulatory overload, hepatitis, transfusion reaction, and other problems related to the administration of whole blood, it usually is transfused only when there has been acute and massive blood loss or when there must be a total blood exchange in a newborn.

Laboratory procedures that separate the various components by centrifuge or other means allow for the administration of only the particular element of blood needed by a particular patient. Among the various blood components that can be given by transfusion are:

- Fresh plasma to expand blood volume.
- Packed red cells for patients with anemia or those who cannot tolerate rapid shifts of blood volume.
- Granulocytes to help patients overcome progressive infections that are not responding well to antibiotics.
- Plasma albumin to expand blood volume.
- Coagulation factors VIII and IX to help manage hemophilia.

Transfusion reactions are discussed in Chapter 8. In general, prevention of reactions depends on properly matching donor and recipient; identifying patients who have an allergy, especially to transfused blood products; maintaining aseptic collection and administration techniques; and keeping the patient who is susceptible to febrile reaction covered and warm during a transfusion.

The recommended procedure for dealing with a severe transfusion reaction once it is recognized is to stop the transfusion and notify the physician.

Bone marrow transplantation has become an alternative treatment for leukemia. The marrow is given by intravenous infusion and offers the possibility of cure for a percentage of patients with certain types of leukemia.

OXYGEN THERAPY

The administration of low concentrations of oxygen may be employed to relieve severe dyspnea and hypoxia during the acute phase of a blood dyscrasia. The treatment is purely symptomatic, but it does offer some relief. The care of a patient receiving oxygen therapy and the need for careful monitoring of blood gases are discussed in Chapter 17.

IRON THERAPY

Iron is one of the principal elements in the production and maturation of red blood cells. When the body lacks iron, the amount of hemoglobin is decreased in the red cells, making them very small and pale in color. In a simple deficiency anemia, the condition is relieved by administering iron salts. The iron preparations most often used are ferrous sulfate and ferrous gluconate.

Iron salts are irritating to the gastrointestinal tract when taken on an empty stomach. There will be fewer gastric upsets if this medication is given in divided doses and immediately after meals. The patient should be warned that the taking of iron salts by mouth produces greenish-black stools and that there is no cause for alarm if he notices this change in the color of his stools. Because iron salts may form deposits on the teeth and gums, causing a discoloration, the liquid forms of this medication should be given through a straw. Following administration of each dose, the teeth should be thoroughly cleansed and the mouth well rinsed.

Some patients suffer such severe gastric disturbances from the oral intake of iron salts that the medication must be given by another route. Patients who are anemic because of gastric or intestinal bleeding cannot take iron by mouth because the irritation aggravates their condition. The drug of choice in these cases is iron dextran (Imferon), an iron preparation that is injected into the muscle. These injections must not exceed 2 mL at each site, and the sites of injection should be rotated to allow for proper absorption and to minimize the hazards of local inflammation. The "Z tract" technique for intramuscular injection is recommended.

Vitamin C is usually given with iron, because it enhances its absorption. If a pharmaceutical preparation of vitamin C is not prescribed, the patient can take the iron salts with orange juice or another juice that is a good source of the vitamin.

VITAMIN B_{12} THERAPY

Vitamin B_{12} has two main functions in the body. First, it is needed for the development of red blood cells into mature, normally functioning cells; second, it is necessary for normal function of nerve cells. Another B-group vitamin, *folic acid*, is also needed for red blood cell maturation, but it has no effect on the nervous system.

Concerns for the Elderly

After age 60, the plasma volume decreases, and there is less blood volume. The bone marrow becomes infiltrated with fat and fibrotic tissue as the years advance, with bone marrow activity eventually decreased by about 50%. The platelets tend to aggregate (clump together) more with advancing age, and because of decreased fibrinogen activity, the blood is more prone to coagulate. This may be a factor in the increased incidence of thrombosis in the coronary and cerebral arteries.

Anemia is not a normal part of aging. In the older age group, anemia is more commonly the result of poor nutrition.

In pernicious anemia, the intrinsic factor is missing from the gastric juices, so the iron and protein taken into the stomach cannot be properly absorbed. The result is that the red cell production is decreased, and those red cells that are produced are abnormal in structure and function. In order to correct this condition, the physician will order the administration of vitamin B_{12}.

These injections are given daily for the first few weeks and later may be spaced a week apart. As the patient improves, the injections may be necessary only once a month.

In addition to administration of supplemental iron and vitamins, the patient with nutritional anemia should eat nutritionally balanced, high-protein meals. Hints for adding protein to the diet are shown in Table 18-4.

BIBLIOGRAPHY

Andreoli, T. E., et al.: Cecil Essentials of Medicine, 2nd ed. Philadelphia, W. B. Saunders, 1990.

American Cancer Society: Cancer Facts & Figures—1990. Atlanta, American Cancer Society, Inc., 1990.

Beare, P. G., and Myers, J. L.: Principles and Practices of Adult Health Nursing. St. Louis, C. V. Mosby, 1990.

Buchsel, P. C., et al.: Bone marrow transplantation. Nurs. Clin. North Am., Dec., 1989, p. 907.

Bullock, B. L., and Rosendalhl, P. O.: Pathophysiology: Adaptations and Alterations in Function, 2nd ed. Boston, Scott, Foresman, 1988.

Cerrato, P. L.: Does your patient need more iron? RN, July, 1990, p. 63.

Consalvo, K., and Gallagher, M.: Winning the battle against Hodgkin's disease. RN, Dec., 1986, p. 20.

Froberg, J. H.: The anemias: Causes and course of action, part 2. RN, March, 1989, p. 52.

Guyton, A. C.: Textbook of Medical Physiology, 8th ed. Philadelphia, W. B. Saunders, 1991.

Ignatavicius, D. D., and Bayne, M. J.: Medical-Surgical Nursing. Philadelphia, W. B. Saunders, 1991.

Konradi, D., and Stockert, P.: A close-up look at leukemia. Nursing 89, June, 1989, p. 34.

London, F.: Nursing diagnoses and caring for patients with sickle cell disease. Adv. Clin. Care, Sept./Oct., 1990, p. 12.

Luckmann, J., and Sorensen, K. C.: Medical-Surgical Nursing: A Psychophysiologic Approach, 3rd ed. Philadelphia, W. B. Saunders, 1987.

Matteson, M. A., and McConnell, E. S.: Gerontological Nursing: Concepts and Practice. Philadelphia, W. B. Saunders, 1987.

McCormac, M.: Managing hemorrhagic shock. Am. J. Nurs., Aug., 1990, p. 22.

Rakel, R. E., ed.: Conn's Current Therapy 1990. Philadelphia, W. B. Saunders, 1990.

Rivers, R., and Williamson, N.: Sickle cell anemia: Complex disease, challenge. RN, June, 1990, p. 24.

Rutman, R. C., et al.: Blood transfusions outside the hospital. Am J. Nurs., April, 1989, p. 486.

TABLE 18-4 **HINTS FOR ADDING PROTEIN TO THE DIET**

Add two tablespoons of dry skin milk to the regular amount of milk in recipes.
Add milk powder to hot or cold cereals, scrambled eggs, soups, gravies; to ground meat for patties, meatballs, and meat loaf; to casserole dishes; and in desserts and baking.
Add diced or ground meat to soups and casseroles.
Add grated cheese or chunks of cheese to sauces, vegetables, soups, and casseroles.
Add cream cheese or peanut butter to butter on hot breads.
Add cooked cubed shrimp, tuna, crab meat, diced ham, or sliced boiled eggs to sauces and serve over rice, cooked noodles, buttered toast, or hot biscuits.
Choose dessert recipes that contain eggs such as sponge cake and angel food cake, egg custard, bread pudding or rice pudding.
Add peanut butter to sauces, use on crackers, waffles, or celery sticks.

Data from Eating Hints. Bethesda, MD, U.S. Department of Health and Human Services, National Institutes of Health, 1982.

Sherman, D. W., et al.: Shalom, Melissa: Comforting the terminally ill leukemia patient. Nursing 88, June, 1988, p. 52.

Simonson, G. M.: Caring for patients with acute myelocytic leukemia. Am. J. Nurs., March, 1988, p. 304.

Taptich, B. J., et al.: Nursing Diagnosis and Care Planning. Philadelphia, W. B. Saunders, 1989.

Ulrich, S. P., et al.: Nursing Care Planning Guides A Nursing Diagnosis Approach, 2nd ed. Philadelphia, W. B. Saunders, 1990.

Wade, T. J., and Coyle, K.: Bone marrow transplant: Today and tomorrow. Am. J. Nurs., May, 1990, p. 48.

STUDENT STUDY AIDS

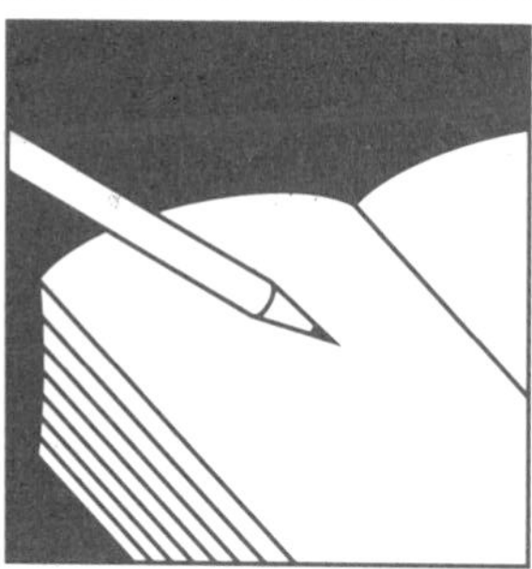

CLINICAL CASE PROBLEMS

Read each clinical case problem and discuss the questions with your classmates.

1. Mrs. Thomas is a young mother who has three small children. She is admitted to the hospital with a severe anemia. Her hemoglobin is 5 g/dL and her red cell count is also very low. Mrs. Thomas confides in you that she has never eaten as she should, especially when she was a teen-ager, and with the added strain of having the children to care for at home, she doesn't take the time to cook the meals she knows they should have because she is so tired all the time.

Her husband makes a fairly good salary, but Mrs. Thomas is under the impression that an adequate diet would cost more than they can afford at present.

- How can you teach the patient the value of nutritious food and help her with shopping practices that would provide her family with food items that are not expensive?
- Which foods that are high in iron would you suggest she include in her diet?
- What practical suggestions could you make to help her with the problem of fatigue?
- What points would your teaching plan include regarding her prescribed prescriptions?

---

2. Mr. Rogers is a 24-year-old who has acute lymphocytic leukemia. He is receiving chemotherapy and is experiencing many of the problems associated with a blood dyscrasia, as well as the problems caused by the side effects of the potent drugs he is receiving.

- Describe the physiologic problems Mr. Rogers is likely to experience as a result of the disease and the therapy.
- Identify psychosocial concerns that Mr. Rogers might have.
- Design a plan of nursing care that would help alleviate or prevent each of the problems and concerns you have identified.

STUDY OUTLINE

I. Pathophysiology

A. Blood is tissue: 45% formed elements, remainder plasma.
  1. Primary function is transportation of gases, nutrients, and wastes.

B. Erythrocytes:
  1. Formed in red bone marrow by erythropoiesis.
  2. Pathologic conditions result from too few, too many, and abnormal shape and function.

C. Leukocytes:
  1. Primary function outside the blood stream.
  2. Protect the body against foreign agents.

D. Platelets (thrombocytes) provide first line of defense against hemorrhage.
E. Plasma: liquid or noncellular portion of blood.
   1. Contains three major kinds of proteins: albumin, globulins, and fibrinogen.
F. Lymphatic system: an accessory system for transport of fluids from tissue spaces to blood.
   1. Lymph vessels and nodes rarely the site of primary disease.
G. Spleen: largest unit of monocyte-macrophage system.
   1. Functions include filtration of blood and tissue fluids, phagocytosis, and production of blood elements.
   2. Traumatic rupture of spleen and splenomegaly most common disorders.

II. Causes of blood dyscrasias
A. Some caused by inherited genes.
B. Some caused by drugs and toxic chemicals that damage the bone marrow.
C. Some of unknown cause.
D. Reaction to blood administration can cause hemolysis.

III. Diagnostic tests and procedures
A. Large quantity of information available from CBC count with differential.
B. Cell counts, differential count of WBCs (see Table 18–1), study of shape and maturity of cells.
C. Types and amount of hemoglobin.
D. Hematocrit: ratio of cells to plasma.
E. Bone marrow biopsy (sternal puncture).
F. Schilling test for pernicious anemia.
G. Sickle cell test; hemoglobin electrophoresis.

IV. Nursing assessment of hematologic status
A. History taking: race, sex, age, ethnic group; history of abnormal bleeding, weakness, fatigue, pain, neurologic symptoms, gastrointestinal problems; inability to tolerate cold; abnormal coloration of urine or stools; repeated infections, swollen lymph nodes.
B. Assessment:
   1. Skin color: pallor, cyanosis, jaundice; bruises and petechiae; plethora.
   2. Mucous membranes; swollen, bleeding gums.
   3. Stools and urine for abnormal color.
   4. Swollen and painful joints.
   5. Lymph node involvement, red streaks.
   6. Mental state: depression, irritability.
   7. Activity intolerance.

V. Common nursing diagnoses related to blood disorders: see Table 18–2.

VI. Anemia: a state in which there are not enough functioning red cells to meet the oxygen demands of the tissues.
A. Classification:
   1. According to cause:
      a. Blood loss.
      b. Failure in production of RBCs.
      c. Excessive destruction of RBCs (hemolytic anemias).
   2. According to laboratory findings in tests for size, shape, and hemoglobin content.
B. Signs, symptoms, and medical treatment
   1. Hypovolemia: hypotension; decreased urine output; pallor; rapid, weak pulse; cool, damp skin; restlessness; stupor.

2. Blood loss treated with blood transfusion and fluids.
3. Other anemias: pallor, fatigue, dizziness, headache, weakness, shortness of breath with exertion.
4. Treated with iron, vitamin B_{12}, folic acid, protein, and nutritious diet, depending on cause.

C. Nursing interventions
1. Assessment of patient's status and determination of nursing diagnosis.
2. Set realistic goals.
3. Intervention to prevent, minimize, or alleviate each problem (see Table 18–2).

VII. **Polycythemia vera**
A. Excessive production of RBCs.
B. Viscosity causes clotting.
C. Signs and symptoms: ruddy complexion, fatigue, weakness, headache, enlarged spleen, bleeding tendency.
D. Treatment primarily by phlebotomy; may use antineoplastic agents and radiation.

VIII. **Idiopathic thrombocytopenia purpura**
A. Disorder of decreased platelets.
B. Signs include bleeding, purpura, and ecchymoses.
C. Treated with blood transfusion; platelets; possibly splenectomy.

IX. **Sickle cell disease**
A. Includes all genetic disorders in which there is abnormal hemoglobin and sickling of cells.
B. Difference between sickle cell trait and sickle cell anemia.
C. Sickle cell anemia is the most common type of sickle cell disease.
D. In addition to the anemia there are complications arising from occlusion of blood vessels.
E. Symptoms of acute sickling episodes include dactylitis, chronic leg ulcers, aplastic anemia crisis, stroke, infarct and aseptic necrosis of bones, and infections.
1. Medical treatment: There is no cure for sickle cell anemia. Antisickling agents are currently under evaluation.
2. Nursing intervention:
a. Education of patient, family, and general public.
b. Prevention of complications: adequate nutrition, increased fluid intake, avoidance and prompt treatment of infections, regular visits to clinic or physician.
3. Genetic counseling.
4. Utilization of available resources for information and support.

X. **Aplastic anemia**
A. Various causes: virus, toxic substance, inherited tendency, radiation exposure.
B. Signs and symptoms: same as other anemias, plus indications of bleeding.
C. Susceptible to infection because of low leukocyte levels.
D. Treatment: eliminate underlying cause; reverse isolation; packed cell and platelet transfusions; oxygen.
E. Bone marrow transplant.
F. Prevent infection and hemorrhage.
G. Psychological support of patient and family.
H. Educate patients and public about substances that can damage bone marrow.

XI. **Leukemia**
A. A malignancy of white blood cells.

B. Classification: acute and chronic; myeloid and lymphoid.
C. Causative factors and effects:
   1. No specific infectious agent or other causative factor known.
   2. Exposure to ionizing radiation and toxic chemicals such as benzene are believed to contribute to development of leukemias.
   3. Three major effects:
      a. Increased numbers of abnormal leukocytes.
      b. Accumulations of masses of white cells in the lymph nodes.
      c. Infiltration of malignant cells throughout the body.
D. Bases for symptoms (see Table 18–3).
E. Treatment: chemotherapy, radiation, transfusions, marrow transplants.
F. Nursing intervention:
   1. Susceptibility to infection. Most common cause of death in leukemia patients.
   2. Abnormal bleeding. Second most common and threatening complication.
   3. Anemia: fatigue, hypoxia, gastrointestinal problems, cardiovascular complications.
   4. Nutritional alteration; common to all malignancies.
   5. Increased levels of uric acid.
   6. Emotional impact and psychosocial needs.

XII. Hemophilia: an inherited disorder in which there is a deficiency of specific clotting factors

A. Classic hemophilia: factor VIII deficiency. Most common of all hemophilias.
B. Three major types: classic hemophilia (hemophilia A), Christmas disease (hemophilia B), and von Willebrand's disease.
C. Symptoms primarily caused by internal hemorrhage involving joints, muscles, and peritoneal and cranial cavities.
D. Medical treatment and nursing intervention:
   1. Transfusions of replacement factors have improved prognosis.
   2. Overprotective attitudes should be avoided. Patient encouraged to live as normal a life as possible within limitations imposed by disease.

XIII. Disorders of the lymphatic system

A. Movement of lymph depends on massage by arteries, skeletal muscles, and intestinal peristalsis.
B. Lymph is fluid drained from interstitial spaces.
C. Diagnostic tests: lymphangiography and physical examination of lymph nodes.
D. Lymphangitis: inflammation of lymph vessels.
   1. Red streaks and tenderness along lymphatic vessels.
   2. Treatment aimed at relieving infection at primary site.
   3. Can lead to septicemia.
E. Lymphedema: swelling of tissues drained by lymphatic vessels.
   1. Usually caused by obstruction to flow of lymph.
      a. Congenital hypoplasia of lymph vessel of lower extremities.
      b. Acquired lymphedema: surgical destruction of lymph nodes and vessels; extensive soft tissue injury; parasites.
   2. Nursing intervention:
      a. Elevate swollen extremity.
      b. Active exercise of skeletal muscles.
      c. Apply full-length elasticized stockings and gloves.
F. Lymphomas.
   1. Malignancy of lymph tissue.

2. Hodgkin's disease.
   a. Affects primarily young adults.
   b. Signs: swollen lymph node, fever, night sweats, weight loss.
   c. Diagnosed by Reed-Sternberg cells in blood; lymphangiography.
   d. Treatment: chemotherapy, radiation, bone marrow transplant.
3. Non-Hodgkin's lymphoma.
   a. Widespread involvement of lymph tissue.
   b. Treatment with chemotherapy and radiation.

XIV. Spleen

A. Rarely the original site of disease.
B. Most common disorders are traumatic rupture and splenomegaly.
C. Splenectomy:
   1. Indicated when there is traumatic injury, degeneration of splenic tissue, and splenomegaly.
   2. Spleen is not indispensable.
   3. Patient is watched postoperatively for signs of infection, abdominal distention, and other problems related to abdominal surgery.
   4. Persons who have had a splenectomy are at higher risk for infections, particularly pneumonia.

XV. Therapies frequently used

A. Transfusions: whole blood, blood components.
   1. Plasma to expand blood volume.
   2. Packed red cells to avoid shifts in blood volume.
   3. Granulocytes for infections.
   4. Coagulation factors.
   5. Preventing transfusion reactions.
   6. Bone marrow transplants.
B. Oxygen therapy: administration of low concentrations for relief of symptoms of hypoxemia.
C. Iron therapy for iron-deficiency anemia.
   1. Iron salts irritating to stomach mucosa. Give oral preparations after meals.
   2. Vitamin C enhances iron absorption.
   3. Vitamin B_{12} for pernicious anemia.

XVI. Concerns for the elderly

A. Decreased plasma volume and blood volume.
B. Bone marrow activity drops 50%; infiltration of fat and fibrotic tissue.
C. Increased platelet aggregation and coaguability of blood.
D. Anemias in elderly mostly a result of poor nutrition.

CHAPTER 19

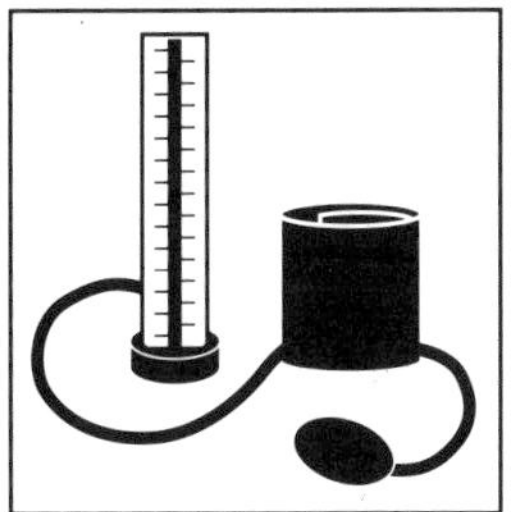

Care of Patients With Hypertension

VOCABULARY

adrenergic
antihypertensive
diastolic
idiopathic
labile
systolic

Upon completion of this part, the student should be able to:

1. List risk factors for the development of hypertension.
2. Describe the complications that can occur as a consequence of hypertension.
3. Perform an assessment, including learning needs, on a patient with a diagnosis of hypertension.
4. Describe conservative measures effective in the management of borderline hypertension.
5. Briefly describe the treatment program for mild, moderate, and severe hypertension.
6. Develop and implement a long-term care plan for a patient who has hypertension.
7. Describe the nurse's role in prevention and control of hypertension.

Hypertension is defined as persistently high blood pressure. In adults, this means a systolic pressure that is equal to or greater than 140 mm Hg and a diastolic pressure that is equal to or greater than 90 mm Hg when taken at least twice and averaged on two different occasions. The diastolic pressure usually is the focus of treatment, because it reflects the amount of pressure being exerted against the vessel walls while the heart is in its phase of relaxation and there is no added pressure from blood being forced out of the left ventricle and into the arteries.

A diastolic pressure of 85 to 89 mm Hg is considered high normal. Diastolic readings of 90 to 104 mm Hg indicate mild hypertension; moderate hypertension patients have diastolic pressures of 105 to 114 mm Hg, and those with severe hypertension have a diastolic pressure greater than 115 mm Hg. A patient has borderline systolic hypertension if his systolic pressure ranges from 140 to 159 mm Hg; a systolic pressure greater than 160 mm Hg indicates systolic hypertension.

There are 65 million Americans who are hypertensive and therefore at increased risk of heart disease, stroke, and kidney disease. Although the disease mainly effects people over 40 years of age, it is not limited to older persons. Screening clinics have detected hypertension in increasing numbers of teenagers. Between 2% and 6% of adolescents have persistent blood pressure elevations. Hypertension is more severe and more prevalent in blacks than in whites by an overall ratio of two to one.

Hypertensive individuals usually die from long-term damage to the so-called end organs or target organs; that is, the brain, heart, and kidney. Over half the deaths associated with persistent and unrelieved hypertension are caused by myocardial infarction. Immediate causes of death related to high blood pressure include cerebral hemorrhage and heart failure.

CAUSATIVE FACTORS AND PREVENTION

The cause of essential hypertension is not known. High blood pressure is a reflection of homeostatic mechanisms that (1) control the caliber of blood vessels and their responsiveness to various stimuli, (2) regulate fluid volume in the intravascular and extravascular compartments, and (3) control cardiac output.

Blood pressure equals the cardiac output multiplied by the peripheral vascular resistance. If the caliber of blood vessels becomes smaller because of atherosclerosis, blood pressure increases in an effort to force the blood through the smaller opening. If there is an increase in the volume of fluid in the blood vessels, the pressure within the vessels increases, and the heart must work harder to pump the increased volume of fluid through the vessels. Angiotensin acts directly on the blood vessels, causing them to constrict, and also stimulates the adrenal gland to release aldosterone. Angiotensin thereby increases resistance to blood flow in the peripheral vessels and causes retention of sodium and water by the renal tubules through the influence of aldosterone. The retained sodium and water increase the blood volume, causing increased cardiac output and elevation of blood pressure.

There are two major types of hypertension: essential (primary or idiopathic) and secondary hypertension. About 90% of all cases of hypertension are classified as essential hypertension. Its cause is unknown, and the goals of treatment are (1) reduction of high blood pressure and (2) long-term control to decrease the risk of stroke, heart attack, and kidney disease.

In the remaining 10% the hypertension is actually a symptom of another disorder; that is, the hypertension is secondary to another disease. If the primary disease can be detected and treated successfully, the problem of hypertension is eliminated. Examples of diseases that can produce secondary hypertension include renal vascular disease (for example, atherosclerosis of the renal artery), dysfunction of the adrenal cortex and medulla, atherosclerosis of the arteries of systemic circulation, and coarctation of the aorta.

Some major factors associated with essential hypertension are age, race, obesity, and sodium intake. Female hormone therapy, nicotine, and caffeine consumption appear to be contributing factors in some people. Persons with a family history of hypertension are also at greater risk for developing essential hypertension.

Blood pressure tends to rise with age. Average blood pressure readings for various age groups are shown in Table 19–1. An elevation above normal limits in either systolic or diastolic blood pressure at any age is not normal and increases the risk for illness and death from a cardiovascular disease.

Obesity is closely associated with an elevation of blood pressure. There is a correlation between

TABLE 19–1 AVERAGE BLOOD PRESSURE READINGS FOR VARIOUS AGE GROUPS

Age (Years)	Average Reading
4	98/60
6	105/60
10	112/64
11 to 16	120/75
Over 18	130/80

an increase in body weight over a period of years and a simultaneous increase in blood pressure. Many times a loss of excess weight alone can return a slightly elevated blood pressure to normal.

Nicotine and caffeine can have immediate effects on the level of blood pressure. Smoking increases the chances of developing cardiovascular disease and also elevates the blood pressure significantly each time a cigarette is smoked.

There is evidence that salt intake is also a factor. Epidemiologic studies have shown that many people who consume large amounts of salt have normal blood pressure. A possible explanation is that sodium brings out an inherent susceptibility to hypertension. At any rate, reduction of salt intake has been effective in lowering the blood pressure of some persons with mild or moderate hypertension.

Essential hypertension cannot be prevented, but it can be managed with diligent therapy and cooperation of the patient. Controlling the factors mentioned above (e.g., obesity, cigarette smoking), increasing the level of physical activity, and improving dietary habits can help in the management of certain kinds of hypertension and in avoiding some of the more serious consequences. Through the efforts of the American Heart Association and the National Heart, Lung, and Blood Institute, the American public is more aware of the risk factors of hypertension and the need to develop more sensible and wholesome habits of daily living.

A major component of the prevention and control of high blood pressure is education. Nurses can play a major role in teaching others about the disease and supporting their efforts to avoid hypertension and its long-term consequences.

Nurses also can contribute to reducing the incidence of the harmful effects of hypertension by participating in community screening programs to detect hypertension in its early stages, confirm its presence, and initiate prompt treatment. Additionally, nurses and other health care professionals have some obligation to serve as models for a healthy lifestyle.

DIAGNOSTIC TESTS AND PROCEDURES

The first step is to conduct a series of blood pressure readings. A single measurement cannot be considered reliable, as emotional state and degree of physical activity can affect blood pressure.

A complete blood cell (CBC) count, urinalysis, cholesterol assessment, and SMA panel of liver and kidney function and electrolyte and general health status are done. Tests of thyroid, adrenal glands, kidneys, and renal arteries are done to rule out the possibility of another disease that is causing secondary hypertension. Hyperthyroidism, Cushing's syndrome, pheochromocytoma, nephrosclerosis, and renal arterial stenosis all elevate blood pressure.

If no underlying disease can be identified as elevating the patient's blood pressure, the patient is said to have "essential" hypertension, meaning hypertension without known cause.

Examination of the blood vessels of the retina will reveal any damage to the retinal vessels. This gives an indication as to how much damage the high blood pressure has done to vessels throughout the body. If damage has occurred, it is an indication that the person's hypertension is moderate to severe. Electrocardiogram (EKG) and cardiac stress testing may be ordered to determine whether any damage has been done to the coronary arteries or heart muscle.

NURSING ASSESSMENT

The nursing assessment for the patient with possible hypertension includes a thorough history taking. The patient is questioned about history of diabetes mellitus; cardiovascular, thyroid, or renal disease; arteriosclerosis; atherosclerosis; or immune disorders, such as lupus erythematosus, which can affect the blood vessels. The patient is also questioned about close relatives who have these diseases, because the tendency to develop these conditions is inherited.

Other subjective data include questions regarding medications taken regularly, both prescription and nonprescription, as many drugs can cause vasoconstriction and elevate blood pressure. Cold remedies, decongestants, and diet pills are particularly noted for having this effect. Questions regarding smoking habits and alcohol consumption should be asked. A careful, specific diet history should be gathered by asking the patient exactly what he eats each day, what snacks he has, what fluids he drinks, and what his favorite foods are. Does he eat "fast foods" or convenience foods regularly? These may be high in fat and sodium. Does he add salt to his food?

Questions regarding problems from damage to the heart, brain, or kidneys should be asked. Has the patient experienced dizziness, headache, blackouts, or vision changes? Has he been getting up to urinate at night? Have there been any changes in urination? Has there been shortness of breath, swelling of the feet and ankles, or chest pain?

Objective measurement of blood pressure (BP) must be done strictly according to correct procedure and with accurate equipment. The cuff must be the correct size, and it must be placed with the middle of the bladder over the artery. A cuff that is the wrong size or placed slightly incorrectly can alter BP readings significantly. Deflation of the cuff must be done slowly and smoothly.

NURSING DIAGNOSES

Nursing diagnoses that may be appropriate for the patient with hypertension include:

- Alteration in tissue perfusion related to vascular damage.
- Knowledge deficit related to medications, diet, and control of disease.
- Body image disturbance related to diagnosis of chronic illness.
- Potential noncompliance related to denial of disease or inability to follow treatment plan.

SIGNS AND SYMPTOMS

Hypertension has been called the "silent killer," because it does not usually cause discomfort or any other subjective signs and symptoms to indicate that it is present. Patients with symptoms may complain of headache, dizziness, blurred vision, blackouts, irritability, fatigue, or nervousness. However, about one third of those who have hypertension are not aware of it. Signs may appear only in the later stages when damage has already been done to the target organs—that is, the kidney (renal ischemia), brain (arteriosclerosis and microaneurysms), and heart (left ventricular hypertrophy and reduced cardiac output). Hypertensive patients develop coronary heart disease at a rate two to three times greater than that of persons with normal blood pressure.

MEDICAL TREATMENT

The goal of treatment is control of blood pressure levels so as to prevent complications and death from cerebrovascular, cardiovascular, and renal damage. For patients with borderline hypertension, reduction of BP to normal is attempted by reducing sodium and fat in the diet, exercising regularly, reducing weight to normal range, decreasing alcohol and tobacco consumption, and utilizing stress reduction techniques.

Individualized treatment has taken the place of the previous stepped-care approach. For mild hypertension, a thiazide diuretic or beta-adrenergic blocking drug is usually prescribed along with the lifestyle modifications used for borderline hypertension. Other drugs are added, if needed, in order to keep the BP consistently within normal limits. Patients with more severe hypertension often require more than two drugs to attain control. Other drug possibilities include calcium channel blocking agents, angiotensin-converting enzyme inhibitors, and adrenergic inhibitors or vasodilators. The dose of each drug is increased as needed to achieve the desired blood pressure level unless side effects occur. In this event, another drug is substituted. A common combination used is a diuretic, a vasodilator, and an adrenergic inhibitor.

If a potassium-wasting diuretic is prescribed, the patient is taught to increase his potassium intake. A potassium supplement may be added to his treatment and electrolyte levels monitored regularly.

The patient is often told to monitor his blood pressure at home and keep records of his readings. He returns to the physician's office for periodic, regular examinations.

The better the blood pressure is controlled within normal limits, the less damage there will be to the target organs.

ANTIHYPERTENSIVE THERAPY

The drugs prescribed to reduce blood pressure work by decreasing blood volume, cardiac output, or peripheral resistance.

Diuretics reduce circulating blood volume. Commonly prescribed diuretics include thiazides, furosemide (Lasix), or spironolactone (Aldactone). Potassium levels of patients taking furosemide must be watched very closely, as this drug causes excretion of a lot of potassium.

Drugs that decrease cardiac output and also decrease peripheral resistance include the beta-adrenergic inhibitors (beta blockers) and calcium channel blockers. Examples of commonly prescribed beta blockers include atenolol (Tenormin), and metoprolol tartrate (Lopressor). The calcium channel blocker most often used for blood pressure control is nifedipine (Procardia).

Adrenergic inhibitor medications decrease peripheral resistance. Examples of these drugs include clonidine (Catapres), methyldopa (Aldomet) and minoxidil (Loniten).

Hydralazine (Apresoline) is a vasodilator. It is most commonly used in combination with a beta-blocking agent and a diuretic.

Captopril (Capoten), an angiotensin-converting enzyme inhibitor, has been quite effective in patients with severe hypertension. It reduces peripheral resistance without lowering cardiac output.

NURSING INTERVENTION

Interventions related to drug therapy include tracking intake and output of patients on diuretics, monitoring electrolyte values and signs and symptoms of hypokalemia, and closely monitoring blood pressure. Because many antihypertensive drugs can also lower heart rate, the pulse rate as well as the blood pressure should be checked before administering each dose of medication. A heart rate below 60 is often an indication to hold the medication until the heart rate is higher. Patients should be cautioned to change positions slowly and to sit a minute before standing to counteract the effect of postural hypotension that occurs with many antihypertensive medications.

The nurse should encourage the patient to take his blood pressure medications at the same time each day. It will be easier to remember to take them if they are linked to some activity that is performed daily, such as taking a shower, brushing the teeth after breakfast, or getting ready for bed.

Patients who are utilizing a drug patch for skin absorption of antihypertensive medication should be checked each day to see that the patch is still intact.

Other nursing interventions are directed toward teaching the patient the things he needs to know to comply with the prescribed medical treatment. These include diet, exercise, stress reduction, and prevention of complications.

Diet changes are often the hardest for the patient. It is best to work within the patient's current diet, his likes and dislikes, modifying methods of food preparation to decrease sodium and fat content. Sources of hidden sodium should be learned, and the patient should become a reader of food labels, looking for the words *salt* and *sodium* and the letters *NaCl*. Canned vegetables are a big source of added sodium, and it is better to use fresh or frozen vegetables whenever possible. However, food companies are beginning to pack some canned goods without added sodium. Smoked or preserved meats are other products that contain a lot of sodium and should be avoided. Those patients who need to increase potassium intake are taught to include fruits and fruit juices, beef and turkey, tomatoes, and potatoes in their diet.

If caffeine restriction is recommended, the patient should be told to gradually decrease his caffeine consumption so that he will not experience withdrawal symptoms such as headache and nervousness.

Nicotine has a major impact on blood vessels and blood pressure, and stopping smoking can be a difficult task for many patients. Referral to a self-help program should be made.

An exercise program that fits the patient's personality, ability, and preference should be designed. Walking to work from a parking lot a few blocks away, climbing stairs instead of using elevators, and a daily walk in the neighborhood often are sufficient. Other patients might prefer to use a stationary bicycle. The object is to work on something that the patient will continue to do the rest of his life.

Weight loss will begin to occur if the patient is faithful to the prescribed diet and exercise program. As the weight decreases, the nurse can remind the patient of the direct effect his efforts have had on his blood pressure. Positive reinforcement should be given for even small decreases.

Stress reduction requires an evaluation of lifestyle. Meditation, yoga, leisure activities, or just saying "no" to extra obligations can all decrease stress. The nurse should help the patient determine where his stressors are and what can practically be done about them.

Lifetime compliance with the diet, exercise, stress reduction and medication plan is the biggest problem for most patients. Many do not understand that it is up to them to control their disease. They do well for several months or a few years, but then, because they feel fine (while their blood pressure has been controlled), they stop taking their medication and gradually return to previous lifestyle patterns. By teaching them what high blood pressure does to the blood vessels and the heart, brain, and kidneys, the nurse can do much to see that patients follow the treatment plan for life. Each patient needs continuing praise for maintaining control of his blood pressure. See Nursing Care Plan 4–1 in Chapter 4 for information on caring for a patient with hypertension.

There are many resources to help hypertensive patients manage their illness more effectively. The American Heart Association has booklets such as "How You Can Help Your Doctor Treat High Blood Pressure," and "About Your Heart and High Blood Pressure." Other resources include the National High Blood Pressure Education Program, Health and Human Services, Washington, DC, and the National High Blood Pressure Committee, National Institutes of Health, Bethesda, MD 20814; (301) 951-3260.

BIBLIOGRAPHY

Andreoli, T. E., et al: Cecil Essentials of Medicine, 2nd ed. Philadelphia, W. B. Saunders, 1990.

Beare, P. G.: Calcium channel blockers: Nursing care for hypertension. Crit. Care Nurs., Feb., 1989, p. 37.

Bullock, B. L., and Rosendalhl P. O.: Pathophysiology: Adaptations and Alterations in Function, 2nd ed. Boston, Scott, Foresman, 1988.

Feury, D., and Nash, D. T.: Hypertension: The nurse's role. RN, Nov., 1990, p. 54.

Guyton, A. C.: Textbook of Medical Physiology, 8th ed. Philadelphia, W. B. Saunders, 1991.

Hahn, K.: Think twice about borderline hypertension. Nursing 88, April, 1988, p. 90.

Hargrove-Huttel, R. A.: CEU program: Arterial hypertension. Adv. Clin. Care, Jan./Feb., 1991, p. 4.

Hill, M. N.: Diuretics for mild hypertension: Still the best choice? Nursing 87, Sept., 1987, p. 62.

Ignatavicius, D. D., and Bayne, M. J.: Medical-Surgical Nursing. Philadelphia, W. B. Saunders, 1991.

Matteson, M. A., and McConnell, E. S.: Gerontological Nursing: Concepts and Practice. Philadelphia, W. B. Saunders, 1988.

Porterfield, L. M.: Pharmacology: Potassium replacement. Adv. Clin. Care, Nov./Dec., 1990, p. 18.

Rakel, R. E., ed.: Conn's Current Therapy 1990. Philadelphia, W. B. Saunders, 1990.
Rodman, M. J.: Hypertension: Step-care management. RN, Feb., 1991, p. 24.
Teplitz, L.: Action STAT! Hypertensive crisis. Nursing 90, April, 1990, p. 33.
Trottier, D., and Kochar, M.: Hypotension—the other side of the coin. RN, March, 1991, p. 38.

STUDENT STUDY AIDS

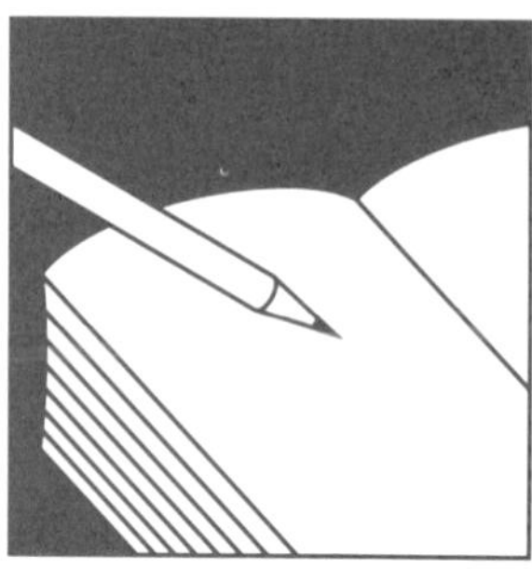

CLINICAL CASE PROBLEMS

Read each clinical case problem and discuss the questions with your classmates.

1. Mrs. Tyson, age 62, has had consistent blood pressure readings between 166/104 and 180/110. Her physician has placed her on a potassium-sparing diuretic and a daily dose of atenolol (Tenormin). Mrs. Tyson is to limit her intake of sodium and should lose 30 pounds of excess weight. In spite of several sessions in which an effort was made to teach Mrs. Tyson about her illness and prescribed therapy, she has had difficulty complying with the physician's orders.

- What specific objectives could be included in Mrs. Tyson's care plan?
- What activities should be included to help her accomplish these goals?

---

2. Mr. Bing and his son and daughter all have recently found out that they have a tendency toward hypertension. They are your neighbors and ask you how they can avoid the problems of high blood pressure. They have many misconceptions about high blood pressure and its long-term effects.

- Where could you find some resources to help this family understand hypertension better?
- How could you follow up or help them in a continuing manner?

STUDY OUTLINE

I. Introduction

A. Hypertension defined as a blood pressure reading equal to or greater than 140/90.
B. Mainly affects people over 40, but is not limited to older adults.
C. Hypertensive persons usually die from damage to one or more of the target organs; that is, the brain, heart, or kidney.

II. Causative factors and prevention

A. There is no single cause of hypertension and no cure.
B. Primary or essential hypertension and secondary hypertension are two major types.
C. Contributing factors include age, sex, race, obesity, sodium intake, cigarette smoking, and family history of hypertension.
D. Preventive measures include eliminating or reducing controllable risk factors, screening for early detection, and prompt and continued treatment.

III. Diagnostic tests and procedures

A. Series of blood pressure readings. The disorder is mostly asymptomatic until its later stages.
B. Testing for underlying disorder (e.g., hyperthyroidism, disorder of adrenal gland).

IV. Nursing Assessment

A. History taking to identify past history of arterial disease, diabetes, or other possible primary diseases causing high blood pressure. Drugs and family history are also important. Data concerning risk factors are gathered.

B. Symptoms of hypertension are notably lacking. Patient may complain of headache, dizziness.
C. History and observations for signs of kidney disease, cardiac involvement, cerebral and neurologic disorders.
D. Accurate measurement of blood pressure.
E. Nursing diagnoses for patient with hypertension may include: alteration in tissue perfusion; knowledge deficit; body image disturbance; potential noncompliance.

V. Medical treatment

A. Goal is control of blood pressure to prevent damage to target organs.
B. Mild hypertension may respond to conservative therapy with weight control, exercise, sodium and caffeine restriction, cessation of smoking, and relaxation techniques.
C. Individualized care has replaced the stepped-care approach and includes a combination of various drugs plus lifestyle changes.
D. Antihypertensive drug therapy includes diuretics, adrenergic inhibitors (beta blockers), calcium channel blockers, and vasodilators.

VI. Nursing intervention

A. Monitor blood pressure and intake and output.
B. Caution patient to change position slowly, as he may become dizzy from postural hypotension.
C. Administer medications and monitor for side effects.
D. Teaching regarding self-monitoring of BP, diet and weight loss, exercise, medications, stress reduction, and signs and symptoms of hypokalemia.
E. Encourage him to stop smoking.
F. Stress importance of lifelong compliance to prevent complications.
G. Refer to community resources.

CHAPTER 20

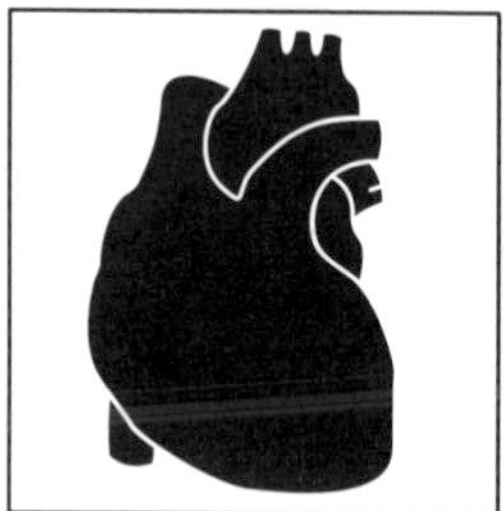

Care of Patients With Disorders of the Heart

VOCABULARY

arteriosclerosis
arrhythmia
asystole
atherosclerosis
bradycardia
defibrillation
endocarditis
fibrillation
infarction
insufficiency
ischemia
oscilloscope
palpitations
paroxysmal nocturnal dyspnea
petechiae
plaque
stenosis
telemetry

Upon completion of this part of the chapter the student should be able to:

1. List avoidable and unavoidable risk factors for the development of heart disease.
2. State ways in which nurses can contribute to the prevention of cardiovascular disease.
3. Describe the more common diagnostic tests and procedures used by cardiologists to diagnose and evaluate cardiovascular diseases.
4. Describe initial and ongoing nursing assessment to evaluate cardiovascular status.
5. List common nursing diagnoses with nursing interventions for patients with angina pectoris, myocardial infarction, cardiac arrythmias, and congestive heart failure.
6. State six nursing responsibilities in the administration of cardiac drugs, dietary control, and oxygen therapy for patients with cardiac disorders.
7. Describe pre- and postoperative problems and nursing care for patients undergoing open heart surgery.

PATHOPHYSIOLOGY

The heart is essentially a four-chambered pump whose function is to receive unoxygenated blood from the systemic circulation, send it to the lungs for exchange of carbon dioxide and oxygen, and return the oxygenated blood to the general circulation. The pumping actions of the heart are performed by muscle tissues that must have their own adequate blood supply. The "motor" of the heart is driven by specialized pacemaker cells and conduction fibers that initiate heart beats and keep them going.

The heart and blood vessels play a major role in distributing oxygen and nutrients to the cells of the body. The cardiovascular system also acts as the transportation system for cellular waste products, carrying these substances to the kidneys and lungs for elimination. When a problem arises within the system, normal functions are disrupted.

The heart's pumping action is sparked by specialized pacemaker cells and conduction fibers that initiate spontaneous electrical activity, causing muscle contractions that result in a heart beat. The sinoatrial (SA) node, which is located in the upper area of the right atrium, normally initiates and regulates the heart beat.

Structural pathologic conditions of the heart or vessels can be either congenital or acquired. Congenital defects occur in the structure of the chambers, valves, septum, or large blood vessels or in the placement of the large vessels. Acquired defects include narrowing or hardening of the blood vessels from arteriosclerosis (loss of elasticity, hardening) or atherosclerosis (formation of fatty plaque in the artery wall); aneurysms of the large vessels; alteration of the valve structure, causing stenosis (narrowing) or insufficiency (incomplete closure); alteration of the myocardial muscle tissue by hypertrophy, ischemia (lack of adequate blood supply), or infarct; deterioration of the pacemaker cells and conduction fibers; or inflammation of the various tissues. An *infarct* is an area of tissue that has died from lack of blood supply.

Any disorder involving either the heart or the blood vessels through which it pumps blood can eventually weaken and exhaust heart muscle and lead to a slowing down or congestion of blood flow. This condition, called *congestive heart failure,* is a complication of many cardiovascular diseases. Another complication that occurs when the heart is greatly stressed by various cardiovascular disorders or is damaged by a virus is cardiomyopathy. *Cardiomyopathy* means that the heart muscle can no longer pump effectively, and heart failure occurs. Severe cardiomyopathy is an indication for a heart transplant.

Infection and inflammation also can take their toll on the structure and function of the heart. *Endocarditis,* inflammation within the lining and valves of the heart, and *pericarditis,* which is inflammation of the sac surrounding the heart, can occur as primary diseases, but they more often are secondary to infection and inflammation elsewhere in the body. An example is rheumatic heart disease following a streptococcal infection.

The rate and rhythm of the heart beat are controlled by an intrinsic nerve supply or conduction system and by an extrinsic nerve supply that is part of the autonomic nervous system. Thus substances in the blood such as excess carbon dioxide and certain drugs can affect the rate and rhythm of the heart. The heart also responds to physiologic changes that indicate a need for more or less oxygen. Disturbances in any part of the heart's conduction system can result in an increase in heart rate *(tachycardia),* a slowing down of the heart rate *(bradycardia),* and disturbances in the rhythm of the heart beat *(arrhythmias).*

PREVENTION OF HEART DISEASE

Heart disease remains the major cause of death in the United States, even though the rate of death due to heart disease has declined since 1970. Cardiovascular diseases do, however, account for a large percentage of the chronic illnesses that disable to some degree a large segment of the population of this country.

Although the statistics about mortality and morbidity of cardiovascular diseases may be somewhat sobering, they should not be interpreted to mean that all such disorders are either fatal or totally disabling. There are many kinds and degrees of heart disease. Advances in medical science have made it possible to either cure or successfully manage a significant number of cardiovascular disorders. Reasons for the decline in the mortality rate of heart disease in the past decade include improved emergency treatment of persons experiencing a coronary occlusion or "heart attack" and improved education of the public regarding ways to prevent heart disease and the warning signs of a heart attack. Every nurse has a responsibility to assist with public education about heart disease.

Controllable risk factors are the major focus in public education. These include obesity, elevated blood lipid levels, lack of regular exercise, hypertension, cigarette smoking, and an excessively stressful lifestyle. Old habits are hard to change, but there is strong evidence that reducing these risk factors can greatly cut down the chance of developing heart disease and thereby improve the quality of an individual's life.

Cocaine use is another controllable risk factor. Cocaine causes vasoconstriction and is thought to speed up the atherosclerosis process. Also, cocaine has been known to cause sudden cardiac death in susceptible individuals. Research is finding that the ingestion of alcohol along with cocaine greatly increases the chance of cardiac death.

Uncontrollable risk factors include birth factors such as race, sex, and family history of heart disease and diabetes or those that result from the aging process such as arteriosclerosis.

Management of hypertension is a very important aspect of heart disease prevention (see Chapter 19).

DIAGNOSTIC TESTS AND PROCEDURES

In addition to a routine physical examination and medical history, the physician has access to a number of both noninvasive and invasive procedures and tests to help in the diagnosis of heart disease. Because of the hazards and risks of invasive procedures that require entry into the cardiovascular system or the injection of substances into the circulating blood, noninvasive procedures usually are performed first.

Among the more common noninvasive diagnostic tests are electrocardiography (resting and ambulatory), exercise stress testing, echocardiography, and chest radiography. More sophisticated testing utilizes injectable radioisotopes, imaging devices, and computers. Invasive procedures include cardiac catheterization, coronary angiography, and electrophysiology studies. Electrolyte assessment, complete blood cell (CBC) count, and blood gas measurements are an integral part of the diagnostic testing done on patients who have a cardiac disorder. Assessment of serum levels is performed for most cardiotonic and antiarrythmic drugs to check for therapeutic level and possible toxicity. Specific diagnostic tests and their nursing implications are listed in Table 20–1.

TELEMETRY

Continuous monitoring of cardiac rate and rhythm is often done by telemetry. Disposable electrodes and wire leads from a bedside monitor (Fig. 20–3) or battery-operated transmitter unit are applied to the patient. The wave pattern signals are sent to a monitor in a central station, where they are continually observed. This allows patients to walk around the unit while being monitored. The wave may also be displayed on a bedside *oscilloscope.* An oscilloscope is a machine that shows a picture of electrical current and its variations. In this instance, the patient's movement is limited by the wire attachments. Modern computerized telemetry monitors can detect specific arrhythmias (abnormal variations of heart rhythm), automatically store the wave pattern, and alert the nurse to the abnormality with sound. Telemetry monitoring is used for patients experiencing an acute cardiac disorder, following cardiac surgery, and after pacemaker insertion.

NURSING ASSESSMENT OF CARDIOVASCULAR STATUS

HISTORY TAKING

Considering the known risk factors for heart disease, the patient's medical history and those of his relatives are important in the medical diagnosis of heart disease and in assessing the current nursing needs of the patient. Significant data include any family history of heart disease, diabetes mellitus, high blood pressure, stroke, gout, or kidney disease. It is helpful, too, to know about the patient's lifestyle; for example, smoking, drinking, and eating habits; weight gains or losses; type and amount of daily exercise; occupation; and sources of stress.

Much of this information is obtained by the physician when he takes a medical history and by the nurse in a comprehensive nursing assessment conducted at the time the patient is admitted to the hospital. There will be some additional information, however, that is gathered in less formal interviews when the patient becomes more relaxed and comfortable with the nurses who care for him.

Information concerning the patient's actual eating habits such as snacking on "junk" food or daily consumption of several drinks containing caffeine is more likely to be obtained during nursing care activities than by initial interview. Data concerning stressors in the patient's life and his response to them are more easily assessed while interacting with the patient over time. An understanding of the patient's perception of his disorder and overall health are necessary in order to plan appropriate teaching for him.

SUBJECTIVE AND OBJECTIVE DATA

Significant subjective data related to cardiac status include chest pain, fatigue, complaints of shortness of breath, cough, hemoptysis, palpitations, and nocturia. Light-headedness, dizziness or fainting also are associated with cardiovascular disease.

Relevant questions in regard to each of these symptoms are as follows:

- Where is the pain? What does it feel like? What, if anything seems to bring it on? What

TABLE 20–1 **DIAGNOSTIC TESTS FOR HEART PROBLEMS**

Test	Purpose	Description	Nursing Implications
Electrocardiography 12-Lead electrocardiogram	Records electrical impulses of the heart to determine rhythm of heart, site of pacemaker, and presence of injury.	Small electrodes are placed on the chest and extremities, and leads are changed to show conduction patterns in different directions of electrical flow. Figure 20–1 shows a basic EKG tracing.	Inform patient that there is no discomfort with this test. Maintain electrical safety. Normal finding: Normal EKG
Exercise EKG—stress test	Record electrical activity of the heart during exercise. Insufficient blood flow and oxygen show up in abnormal wave forms.	Small electrodes are placed on the chest, and a tracing is made while the patient exercises on a treadmill, bicycle, or stairs (Fig. 20–2). The degree of difficulty of the exercise is increased as the test continues to see how the heart reacts to increasing work demands. Vital signs are continuously recorded.	Requires a signed consent form. Have patient wear comfortable clothes and walking shoes. Light meal 2 to 3 hours prior, then NPO. Regular medications are given. Chest is shaved as needed for electrode placement. Inform patient that the test will be stopped if he experiences chest pain, severe fatigue or dyspnea. Test takes approximately 30 minutes. Normal finding: No ST segment depression with exercise.
Ambulatory EKG—Holter monitor	Correlate normal daily activity with electrical function of the heart to determine if activity causes abnormalities.	Patient wears a small EKG recorder for 6, 12, or 24 hours while he goes about his usual tasks. He keeps a diary showing at what time he performs different activities. The tape is analyzed to correlate any arrhythmia with the activity that caused it.	Remind patient that all activities must be recorded in the diary: brushing teeth, climbing stairs, sexual intercourse, bowel movements, sleeping, etc. Caution him not to remove the electrodes and not to get the recorder or wires wet. Have patient wear a loose shirt during test.
Echocardiography	Useful in evaluating size, shape, and position of structures within the heart. Test of choice for valve problems.	A metal wand that emits sonar waves is guided over the chest wall while the patient is supine or turned on his left side. Takes 30 to 60 minutes. May be done in combination with the exercise (stress) test.	Inform patient that there is no discomfort, although conduction jelly may feel cool. Normal finding: No abnormalities of size or location of heart structures; normal wall movement.
Cardiac catheterization	Assesses pumping action of both sides of the heart. Measures pressure within the heart chambers. Measures cardiac output. Calculates differences in oxygen content of arterial and venous blood.	Requires a signed consent form, as it is not without risk. Catheter is inserted into vein or artery, depending on which side of the heart is to be tested. Femoral artery or brachial vein is often used. With local anesthetic, the catheter is threaded up into the heart, and pressure readings and oxygen saturation determinations are taken. Contrast media	Patient is NPO for 6 to 8 hours prior to test. Assess for allergy to iodine, shellfish, or contrast dye. Have patient void before giving preop medications. Record baseline vital signs and mark location of pedal pulses. Inform patient that he will be strapped to a table that tilts and that he must lie still during the test. EKG leads will be in place dur-

Table continued on following page

TABLE 20-1 **DIAGNOSTIC TESTS FOR HEART PROBLEMS** *Continued*

Test	Purpose	Description	Nursing Implications
		may be injected to visualize the size and shape of the chambers and structures. Takes 1½ to 3 hours. Fluoroscopy is used during the procedure.	ing the test. If dye is injected, patient will feel a hot flush for about a minute. He may be asked to cough during the procedure. Posttest: Vital signs q 15 min × 4, q 30 min × 4, then q 1 h × 4 or until stable. Assess peripheral pulses with vital signs, and question patient about numbness or tingling. Inspect insertion site for bleeding or sign of hematoma. Pressure dressing and sandbag weight are left in place for 1 to 3 hours. If femoral insertion site was used, keep patient flat and leg extended for 6 hours. If brachial site was used, immobilize arm for 3 hours. If dye was used, encourage fluids unless contraindicated.
Coronary angiography	Determines patency of coronary arteries and presence of collateral circulation.	Performed by dye injection during cardiac catheterization. Video recording made during procedure for later review.	Same as for cardiac catheterization.
Electrophysiology studies	Measures and records electrical activity from within the heart to determine the area of origin of the arrhythmia and the effectiveness of the antiarrhythmic drug for the particular arrythmia.	Three to six electrodes are placed in the heart through the venous system. They are attached to an oscilloscope that records the intracardiac and EKG waveforms simultaneously. After baseline tracings are taken, the cardiologist tries to trigger the arrhythmia that is to be studied by programmed electrical stimulation through the electrodes. Once the arrythmia is triggered, an antiarrhythmic drug is administered to determine its effectiveness in stopping the abnormal rhythm. Studies may take from 1½ to 4 hours; serial studies may be done on different days.	Provide psychological support for the patient, who is often scared of having arrhythmias induced. Antiarrhythmic drugs are stopped 24 hours or more before the test to eliminate them from the patient's system. Assure the patient that he will be monitored constantly and that emergency equipment and staff will be on hand. Keep patient NPO after midnight. Patent IV line is maintained. Electrodes are placed using fluoroscopy. Patient will be supine on an x-ray table. Chest surface electrodes will be placed before the electrodes are threaded into the heart. The femoral vein is most commonly used; the groin is shaved, and local anesthesia is used. Posttest care: Much the same as for cardiac catheterization.

TABLE 20-1 **DIAGNOSTIC TESTS FOR HEART PROBLEMS** *Continued*

Test	Purpose	Description	Nursing Implications
Nuclear imaging			
Thallium perfusion imaging	Evaluates blood flow in various parts of the heart; determines areas of infarction.	Thallium 201 is injected IV; radioactive uptake is counted over the heart by a gamma scintillation camera. May be done in conjunction with an exercise EKG stress test.	Explain that the radioactivity used is a very small amount and lasts only a few hours. Explain that a camera will be positioned over the heart. EKG electrodes are placed on the chest; scanning is done 10 to 15 minutes after injection; can be done as an outpatient procedure.
Technectium pyrophosphate scan	Determine area and extent of myocardial infarction.	Technetium Tc 99m is injected IV and is taken up by areas of infarction, producing hot spots when scanned. Best results occur when done 1 to 6 days after a suspected MI.	Inform patient that scan is done 1½ to 2 hours after injection of the technectium. Explain that it will determine if he actually suffered damage from MI.
Laboratory Tests			
Cardiac serum enzymes	Measures specific enzyme levels to determine what type of cells have been injured and to what extent.	Creatine kinase (CK) is found in the heart, skeletal muscle, and brain cells. It rises within 6 hours of MI and returns to normal within 48 to 72 hours. CK-MB is a fraction of the enzyme, or isoenzyme, that is specific to heart muscle cells. Lactic dehydrogenase (LDH) rises following MI but is not specific. LDH_1 and LDH_2 are the isoenzymes contained in heart muscle. If $LDH_1/LDH_2 > 1$, it indicates MI has occurred. Aspartate aminotransferase (AST) rises 6 to 8 hours after MI, peaks within 24 to 48 hours, and returns to normal in 4 to 8 days but is not specific to heart damage. Table 20-2 summarizes serum enzyme data with regard to acute myocardial infarction.	Explain purpose of lab work. Inform patient that blood will be drawn at intervals to check enzyme levels.
CK	Normal Values: Female: 5-35 mU/mL Male: 5-50 mU/mL		
CK-MB	<5% total CK		
LDH	150-450 U/mL		
LDH_1	17%-27%		
LDH_2	27%-37%		
AST	5-40 U/mL		
Serum lipids	Determines level	Elevation of cholesterol is a risk factor for atherosclerotic heart disease.	Patient is NPO except for noncaloric liquids for 12 hours.
	Normal Values:		
Cholesterol	150-200 mg/dL		
HDL	32-75 mg/dL		
LDL	73-200 mg/dL		
Triglycerides	50-250 mg/dL	Triglycerides contribute to arterial disease. As triglycerides rise, so do low-den-	

Table continued on following page

TABLE 20-1 **DIAGNOSTIC TESTS FOR HEART PROBLEMS** *Continued*

Test	Purpose	Description	Nursing Implications
		sity lipoproteins, which are a factor in atherosclerosis. The lipoproteins (LDL, VLDL, and HDL) are increased in hyperlipidemia. Lipoprotein fractions are determined by electrophoresis and are used to assign a "risk" factor in cardiovascular disease. High levels of HDL appear to be protective against coronary artery disease and MI, whereas increased levels of LDL are associated with increased atherosclerosis and MI.	

makes it worse? What gives relief? Does the pain radiate (spread) to other parts of the body, for example, down the arm, upward to the neck and jaws, to the upper abdomen? Is it localized or does it cover a large area? On a scale of 1 to 10, with 10 being the worst and 1 being the least, how do you rate your pain?

- When do you notice shortness of breath? Do you sleep on more than one pillow? Is your shortness of breath worse after physical activity? What kind of activity? Walking up steps? Does it occur when you are at rest? Does resting relieve it? Do you wake up at night short of breath or feeling like you are suffocating? Does sitting up on the side of the bed or getting up give you relief?
- What kind of cough do you have—dry and hacking or wet and productive? What does the sputum look like? Is there ever any blood in your sputum?

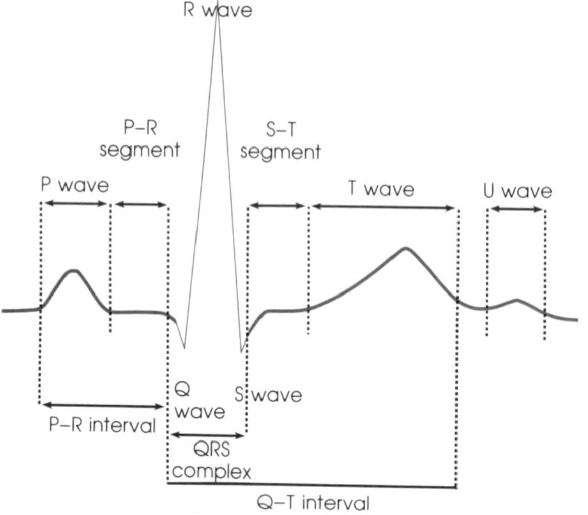

Figure 20-1 Basic EKG tracing.

- Do you notice your heart beating very fast or pounding in your chest? Does it skip a beat?
- Do you get up in the night to urinate? How many times do you get up each night?
- Do you ever feel light-headed or faint?

Objective data obtained from physical assessment include vital signs; heart sounds; apical pulse rate; breath sounds; quality of pulses; skin color, temperature, and texture; shape of fingers; appearance of neck veins; abdominal distention; facial expression; and degree of body tension. Significant findings include abnormal or extra heart sounds; crackles in the lungs; orthopneic position (sitting up in bed with two or three pillows behind the back) to ease breathing; placement of hand on chest, indicating pain; a blueish cast to skin or pallor; diaphoresis; clubbing of the fingers; pitting edema of the feet, ankles, or sacral area; distended jugular veins; and abnormal rate or volume of pulses or a pulse deficit. A pulse deficit is the difference between the apical and radial pulse when counted at the same time.

An apical pulse rate should be taken on all patients on admission. Heart sounds are auscultated at least every 24 hours on all patients who have a known arrhythmia or a potential for arrhythmia, a valve problem, or congestive heart failure. The diaphragm of the stethoscope is placed over the bare skin at the mitral area to listen to the apical pulse. S_1 (lub) and S_2 (dub) should be distinguished. The pulse should be counted for a full minute.

The bell of the stethoscope is used to listen for heart murmurs. It must be placed very lightly on the skin for the sounds to be audible. Aortic valve sounds are heard in the second right intercostal space close to the sternum. The pulmonic valve is auscultated in the left second intercostal space close to the sternum. The tricuspid valve sounds are heard at the left lower sternal border,

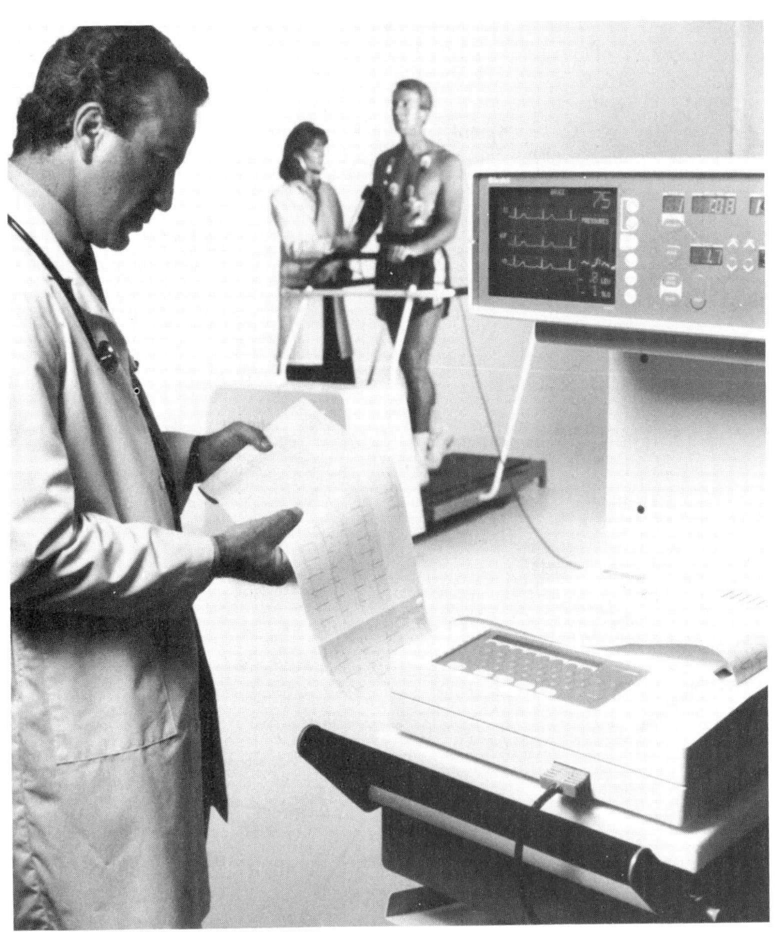

Figure 20-2 Stress EKG test.
(Courtesy of Siemens Burdick Inc., Schaumburg, IL.)

TABLE 20-2 SERUM ENZYME DATA AND EVALUATION OF ACUTE MYOCARDIAL INFARCTION

Type of Enzyme	Onset of Rise	Peak of Rise	Return to Normal	Comments
CK (also called CPK)	3-6 hr after onset of chest pain	12-24 h	3-5 days	Can reach 5 to 10 times the upper limit of normal.
CK-MB	4-6 h	12-20 h	2-3 days	CK-MB is the fraction of the enzyme found only in the heart. It is the most reliable indicator of acute MI when other enzymes can be elevated from different causes.
LDH	8-12 h	24-48 h	10-14 days	Helpful in diagnosing acute MI in patients whose diagnosis and treatment were delayed.
LDH_1 and LDH_2	4 h	48 h	10 days	Normal ratio is <1%-25% LDH_1 to 35% LDH_2. If LDH_1 levels exceed LDH_2 levels, the patient has a "flipped LDH profile." In about 80% of patients this indicates an acute MI, but it also is present in patients with liver engorgement and congestive heart failure.
AST	12 h	24-48 h	5-6 days	Peak levels can be up to 10 times the upper limit of normal within 24 to 36 hours after acute MI and are roughly proportional to extent of myocardial damage; however, lower elevations do not necessarily mean a favorable prognosis.

Data from Ryan, A. M.: What cardiac enzymes tell you about acute MI, RN, March, 1984, p. 46.

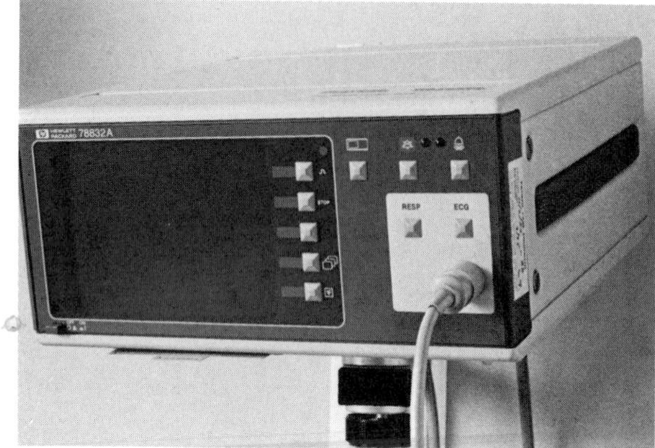

Figure 20-3 Bedside EKG monitoring.

and the mitral valve sounds are found in the apical area at the left fifth intercostal space at the midclavicular line. Figure 20-4 shows the locations for auscultation of heart sounds. As heart sounds are often very soft, ask the patient to refrain from talking and turn off the television or radio while auscultating.

NURSING DIAGNOSES

Appropriate nursing diagnoses for patients experiencing cardiac problems include:

- Decreased cardiac output related to pump failure.
- Alteration in tissue perfusion related to decreased cardiac output.
- Fluid volume excess related to pump failure and fluid retention.
- Impaired gas exchange related to inadequate pumping and fluid congestion in lungs.
- Activity intolerance related to dyspnea on exertion.
- Potential for injury related to inflammation of the lining of the heart.
- Potential for injury related to abnormal rhythm of the heart.
- Pain related to cardiac ischemia.
- Potential for infection related to abnormality of lining of heart structures.
- Impairment of tissue integrity related to cardiac surgical incisions.
- Knowledge deficit related to lack of information about disease process, proper self-care, diet, or medications.
- Self-care deficit related to fatigue, pain, or dyspnea.
- Body image disturbance related to disease of heart and inability to maintain former lifestyle.
- Impaired home maintenance management related to fatigue, dyspnea, and activity intolerance.

CORONARY ARTERY DISEASE

The coronary arteries supply the heart muscle with the oxygen and nutrients needed to carry out the heart's pumping action (Fig. 20-5). A sudden obstruction to blood flow through one or more major coronary arteries (coronary occlusion) results in what is commonly known as a heart attack. If tissue damage results from the lack of blood flow to the heart muscle, the patient suffers a myocardial infarction. Obstruction to blood flow is usually caused by atherosclerosis and thrombus formation but can also result from embolus or arterial spasm.

Coronary artery disease (CAD) is the leading cause of death in the United States.

ATHEROSCLEROSIS

The term *atherosclerosis* refers to a disease process within the arteries. It can affect the cerebral vessels and the aorta and other arteries as well as the coronary arteries. It is one form of arteriosclerosis.

The process of atherosclerosis begins during childhood, when streaks or islands of fatty material are laid down on the inner walls of the arteries. Later, fibrinous plaques are formed as a result of inflammation and healing. The plaque area protrudes into the artery, decreasing the vessel's size. Narrowing of the coronary arteries causes coronary insufficiency (decreased or insufficient blood flow). Obstruction occurs from this process and from thrombosis. The plaque areas eventually rupture, causing platelet aggregation and thrombosis. Spasm of the artery may contribute to occlusion and consequent infarction also.

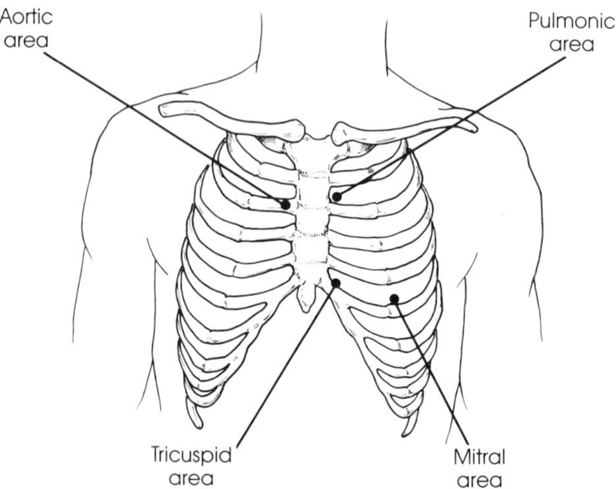

Figure 20-4 Anatomic sites for auscultation of heart sounds.

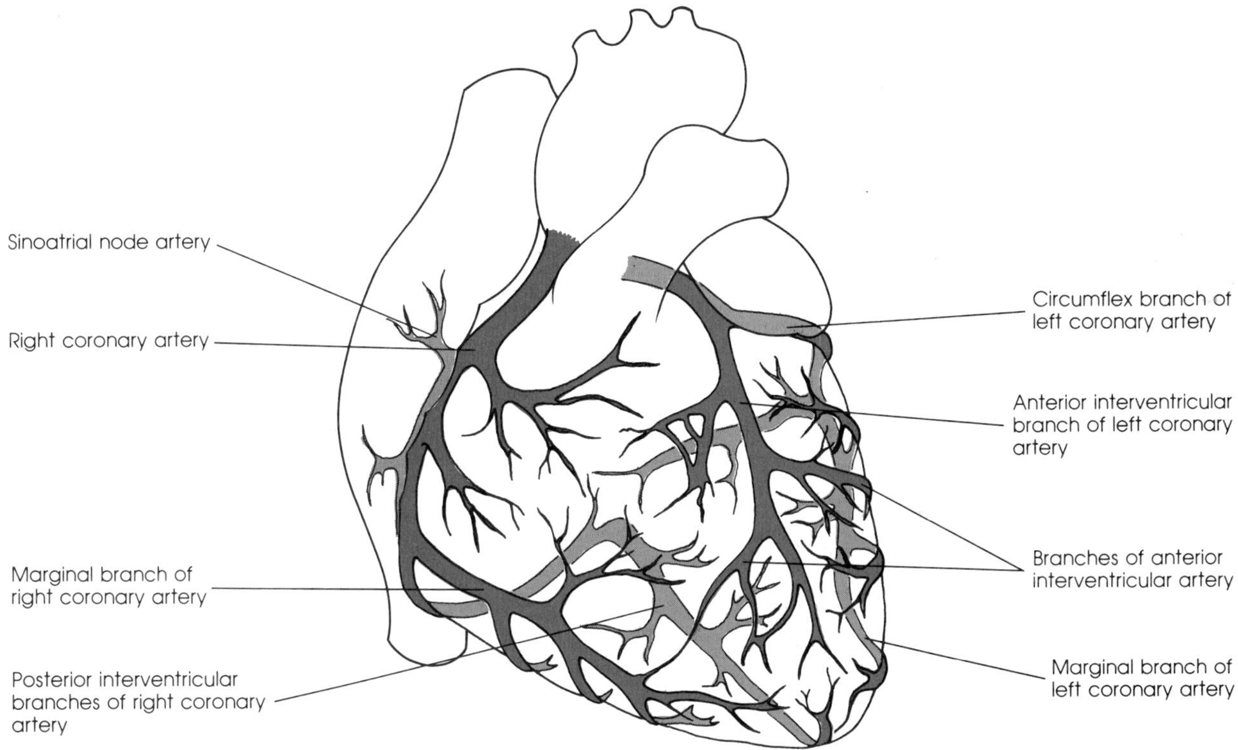

Figure 20-5 A view of the coronary arterial system. The arteries serving the posterior aspect of the myocardium are shown here in a lighter shade.

Causative Factors

Experts do not agree completely on the causative factors responsible for the development of atherosclerosis and coronary artery disease. Atherosclerosis occurs from childhood on and affects all people to some degree. There is a proven link between high serum cholesterol or high levels of low-density lipoproteins and coronary artery disease. There also seem to be many environmental and genetic factors involved. Patients with diabetes and hypertension appear to develop arteriosclerosis at an earlier age.

Environmental factors that are most strongly suspected include emotional stress, heavy smoking, obesity or a diet high in saturated fats, and lack of physical exercise. Genetic factors include such familial diseases as diabetes, hypertension, and abnormal fat metabolism (hyperlipidemia). Those who have had one or more immediate family members die of coronary artery disease during their middle years are considered to be at high risk for the disorder.

Atherosclerosis is indirectly diagnosed by blood lipid levels and by arteriography. If elevated cholesterol and triglyceride levels cannot be lowered by a low-fat diet, then drugs that have been found to lower blood lipids are prescribed. Examples include cholestyramine (Questran), gemfibrozil (Lopid), lovastatin (formerly called *mevinolin*), and nicotinic acid (niacin).

ANGINA PECTORIS

The decreased blood flow that occurs with coronary insufficiency causes pain in the heart muscle, known as *angina pectoris*, or "strangling pain in the chest." Any activity that increases the heart's workload increases its need for oxygen. When the occluded coronary arteries cannot deliver adequate amounts of blood to meet these needs, the patient experiences an angina attack. Attacks can be brought on by physical exertion, emotional excitement, eating a heavy meal, or exposure to cold.

When the patient's angina is no longer adequately controlled by medication and his attacks become more frequent or severe, surgery is indicated to prevent a life-threatening myocardial infarction (MI).

Symptoms and Medical Diagnosis

The type of pain or discomfort may vary in individuals, but in most cases it is described as a dull pain or tightness under the sternum or pain that goes up into the neck and jaw. It may or may not radiate down one or both arms. Sometimes the patient experiences dyspnea, and there may be pallor or flushing of the face, profuse perspiration, and apprehension.

Medical diagnosis is established on the basis of clinical manifestations and whether nitroglycerin provides relief during an acute attack. Response of the heart muscle to increased oxygen demands can be determined by exercise stress testing.

Medical Treatment

The treatment of angina pectoris is mostly symptomatic, with emphasis on eliminating those factors that are known to precipitate an attack in the individual patient. With guidance and teaching, the patient may soon be able to correlate certain activities with an attack and thereby learn to avoid them whenever possible.

Medications

The most specific type of medications used for angina pectoris is the *vasodilators,* the drugs that expand the blood vessels and allow a more rapid flow of blood. The drug of choice during an attack is sublingual nitroglycerin. Common long-acting vasodilators include other forms of nitroglycerin (NitroBid, Transderm-Nitro), pentaerythritol tetranitrate (Peritrate SA), and erythrityl tetranitrate (Cardilate). A calcium antagonist (blocker) may also be prescribed. Calcium channel blockers cause vasodilation and decreased heart rate and contractility, bringing about a drop in oxygen demand by the heart. Examples of calcium channel blockers include diltiazem hydrochloride (Cardizem) and nifedipine (Procardia). If relief from anginal attacks is not obtained, the physician may prescribe a beta-adrenergic blocking agent such as nadolol (Corgard) or propranolol hydrochloride (Inderal). Agents of this kind block sympathetic nerve impulses to the heart, which decreases heart rate and contractility and reduces work load, thereby lowering oxygen use. A low daily dose of aspirin has been added to the treatment of CAD in the past few years. Aspirin decreases platelet aggregation and helps prevent thrombosis.

Effects of the Cold

Cold has a direct effect on the blood vessels, causing them to constrict. The patient with angina pectoris is already suffering from a narrowing of the arteries, and thus he must avoid exposure to cold, which will further aggravate the condition. He should be instructed to wear warm clothing and stay indoors when the weather is extremely cold.

Patient Teaching

Patients who experience anginal attacks are taught to:

- Avoid eating heavy meals.
- Avoid physical activity for an hour after meals to prevent excessive oxygen demands.
- Take nitroglycerin before heavy physical activity such as intercourse or sports activities.
- Avoid exposure to cold; do not walk into a cold wind.
- Decrease controllable risk factors such as lifestyle stress, obesity, and improper diet.
- Adopt a regular, graduated exercise program.
- Stop smoking.
- Learn meditation or other deep relaxation techniques.
- Take a sublingual nitroglycerin tablet and lie down at the beginning of an anginal attack. Nitroglycerin may be repeated twice at 5-minute intervals if the pain persists. If the pain has not eased within 20 minutes, he should notify his physician and have someone drive him to the emergency department.
- Check pulse rate once daily if taking a calcium channel blocker or a beta-adrenergic blocker. These drugs should never be stopped abruptly.
- Rise slowly from a supine or sitting position because of potential postural hypotension.
- Cleanse the area of previous application of nitroglycerin paste when applying a new dose.
- Keep appointments with his physician for regular checkups.
- Obtain sufficient rest daily.

Nursing interventions for selected problems in a patient with angina pectoris are summarized in Nursing Care Plan 20–1.

ACUTE MYOCARDIAL INFARCTION (ACUTE MI)

An *infarction* is an area of dead tissue caused by an obstruction to the flow of blood to that area for a prolonged period (Fig. 20–6). *Myocardial* means "pertaining to the heart muscle." Thus in a myocardial infarction, there is an area of *necrosis* (cell death) in the heart muscle. The prognosis of the patient who suffers an acute myocardial infarction depends on the size of the artery plugged by a clot and the amount of heart tissue that the artery had formerly supplied with blood. If a large area of the heart is affected, instant death may occur. Smaller areas may heal if treated promptly and effectively. Most MIs occur in the left ventricle, the main "pump."

Cardiopulmonary resuscitation of an acute MI victim is discussed in Chapter 36.

Symptoms and Medical Diagnosis

The clinical picture presented by the patient with an acute myocardial infarction is one that most people recognize as a "heart attack." There is a sudden, severe pain in the chest, usually described as crushing or burning. Sometimes the

NURSING CARE PLAN 20–1

Selected nursing diagnoses, goals/outcome criteria, nursing interventions, and evaluations for a patient with angina pectoris (coronary insufficiency)

Situation: Patient is a 63-year-old female with a history of chest pains and dyspnea brought on by physical or emotional exertion. She is 55 pounds overweight and has smoked "about two packs" of cigarettes each day since she was 17 years old. She is admitted for diagnostic tests to evaluate the presence and extent of coronary atherosclerosis.

Nursing Diagnosis	Goals/Outcome Criteria	Nursing Intervention	Evaluation
Pain related to cardiac ischemia. SUPPORTING DATA Clutching hand to center of chest, states "I'm having chest pain."	Pain will be relieved within 20 minutes by sublingual nitroglycerin. Patient will identify any precipitating cause for pain.	Teach to lie down and rest when pain appears. Assess pulse, blood pressure, and respirations and administer sublingual nitroglycerin. Assess vital signs in 5 minutes; assess degree of continuing pain; administer another nitroglycerin tablet if needed. When pain has subsided and patient is stable and calm, explore possible causes of onset of pain.	Chest pain at 11:30 relieved after two nitroglycerin tablets; son had just visited; became upset over financial problem; continue plan.
Anxiety related to diagnostic tests and recurrent chest pain. SUPPORTING DATA "I don't want to die. Isn't a cardiac catheterization dangerous?"	Patient will verbalize understanding of procedure for anginal attack to help diagnose cause of pain. Patient will verbalize that anxiety has decreased within 12 hours.	Explain that EKG is to be done each time she has severe chest pain. Ask patient to report onset of pain promptly so that medication can be given and EKG can be done. Establish trusting relationship and allow patient to ventilate fears and concerns. Assure her that she will be monitored closely. Prepare her for stress test and cardiac catheterization and have other patients who have had these tests talk with her. Answer her questions and help her prepare a list of questions she wishes to ask her physician.	Teaching for diagnostic tests done; spoke with patient who had had cardiac catheterization; states she is less anxious about it; continue plan.
Lack of knowledge about low-fat, low-calorie diet and exercise program. SUPPORTING DATA Cannot describe ways to cut fat in diet and is unaware of calorie content of various foods. Does not exercise regularly.	Within 1 week patient will be able to verbalize ways to cut amount of fat in diet. Patient will express commitment to low-calorie diet and desire to lose 55 pounds over the next 6 months by discharge. Patient will design regular exercise program before discharge. Patient will stick to exercise and diet program at end of 2 months. Patient will reach and maintain normal weight. Cholesterol will be within normal limits at end of 6 months.	Perform a dietary assessment with 24-hour food intake history of usual diet. Provide consult with dietitian. Provide materials from American Heart Association and telephone numbers for local support groups such as Weight Watchers, Overeaters Anonymous, or TOPS. Provide emotional support for patient and praise all efforts to learn about needed lifestyle changes. Help her to design an exercise program that fits into lifestyle and that she will be willing to continue.	Met with dietitian; states that a neighbor goes to Weight Watchers and that she will consider that; she could walk in the evenings with her husband; is considering options; continue plan.
Potential for injury related to cigarette smoking. SUPPORTING DATA Has smoked 2 packs of	Patient will decrease smoking to ½ pack per day by discharge. Patient will state desire to	Explain that nicotine causes vasoconstriction, which further compromises oxygen supply to the	Discussed action of nicotine in body; given AHA literature on quitting smoking; cut back to 1 pack yesterday, ¾ pack today; continue plan.

Nursing Care Plan continued on following page

NURSING CARE PLAN 20–1, *Continued*

Nursing Diagnosis	Goals/Outcome Criteria	Nursing Intervention	Evaluation
cigarettes per day for 46 years; is craving cigarettes constantly.	quit smoking by discharge. Patient will stop smoking within 3 weeks.	heart; explain danger of coronary occlusion. Allow patient to ventilate her anxiety and concerns over trying to quit smoking. Obtain American Lung Association literature for her on quitting smoking. Help her design realistic plan for quitting smoking, including support from significant others.	

pain is mistaken for a symptom of acute indigestion. The patient also shows symptoms of shock with pallor, profuse sweating, anxiety, and often nausea and vomiting.

Although these symptoms are usually present in an acute myocardial infarction, they are not always severe, and in some cases patients have described their pain as mild. Sometimes the patient only experiences left arm, jaw, or back pain. The electrocardiogram (EKG) may or may not show evidence of an MI initially. For this reason EKGs are repeated every 24 hours for 3 days. The severity of the symptoms will depend on the size of the area of ischemia or infarction.

Whenever there is necrotic tissue anywhere in the body, the white cell count increases and the sedimentation rate rises. Within 24 hours of an acute attack, the temperature of the patient with myocardial infarction rises slightly, and mild leukocytosis appears.

In addition to the clinical manifestations, EKG changes, and other diagnostic tests, laboratory determinations of specific enzymes are used to establish a diagnosis of myocardial infarction and evaluate the extent of damage done to the heart muscle. (See Table 20–1 for information on diagnostic tests.)

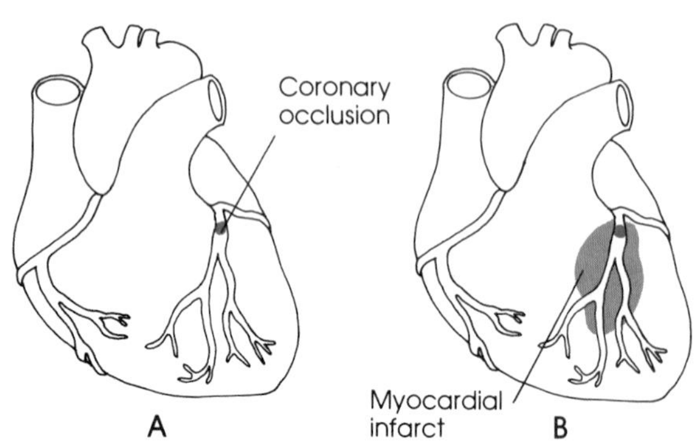

Figure 20–6 Occlusion of a major coronary artery *(A)* leads to a region of infarct *(B)* because of ischemia.

Medical Treatment

As soon as a patient with acute MI is brought to the emergency room, measures are taken to relieve pain, decrease ischemia, and prevent further circulatory collapse and shock. In many large cities and some rural areas of the United States, there are specially designed and equipped mobile units staffed with trained personnel to give immediate care to the patient who has had a heart attack. This care is given while the patient is in transit to the hospital.

Drugs administered for the control of pain in a patient with acute MI usually are morphine sulfate, meperidine hydrochloride (Demerol), or hydromorphone hydrochloride (Dilaudid). They are given intravenously to provide immediate relief. Antianxiety agents such as diazepam (Valium) are administered to relieve anxiety. Intravenous fluids are started, oxygen is administered, and the patient's condition is stabilized. Close assessment of respiration is essential, as these drugs can depress respiration at a time when the heart needs all the oxygen it can get.

Acute Care

On admission to the coronary care unit (CCU), the patient is placed in bed and kept on bed rest with bedside commode privileges for 1 to 3 days. Physical activity is gradually increased according to the patient's individual condition and response to therapy. IV lines or a PRN IV cannula are inserted to provide a route for administration of emergency drugs should they be needed.

Vital signs are continuously monitored by electronic means and are assessed by the nurse every 1 to 2 hours. Mean arterial pressure is often provided by a Dinamap machine. This machine electronically reads blood pressure, tracks heart rate and systolic and diastolic pressure, and calculates mean arterial pressure, which is an indicator of changes in heart function. A *pulse oximeter* is used to monitor oxygenation. This is an electronic device that, with the use of light and a sensor, measures oxygen saturation of the blood. The sensor is placed on the fingertip, ear, or tip of the nose. Abnormal values are rechecked by arterial blood gas measurements, which are more accurate. Continuous EKG (cardiac telemetry monitoring) is essential to accurate evaluation of the status of the heart.

The critically ill patient will have more sophisticated monitoring done in the CCU. A pulmonary artery flow-directed catheter (Swan-Ganz type) will be inserted for readings of central venous pressure (CVP), pulmonary artery pressure (PAP), and pulmonary capillary wedge pressure (PCWP), which give a better picture of the injured heart's ability to pump. Data for calculating cardiac output can also be obtained.

A low-sodium, low-fat diet is ordered when the patient's vital signs have stabilized. Medication to correct arrhythmia is ordered as needed. Measures to correct acid-base imbalance are begun. A beta-adrenergic blocker such as propranolol (Inderal) may be ordered to ease the heart's workload, or a calcium channel blocker such as diltiazem (Cardizem) may be used. Continuous oxygen via mask or nasal cannula is begun at a rate of 2 to 5 L/min. Various IV drugs may be used to regulate blood pressure or to control arrhythmias; these include nitroglycerin (Nipride) to lower blood pressure and dopamine (Intropin) to raise blood pressure.

If the patient's heart rate drops below 40 and stays there or if he experiences complete heart block (the electrical impulse does not go through the atrioventricular [AV] node to the ventricles and the ventricles are not signaled to contract), a temporary pacemaker may be inserted. (See "Disorders of the Heart's Conduction System" for information on pacemaker insertion.)

If the patient sought immediate medical attention upon experiencing the symptoms of MI, he may be given thrombolytic agents in an attempt to dissolve the clot obstructing the coronary artery. Thrombolytic therapy must be started within 4 to 6 hours in order to prevent necrosis of the myocardium. Agents used intraarterially to dissolve the clot include tissue plasminogen activator (TPA), streptokinase, urokinase, and anistreplase (APSAC). After infusion of one of these agents, a heparin drip is started to prevent reocclusion. Heparin is continued for 3 to 4 days until the patient is stabilized on warfarin sodium (Coumadin), an oral anticoagulant.

When the patient is stabilized, he may undergo cardiac catheterization and coronary angiography. If only a couple areas of stenosis are identified, he may have a percutaneous transluminal coronary angioplasty (PTCA) or coronary artery bypass graft surgery (CABG) to improve blood flow. PTCA is a nonsurgical technique to open blocked coronary arteries. It is performed in the cardiac catheterization laboratory using fluoroscopy. A catheter with a balloon attachment is threaded into the blocked artery, and when the narrowed area is reached, the balloon is inflated repeatedly, flattening the plaque and widening the interior of the artery. Experimentation is under way with a new procedure using a laser to vaporize and extract the plaque from the artery. This is done with a similar type catheter and avoids open heart surgery. CABG surgery is covered in the section on cardiac surgery.

Studies are presently being conducted to determine whether a regimen consisting of a very low fat diet, regular exercise, reduction of stress, and practice of relaxation techniques can reverse coronary artery disease without surgery. These methods have been effective in some people (Siberner, 1990). However, more data are needed before PTCA and CABG will be used less frequently.

If the left ventricle is badly damaged, the intraaortic balloon pump (IABP) may be used to ease the heart's workload while it begins to heal. This device is a highly technical machine utilizing a balloon catheter positioned in the aorta that inflates during diastole and deflates during systole, effectively decreasing the workload of the heart and increasing blood flow through the coronary arteries.

Patient Teaching and Nursing Intervention

Nursing care is directed at promoting rest, administering ordered medical therapy and observing for side effects, assisting with activities of daily living (ADL) and ambulation, constantly monitoring physical status by performing a good cardiovascular assessment every 4 to 8 hours and monitoring vital signs every 2 to 4 hours. Daily weight is recorded. Intake and output are accurately recorded and compared, and urine output is closely monitored. A patent IV access is maintained at all times. The nurse closely watches for signs of complications of MI such as arrhythmia, congestive heart failure, pulmonary edema, cardiogenic shock, or cardiac arrest.

A very important nursing measure is to decrease anxiety and stress for the patient. It is helpful to explain the function of all equipment and tests in simple terms and to explain the routine of frequent assessment and tests so the patient will know what to expect. Visitors are restricted to immediate family for the first few days, and no phone calls are allowed. The nurse will need to help decrease the family's anxiety by reinforcing what the physician has told them about the patient's condition and treatment.

The American Heart Association, through its local chapters, provides an abundance of written material designed for the person recovering from an MI. Patients and their families should know about this valuable source of information and support as they work toward the goals of rehabilitation.

Intermediate Care

As the patient recovers from the acute phase of his illness, he is gradually weaned away from intensive care. When the physicians feel that continuous monitoring is no longer essential and that the patient is able to participate in his own personal hygiene activities without detrimental effects on the healing heart tissues, he is transferred out of the CCU into a telemetry or "step-down" medical unit. For some patients, this move is frightening, because they have become dependent on the nurses and other staff members in the CCU. Every effort is made to assure the patient that he is making progress toward recovery and is no longer in need of intensive care.

During the time the patient is in the general medical care unit, his physical activities are gradually increased according to his ability to tolerate exercise. He is watched closely for subjective and objective symptoms of excessive strain on the heart or the development of complications. The most common complications of MI are congestive heart failure, pulmonary embolism, arrhythmias, pericarditis, and recurrent myocardial infarction.

Rehabilitation

As the patient gains an understanding of his illness and ways in which he can help himself toward recovery, he should become more confident and optimistic about his condition. Realization that one has suffered a serious heart attack is a frightening experience. The patient and his family will need much help and support as they work to make the necessary adjustments. One area of major concern is sexuality. The patient may be fearful of resuming intercourse, thinking that it may cause a heart attack. The spouse, too, often has these fears. Both partners need reassurance that resumption of normal sexual activities will be possible. The patient may need to take a more passive role during intercourse, at least for a while, using alternate positions that cause less strain and less oxygen demand. The physician should cover this area with the patient and his spouse, but if he does not, the nurse should see that the patient gets the proper information.

Patients need to be taught to plan sexual activity for times when they are well rested and to avoid an environment that is too hot or too cold. It is best to space such activity at least 2 hours after eating a meal or drinking any alcohol. Nitroglycerin should be used prophylactically if intercourse causes angina symptoms. If angina does occur, the patient should cease activity, place a nitroglycerin tablet under his tongue, lie down, and rest. Intercourse may be resumed 3 to 6 weeks after an MI and 6 to 8 weeks after open heart surgery, depending on the patient's exercise tolerance as determined by stress testing. Sexual dysfunction may occur at first, but with patience on the part of both partners, this usually passes.

Rehabilitation involves three major aspects: (1) a program of increasing activity based on the patient's individual progress and needs, (2) instruction of the patient and his family about the nature of his illness and the rationale for every aspect of its management, and (3) assistance to the patient and his family as they work toward the goal of accepting the limitations imposed and the changes in lifestyle that may be required.

In spite of all efforts to educate the post–myocardial infarction patient about his illness and the need to continue his exercise program and modify his lifestyle, compliance with the prescribed regimen remains low. The main purpose of instruction is to provide the patient with the information he needs to avoid the problems and complications that can occur once he leaves the hospital.

The patient's perception of his own situation greatly influences whether he will comply with the instructions he has received for continued treatment and preventive therapy. He may not follow instructions if he does not see himself as particularly susceptible to a condition—that is, if he doesn't think he is at risk for complications or further damage.

The patient is taught to:

- Recognize the signs of recurrent MI and to seek immediate medical attention should they occur. These are: chest pain, diaphoresis, nausea, and anxiety.
- Adopt a regular, graduated exercise program.
- Alter controllable risk factors: reach and maintain a normal weight; cease smoking; keep alcohol consumption at a moderate level; keep cholesterol within normal limits.
- Reduce stress and learn relaxation techniques.
- Observe for complications such as irregular pulse rate, dypsnea and fatigue, chest pain, and fever.
- Control hypertension.
- Continue on a low-fat, low-sodium diet individualized to his taste.

It is important to stress to the patient that he has control over his rehabilitation and his prognosis. He and his physician and other health

NURSING CARE PLAN 20-2, *Continued*

Nursing Diagnosis	Goals/Outcome Criteria	Nursing Intervention	Evaluation
Knowledge deficit related to disease and various therapies. SUPPORTING DATA "Doesn't heart failure mean that my heart is worn out and going to quit?" What do these medicines do?	By time of discharge patient will verbalize simple explanation of congestive heart failure. By time of discharge patient will verbalize purpose of each medicine, how to take it, and side effects to watch for.	Teach what happens in congestive heart failure. Teach patient, husband, and daughter how to measure pulse rate and rhythm; symptoms of digitalis toxity; purpose of watching for symptoms of hypokalemia; foods high in potassium content; purpose of low-sodium diet; importance of daily weight record; importance of keeping appointments for follow-up; symptoms that indicate a worsening of heart failure and the need to seek medical help promptly.	Teaching session no. 2 completed; can verbalize simple explanation of heart failure; measures own pulse accurately; can pick foods high in potassium from list; recording daily weight in notebook; continue plan.

tract too fast to allow time for adequate filling with blood; cardiac output falls drastically, and death may occur.

- *Ventricular fibrillation*. The ventricles quiver rather than contract; there is no effective cardiac output, and without CPR, death will occur.
- *Premature ventricular contractions* (PVC). The ventricular impulse causes ventricular contraction before impulse and contraction of atria is complete. Blood is not received from the atria to be pumped out to body. A few PVCs are not abnormal, but when there are more than six to seven in a minute, cardiac output falls. This arrhythmia also makes the heart more likely to develop ventricular tachycardia or ventricular fibrillation.
- *Complete heart block* (third-degree heart block). Separate impulses cause contraction in the atria and in the ventricles; contraction is uncoordinated, and blood is not received normally from the atria, which decreases the amount of blood available to be pumped out to body; cardiac output falls drastically. This is a life-threatening arrhythmia.

There are many other types of cardiac arrhythmias. Nurses assigned to a coronary care unit take a special course in arrhythmias to learn the patterns, significance, and treatment of each type.

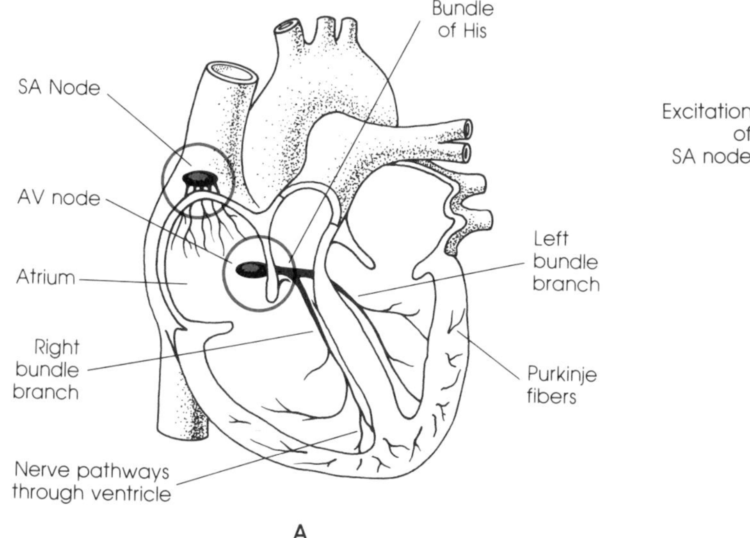

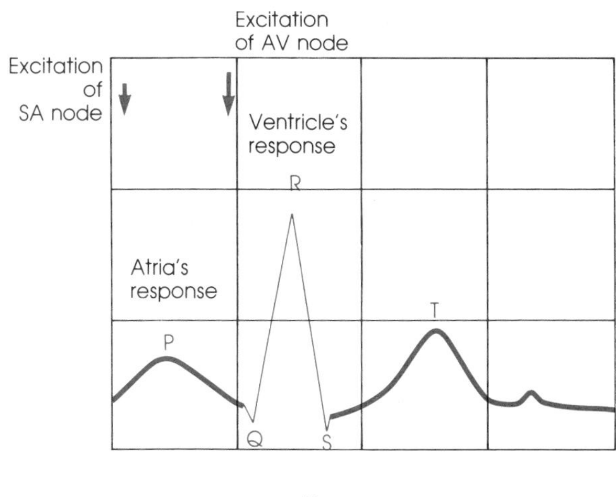

Figure 20-7 Conducting system of the heart *(A)* and impulses it produces on electrocardiogram *(B)*. Electrical impulses that excite the heart muscle to contract originate in the sinoatrial (SA) node and spread through the atrium (P wave on the EKG). They then pass through the atrioventricular (AV) node (Q wave) to the bundle of His, which divides into a left and right branch. The impulses travel along these branches and excite the ventricle (S wave). The smaller fibers that branch into the myocardium are called the *Purkinje fibers*.

DIAGNOSIS AND MEDICAL TREATMENT

Disorders of the cardiac conduction system are diagnosed by a 12-lead EKG, continuous EKG monitoring (Holter monitoring), patient history, and electrophysiology tests, which can be performed during cardiac catheterization.

Drug therapy is effective in correcting arrhythmias in many cases. A variety of antiarrhythmic agents may be used alone or in combination to regulate the heart beat (Table 20–3).

When drug therapy does not control a life-threatening arrhythmia, surgical destruction (ablation) of the tissue initiating the abnormal impulse can sometimes correct the problem if such an area can be located with electrophysiology tests.

Artificial cardiac pacing can be a temporary measure if the problem is an emergency, as in a transient condition such as drug toxicity. A temporary pacemaker is used if transient complete heart block (i.e., no impulse travels from the atria to the ventricles) develops after a myocardial infarction. Pacemaker wires are always placed during cardiac surgery for quick use should the patient need to be "paced" in the postoperative period. When the need for the wires is past, the surgeon will pull them out.

A permanent pacemaker is indicated if the cardiac arrhythmia is the result of an irreversible disorder, as in failure of the SA node. Other conditions in which a permanent pacemaker is inserted include pathologic complete heart block, secondary AV block, supraventricular tachycardia, and bradytachycardia, in which the SA node alternates between firing too slowly and firing too rapidly.

Transvenous pacemakers are inserted using fluoroscopy with local anesthesia. Patient consent is required, and a sedative is given to the patient before the procedure. Insertion of a permanent pacemaker is done in the operating room to ensure an aseptic environment, even though it is a relatively minor procedure (Fig. 20–8).

The newer types of pacemakers can sense and pace in both the atrium and the ventricle, thus making the heart function in a more natural way and giving the patient better cardiac output. Another type of pacemaker is so sophisticated that it can speed up and slow down the heart rate according to the patient's activity needs, much as a normal heart does.

Patients who experience supraventricular tachycardia or atrial fibrillation that does not respond to drug therapy may be treated with *cardioversion*. A mild electrical shock is delivered to the heart at a specific time in the cardiac cycle to interrupt the abnormal rhythm and begin a new, normal rhythm of electrical impulse and contraction.

Frequent PVCs (more than 6 to 7 per minute) and ventricular tachycardia are treated with IV lidocaine. If ventricular tachycardia is not responsive to the lidocaine, cardioversion is performed to restore a more normal rhythm. Ventricular fibrillation is treated by starting CPR and performing defibrillation as soon as possible. Defibrillation means to "get the heart to stop fibrillating." This procedure is covered in Chapter 36.

Automatic implantable cardiac defibrillators (AICD) are used for patients who have repeated episodes of life-threatening ventricular fibrillation or cardiac asystole (arrest). This device has saved many lives by monitoring the heart beat and providing an electrical shock similar to that

TABLE 20–3 COMMON ANTIARRYTHMIC DRUGS

Drug	Use
Digoxin (Lanoxin)	Atrial arrhythmias; fibrillation and flutter
Verapamil HCL (Calan, Isoptin)	Supraventricular tachycardia
Quinidine sulfate (Quinaglute)	Atrial and ventricular arrhythmias
Propanolol HCL (Inderal)	Atrial arrhythmia; paroxysmal atrial tachycardia
Phenytoin (Dilantin)	Digitalis-induced ventricular arrhythmia
Xylocaine (Lidocaine) (IV)	Ventricular arrhythmias; PVCs Ventricular tachycardia
Procainamide (Pronestyl)	Ventricular arrhythmias
Encainide (Enkaid)	Ventricular arrhythmias
Disopyramide (Norpace)	Ventricular arrhythmias
Flecainide acetate (Tambocor)	Ventricular arrhythmias
Amiodarone HCL (Cordarone)	Refractory ventricular arrhythmias
Mexiletine HCL (Mexitil)	Ventricular and supraventricular arrhythmias
Atropine sulfate (IV)	Symptomatic bradycardia
Isoproterenol (Isuprel) (IV)	Bradycardia unresponsive to atropine

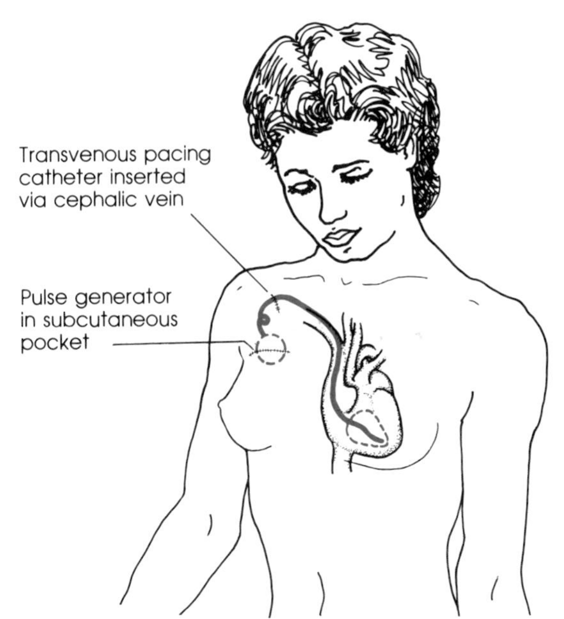

Figure 20-8 Thoracic placement of permanent pacemaker and transvenous pacing catheter.

delivered in cardiac defibrillation when a life-threatening rhythm is detected.

NURSING INTERVENTION

If insertion of a pacemaker is not an emergency procedure, the nurse will have opportunities to assess her patient's knowledge of and feelings about having a pacemaker to regulate his heart beat. While the physician is responsible for explaining the purpose of the pacemaker and its benefits to the patient, these explanations can raise more questions and possibly create fears and anxiety. The nurse should assess the patient's learning needs and seek to identify the source of his fear and the level of his anxiety.

The American Heart Association and the manufacturers of pacemakers both provide illustrated booklets to help patients learn more about their cardiac pacers. The nurse can go over these booklets with her patient and perhaps show him a demonstration model and explain how it works to his advantage. Care of the patient who has a temporary pacemaker includes checking the connections of the lead wires to the pulse generator, keeping the device and wires dry, checking the control settings, and protecting the patient from electrical shock. For protection the pulse generator and exposed wires are placed in a rubber glove, and contact is avoided with all electrical apparatus (e.g., unplug bed; do not use an electric razor). Other care is identical to that of the patient with insertion of a permanent pacemaker.

Postoperative nursing care for the permanent pacemaker patient includes continuous monitoring of heart rate and rhythm, dressing changes, and care of the insertion site according to the protocol of the nursing care unit. Vital signs, especially peripheral pulses distal to the insertion site, and level of consciousness are checked regularly during the immediate postoperative period.

Discharge instruction for the patient with a permanent pacemaker should include amount of physical activity allowed until the electrode is securely in place. This usually is no more than 6 weeks, after which time the patient can be as physically active as he wishes, but he is warned not to engage in contact sports or other activities that may result in injury to the chest.

Although the newer pacemakers have a shield to protect them from electromagnetic signals from machinery, the patient should be cautioned not to expose his pacemaker unnecessarily to high-voltage equipment. Faulty microwave ovens and other sources of electromagnetic signals can "confuse" a pacemaker with impulses that could cause it to malfunction. Should this occur, function will return to normal as soon as the patient moves away from the source of electromagnetic signals. The battery in a pacemaker should last 15 to 30 years, depending on the type, but it could weaken prematurely. This results in a drop in pulse rate, which should be reported to the physician immediately.

The patient will need to know how to take his pulse so that he can regularly evaluate the performance of his pacemaker. He should take his pulse for 1 full minute while he is in a resting position.

A patient with a pacer should wear some form of identification such as a bracelet or necklace at all times and carry an identification card stating that he is wearing a pacemaker. Follow-up care is an essential part of the life of every person with a pacemaker. He must understand the importance of periodic evaluations of his condition for the rest of his life. Some types of pacemakers have a telephone monitoring device that allows the patient to call a monitoring station and have his pacemaker checked. Instructions for the use of the pacemaker and monitoring device are included in the owner's manual.

Because of the sensors planted in the chambers of the heart, this patient is at risk for infection of the lining of the heart (*endocarditis*). He should be given prophylactic antibiotics before any invasive medical or dental procedure.

INFLAMMATORY DISEASES OF THE HEART

The tissues of the heart are subject to the same inflammatory conditions that may affect other parts of the body. The inflammation may be present in the inner lining *(endocarditis)*, the heart muscle *(myocarditis)*, or the sac surrounding the heart *(pericarditis)*. The process may also involve the valves between the heart chambers or those located at the base of the major vessels leading from the heart (Fig. 20–9).

Bacterial infection of the heart can result from an acute infection elsewhere in the body, such as those caused by staphylococci, pneumococci, and gonococci. This condition is called *infective endocarditis* (IE), *bacterial endocarditis* (BE), or *subacute bacterial endocarditis* (SBE). In adults the introduction of bacteria during dental procedures is a frequent cause of endocarditis.

In the past, the most common cause of heart inflammation was damage resulting from rheumatic fever. Although antibiotics, particularly penicillin, have decreased the incidence of rheumatic fever, the danger is still present. Today, untreated strep throat is the most common cause of cardiac inflammation in children who do not have congenital cardiac abnormalities. This is a common disease of childhood caused by group A streptococcus. If the streptococcal infection is treated early, inflammation in the heart can be avoided.

The invading microorganisms grow on the heart valves or in areas of the endocardium that are congenitally abnormal. The mitral valve is the most frequent location of infection.

SYMPTOMS

The signs and symptoms of infective endocarditis vary considerably. The sedimentation rate and leukocyte count are elevated, and signs of low-grade intermittent fever are evident. The spleen becomes enlarged. Splinter hemorrhages (thin black lines) can occur under the nails, and there may be petechiae inside the mouth. Cardiac inflammation (endocarditis) may be recurring. Each instance of endocarditis further damages the heart valves. The scar tissue that occurs as the inflammation subsides may cause the valve to leak, resulting in insufficiency, or the valve leaflets may become thickened and calcified, causing narrowing or stenosis. An existing cardiac murmur may worsen or a new murmur may appear as a valve is damaged. The mitral and aortic valves are most often affected. When mitral or aortic stenosis or insufficiency cause symptoms sufficient to interfere with the patient's usual lifestyle, surgery becomes necessary (See section on cardiac surgery.) Both stenosis and insufficiency of cardiac valves eventually cause congestive heart failure.

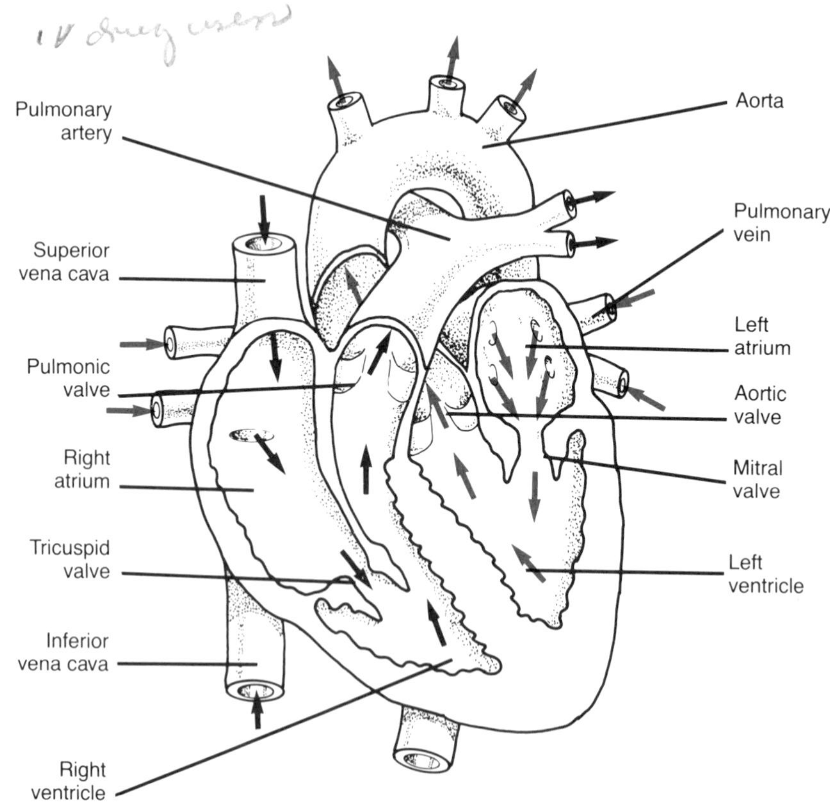

Figure 20–9 Major vessels and valves of the heart.

MEDICAL TREATMENT

Rest

Inflammatory conditions are primarily treated with rest of the affected part, and the same is true of inflammatory diseases of the heart. Treatment consists of measures intended to decrease the workload of the heart. The patient is placed on bed rest with bathroom privileges during the acute stage of the infection.

Medications

Specific medications for the treatment of inflammatory conditions of the heart include the antiinflammatories used for pericarditis and antiinfectives used for infective endocarditis. Choice of drug is determined by blood culture for the particular organism responsible for the infection and sensitivity testing for the drug that kills it best. Often a combination of at least two antibiotics is given intravenously through a central line for 4 to 6 weeks, with further oral therapy thereafter. After the first 2 to 3 weeks, the patient is often discharged home, and the medications are administered by visiting nurses.

Surgery

Pericarditis may be surgically treated by *pericardotomy* or *pericardiocentesis.* Repair of congenital cardiac problems such as atrial or ventricular septal defect is performed. *Balloon valvuloplasty* is a relatively new procedure that is used to open stenosed valves. It is performed with a balloon-tipped catheter much like the one used for PTCA. However, it is questionable as to whether the valve will close again with time. *Valve replacement* is an open heart surgical procedure in which the valve is replaced with either a porcine (pork) or synthetic valve. (See section on specific cardiac surgeries.) When a synthetic valve is used, the patient must be on anticoagulant therapy for the rest of his life, as the synthetic material tends to cause breakup of blood cells and clumping of platelets, which in turn cause emboli.

COMMON PROBLEMS RELATED TO CARDIAC DISEASE

FATIGUE AND DYSPNEA

In the early stages of heart disease, the patient may be only slightly aware of his inability to do as much physical work as he formerly could. He may attribute this to "just getting old," or he may have some vague idea that something more is wrong and that one of these days he will get around to seeing a physician. If he procrastinates too long, he will find that his physical activities are becoming increasingly restricted, because he lacks the energy to perform the simplest of tasks and becomes short of breath after the slightest exertion.

The coronary arteries supply the heart muscle with the oxygen it needs to work continuously as a pump for the circulatory system. When these arteries fail to supply adequate oxygen to the cells of the heart muscle, the heart is unable to perform as it should when extra demands are placed on it. The result is a general hypoxia of the tissues throughout the body, which causes fatigue and dyspnea on exertion.

Nursing Intervention: Rest and Exercise

Traditionally, prolonged bed rest was prescribed for every patient with a heart condition. Currently, bed rest with bedside commode privileges is ordered for the first 24 to 72 hours. The patient may feed himself and assist with his sponge bath. He is cautioned against any isometric activity such as pushing himself up in bed. Stool softeners are given to prevent straining (Valsalva maneuver). Activity progresses to chair sitting, ambulating to the bathroom, and then down the hall. Patients are monitored by telemetry units in order to watch for arrhythmias or excessive heart rate changes during ambulation. The amount of energy utilized in activity is expressed in *metabolic equivalents* (METs). The patient is guided from 1 to 3 METs before discharge.

Because patients are being discharged much earlier in their course of recovery, outpatient rehabilitation units are using telemetry and monitoring their patients during the first stages of their exercise programs. Physicians and nurses are available in case a problem arises.

Criteria used to determine whether the patient is tolerating the activity include the following:

1. The heart rate does not rise more than 20 beats per minute.
2. Systolic blood pressure does not drop.
3. There is no complaint of chest pain, dyspnea, or severe fatigue.
4. There is no abnormal heart rate or rhythm.

Activity progression is often jointly supervised by a physical therapist and a nurse.

The physical and emotional benefits of exercise in cardiac rehabilitation are well documented. Many patients who have coronary artery disease feel that they have been doomed to a life of invalidism and are hesitant to undertake any kind of exercise. If a patient is closely monitored while he is exercising in the initial stages of rehabilitation and a positive outlook for his full recovery is conveyed by members of the health care team, he will gain confidence.

EDEMA

As explained in Chapter 8, edema is an accumulation of fluid in the interstitial fluid compartment. It becomes a problem in heart disease when the blood flow into or out of the heart is inhibited, causing a slowing down of the normal movement of body fluids and their eventual excretion.

Nursing Intervention

The nurse continually assesses the fluid balance of a patient with cardiac disease by looking for signs of abnormal collections of fluid in the body tissues. Daily weight change is considered the best indicator of fluid buildup. The feet and ankles of ambulatory patients are checked for signs of dependent edema, and bed rest patients are watched for signs of swelling in the area of the sacrum, buttocks, and thighs. The patient is observed for progressive signs of shortness of breath, and lung fields are auscultated each shift to detect crackles, a sign of beginning pulmonary congestion.

Nursing responsibilities include recording the patient's weight daily before breakfast, supervising fluid restriction, accurately measuring intake and output, and assessing for signs of fluid deficit as well as fluid overload. Elderly patients on fluid restriction and diuretics can easily become dehydrated.

Therapeutic measures to control edema include administration of diuretics and restriction of sodium and possibly fluids. The nurse must observe for adverse effects of medication such as electrolyte imbalance and postural hypotension. Potassium supplementation may be ordered for patient's experiencing hypokalemia. Foods high in potassium such as bananas, orange juice, avocados, potatoes, and meat should be encouraged.

PAIN

Severe pain is most often associated with heart disease of an acute nature (e.g., myocardial infarction). The analgesic drugs used most often are morphine sulfate and meperidine hydrochloride (Demerol). These are given intravenously initially for quick pain relief. As the acute phase and severe pain subside, these drugs may be replaced with oral dosages or milder sedatives that promote relaxation and freedom from anxiety. Anginal pain can interfere with the patient's lifestyle, as well as cause discomfort.

Nursing Intervention

Much of the patient's pain may be caused by his nervousness and anxiety, and the nurse can do much to help relieve his pain by providing a restful environment, interacting therapeutically with "active listening," and balancing rest with prescribed physical activity.

Sleep deprivation and fatigue can increase the pain. Turning, administration of medications, exercise, and other procedures should be coordinated so that the patient is not disturbed more than necessary.

Anginal pain is treated with sublingual nitroglycerin, reassurance, and careful monitoring for relief. Assessment for things that seem to trigger an attack can identify stressors that the patient may be able to avoid.

Relaxation and other noninvasive techniques for the management of pain are discussed in Chapter 10.

COMMON THERAPIES AND THEIR NURSING IMPLICATIONS

The medical treatments most commonly used in the management of heart disease include (1) pharmacologic agents, (2) dietary controls, and (3) oxygen therapy. Patient education and rehabilitation of the cardiac patient must also be included.

Surgical treatment of cardiac conditions most often is employed for correction of structural defects of the heart and great vessels and for bypassing or enlarging the lumen of occluded coronary arteries in order to give the heart muscle a more reliable supply of blood.

PHARMACOLOGIC AGENTS

Cardiotonics (Cardiac Glycosides)

These drugs are used to (1) strengthen contractions of the heart muscle, thereby providing more blood to body tissues and (2) decrease the heart rate by slowing conduction of the cardiac impulse through the atrioventricular node. They are especially effective in the treatment of congestive heart failure and the control of atrial fibrillation, atrial flutter, and tachycardia.

The most frequently used cardiotonics are digitalis preparations derived from the foxglove plant. They include digoxin (Lanoxin) and digitoxin. Of the two, digitoxin has a slower and more prolonged action and is 10 times more potent than digoxin.

Digitalis in its various forms is a widely prescribed drug in the United States. However, it is a potent drug that can produce serious problems of toxicity. It can be very effective in the treatment of certain kinds of cardiac disorders, but its therapeutic range is quite narrow. A therapeutic dose is only about one third less than the dose that will induce toxicity. Moreover, physiologic changes resulting from age, electrolyte imbalances (particularly hypokalemia or hypercalcemia), renal impairment, metabolic disturbances, and certain heart conditions can predispose a patient to digitalis toxicity. Other drugs given simultaneously also can alter the effects of digitalis and make it more toxic.

The apical pulse must be counted for 1 full minute before administering each dose of a digitalis preparation. If the pulse is lower than 60 per minute or newly irregular, the drug is held and the physician notified. The digitalis serum level is checked, and the patient is assessed for signs of digitalis toxicity: fatigue, anorexia, nausea, diarrhea, blurred vision or yellow-green halos around objects, and dysrhythmias. If there are no signs of toxicity, the digitalis serum level is within therapeutic range, and the patient has signs of adequate perfusion, the dose is usually given unless orders have been written to "hold if apical rate is below 60 bpm." Signs of adequate perfusion include alertness, no dizziness or palpitations, and skin that is warm, dry, and either pink or a normal color. Careful documentation of assessment findings in the nurse's notes should be done whenever the apical pulse is below 60 and digitalis is given. While decreased pulse rate is the most typical sign of digitalis intoxication, there are earlier signs that should be watched for. These include nausea, blurred vision, mental depression, disorientation, and malaise.

Because digitalis is so often prescribed for self-medication by the patient, it is imperative that he be taught safe administration of the drug. He should know about the early signs and symptoms of toxicity and the dangers of taking digitalis with over-the-counter drugs such as antacids. If he does not know how to check his pulse for rate and rhythm, he will need to learn how to do this and why he should notify his physician if his pulse becomes unusually irregular or if the rate falls below his normal range. Written information usually is the best way to help remind the patient of his responsibilities in administering his own medication safely.

Antiarrhythmic Agents

Changes in the heart's rate and rhythm can result from any condition that affects its sensitivity to nerve impulses—for example, electrolyte imbalance, ischemic heart disease, or stimulation of the autonomic nervous system. Antiarrhythmic agents help change the heart rate to more normal values and restore the origin of the heart beat to its natural pacemaker. The drugs most often used to accomplish this action are listed in Table 20–3.

Diuretics

Diuretics are given to increase urinary output and thereby help rid the body of excess water and sodium. In the treatment of cardiovascular disease, diuretics are most often used to help control hypertension and manage a complication of the disease process such as congestive heart failure.

The thiazide diuretics act directly on the kidney to block tubular reabsorption of water, sodium, and chloride and tend to promote excretion of potassium. Chlorothiazide (Diuril) and chlorthalidone (Hygroton) are examples of thiazide diuretics. Thiazides are potent drugs capable of causing a serious depletion of potassium, especially in patients receiving digitalis.

The loop diuretics depress sodium and chloride reabsorption in the ascending loop of Henle. They also cause potassium loss in the urine. Furosemide (Lasix) is a commonly used loop diuretic. It is a potent, rapidly acting diuretic of short duration. The side effects of both thiazide and loop diuretics are hypokalemia, hyperuricemia, and hyperglycemia.

Potassium-sparing diuretics inhibit reabsorption of sodium and water in exchange for potassium and hydrogen. Their main value is in maintaining normal levels of serum potassium. Examples include spironolactone (Aldactone), which is an aldosterone antagonist, and triamterene (Dyrenium).

Diuretics scheduled for once a day should be given in the early morning to prevent diuresis during the night, which would interfere with sleep. Potassium levels should be checked before giving a diuretic dose while the patient is in the hospital.

All diuretics are potentially dangerous and some are especially toxic. Patients who receive diuretics should be weighed daily, have their fluid intake and output carefully measured and recorded, and have their serum electrolytes periodically evaluated.

When patients take diuretics at home, they should receive detailed instructions before starting to take the medication on their own. Instructions should include (1) the purpose and desired effects of the drug, (2) the importance of taking the medication exactly as prescribed, (3) signs of side effects and toxicity that should be reported immediately to the physician, and (4) symptoms of potassium and sodium depletion.

Anticoagulants

Anticoagulants are prescribed to inhibit the formation of clots within blood vessels. Anticoagulants do not dissolve clots that have already formed, but they can prevent existing ones from growing larger and also interfere with the development of new clots.

Examples of anticoagulant agents include coumarin compounds such as dicumarol and warfarin sodium (Coumadin and Panwarfin). These drugs can be given orally. Another commonly used anticoagulant is heparin, which inhibits blood clotting and the ability of platelets to agglutinate. Heparin blocks the conversion of prothrombin to thrombin and fibrinogen to fibrin. Heparin is ineffective when given orally and so must be administered intravenously or subcutaneously.

Whenever a patient is on anticoagulant therapy, his clotting time must be carefully monitored. Prothrombin time (PT, or pro time) is used to monitor response to oral anticoagulant therapy. Heparin therapy is monitored by activated partial thromboplastin time (APTT, PTT). See Table 20–1 for information on these tests.

When a patient is on anticoagulant therapy there is the potential for a dangerous delay in the clotting of blood. Nursing observations for abnormal bleeding include periodic checking of vital signs, monitoring urine and stools for signs of internal bleeding, and inspection of the skin for bruises and petechiae.

In addition to the obvious problem of hemorrhage, there are other problems associated with the administration of anticoagulants. Drug interactions can either enhance or counteract the physiologic effects of coumarin. Aspirin and other salicylates, when taken with anticoagulants, can predispose the person even more to abnormal blood loss. Patients receiving long-term anticoagulant therapy should be monitored periodically for signs of toxicity by obtaining prothrombin time evaluations. Some patients may complain of fatigue when on oral anticoagulants.

Patients who are treated with anticoagulant therapy on an outpatient basis should receive thorough instruction in the effects of the drug they are taking and its special hazards in regard to hemorrhage. This instruction should include the action of the drug prescribed, the purpose of frequent blood tests, the dangers of anticoagulant therapy, safety precautions, foods that affect clotting, and over-the-counter drugs that can increase or decrease the anticoagulant effect.

Vasodilators

Drugs of this kind dilate or enlarge the blood vessels. They are prescribed for patients who have chest pain due to insufficient blood supply to the myocardium (myocardial ischemia). The most frequently prescribed vasodilator is nitroglycerin. Long-acting nitrates such as isosorbide dinitrate (Isordil) are also prescribed.

When sublingual nitroglycerin (NTG) is given for an anginal attack, baseline pulse and blood pressure should be recorded and then taken again every 5 minutes to determine the effectiveness of the medication. If relief is not obtained after three tablets, each given 5 minutes apart, the doctor should be immediately notified.

Nitroglycerin ointment should be applied to a hairless part of the body. Rotation of sites helps eliminate minor skin irritation. The previous site should be washed to eliminate any residue of the ointment. The nurse must be careful not to get the ointment on her hands, as it can cause a throbbing headache. The ointment is applied using a measured-dose paper applicator supplied by the manufacturer. A time-release form is available as a patch resembling an oval adhesive bandage. Some patients develop tolerance to nitroglycerin. Removing the patch for 8 hours during the night when the heart is at rest will sometimes help this problem.

The most common side effect of nitroglycerin and other nitrates is headache, which usually can be prevented by decreasing the dosage or having the patient take a mild pain reliever (Tylenol) with his dose of NTG or Isordil. Although the drugs are relatively safe, they can produce potentially harmful side effects. Hypotension is particularly likely to occur; therefore ambulatory patients, especially the elderly, should be watched carefully for significant drops in blood pressure, which can produce syncope and falls. Patients who have orthostatic hypotension should not be given nitroglycerin because of the danger of sudden and serious drops in blood pressure during position changes.

Dipyridamole (Persantin) inhibits platelet adhesion, helping to prevent thrombosis and to keep the blood fluid. It is prescribed for patients who have coronary insufficiency, and after coronary artery bypass.

Aspirin is administered after an MI to prevent platelet aggregation and clot formation.

Calcium Channel Blockers

These agents, also called slow channel-blocking agents and calcium antagonists, have improved medical treatment of coronary heart disease and other cardiovascular disorders. At the present time calcium channel–blocking agents have been approved by the Federal Drug Administration for treatment of angina pectoris, hypertension, and cardiac arrhythmias. Although all of the compounds that act as calcium antagonists differ widely in chemical structure, they have in common the basic action of inhibiting the flow of calcium across the cell membrane.

The general physiologic effect of drugs in this group is to increase the flow of blood through the coronary arteries by relaxing smooth muscle in these vessels. This has the effect of enlarging the openings in the arteries, thus reducing resistance to blood flow and improving oxygen supply to the myocardium.

Examples of slow channel-blocking agents include nifedipine (Procardia), verapamil (Calan and Isoptin), and diltiazem (Cardizem).

Because of the nature of their physiologic effects, the most serious effects of calcium antagonists are hypotension and bradycardia. Dizziness, headache, and flushing also can occur. Constipation can be a problem when verapamil is taken; nifedipine can cause pedal edema.

The calcium antagonists complement the action of other drugs and enhance the effectiveness of such nonchemical therapies as relaxation, moderate exercise, quitting smoking, and modifying the diet.

Analgesics

As previously explained, severe chest pain accompanying acute heart attack is relieved by morphine sulfate or meperidine hydrochloride (Demerol). Other drugs that may be prescribed for the cardiac patient to relieve discomfort include mild sedatives and tranquilizers to reduce anxiety.

DIETARY CONTROL

Contrary to popular opinion, obesity itself is not a direct cause of heart disease. However, the National Heart, Lung and Blood Institute lists obesity as a risk factor for cardiac disorders. When obesity is present in conjunction with other factors such as hypertension, diabetes mellitus, smoking, and family history of heart disease, the likelihood of cardiovascular problems is increased.

For the prevention of heart disease and mitigation of the factors that predispose one to cardiovascular disease, the American Heart Association recommends the following "prudent" measures:

- A caloric intake to achieve or maintain ideal body weight.
- Ingestion of a 2:1 ratio of polyunsaturated to saturated fat up to about 10% of the total calories.
- A reduction in total fat calories from 45% (the national daily average for Americans) to 30% of total calories.
- A reduction in dietary cholesterol to 300 mg per day.
- An increase in complex dietary carbohydrates, particularly those with fiber (*not* simple sugars), to replace calories from fats.
- Reduction of refined sugar intake to about 10% of total calories.
- Limitation of sodium intake to no more than 5 gm per day.
- Consumption of alcohol in moderation.

There are excellent resources for information and support for patients who have a cardiovascular disease and are attempting to follow a dietary regimen as part of their overall treatment plan. Many community hospitals sponsor weight loss programs. Local chapters of the American Heart Association provide pamphlets and other sources of information about diet.

Although there are some persons who are more susceptible to hypertension than others, a high intake of sodium is thought to contribute to the development of high blood pressure. Limiting sodium intake is an important part of prevention and treatment of hypertension. Instruction of the patient should recognize his willingness to change his eating habits and the support and encouragement he receives from his family. There are several cookbooks sponsored by the American Heart Association and others that make low-sodium, low-cholesterol meals easier to plan and prepare and more palatable. The fact that the tendency to develop cardiovascular disease runs in families gives the patient and his whole family good reason to develop good eating habits and to change to more wholesome foods.

Many health professionals consider the self-help groups to be most successful in assisting persons to lose pounds and then to keep their weight within normal range once the excess is lost. These groups include TOPS (Take Off Pounds Sensibly), Overeaters Anonymous, and Weight Watchers. Results of studies have shown that the behavior modification techniques employed by these groups are very successful.

Restriction of sodium, prescribed because of sodium's association with retention of water in the tissues, is discussed in Chapter 8. Patients who are on sodium-restricted diets require special encouragement and instruction in the ways to avoid an intake of sodium that would be harmful and contribute to their discomfort.

OXYGEN THERAPY

The administration of supplemental oxygen to relieve the dyspnea and hypoxemia of a cardiac patient is a routine therapeutic measure. Any patient experiencing chest pain is started on oxygen. This form of therapy is discussed earlier in this chapter and in Chapter 17. The responsibilities of the nurse in regard to oxygen therapy for a cardiac patient are primarily concerned with observation to determine a patient's need for supplemental oxygen, maintenance of the ordered flow rate, and his response to this therapy once it has been initiated.

> ***As previously explained, cyanosis is a*** **late** ***symptom of hypoxemia and oxygen need. It is important, therefore, that the nurse be alert to earlier signs such as increase in pulse rate and symptoms of cerebral anoxia such as irritability and disorientation.***

The response of the patient to the administration of oxygen is best determined by blood gas analysis and pH determination.

CARDIAC SURGERY

Until the 1950s, there was little that could be done in the way of surgical procedures involving the heart itself, because prolonged interruption of circulation meant certain death for the patient. However, with the advent of the heart-lung machine and hypothermic techniques, surgeons can now repair or replace damaged valves, correct many congenital heart defects, and bypass clogged coronary arteries.

The heart-lung machine, which has many variations in design and appearance, functions as an artificial heart (pump) and lungs (oxygenator). For this reason, it is sometimes called a *pump-oxygenator.* Because all of this is done outside the patient's body, the procedure is called *extracorporeal circulation.* The surgeon inserts large tubes in the venae cavae and reroutes the unoxygenated venous blood through the heart-lung machine. There, the blood is exposed to an atmosphere of oxygen in which an exchange of gases takes place—carbon dioxide is released and oxygen is taken up—and the oxygenated blood is returned to the patient via the femoral artery. The blood also may be cooled so that the patient's body temperature is lowered (hypothermia), thereby reducing the body's metabolic needs during surgery.

Specific Types of Cardiac Surgery

Open heart surgery is performed using extracorporeal circulation and hypothermia. Hypothermia decreases the metabolic rate and lowers the oxygen need of the body. Congenital heart defects, valve replacements, and bypass of clogged coronary arteries are accomplished by open heart techniques.

Coronary artery bypass surgery (CABG) is done when angina cannot be controlled medically. CABG surgery bypasses the artery that is blocked, replacing it with sections of a vein or artery taken from another part of the patient's body. Usually sections of saphenous vein are used, or the mammary artery is moved to supply the area. The transplanted vessel is sewn into the heart muscle and attached to another artery so that an adequate supply of blood will reach the heart muscle. Figure 20–10 shows one of the procedures to bypass the coronary arteries. Coronary bypass surgery is expensive, averaging $75,000 to $100,000 dollars for the surgery, anesthesia, and hospital costs. Chest pain disappears in about 65% of patients, and another 25% show improvement. There are still some who question the benefits of such surgery compared with the cost and effectiveness of more conservative medical therapies. Presently, many of those patients who had a coronary artery bypass in the early to mid 1980s are returning for a second operation, because the new arteries have become occluded.

The CABG patient will have a midsternal incision and, if saphenous veins were used for the grafts, will have leg incisions as well.

Mitral or aortic valve replacement is done when the patient's condition prevents him from going about his usual daily activities, whether the problem is stenosis or insufficiency. Replacement is done as an open heart procedure using extracorporeal circulation and hypothermia. Pre- and postoperative care are much the same as for CABG patients.

Open heart surgeries usually take between 3 and 6 hours, depending on the amount of repair or replacement necessary. The patient returns to the cardiac surgical intensive care unit and remains on a ventilator for 8 to 24 hours. Patient care requires highly skilled nurses, as there are multiple tubes and lines for monitoring physiologic status and for delivering drugs to control blood pressure and arrhythmias. If the patient's recovery is uncomplicated, he will be transferred to a step-down telemetry unit 2 to 3 days after surgery.

Heart Transplant

Heart transplants are performed for selected patients who have end-stage left ventricular failure resulting from cardiomyopathy. Candidates for heart transplant undergo an extensive psychological evaluation and thorough physical assessment. Very few donor hearts are available, and the waiting lists are long. Patients who do receive a heart transplant face considerable financial burdens, a life of taking immunosuppressive drugs that have many serious side effects, and the constant threat of organ rejection. However, the benefits are considerable with a 1-year survival rate of 80% to 90% and a 3-year survival time of about 70%. Heart transplants are performed in highly specialized medical centers.

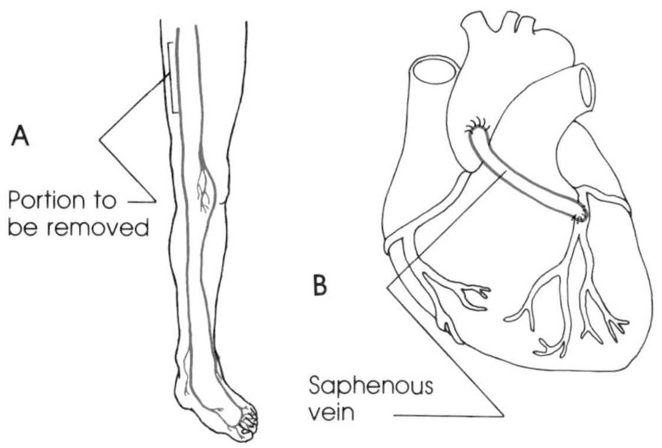

Figure 20-10 *A*, Saphenous vein, which is removed and grafted onto the heart and aorta to provide adequate coronary circulation. *B*, Bypass graft from the aorta to one of the coronary arteries.

Preoperative Care

Before cardiac surgery, the patient undergoes a series of diagnostic tests and examinations such as those presented in Table 20-1. Once a decision is made to undergo surgery, measures are taken to ensure that the patient is in the best possible condition. Psychological preparation is largely the responsibility of the nurse. There is considerable apprehension on the part of the patient and the family when faced with open heart surgery.

The patient is given information about the procedure, explaining what he can expect and the kind of equipment he will see.

Postoperative Care

During the early postoperative period, the patient is kept in an intensive care unit (ICU), where specialized monitoring equipment is used and highly trained personnel are in constant attendance. Thoracotomy tubes for drainage and proper re-expansion of the lungs will need special attention. Chest tubes are removed before the patient is moved out of the ICU. (See Chapter 17 for details.) After the first 48 hours, the surgeon will assess the patient's condition and decide whether he can be transferred to a general surgical unit. The patient will continue to need very special nursing care. His vital signs must be taken and recorded at frequent intervals. His urinary output must be measured and recorded every 2 to 8 hours, and his fluid intake may be restricted for a period. Daily weight is monitored to assess fluid balance also.

Coronary bypass surgery can produce many special problems related to physical and emotional disability and rehabilitation of the patient. Among the physiologic symptoms that can persist into the home recovery period are fatigue and weakness, incisional discomfort, edema in the donor leg, arrhythmias, loss of appetite, depression, and unusual physical sensations. There also is the possibility of closure of the graft and the reappearance of symptoms. Often the patient develops Dressler's syndrome, a type of pericarditis. This is treated with nonsteroidal antiinflammatory drugs such as indomethacin (Indocin).

Depression for weeks to months is not uncommon after open heart surgery. Patients should be alerted to this possibility and referred for assistance if this occurs.

Most patients do not experience all of these problems during the home recovery period after coronary artery bypass surgery, and some have relatively trouble-free recovery periods. It is important, however, that health care professionals not directly involved in this kind of surgery, as well as bypass surgery patients and their families, realize that it is not a cure for coronary artery disease. It is simply one form of therapy for a chronic condition that will require continued management to slow the disease process and reduce the incidence of life-threatening events in the person's life.

Other specific postoperative care is directed toward preventing infection, monitoring for complications, and promoting rehabilitation. Usually after the first 48 hours, minimal medication is needed for pain. The patient is often quite fatigued and tends to have mood swings. With an uncomplicated recovery, the patient is usually discharged home within a week.

Concerns for the Elderly

With age there is thickening of the left ventricle and cardiac valves and an increase of fibrous tissue and fat in the SA node, which decreases the number of pacemaker cells it contains. These changes make those over 75 more prone to cardiac arrythmias as changes occur in the conduction system. Failure of the SA node and the need for a pacemaker occur fairly frequently. The thickening of valve leaflets gives rise to the common systolic murmur heard in persons over age 80.

At 60 years of age, coronary blood flow is about 35% of the amount of flow in a 25-year-old. The heart's stress response is less efficient in the older adult; the heart rate does not elevate as much with stress and takes longer to return to a normal resting level. Use of oxygen by the heart is less efficient with increasing years, and the heart does not tolerate tachycardia well. Tachycardia brought about by fever from infection can give rise to heart failure rather quickly in the older adult. Nurses in long-term-care settings and in the community should be especially vigilant for beginning signs of heart failure in elderly patients who have an increased metabolic rate and an accompanying increase in heart rate, regardless of the cause.

BIBLIOGRAPHY

Andreoli, T. E., et al: Cecil Essentials of Medicine, 2nd ed. Philadelphia, W. B. Saunders, 1990.

Bailey T., et al.: Last hope for a failing heart. Am. J. Nurs., May, 1989, p. 672.

Barbiere, C. C.: PTCA: Treating the tough cases. RN, Feb., 1991, p. 38.

Barden, C., et al.: Balloon aortic valvuloplasty: Nursing care implications. Crit. Care Nurs., June, 1990, p. 22.

Becker, K. L., et al.: Get in touch and in tune with cardiac assessment, part 1. Nursing 88, March, 1988, p. 51.

Boyd, M. D., and Citro, K. M.: Is your MI patient too scared to recover? RN, May, 1988, p. 50.

Braun, A. E.: Drugs that dissolve clots. RN, June, 1991, p. 52.

Braun, A. E.: What to do when a patient needs defibrillation or cardioversion. Nursing 91, July, 1991, p. 50.

Bruna-Senerchia, C.: Thrombolytic therapy: A review of the literature on streptokinase and tissue plasminogen activator with implications for practice. Crit. Care Nurs. Clin. North Am., June, 1989, p. 359.

Caplan, M., et al.: What's the ECG telling you? A guide for nurses. RN, Feb., 1989, p. 42.

Dennison, R. D.: Understanding the four determinants of cardiac output. Nursing 90, July, 1990, p. 34.

Dugan, L.: What you need to know about permanent pacemakers. Nursing 91, June, 1991, p. 46.

Ehrhardt, B. S., and Graham, M.: Pulse oximetry: An easy way to check oxygen saturation. Nursing 90, March, 1990, p. 50.

Eiken F.: How to care for patients with temporary cardiac pacemakers. Adv. Clin. Care, Nov./Dec., 1989, p. 18.

Fulterman, L. G.: Cardiac transplantation: A comprehensive nursing perspective. Heart Lung, Nov., 1988, p. 631.

Gleeson, B.: Loosening the grip of anginal pain. Nursing 91, Jan., 1991, p. 33.

Gleeson, B.: Teaching your patient about his antianginal drugs. Nursing 91, Feb., 1991, p. 65.

Green, E.: Clues to a code: Subtle signs can help you save a life. RN, July, 1990, p. 26.

Guyton, A. C.: Textbook of Medical Physiology, 8th ed. Philadelphia, W. B. Saunders, 1991.

Higgins, C. A.: The AICD: A teaching plan for patients and families. Crit. Care Nurs., June, 1990, p. 69.

Huang, S. H., et al.: Coronary Care Nursing, 2nd ed. Philadelphia, W. B. Saunders, 1989.

Ignatavicius, D. D., and Bayne, M. J.: Medical-Surgical Nursing. Philadelphia, W. B. Saunders, 1991.

Juleff, G. L.: Cracking open a blocked heart valve. Nursing 89, July, 1989, p. 58.

Lazarus, M., et al.: Cardiac arrhythmias: Diagnosis and treatment. July, 1988, p. 57.

Lubliner, C.: When to expect heart block. RN, Jan., 1990, pp. 28–36.

Marrie, T. J.: Infective endocarditis: A serious and changing disease. Crit. Care Nurs., Feb., 1987, p. 31.

Matteson, M. A., and McConnell, E. S.: Gerontological Nursing: Concepts and Practice. Philadelphia, W. B. Saunders, 1987.

McCann, M. E.: Sexual healing after heart attack. Am. J. Nurs., Sept., 1989, p. 1132.

Mercer, M. E.: The electrophysiology study: A nursing concern. Crit. Care Nurs., March/April, 1987, p. 58.

Miller, K.: When your patient has an implanted defibrillator. RN, June, 1990, p. 32.

Miracle, V. A.: Understanding the different types of MI. Nursing 88, Jan., 1988, p. 53.

Miracle, V. A.: Get in touch and in tune with cardiac assessment, part 2. Nursing 88, April, 1988, p. 41.

Monticco, L. M., and Hill, K. M.: EP studies: When they're called for, what they reveal. RN, Feb., 1989, p. 54.

Porterfield, L. M.: Digitalis. AD Nurse., Nov./Dec., 1988, p. 14.

Purcell, J. A.: Cardiomyopathy. Am. J. Nurs., Jan., 1989, p. 57.

Rakel, R. E. ed.: Conn's Current Therapy 1990. Philadelphia, W. B. Saunders, 1990.

Roberts, P. J.: Caring for patients undergoing therapeutic cardiac catheterization. Crit. Care Nurs. Clin. North Am., June, 1989, p. 275.

Siberner, J.: Reversing heart disease. U.S. News and World Report, Aug. 6, 1990, p. 55.

Thompson, V. C.: Chest pain: Your response to a classic warning. RN, April, 1989, p. 32.

Ulrich, S. P., et al.: Nursing Care Planning Guides: A Nursing Diagnosis Approach, 2nd ed. Philadelphia, W. B. Saunders, 1990.

Verani, M. S.: Recent advances in cardiac nuclear imaging. Houston Heart Bulletin, Issue 4, 1989, p. 9.

Zimmaro, D. M.: Catheter ablation of ventricular tachycardia and related nursing interventions. Crit. Care Nurs., July/Aug., 1987, p. 20.

STUDENT STUDY AIDS

CLINICAL CASE PROBLEMS

Read each clinical case problem and discuss the questions with your classmates.

1. Mrs. Wolfe is admitted to the hospital with a medical diagnosis of congestive heart failure (CHF) resulting from mitral stenosis. She has a history of atherosclerotic heart disease (ASHD) and angina pectoris. Her chief complaints on admission are dyspnea on exertion, fatigue, and palpitations.

- What disease processes probably have led to the development of Mrs. Wolfe's mitral stenosis and CHF?
- List three nursing diagnoses with interventions in your care plan for her.
- What should be included in the preoperative teaching plan for her mitral valve replacement?

---

2. Mr. North, aged 54, is admitted to the coronary care unit after having suffered an acute myocardial infarction while shoveling snow at his home.

- What disease processes probably led to Mr. North's MI?
- Describe the diagnostic tests that will most likely be ordered for Mr. North.

- After Mr. North is transferred from the CCU to the telemetry step-down unit, how would you go about assessing his status and identifying his specific problems and nursing care needs?
- Prepare a plan of care to help alleviate the problems you have identified and to avoid others that might develop.
- Make a discharge teaching plan for Mr. North that includes rehabilitation activities.

STUDY OUTLINE

I. **Pathophysiology**
   A. Structural defects: congenital and acquired.
   B. Coronary artery disease leading to myocardial ischemia.
   C. Weakness of heart muscle and congestion of blood flow: congestive heart failure.
   D. Infection and inflammation of heart structures.
   E. Disturbances of heart conduction systems: arrhythmias.
   F. Cardiomyopathy

II. **Prevention of heart disease**
   A. Heart disease remains leading cause of death in the United States.
   B. Mortality rate for heart disease has declined in recent years.
   C. Risk factors: avoidable and unavoidable.
      1. Avoidable (can be controlled or corrected): elevated blood lipids, obesity, habitual dietary excesses, lack of exercise, hypertension, cigarette smoking, cocaine use.
      2. Unavoidable: age or aging, sex, race, ethnic origin, environment in early childhood, heredity.

III. **Diagnostic tests and procedures** (see Table 20–1)

IV. **Nursing assessment of cardiovascular status**
   A. History taking: medical history of patient and his family.
      1. Exposure to known high-risk factors.
   B. Subjective data: chest pain, fatigue, complaints of shortness of breath, cough, hemoptysis, palpitations of the heart, and nocturia.
   C. Objective data: patient's posture in bed, color and temperature of skin, diaphoresis, pitting edema, abnormal breathing patterns, distended neck veins, heart sounds, apical pulse, distended neck veins, and peripheral pulses.

V. **Coronary heart disease (CHD), also called coronary artery disease (CAD)**
   A. Atherosclerosis: deposits of fibrous plaque on the inner lining of the arteries.
      1. Major forms: coronary insufficiency, angina pectoris, acute myocardial infarction.
      2. Causative factors:
         a. Environmental: emotional stress, heavy cigarette smoking, high-fat diet, lack of physical exercise.
         b. Genetic: familial tendency, diabetes mellitus, hypercholesteremia.
   B. Angina pectoris:
      1. Cardiac pain of effort and emotion.
      2. Medical diagnosis based on symptoms: chest pain, dyspnea, pallor or flushing of face, diaphoresis. Exercise stress testing and coronary angiography aid diagnosis.
      3. Medical treatment aimed at relief of symptoms, avoidance of factors that precipitate attacks.
         a. Medications include vasodilators (e.g., nitroglycerin, calcium

channel blockers, and beta-adrenergic blockers, which block sympathetic impulses to heart).

b. Aspirin decreases platelet aggregation and helps prevent thrombosis.

c. Avoid or minimize effects of environmental cold.

4. Patient teaching is an important aspect of nursing care.

C. Acute myocardial infarction:

1. Area of necrosis in heart muscle resulting from ischemia of affected part.

2. Symptoms and medical diagnosis:

a. Sudden, severe pain in the chest, arm, or jaw, sometimes mistaken for indigestion; pallor, symptoms of shock.

b. Within 24 hours there is leukocytosis.

c. Serum enzymes and isoenzymes elevated (AST, CK, CK-MB, LDH, LDH_1, LDH_2).

3. Medical treatment:

a. Pain relief: IV morphine or Demerol initially; then oral analgesia.

b. Sedatives to reduce anxiety.

c. Patent IV access for emergency drugs if needed.

d. Oxygen therapy.

e. Rest and gradual increase in physical activity.

f. Avoidance of Valsalva maneuver.

g. Intensive monitoring; hemodynamic monitoring with pulmonary artery flow-directed catheters for CVP, PAP, PAWP; arterial line; oximeter; cardiac output.

h. Thrombolytic therapy if patient seeks help within 4 to 6 hours of onset of pain.

i. Percutaneous transluminal coronary angioplasty (PTCA): nonsurgical method of improving coronary blood flow.

j. Intraaortic balloon pump (IABP) may be used for seriously damaged left ventricle and low cardiac output.

k. Low-sodium, low-fat diet.

l. Treatment of arrhythmias.

4. Nursing intervention and patient teaching

a. Promote rest, relieve pain, decrease stress and anxiety.

b. Monitor for arrhythmias and complications: CHF, pericarditis, cardiogenic shock.

c. Constant, thorough assessment.

d. Record daily weight and intake and output; check for edema.

e. Supervise progressive activity.

f. Discharge teaching regarding disease, diet, medications, activity.

5. Rehabilitation

a. Teach patient about nature of disease and rationale for prescribed regimen.

b. Attention to psychosocial concerns; issues of sexuality.

c. Put patient in control of his disease and prognosis.

d. Referral to community agencies such as American Heart Association.

VI. Congestive heart failure (CHF)

A. Chief complication in 70% of all cardiac patients.

B. Pathophysiology: Heart fails to pump as it should, and flow of blood becomes sluggish, backing up into lungs and/or systemic circulation. Fluid moves from intravascular compartment to tissue spaces, producing generalized or localized edema and lung congestion.

C. Symptoms depend on whether the left or right side of the heart fails.
   1. Left-sided symptoms: dyspnea, cough, decreased urinary output, weight gain.
   2. Right-sided symptoms: pitting peripheral edema, abdominal distention, weight gain.

D. Medical treatment:
   1. Bed rest or limited physical activity.
   2. Oxygen therapy.
   3. Digitalization.
   4. Administration of "unloading" agents; morphine.
   5. Limitation of sodium and fluid intake.
   6. Rotating tourniquets.

E. Nursing assessment:
   1. Subjective data: increasing fatigue, shortness of breath; feeling bloated, loss of appetite, complaints of feeling warm, anxiety and depression, difficulty in concentrating or remembering.
   2. Objective data: pale, cool, dry skin; cyanosis; dependent, pitting edema; fleeting or absent peripheral pulses; crackles in lung fields; distended neck veins; extra heart sound; increased heart rate; reduced urinary output.

F. Nursing intervention: planned according to specific problems identified and whether patient is in mild, moderate, or acute congestive failure with pulmonary edema.
   1. Careful, thorough ongoing assessment.
   2. Administer oxygen; assist with ADL.
   3. Promote rest; position patient upright with pillows behind back to ease breathing.
   4. Record daily weight and intake and output.
   5. Careful skin care to prevent breakdown.
   6. Prevent deep vein thrombosis with elastic stockings and leg exercises.
   7. Observe for side effects of medications.
   8. Discharge and self-care teaching.

VII. Disorders of the heart's conduction system

A. Heart's natural pacemaker fails, must be replaced by artificial pacemaker.
   1. Artificial pacing can be temporary or permanent.
   2. Indications for insertion of permanent pacemaker include sinus bradycardia, atrial fibrillation, complete heart block, secondary AV block, and bradytachycardia.
   3. Cardioversion: treatment for atrial fibrillation uncontrolled by medication.
   4. Life-threatening arrhythmias: ventricular tachycardia, ventricular fibrillation, third-degree heart block, asystole.
   5. Antiarrhythmic drugs used for control of conduction disorders (Table 20–3).
   6. CPR and defibrillation covered in Chapter 36.
   7. Automatic implantable cardiac defibrillators (AICDs) used in patients with repeated episodes of ventricular tachycardia, ventricular fibrillation, or asystole.

B. Nursing assessment and intervention:
   1. Preoperative care includes teaching patient about pacemaker, its purpose and benefits.
   2. Postoperative care: continuous heart monitoring; dressing changes and care of wound site; peripheral pulses and vital signs.

3. Discharge instruction to help patient live with his pacemaker or AICD.

VIII. Inflammatory diseases of the heart: myocarditis, endocarditis, pericarditis.

A. Symptoms vary according to site of inflammation.
   1. Symptoms of infective endocarditis: intermittent fever, spleen enlargement, splinter hemorrhages under the nails, heart murmur, or petechiae inside the mouth.

B. Medical treatment includes rest to reduce workload of heart; antiinfectives to control infection; surgery to replace or repair valves damaged by the inflammatory process.

IX. Common problems related to cardiac disease

A. Fatigue and dyspnea:
   1. Program of rest and exercise.
   2. Stool softeners; prevent Valsalva maneuver.
   3. Telemetry monitoring.
   4. Progressive activity measured by metabolic equivalents (METs).
   5. Outpatient rehabilitation programs.
   6. Psychological support important.

B. Edema:
   1. Weigh daily.
   2. Measure fluid intake and output.
   3. Limit sodium intake.
   4. Watch for skin breakdown in dependent areas of body.
   5. Be alert for early signs of pulmonary edema.

C. Pain:
   1. Administer analgesic or vasodilator.
   2. Provide restful environment.
   3. Relieve anxiety.
   4. Teach patient noninvasive relaxation techniques.

X. Common therapies and nursing implications

A. Medical treatment with drugs, dietary control, oxygen to combat hypoxemia.

B. Pharmacologic agents:
   1. Cardiotonics slow and strengthen heart beat.
      a. Digitalis preparations: Patient must be watched for signs of toxicity. Therapeutic dose is only about one third less than toxic dose. Apical pulse must be counted for 1 full minute before each dose. Patient education must prepare patient to administer his own medication safely at home.
      b. Signs of digitalis toxicity: fatigue, anorexia, nausea, diarrhea, blurred vision or yellow-green halos around objects, new arrhythmia.
      c. Hypokalemia can cause digitalis toxicity.
   2. Antiarrhythmic agents restore rhythmic movements of heart to normal or near normal. Overdosage can cause severe arrhythmias and cardiac arrest.
   3. Diuretics to increase water and sodium loss and correct edema; potassium may be lost; watch for hypokalemia.
   4. Anticoagulants to treat abnormal clot formation. Patient monitored by laboratory tests to evaluate effective dose. Patient education important for safe self-administration of anticoagulants.
   5. Vasodilators dilate or enlarge blood vessels to improve circulation of blood to heart muscle.
      a. Nitroglycerin: administered sublingually or topically.

b. Long-acting nitrates (e.g., Isordil).

6. Calcium channel blockers increase flow of blood through coronary arteries by relaxing smooth muscle in vessels and decreasing resistance to blood flow. Not intended to replace other modes of therapy, but as a complement to them.
7. Analgesics: Morphine or meperidine for acute pain associated with coronary occlusion and ischemic heart disease.

C. Dietary control to restore or maintain normal body weight, reduce intake of fats, limit sodium intake. "Prudent" diet recommended by Heart Association can be beneficial to family members as well as patient.

D. Oxygen therapy. Observe patient for early signs of hypoxemia and oxygen lack.

E. Cardiac surgery.
1. Correct structural defects.
2. Replace defective valves.
3. Coronary artery bypass surgery.
4. Heart transplant.
5. Preoperative care:
   a. Support during diagnostic testing.
   b. Teaching for preoperative measures and postoperative care: what to expect; ventilator and other equipment; frequent monitoring; alarm sounds.
6. Postoperative care: ICU then telemetry step-down unit.
   a. Prevent infection.
   b. Promote balanced rest and activity.
   c. Monitor for complications.
   d. Psychosocial support and preparation for discharge.

XI. Concerns for the elderly

A. Thickening of left ventricle and valves; fibrosis of SA node; prone to cardiac arrhythmias.

B. Systolic ejection murmur common after age 80.

C. Tachycardia from fever or infection may cause CHF.

CHAPTER 21

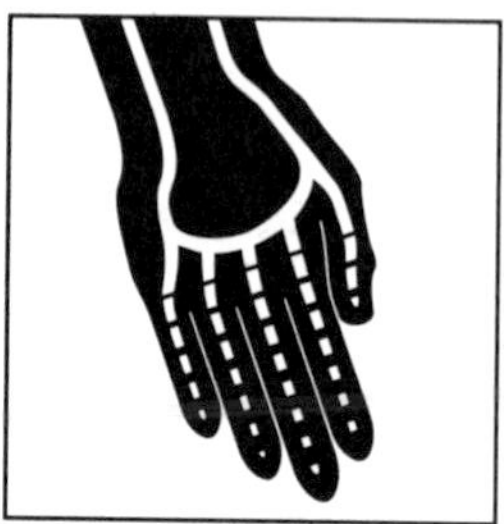

Care of Patients With Peripheral Vascular Disorders

VOCABULARY

atherosclerosis
claudication
embolus
endarterectomy
ischemia
perfusion
thrombus
thrombophlebitis

Upon completion of this chapter, the student should be able to:

1. List four factors that contribute to peripheral vascular disease.
2. Describe specific factors and techniques for assessment of the peripheral vascular system.
3. Identify three likely nursing diagnoses for patients who have peripheral vascular disease and list the appropriate nursing interventions for each.
4. Describe the points to be included in the teaching plan for the patient who has experienced thrombophlebitis and has vascular insufficiency.
5. List types of surgery performed for problems of the peripheral vascular system.
6. List four nursing interventions for the patient undergoing anticoagulant therapy.

PATHOPHYSIOLOGY

The peripheral blood vessels are those situated some distance from the heart. Disorders of the peripheral veins and arteries are almost always chronic, affect people in older age groups, and are associated with other diseases of the cardiovascular system. For example, atherosclerosis affects the aorta as well as the arteries branching from it.

In order for the arteries to carry out their function of circulating oxygenated blood throughout the body, they must be *patent* (unobstructed), and they must be able to dilate and constrict as necessary to regulate the blood flow. Veins also must be patent, their valves must function normally, and surrounding muscles must contract so that venous blood is continually being moved in the direction of the heart.

Diseases of the peripheral arteries, whatever the specific disease process, invariably lead to *ischemia* of the tissues. You will recall that ischemia is defined as *a localized deficiency of blood to the tissues.* If the ischemia is not relieved, the ultimate outcome is tissue necrosis and gangrene.

Interruptions to the flow of blood through the veins lead to increased pressure within the walls of the vessel. When blood is not moved out of the veins of the lower extremities, it accumulates there and provides a medium for the growth of bacteria and contributes to the formation of leg ulcers.

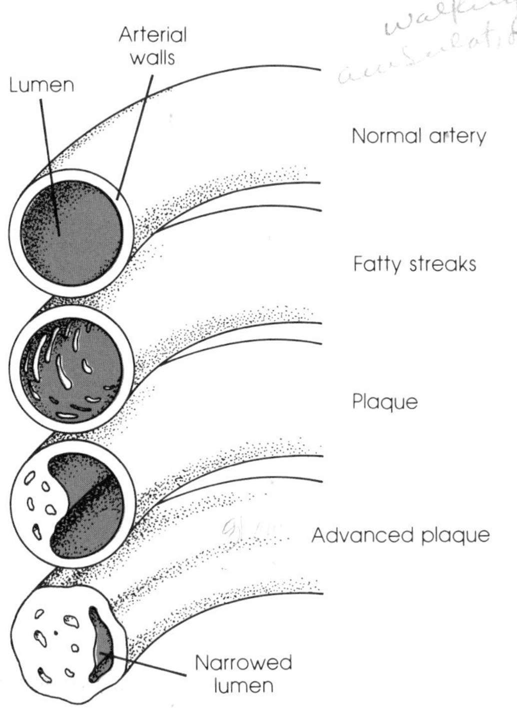

Figure 21–1 Cross section of an artery showing progressive narrowing of the diameter of the artery as a result of atherosclerosis and plaque formation.

The treatment of peripheral vascular disease is concerned with maintenance of adequate circulation and prevention of the natural outcome of diminished blood flow to and from the tissues.

CAUSATIVE FACTORS

The most common cause of peripheral arterial disorders is atherosclerosis (Fig. 21–1). Other causes of problems include spasm of the smooth muscles in the arterial walls, structural defects in the arteries, trauma, or embolus (blood clot or debris that travels and lodges in a blood vessel) that occludes a vessel. Peripheral venous problems are caused by defective valvular function and formation of blood clots (venous thrombosis), which may be accompanied by inflammation (thrombophlebitis).

NURSING ASSESSMENT OF PERIPHERAL CIRCULATION

ASSESSMENT OF ARTERIAL BLOOD FLOW

Pain

The patient with diminished arterial blood flow experiences two characteristic kinds of pain. The first, which is the most common subjective symptom of arterial insufficiency, is called *intermittent claudication.* This is defined as a "cramping" pain in the muscles brought on by exercise and relieved by rest. The pain occurs most often in the calves of the legs, but it also can affect the muscles in the thighs and buttocks.

The second type of pain is characteristic of advanced chronic occlusive arterial disease. It is called *rest pain* because it occurs even when the patient is resting. Rest pain is particularly noticeable at night when the patient is in bed. The sensation is described as burning and tingling, with numbness of the toes.

Color

Tissues that are receiving an adequate supply of oxygenated blood appear pink and rosy, whereas those deprived of normal amounts of arterial blood appear pale and mottled. However, the environment must be taken into account. Pale and mottled skin can also indicate that the patient is just cold. Reddish-blue color can indicate severe ischemia.

One way to assess arterial blood flow more accurately is by having the patient elevate the feet and legs above the level of the heart for 2 to 3 minutes and then lower them to a dangling position. Return of color to the

lowered feet is delayed in arterial insufficiency. If there is severe ischemia, the dangling feet soon take on a reddish-blue color. This indicates permanent dilation of the vessels; they are no longer able to constrict as they should. In addition to being reddened, the feet and ankles may appear swollen and edematous.

Skin Temperature

A cold environment and immobility will cause the extremities to feel cold to the touch. However, when a patient experiences persistent coldness of an extremity in a warm environment, arterial insufficiency should be suspected.

When observing a patient for signs of arterial disease, the nurse should note differences in skin temperature in various areas of the same limb, as well as differences between limbs.

Trophic Changes

The word *trophic* refers to nutrition. Epidermoid tissues that are chronically malnourished because of decreased blood supply have a characteristic appearance: the skin appears smooth, shiny, and thin, and there is little or no hair on its surface. The nails are thick with deposits of viscous, cornlike material under them.

If there is severe malnutrition of the tissues for several days, they become necrotic. This causes the skin to assume a purple-black color. This is a deep cyanotic condition indicative of gangrene.

Peripheral Pulses

Whenever other signs and symptoms indicate that the patient may have an arterial insufficiency, the nurse checks blood flow through the arteries to determine the rate, rhythm, and force of the pulse at various sites. These sites are depicted in Figure 21–2. The pulse may be described as *normal, impaired,* or *absent.*

If pulsations are weak or undetectable, the nurse uses a Doppler device to check them. A Doppler device measures the velocity of blood flow through a vessel with ultrasound waves. It can sense weak pulsations even in severely narrowed arteries.

Bruits

A whooshing or purring sound is made when blood passes through a partially obstructed artery. To detect bruits, listen with the bell of the stethoscope applied lightly over the skin of the carotid, abdominal aorta, and femoral arteries.

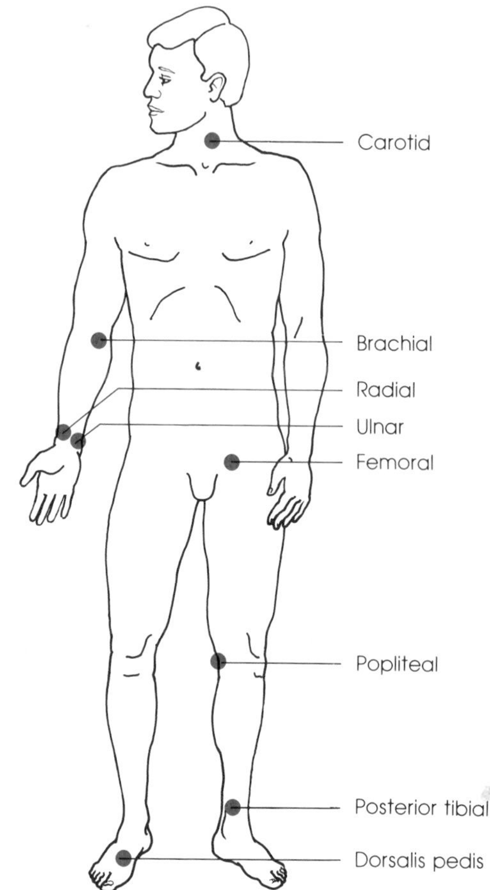

Figure 21–2 Pulses palpated during assessment of the arterial system.

ASSESSMENT OF VENOUS BLOOD FLOW

The most common incidences of venous insufficiency occur in one or both lower extremities. The condition is characterized by changes in the hydration status (edema) and altered pigmentation of the skin. The most common disorders of this type are varicose veins, thrombosis, and thrombophlebitis.

Edema and Cellulitis

Chronic venous insufficiency is accompanied by chronic edema. This in turn leads to inflammation of the tissues (cellulitis) and eventually to the formation of ulcers.

Increased pigmentation of the skin, dryness and scaling, and excoriations are objective signs of venous insufficiency.

Trendelenburg Test

This test, also called the *retrograde filling test,* is an assessment of the ability of the valves to prevent the backflow of blood in the veins. The patient is placed in a recumbent position with the affected leg elevated above the level of the heart. A tourniquet is applied below the knee to compress the superficial veins. The patient is then asked to stand up, and the tourniquet is removed. If the valves are incompetent, the veins will quickly become engorged with blood.

NURSING DIAGNOSES

Nursing diagnoses for the patient with peripheral vascular disease could include:

- Altered peripheral tissue perfusion related to vessel occlusion.
- Pain related to decreased blood flow.
- Activity intolerance related to pain in the legs when walking.
- Sleep pattern disturbance related to pain in the legs while at rest.
- Body image disturbance related to edema and dilated veins in the legs.
- Body image disturbance related to a loss of limb by amputation.
- Knowledge deficit related to causes of peripheral vascular disease, treatment, and proper self-care.
- Potential for injury related to potential for embolus or bleeding from anticoagulant medication.
- Potential for infection related to impaired skin integrity.
- Self-esteem disturbance related to the inability to perform usual roles because of chronic leg ulcers.

DIAGNOSTIC TESTS

Ultrasound

Doppler flow studies of vessels suspected of containing a blood clot are performed on patients who have signs of venous thrombosis. This is most commonly done for problems in the lower extremities. Carotid flow studies and studies of the circle of Willis in the brain can even detect arterial spasm. There is no special preparation for the patient except that the skin should be clean and dry without lotions or powder. The study takes about 15 to 30 minutes.

Radiologic Studies

Venogram

Venography involves injecting a radiopaque substance into the vein and taking radiographs of the area. Veins that are tortuous and engorged will appear so on the film. A lack of filling of the vein indicates a thrombus. This procedure is somewhat uncomfortable, as the dye can be irritating to the vessels.

Angiogram

Angiography is performed on arteries with a radiopaque dye to determine areas of narrowing, structural changes such as an aneurysm (bulging of the vessel wall), or the presence of an embolus. These can be done on arterial systems anywhere in the body but are most commonly used for the aorta and for vessels in the lungs and head. These tests are also called *arteriograms*. A signed consent form is required for an angiogram, and the patient is prepared the same as for surgery. Preoperative medication may be ordered. After the procedure the patient is closely watched for signs of bleeding from the catheter insertion site. Vital signs are taken very frequently to detect any internal bleeding from perforation of a vessel. A neurologic examination is performed along with vital signs to detect any complications from an embolus.

Nuclear Medicine Scan

This technique involves injecting a radioisotope and then using a scanning camera to assess the amount of radioactivity concentrated at the site of blood clots. A lung scan, used to identify the presence of pulmonary emboli, is an example of this technique. After the test, the patient is encouraged to drink a lot of fluid, unless this is contraindicated, to flush the dye through the kidneys.

COMMON PROBLEMS AND THERAPIES AND THEIR NURSING IMPLICATIONS

DECREASED BLOOD FLOW

The smooth muscles of the arterial walls respond to temperature by constricting in the presence of cold and extreme heat, and relaxing in the presence of warmth. Therefore the nurse's care plan should include (1) providing a warm environment for the patient, (2) covering the hospitalized patient with warm blankets and dressing him in warm clothing, and (3) instructing the patient in the need for avoiding extremes of cold and heat.

The constricting effect of extreme heat rules out the use of local applications in the form of hot water bottles and electric heating pads. Although moderate heat causes dilation of blood vessels, very high temperatures cause constriction. In addition to the danger of burning the patient because of decreased sensitivity to extremes of temperature, local heat increases metabolic activity in the tissues to which it is applied and therefore upsets even more the balance of supply and demand for blood flow to all of the tissues.

The goal in application of additional warmth is even distribution throughout the body.

A second consideration is that of *pressure* against the walls of the blood vessels. Constricting clothing is avoided, particularly circular garters and elastic materials in underclothing. Frequent position changes also are essential.

The patient with poor venous circulation can benefit from periodic elevation of the lower extremities to facilitate venous return of blood to the heart.

Even, well-distributed *support* of the vessels near the surface of the body will help improve venous return. To provide this kind of support, the physician may prescribe an elastic bandage or fitted elastic stockings. The hose or elastic bandage should be applied early in the morning, before the patient gets out of bed, because the blood vessels are less congested after a prolonged rest. Bandages and hose should be applied by beginning at the feet and working upward to avoid trapping blood in the lower leg.

Exercise is especially beneficial to patients with decreased blood flow. Walking is ideal exercise for the ambulatory patient. Bed-ridden patients will need range-of-motion exercises and the other kinds of muscular movements described in Chapter 9.

Buerger-Allen exercises (Fig. 21–3) are often prescribed for the patient who is able to move about on his own. The patient is instructed to do the following:

1. Lie down in a supine position and elevate the lower extremities at an angle of 45 to 90 degrees. Support them in this position until the skin of the extremities turns dead white.
2. Lower the feet and legs so that they are below the level of the rest of the body, being careful that there is no pressure on the backs of the knees.
3. When redness appears in the lower extremities, place them flat on the bed for 3 to 5 minutes.

VASOCONSTRICTION

In addition to the mechanical factors, certain chemical factors affect the constriction of blood vessels. *Nicotine*, which is inhaled with tobacco smoke, has the effect of producing spasmodic narrowing of the peripheral arteries. Patients with arterial insufficiency are therefore encouraged to stop smoking.

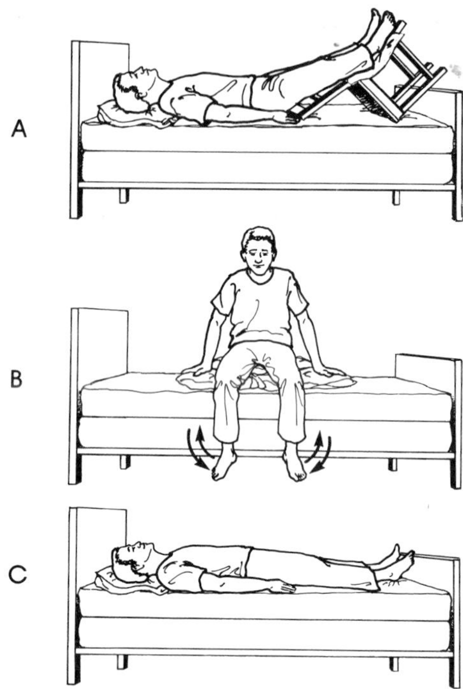

Figure 21–3 Exercises for a patient with peripheral arterial insufficiency. *A*, The legs are elevated to a 45- to 90-degree angle and supported in this position until the skin blanches (usually 2 to 3 minutes). *B*, The feet and legs are then lowered below the level of the rest of the body until color returns (usually 5 to 10 minutes). Care must be taken to avoid pressure on the backs of the knees during this phase. *C*, The legs are placed flat on the bed for about 10 minutes. Actual length of time for each position depends on the patient's tolerance and the speed with which color changes occur.

Alcohol is a mild vasodilator when taken in moderate amounts. Unless the patient has moral or religious convictions against its use, the physician may approve daily intake of small amounts of wine or liquor.

Drugs that are helpful in relief of vasoconstriction and improving blood flow by lowering viscosity include such peripheral dilators as papaverine hydrochloride, tolazoline (Priscoline), phenoxybenzamine (Dibenzyline), and pentoxifylline (Trental), which makes red cells more flexible. These drugs are of value only when the arteries are still capable of dilating. Severely sclerosed vessels respond very poorly to therapy of this kind. Cyclandelate (Cyclospasmol) is another agent thought to be useful in vasodilator therapy. However, some think that vasodilators may actually be harmful in that they shunt blood away from the zone of ischemia to well-perfused tissues.

Sympathectomy is a surgical technique that may be used to relieve vasoconstriction. Because this procedure severs sympathetic nerve fibers supplying the peripheral vessels so that the arterioles will relax, it is of benefit only to those patients who do not have advanced pathologic changes in these vessels.

TISSUE DAMAGE AND ULCERATION

Tissues that have a diminished blood supply are subject to severe and permanent damage from the slightest injury, because the normal processes of healing and repair are impaired. When efforts to restore arterial circulation are unsuccessful, the limb may become gangrenous, necessitating amputation.

Arterial and venous stasis often lead to chronic ulcers of the leg.

These ulcers are particularly distressing to the patient, because they heal very slowly, and many never completely heal. Patients must be taught to avoid conditions that contribute to injury of the extremities and to report any injury, no matter how minor. The kind of information usually given to a patient is shown below.

INFORMATION FOR PATIENTS WITH PERIPHERAL VASCULAR DISEASE

- Keep warm; avoid extreme heat or cold. If the feet become cold, soak them in lukewarm water.
- Do not use tobacco in any form.
- Take great care that the foot and lower leg are not injured; avoid crowded places.
- Never go barefoot. Wear shoes that are wide-toed and thick-soled with soft tops and cause no pressure at any point.
- Wear only clean, cotton socks.
- Do not wear circular garters or trousers with legs that constrict when sitting.
- Do not sit for long periods; never cross the legs at the knee.
- If the weight of the bed linens is uncomfortable, use a pillow to hold them off the feet.
- Perform daily foot care by washing with mild soap and water. Inspect for cuts, blisters, ulcers, or infections. Dry thoroughly by blotting, not rubbing. If the feet are sweaty, lightly powder them with talc. If the feet are dry and scaly, apply lanolin or a similar cream.
- Have nails trimmed by a doctor or podiatrist and let him treat calluses and corns; never shave these yourself.
- For foot pain at night, elevate the head of the bed on 15- to 30-cm blocks to increase blood flow to the legs and feet.
- For exercise, walk 1 to 2 miles each day in short segments. Stop if leg pain develops, rest, and then continue.
- Drink the equivalent of 10 to 15 glasses of water every day.

Prevention of leg ulcers includes (1) wearing elastic bandages or support hose, (2) proper positioning and exercise, and (3) avoiding extremes of heat and cold and other mechanical and chemical factors that contribute to obstruction of blood flow. Nursing interventions for selected problems in a patient with a venous stasis ulcer are summarized in Nursing Care Plan 21–1.

SPECIFIC DISORDERS

Among the more common disorders affecting the arteries and veins and causing interruption of the flow of blood are thrombosis, embolism, aneurysm, peripheral arterial occlusive disease, venous insufficiency, and varicose veins.

THROMBOSIS AND EMBOLISM

Thrombosis is the formation, development, or presence of a clump of blood elements, particularly platelets and fibrin, that form a clot in a blood vessel and diminish or completely obstruct the flow of blood. A thrombus can occur or develop as a result of injury to vascular endothelium, sluggish flow of blood, or changes in the number of blood elements (for example, an increase in the number of red blood cells or platelets). Thrombosis can be present in either veins or arteries, but because the flow of blood is slower through the veins than through the arteries, venous thrombosis is more common. Venous thrombosis in which there is an inflammation of the vein wall is called *thrombophlebitis.*

The effects of thrombosis depend on (1) the location and size of the thrombus, (2) whether it completely or only partially blocks blood flow through a vessel, and (3) whether the body is able to establish collateral circulation to prevent ischemia in the area formerly served by the obstructed vessel.

An *embolism* is the sudden obstruction of an artery by a mass of foreign material that has been brought to the site by the blood current. The embolus usually is a blood clot that has broken off from a thrombus. However, it can be a globule of fat, air bubble, piece of tissue, clump of bacteria, or bolus of liquid that is not dissolved in the blood.

The effects of an embolism depend on the site at which it is lodged, and its size compared with the caliber of the blood vessel in which it is located.

Deep Vein Thrombosis

A clot in a deep vein, or *deep vein thrombosis* (DVT), most often occurs in the lower leg, although it can occur in any vein in the body. A great many factors contribute to the formation of a deep vein thrombosis. Immobility, trauma,

NURSING CARE PLAN 21-1

Selected nursing diagnoses, goals/outcome criteria, nursing interventions, and evaluations for a patient with a venous stasis ulcer

Situation: A male patient, age 52, with chronic peripheral vascular disease (PVD) has a large stasis ulcer on the inner aspect of the lower third of his left leg. His lower right leg shows some edema; dry, scaly skin; and brownish coloration. The ulcer is being treated with wet-to-dry dressings and Elase ointment bid, bed rest, and elevation of the leg. Duoderm will be applied, beginning in another 3 days.

Nursing Diagnosis	Goals/Outcome Criteria	Nursing Intervention	Evaluation
Impaired skin integrity related to decreased peripheral circulation and abrasion. SUPPORTING DATA Ulcer on anterior lower third of left leg 2½ cm × 4 cm; history of chronic PVD.	Ulcer will heal completely.	Apply wet to dry dressings bid; dress with Elase ointment as ordered. Inspect for signs of infection: purulent drainage, elevated WBC count, increased size of wound.	Wet-to-dry dressing, 10:30 A.M.; Elase used on wound; serosanguinous drainage; edges less reddened; WBC count, 12,800; continue plan.
Noncompliance as evidenced by continued smoking. SUPPORTING DATA Quit smoking for 3 months; has resumed smoking ½ pack per day.	Patient will quit smoking and not smoke again.	Obtain literature on the smoking cessation program from American Lung Association. Re-explain what smoking does to decrease peripheral circulation. Teach relaxation exercises.	Began teaching relaxation exercises; gave ALA literature on quitting smoking; discussed smoking effects on vessels again; continue plan.
Knowledge deficit related to care of skin and ways to prevent ulceration. SUPPORTING DATA Has not been wearing support hose; obtaining little exercise; cannot verbalize points of proper self-care.	Patient will verbalize six points in proper self-care. Patient will not cross legs or ankles when sitting. Patient will wear support hose daily.	Explain how sluggish circulation contributes to breakdown of skin and tissues. Encourage active exercise: ankle rotation and leg bending while on bed rest; walking when ambulatory. Teach patient and wife how to apply elastic stockings before patient arises in A.M. Teach him to inspect feet and legs each day after bath; use lotion bid to decrease drying and scaling. Teach him to report any sign of reddening or break in skin to doctor immediately. Teach him not to cross ankles or legs at knee when sitting and to avoid prolonged standing. Teach patient to place wedge under foot of mattress at home to raise the legs above the level of the heart. Teach him to elevate legs when sitting.	Catches self when crosses legs while sitting; performing foot and ankle exercises each day; demonstrated proper application of elastic stockings; legs elevated when not standing; continue plan.
Depression related to repeated leg ulceration; inability to work because of hospitalization. SUPPORTING DATA Third hospitalization for leg ulcers; works as a car salesman; acts withdrawn and is having difficulty sleeping; states he is depressed.	Patient will express that he is less depressed. Patient will be able to sleep all night. Patient will talk about taking charge of his own self-care and returning to work.	Establish trusting relationship. Encourage him to ventilate feelings. Assist him to set small goals for self. Assure him that condition can be improved with proper self-care. Give praise for each effort at self-care and for efforts to quit smoking.	Verbalizing discouragement about wound not healing and interference with work; encouraged to set small goals so he can see progress; planned to work on this together tomorrow; praise given for doing own foot care today; continue plan.

sepsis, clotting problems, surgical procedures, dehydration, cancer, or any condition that causes slowing of venous flow can cause a clot to form.

The main sign of a DVT is edema in one extremity. There may be pain in the calf of the leg when the foot is dorsiflexed (Homans' sign). The area over the thrombosis may feel warm. The nurse should never rub or vigorously palpate the area, as this can dislodge the clot and send it into the circulation, which can cause severe damage or death. Encouraging patients on bed rest to perform leg and ankle exercises each hour while awake can do much to decrease the incidence of deep vein thrombosis.

Medical treatment usually consists of IV heparin and then oral warfarin sodium (Coumadin) with good hydration. Anticoagulants will not dissolve the clot but will prevent it from growing larger. The body dissolves the clot on its own over time. Thrombolytic therapy may be used to dissolve the thrombus; streptokinase, urokinase, or tissue plasminogen activator (TPA) are the agents used. There is a high risk of bleeding with these drugs. A thrombolytic agent is followed by a few additional days of heparin while the patient is started on warfarin. Warfarin takes at least 3 days to build up to an effective blood level. Elastic hose are prescribed for continuous use thereafter. Nursing care of the patient with a deep vein thrombosis and thrombophlebitis is presented in Nursing Care Plan 21–2.

Thrombophlebitis

Thrombophlebitis is inflammation of a superficial vein caused by a blood clot. It occurs from trauma or irritation to the vein or from infection from an IV line or dirty IV drug needles. Signs include swelling, redness, warmth, and considerable tenderness and pain when touched.

Treatment includes discontinuing the source of irritation; applying warm, moist heat; elevating the extremity; and administering aspirin and sometimes antibiotics.

Embolism

Embolism is most often caused when a portion of a deep vein thrombus in a leg breaks loose and travels to the lungs, heart, or brain. Cardiac arrhythmias also cause emboli. Release of fat droplets from a long-bone fracture and amniotic fluid introduced into a vein during the birthing process can also result in embolus. Cancer patients often die from pulmonary embolus. The National Institutes of Health estimate that 50,000 people die as a result of pulmonary embolus each year (Beare and Myers, 1990).

Signs and symptoms of pulmonary embolus are dyspnea, hemoptysis, a feeling of impending doom, cyanosis, and chest splinting. These signs indicate an emergency situation. Supportive treatment during diagnostic testing consists of providing a calm atmosphere, oxygen, and anticoagulants. Cardiac and ventilatory support is often necessary. Treatment may consist of thrombectomy (excision of the clot) or thrombolytic therapy.

If a patient is considered at risk for further embolus formation from deep venous thrombosis, a vena caval umbrella may be inserted to prevent damage from emboli. This is a strainerlike device positioned in the vena cava that catches the emboli, preventing them from traveling further.

The outcome of thrombosis or embolus can range from mild local congestion and edema to sudden death from occlusion of a major artery in the brain, lungs, or heart.

PERIPHERAL ARTERIAL OCCLUSIVE DISEASE (ATHEROSCLEROSIS OBLITERANS)

As previously stated, a diminished flow of blood through the arteries is caused by atherosclerosis. Atherosclerotic changes can affect any large artery of the body, but when the peripheral arteries are involved, the arterial insufficiency usually affects the lower extremities. Smoking causes vasoconstriction, further narrowing the vessels and causing worsening of the condition. Although arterial perfusion can be impaired in both legs, one extremity is often more severely involved than the other.

Signs and symptoms of peripheral arterial insufficiency of the lower extremities include intermittent claudication, rest pain, and ischemic changes. The severity of these symptoms depends on the extent of the lesion, degree of occlusion, and amount of collateral circulation that has been established.

If severe ischemia occurs from occlusion of arterial blood flow, tissue distal to the occlusion blanches, becomes cold, hurts, and eventually becomes numb as necrosis occurs. Eventually the affected part becomes gangrenous, necessitating amputation.

Surgical treatment of peripheral arterial insufficiency is a palliative measure only. It does not cure the disease or halt the atherosclerotic process. It can, however, relieve ischemic pain, help avoid amputation, and add years to a patient's life. The purpose of vascular surgery of this kind is to provide a means for revascularization and nourishment of cells in the affected area.

Pentoxifylline (Trental), a drug that reduces blood viscosity, may be prescribed for patients who have claudication but are not yet candidates for reconstructive surgery. Because the medication acts on the cell wall during its formation, it has to be taken for at least 4 months before its

NURSING CARE PLAN 21–2

Selected nursing diagnoses, goals/outcome criteria, nursing interventions, and evaluations for a patient with a deep vein thrombosis and thrombophlebitis

Situation: Mrs. Hanson, age 72, sustained multiple bruises and a concussion in an automobile accident. She has cardiac arrhythmias and was admitted 4 days ago for observation and recuperation. She has now developed pain in her right calf, and her lower leg is swollen, with a hot, tender area in the midcalf region. She has been placed on a continuous heparin drip.

Nursing Diagnosis	Goals/Outcome Criteria	Nursing Intervention	Evaluation
Alteration in peripheral tissue perfusion related to deep vein thrombosis and thrombophlebitis. SUPPORTING DATA Thrombus in saphenous vein, right calf. Reddened, warm, tender area on midcalf. Temperature, 101.2°F.	Thrombus will resolve within 2 weeks as evidenced by Doppler flow studies. Thrombophlebitis will resolve by discharge as evidenced by normal temperature and no calf tenderness, redness, or swelling.	Maintain on bed rest with bathroom privileges; keep right lower leg elevated. Active ROM of left ankle, knee, and hip. Elastic stocking on left leg. Warm packs to right leg; handle right leg gently. Maintain heparin drip on IV pump at ordered rate; assess IV site q h for infiltration. Assess legs q shift for status of thrombus and development of other problems.	Heparin drip continuous; IV site without redness or swelling; right leg elevated; active ROM on left leg at 8, 10, 12, and 2; moist heating pad to right calf for 30 minutes each hour; swelling down slightly; continue plan.
Potential for injury related to heparin drip and to possibility of embolus. SUPPORTING DATA Heparin drip 50,000 U in 500 mL at 50 mL per hour. Deep vein thrombosis in right leg.	Patient will not experience embolus during hospitalization. No hemorrhage from heparin as evidenced by no sign of bleeding internally or externally.	Auscultate lung sounds q shift; be alert for signs of pulmonary emboli. Monitor level of consciousness (LOC) and neurologic status q shift. Observe for bleeding of gums, excessive bruising, blood in urine or stool, nosebleeds, and abdominal pain and rigidity. Monitor Hgb and hematocrit to detect blood loss. Monitor PTT and advise physician immediately if it rises above 2½ times the control value. Begin Coumadin therapy as ordered 3 days before heparin is stopped. Handle patient very gently.	Lungs clear to auscultation: PEARL without headache, alert and oriented; PTT 2 × control value; no change in Hgb and hematocrit; no evidence of blood in urine or stool; bowel sounds present all 4 quadrants, abdomen soft; bruising from previous needle sticks; buttocks bruised from bed rest; continue plan.
Knowledge deficit related to precautions necessary when taking Coumadin. SUPPORTING DATA Will go home on Coumadin for at least 6 to 12 months; has never taken this medication.	Patient will verbalize danger signs to report to physician and proper dosage schedule before discharge. Patient will verbalize understanding of need for regular medical follow-up and periodic clotting times before discharge.	Teach the following: • Avoid foods high in vitamin K (give list). • Avoid over-the-counter medications and drugs that might extend clotting time or interfere with action of Coumadin (e.g., aspirin, etc.) • Move around carefully, trying not to hit head on anything or bump into things, as internal hemorrhage is a threat. • Observe urine and stool for signs of bleeding. • Maintain good hydration by drinking at least 10 glasses of fluid a day. Instruct her to maintain close contact with physician to monitor clotting times, as many things can alter it when on Coumadin. Explain dosage schedule. Give written instruction sheet.	Began teaching regarding dangers of Coumadin; needs time to absorb information; will continue teaching tomorrow; gave written instruction sheet; continue plan.

effect on all circulating red blood cells can be determined. It is not effective for patients with severe occlusion. Other drugs that act as vasodilators are isoxsuprine (Vasodilan), tolazoline (Priscoline), or cyclandelate (Cyclospasmol). These are effective in some patients.

Laser angioplasty is now used more commonly to open up clogged arteries. This procedure is done in a fashion similar to percutaneous balloon angioplasty. The surgeon enters the artery with a catheter and uses the laser to destroy the plaque buildup that is occluding the artery.

Percutaneous transluminal angioplasty may be done to open an occluded artery. A catheter is introduced into the artery, and when the proper spot is reached, a balloon is inflated multiple times to dilate the vessel, promoting better blood flow.

An aorto-iliac bypass or a femoral-popliteal bypass is performed to correct arterial occlusion of the leg in an attempt to prevent the need for amputation. A synthetic graft is placed to divert blood around the obstructed area, or the occluded portion is dissected and replaced by a graft.

A hyperbaric oxygen chamber is also sometimes used to increase tissue oxygen and avoid amputation.

The major nursing care goals following peripheral arterial surgery are (1) maintaining arterial blood flow to the lower extremities, (2) protecting tissues from further injury due to pressure and constriction of blood flow, and (3) preventing wound infection. Rehabilitation of the patient requires instruction and guidance in special exercises to increase collateral circulation to the legs.

ANEURYSM

An aneurysm can occur along any artery. It is an out-pouching of the wall of the artery due to a structural defect in the layers of the arterial wall. Blood flow is stagnant along the wall of the aneurysm, and clots can form, causing either thrombosis or embolus. Once an aneurysm develops, it continues to grow larger. Aneurysms eventually rupture if not repaired.

Congenital malformations cause many types of aneurysm. However, atherosclerosis and hypertension are thought to be major factors in their development. Atherosclerotic plaque weakens the vessel wall, and hypertension puts extra pressure on the weakened walls. Diabetes mellitus and hyperlipidemia are two other conditions that contribute to the development of vessel problems.

Aneurysm rupture is common in the cerebral vessels, causing intercerebral bleeding and stroke. Aortic aneurysms can occur along either the thoracic or the abdominal portion of the vessel. A ruptured aneurysm often causes sudden death. However, if an aneurysm is detected early, it can often be surgically repaired before it ruptures. Aneurysms often cause no obvious symptoms, although cerebral aneurysms may cause headaches or blurred vision, and an aortic aneurysm may cause back pain or a feeling of pressure.

The surgical procedure and nursing care depend on the location of the aneurysm. Cerebral aneurysm is treated by craniotomy; this is covered in Chapter 15. Aortic aneurysm is treated by thoracotomy or abdominal surgery, and the care is similar to that of other types of thoracic and abdominal surgery. The main difference is that the nurse must also carefully assess pulses and function distal to the repair site.

CAROTID OCCLUSION

When atherosclerosis has narrowed the carotid arteries leading to the brain, the signs and symptoms include carotid bruit (a purring sound heard with a stethoscope), confusion, visual abnormality in one eye, fainting, extremity weakness or paralysis, or other signs of decreased blood flow to the brain. The condition is treated by *carotid endarterectomy*, which surgically removes the atherosclerotic plaque, or by bypass surgery, which connects an artery from outside the cranium to an area on the cerebral artery beyond the obstruction. Both procedures are done to prevent the occurrence of stroke.

Specific postoperative care includes assessing for signs of bleeding, for pressure from hematoma on the trachea, and for neurologic problems caused by thrombosis or embolus.

RAYNAUD'S DISEASE

Raynaud's disease is characterized by spasm of the arteries. The disease is seen more often in women than in men. It mostly affects the fingers and toes and can be a primary disorder or occur secondary to another disease. In the latter instance it is known as *Raynaud's phenomenon*. The arterial spasm occurs in response to emotional stress or exposure to cold. The affected body part changes color, ranging from white to red to blue. When the spasm stops, there is often burning pain and throbbing. In about 10% of those affected, the disease progresses to the point where ischemia from arterial spasm is so severe that gangrene occurs and amputation is necessary. Medical therapy consists of stress control, avoidance of exposure to cold, cessation of smoking, and the use of calcium channel blockers to prevent arterial spasm.

THROMBOANGIITIS OBLITERANS

Thromboangiitis obliterans, or *Buerger's disease*, involves the small- and medium-sized arteries. Inflammation, thickening of the arterial walls, and occlusion of the vessels occur. The disease occurs more often in men than women and is commonly found in people from Eastern countries, particularly those of Jewish descent. Smoking is directly linked to progression of the disease. The signs and symptoms include numbness and tingling of the toes or fingers in cold weather, pain in the feet, and intermittent claudication that progressively becomes more severe. If ischemia causes gangrene, amputation is performed. Cessation of smoking is the single most important treatment factor.

VARICOSE VEINS

These are enlarged and tortuous veins that are distorted in shape by accumulations of pooled blood. Veins that develop varicosities have incompetent valves that allow reflux of blood from the deep to the superficial veins. The increased blood flow and resultant pressure on the vein walls cause the vessel to dilate and become tortuous. Heredity, standing for long periods of time, obesity, and pregnancy all contribute to the formation of varicose veins.

Signs and symptoms include dilated, twisted-appearing, superficial vessels on the legs. Swelling of the foot and ankle on the affected leg may occur by the end of the day and is often accompanied by aching.

Treatment includes the use of elastic support hose, exercising the legs and feet periodically throughout the day, and elevating the legs whenever possible. Prolonged standing, sitting, or crossing the legs is to be avoided. Weight reduction is recommended for obese patients. Exercises such as walking or swimming are beneficial, because the muscle contraction encourages venous return to the heart.

Small varicosities can be treated by scleropathy, which involves injection of an agent that will sclerose the vessel, causing thrombosis, which prevents further blood from filling the area. Veins with multiple, severe varicosities are treated by vein stripping, done as an outpatient procedure.

VENOUS STASIS ULCERS

Chronic venous insufficiency causes chronic skin and tissue lesions on the lower extremities, especially around the ankle. The ulcers may extend deeply into the tissue and are very slow and difficult to heal because of the poor blood supply. The ulcer may begin as a small, tender, inflamed area. With the slightest trauma, the skin breaks and the ulcer grows. Any skin trauma to the lower extremity may cause an ulcer to form, and it is imperative that the patient with venous insufficiency be taught the extreme importance of good foot and leg care. An inflamed area discovered by the nurse can be preventively treated with a clear occlusive dressing such as Tegaderm.

Treatment for the hospitalized patient with an open ulcer consists of leg elevation and either a dry or wet-to-dry dressing. Dressings are changed several times a day, helping to débride the area (i.e., peel away dead tissue). Often the wound needs a graft in order to heal completely. Venous stasis ulcers can take weeks to months to heal. Ambulatory patients are treated with compression dressings. An Unna boot may also be applied; this consists of gauze saturated with zinc oxide and calamine lotion in a glycerine base. This is covered with outer gauze, and then an elastic bandage is applied from the foot to the knee.

NURSING INTERVENTIONS

Decreased Blood Flow

The nurse can encourage blood flow by keeping the patient and the environment warm. Although moderate heat causes dilation of blood vessels, very high temperatures cause constriction. In addition to the danger of burning the patient because of decreased sensitivity to extremes of temperature, local heat increases metabolic activity in the tissues to which it is applied and therefore upsets even more the balance of supply and demand for blood flow to all of the tissues.

The goal in application of additional warmth is even distribution throughout the body.

Constricting clothing is to be avoided, and the leg gatch on the bed should never be used, as it puts added pressure on the back of the knees and further occludes blood flow. The nurse should encourage the patient to change his position while awake frequently. The lower legs should be elevated at every opportunity.

Support stockings, thromboembolic disease (TED) hose, or Jobst hose should be applied in the morning before the legs have been dependent. Hose should be checked and straightened frequently so that they do not bunch up and put pressure on the back of the knee.

Exercise is especially beneficial to patients with decreased blood flow. Walking regularly every day is best for the ambulatory patient. Swimming is also good, as it applies light pressure to the surface of the legs and requires muscle action that encourages venous return. Bed rest patients should be encouraged to do foot and leg exercises at least once an hour. The nurse can encourage those who watch television to do the exercises during each commercial.

Vasoconstriction

Patients with arterial insufficiency are to be very strongly encouraged to quit smoking. Nicotine is a potent vasoconstrictor and has the effect of producing spasmodic narrowing of the peripheral arteries.

Alcohol is a mild vasodilator when used in moderate amounts. The doctor may suggest daily intake of small amounts of wine or liquor if the patient has no objection.

Administration of pentoxifylline (Trental) may be of benefit to patients with chronic vasoconstriction, as it reduces blood viscosity, making the blood move more easily through narrowed vessels. The patient should also be kept well hydrated at all times.

Thrombosis

The patient with thrombosis is taught not to rub his extremity. The nurse encourages high fluid intake to reduce blood viscosity. Elastic hose or inflatable pressure devices are applied correctly, and the procedure for use is explained to the patient. The nurse administers anticoagulant therapy and monitors for adverse side effects, checking for bleeding and monitoring coagulation times. The patient receiving IV heparin should be placed on a Biofoam or similar pad beforehand to reduce bruising. The patient must be cautioned to move cautiously, avoiding hitting his head or injuring himself on furniture, doors, or other objects. The IV site should be monitored closely, as heparin can be irritating to the vessel in some people. At the first sign of inflammation, the IV site should be changed. Firm pressure should be applied to any needle stick for at least 5 minutes to prevent hematoma formation. The nurse must be alert for signs of pulmonary embolus.

The patient with deep vein thrombosis is taught to prevent venous stasis by exercising, keeping well hydrated, quitting smoking, avoiding substances that cause the blood to coagulate more easily (e.g., hormones), and avoiding sitting for long periods. The legs should never be crossed.

Venous Insufficiency and Stasis Ulcers

Thorough teaching is done to alert the patient to proper self-care and to signs of beginning skin breakdown. The slightest injury to an ischemic area can take a very long time to heal and can easily become infected, as the blood supply is inadequate to provide the usual leukocyte defenses. Any injury to an affected extremity should be reported to the doctor immediately, no matter how minor it is.

The nurse can give the patient considerable support, as treatment is long, recurrent, and tedious. Patients with stasis ulcers frequently become depressed. Praise for compliance with instructions and for any small gain made toward healing can do much for their morale.

Concerns for the Elderly

The main cause of peripheral vascular disease in the elderly is atherosclerosis. Early recognition of decreased peripheral circulation, combined with teaching about proper self-care can prevent problems with ulceration, gangrene, and possibly amputation.

Varicose veins develop in the elderly as the veins lose their elasticity and the leg muscles weaken and atrophy from decreased exercise. The occurrence of thrombophlebitis increases with advanced age. Factors that contribute to deep vein thrombosis include venous stasis, changes in the lining of the veins, and increased ease of clotting. Dehydration and immobility are added causes of thrombosis during hospitalization.

Many elderly persons become less active as they advance in years as a result of decreasing eyesight, arthritis, obesity, heart problems, or fatigue from nutritional anemia. The nurse should encourage each patient to regularly exercise within his ability in order to improve peripheral circulation and decrease the problems of peripheral vascular disease.

BIBLIOGRAPHY

Andreoli, T. E., et al.: Cecil Essentials of Medicine, 2nd ed. Philadelphia, W. B. Saunders, 1990.

Beal, K.: Lasers in vascular surgery. Nurs. Clin. North Am., Sept., 1990, p. 711.

Beare, P. G., and Myers, J. L.: Principles and Practices of Adult Health Nursing. St. Louis, C. V. Mosby, 1990.

Dickinson, R.: Our way, VI ulcers heal. RN, July, 1990, p. 32.

Fahey, V. A.: Vascular Nursing. Philadelphia, W. B. Saunders, 1988.

Fahey, V. A.: An in-depth look at deep vein thrombosis. Nursing 89, Jan., 1989, p. 84.

Fellows, E., and Jocz, A. M.: Getting the upper hand on lower extremity arterial disease. Nursing 91, Aug., 1991, p. 34.

Guyton, A. C.: Textbook of Medical Physiology, 8th ed. Philadelphia, W. B. Saunders, 1991.

Herman, J. A.: Nursing assessment and nursing diagnosis in patients with peripheral vascular disease. Nurs. Clin. North Am., June, 1986, p. 219.

Matteson, M. A., and McConnell, E. S.: Gerontological Nursing: Concepts and Practice. Philadelphia, W. B. Saunders, 1988.

McMahan, B. E.: Why deep vein thrombosis is so dangerous. RN, Jan., 1987, p. 20.

Price, S., and Wilson, L.: Pathophysiology, 3rd ed. New York, McGraw-Hill, 1986.

Rakel, R. E., ed.: Conn's Current Therapy 1990. Philadelphia, W. B. Saunders, 1990.
Schulze, C.: Aortic dissection—an ICU crisis. RN, Aug., 1990, p. 42.
Springhouse Company: Nurse Review: Vascular Disease. Springhouse, PA, 1988.
Ulrich, S. P., et al.: Nursing Care Planning Guides: A Nursing Diagnosis Approach, 2nd ed. Philadelphia, W. B. Saunders, 1990.
Wagner, M. M.: Pathophysiology related to peripheral vascular disease. Nurs. Clin. North Am., June, 1986, p. 195.

STUDENT STUDY AIDS

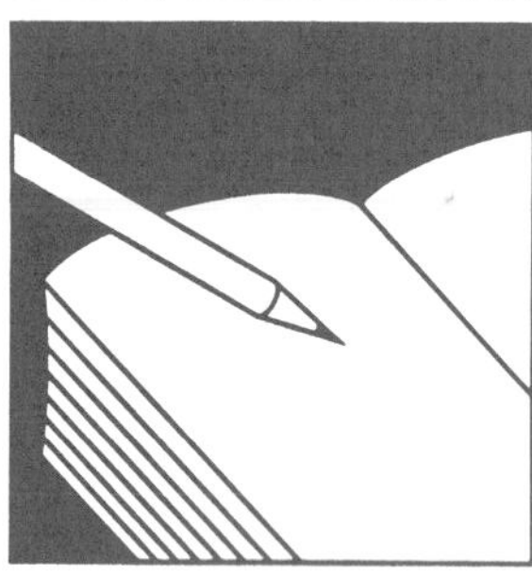

CLINICAL CASE PROBLEMS

Read each clinical case problem and discuss the questions with your classmates.

1. Mr. Dalino is being discharged from the hospital after treatment for arterial insufficiency in both lower extremities. His physician requests that Mr. Dalino receive instruction in the care of his feet and legs before the patient is permitted to leave.

- What are some problems you might expect Mr. Dalino to have because of his peripheral vascular disease?
- What kinds of information would Mr. Dalino need in order to alleviate these problems and prevent others?
- What would you include in your teaching plan to help him alleviate these problems and to prevent others?

---

2. Mrs. Hart is 83 years old and is hospitalized with congestive heart failure. She has a history of deep vein thrombosis in the lower extremities.

- What techniques would you include in your assessment, considering her history?
- What would you include in the care plan to try to prevent further DVT?

STUDY OUTLINE

I. Pathophysiology
- A. Disorders of peripheral blood vessels almost always chronic in nature and mainly affect older age groups.
- B. Disorders of peripheral arteries invariably lead to ischemia.
- C. Disorders of peripheral veins lead to increased pressure within the vessel.

II. Causative factors
- A. Peripheral arteries:
  1. Atherosclerosis.
  2. Embolus.
  3. Trauma.
  4. Smooth muscle spasm.
  5. Congenital defects.
- B. Peripheral veins:
  1. Defective valvular function.
  2. Thrombosis and thrombophlebitis.

III. Nursing assessment of peripheral circulation
- A. Assessment of arterial blood flow:
  1. Pain: intermittent claudication and rest pain.
  2. Color:
     - a. Have patient elevate feet and legs above level of heart for 2 to 3 minutes, then dangle legs.
     - b. Delayed return of color to feet indicates arterial insufficiency.
     - c. Pale, mottled appearance may indicate only that patient is cold.

d. Reddish-blue color indicates severe ischemia.
3. Skin temperature:
   a. Note coldness of extremity when environment is warm.
   b. Compare temperature of limbs.
4. Trophic changes resulting from malnutrition of tissues:
   a. Skin smooth, shiny, without hair.
   b. Nails are thick.
   c. Necrosis and gangrene after prolonged malnutrition.
5. Peripheral pulses:
   a. Noted at various sites (Fig. 21–2).
   b. May be normal, impaired, or absent.
6. Bruits: whooshing or purring sound heard over partially occluded arteries.

B. Assessment of venous blood flow:
1. Edema and cellulitis: increased pigmentation, dry and scaly skin, excoriations, and ulcers.
2. Trendelenburg test.

C. Nursing diagnoses for patients with peripheral vascular disease:
1. Altered peripheral tissue perfusion related to vessel occlusion.
2. Pain related to decreased blood flow.
3. Activity intolerance related to pain in legs when walking.
4. Sleep pattern disturbance related to pain in legs while at rest.
5. Body image disturbance related to edema and dilated veins on legs.
6. Body image disturbance related to loss of limb by amputation.
7. Knowledge deficit related to causes of peripheral vascular disease, treatment, and proper self-care.
8. Potential for injury related to potential for embolus or bleeding from anticoagulant medication.
9. Potential for infection related to impaired skin integrity.
10. Self-esteem disturbance related to inability to perform usual roles because of chronic leg ulcers.

D. Diagnostic tests:
1. Doppler ultrasound flow studies.
2. Radiologic studies: venogram, angiogram, or arteriogram.
3. Nuclear medicine scan to detect clots: lung scan.

IV. Common problems and therapies and their nursing implications

A. Decreased blood flow:
1. Smooth muscles of arterial walls constrict in presence of cold and extreme heat, relax when warm.
2. Pressure against vessel walls.
   a. Avoid constricting clothing.
   b. Change position frequently.
   c. Elevate extremities periodically to increase venous return.
   d. Support hose or elastic bandages.
   e. Walking and exercise.

B. Vasoconstriction:
1. Chemical factors: nicotine is a vasoconstrictor.
2. Alcohol in moderate amounts is a vasodilator.
3. Vasodilating drugs.
4. Sympathectomy.

C. Tissue damage and ulceration:
1. Chronic leg ulcers.
2. Gangrene.
3. Patient education in care of feet and legs.

V. Specific disorders

A. Thrombosis: formation of clot within blood vessel.

1. Effects depend on:
   a. Location and size of clot.
   b. Degree of obstruction to blood flow.
   c. Whether body can establish collateral circulation.

B. Embolism: sudden obstruction caused by mass floating in blood stream.
   1. Effects depend on site at which it is lodged, and size.
   2. May cause severe disability or death.

C. Peripheral arterial occlusive disease (atherosclerosis obliterans).
   1. Usually affects lower extremities.
   2. Signs and symptoms include intermittent claudication, rest pain, and ischemic changes.
   3. Peripheral vasodilators and medication to decrease blood viscosity are given to improve blood flow.
   4. A hyperbaric oxygen chamber sometimes is used to increase oxygen in tissues and avoid amputation.
   5. Surgical treatment helps relieve ischemic pain, avoid amputation, and add years to patient's life.
      a. Laser angioplasty.
      b. Percutaneous transluminal angioplasty.
      c. Bypass procedure with synthetic arterial graft.
      d. Aneurysm repair.
      e. Carotid endarterectomy.

D. Deep vein thrombosis: clot in deep vein occluding blood flow.
   1. Causes: immobility, trauma, surgery, dehydration, abnormal clotting.
   2. Signs and symptoms: edema in one extremity, positive Homans' sign, warmth over area.
   3. Treatment: IV heparin, oral warfarin (Coumadin), and hydration; thrombolytic therapy may be used.

E. Thrombophlebitis: clot and inflammation of vessel.
   1. Symptoms: vein appears distended; tenderness; redness.
   2. Medical management: elevation of part, support hose, warm packs, aspirin and sometimes antibiotics.
   3. Surgical treatment: vein ligation.

F. Embolism: thrombus lodges in a vessel, blocking blood flow beyond it.
   1. Causes: DVT of lower leg the most common cause; fat droplets from fracture, clots formed from cardiac arrhythmias, and amniotic fluid also cause emboli.
   2. Signs and symptoms of pulmonary embolus: dyspnea, hemoptysis, feeling of impending doom, cyanosis, chest splinting.
   3. Treatment: oxygen, thrombolytic therapy, anticoagulants, or thrombectomy; vena caval umbrella insertion.

G. Raynaud's disease: spasm of small arteries; mostly affects fingers and toes.

H. Thromboangiitis obliterans (Buerger's disease): inflammation and thickening of small- and medium-sized arteries; smoking is a major factor.

I. Varicose veins: enlarged, tortuous veins engorged with pooled blood.
   1. Symptoms: fatigue, feeling of heaviness in legs after prolonged standing or sitting, pain, itching along course of blood vessel.
   2. Medical management: support hose, treatment of obesity, exercise.
   3. Surgical treatment: scleropathy, vein stripping, or ligation.

J. Venous stasis ulcers: skin lesion, usually on lower leg, from venous insufficiency.

1. Occur with slightest trauma.
2. Difficult to treat and slow to heal.
3. Treatment: débridement and prevention of infection.

VI. Nursing interventions

A. Decreased blood flow:
   1. Slightly warm environment; not hot.
   2. No constricting clothing.
   3. No pressure on back of knees.
   4. Elevate lower legs.
   5. Support hose.
   6. Exercise: walking regularly; swimming.

B. Vasoconstriction:
   1. Encourage patient to stop smoking.
   2. Light alcohol intake, if acceptable, for vasodilation effect.

C. Thrombosis:
   1. Instruct patient not to rub extremity.
   2. Encourage increased fluid intake if permitted.
   3. Apply elastic hose or inflatable pressure boots.
   4. Monitor anticoagulant therapy: check clotting times; assess for bruising and bleeding.
   5. Observe for signs of embolus.
   6. Encourage exercise to decrease venous stasis in other leg.

D. Venous insufficiency and stasis ulcers:
   1. Teach proper self-care.
   2. Attention to psychological support and psychosocial concerns.
   3. Wet-to-dry dressings; Elase ointment, Duoderm for healing.

VII. Concerns for the elderly

A. Atherosclerosis is main cause of PVD in elderly.
B. Varicose veins: vessels lose elasticity; muscles weaken.
C. Thrombophlebitis more frequent in elderly, who have altered coagulation and are quick to dehydrate and less mobile.
D. Lessened activity as a result of arthritis and other conditions predisposes patients to problems with PVD.
E. Nurse should encourage as much physical activity as possible within patient's limitations.

CHAPTER 22

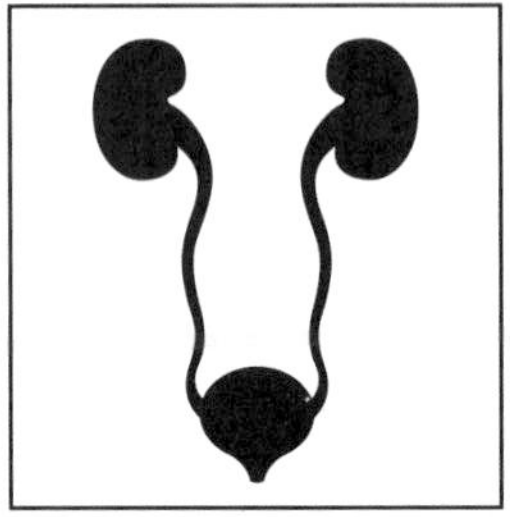

Care of Patients With Urologic Disorders

VOCABULARY

anuria
cystitis
cystoscopy
dysuria
glycosuria
hematuria
hydronephrosis
hyperlipidemia
hypervolemia
hypoalbuminemia
ketonuria
nephrostomy
nocturia
oliguria
percutaneous
polyuria
proteinuria
pyuria
residual
retrograde
uremia

Upon completion of this chapter the student should be able to:

1. Identify nursing responsibilities in the pre- and posttest care of patients having urologic diagnostic studies.
2. Describe initial and ongoing nursing assessment of a patient's urologic status.
3. List four nursing responsibilities in maintaining urinary flow via an indwelling catheter.
4. Describe nursing assessment and interventions for patients with selected urologic inflammatory disorders (e.g., cystitis, urethritis, nephritis, and pyelonephritis).
5. Devise a nursing care plan, including preparation for home care, for the patient with renal failure.
6. Describe the special needs of patients on long-term hemodialysis.
7. List specific nursing responsibilities in the care of patients receiving peritoneal dialysis.
8. Discuss the benefits and special problems associated with kidney transplantation.
9. List five specific nursing responsibilities in the care of patients with renal calculi.
10. Describe the pre- and postoperative nursing care of patients having surgery of the kidney.

The urinary system is composed of the kidneys, ureters, urinary bladder, and urethra (Fig. 22–1). Their functions are secretion, storage, and excretion. The kidneys are two bean-shaped organs that lie on either side of the vertebral column at the level of the last thoracic and first lumbar vertebrae. They are richly supplied with blood from branches of the aorta and vena cava.

The need for an abundant supply of blood to the kidneys becomes apparent when one realizes that nearly one fourth of the body's blood is filtered by the kidneys at one time. Waste products are retained in the kidneys in urine to be excreted, while the remainder of the fluid is returned to the blood. During a 24-hour period, the kidneys handle approximately as much as 200 liters of liquid, excreting only 1.5 to 2 liters as urine.

The *nephron* is the functional unit of the kidney (Fig. 22–2). Each kidney is composed of about 1 million nephrons, and each nephron can form urine by itself. Thus to understand the function of the nephron is to understand the function of the kidney. The basic function of the nephron is to filter a large portion of the blood plasma out of the blood stream and through the glomerular membrane. Unwanted substances such as urea, creatinine, uric acid, and other wastes are retained in the tubules, whereas water and some electrolytes are allowed to reenter the blood stream. The water and wastes remaining in the tubules are excreted as urine.

The ureters, one from each kidney, convey the urine by *peristaltic* action from the kidney to the urinary bladder. The bladder serves as a reservoir and holds the urine until it is distended with 300 to 400 mL; then the urge to urinate compels emptying the bladder. The urine passes from the bladder through the urethra to the outside. The urethra is approximately 3 to 5 cm long in women and 20 cm in men.

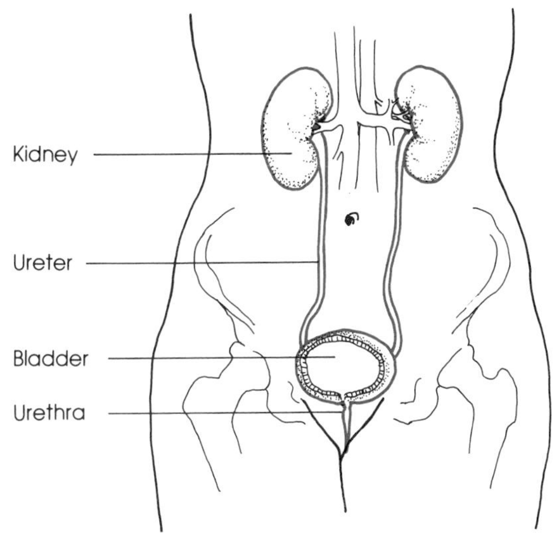

Figure 22–1 Structures of the urinary system.

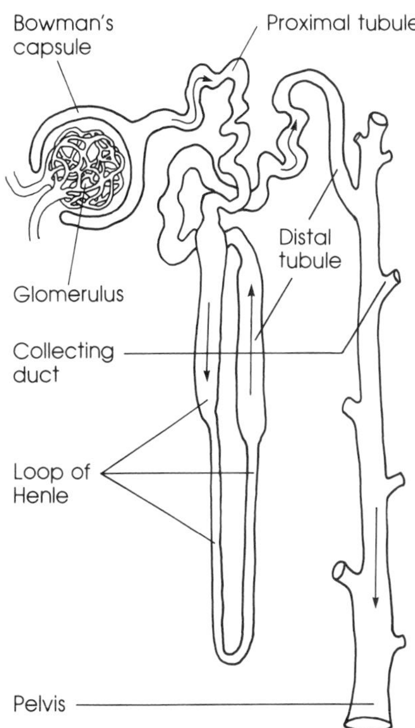

Figure 22–2 The nephron.

The kidneys and urinary tract are responsible for maintaining the proper balance of fluids, minerals, and organic substances necessary for life. In view of this, it is not surprising that a diseased condition of any one system of the body may have a direct effect on the kidneys and urinary tract. Generalized diseases such as atherosclerosis, other circulatory lesions, infections, or disturbances in the metabolic processes may very seriously impair the proper functioning of the kidneys. Similarly, involvement of the heart, lungs, or circulatory system can arise from kidney failure.

Diseases do not always conveniently fit into clearly defined categories. The body functions as a whole, and the systems are interdependent. This chapter will be concerned primarily with diseases of the urinary system; however, it should be remembered that the nurse will frequently have need for a good working knowledge of the basic principles of urologic nursing in a wide variety of nursing care situations.

DIAGNOSTIC TESTS AND PROCEDURES AND NURSING IMPLICATIONS

Patients experiencing problems with the urinary system undergo general systems tests, including a complete blood cell (CBC) count and chemistry panel and other diagnostic tests or procedures specific to the problem. Table 22–1

Text continued on page 526

TABLE 22-1 **DIAGNOSTIC TESTS FOR UROLOGIC PROBLEMS**

Test	Purpose	Description	Nursing Implications
Urinalysis	Detects bacteria, blood, casts, and other abnormalities of the urine.	The urine is observed for color and clarity; the pH and specific gravity are determined; tests are performed to detect blood, protein, sugar, bilirubin and acetone; a microscopic exam is performed to detect the presence of red and white blood cells, casts, and crystals.	Obtain a urine specimen of at least 10 mL. A fresh morning specimen is preferred. Send specimen to lab immediately. Normal urine is clear, straw to dark amber in color, has a pH of 4.5 to 6.0, a specific gravity of 1.010 to 1.030, and is negative for protein, glucose, ketones, and bilirubin. It should have only a rare RBC, no more than 0 to 4 WBCs, and occasional cast.
Fractional urine (two- to three-bottle routine)	Determines site and degree of bleeding after prostate surgery.	Patient voids into one urine container and then, without stopping the stream, continues to void into another container. The amount of blood in each container gives an indication of degree and site of bleeding.	Provide two or three urine containers and instruct patient to switch containers midway through the voiding without stopping the stream.
Urine culture and sensitivity	Verifies urinary tract infection (UTI) and determines type of organism responsible. Usually done in conjunction with an antiinfective sensitivity screen.	A midstream clean catch or sterile catheterized specimen is obtained, and the urine is placed in a culture medium for growth of bacterial colonies. After incubation, the colonies are counted. If more than 100,000 organisms per milliliter are counted, there is a urinary tract infection. The organisms are then identified as to type. Gram-negative bacilli are the most common cause of UTIs. *Escherichia coli (E. coli)* found in the intestinal tract is a frequent cause of UTI. Sensitivity tests involve exposing the bacteria to various antiinfectives to see which most effectively kills the organism.	Instruct patient in method for collection of a "clean catch" specimen. Instructions come with the specimen container. Allow time for questions after patient is familiar with directions. A sterile speciment can also be obtained via urinary catheterization. Send specimen to lab immediately to prevent change in pH, which can affect bacterial growth.
Urine osmolality	Determines whether the kidneys can concentrate urine normally.	The patient is either placed on fluid restriction or given a specific amount of fluid to drink before the test. Normal range for urine osmolality is 300 to 1,200 mOsm/kg.	Give a high protein diet for 3 days prior to the urine collection. Restrict fluids for 8 to 12 hours before obtaining specimen. Collect a random urine specimen, preferably in the morning, label it (including the time), and send to lab.
Protein metabolites Blood urea nitrogen (BUN)	Determines ability of the kidneys to filter and excrete end products of metabolism.	Urea is the main protein metabolite excreted. Blood urea nitrogen (BUN) is measured to help evaluate kidney function, extent of renal disease, and hydra-	Usually done with patient NPO for 8 hours. Requires 5 mL of venous blood.

TABLE 22-1 DIAGNOSTIC TESTS FOR UROLOGIC PROBLEMS *Continued*

Test	Purpose	Description	Nursing Implications
		tion status. Increased BUN can indicate poor kidney function, dehydration, or increased breakdown of body protein such as occurs with severe burns or excessive exercise. A depressed BUN is found in severe liver damage, excessive hydration, and protein deficiency. Normal BUN levels average 8 to 20 mg/dL, depending on sex and age.	
Serum creatinine	Evaluates kidney function.	Creatinine is produced in fairly constant amounts in the body in proportion to muscle mass. The measurement of the amount of creatinine in the blood makes it a good estimator of kidney function. Serum creatinine is measured first, and if it is elevated, then urine creatinine is assessed. Urine creatinine helps assess glomerular filtration and goes up when renal perfusion is lessened or when the glomeruli cannot function properly. Normal serum creatinine is 0.4 to 1.2 mg/dL.	No food or drink restriction, but patient should not eat large amounts of meat beforehand. Requires 5 to 10 mL venous blood. List drugs patient is taking on lab slip, as certain drugs affect the test.
Creatinine clearance	Determines how well kidneys can excrete creatinine by examining both blood and urine.	A 12- to 24-hour urine specimen is obtained, and a blood specimen is drawn. Elevated serum creatinine with decreased urine creatinine indicates decreased kidney function. Normal creatinine clearance is 15 to 25 mg/kg body weight in 24 hours.	A 5-mL venous blood sample is collected before the test begins. Place a sign on the patient's door and over the toilet stating "24-hour urine test in progress" so that everyone will save the urine properly. Collect a 12- or 24-hour urine specimen: have patient void and discard the urine: note the time on the lab slip; put each successive voiding into the collection container. Check with lab as to whether the container must be kept on ice. At the time the test is to end, ask the patient to void and add this last urine to the collection bottle. Send the specimen to the lab.
Radiologic studies KUB (Kidneys, ureters, bladder)	Visualizes the structures of the urinary tract; locates stones or abnormalities.	Radiograph of the lower abdomen done without contrast medium.	Explain purpose and procedure; have patient put on x-ray gown.
Intravenous pyelogram (IVP)	Visualizes the kidneys and ureters. Detects impairment of kidney function	After intravenous injection of an iodine-based dye, multiple radiographs are	Explain purpose and procedure; check for allergy to iodine or shellfish and

Table continued on following page

TABLE 22-1 **DIAGNOSTIC TESTS FOR UROLOGIC PROBLEMS** *Continued*

Test	Purpose	Description	Nursing Implications
	resulting from obstruction, stones, or tumor in the kidneys, ureters, or prostate.	taken at 5 or more minutes apart, showing the flow of the dye through the renal system. A retrograde pyelogram is done during cystoscopy. Catheters are threaded into the ureters for injection of the dye into the kidneys.	consult with physician if one exists. Patient may feel a hot flush when dye is injected; nausea sometimes occurs. Inform patient that the test takes 30 to 60 minutes.
Cystogram	Visualizes the contour of the bladder.	X-ray films are taken before and after sodium iodide is injected into the bladder through a urethral catheter.	Inform patient that the bladder may feel very full and he may feel like he needs to void after the dye is instilled. A Foley catheter is usually inserted prior to the procedure. The bladder is drained after the radiographs are taken.
Computed tomographic (CT) scan	Determines presence of a cyst or tumor in the kidney.	A combination of x-ray and computer techniques yields cross-sectional information and indicates the density of tissues.	Explain the purpose and procedure. Contrast medium may be given; check for allergy to iodine. Describe the CT scan machine and the sounds he might hear (clicking and whirring).
Renal ultrasonography	Determines size, shape, and location of each kidney, the ureter, and the bladder; indicates tumors and obstructions to urine flow.	Uses high-frequency sound waves and an oscilloscope screen. A probe is passed over the surface of the flank while the patient is positioned on a table.	Explain the purpose and procedure. Patient may be asked to drink fluid to fill bladder prior to sonogram. Test takes approximately 30 minutes.
Renal angiography	Assesses renal arterial system function and identifies areas of obstruction to blood flow.	Under local anesthesia, a catheter is threaded through the femoral artery, up the aorta to the renal artery, and a contrast agent is injected. Fluoroscopic examination is done while the agent enters and fills the blood vessels. Angiography is performed to detect complications in a transplanted kidney, to evaluate a kidney mass, or to determine the extent of kidney trauma.	Requires a signed permission form. Check for allergy to iodine-based dye. Pressure is applied to the entrance site for 20 minutes after procedure, a pressure dressing and a sandbag are applied, and the patient is kept flat in bed for 4 to 12 hours, assessed frequently for signs of bleeding, shock, or other complications, and kept on bed rest for 24 hours. Vital signs are taken q 15 to 30 min until stable, and popliteal and pedal pulses are checked at least q 4 h to evaluate peripheral circulation. The puncture site is watched for bleeding or hematoma formation.
Radionuclide renal scan	Studies renal blood flow or detects abnormal areas of kidney tissue (i.e., tumors or cysts).	A radioisotope is injected into the blood, and a scintillation scanner is passed over the area of the kidney. This yields a pattern of areas in which the isotope has been taken up. An interval of about 30	Explain that the isotope used is low-dose radiation and is quickly eliminated from the body. There is usually no danger to the patient or others from it. Describe the clicking sounds the scanner makes; test takes

TABLE 22–1 DIAGNOSTIC TESTS FOR UROLOGIC PROBLEMS *Continued*

Test	Purpose	Description	Nursing Implications
		min is allowed before scanning if a tumor or cysts are suspected.	approximately 45 to 90 min.
Cystoscopy	Examines the interior of the bladder.	Under short-acting anesthesia, a cystoscope is passed up the urethra into the bladder. The scope can be guided into a ureter to extract a stone or to biopsy lesions in the bladder.	Requires a signed permission form, as it is a surgical procedure. Explain the purpose and procedure. Unless general anesthesia is to be used, a full liquid breakfast is given. A preoperative sedative/tranquilizer and analgesic is given 1 hour prior to the procedure. The patient will be placed in the lithotomy position on the operating table. Water may be instilled into the bladder to promote better visualization. Test takes about 1 hour. After the procedure, burning, frequency, and pink-tinged urine are normal. Warm sitz baths and mild analgesics are given for voiding discomfort. Urine is monitored for 24 hours for signs of frank bleeding.
Renal biopsy	Obtains tissue for pathologic study.	With local anesthetic, the patient is placed in the prone position, and a biopsy needle is inserted into the lower lobe of the kidney. A tissue sample is extracted and sent to the lab.	The patient is placed in a prone position with a pillow wedged under the abdomen at the level of the kidney. The results of IVP or ultrasound are used to precisely locate the kidney, a local anesthetic is given, and a biopsy needle is inserted below the 12th rib. The patient must hold his breath while the needle is inserted and withdrawn. Afterward a pressure dressing is applied, and the patient is kept prone for 30 to 60 minutes. He is usually on bed rest for 24 hours. Vital signs are taken every 5 to 10 minutes for 1 hour and then with decreasing frequency until stable. The patient is assessed for flank pain and for gross and microscopic hematuria (blood in the urine). He is not to lift heavy objects for 5 to 7 days. WBCs and temperature are monitored for signs of infection.

lists the diagnostic tests and procedures most commonly performed, along with their nursing implications. Other tests may also be ordered. A magnetic resonance imaging (MRI) scan is sometimes done to detect a kidney tumor, but because it is very expensive, other methods of diagnosis are usually used first.

NURSING ASSESSMENT OF RENAL FUNCTION AND THE URINARY DRAINAGE SYSTEM

DEFINITION OF TERMS

The following terms are commonly used to describe various kinds of abnormal flow of urine.

- *anuria*—absence of urine. This rarely occurs, but can be due to renal failure, usually acute.
- *oliguria*—diminished or abnormally decreased flow of urine. It may be dehydration, renal failure, or obstruction to the flow of urine somewhere in the drainage system.
- *polyuria*—abnormally high urinary output; the result of excessive reabsorption of solutes and increased excretion of water. Therefore urine is very dilute. Possible causes include hypercalcemia, diabetes insipidus, uncontrolled diabetes mellitus, and increased fluid intake.
- *urinary retention*—retaining or holding urine in the bladder. This can be due to anxiety; postoperative swelling; fear of pain on voiding, particularly following surgery; neurologic disorders; and obstruction to flow of urine through the urethra, as in enlargement of the prostate gland. If a catheter is not passed to relieve urinary retention and bladder distention, the bladder will not rupture, but urine will begin to dribble out the urethra. Retention of urine stretches the bladder walls, causing extreme discomfort. Nursing measures to induce voiding may be effective in some cases, thereby avoiding the danger of introducing infectious organisms by catheterization.
- *residual urine*—that which is left in the bladder after voiding. Poor bladder tone or partial obstruction of the urethra can result in dribbling of urine or passing only the overflow, leaving the bladder partially full. Residual urine is measured by having the patient void as much urine as possible and then inserting a catheter immediately after. Fifteen milliliters is considered a normal amount of residual urine. Any amount over this can become more and more stagnant and concentrated over a period of time, predisposing the patient to bladder infection and stones.
- *suppression of urine*—inability of the kidney to produce urine. This is due to renal failure and results in oliguria or anuria.

HISTORY AND PRESENT ILLNESS

At the time of admission the nurse will try to obtain background data related to urinary problems so as to establish a nursing data base for intervention. Because of the kidney's response to pathologic conditions in virtually every other system of the body, a personal history of illness or injury to any system could be relevant to an assessment of kidney function. Previous disorders of the urinary tract, especially those that required surgery, are particularly relevant.

Family history of cardiovascular disease, diabetes, and kidney stone formation is pertinent to assessment of a patient's renal status. These diseases can adversely affect the kidney, and they tend to occur more often in family members than would be expected by chance.

Sexually transmitted diseases and other genital and reproductive disorders frequently have a negative impact on the urinary drainage system by interfering with normal urination. Examples include herpetic inflammation of the urethra and benign or malignant enlargement of the prostate gland.

Many drugs can be toxic to the kidney (i.e., nephrotoxic). Therefore the nursing history should include any drugs recently or currently being taken by the patient.

Information from the patient about his present illness should include observations of changes in urinary output, including amount and character of urine, pain or discomfort in either the bladder or the kidney region, and abnormal patterns of voiding. These kinds of data pertinent to assessment of urologic status are discussed in detail below.

ONGOING ASSESSMENT

Nursing responsibilities in the daily assessment of urinary function include (1) measuring intake and output; (2) assessing abnormal flow of urine; (3) noting the character of urine—color, odor, clouding; (4) noting changes in the pattern of voiding; and (5) assessing pain and discomfort.

Intake and Output

The quantity of fluids entering the body, by whatever route, has a direct bearing on fluid balance. The importance of maintaining a normal fluid balance is covered in Chapter 8. Patients with urologic disorders are very likely to suffer fluid imbalances, and therefore their intake and output should be measured and the totals recorded every 8 hours during hospitalization.

In critically ill patients the urinary output is sometimes measured hourly. Specially designed urine meters, combined with drainage bags, are used to obtain accurate readings of small quantities of urine and to avoid contamination of the urinary tract. If measurement of the *total urinary output* is required, the nurse must make sure that urine from all points of drainage is measured and the exact amount recorded. For example, urine from a ureterostomy tube and from a urethral catheter should both be included. When *total output* is to be measured, this must include vomitus, watery stools, urine excreted, and an estimate of the amount of fluid lost through perspiration. Any fluid used to irrigate urinary catheters and tubing must be measured and the amount subtracted from the *total* output to measure the total *urinary* output.

Characteristics of Urine

The color of urine can give helpful information about the status of the patient and the functioning of the kidney. Table 22-2 shows color variations in urine and the significance of abnormal coloration.

Another characteristic that should be noted is *odor*. Normal urine develops an ammonia-like odor after it has stood for a length of time, but this odor should not be present in freshly voided urine. A foul smell indicates infection. Acetone in the urine causes it to have a sweet, fruity odor.

Hematuria means blood in the urine. Microscopic hematuria usually is not indicative of any abnormality in the urinary system. Gross hematuria, a common cause of abnormal changes in urine color, is a sign of continued bleeding from some point in the urinary tract. Red blood in the urine is not easily missed, but if the blood has been in the bladder or kidney for a period of time, it could have deteriorated and will cause the urine to be a smoky gray or dark brown.

When assessing a patient with hematuria, the nurse should try to find out at what point during the act of urinating the blood is noticed. This information can help locate the source of bleeding. If the blood is noticed as soon as voiding starts, it is likely that the bleeding is from somewhere in the urethra. If it is noticed at the end of urination, the site probably is near the neck of the bladder. Bleeding throughout voiding indicates that the blood is coming from a site above the neck of the bladder, because the blood has been well mixed with the urine in the bladder.

Changes in Voiding Pattern

These changes include the number of times during the day and night the patient has the urge to urinate (frequency). Other alterations could be in the size and force of the urinary stream,

TABLE 22-2 COMMON CAUSES OF VARIATIONS IN COLOR OF URINE

Coloration	Possible cause
Colorless	Dilute urine, high fluid intake, diabetes insipidus, inability of kidney to concentrate urine.
Dark yellow or yellow-orange	Concentrated urine, low fluid intake, dehydration, inability of kidney to dilute urine. Fluorescein causes the urine to be bright yellow.
Smoky or with grayish cast	Hemoglobin and remnants of old red blood cells, chyle, prostatic fluid, yeasts.
Red or red-brown	Fresh blood, porphyrin, menstrual contamination, pyrvinium pamoate (Povan), sulfonamides.
Bright orange red	Pyridium.
Yellow-brown (dull amber) or green-brown	Bile in urine, phenol poisoning.
Dark brown or black	Methylene blue medication, typhus.
Cloudy	Phosphate precipitation (normal after sitting for a while), urates, leukocytes, pus, blood, epithelial cells, fat droplets, strict vegetarian diet.

feeling of fullness even after voiding, and change in the amount urinated each time.

Increased frequency can be a manifestation of some abnormality in the urinary draining system, particularly in the bladder and urethra. The frequency with which a person feels the urge to urinate can be related to psychological as well as physiologic factors. Excitement, anxiety, and fear can produce increased frequency of urination. Caffeine and other diuretics found in foods and drinks and simply an increased intake of water can increase the number of times a person must urinate. Pathologic conditions that can cause increased frequency include inflammation of the bladder (cystitis) or urethra (urethritis).

Urgency also is symptomatic of inflammation. Urgency refers to an almost uncontrollable desire to void. Sometimes it causes incontinence, because it is not possible to get to a bathroom as soon as the urge to urinate is felt.

Pain and Discomfort

In general, the locations in which the patient with a urinary problem is most likely to experience discomfort are either the bladder or suprapubic area or the region over the kidney (flank pain). The third kind of discomfort may be painful urination or dysuria.

Bladder pain can be due to an overfull bladder and stretching of its walls. Assessment of the size and location of the bladder may be indicated when a patient reports pain in the bladder region. Normally the bladder cannot be felt. If a smooth, rounded mass is felt on palpation in the area above the pubic bone, the bladder is distended.

Bladder pain also can be caused by spasms of the bladder musculature as it attempts to empty itself of clots, bits of tissue, and other cellular debris. This can occur postoperatively or when there is moderate to severe inflammation and bleeding in the urinary tract. Relief sometimes can be obtained by irrigating the bladder and tubing to remove the clots and debris. Belladonna and opium (B & O) suppositories are often ordered for bladder spasms.

Flank pain also can be due to obstruction and distention; in this case the affected organs are the ureters and kidney pelvis. Spasmodic peristaltic contractions along the ureter can be caused by stones, clots, a tumor, inflammatory swelling, or any other condition that prevents the flow of urine from the kidney to the bladder. In her evaluation of flank pain the nurse should ask the patient the location of the pain, as it tends to radiate from the kidney or ureter to the genitalia and thigh.

Dysuria usually is caused by inflammation in either the bladder or the urethra. It is often described as burning and can range from mild to moderate to severe. In addition to determining where the pain is and how it feels, the nurse also should ask the patient when the pain occurs and if it is related to and felt immediately before, during, or after voiding.

Nursing diagnoses frequently associated with kidney disease and disturbances in urinary flow include the following:

- Altered pattern of urinary elimination related to oliguria or anuria.
- Fluid volume excess related to decreased kidney function.
- Pain related to ureteral spasm, bladder spasm, or inflammation.
- Activity intolerance related to fatigue.
- Sleep pattern disturbance related to nocturia.
- Knowledge deficit related to management of disease and means of prevention.
- Fear related to cause of hematuria, possibility of malignancy, or dialysis.
- Body image disturbance related to maintenance of life by dialysis.
- Potential sexual dysfunction related to manifestations of kidney failure.

MAINTAINING URINARY FLOW

Urinary stasis is a major cause of infection and leads to the formation of stones in the urinary tract. When urine does not flow freely, it forms stagnant pools that are excellent media for the growth of bacteria. This stagnant urine also allows for the settling out of crystals and other substances that are the beginnings of urinary stones.

An interruption in the flow of urine can occur anywhere in the system. If, for example, a ureter is blocked, urine that is continually being formed by the kidneys begins to accumulate in the ureter above the site of the obstruction. If the obstruction is not relieved, the urine continues to back up into the kidneys, causing *hydronephrosis.*

Another point at which urine accumulates is in the bladder. This is a natural reservoir; the normal function of the bladder is to hold urine until it is voided during urination. If, for some neurologic or mechanical reason, the bladder is not emptied completely and regularly, the urine remaining in the bladder becomes a source of infection and stones. In order to avoid these problems, the urine flow sometimes must be maintained artificially.

The tubes used to draw urine from any point along the urinary tract are called *urinary catheters.* Catheterization should *never* be done solely because it is quicker or more convenient for the nurse than noninvasive nursing measures.

Various types of tubes that may be used are

described in this chapter. However, no matter what type of catheter is used, there are some general principles that apply in every case. These are presented in the following section.

PRINCIPLES OF CATHETER CARE

Although urinary stasis is a cause of infection and catheters are inserted to prevent infection, it is an unfortunate fact that catheter-associated urinary tract infections are the most common kinds of hospital-acquired infections.

Urinary tract infections account for about 40% of all nosocomial infections, and about three fourths of these are related to indwelling bladder catheters. Thus the use of a catheter to prevent infection from stasis is very likely to be self-defeating, because the catheter itself serves as an excellent avenue for the entry of infectious organisms.

Indwelling catheters are inserted with the intention of leaving them in place for an extended period, in some cases for several hours and in others for a longer time. Because of the many problems they can cause, indwelling catheters should be used only after all other alternatives have failed. Indwelling catheters are inserted when the patient has (1) an obstruction in the lower urinary tract, (2) blood clots in the bladder, (3) urinary incontinence or neurologic dysfunction, or (4) surgical repair of the urethra or surrounding tissues. Sometimes an indwelling catheter is used when careful monitoring of urinary output is essential to deciding modes of treatment.

In order to avoid catheter-related infection insofar as is possible, the nurse must exercise extreme care in handling these catheters. They usually are inserted into the bladder via the urethra and are called *urethral catheters.*

Before insertion of a urethral catheter, the urinary meatus must be cleansed thoroughly. Catheter insertion must be performed under sterile conditions. An exception is self-catheterization, in which the patient is taught a "clean" technique to avoid infection. During insertion, trauma to the mucosa of the urethra must be avoided.

Once an indwelling catheter is in place, it is connected to a closed drainage system for the collection of urine. The point at which the catheter enters the urinary meatus must be kept extremely clean.

The area should be kept as dry as possible; creams and powders are avoided, because they tend to cake and further irritate the mucosa and promote bacterial growth. Soap and water, gently applied, will do much to prevent odors, irritation, and discomfort. Antibacterial ointments, if used at all, are applied according to hospital policy.

The drainage tubing leading from the catheter must be kept patent so that urine can drain freely at all times. Tension on the tubing traumatizes the bladder, urethra, and meatus. The collecting bag is kept below the level of the bladder; raising it above this level will cause a flow of urine from the bag back into the bladder. The same thing will happen if the bag is inverted.

The point or points at which there are connections between (1) the catheter and the tubing and (2) the tubing and the collection bag are sites at which bacteria are most likely to enter the system (Fig. 22–3). The best system is a *closed* system. If at any time the tubing must be disconnected, as in changing a catheter or irrigating the bladder, care must be taken to avoid contamination.

The physician may order either periodic or continuous irrigation of the bladder to remove clots, mucus, or bits of tissue that may interfere with the flow of urine. The nurse must have specific orders about the type of fluid to be used and the rate of flow for continuous irrigations. When intermittent irrigations are prescribed, the nurse should realize that each time the system is opened, the possibility of introducing infectious agents is increased. Some authorities feel that the best way to irrigate a bladder and keep a catheter open is by forcing fluids and increasing urinary flow.

A *retention catheter* in the urethra should always be kept open and draining freely unless there are specific orders to clamp it off. Clamping is sometimes done as part of a bladder training program. Incontinence of urine and techniques to overcome this problem due to neurologic dysfunction are discussed in Chapter 15.

When the physician orders removal of the retention catheter, the nurse accepts responsibility

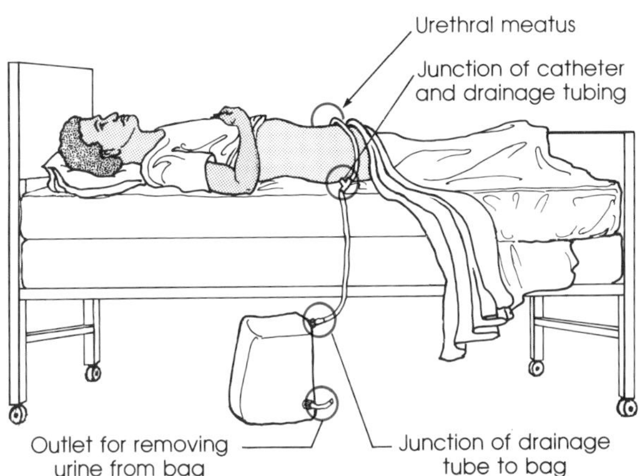

Figure 22–3 Potential portals of entry for bacteria in a patient with a retention catheter.

for removing the catheter and carefully observing the patient for signs of retention of urine. The time of removal of the catheter is recorded, and the patient is observed for signs of difficulty in voiding. Any bleeding, dribbling, or incontinence of urine should be reported as possible signs of an excessive amount of residual urine or bleeding from the bladder or urethra.

Alternatives to indwelling urethral catheters should always be considered when there is evidence that the patient cannot remain continent of urine. Such alternatives can be used temporarily, as in a bladder control program, or permanently. They include condom (external) drainage for males (Fig. 22–4), drainage by suprapubic catheter, and self-catheterization.

When one of these alternatives is used, precautions against introducing infectious agents into the urinary system and assurance of continuous drainage of urine are as important as they are for an indwelling urethral catheter.

TYPES OF CATHETERS

The *urethral catheter* is the most commonly used means of establishing and maintaining urinary flow. Figures 22–5 and 22–6 show various kinds of catheters that are inserted into the bladder by way of the urethra. The *self-retaining catheters* are also called *indwelling* and *retention catheters.* They are used when there is need for continuous drainage from the bladder.

Suprapubic catheters are inserted directly into the bladder, usually during a surgical procedure

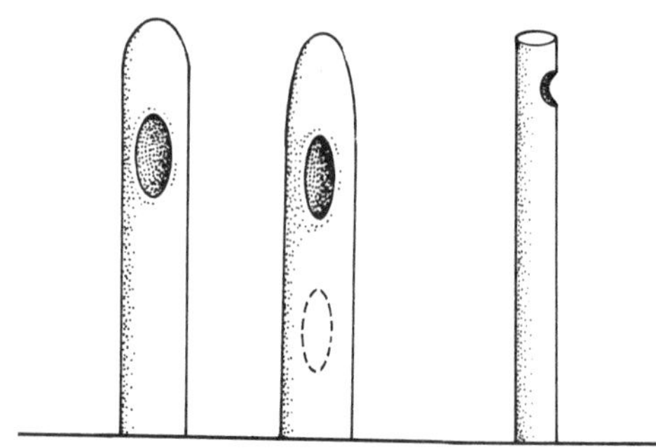

Figure 22–5 Straight catheters. These may have one or two eyes, a round tip, or a "whistle" tip and are not self-retaining.

while the patient is under anesthesia. A surgical incision is made, or the catheter may be threaded through a large trocar or needle that has been inserted through the bladder wall. A suprapubic catheter is *not* self-retaining and therefore must be sutured in place.

The patient with a suprapubic catheter in place is checked at least hourly during the first 24 hours after insertion. The catheter and drainage tubing are checked for signs of obstruction, and the bladder is examined for distention. A decrease in urinary output through the catheter and into the collection bag and a distended and tender bladder indicate obstruction. These signs

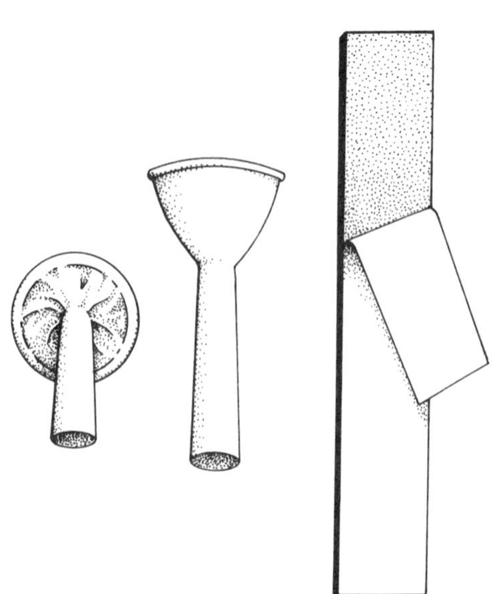

Figure 22–4 External (condom, or sheath) catheter. Rubber condom with adapter and one-piece molded latex sheath are shown.

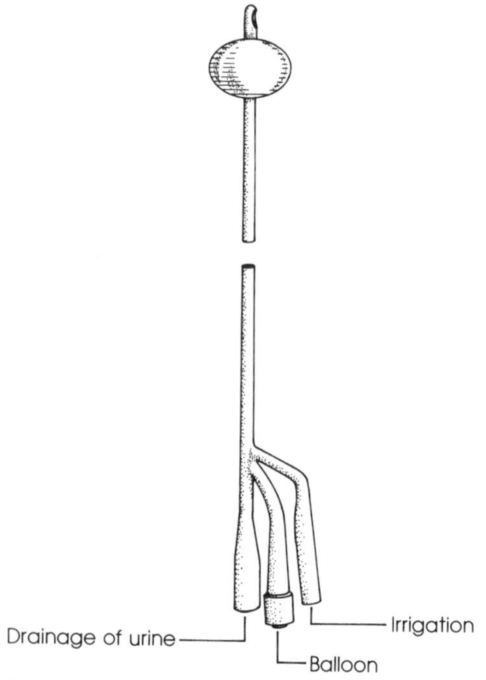

Figure 22–6 Foley catheter. Three separate lumens are incorporated within the round shaft of the catheter for drainage of urine, inflation, and introduction of irrigating solutions into the bladder.

must be reported immediately. An obstruction will continue to cause symptoms that only increase in severity if the obstruction is not relieved.

If the patient complains of pain but the output continues to flow as expected, the patient is probably experiencing bladder spasms that will subside within 48 hours after insertion of the catheter.

Before a suprapubic catheter is removed, it is clamped off periodically to encourage normal voiding. Unlike a urethral catheter, a suprapubic catheter does not interfere with voiding through the urethra.

Suprapubic catheters usually have a very small, narrow diameter. When they are removed, the site is covered with a small bandage. Healing takes place very rapidly, sealing over the site of insertion. If a catheter with a larger bore is inserted, the insertion wound may take much longer to heal.

Ureteral catheters are very small and narrow in gauge. They are inserted by the urologist directly into the ureter, usually with the aid of a cystoscope. The ureteral catheter may be attached to a urethral catheter.

Ureteral catheters are used to drain urine directly from the ureter or kidneys. They are used either to prevent or to treat hydronephrosis when an obstruction of the ureter impedes the flow of urine from the kidney pelvis. A ureteral stent (a small tube placed inside the ureter) may be inserted during cystoscopy or after surgery to maintain urine flow through the ureter and promote healing. This should be labeled "ureteral stent" so that it is not mistaken for a bladder catheter. If it is to be slowly irrigated, no more than 5 mL of lukewarm sterile saline is used.

Nephrostomy and *pyelostomy* tubes are placed directly into the kidney pelvis by way of a surgical incision over the kidneys. A nonsurgical technique for insertion of a catheter into the kidney can be done with use of local anesthesia. The tube that is used is called a *percutaneous nephrostomy tube*. As the name implies, the tube is inserted through the skin (percutaneous) and directed into the kidney to allow for drainage of urine (nephrostomy). The physician uses either fluoroscopy or ultrasonography to guide the tube to its correct location.

No large surgical incision is required, which makes this technique ideal for patients who are poor surgical risks but need urinary diversion to prevent damage to the kidney from hydronephrosis.

It should be remembered that all these tubes and catheters share a common purpose—the drainage of urine. Observations made by the nurse caring for a patient with artificial urinary drainage must include noting whether this purpose is being accomplished.

Signs of a decrease or complete cessation of urine flow and extreme discomfort from bladder distention should be reported promptly.

URINARY INCONTINENCE

Urine flow out of the bladder is controlled by two circular muscles called *sphincters*. The internal sphincter lies close to the lowermost part of the bladder, and the external sphincter surrounds the urethra. Many factors can cause loss of sphincter control. Unconsciousness, urinary tract infection, paralysis, interference with nerve transmission to and from the brain, and loss of muscle tone of the bladder and sphincters are some of the conditions that frequently cause patients to become incontinent.

Nursing Intervention

When incontinence is not remedied by correction of an underlying cause, the nurse attempts to help the patient by setting up a voiding schedule. The nurse first assesses when the patient is experiencing incontinence. By tracking the times when this occurs, she can then begin to offer a bed pan or assist the patient to the bathroom to void at set times just prior to when he is usually incontinent.

Spacing fluid intake, with the majority of fluids taken during the day, can assist in keeping the patient dry at night and make his voidings more predictable.

Getting the patient onto a voiding schedule takes a great deal of patience and persistence on the part of the nurse and the patient. However, the patient's joy at being dry is more than enough reward for the effort.

Patients often experience transient incontinence after removal of an indwelling catheter that has been in place for several days. Usually the catheter is clamped for intervals and then opened to drainage before it is removed to help rebuild bladder muscle tone. After this has been done for 12 to 24 hours, the catheter is removed. The patient should then be instructed to void every hour in order to prevent incontinence. It takes time to retrain the bladder to hold greater capacity. Gradually the interval between voidings is lengthened to 2, 3, or 4 hours. Because it is not practical to continue a frequent voiding schedule at night, external drainage is used. A condom catheter is used for males, and absorbent pads and moisture-proof pants or adult diapers can be used for women. Accidents will happen during the retraining period, and patients need to be assured that this is expected. They should be treated with kindness, not scolding.

Details of bladder training for the patient who has a neurologic problem are given in Chapter 15.

INFLAMMATORY DISORDERS OF THE URINARY TRACT

CYSTITIS

Cystitis is an inflammation of the urinary bladder. It is one of the most common urinary tract infections, especially in women, probably because the urethra is shorter in women and the urinary meatus is in proximity to the vaginal and anal areas. The *Escherichia coli* bacterium, which normally resides in the intestinal tract as a nonpathogenic microorganism, accounts for about 80% of all urinary tract infections in females.

Cystitis and urethritis are most often seen in women after they have become sexually active. It is more common in older women, its incidence increasing with age as the decreased muscle tone in the urinary tract prevents complete emptying of the bladder.

Assessment

The most common symptoms of cystitis are painful urination, frequent and urgent urination, and low back pain. The urinary meatus may appear swollen and inflamed. Cystitis has a tendency to recur, producing less acute symptoms such as fatigue, anorexia, and a constant feeling of pressure in the bladder region between flare-ups. The urine may appear cloudy or even bloody.

Urinalysis and urine cultures are used to establish a definite diagnosis and to identify the specific causative organism in cystitis.

Nursing Intervention

No one has yet found definitive proof as to how infectious organisms enter the bladder and cause cystitis. Some authorities believe the organisms travel upward through the urethra from the perineal region. Others believe that they enter the bladder via the lymphatics and blood vessels. In any case, there are some measures that can be taken to reduce the possibility of bacterial growth and resultant cystitis:

- Always wipe the anus from front to back after a bowel movement.
- Avoid wearing nylon pantyhose, tight slacks, or any clothing that increases perineal moisture.
- Do not wash underclothing in strong soap powders or bleaches; rinse clothing repeatedly until water is clear.
- Do not sit around in a wet bathing suit for long periods of time.
- Do not use bubble bath, perfumed soap, feminine hygiene sprays, or products containing hexachlorophene.
- Prolonged bicycling, motorcycling, horseback riding, or traveling involving prolonged sitting can contribute to urethritis and cystitis.
- Get into the habit of drinking at least 8 full glasses of water each day.
- Do not ignore vaginal discharge or other signs of vaginal infection. *Candida* and *Trichomonas* infections should be treated promptly to prevent their spread to the bladder.
- Empty the bladder promptly after sexual intercourse and then drink two glasses of water to help flush out microorganisms that may have entered the urethra and bladder during intercourse.

Measures to relieve the discomfort of cystitis include the application of heat in the form of sitz baths and hot water bottles on the back or directly over the bladder region.

Medical Treatment

Treatment of cystitis includes administration of either urinary antiseptics or antibacterial drugs. Table 22–3 lists the most commonly used drugs and their implications for nursing. The patient is encouraged to drink large amounts of fluids during treatment and to continue the habit once the acute symptoms subside. Vitamin C can help acidify the urine and decrease the frequency of cystitis. Drinking cranberry juice is also thought to be beneficial, as it alters urine pH.

URETHRITIS

Urethritis is an inflammation of the urethra and can be caused by many different organisms. Urethritis is one of the most common symptoms of gonorrhea, however, and should be investigated as soon as it is first noticed. Nonspecific urethritis (NSU) is a sexually transmitted inflammation of the urethra caused by a variety of organisms other than gonococci. It is thought to be the most common sexually transmitted urethritis in males in the United States, but this cannot be validated because NSU is not a reportable disease in this country. NSU usually responds to treatment with antibiotics.

Inflammatory involvement of the urethra from the herpes virus is found in males and females. In women, trauma during childbirth and the proximity of the urethra to external genitalia and the anus predispose the urethra to infection and inflammation.

TABLE 22-3 DRUGS USED FOR URINARY TRACT INFECTIONS

Drug	Features and Action	Nursing Implications
Urinary Antiseptics		
Methenamine (Cystamin, Cystogen, Urotropin, Mandelamine)	Bacteriostatic compounds of ammonia and formaldehyde.	Needs acid urine. Fluids encouraged.
Nalidixic acid (NegGram)	Effective against gram-negative organisms.	Give 1 hour a.c. to maximize blood levels.
Nitrofurantoin (Macrodantin, Furadantin)	Wide range of antibacterial action against both gram-negative and gram-positive organisms.	Tints urine brown. Give with food.
Phenazopyridine (Pyridium)	Mildly antiseptic. Has analgesic effect on urinary mucosa.	Colors urine orange.
Antiinfectives: sulfonamides		Sulfonamides potentiate oral anticoagulants, methotrexate, and hypoglycemic agents that are sulfonylureas. Force fluids.
Sulfisoxazole (Gantrisin)	Short-acting antiinfective	Protect preparations from light and moisture.
Sulfamethoxazole (Gantanol)	Intermediate-acting antiinfective.	Maintain fluid intake at minimum of 3,000 mL daily.
(Azo Gantanol)	Sulfamethoxazole combined with phenazopyride provides analgesic action.	Colors urine orange-red.
Sulfamethoxazole-trimethoprim (Bactrim, Septra)	Active against gram-negative and gram-positive organisms.	Maintain fluid intake at minimum of 3,000 mL daily. Stress need to take all of medication. Repeat urinalysis after course of medication.
Penicillins		
Ampicillin (Omnipen, Polycillin) Carbenicillin (Geocillin)	Bacteriostatic and bactericidal	Watch for signs of hypersensitivity. Do not give to patients with known allergy to penicillin.
Tetracycline Vibramycin Minocin	Long-acting antiinfective	Avoid prolonged exposure to sunlight. Do not take with milk or milk products.
Cephalosporins		
Cephalexin monohydrate (Keflex)	Well absorbed from intestinal tract and excreted 90% unchanged in the urine in 8 hours.	Used to treat infections that do not respond to other, less expensive drugs. Candidal (yeast) vaginitis is common side effect of all drugs that destroy normal vaginal flora.
Aminoglycosides (tobramycin, gentamicin)	Effective against resistant infections; used cautiously, as they are nephrotoxic.	Monitor BUN and creatine levels. Monitor for signs of ototoxicity.

Assessment

The chief symptoms of urethritis are burning, itching, frequency in voiding, and painful urination. There is a discharge, which becomes increasingly more purulent if gonorrhea is present. The urinary meatus is swollen and inflamed.

Medical Treatment and Nursing Intervention

Treatment of urethritis begins with determination of the causative organism by smear and Gram stain or culture of the discharge, and the administration of specific drugs to combat the infection. The nursing care is similar to that for the patient with cystitis. The nurse should be especially aware of the possibility of a gonorrheal infection until a definite diagnosis has been established and should carry out the necessary teaching to prevent spread of the infection to the eyes.

NEPHRITIS

Nephritis, sometimes called *Bright's disease*, refers to a general inflammation of the kidneys and the resultant degeneration of the cells. The inflammation is not the result of an invasion of bacteria and is therefore classified as a *noninfectious disease*.

Acute Glomerulonephritis

Glomerulonephritis is an immunologic problem caused by an antigen-antibody reaction and results from a variety of diseases. It most commonly occurs about 2 to 3 weeks after a group A beta-hemolytic streptococcal infection such as "strep throat" or impetigo. It is primarily seen in children and young adults and affects males more than females. The glomerular basement membrane is damaged, causing altered permeability.

Assessment

The patient with acute glomerulonephritis usually becomes ill suddenly with fever, chills, flank pain, widespread edema, puffiness about the eyes, visual disturbances, and marked hypertension. The urine may be smoky, contains red blood cells and protein, and has an increased specific gravity. The serum BUN and creatinine will rise above normal. If treatment is not successful, the disease will rapidly progress to uremia and death.

Medical Treatment and Nursing Intervention

The nurse's first responsibility in the treatment of acute glomerulonephritis is to provide rest for the kidney. Absolute bed rest is usually ordered until the clinical signs are gone. If the patient responds quickly to treatment, he may wish to be more active, and the nurse must emphasize the need for continued rest.

A sodium-restricted diet is indicated if edema is present, and fluids may be limited if there is oliguria or anuria. A low-protein, high-carbohydrate diet may be ordered. The nurse should be sure the patient understands the importance of these factors in the treatment of the disease and should do all she can to encourage his cooperation.

Edema that is obvious from external signs may very well be present in the internal organs. For this reason, the blood pressure and pulse must be checked frequently for indications of cerebral edema with increased *intracranial* pressure. Cardiac failure or pulmonary edema may also develop, and the patient must be watched closely for extreme restlessness, increased respiratory difficulty, or cyanosis. Antihypertensives and diuretics are ordered to control the hypertension and edema.

The prognosis for acute glomerulonephritis varies, depending on the extent of permanent damage done to the kidneys or other vital organs.

Chronic Glomerulonephritis

Chronic glomerulonephritis may develop rapidly or progress slowly over several years.

Assessment and Prognosis

Insidious edema, headache associated with hypertension, fatigue, and dyspnea accompany glomerulonephritis. The prognosis for this disease is ultimately poor. However, the speed with which it progresses to renal failure and uremia varies with the individual. The exact reason for this is not known. Some patients who develop chronic glomerulonephritis may have acute exacerbations (flare-ups) that subside. They may live for several years before damage to the glomeruli of the kidneys brings about the symptoms of renal failure.

Medical Treatment and Nursing Intervention

The treatment for chronic glomerulonephritis in the latent stage is primarily *symptomatic*, with emphasis on avoiding fatigue and infections, particularly of the upper respiratory tract. When renal failure develops, dialysis and possibly a kidney transplant are the only alternative modes of therapy. Chronic renal failure is discussed later in this chapter.

Nephrotic Syndrome

Nephrotic syndrome sometimes occurs after the glomeruli have been damaged by glomerulonephritis or some other disease. It is characterized by extensive proteinuria, hyperlipidemia (elevated blood lipids), hypoalbuminemia (low blood albumin), and severe edema. The outcome is variable, with some patients recovering without further incidence and others experiencing repeated episodes and eventual kidney failure.

Medical Treatment and Nursing Intervention

Treatment consists of a high-protein, low-sodium diet; diuretics; and antibiotics if infection is present. Some patients are treated with cortisone and cyclophosphamide (Cytoxan).

Nursing care includes monitoring intake and output, recording daily weight, encouraging rest, and providing excellent skin care.

Nephrosclerosis

The primary causes of nephrosclerosis are hypertension and atherosclerotic disease of the small arteries in the kidneys. As the blood supply decreases, the kidney cells degenerate and lose their ability to function. Nephrosclerosis is classified as benign or malignant, depending on the severity of the disease and the speed with which hypertensive and atherosclerotic changes occur.

Assessment

The symptoms of nephrosclerosis are similar to those of chronic glomerulonephritis and renal failure. Treatment is the same as for hypertension.

PYELONEPHRITIS

Acute pyelonephritis is an infection of the kidneys. It is thought to occur when bacteria from a bladder infection travel up the ureters to infect the kidneys. A frequent cause of pyelonephritis is an obstruction causing stasis of urine and stones that cause irritation of the tissue. Both situations provide an environment in which bacteria can grow.

Assessment

In the acute state of pyelonephritis, the symptoms include fever, chills, headache, malaise, nausea and vomiting, and pain in the flank radiating to the thigh and genitalia. The chronic phase is more often insidious, with gradual scarring of the kidney tissues. This results in loss of weight, low-grade fever, and weakness. Eventually the urine becomes loaded with bacteria and pus.

Medical Treatment and Nursing Intervention

Prompt treatment of cystitis and prevention of recurrence can help prevent acute pyelonephritis. Correction of obstruction, removal of stones, and prevention of stone formation are essential to correct chronic pyelonephritis. Bed rest, analgesics, and antipyretics are prescribed. The nurse encourages high fluid intake, records intake and output, monitors the urine for changes, and keeps the patient comfortable. Intravenous fluids may be given to flush the kidneys, especially if the patient is nauseous and vomiting.

Special diagnostic tests may be done to determine the location of the obstruction if one is suspected.

Specific drugs to destroy the bacteria are usually chosen according to the sensitivity of the causative organism, so that the most effective antibiotic is given (see Table 22–3).

The prognosis of the patient depends on the success of the treatment of the active infection before destruction and scarring of the kidney cells can occur. With chronic pyelonephritis, the patient may live for years without significant symptoms before renal damage leads to hypertension or uremia.

RENAL FAILURE

Renal failure is the inability of the kidneys to maintain normal function. Impairment of renal function affects most of the body's major systems because of the role the kidneys play in maintaining fluid balance, regulating the electrochemical composition of body fluids, providing protection against acid-base imbalance, and eliminating waste products. The kidneys also take part in red blood cell formation and regulating calcium levels and, in conjunction with the endocrine system, controlling blood pressure.

Renal failure is classified as acute or chronic. The final stages of chronic and irreversible renal failure is called *end-stage renal disease* (ESRD).

Acute renal failure occurs suddenly as a result of physical injury, infection, inflammation, or damage from toxic chemicals. Nephrotoxic agents are those that are poisonous to kidney cells and include many drugs, radiographic iodine substances used as contrast media, and heavy metals. These toxins may inflict damage on the renal tubules, causing necrosis and loss of function. They also can indirectly harm the tubules by causing severe constriction of blood vessels that serve the kidney, producing renal ischemia. Other causes of renal ischemia include circulatory collapse, severe dehydration, and prolonged hypotension in certain compromised surgical or trauma patients. Acute renal failure is potentially reversible. Often the patient regains kidney function.

Chronic renal failure is a progressive loss of kidney function that develops over the course of many months or years. In the early stages of the disease renal function can remain adequate, but the waste products normally filtered out by the kidney and excreted in the urine begin to accumulate in the plasma. The patient does not experience symptoms until about 65% of the kidney tissue is damaged. As the disease progresses, nitrogenous waste products such as urea nitrogen and creatinine build up to higher levels in the blood. In the final or end stage of renal failure,

90% or more of kidney function is lost. Chronic renal failure indicates permanent renal damage.

CAUSES OF RENAL FAILURE

Causes of renal failure can be divided into three major groups: (1) those that directly affect kidney cells by infection, inflammation, and upper urinary tract obstruction; (2) those in which there is an obstruction in the lower urinary tract; and (3) systemic diseases and toxic states such as hypokalemia, hypercalcemia, hypertension, diabetes mellitus, heart failure, and cirrhosis of the liver. The most common causes of chronic renal failure are glomerulonephritis and nephrosclerosis. Diabetic nephropathy (pathologic condition of the kidney associated with diabetes mellitus) is the third major cause of chronic renal failure and the most common cause of death in patients with diabetes mellitus.

MEDICAL DIAGNOSIS

The physician uses a variety of diagnostic tests and procedures to establish a diagnosis of renal failure. A renal biopsy sometimes is done to identify the specific cause, because there are some patients in whom the original cause cannot be identified in any other way.

Evaluation of kidney function is usually based on measurements of creatinine clearance. Clearance is the volume of plasma that can be cleared of a substance by the kidneys in a given period of time. It is also a reflection of the flow of plasma through the renal circulation, which can be severely impeded by narrowing of the renal arterioles. Effective clearance depends on the ability of the renal tubular cells to handle substances that have been filtered by the glomeruli. Determining the blood urea nitrogen (BUN) level and the serum creatinine are the two tests most often used to screen for kidney problems. Measurement of creatinine clearance involves collection of a 12-hour or 24-hour urine specimen.

The symptoms of chronic renal failure do not appear early in the disease. Renal insufficiency, which occurs before renal failure, can produce occasional headaches and fatigue, but these symptoms usually either go unnoticed or are not reported by the patient. At this point in the process kidney function is about 75% of normal. When symptoms do become apparent, kidney function can be as little as 5% to 10% of normal.

The symptoms of end-stage renal disease constitute a syndrome called *uremia*. Clinical signs and symptoms of uremia are manifestations of pathologic changes in the various body systems and depend on the extent of these changes and the degree of renal impairment.

One of the earliest signs of renal impairment is inability of the kidneys to concentrate urine. This produces polyuria and a very dilute urine. The patient may complain of having to get up frequently during the night to urinate (nocturia). Later on, as renal insufficiency progresses, the kidneys may not be able to produce much urine at all. This causes oliguria and eventually anuria.

The systemic effects of uremia are manifested in virtually every body system. These effects and some of their clinical manifestations are shown in Figure 22-7.

MEDICAL TREATMENT

The major goal of treatment in cases of* acute *renal failure is to restore and maintain a tolerable internal environment until the kidneys are able to recover and resume their normal functions.

Symptomatic treatment includes measures to maintain fluid and electrolyte balances, manage the accompanying anemia and hypertension, and cleanse the blood and tissues of uremic waste products with peritoneal dialysis or hemodialysis.

Management of chronic renal failure is highly complex because of the impact kidney failure has on homeostasis and major body systems. Medical treatment and nursing intervention include measures to correct fluid and electrolyte imbalance and acid-base imbalance whenever possible. Renal dialysis, which is discussed later, and kidney transplant are two major alternatives that offer hope to the patient with end-stage renal failure.

NURSING ASSESSMENT AND INTERVENTION

Appropriate medical and nursing intervention for the management of renal insufficiency and renal failure can help patients remain relatively free of symptoms until the final stages of renal failure. The accomplishment of this goal requires cooperative effort on the part of every person on the health care team, including the patient and his family.

A major role of the nurse is assessment of the patient's health status throughout the course of his illness and of his learning needs to help him manage his symptoms and prevent further damage whenever possible. A thorough and careful nursing assessment can lead to accurate identification of specific nursing diagnoses. Some of the nursing care problems likely to occur with renal insufficiency and failure are summarized in Nursing Care Plan 22-1. Assessment and nursing intervention for many of these nursing diagnoses have already been covered earlier in this text. For example, anemia, bleeding tendency, and susceptibility to infection are discussed in Chapter 18; nausea, vomiting, anorexia, gastrointesti-

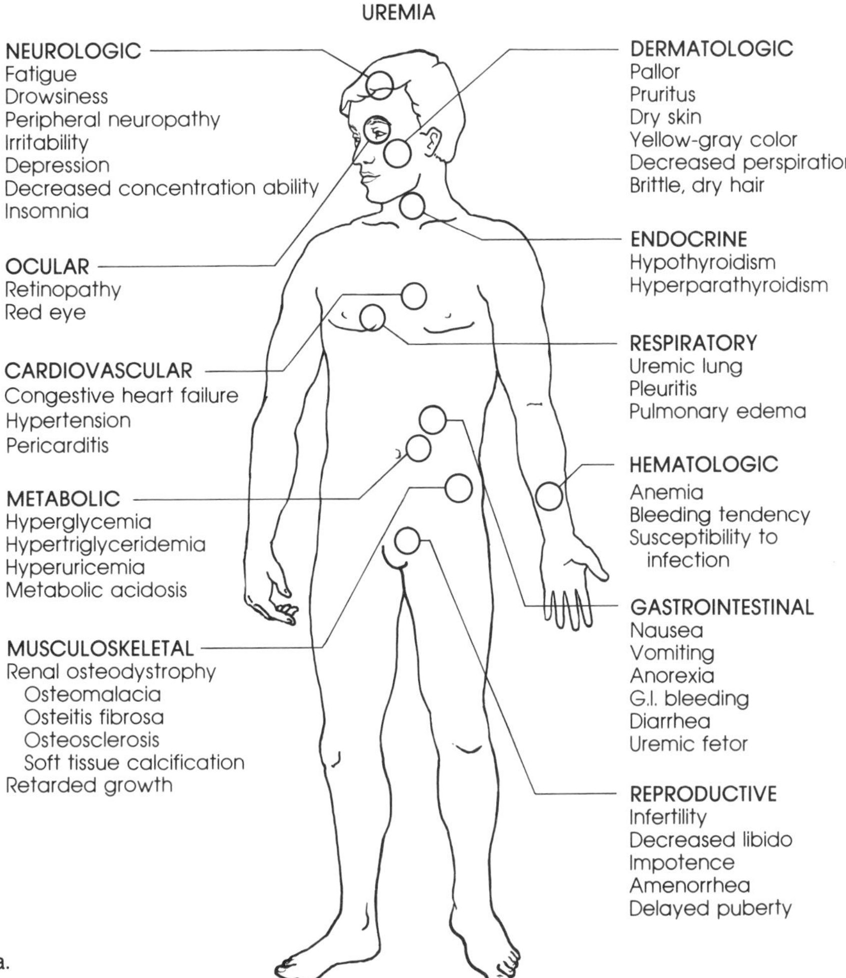

Figure 22-7 Systemic effects of uremia.

nal bleeding, and other gastrointestinal problems are covered in Chapter 23.

Because fluid and electrolyte balance are major concerns in the management of renal failure, the nurse must be especially aware of hydration status. Daily weight, measurement of intake and output, determining the pattern of urination, and restricting fluid are essential to the well-being of the patient with renal damage.

In addition to these rather basic procedures, the nursing care plan should include monitoring the serum levels of electrolytes, blood urea nitrogen, and creatinine. The presence of accumulations of these nitrogenous products is called *azotemia*. This condition requires frequent monitoring of the patient for nausea and vomiting and changes in mental awareness and levels of consciousness.

High levels of serum potassium (5 to 7 mEq/L) can adversely affect the heart, causing arrhythmia and arrest. By watching for earlier signs of hyperkalemia and promptly reporting them, the nurse can help avoid serious cardiovascular problems.

The patient with end-stage renal disease does not absorb calcium from the intestinal tract. This causes a loss of calcium from the body and a corresponding drop in serum calcium. If the hypocalcemia is not corrected, the patient will eventually suffer from muscle cramps, twitching, and possibly seizures.

As kidney cells cease to function they are less and less able to secrete phosphorus in the urine. This results in an elevated serum phosphate level (hyperphosphatemia), which only serves to exaggerate the problem of inadequate calcium absorption. That is because phosphate binds with the calcium, making its absorption from the intestinal tract even less likely to occur.

Specific electrolyte imbalances, their symptoms, and nursing intervention for imbalances are discussed in Chapter 8.

Maintaining adequate nutrition for the patient with chronic renal failure is a very real challenge. Because of the buildup of nitrogenous wastes from protein metabolism, restriction of protein intake is necessary. The reduced intake of protein requires that only high-quality protein

NURSING CARE PLAN 22–1

Nursing diagnoses, goals/outcome criteria, nursing interventions, and evaluations for a patient with chronic renal disease

Situation: Mrs. Chavez, age 55, is admitted to the hospital for renal evaluation after having noticed blood in her urine and a feeling of abdominal fullness and "bloating." Her mother died of kidney disease, and her older brother is currently on dialysis for renal failure.

During nursing assessment the patient stated that she felt "tired all the time," had shortness of breath and swelling in her feet and ankles, awakened frequently at night to urinate, and had many headaches. She said that she was "worried that I've got the same thing that killed my mother and has made my brother sick."

At the time of admission her blood pressure was 180/120, her hemoglobin was 8 gm per 100 mL, and her hematocrit was 20%.

Nursing Diagnosis	Goals/Outcome Criteria	Nursing Intervention	Evaluation
Potential for injury related to abnormal blood pressure. SUPPORTING DATA BP, 180/120; headaches; fatigue.	Blood pressure will be reduced to 150/88 within 36 hours. Blood pressure will be maintained at 140/80 within 7 days.	Take vital signs q 2 h in sitting, lying, and standing positions until diastolic is below 100, then q 4 h. Administer antihypertensive as ordered. Teach her to take own blood pressure. Observe for adverse side effects of medications.	BP still 160/108 at 2 P.M.; antihypertensive and diuretic given this A.M.; began instruction on taking BP; discussed side effects of medications; continue plan.
Fluid imbalance, excess, related to retention of sodium and water. SUPPORTING DATA Edema of feet and ankles; shortness of breath and crackles in lungs; weight up 7 lb in 1 week.	Lungs will be clear to auscultation within 36 hours. Weight will return to previous level (136 lb) within 10 days. Foot and ankle edema will show decrease by measurement within 24 hours. No evidence of foot and ankle edema within 7 days.	Record objective assessment of foot and ankle edema. Administer diuretic as ordered. Restrict fluid intake to 1,200 mL/24 hours as ordered. Restrict sodium to 2 gm/day as ordered. Obtain daily weight before breakfast and record. Auscultate lungs q shift. Assess for shortness of breath q shift. Assist her to establish acceptable schedule for restricted fluids. Explain reason for fluid restriction. Provide hard candy and gum; give mouth care q 2 h. Carefully measure and record intake and output.	Edema of feet and ankles, 2+; weight down 1.5 lb; lungs: few crackles in right base; complaining about fluid restriction but intake = 400 mL this shift; using hard candy; intake, 400 mL; output, 1,200 mL; continue plan.
Activity intolerance related to decreased hemoglobin and hematocrit. SUPPORTING DATA Hemoglobin, 8 gm/100 mL; hematocrit, 20%; states she is tired all the time.	Hemoglobin will increase to 11 gm/100 mL by discharge. Hematocrit will increase to 28% by discharge. Fatigue will be lessened as judged by patient.	Transfuse with blood product if ordered; monitor for adverse effects. Administer ferrous sulfate and folic acid as ordered. Instruct about foods with high iron content. Monitor urine for blood. Alternate periods of activity with adequate rest.	Order changed from blood transfusion to Epogen injections; instructed regarding foods high in iron; trace blood in urine; Hgb, 8.2 gm/100 mL; hematocrit, 26%; still tired; plan: give Epogen as ordered, monitor Hgb and hematocrit.
Knowledge deficit related to scheduled diagnostic tests and side effects of drugs ordered. SUPPORTING DATA Cannot identify side effects of drugs ordered; unfamiliar with diagnostic tests ordered.	Patient will be able to identify common side effects of drugs prescribed by time of discharge. Patient will verbalize purpose of each diagnostic test and the preparation requirements before the test is performed.	Create teaching plan for side effects and purpose of each drug prescribed; perform teaching in short sessions; obtain feedback for evaluation of comprehension. Explain the purpose and preparation requirements for each diagnostic test ahead of time. Obtain feedback for evaluation of comprehension.	Began teaching regarding medications; prepared for cystoscopy and IVP; verbalizes purpose and what she will experience during diagnostic tests; continue plan.

NURSING CARE PLAN 22–1, *Continued*

Nursing Diagnosis	Goals/Outcome Criteria	Nursing Intervention	Evaluation
Fear of malignancy, renal failure, and death. SUPPORTING DATA States she is afraid she has malignancy and renal failure and that she will die.	Patient will begin to talk about her fear of renal failure and death within 36 hours. Patient will verbalize her specific fears about dialysis, before it is instituted.	Establish trusting relationship. Encourage verbalization of feelings. Provide information on chronic renal failure and treatment options—peritoneal dialysis, hemodialysis, renal transplant. Emphasize that good quality of life can be attained with dialysis.	Verbalizing fears of becoming dependent on dialysis and of death from renal failure; discussed options if dialysis is necessary; continue plan.

foods be used in the diet. These include meat, eggs, milk, and cheese, which provide all of the essential amino acids in relatively small servings.

Potassium restriction is also necessary because of the inability of the kidney to excrete it. Sodium is often restricted, especially if the patient is hypertensive. Phosphate binders (basic aluminum carbonate [Basalgel]) are given with meals to prevent the absorption of phosphorus.

The multiplicity of diet restrictions and modifications makes understanding and compliance very difficult for the patient. The expertise of nutritionists and other professionals is needed to help accomplish the goals of (1) minimizing uremic toxicity, (2) maintaining acceptable electrolyte levels, (3) controlling hypertension, (4) providing sufficient calories, and (5) maintaining good nutritional status.

RENAL DIALYSIS

Hemodialysis and peritoneal dialysis are two procedures commonly used to remove waste products normally excreted by the kidneys.

Both procedures employ the effect of diffusion to remove elements normally excreted in the urine. The principle of diffusion states that *solute* molecules that are in constant motion tend to pass through a semipermeable membrane from the side of higher concentration to the side of lower concentration.

Hemodialysis

Hemodialysis removes nitrogenous waste products from the blood by pumping the blood from the arterial circulation through a dialysate bath and back to the venous circulation. A dialysis membrane separates the blood from the dialyzing solution. The molecules of waste pass through this membrane out of the blood and into the dialyzing solution until the two solutions are equal in concentration (Fig. 22–8).

Two kinds of shunts are used to withdraw arterial blood, bathe it in dialyzing solution, and return it to the venous system. In one, an external cannula is inserted into an artery, and a similar cannula is inserted into a vein. The tips of both are sutured in place. A part of each cannula is tunneled into the blood vessel. Between dialysis treatments, the tubes are joined by a connector (Fig. 22–9). This external shunt can only be used for 6 to 9 months.

A temporary access for hemodialysis can be achieved by insertion of a subclavian or femoral vein dialysis catheter and is more commonly used than an external shunt.

The second kind of arteriovenous (AV) shunt is accomplished by anastomosing a vein to an artery. In other words, the vein is "arterialized"; that is, it is made into a large superficial vein with an arterial supply that is easily accessible by venipuncture (Fig. 22–10). If the veins are not strong enough for arterialization, natural or synthetic materials can be used as a graft to strengthen the anastomosis. This kind of shunt is more permanent than the external shunt and is usually the type used because of its advantages over the use of cannulas.

When caring for the hospitalized patient who has an arteriovenous graft, it is important to protect the graft from injury and check its status. The site should be observed at least four times a day for signs of clotting or infection, and the fingers of the arm with the graft should be checked for adequate circulation. The arm or leg in which the arteriovenous shunt has been created should not be used for checking blood pressure or performing venipuncture.

The scheduling of hemodialysis sessions varies from patient to patient, but treatments usually are done two to three times a week. The problems that a patient on hemodialysis may experience include fluid overload (hypervolemia), electrolyte imbalance, alterations in blood components leading to anemia, and platelet abnormalities that produce a tendency to bleed abnormally. Other major problems are infection in either the access site or the blood.

Medications frequently prescribed for the dial-

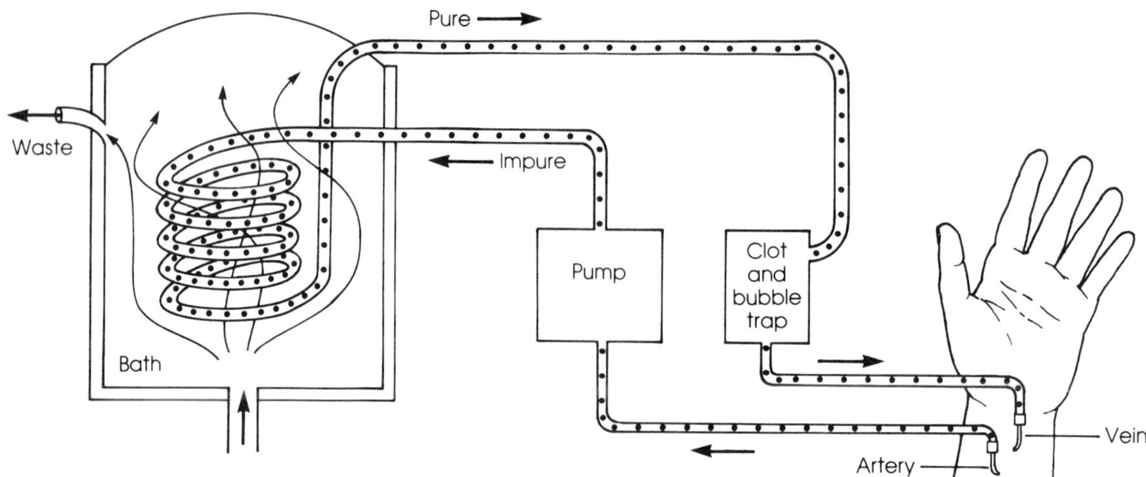

Figure 22-8 Schematic diagram of hemodialysis.
(From Jacob, S. W., and Francone, C. A.: Structure and Function in Man, 4th ed. Philadelphia, W. B. Saunders, 1978.)

ysis patient include multivitamins, antacids, iron supplements, antihypertensives, digitalis, vasodilators, cimetadine, and phosphate binders. A new drug, Epogen, is a synthetic substance that stimulates red blood cell production. It is given to combat the suppression of natural erythropoietin that occurs in renal failure. Antihypertensive drugs are not given the morning of dialysis, as they can cause severe hypotension during the treatment.

Patients who depend on hemodialysis for survival require extensive instruction in the care of their cannulas and access sites. They also must understand the rationale for various fluid and food restrictions and the medications prescribed. Patient compliance is a major challenge to nurses who care for patients on dialysis.

Hepatitis and acquired immunodeficiency syndrome (AIDS) are constant dangers because of the number of transfusions needed and because of the exposure to multi-user dialysis machines. Patients who had multiple transfusions before the time when reliable testing of blood for the human immunodeficiency virus (HIV) may have been exposed to the virus. It can take 5 years or more before signs of infection with HIV is detectable.

Perhaps an even greater challenge for the nurse is helping dialysis-dependent patients cope with the stress of prolonged intensive treatment and the frustrations of dealing with an incurable illness. Rigid dietary restrictions, limited mobility, and possibly sexual difficulties take their toll on the patient as well as his significant others.

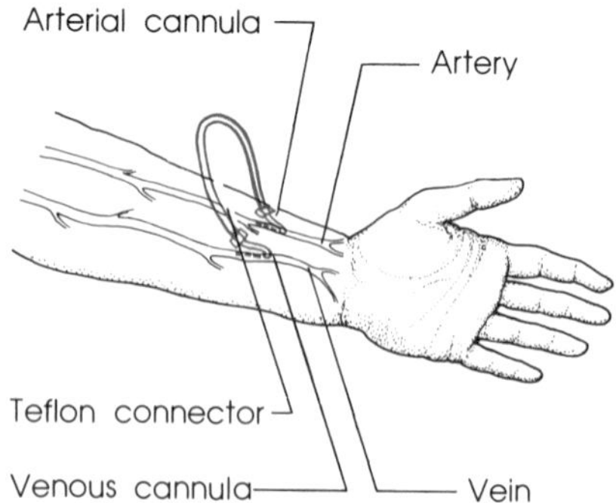

Figure 22-9 Arteriovenous shunt provides a means for drawing blood directly from an artery and returning the dialyzed blood to a vein in a similar manner. A portion of each cannula is tunneled under the skin, with the remainder exposed outside the skin. Between dialysis treatments the two cannulas are joined by a Teflon connecting tube. Because of its potential for complications, an arteriovenous shunt is a temporary measure, as for acute dialysis or while waiting for maturation of an arterialized vein.

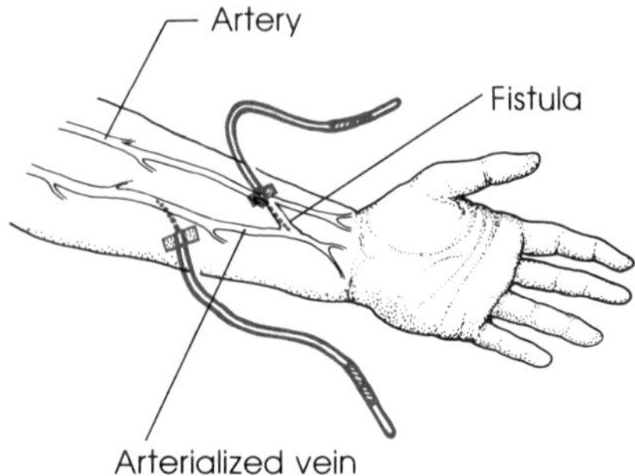

Figure 22-10 Arterialized vein (arteriovenous fistula). An internal shunt is created by anastomosing an adjacent vein and artery. This provides an enlarged superficial vein with an arterial blood supply that is easily accessible by venipuncture. Two catheters may be used: one for the flow of blood to the dialyzer and the other for return of dialyzed blood. The arterialized vein is more satisfactory for chronic dialysis than is the arteriovenous shunt.

Family members usually are profoundly affected by the patient's chronic illness and the demands long-term dialysis places on them. Their needs, as well as the patient's, are part of planning nursing intervention. The major goals of nursing care are to facilitate acceptance of the diagnosis of chronic renal failure and adaptation to dialysis treatment.

Guidelines for facilitating positive adaptation to dialysis are as follows:

- Enhance nursing assessment and observation skills and keep abreast of all aspects of dialysis treatment.
- Genuinely care for the patient, accepting him as an individual and allowing him to realize his full human potential.
- Practice empathetic listening and provide opportunities for the patient to express his feelings.
- Monitor verbal and nonverbal behavior that might indicate depression or suicidal behavior.
- Work closely with the family to assess the impact the patient's illness and treatment is having on them. Encourage them to achieve a balance between supporting the patient and allowing him to remain as independent as possible. Encourage communication between patient and spouse to express feelings about changes in sexual activities, role reversal, and family responsibilities.
- Examine personal feelings about patient rights, adaptation to stress, and allowing a patient to die with dignity.

Postdialysis nursing care includes monitoring the access site for bleeding, assessing the patient for signs of confusion or disorientation, monitoring vital signs, and continuing assessment of the access site for patency and signs of infection.

Peritoneal Dialysis

Peritoneal dialysis is an alternative procedure that can be used instead of hemodialysis to remove waste products or toxins that have accumulated as a result of renal failure. Peritoneal dialysis operates on the same principles as hemodialysis, the difference being that in this procedure the semipermeable membrane is in the peritoneum and the dialyzing solution is introduced into and withdrawn from the peritoneal cavity.

Peritoneal dialysis has the advantages of being initiated more quickly than hemodialysis because there is no need for a dialyzing apparatus, anticoagulants are not necessary, and cannulization of blood vessels is not required. And, because chemical and fluid exchanges occur more slowly in peritoneal dialysis, there is less stress on the cardiovascular system.

Acute and chronic renal failure can both be treated with peritoneal dialysis. Some patients with renal failure fare better on a gentler dialytic therapy. With new developments in equipment, it is possible for a patient to have intermittent or continuous peritoneal ambulatory dialysis or continuous cycling peritoneal dialysis at night. The patient is taught to operate a portable, manual device, and to perform his own dialysis as often as necessary to manage his disease and prevent symptoms. Figure 22-11 shows the basic steps of continuous ambulatory peritoneal dialysis.

Peritoneal dialysis cannot be done when there

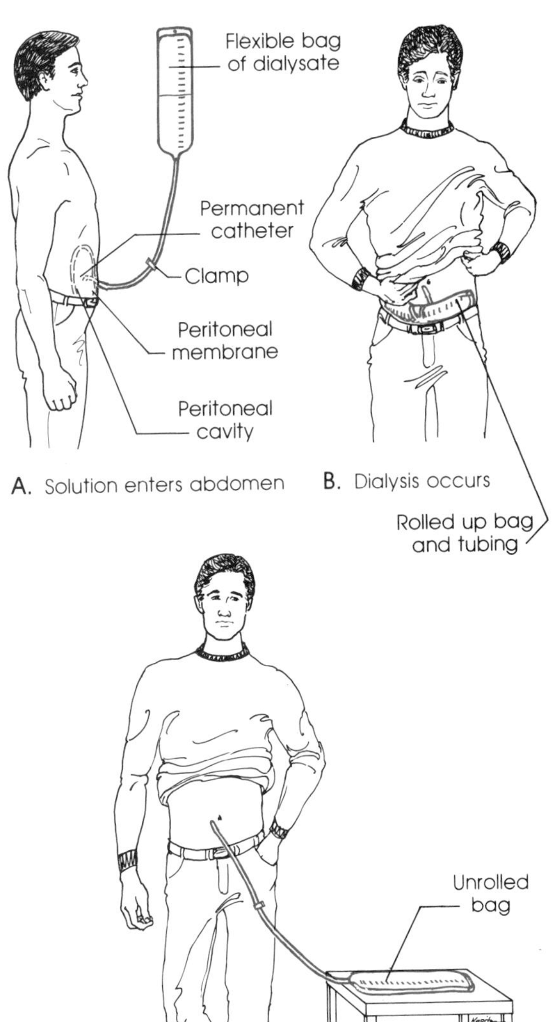

Figure 22-11 Basic steps for continuous ambulatory dialysis. *A*, The bag of dialyzing solution is suspended above the level of the abdomen. The clamp on the tubing attached to a permanent catheter in the abdomen is opened, allowing the solution to enter the abdominal cavity by gravity flow. *B*, After the solution is deposited in the abdomen, the bag can be rolled up and secured during the "dwell time." The patient is then free to move about while dialysis occurs. *C*, At the end of the dwell time, the bag is unrolled and placed below the level of the abdomen. This permits drainage of the dialysate (which now contains waste products) from the abdominal cavity.

is severe trauma to the abdomen, after multiple abdominal procedures have been done, if there are adhesions in the abdominal cavity, or if the patient has a severe coagulation defect, paralytic ileus, or diffuse peritonitis.

During the procedure, fluid equal in osmolarity and similar in composition to normal body fluid is introduced into the peritoneal cavity via a catheter. The fluid infuses by gravity; its rate of flow can be controlled by lowering or raising the container of dialysate or by manipulating a clamp on the tubing.

The solution is left in the peritoneal cavity a specified period of time (dwell time) until the concentrations of the solutions on either side of the membrane are equalized. After the solution has remained in the peritoneal cavity the correct period of time, the fluid is drained from the cavity. This either completes the dialysis or prepares the cavity for instillation of fresh dialysate.

Complications such as peritonitis, leakage, obstruction or other problems with the catheter, respiratory problems, and fluid overload can occur.

Specific nursing care for the patient having peritoneal dialysis includes obtaining the patient's weight before and after the treatment; maintaining careful intake and output records; maintaining strict aseptic technique in handling the dialysate bags, peritoneal catheter, and all equipment; monitoring vital signs; observing for complications such as peritonitis; and keeping the patient as comfortable as possible. The solution should be at room temperature and must be instilled slowly. The patient and family are taught all the steps of the procedure before discharge.

Continuous Hemofiltration

Another method of treatment for renal failure is continuous arteriovenous hemofiltration (CAVH). The patient's own blood pressure gradient is used for filtration. The same type of access is used as for hemodialysis, but no special dialysis machine is needed. The arterial blood passes through a special hollow-fiber filter and returns to the vein. This method filters out wastes much more slowly than hemodialysis but does not cause such rapid fluid and electrolyte shifts. CAVH may be used for 30 to 40 days.

KIDNEY TRANSPLANTATION

Currently, the expected life span for many patients on chronic dialysis is about 12 years. An alternative to this form of treatment for renal failure is to transplant a kidney from a relative of the patient or from a cadaver whose kidney tissue is compatible with that of the recipient.

Tissue typing to determine donor-recipient compatibility is done along with extensive psychological assessment and counseling for both the live donor and the recipient. The closer the tissue match, the greater the chance of successful retention of the kidney.

Hypertension is brought under the best possible control, any infection is treated, and the patient is dialyzed immediately before transplantation. Immunosuppressive drugs are started and are continued postoperatively in decreasing dosages to prevent rejection of the organ. Long-term problems for transplant patients are increased susceptibility to infection and a 35% higher risk of malignancy, both directly related to the necessary immunosuppressive therapy.

Renal transplant patients are transferred to critical care or specialty units after surgery, where they are closely monitored for signs of rejection: fever, increased blood pressure, and pain over the iliac fossa where the new kidney was placed. Ongoing assessment includes watching for the signs of renal failure, particularly oliguria, anuria, and rising BUN levels and serum creatinine. Protection from sources of infection is a top priority. Once the new kidney is functioning properly, the primary physician may lift the previous dietary restrictions.

Renal failure and dialysis are very expensive for the patient and his family. However, lack of funds does not exclude anyone from needed care. Since July, 1973, an amendment to the Social Security Act allows Medicare to pay 80% of the cost of treating end-stage renal disease including dialysis and renal transplant.

OBSTRUCTIONS OF THE URINARY TRACT

HYDRONEPHROSIS

Whenever the normal flow of urine is obstructed, there follows a backward flow of fluid into the renal pelvis. If this condition is not relieved by removal of the obstruction, the kidney will become dilated and continue to fill with fluid. Soon, the kidney cells will atrophy until all normal function ceases and the kidney becomes merely a thin, walled cyst. This condition is known as *hydronephrosis*. It can eventually result in complete destruction of the kidneys. Hydronephrosis may be *unilateral* or *bilateral* (one or both kidneys). If it occurs only on one side, the other kidney may enlarge and efficiently carry on the work of two kidneys. This is called *compensatory hypertrophy*.

Symptoms and Medical Diagnosis

Severe pain is present only if hydronephrosis develops rapidly. Otherwise, there are no outstanding symptoms, and the patient may develop signs of uremia only after serious damage has occurred. A definitive diagnosis is obtained by extensive urologic examination and detailed radiologic studies of the kidney and ureters, which usually reveal the site and cause of obstruction and distention of the renal pelvis.

Surgical Treatment and Nursing Intervention

The primary goal of treatment for hydronephrosis is removal of the obstruction so the kidney may drain properly. The ideal remedy is to drain the kidney in the early stages with a nephrostomy tube. If the damage is irreparable, surgery is necessary to remove the damaged kidney (nephrectomy).

Nursing care of the patient with hydronephrosis is concerned with close observation and accurate reporting of urinary output and early signs of impending uremia. If nephrectomy is performed, the nursing care is the same as for any patient with kidney surgery.

RENAL STONES

A renal or kidney stone is a crystalline mass that forms in the urinary system. Stones can be as small as a grain of sand or quite large. Renal stones also vary in composition and in the environment in which they form. Some stones form more readily in an acid urine, whereas others occur in alkaline urine.

There are four major types of renal stones. Table 22-4 shows a description of each type, whether they are radiopaque (that is, will show up on radiographs), and the effect urinary pH has on their formation.

Identifying the type and cause of particular kinds of stones can be very effective in preventing further formation and deciding the appropriate method of treatment for each patient. However, in about half the cases the precise cause of stone formation cannot be identified. It is known, however, that certain conditions predispose a person to renal calculi.

Causative Factors

Among the most common causative factors are: (1) supersaturation of the urine with crystalloids that do not readily dissolve (for example, calcium, uric acid, and cystine); (2) urinary infections, which produce bacteria and other debris in the urine that form the core around which a stone can form; (3) inadequate fluid intake, which leaves the urine concentrated and does not allow for adequate flushing of the urinary tract; (4) sluggish flow of urine; and (5) certain substances in the urine (for example, urate, which encourages the formation of crystals of calcium oxalate or calcium phosphate).

Prevention

An essential factor in preventing stone formation is high fluid intake to prevent urinary stasis. A continuous flow of dilute urine flushes the tract and removes substances that could form stones. In order to prevent stone formation by diluting the urine, the adult must put out almost 4,000 mL of urine every 24 hours.

Prevention of urinary infections and maintaining adequate drainage when tubes and catheters

TABLE 22-4 COMPARISON OF TYPES OF RENAL STONES

Type	Appearance	Radiopacity	Urinary pH
Calcium stones			
Calcium oxalate	Small, rough, dark in color; covered with sharp spicules	Opaque	Formation not dependent on pH
Calcium phosphate	Soft or hard; yellow-brown; often form staghorn masses	Very opaque	Soluble in acidic urine
Struvite stones	Yellowish; break apart easily	Moderately opaque	Maintain urine pH below 6.5
Uric acid stones	Small, hard; yellow to reddish brown; may be multiple	Nonopaque on plain films; show as filling defect on IVP	Form only in acid urine
Cystine	Light yellow or yellow-brown	Slightly opaque	Form only in acid urine

Adapted from Metheny, N.: Renal stones and urinary pH. Am. J. Nurs., Sept., 1982, p. 1372.

are in place also can help prevent stone formation. In those cases in which the urine pH is crucial to stone formation, changing the pH to a less favorable level can prevent or reduce the incidence of renal calculi.

A very small percentage of patients with calcium stones have a tumor of the parathyroid. This gland produces a hormone that raises the level of serum calcium and thus calcium in the urine. Treatment of the parathyroid condition removes the cause of the stones.

Treatment and prevention of the recurrence of renal stones must be based on identification of the specific type of stone being produced.

Symptoms and Medical Diagnosis

Some renal stones do not cause noticeable symptoms and can be passed without the person being aware of them. Others may lodge in the renal pelvis and cause symptoms only after they begin to destroy kidney cells. The stones that cause the severe pain typically associated with kidney stones are those that are small enough to be moved along the ureter with the urine. Moving stones can get trapped somewhere along the ureter, causing obstruction to the flow of urine and swelling of the ureter.

Many renal stones have sharp little spikes, or spicules, on their surface. As a stone rolls along the ureter, it can scrape the ureteral lining, causing excruciating pain and bleeding. The pain is typically felt in the flank over the affected kidney and ureter, and radiates downward toward the genitalia and inner thigh. Nausea and vomiting often occur because of the severity of the pain.

Diagnostic tests include urinalysis and x-ray studies to locate stones that are radiopaque and an intravenous pyelogram (IVP) to find those that are not. The IVP will not show the stone itself, but there will be gap in the stream of dye being excreted in the urine. Once the stone has been found and dealt with, further studies of the blood and urine might be done to determine the levels of substances such as calcium, uric acid, and cystine that can form stones.

Medical and Surgical Treatment

At first, the physician may try to flush the stone out by increasing the patient's fluid intake and managing pain by prescribing analgesics and antispasmodics such as propantheline bromide (Pro-Banthine) or oxybutynin chloride (Ditropan). Fluids may be administered intravenously to augment oral intake. If there are pus cells in the urine, an antibiotic is prescribed to deal with infection.

When the stone is not passed spontaneously, surgical intervention is necessary. Some stones can be broken up and dissolved by irrigation through a ureteral catheter or percutaneous nephrostomy tube or crushed by use of ultrasound. Extracorporeal shock wave lithotripsy (ESWL) has largely replaced surgery for renal stones. Newer refinements of this form of ultrasound are occurring frequently. The latest technique is percutaneous ultrasonic lithotripsy, which can pulverize larger stones than can ESWL. Others require cystoscopy and surgical removal of the stone. Extremely large stones in the renal pelvis require surgical excision from the kidney.

Once stones have been removed, chemical analyses of the urine, blood, and the stone itself are necessary to plan effective preventive measures for the future.

Nursing Assessment and Intervention

Patients most at risk for kidney stone formation include:

- Males, who are much more at risk than women for development of calcium stones.
- Those who have a family history of renal stones.
- Those who have had intestinal bypass surgery for obesity. They absorb too much oxalate from foods; this oxalate is excreted in the urine and sets up conditions for formation of calcium oxalate stones.
- Those who are immobilized for any reason and are in danger of urinary stasis.
- Those who have recurrent urinary infections. During initial assessment of a patient with kidney stones, the nurse will need to gather information about changes in urinary output, characteristics of the urine, and other assessment data presented earlier in this chapter.

While attempts are made to have the patient pass the stone spontaneously, all urine is strained to recover the stone or fragments of it for analysis. Fluids are forced during this time to encourage removal of the stone without surgery.

Nursing interventions for selected problems in a patient with a renal stone are summarized in Nursing Care Plan 22–2. Nursing measures to prevent further stone formation include the following:

- Teach the patient the reason for forcing fluids to the point that 4,000 mL (about 4 quarts) of urine are excreted every 24 hours.
- Explain the reason for dietary restrictions to alter urinary pH or minimize the intake of substances that encourage a particular kind of stone to form.
- Encourage patient to take daily medication if one is prescribed; for example, allopurinol to decrease formation of uric acid or potassium citrate (Urocit) to alter urine pH.

NURSING CARE PLAN 22–2

Selected nursing diagnoses, goals/outcome criteria, nursing interventions, and evaluations for a patient with a renal stone

Situation: Herbert Simpson, 29 years old, has been admitted with severe flank pain radiating downward into the scrotum, a history of renal stone formation, and blood-tinged urine.

Nursing Diagnosis	Goals/Outcome Criteria	Nursing Intervention	Evaluation
Pain related to ureteral spasm. SUPPORTING DATA Severe flank pain.	Pain will be controlled with analgesia within 2 hours. No pain at time of discharge as verbalized by patient.	Administer analgesic as ordered; assess for effectiveness within 30 to 60 minutes; assess for side effects.	Obtaining good pain control with analgesic; Demerol 50 mg IM at 8 A.M., 11 A.M., and 2:20 P.M.; continue plan.
Potential alteration in urinary elimination related to obstruction of flow. SUPPORTING DATA Flank pain indicative of ureteral stone; history of stone formation; blood-tinged urine.	Stone will be passed within 24 hours. No signs of hydronephrosis evident at time of discharge.	Force fluids to 3,000 to 4,000 mL in each 24 hours. Strain all urine. Send any stones to laboratory for analysis. Assess characteristics of urine; have patient stand to void.	Taking 8 oz fluids q h; straining urine; no sign of stone yet; urine dark amber; continue plan.
Potential for urinary tract infection related to disruption in urinary system. SUPPORTING DATA Blood-tinged urine; flank pain indicative of stone.	Urinalysis will show no abnormality at discharge. Temperature will be within normal limits at discharge.	Force fluids. Administer prophylactic antimicrobial agent as ordered. Monitor temperature; instruct to report chills or dysuria.	Forcing fluids; temperature normal; urine not cloudy; odor normal; continue plan.
Knowledge deficit related to prescribed regimen to prevent renal stone formation. SUPPORTING DATA Cannot verbalize need for increased fluids daily, foods to avoid in diet.	Patient will verbalize rationale for intake of 3,000 to 4,000 mL of fluid per day within 24 hours. Patient will verbalize foods to avoid in diet before discharge. Patient will not experience stone recurrence in next 5 years.	Explain rationale for high fluid intake. Reinforce dietitian's dietary instructions to alter urine pH and prevent stone formation. Explain rationale and action of medication ordered to alter urine pH.	Discussed need for continuous high fluid intake after discharge; dietitian to see patient; continue plan.

- Prevent urinary tract infections by meticulous catheter care, adequate fluid intake in immobilized patients, and maintenance of urinary flow in patients with urinary diversion appliances.
- Encourage prompt reporting and treatment of urinary tract infections.

NEOPLASMS OF THE KIDNEY

Neoplasms of the kidney are fairly uncommon, actually constituting less than 1% of all malignant tumors of the body. They are, however, nearly always cancerous and are extremely difficult to treat in the later stages. Except for Wilms' tumors, which occur in infants and small children, neoplasms of the kidney occur mostly in middle life.

SYMPTOMS AND MEDICAL DIAGNOSIS

The principal symptom of malignant tumors of the kidney is *hematuria* (blood in the urine), which is usually not accompanied by pain in the early stages. The affected kidney may be enlarged. Tests such as the renal angiogram, arteriogram, computed tomographic and MRI scans and those using ultrasound are performed to determine whether the symptoms are being caused by a cyst (nonmalignant) or a tumor.

TREATMENT AND NURSING INTERVENTION

The only treatment that has met with any degree of success is surgical removal of the affected kidney before *metastasis* has occurred. Unfortunately, this is difficult to achieve, because the patient usually does not have symptoms severe enough to send him to the doctor until metastases have occurred. Postoperative radiation is sometimes used to deter further involvement after nephrectomy.

Nursing care of the patient is the same as that for patients receiving radiation therapy and postoperative care following nephrectomy, as discussed in the following section.

CARE OF THE PATIENT WHO HAS HAD SURGERY OF THE KIDNEY

TYPES OF SURGERY

The two main types of surgical procedures that may be performed on the kidney are *nephrectomy* and *nephrostomy.*

Nephrectomy is the surgical removal of the kidney. Although this is always a serious operation, a person may live with only one kidney. The remaining kidney enlarges and is usually able to carry on the work formerly done by two kidneys.

Nephrostomy is a surgical incision into a kidney for the purpose of providing an artificial means of draining the kidney. This procedure may be done in the treatment of obstructions from large stones or strictures of the ureter or to drain purulent material from an infected kidney.

NURSING ASSESSMENT AND INTERVENTION

In both nephrectomy and nephrostomy, the surgical incision may be lumbar, transabdominal, or thoracic. When the patient returns from surgery, the nurse must check carefully for the location of the surgical wound and the presence of any drains or tubes that may have been inserted during the operation.

Dressings over the surgical wound may be reinforced. The drainage on these dressings will be blood-tinged at first, but it should gradually become clearer. If bright red blood appears or there is a sudden change in the amount of drainage, the doctor should be notified. Extreme care must be taken during the changing of dressings to ensure that the drains or tubes are not dislodged or pulled from the surgical incision.

Positioning of the patient depends on the wishes of the surgeon. He may prefer to have the patient lie only on the affected side. Turning the patient may be difficult at first, because it is usually quite painful for him to move about. The nurse should explain the need for frequent turning and deep breathing so that complications may be prevented.

Hemorrhage is always a danger after surgery of the kidney. It will be remembered that the kidneys have a very rich supply of blood directly from the aorta and vena cava. The vital signs are carefully checked and any indication of shock or hemorrhage reported immediately.

Adequate drainage from the opposite kidney after surgery is of great importance. Urinary output must be very carefully measured and recorded. Fluids are usually restricted immediately after surgery and then gradually increased as the remaining kidney compensates for the loss of its partner. If a nephrostomy has been done, fluids are restricted until the affected kidney can recover sufficiently and resume its functions.

TUMORS OF THE BLADDER

Most tumors of the bladder are malignant, and the prognosis for cure is generally not good. However, superficial tumors, if detected in the early stages, have a more favorable prognosis. Bladder cancer usually occurs in people over 50 years of age and is most often seen in men. Exposure to tobacco smoke is thought to be one of the key factors in the development of bladder cancer. Other carcinogenic factors are coffee, nitrates, and various industrial dyes and solvents.

SYMPTOMS AND MEDICAL DIAGNOSIS

Frequency of urination, or *dysuria,* and painless hematuria are the most common symptoms of a bladder tumor. In the later stages, as the tumor becomes larger, there may be an obstruction of the flow or urine. Biopsy and cytologic studies establish the diagnosis of malignancy.

TREATMENT

The treatment for a bladder tumor is complete or partial removal of the bladder with transplantation of the ureters to the outside or to the intestinal tract, as discussed in the following section.

CARE OF THE PATIENT HAVING SURGERY OF THE BLADDER AND URETERS

TYPES OF SURGERY

Cystectomy is the surgical removal of the bladder. *Ureterostomy* is a surgical incision into the ureter for the purpose of diverting the flow of urine. If the bladder is removed, there obviously must be some means of diverting the flow of urine that normally would pass through the ureters and into the bladder. One procedure is a *cutaneous ureterostomy,* in which the ureters are transplanted to the skin on the abdomen (Fig. 22–12). This is a relatively safe procedure, but it is frequently complicated by stricture of the ureter at the point where it joins the skin or fascia.

Another surgical procedure necessitated by cystectomy is ureterosigmoidostomy, in which the ureters are attached to the sigmoid colon, which then acts as a reservoir for the urine.

A third procedure (Bricker's procedure) involves suturing the ureters to an isolated section of ileum that is connected to an opening in the skin, forming an ileal conduit. The open ends of the intestines where the section of ileum was removed are rejoined by anastomosis.

A fourth procedure has recently been devised that creates a continent internal ileal reservoir (Kock pouch). The ureters are implanted into a segment of ileum that has been isolated. Special nipple valves connect the pouch to the exterior of the skin. The pouch can then be catheterized by the patient, providing continence with no exterior collection device.

A new treatment for bladder cancer, still experimental, provides an alternative to cystectomy. It involves treating the bladder tissue with a substance that makes the tumor cells photosensitive and then introducing laser beams through a cystoscope, which alters cell structure, preventing further tumor growth.

Psychological care of the patient facing malignancy and an operation that will radically change his body image should be a primary nursing concern. The nurse must encourage the patient to talk about his fears and concerns. The spouse must be encouraged to share feelings There are always sexual concerns when cystectomy and urinary diversion are performed. Some of the more radical procedures will produce impotence in the male. The caring nurse will not leave the patient and family to sort out these concerns alone.

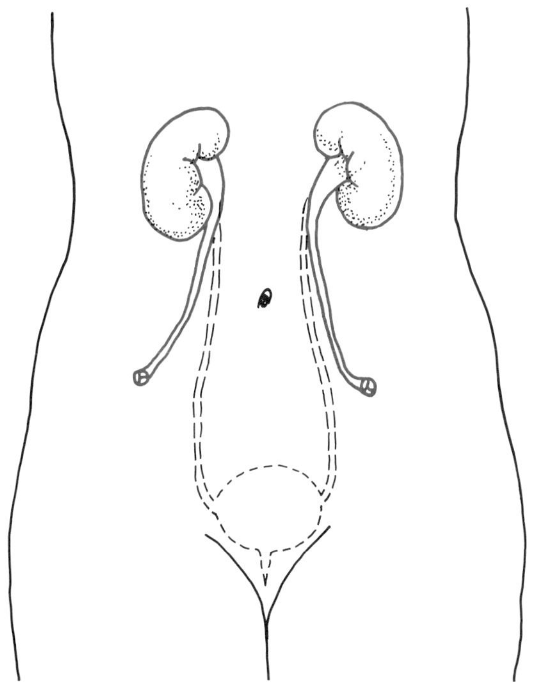

Figure 22–12 Cystectomy and cutaneous ureterostomies.

Nursing care following cystectomy is always difficult because of the danger of hemorrhage and infection. There are also problems involved in devising a satisfactory arrangement for the collection of urine. Care of a patient with a ureterostomy is discussed in Chapter 25.

TRAUMA TO THE KIDNEYS AND URETERS

Accidental injury to the kidneys, ureters, bladder, or urethra occurs frequently and should always be considered a possibility whenever there has been trauma to the abdominal cavity or thoracic cage.

SYMPTOMS AND DIAGNOSIS

Signs and symptoms characteristic of trauma to the kidneys include massive hemorrhage, hematuria, abdominal or flank pain, and possibly an enlarged mass in the kidney area. Diagnostic tests include serial urinalyses, hemoglobin and hematocrit tests, and measurements of electrolytes. Rising levels of blood urea nitrogen and creatinine indicate diminishing renal function. Radiologic studies including films of the kidney, ureters, and bladder, and IVP can demonstrate the extent of damage to the urinary system.

Hourly measurements of urinary output and observation of the characteristics of the urine can help determine the type and extent of injury.

MEDICAL TREATMENT AND NURSING INTERVENTION

Bleeding in the kidney often is self-limiting. Lacerations and contusions without interruption of urinary function usually can be treated conservatively by bed rest. For this reason the urologist may advocate a period of watchful waiting to see if the kidney can be saved.

During this time the patient is monitored closely for signs of hypovolemic and traumatic shock, cardiovascular changes, urinary output, and size of the flank mass.

Nursing intervention in the care of all patients with trauma to the kidney must not be focused only on renal function. Most patients with injuries of this kind also have had damage to the colon, spleen, or pancreas. A comprehensive plan for dealing with problems associated with multiple trauma is usually necessary.

TRAUMA TO THE BLADDER

Any violent blow or crushing injury to the lower abdomen may result in rupture or perforation of the bladder wall with resulting leakage of the urine into the pelvic tissues or peritoneal cavity. This brings about a severe inflammation in these areas.

SYMPTOMS AND MEDICAL DIAGNOSIS

Early symptoms of bladder injury are painful hematuria or inability to void, marked tenderness and spasm in the suprapubic area, or the development of a large mass in that area.

SURGICAL TREATMENT AND NURSING INTERVENTION

If the bladder has ruptured or is perforated, treatment consists of a suprapubic cystostomy for the purpose of providing drainage of blood and urine. Care of the patient demands meticulous attention to drains and dressings in order to avoid infection and to maintain good drainage. Cold applications to the surgical site both before and after surgery may be ordered.

The nurse should observe the patient carefully for postoperative shock and massive hemorrhage. Any formation of a mass in the suprapubic area before or after surgery or any change in the vital signs should be reported immediately.

In addition to physical distress, the patient with bladder injuries is likely to have emotional difficulties in dealing with the problems arising from the sudden loss of control over the urinary flow and the intimate procedures and treatments necessary. The nurse must be prepared for this and do all she can to encourage and help the patient through this difficult period of adjustment.

Concerns for the Elderly

Kidney function begins to lessen after age 45 and gradually decreases to a point where renal blood flow and glomerular filtration rate are about half that of a young adult. Essentially this means that the elderly patient has less renal reserve, and if he experiences infection or trauma of the renal system, acute renal failure may result.

The aged kidney has less ability to concentrate the urine, and this predisposes the patient to dehydration when fluid intake is restricted for diagnostic tests. The contrast agents used for x-ray tests, in conjunction with dehydration, can cause acute renal failure in the elderly patient. The nurse should pay particular attention to rehydration as soon as the test is finished to prevent this problem.

In males the prostate gland hypertrophies with age and causes varying degrees of obstruction to the normal flow of urine. This predisposes patients to stasis, reflux, infection, and eventual kidney damage.

Degenerative changes in the bladder muscles lead to incomplete emptying and constant residual urine, which predispose to infection. Elderly women often have stress incontinence. Less fluid is consumed as a way to diminish the incontinence problem, and this increases the incidence of urinary tract infection.

BIBLIOGRAPHY

Baer, C. L.: Acute renal failure: Recognizing and reversing its deadly course. Nursing 90, June, 1990, p. 34.

Cameron, V.: A dialysis catheter with staying power. RN, July, 1990, p. 56.

Coco, P.: When kidneys fail: Nursing management of acute renal failure. A.D. Nurse, July/Aug., 1988, p. 16.

Dirkes, S. M.: Making a critical difference with CAVH. Nursing 89, Nov., 1989, p. 57.

Erlich, L.: Use of Epogen for treatment of anemia associated with chronic renal failure. Crit. Care Nurs. Clin. North Am., March, 1990, p. 101.

Fedric, T. N.: Immunosuppressive therapy in renal transplantation. Crit. Care Nurs. Clin. North Am., March, 1990, p. 123.

Ghiotto, D. L.: A full range of care for nephrostomy patients. RN, April, 1988, p. 72.

Greig, B.: A new option for cystectomy patients. RN, Sept., 1990, p. 34.

Harasyko, C.: Kidney transplantation. Nurs. Clin. North Am., Dec., 1989, p. 851.

Jameson, M. D., and Wiegmann, T. B.: Principles, uses and complications of hemodialysis. Med. Clin. North Am., July, 1990, p. 945.

Jones, A., and Hoeft, R.: Cancer of the prostate. Am. J. Nurs., May, 1982, p. 826.

Levine, D. I.: Care of the Renal Patient. Philadelphia, W. B. Saunders, 1983.

Maldonado, M. M., and Kumjian, D. A.: Acute renal failure due to urinary tract obstruction. Med. Clin. North Am., July, 1990, p. 919.

Mallette, C.: What those "difficult" renal patients need from you. RN, April, 1990, p. 25.

Malti, J., and Wellons, D.: CAPD: A dialysis breakthrough with its own burdens. RN, Feb., 1988, p. 30.

Metheny, N.: Renal stones and urinary pH. Am. J. Nurs., Sept., 1982, p. 1372.

Miller, L. A.: At-home help for the CAPD patient. RN, Aug., 1990, p. 77.

Pritchard, V.: Geriatric infections: The urinary tract. RN, May, 1988, p. 36.

Reilly, N. J., and Torosian, L. C.: The new wave in lithotripsy: Implications for nursing. RN, March, 1988, p. 44.

Strangis, L.: Peritoneal dialysis made easy. Nursing 88, Jan., 1988, p. 43.

Webber-Jones, J. E.: Performing clean intermittent self-catheterization. Nursing 91, Aug., 1991, p. 56.

STUDENT STUDY AIDS

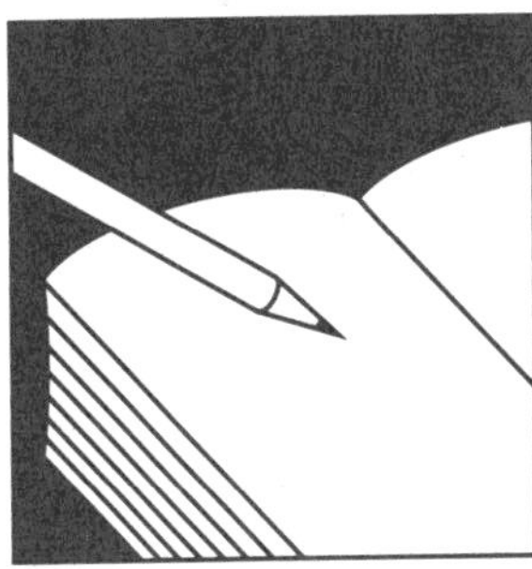

CLINICAL CASE PROBLEMS

Read each of the clinical situations and discuss the questions with your classmates.

1. A friend of yours tells you that she has been very uncomfortable during the past week because of frequency of urination and burning when she voids. Last night, she had a severe chill and some elevation of temperature. She has been told that she probably has a very common ailment in women and that if she drinks a lot of fluids, it will probably go away.

- What would be your advice to your friend?
- How would you explain the need for her to follow your advice?

---

2. Mrs. Spence, age 54, has had hypertension since her early 20s. She now has developed symptoms of chronic renal failure. She was referred to a nephrologist who, after a series of diagnostic tests, recommended hemodialysis and kidney transplant when an organ is available.

- What diagnostic tests do you think the nephrologist would have ordered for Mrs. Spence?
- Why might Mrs. Spence's renal disease not have been diagnosed earlier?
- If Mrs. Spence does not agree to renal dialysis, what symptoms is she likely to experience eventually?
- What psychosocial problems would you expect Mrs. Spence to have? Write specific nursing diagnoses for each and list nursing interventions that might be effective in helping her deal with them.

---

3. Mrs. Downs is a 35-year-old patient who has had a nephrostomy for treatment of hydronephrosis resulting from obstruction by a renal stone in the pelvis of the kidney. She returns from surgery with a nephrostomy tube, a urethral catheter, and a rubber Penrose drain in place.

- How would you explain the purpose of the nephrostomy tube?
- What is the specific nursing care for these tubes and the drain?
- What is the likely treatment for the renal stone?

STUDY OUTLINE

I. Introduction

A. Urinary system composed of kidneys, ureters, urinary bladder, and urethra.

B. Urinary system maintains proper balance of fluids, minerals, and vital organic substances.

C. Systemic diseases such as cardiovascular disorders and metabolic disturbances can affect renal function.

II. Diagnostic tests and procedures and nursing implications (see Table 22–1)

III. Nursing assessment of renal function and the urinary drainage system

A. Definition of terms:

1. Anuria: absence of urine.
2. Oliguria: decreased flow of urine.
3. Polyuria: increased flow of urine.
4. Urinary retention: urine held in bladder.
5. Residual urine: that left in the bladder after voiding.
6. Suppression of urine: inability of the kidney to produce urine.

B. History and present illness:
   1. Previous illness affecting any of the major systems.
   2. Previous surgery involving the urinary system.
   3. Family history of cardiovascular disease, diabetes, and kidney stone formation.
   4. Sexually transmitted diseases.
   5. Drug history to identify nephrotoxic drugs.

C. Ongoing assessment:
   1. Fluid intake and output.
   2. Character of urine: abnormal color, odor, clarity.
   3. Changes in voiding pattern: frequency, urgency.
   4. Pain and discomfort.

D. Associated nursing diagnoses:
   1. Fluid imbalance, excess.
   2. Altered patterns of urinary elimination.
   3. Urinary retention.
   4. Pain.
   5. Sleep pattern disturbance.
   6. Fear.
   7. Body image disturbance.
   8. Knowledge deficit.
   9. Potential for sexual dysfunction.

IV. Maintaining urinary flow

A. Introduction:
   1. Urinary stasis a major factor in infection and stone formation.
   2. Blockage of urine flow can occur anywhere in urinary tract.
   3. Catheterization never done for convenience of staff.

B. Principles of catheter care:
   1. Catheter-associated infections most common type of nosocomial infections.
   2. Strict asepsis required. Exception is self-catheterization in which patient is taught "clean" technique.
   3. Catheter and tubing must be kept open and draining freely.
   4. Best kind of irrigation is forcing fluids.
   5. Each time system is opened, chance of contamination is increased.
   6. Drainage bag is kept below level of bladder.

C. Indications for insertion of indwelling catheter:
   1. Obstruction in lower urinary tract.
   2. Blood clots and debris in bladder.
   3. Neurogenic incontinence.
   4. Surgical removal of urethra or surrounding structures.
   5. Sometimes used when urinary drainage critical to deciding mode of therapy.

D. Alternatives to indwelling urethral catheter: condom drainage for males, suprapubic catheter, intermittent self-catheterization.

E. Types of catheters:
   1. Urethral.
   2. Ureteral: passed into ureter (stent).
   3. Suprapubic: tube is inserted directly into bladder through incision in bladder wall.
   4. Nephrostomy tubes.

V. Inflammatory disorders

A. Cystitis: more common in females.
   1. Preventive measures aimed at reducing contamination of urinary meatus, especially by intestinal bacteria.

2. Medical treatment includes urinary antiseptics and systemic anti-infectives.

B. Urethritis: may be associated with sexually transmitted disease, especially gonorrhea. Nonspecific urethritis caused by a variety of organisms.

C. Nephritis: general inflammation and resulting degeneration of the renal cells.
   1. Acute glomerulonephritis is an immunologic disorder most often associated with systemic streptococcal infections.
      a. Assessment: widespread edema, visual disturbances, marked hypertension.
      b. Medical treatment and nursing intervention: rest, low-sodium diet, and observation for signs of increased intracranial pressure, cardiac failure, or pulmonary edema.
   2. Chronic glomerulonephritis can develop rapidly or over a period of years.
      a. Assessment: observe for insidious edema, headache associated with hypertension, and dyspnea.
      b. Medical treatment and nursing intervention as for patient with chronic kidney failure.
   3. Nephrosclerosis: hardening and narrowing of renal arterioles, leading to degeneration of renal cells.
      a. Symptoms and treatment similar to those of chronic renal failure.
   4. Nephrotic syndrome sometimes occurs after glomerulonephritis.
      a. Signs and symptoms: severe edema, proteinuria, hyperlipidemia, hypoalbuminemia.
      b. Treatment: diuretics, bed rest, high protein diet; sometimes cortisone and cyclophosphamide (Cytoxan).
      c. Excellent skin care required because of edema.

D. Pyelonephritis: infection of the kidney caused by bacterial invasion.
   1. Causes:
      a. Bacteria from bladder travel up ureters to kidneys.
      b. Increase in strength and number of bacteria in blood stream.
      c. Back pressure of urine because of obstruction to drainage.
   2. Assessment: fever, chills, nausea and vomiting, and pain in flank radiating to the thigh and genitalia. Later symptoms: weight loss, weakness, and bacteria and pus in the urine.
   3. Medical treatment and nursing intervention: bed rest, fluids, careful observation of urine for amount, color, and odor; administer urinary antiseptics and antibiotics.

VI. Renal failure: failure of the kidneys to function normally

A. Classified as acute or chronic renal failure.

B. Causes:
   1. Infection, inflammation, and upper urinary tract obstruction.
   2. Obstruction in lower urinary tract.
   3. Systemic diseases and toxic states, such as hypercalcemia, hypokalemia, hypertension, heart failure, cirrhosis of the liver and diabetes.
      a. Diabetic nephropathy is the third major cause of chronic renal failure and the most common cause of death in persons with diabetes.

C. Medical diagnosis:
   1. Renal biopsy.
   2. Evaluation of BUN, serum creatinine, and creatinine clearance.

3. Clinical manifestations usually do not appear until large percentage of renal function is lost.
4. Symptoms of end-stage renal disease comprise the syndrome known as uremia.

D. Systemic effects of renal failure (see Fig. 22–7).

E. Medical treatment:
1. In acute renal failure, goal is to restore and maintain tolerable internal environment until kidneys resume normal function. Peritoneal dialysis used in some cases.
2. In chronic renal failure, management is highly complex. Patient has two major alternatives to sustain life: renal dialysis and kidney transplant.

F. Nursing assessment and intervention:
1. Patient and family will need help in learning to manage the symptoms of renal failure.
2. Fluid and electrolyte balance and acid-base balance of major concern.
3. Symptoms of azotemia require careful monitoring of patient for changes in level of consciousness, nausea and vomiting, fluid and electrolyte imbalance.
4. Relevant laboratory data to plan nursing care include serum levels of calcium, potassium, and phosphorus.
5. Maintaining nutritional status very difficult.

G. Renal dialysis: removal of waste products normally excreted in urine.
1. Hemodialysis utilizes the principle of diffusion to remove from the blood those waste products normally excreted by the kidneys. It does this by pumping blood from arterial circulation through a dialysate bath and back to the venous circulation.
2. Long-term hemodialysis creates many difficulties for patient and family. Goals of nursing are to facilitate acceptance of the diagnosis of chronic renal failure and adaptation to continued dialysis treatment.
3. Peritoneal dialysis uses the peritoneal lining as the semipermeable membrane. Dialyzing solution is instilled via catheter into peritoneal cavity, left in the cavity for a period of time, and then removed.

H. Kidney transplantation:
1. Most successful of all organ transplants.
2. Major problem is organ rejection by recipient's immune response system.
   a. Immunosuppression can help avoid rejection of organ, but carries the risk of increased susceptibility to infection and the development of cancer.
3. Renal transplant patients require close monitoring for signs of rejection: elevated BP, fever, pain over transplant, fatigue, oliguria, increased BUN, creatinine.
4. Dietary restrictions may no longer be necessary once donor kidney begins to function.
5. Medicare can pay for 80% of cost of treating end-stage renal disease.

VII. Obstructions of the urinary tract

A. Hydronephrosis: flow of urine from the kidney is obstructed; kidney dilates and fills with fluid.
1. Symptoms and medical diagnosis:
   a. Severe pain occurs only if condition develops rapidly; other-

wise, symptoms are mild and patient may not be aware of condition until uremia develops.
      b. Definitive diagnosis made by radiologic studies.
   2. Surgical treatment and nursing intervention:
      a. Aimed at removal of obstruction.
      b. Patient observed for signs of impending uremia, urinary output noted and recorded; nephrectomy may be necessary if damage is extensive.
B. Renal stones: types: listed in Table 22–4.
   1. Causative factors:
      a. Supersaturation of urine with crystalloids that do not dissolve easily.
      b. Urinary infection.
      c. Inadequate fluid intake and concentrated urine.
      d. Urinary stasis.
      e. Urate and other substances in the urine.
   2. Prevention:
      a. High fluid intake.
      b. Prevention and prompt treatment of urinary infections.
      c. Removal of parathyroid tumor.
      d. Identification of specific kind of stone so as to change urinary pH to one less favorable to stone formation.
   3. Symptoms and medical diagnosis:
      a. Clinical manifestations include pain, blood in urine, and nausea and vomiting.
      b. Radiologic studies include radiographs and IVP.
   4. Medical-surgical treatment:
      a. Force fluids to encourage spontaneous passing of stone.
      b. Analgesics and antispasmodics to manage pain.
      c. Break up stones with irrigation or ultrasound.
      d. Surgical removal.
   5. Nursing assessment and intervention:
      a. Identify patients most at risk.
      b. Gather data about changes in urinary output, etc.
      c. Strain all urine to recover stone.
      d. Encourage increased fluid intake.
      e. Education of patient to prevent further stone formation.

VIII. Neoplasms of the kidney

A. Neoplasms fairly uncommon but nearly always malignant.
B. Symptoms and medical diagnosis:
   1. Hematuria and enlargement of affected kidney major signs.
   2. Diagnosis confirmed by radiologic studies, renal ultrasonography, and MRI.
C. Surgical treatment and nursing intervention:
   1. Surgical removal of affected kidney before metastasis has occurred.
   2. Nursing care as for patient having kidney surgery, malignancy, or radiation therapy.

IX. Care of patient who has had surgery of the kidney

A. Types of surgery: nephrectomy and nephrostomy.
B. Nursing assessment and intervention:
   1. Flow of urine through catheters and drains checked frequently.
   2. Dressings may be reinforced but usually are changed by surgeon during immediate postoperative period.
   3. Some blood-tinged drainage expected, but bright red drainage may signal an emergency.

4. Most common complication is hemorrhage.
5. Urinary output measured; fluids may be restricted.

X. Tumors of the bladder

A. Usually malignant.
B. Symptoms and medical diagnosis: intermittent, gross hematuria. Diagnosis confirmed by cystoscopy and biopsy.
C. Treatment: surgical removal of all or part of the bladder.

XI. Care of the patient having surgery of the bladder

A. Cystectomy: surgical removal of the bladder.
B. Ureterostomy: surgical incision into the ureter for the purpose of providing drainage.
C. Surgical procedures to provide for diversion of flow of urine are discussed in Chapter 25.

XII. Trauma to the kidney and ureters

A. Always a possibility when there has been injury to the abdominal cavity or thoracic cage.
B. Symptoms: gross hematuria, pain and tenderness in renal area, enlarged mass in flank.
C. Medical treatment and nursing intervention:
   1. Observe for signs of shock and hemorrhage.
   2. Strict bed rest.
   3. Surgical intervention, usually nephrectomy.

XIII. Trauma to the bladder

A. Caused by violent or crushing blow to lower abdomen.
B. Symptoms and medical diagnosis: painful hematuria, spasm or large mass in suprapubic area.
C. Surgical treatment and nursing intervention:
   1. Suprapubic cystostomy to provide drainage.
   2. Meticulous care of drains and dressings to avoid infection and maintain good drainage of urine.

XIV. Concerns for the elderly

A. Elderly patient has less renal reserve.
B. Less ability to concentrate urine, which can lead to dehydration and potential acute renal failure in the event of serious illness.
C. In the male, prostate gland hypertrophies and can cause obstruction to urine flow.
D. Degenerative changes in the bladder muscles lead to incomplete emptying and predispose patient to infection.
E. Elderly women prone to stress incontinence; decreased fluid intake predisposes them to urinary tract infection.

CHAPTER 23

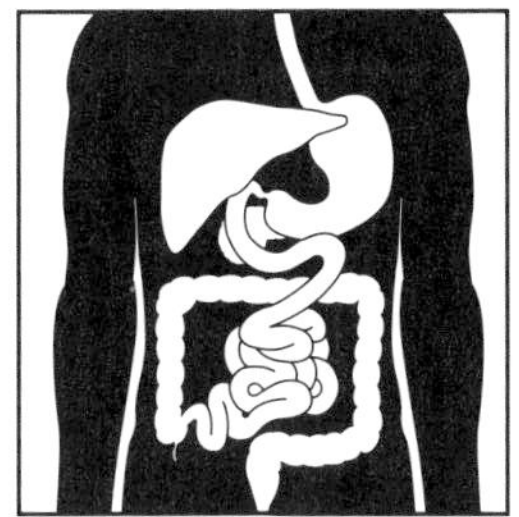

Care of Patients With Disorders of the Digestive Tract

VOCABULARY

adhesion
anorexia
diverticulosis
epigastric
flatus
gastritis
hematemesis
hernia
melena
volvulus

Upon completion of this part the student should be able to:

1. Identify three major causative factors and preventive measures in the development of disorders of the digestive system.
2. List nursing responsibilities in the pre- and posttest care of patients having diagnostic tests for disorders of the intestinal tract.
3. Demonstrate assessment of gastrointestinal status.
4. Describe nursing interventions for patients with gastrointestinal bleeding.
5. Describe the pathophysiology, means of medical diagnosis, and treatment for stomatitis, gastritis, ulcerative colitis, appendicitis, and peritonitis.
6. Devise a nursing care plan for the patient with peptic ulcer.
7. Write a nursing care plan for the patient with cancer of the colon with intestinal obstruction.
8. List nursing interventions for the patient with ulcerative colitis or irritable bowel syndrome.
9. Devise a nursing care plan for the patient having surgery of the lower intestine and rectum.

The main portion of the digestive system is actually one long tube that extends from the mouth to the rectum. This tube is known as the *alimentary tract* or *intestinal tract.* For the sake of clarity, the various sections of this tract are considered as organs. Thus the large bulge just below the esophagus is known as a separate organ, the stomach, even though it is only a continuation of the same tube that forms the esophagus above it and the small intestine below it.

As food enters the alimentary tract by way of the mouth, it immediately begins to undergo physical and chemical changes; that is, it is not only changed in appearance, but new substances are formed from the original material. These changes are the first stages of *digestion.* The food is propelled downward through the alimentary tract by wavelike motions of involuntary muscles within the walls of the alimentary tract. This rhythmic squeezing action is called *peristalsis.* As the food passes down the digestive tube, it continues to undergo changes until it reaches a liquid state and can then be taken into the blood stream. The transfer of nutrients from the intestines into the blood is referred to as *absorption.* Substances such as food fiber that are not digested and absorbed continue through the tube and add bulk to the stool (Fig. 23–1).

Metabolism is the sum of all the many physical and chemical processes concerned with the disposition of nutrients absorbed into the blood stream after digestion has taken place. Metabolic activities involve the synthesis of substances needed to build, maintain, and repair body tissues *(anabolism),* and the breakdown of larger molecules into smaller molecules so that energy is available *(catabolism).*

The central role of the intestinal tract and accessory organs of digestion is the intake, absorption, and assimilation of food to provide nourishment for the body. Hence pathologic conditions of the intestinal tract and accessory organs of digestion ultimately lead to malnutrition and a weakening of the body's defenses. The morbidity and mortality rates for almost all diseases, regardless of their primary site, are higher when these diseases are associated with inadequate nutrition.

Mechanical obstruction to the movement of food through the intestinal tract (as in intestinal obstruction) or to the flow of digestive juices and enzymes (as in blockage of the bile ducts) can give rise to serious disorders of digestion and absorption and can be life threatening. Continued irritation and inflammation of the gastrointestinal mucosa can lead to intestinal bleeding and to increased peristalsis and inadequate absorption of nutrients.

Stress and emotional states such as fear, anxiety, depression, and hostility also can affect the function of the gastrointestinal tract and lead to ulceration, diarrhea, and other dysfunctions. The discomfort associated with gastrointestinal disorders is associated with inflammation, diminished blood supply to the gastrointestinal mucosa, and stretching of smooth muscles and the capsules of internal organs.

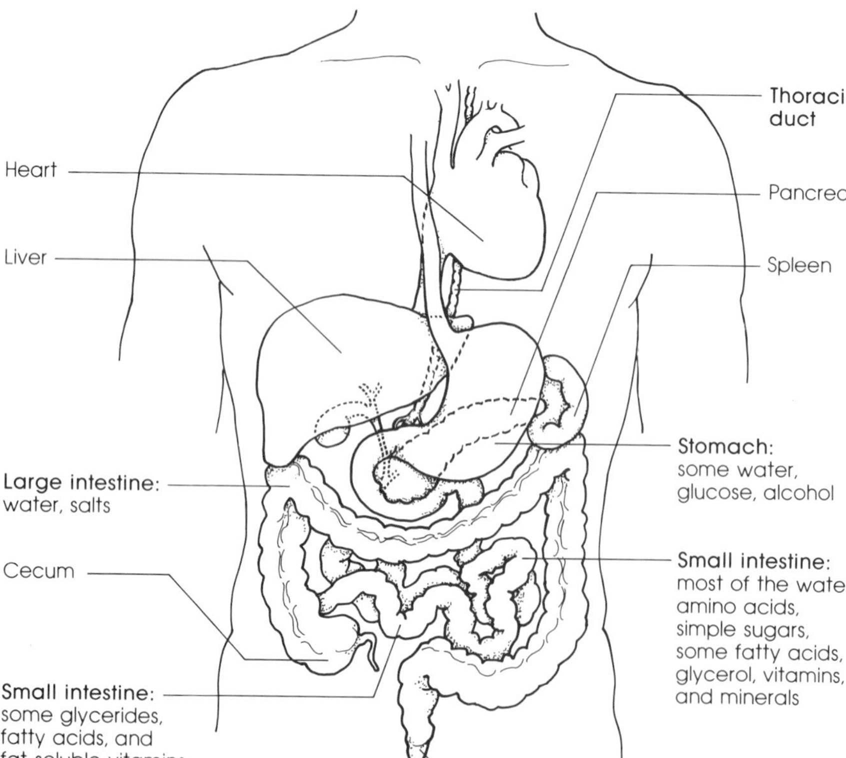

Figure 23–1 Absorption of products of digestion in stomach and intestines. (Redrawn and adapted from Jacob, S. W., et al.: Structure and Function in Man, 5th ed. Philadelphia, W. B. Saunders, 1982.)

CAUSATIVE FACTORS AND PREVENTIVE MEASURES

As with all other tissues of the body, those of the digestive tract are subject to infection, inflammation, physical and chemical trauma, and structural defects. Factors that contribute to these pathologic conditions include the more obvious physical ones, such as exposure to infectious agents (as in food poisoning), and the less apparent psychosocial factors.

Psychological and emotional stresses greatly influence appetite and motility of the stomach and intestines. The secretion of digestive juices in amounts sufficient for the breakdown of food is regulated in large part by the emotions. Excessive stimulation and release of digestive acids and enzymes can cause a breakdown in the integrity of the mucous membrane lining the digestive tract and can bring about such disorders as gastric and duodenal ulcer and chronic colitis.

Prevention of intestinal disorders associated with stress and tension is difficult, because there usually are other factors involved. Stress is not necessarily harmful; and its effects are not always manifested in only one organ or even one system in the body. Teaching patients ways to relax and to cope with undue stress can be helpful, but it does not guarantee freedom from disorders that usually have multiple causes.

Mechanical and chemical irritants that produce inflammation often can be identified by elimination diets to determine the foods that cause gastrointestinal upsets. Once the offending foods are identified, efforts are made to help the patient avoid these foods and at the same time maintain adequate nutrition.

Prevention of infections of the intestinal tract is similar to prevention of infections elsewhere in the body. Washing the hands before eating, care in the cleaning of cooking and eating utensils, and following general rules of good hygiene and sanitation can prevent many infectious gastrointestinal upsets. Food poisoning often can be prevented by adequate refrigeration and proper canning and freezing methods. Botulism and other types of food poisoning are discussed in Chapter 36.

DIAGNOSTIC TESTS AND PROCEDURES AND NURSING IMPLICATIONS

Diagnostic tests for disorders of the intestinal tract consist of radiographs, ultrasound studies, endoscopy, complete blood cell (CBC) count, tests of gastric secretions, and stool studies.

The patient is often scheduled for a series of tests, some of which utilize a contrast media. It is important that gastrointestinal (GI) tests be done in the correct order so that the contrast media don't interfere with other tests. For example, if the patient is scheduled for an upper GI series, a gallbladder sonogram, and a barium enema, he should have them done in this order: sonogram, barium enema, and then the upper GI series.

The nurse should pay particular attention to patient comfort during the preparation phase of diagnostic testing. Many of the studies require cleansing of the GI tract. When laxatives are administered in liquid form, the patient can drink them more easily if they are chilled or poured over ice. If a patient has trouble with nausea, have him suck on an ice cube first and then use a straw to drink the solution. This will decrease taste sensation.

Frequent, loose bowel movements cause rectal irritation. Application of a lubricant such as A and D ointment or petroleum jelly (Vaseline) prior to action of the laxatives can protect this area and make the patient much more comfortable.

For many GI tests, the patient is kept NPO the night before. Mouth care should be offered in the morning, and the door of his room should be kept closed so that food odors do not enter his room and increase his hunger. A food tray should be obtained immediately on his return to the floor, as long as he is no longer scheduled to be NPO. The nurse can provide juices and coffee or tea while waiting for the meal tray to be delivered.

Frequent assessment for signs of dehydration is necessary, as cleansing enemas and lack of oral intake can quickly dehydrate a patient who has already been ill with nausea, vomiting, or diarrhea. The older patient is especially at risk for problems of electrolyte imbalance and dehydration when undergoing preparation for diagnostic tests.

The purpose, description, and nursing implications for the diagnostic tests of the gastrointestinal system are listed in Table 23-1.

SPECIFIC PROBLEMS RELATED TO INGESTION, DIGESTION, AND BOWEL ELIMINATION

If the cells of the body are to receive an adequate supply of nutrients, a series of complex events must take place. These events normally include such activities as (1) voluntarily eating and drinking the foods and liquids necessary for adequate nutrition; (2) the mechanical breakdown of foodstuffs by chewing, swallowing, and peristalsis; and (3) their dissolution and chemical breakdown by enzymes and other chemicals. Once the nutrients are absorbed from the intes-

TABLE 23-1 DIAGNOSTIC TESTS FOR GASTROINTESTINAL PROBLEMS

Test	Purpose	Description	Nursing Implications
Radiologic exams Upper GI series (UGI)	X-ray examination with fluoroscopy to locate obstruction, ulceration, or growths in the esophagus and stomach.	Patient drinks a contrast medium and is placed in various positions on the x-ray table (Fig. 23-2).	Keep patient NPO for 8 to 12 hours prior to the test. Explain what happens during test. After radiographs, increase fluids and give ordered laxatives to clear GI tract of contrast medium and prevent impaction. Stool may be white up to 3 days after test.
Barium enema (BE)	X-ray examination of the colon using fluoroscopy to locate tumors, obstruction, and ulceration.	A radiopague substance is instilled in the colon by enema. After evacuation of this substance, air may be instilled for contrast studies (Fig. 23-3).	Keep patient NPO for 8 hours prior to test. Give ordered laxatives and enemas. Bowel must be clear of stool. Explain what will happen during the test. Posttest care is same as for UGI.
Endoscopic studies Esophagogastroduodenoscopy	Visualizes the esophagus, stomach, and duodenum with a lighted tube (endoscope) to detect tumor, ulceration, or obstruction. Separate study of esophagus, stomach, or stomach duodenum may be done.	Patient is given preoperative sedation. IV sedation may be used for the test. A local spray or gargle may be used to anesthetize the throat. The patient lies on a table, and the endoscope is introduced through the mouth (Fig. 23-4).	Keep patient NPO for 8 hours. Obtain signed consent. Explain what he will experience during the test. Give preoperative medication. After procedure, keep patient NPO until gag reflex has returned. Take vital signs q 15 to 30 minutes as ordered. Watch for signs of perforation: rising temperature, pain, changes in vital signs.
Proctoscopy and sigmoidoscopy	Examination of the lining of the rectum and sigmoid colon to detect polyps, tumor, obstruction, or ulceration.	The patient is placed in the knee-chest position, often on a special table. A sigmoidoscope is introduced through the anus. Biopsies can be taken of suspicious areas; polyps can be removed. The patient will experience some cramping during the procedure.	Give laxatives and enemas the evening before as ordered. Give clear liquids for dinner the night before, then keep patient NPO until after exam. Explain what he will experience. Encourage use of deep breathing and relaxation techniques to decrease cramping. Observe for rectal bleeding after biopsy or polyp removal.
Colonoscopy	Direct visualization of the lining of the colon with a flexible endoscope.	Patient is moderately sedated for this procedure, which takes about 1½ to 2 hours. Polyps can be removed or biopsies taken.	Give clear liquid diet 1 to 3 days prior to test. Patient is NPO for 8 hours prior. Give laxatives for 1 to 3 days prior to test and enemas the night before. Explain procedure and what he will experience. Obtain signed consent. Give preoperative sedation. After procedure, observe for rectal bleeding and signs of perforation: abdominal distention, pain, elevated temperature.
Gastric analysis	Determines the rate of secretion of gastric juices and degree of acidity.	A nasogastric tube is inserted, and stomach contents are aspirated. A substance may be given to stimulate the	Withhold drugs affecting gastric secretion for 24 to 48 hours prior to test. No smoking the morning of test

TABLE 23-1 DIAGNOSTIC TESTS FOR GASTROINTESTINAL PROBLEMS *Continued*

Test	Purpose	Description	Nursing Implications
		flow of gastric secretions, and another sample is aspirated in 30 minutes. Increased secretion can indicate peptic ulcer or pancreatic tumor. A low degree of acidity may indicate gastric ulcer. An absence of acid can accompany cancer of the stomach or pernicious anemia.	(nicotine stimulates secretions). Keep patient NPO for 8 hours prior to test. Explain use of NG tube and procedure.
Tubeless gastric analysis	Determination of presence or absence of hydrochloric acid in the stomach secretions.	The patient is given special granules in 240 mL of water. Urine specimens are collected at specific intervals. If HCl is present in the stomach, the urine will be blue; if none is present, the urine will be normal color.	Explain test and procedure to patient.
Fecal analysis (stool exam)	Analysis for presence of mucus, elevated fat content, blood (guaiac), bacteria, or parasites.	Stool specimen is obtained in bed pan or container in commode. Small smear is made on special paper and tested with special solution for guaiac or Hemoccult test.	Explain test to patient. Provide means for collection of stool. Promptly retrieve stool, obtain sample for guaiac test, place specimen in lab container, and dispatch to lab *immediately*. (Bacteria can multiply if specimen is left at room temperature for extended period; parasites may disintegrate.) Patient must have red meat–free diet for at least 3 days before a stool guaiac test can be considered accurate.

tinal tract, the solid and liquid waste must be eliminated.

Voluntary intake of foodstuffs is related to appetite and hunger. The patient who is anorexic has no appetite and no interest in eating. Hunger has more to do with the unavailability of food than with a lack of desire to eat. The person desires to eat, so he is not anorexic, but because of dietary restrictions, inability to feed himself, poverty, or some other factor, he experiences hunger.

In addition to the problems related to loss of appetite or the unavailability of food, the nurse might also encounter patients who have difficulty chewing because of inflammation and soreness of the gums, tongue, and mouth, or who cannot swallow normally (dysphagia). Another difficulty common to irritation and damage to the intestinal mucosa and erosion of blood vessels is gastrointestinal bleeding.

Surgical intervention, mechanical obstruction, and accidental injury to the intestinal tract can cause disturbances in the passage of material through the intestinal tract, leading to the accumulation of fluids and gases. Severe trauma to the alimentary canal presents serious long-term nutritional deficits that can be treated only by administration of nutrients by the parenteral route.

Nausea and vomiting related to illness, effects of cancer treatment, or stress can also interfere with nutrition.

ANOREXIA

Anorexia is the absence of appetite. The enjoyment and intake of food is partially dependent on one's having an appetite. Physical causes for a diminished interest in eating include poorly fitting dentures, stomatitis, decaying teeth, and halitosis and a bad taste in the mouth.

Psychosocial factors have a significant impact on one's desire for food. Appetite depends on complex mental processes having to do with

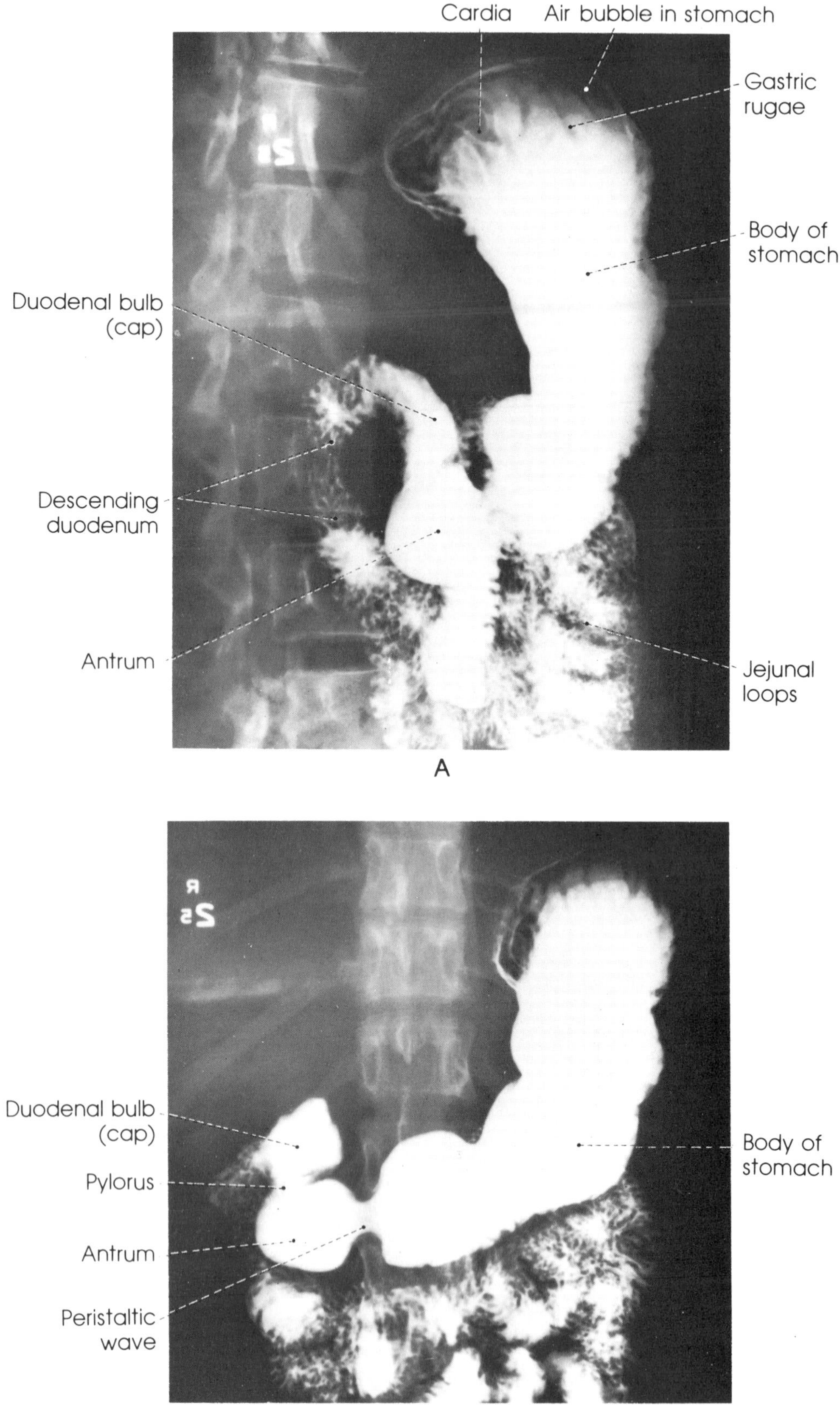

Figure 23-2 Radiographs of stomach and duodenum.
(From Langman, J., and Woerdeman, M. W.: Atlas of Medical Anatomy. Philadelphia, W. B. Saunders, 1982.)

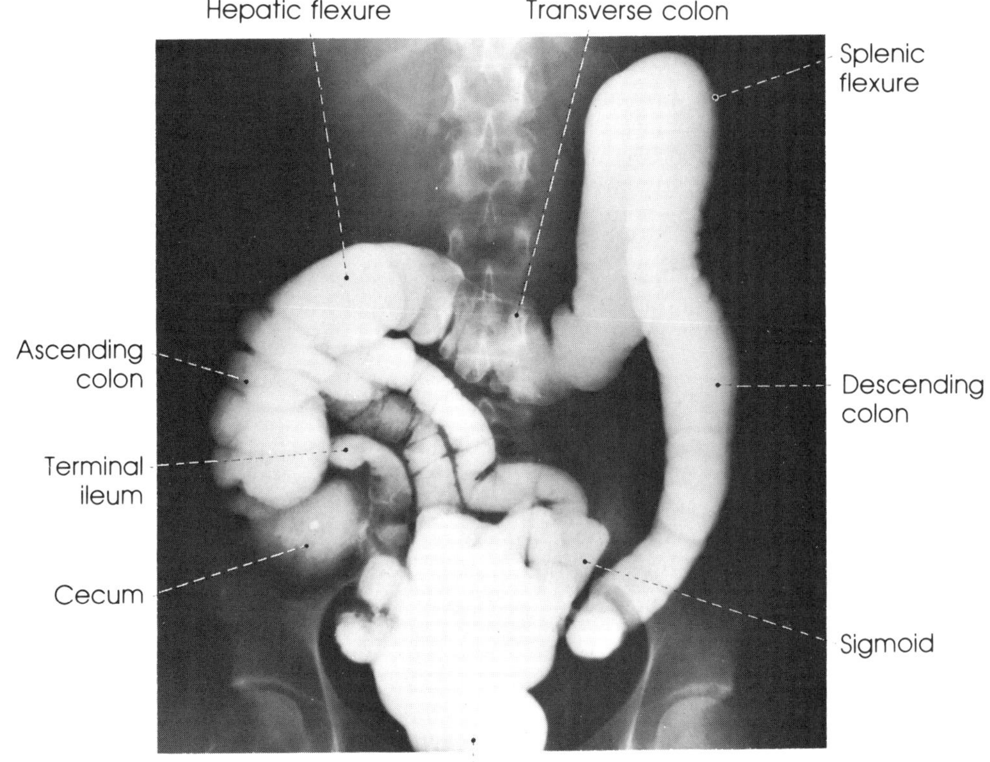

Figure 23-3 Radiograph of colon after barium enema. Note reflux of barium into ileum. (From Langman, J., and Woerdeman, M. W.: Atlas of Medical Anatomy. Philadelphia, W. B. Saunders, 1982.)

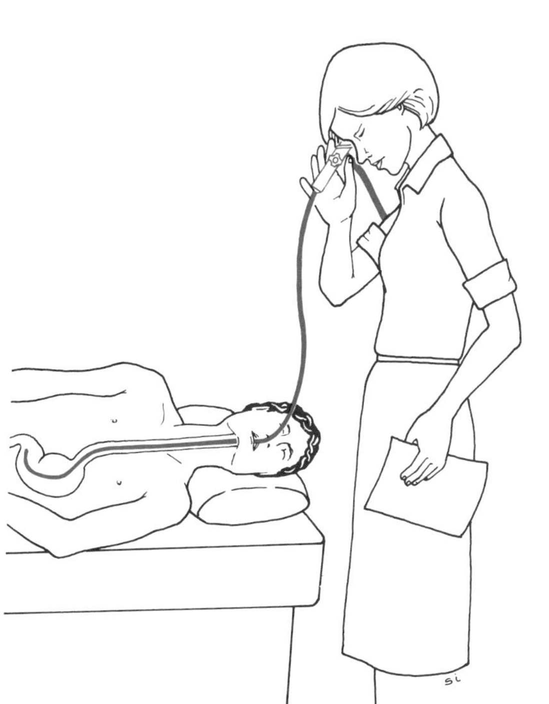

Figure 23-4 Endoscope inserted through patient's mouth for gastroscopy.

memory and mental associations that can be pleasant or extremely unpleasant. Appetite is stimulated by the sight, smell, and thought of food; hence it is influenced by the physical and social environment in which a person is eating. The enjoyment of eating can be inhibited by unattractive or unfamiliar food, surroundings, or company, and by emotional states such as anxiety, anger, and fear. Mental depression can also be a cause of anorexia.

Assessment

Because of the complex nature of anorexia, it may be necessary for the nurse to talk with the patient, his family, and significant others in her effort to learn why he has lost his appetite. She also may need to consult the patient's chart to try to find some physiologic, social, or psychological reason why a patient does not eat as he should. Once the apparent cause of anorexia is discovered, nursing intervention is aimed at minimizing or alleviating those factors that inhibit appetite.

Nursing Intervention

Loss of appetite is to be expected when a person becomes ill. However, persistent anorexia must be dealt with to avoid the consequences of inadequate nutrition. Nursing interventions include mouth care before each meal to eliminate or minimize physical causes of poor appetite.

If psychosocial factors are involved, the nurse might try offering the patient foods that he prefers whenever this is possible and not detrimental to his health. Meals that are planned to include a variety of colors, textures, and tastes are more appealing and enjoyable than those that are monotonous and bland. The patient should be given ample time to eat and encouraged to eat slowly and enjoy his meal. If it is necessary to feed the patient, this should be done cheerfully and in a manner in which the nurse herself would eat a meal.

Eating is a social event, and very few people get as much pleasure eating alone as they would in the company of someone else. The nurse, a family member, or a friend can provide companionship while a patient eats. If there is a patient cafeteria or gathering place for patients to eat together, and the patient is able to go there for meals, this can sometimes alleviate or minimize a problem of anorexia.

Food from home is often a welcome addition to institutional fare. The person bringing the meal will need to be advised of any restrictions on the patient's dietary intake and the importance of reinforcing the nurse's instruction of the patient on dietary limitations.

EATING DISORDERS

Anorexia Nervosa

Anorexia nervosa is a disorder in which the patient is preoccupied with eating but has a morbid fear of becoming fat. Excessive exercise is commonly used by these patients as another means of staying thin. Because the patient refuses to eat adequate quantities of food, rather than suffering from true anorexia, the name *anorexia nervosa* is a misnomer. The cause is unknown, but it is thought to be an inappropriate coping mechanism in response to excessive expectations and controls imposed on the patient by parents or others. It most commonly is seen in females from early teens to 30 years old, although it does occur in males also.

Anorexia nervosa is a dangerous disorder, because the patient can literally starve to death. Although it is a psychiatric disorder, the patient may be admitted to the medical floor for treatment of malnutrition by parenteral therapy. Behavior modification is the focus of treatment.

Bulimia

Bulimia is the practice of inducing vomiting after binge eating. Laxatives may also be taken to purge the system after an eating binge. The patient consumes large quantities of food and then gets rid of it so that weight is not gained. Some patients with anorexia nervosa are also bulimic.

Some individuals practice bulimia occasionally without harm. When it is practiced frequently, it can lead to severe fluid and electrolyte imbalances, starvation, and death.

Treatment of bulimia includes psychotherapy and behavior modification. Both bulimia and anorexia nervosa are difficult to cure.

Obesity

People overeat for a variety of reasons. For some it is a reaction to stress; for others it is a substitute for absent pleasures. For many, overeating is simply habit. A person is considered obese if he weighs more than 20% above the ideal weight for his height, age, and body type.

Obese patients should be counseled by the nurse to lose weight in order to prevent developing one or more of the many diseases in which obesity is a contributing factor. Diabetes and hypertension are particularly correlated to obesity.

Weight that is lost slowly is more likely not to be regained. The patient should have a physical examination with testing for thyroid abnormality and other problems before beginning a weight reduction diet. Physician supervision is the best and safest way to treat obesity. Usually a lower-calorie diet and exercise are prescribed, and the patient is taught ways to change his thinking about food and his weight.

The nurse can offer considerable support for the patient who is dieting by giving praise for pounds lost and by being available to talk about the frustrations of staying on the diet. The nurse should discourage fad diets and emphasize the importance of a well-balanced, nutritious, low-calorie diet.

Weight Watchers is the only commercial program to date that has shown good results with safe weight loss and maintenance of normal weight over a period of years.

DYSPHAGIA

Dysphagia means difficulty in swallowing. It is the most common symptom of disorders of the esophagus, and varies from a mild sensation that something is sticking in the throat to complete inability to swallow solids or liquids.

Assessment

The nurse can aid in the diagnosis of the specific cause of dysphagia by observing carefully the kinds of food the patient can tolerate and the conditions under which he experiences difficulty. Knowing the consistency and temperature of the foods most easily ingested by the patient is helpful. Some patients may strangle on liquids, tolerate soft and semi-solid foods, and have the feeling that high-fiber foods are not moving past a certain point in the esophagus.

Nursing Intervention

Measures that may be helpful in relieving dysphagia include instructing the patient to chew his food more thoroughly, to eat semi-solid foods, to drink liquids throughout the meal, and to assume a more erect posture while eating.

Other factors may be related to the physical and social environment in which meals are eaten. Meals should be served in a relaxing atmosphere, with pleasant surroundings and relief from emotional stress.

Patients with chronic dysphagia are subject to respiratory problems resulting from the aspiration of food into the respiratory tree. Both acute and chronic dysphagia are likely to produce nutritional deficiencies and electrolyte imbalances. If the dysphagia is such that the patient cannot swallow sufficient amounts of food for adequate nutrition, tube feeding may be indicated. This sometimes is necessary when the dysphagia is the result of cerebral damage, as in cerebrovascular accident (CVA).

If the patient cannot swallow anything because of a neurologic condition or if the esophagus is obstructed and cannot be corrected surgically, then the patient must have a gastrostomy. An opening in the wall of the stomach is created, and a permanent feeding tube is sutured in place.

Nursing interventions for the patient with a gastrostomy tube include aspirating for residual contents before each feeding, keeping the skin clean and dry around the tube, and changing the dressing every 24 hours or prn until the site is healed.

NAUSEA AND VOMITING

Interference with comfort and nutrition occur when nausea and vomiting are persistent. A transient problem is not treated, but when the disorder persists, medication with antiemetics, gastrointestinal intubation, and administration of IV fluids are necessary.

Nursing interventions for the patient with nausea and vomiting are discussed in Chapter 8.

ACCUMULATION OF FLUID AND GASES

Whenever ingested material cannot pass through the intestinal tract as it should, it accumulates in the stomach and the intestines, creating problems of pressure and distention. This can occur when peristalsis is decreased or the flow of chyme is inhibited by an obstruction. Gases are formed by the action of digestive juices and bacteria on the ingested material.

Medical Treatment

Abdominal distention with increased pressure within the abdominal cavity is very uncomfortable. Excess fluids and gases also interfere with ventilation of the lungs and normal function of other nearby organs.

Measures to relieve distention include insertion of a rectal tube, suppositories, and enemas to stimulate peristalsis and evacuation of the bowel. If these measures cannot be used or are ineffective, the physician may choose to use gastrointestinal intubation and removal of the intestinal contents by suction. Intubation and decompression also are used as preventive measures following abdominal surgery.

Gastrointestinal tubes vary in length, design, and purpose. The Levin tube and gastric sump tube are shorter, because they are intended to reach only as far as the stomach (Fig. 23–5). The Miller-Abbott, Cantor, and Harris tubes are longer tubes that are directed past the stomach and into the small intestine (Fig. 23–6).

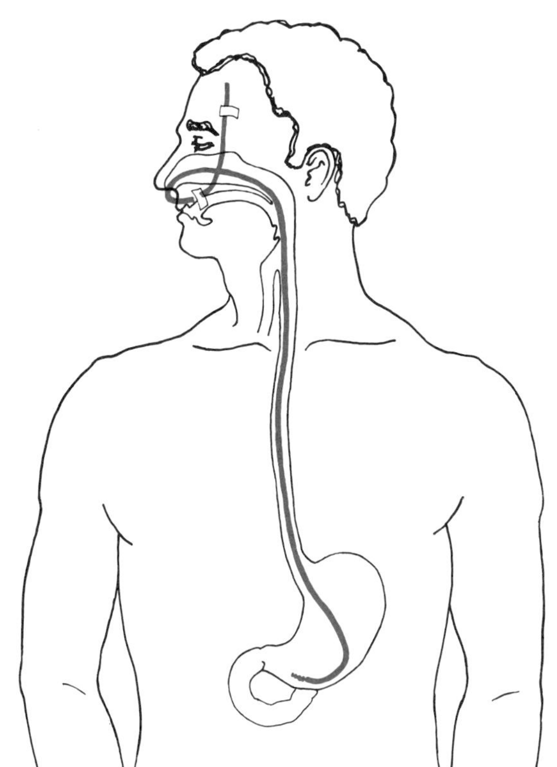

Figure 23–5 A Levin tube in place. The Levin tube is used to aspirate gastric contents or to convey liquids to the stomach.

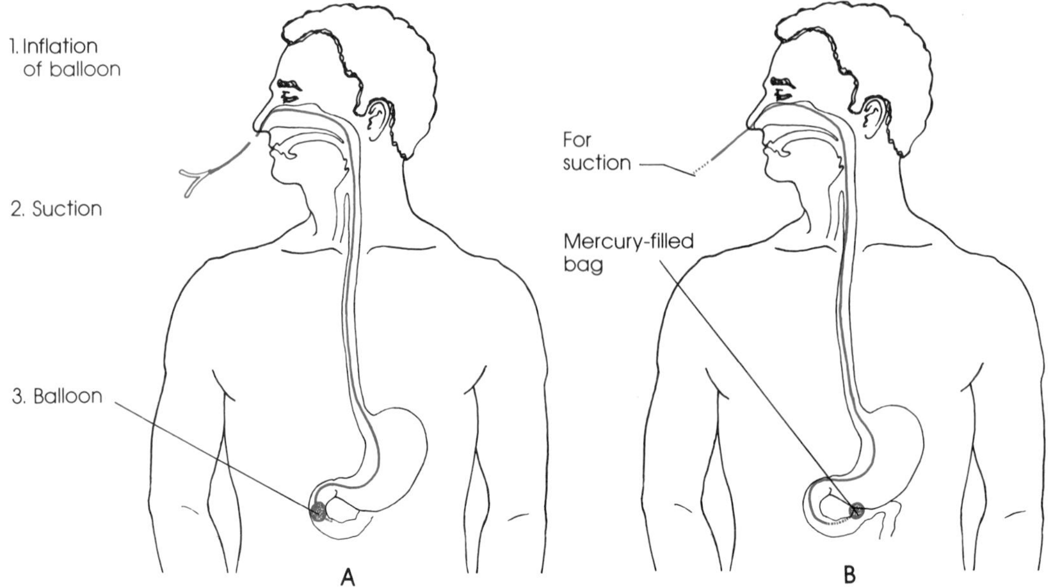

Figure 23-6 *A*, Miller-Abbott tube in place. It is advanced through the intestines to the prescribed point. The Miller-Abbott tube has a double lumen. 1, Portion of the metal tip leading to the balloon. 2, Portion of the metal tip leading to the lumen that can be suctioned. 3, Balloon inflated with air. *B*, Cantor tube in place. This intestinal tube ends in a bag that is filled with mercury to help it to pass along the gastrointestinal tract to the point prescribed by the physician. Intestinal tubes are not taped in place until they have advanced fully. The holes for suctioning are behind the balloon.

Nursing Assessment and Intervention

During gastrointestinal decompression the patient is observed for signs of abdominal distention, which would indicate that excess fluids and gases are not being removed as intended. Nausea, vomiting, complaints of feeling full or bloated, increasing shortness of breath, and increase in the girth of the abdomen are signs that the stomach and intestines are not being decompressed adequately.

Applying too much suction can pull the gastric mucosa into the drainage openings or "eyes" of the tube, causing damage to the mucosa and traumatic ulceration. Using a gastric sump tube (Salem, Ventrol) that has an air vent can help prevent this problem.

Unless ordered otherwise, the low setting is used for suction. The tubing should be kept above the level of the stomach. The connecting tubing leading to the suction machine works best if it is kept above the height of entry into the drainage container.

Irrigations with normal saline are usually ordered to keep the tube patent. The amount instilled should be added to the patient's intake count, and the amount of drainage is recorded as output for each shift. If the patient has had surgery on the intestinal tract, the irrigation procedure should be done with aseptic technique rather than clean technique.

The characteristics of the drainage are charted each shift. If the nurse notices coffee ground–like material in the tube, she should test the drainage for blood, as blood that has been in contact with gastric juices has this appearance. If blood unexpectedly appears in the drainage, the physician should be notified.

Fluid and electrolyte imbalance problems that can be caused by continuous suction and irrigation are discussed in Chapter 8.

A nasogastric (NG) tube is uncomfortable for the patient. The nostril must be checked for signs of pressure, and the tube may need to be retaped to relieve the problem. Common complaints are sore throat, dry mouth, earache (from congestion of the eustachian tube), and dry lips and nasal mucosa. Frequent mouth care and application of a lubricant to the lips and nostril will help. A room humidifier can also be helpful, but this requires a doctor's order. The physician may allow the patient to have limited amounts of ice chips, hard candy, or chewing gum to decrease the problem.

After the tube is removed, the patient is monitored for further nausea and vomiting and for abdominal distention. Sometimes it is necessary to insert the tube again.

GASTROINTESTINAL BLEEDING

Bleeding from the intestinal tract can be acute and profuse or chronic and gradual. GI bleeding usually is referred to as either *upper GI bleeding* or *lower intestinal bleeding,* depending on the source. The most common causes of upper GI bleeding are gastric and duodenal ulcers, varicose veins of the esophagus (esophageal varices), and erosive gastritis. Patients most at risk for blood loss resulting from gastritis are those who have ingested drugs (for example, large doses of unbuffered aspirin) or consumed excessive amounts of alcohol. Tumors, trauma, and foreign bodies also can lead to bleeding anywhere in the GI tract.

Bleeding from a source in the lower intestinal tract usually is more chronic and gradual in nature. Possible causes include tumors and polyps in the lower intestines, chronic colitis, and diverticulosis. Hemorrhoids also can break down and bleed, in which case bright red blood is noticed in the stools.

Nursing Assessment

During history taking, the nurse should inquire about the ingestion of any substance that might cause inflammation of the intestinal mucosa. She should also inquire about signs of weakness and fatigue that could indicate anemia from blood loss. The patient is asked about any changes in the color or character of his stools or in the pattern of bowel elimination. Has he had any persistent nausea, vomiting, or indigestion that might indicate gastrointestinal irritation?

Subjective signs of acute gastrointestinal bleeding include complaints of weakness and feeling faint, nausea and vomiting, restlessness, thirst, and mental confusion. Objective signs include the presence of bright red blood in either the emesis or stool; "coffee ground" emesis (hematemesis) or maroon or tarry stools (melena); diarrhea (blood acts as a cathartic); and decreased blood pressure, rapid pulse, and other signs of hypovolemic shock.

If bleeding from the upper GI system is profuse, maroon or bright red blood can be noted in the stools because of the rapid transit of the blood through the intestinal tract. Black stools almost always indicate the presence of digested blood, which means that the source of bleeding is in the upper gastrointestinal tract. It is well to remember that iron salts can cause the stool to be black. The ingestion of beets can cause the stool to be bright red in color.

Estimates of blood loss from the alimentary canal are based in part on blood pressure readings and pulse rates. Hence blood pressure and pulse rate should be monitored every 15 to 30 minutes when there is evidence of extensive gastrointestinal hemorrhage. Changes in the vital signs that signal hypovolemic shock do not appear until after the patient has lost 20% or more of his blood volume.

Central venous pressure readings also are helpful in determining the amount of blood lost, especially in hypertensive patients, whose blood pressure may not reflect hypovolemia.

Additional data useful in determining the status of patients with GI bleeding include hematocrit and hemoglobin levels. These levels can be normal or even slightly elevated at the beginning of a bleeding episode, because it takes 4 to 6 hours for the body to shift fluids from other compartments to the intravascular compartment and thereby change the ratio of formed elements to fluids in the blood.

The white cell count may be elevated in massive GI bleeding, probably because of the body's response to injury or hypovolemia. An elevated level of blood urea nitrogen (BUN) can indicate digestion of large amounts of blood.

Medical Treatment and Nursing Intervention

The major concerns in the treatment of acute gastrointestinal hemorrhage are replacement of the blood and fluids lost and stoppage of the bleeding. If there is major blood loss, transfusions of whole blood, packed cells, or fresh frozen plasma may be necessary. Normal saline, Plasmanate (plasma protein fraction), and Ringer's solution may be administered until blood is available. Maintenance of fluid balance is of extreme importance. Intake and output must be measured and recorded accurately. Oxygen therapy is often begun.

Once the patient's condition is sufficiently stabilized, diagnostic procedures are done to locate the source of bleeding. These procedures include endoscopic examination of the esophagus, stomach, and small intestine. Barium studies also may be done.

Treatment of gastric bleeding is begun by inserting a large-bore NG tube and using tap water lavage to monitor the quantity of bleeding and evacuate the blood, clots, and stomach contents. This allows the stomach to constrict, halting the blood flow. Antacids are given via the tube to neutralize pepsin and help stop the bleeding. Cimetadine (Tagamet) is given intravenously to decrease stomach acid secretion. Eighty percent of gastrointestinal bleeding will stop spontaneously (Andreoli et al., 1990).

Once the patient has stabilized, diagnostic procedures are done to locate the source of bleeding. Electrocauterization or laser photocoagulation of a vessel can be done through the endoscope. If endoscopy and barium radiographs are unsuccessful in locating the area of bleeding, angiography of the vessels supplying the intestinal tract is performed and embolization done to stop the bleeding. Surgery may be required if the bleeding cannot be stopped by any other means.

Bleeding from esophageal varices, usually caused by cirrhosis of the liver, is controlled by injections of vasopressin (Pitressin) directly in the bleeding artery to stimulate contraction of the vessel and by use of a Sengstaken-Blakemore

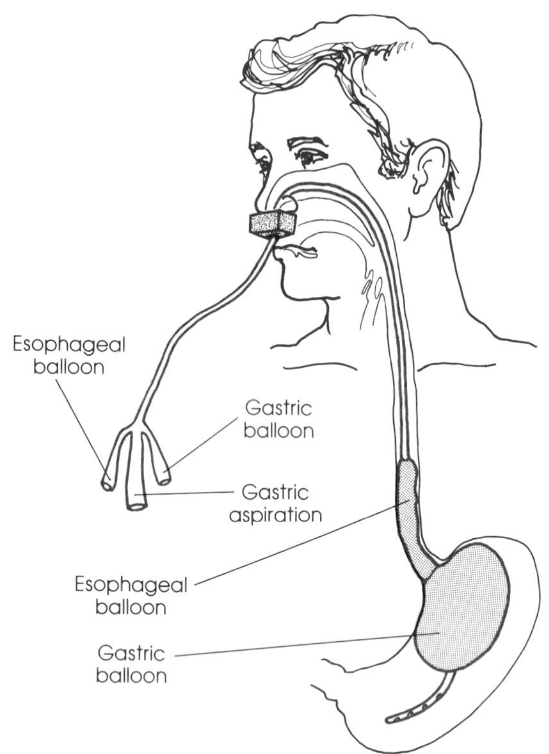

Figure 23-7 Sengstaken-Blackmore tube. If the bleeding site is in the esophagus, as from esophageal varices, the esophageal balloon is inflated. If the bleeding site is in the stomach, the gastric balloon is inflated. Inflation of the balloon creates pressure against bleeding vessels.

tube, which compresses the vessels by inflation of balloons (Fig. 23-7). The tube has three lumens: one for the esophageal balloon, one for the gastric balloon, and one through which saline can be instilled and blood and stomach secretions can be evacuated.

Nursing intervention in the care of a patient with GI bleeding must include consideration for the patient's fear and anxiety. Many times these patients are afraid they are going to die. The sight of so much blood loss is frightening to the patient, to whom it usually appears more profuse than it actually is. Whatever procedures are used, the patient and his family deserve an explanation and reassurance that everything is being done to control the hemorrhage.

After the bleeding has apparently stopped and the patient's vital signs have stabilized, there must be continuous monitoring for signs of persistent or renewed bleeding. Blood pressure and pulse rate are measured regularly; skin color, diaphoresis, thirst, and other signs of continued blood loss and impending hypovolemic shock must be watched for; intake and output are measured and the character of vomitus, aspirated gastric fluid, and stools noted; and the patient's daily weight is taken and recorded.

HIATAL HERNIA (DIAPHRAGMATIC HERNIA)

Hiatal hernia is the result of a defect in the wall of the diaphragm where the esophagus passes through. A hiatal hernia is formed by protrusion of part of the stomach into the esophagus; it is a common disorder in older people, especially women. Loss of muscle strength and tone, factors that cause increased intraabdominal pressure (such as obesity or multiple pregnancies), and congenital defects contribute to the formation of the hernia.

Signs and symptoms include indigestion, belching, and substernal or epigastric pain or feelings of pressure after eating. The symptoms are more severe when the patient lies down. The problem can be visualized on an upper GI series.

Treatment includes weight reduction, administration of antacids, and elevation of the head of the bed on 4-inch to 6-inch blocks. The patient is instructed not to eat within an hour of going to bed.

Occasionally a patient with reflux esophagitis, which is caused by the hernia, may bleed extensively. If bleeding or discomfort cannot be controlled, surgical correction of the hernia is required.

LONG-TERM AND SEVERE NUTRITIONAL DEFICIT

If a patient has long-term difficulty taking in food orally, as when in a coma, enteral feeding is indicated. Current practice calls for a nasoduodenal tube, frequently the Dobhoff tube (Fig. 23-8), to deliver special formula liquid feedings to the gastrointestinal system. The feedings can be given at specified times throughout the day or on a continuous basis. If continuous tube feedings are ordered, they frequently are administered with a feeding pump.

When, for any reason, a patient cannot ingest foods and liquids normally and continues to have weight loss and a negative nitrogen balance, *total parenteral nutrition* (TPN) is indicated. The word *hyperalimentation*, though not technically correct, is frequently used as a synonym for total parenteral nutrition.

Conditions that could warrant TPN include severe trauma to the intestinal tract, as in a gunshot wound, and chronic inflammatory conditions such as regional ileitis that prevent absorption of nutrients. Other conditions not related to the intestinal tract but nevertheless capable of seriously interfering with normal nutrition over a period of time include prolonged sepsis, fever, extensive burns, and cancer.

Total parenteral nutrition is essentially a form of intravenous feeding. However, because the amounts and kinds of nutrients needed for long-

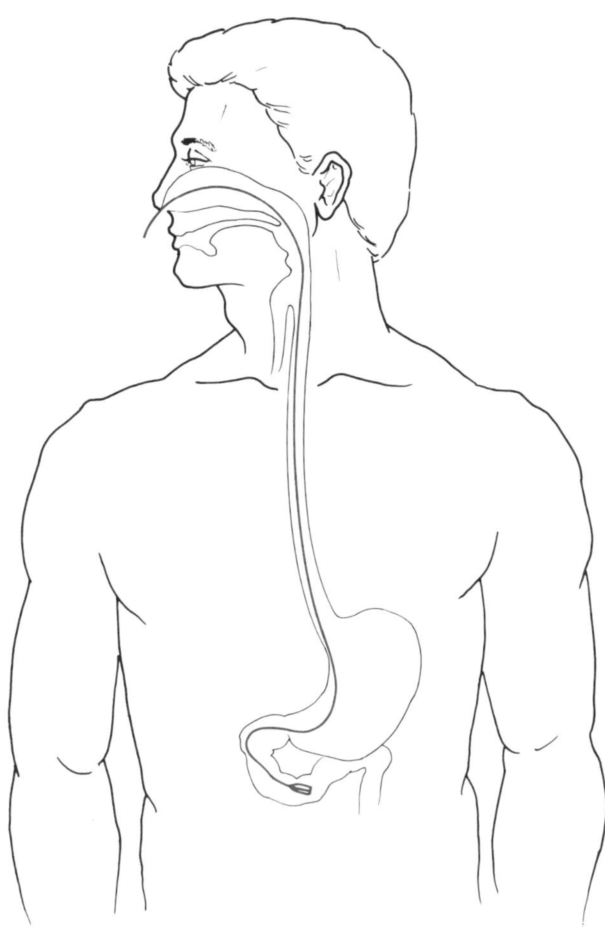

Figure 23-8 Dobhoff-nasoduodenal feeding tube.

term nutritional maintenance usually cannot be handled by peripheral veins, the nutrient mix is given into a larger central vein such as the superior vena cava. To accomplish this the physician may choose a direct central line into the vena cava, or he may use the jugular vein. Lipids may be given via a peripheral vein (Fig. 23-9).

The solution used for TPN includes 50% dextrose in water, amino acids, and such additives as electrolytes, vitamins, and trace minerals. The basic TPN solution is hypertonic but is rapidly diluted by the large amount of blood in the vena cava.

If a patient needs calories and cannot tolerate high concentrations of dextrose, or if he needs amino acids and essential fatty acids and additional protein, a fat emulsion may be given in addition to the main glucose solution.

Administration of a TPN solution is never "speeded up" if it falls behind schedule, as this can cause a dangerous glucose load.

The most obvious danger is infection, because the insertion site and indwelling venous catheter provide infectious agents an open door and direct pathway to the blood. Other problems arise from sensitivity to components of the mix. Phlebitis and thrombosis of the vena cava, elevated blood sugar, cardiac overload and other kinds of trauma to the heart, and fluid and electrolyte imbalances are all possible during TPN.

Care of the patient must be a team effort on the part of physicians, pharmacists, dietitians, and nurses. Nursing care includes assisting with the insertion of the intravenous line, changing the tubing with each new bag or bottle, changing the dressing, and removing the tubing when TPN therapy is discontinued. Some institutions have specially prepared TPN nurses to give direct care to these patients and supervise that given by general duty nurses. However, day-to-day care, including monitoring vital signs and fluid and electrolyte balance, daily weighings, frequent mouth care, and dressing changes and observation of the insertion site, is the responsibility of the staff nurse to whom the patient has been assigned.

INFLAMMATORY DISORDERS OF THE INTESTINAL TRACT

STOMATITIS

Stomatitis is a generalized inflammation of the mucous membranes of the mouth. Causes include trauma from ill-fitting dentures or malocclusions of the teeth, poor oral hygiene, nutritional deficiencies, excessive smoking, excessive

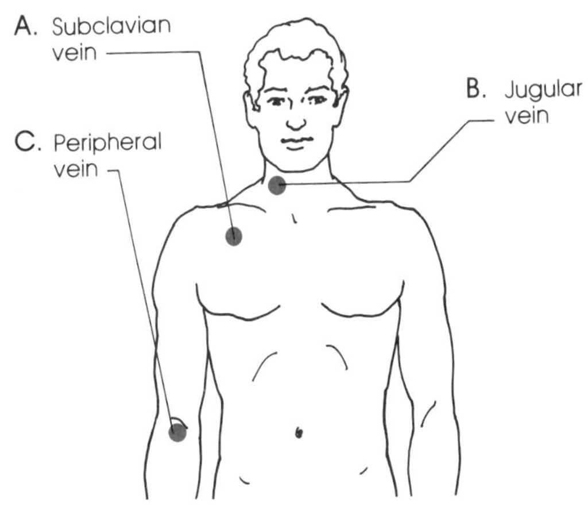

Figure 23-9 Sites for insertion of a line for total parenteral nutrition (TPN). In site A a direct central line is established in the subclavian vein. Selection of this site allows the patient more freedom of movement and provides easier access for dressing and tubing changes. However, it does carry the risk of pneumothorax during insertion. A second choice is the jugular vein (B), which gives access to the subclavian vein. Major disadvantages of this site are limitation of motion of the head and neck and relative inaccessibility for assessment and dressing changes. Lipids can also be infused through a peripheral vein (C).

drinking of alcohol, pathogenic microorganisms, radiation therapy, and drugs (especially those used in chemotherapy for malignancies).

Assessment

Common symptoms of stomatitis include pain and swelling of the oral mucosa, increased salivation or excessive dryness, severe halitosis, and sometimes fever and small, craterlike ulcers in the mouth.

Nursing Intervention

Treatment of stomatitis is chiefly symptomatic, unless a specific infectious causative agent is identified. Nursing measures to control the symptoms of stomatitis, including special mouth care, artificial saliva, and diet, are discussed in Chapter 14.

GASTRITIS

Gastritis is an inflammation of the mucous membrane lining the stomach and may be acute or chronic in nature. *Atrophic* gastritis involves all layers of the stomach and is seen in association with gastric ulcer and malignancies of the stomach. Gastritis associated with uremia is common in the patient with kidney failure. Chronic gastritis frequently progresses to ulcer formation and upper GI hemorrhage.

The main causes of acute gastritis are drinking excessive amounts of alcohol, eating contaminated food, and ingestion of drugs such as unbuffered aspirin, corticosteroids, or nonsteroidal antiinflammatory agents.

Assessment

In both acute and chronic gastritis, the main symptoms are nausea, vomiting, pain and tenderness in the stomach region, and sometimes diarrhea. The patient with chronic gastritis may also have massive hemorrhage from the stomach.

Nursing Diagnosis

Nursing diagnoses for patients with gastritis might include the following:

- Pain related to stomach irritation.
- Fluid volume deficit related to nausea and vomiting.
- Alteration in nutrition, less than body requirements, related to inability to eat or retain food because of stomach pain, nausea, and vomiting.
- Sleep pattern disturbance related to need for frequent medication and nausea and vomiting.
- Knowledge deficit related to eating habits or drug intake that is causing stomach irritation.
- Self-care deficit related to weakness and nausea.

Medical Treatment and Nursing Intervention

Acute gastritis is usually of very short duration. Treatment consists of withholding all foods by mouth and administering drugs that slow down the peristaltic action of the alimentary tract. If severe dehydration or nausea and vomiting occur, fluids may be given intravenously.

The patient with gastritis must be watched closely for signs of fluid and electrolyte imbalance.

Chronic gastritis is not as easily treated as acute gastritis. Diet therapy is of primary importance in chronic gastritis, because the patient frequently admits to indiscretion in his dietary and drinking habits and finds it difficult to change. The diet for these patients is basically bland, devoid of those foods known to produce attacks in an individual patient. It is always difficult to change eating habits of long standing, and the nurse must use tact and patience in encouraging the patient to follow the prescribed diet faithfully.

Treatment consists of antispasmodics to decrease the pain of stomach spasms, antacids, and cimetidine to decrease acid secretions and change pH.

ULCERATIVE COLITIS AND CROHN'S DISEASE

Ulcerative colitis is an inflammation, with the formation of ulcers, of the mucosa of the colon. It is often a chronic disease, and the patient is usually free from symptoms between acute flare-ups.

The exact cause of ulcerative colitis is not known. Infections and emotional tension frequently bring about acute attacks.

Ulcerative colitis and regional ileitis (Crohn's disease) share many of the same characteristics. One difference is that the inflammatory changes in ulcerative colitis are nonspecific, whereas those in Crohn's disease are granulomatous. Another very important difference is that the patient with long-standing chronic ulcerative colitis is at 10 to 20 times greater risk for developing cancer of the colon than one with Crohn's disease. Crohn's disease can affect any area of the intestine.

There is a growing tendency to include both disorders under the title of inflammatory bowel disease (IBD). It is suspected that ulcerative colitis and Crohn's disease are immunologic responses to the same as yet unknown etiologic agent.

Medical Diagnosis

The patient with inflammatory bowel disease suffers from attacks of bloody, mucoid diarrhea that are often precipitated by events that cause undue physical or emotional stress. An acute attack can last for days, weeks, or even months, followed by periods of remission extending from a few weeks to several decades. Some few patients experience only one attack and then remain free of symptoms for the rest of their lives. Others suffer such profound disturbances during the first attack that their lives are in danger if they do not receive prompt treatment to stop intestinal hemorrhage and correct fluid and electrolyte imbalances.

Medical diagnosis usually is based on the patient's medical history and presenting symptoms. Colonoscopy, barium enema, and stool analysis may be used to confirm the diagnosis.

Nursing Diagnosis

Assessment of the patient with inflammatory bowel disease commonly supplies data that support the following nursing diagnoses:

- Diarrhea related to intestinal irritation.
- Fluid volume deficit related to persistent diarrhea.
- Pain related to intestinal cramping from mucosal irritation.
- Sleep pattern disturbance related to constant need to evacuate bowel.
- Potential impaired skin integrity related to irritation of anal area from diarrhea.
- Fatigue related to fluid and electrolyte loss.
- Anxiety related to deteriorating physical condition.

Medical and Surgical Treatment and Nursing Intervention

Treatment for either ulcerative colitis or Crohn's disease varies according to severity of symptoms and whether the condition becomes chronic. Conservative approaches to medical treatment include administration of antidiarrheic drugs, long-term sulfasalazine therapy, medications to relieve abdominal cramps, and a diet of low-residue, bland foods that have a high protein and caloric content. Corticosteroids are used for moderate to severe cases. During acute attacks replacement of fluids may be necessary.

Surgical intervention is an alternative treatment for some patients. The surgical procedure usually involves removal of the affected portion of the bowel and creation of an ileostomy.

The nursing care plan for a patient experiencing an acute attack should include such observations as number and character of stools, periodic auscultation of bowel sounds, measurement of intake and output, daily weighings, checking for signs of internal bleeding and anemia, and monitoring laboratory data for evidence of electrolyte imbalances.

Long-term goals may be concerned with helping the patient adhere to his prescribed regimen, teaching him effective coping mechanisms, and instruction and encouragement in relaxation techniques. The frequent bouts of diarrhea and abdominal cramping can be embarrassing and depressing for the patient. He will need emotional support, empathetic listening, and encouragement to take part in cooperative planning for his care.

APPENDICITIS

Appendicitis is an inflammation of the vermiform appendix. It is called *vermiform* because it is wormlike, and *appendix* because it is an appendage of the cecum. The appendix is a blind pouch and is therefore easily infected by bacteria passing through the intestinal tract.

Assessment

Pain in the lower right side, halfway between the umbilicus and the crest of the ileum, is the best-known symptom of appendicitis. However, the location of the pain may, and often does, vary among individuals. An elevated temperature, nausea and vomiting, and an increase in the white cell count are also characteristic of appendicitis.

Nursing Intervention

Appendicitis is treated by surgical removal of the appendix (*appendectomy*). Before surgery, the patient is allowed nothing by mouth, and an ice bag may be placed on the abdomen to slow down localization of the inflammation and thus avoid rupture of the swollen and inflamed appendix.

Under no circumstances should laxatives be given when appendicitis is suspected. Hot water bottles to relieve abdominal pain are also forbidden.

The patient is usually allowed out of bed the day after surgery if there are no complications. The convalescent period is most often uneventful, and the patient may return to his former activities within 2 or 3 weeks.

PERITONITIS

The peritoneum is a serous sac that lines the abdominal cavity and encloses the intestines, stomach, liver, and spleen and partially encloses the uterus and uterine tubes. Peritonitis is an inflammation of the peritoneum. It usually occurs when one of the organs it encloses ruptures or is perforated so that the organ's contents (including bacteria) are spilled into the abdominal cavity. Examples of common causes of peritonitis are ruptured appendix, perforated duodenal or gastric ulcer, ruptured ectopic (tubal) pregnancy, and traumatic rupture of the spleen or liver.

Assessment

As the peritoneum becomes inflamed, there is local redness and swelling of the membrane with production of serous fluid that becomes more and more purulent as the bacteria multiply. Normal peristaltic action of the intestines slows or ceases altogether, and the symptoms of intestinal obstruction occur. The patient experiences nausea, vomiting, severe abdominal pain and distention, high fever, tachycardia, pallor, and other symptoms of shock. Unless the condition is treated promptly and successfully, peritonitis can be fatal.

Medical Treatment and Nursing Intervention

Antibiotics are given in massive doses to combat infection, fluids and electrolytes are administered to restore a normal balance, and gastric or intestinal suction is initiated to relieve distention. Surgical procedures needed to repair a ruptured organ are done as soon as the patient's condition will permit.

Nursing care is primarily concerned with close, intelligent observation of the patient and prompt and accurate reporting of unexpected changes in his condition. He is usually placed in the semi-Fowler's position to facilitate breathing, prevent respiratory complications, and aid in localizing the purulent material in the lower abdomen or pelvis. His vital signs are noted and recorded every 4 hours during the critical stage. If he vomits, the characteristics and amount of vomitus are noted. The emesis of fecal material indicates complete intestinal obstruction.

A common complication of peritonitis is paralytic ileus. If the patient passes flatus or feces rectally, this should be recorded on his chart, as it indicates return of peristalsis.

Because of the high fever and toxicity that accompany peritonitis, the patient may be delirious or disoriented, and he must be protected from self-injury. This includes putting siderails on the bed and supervising the patient at all times. The patient should be turned *very gently* and moved in the bed with care because of extreme tenderness in the abdominal region. A high fever and the presence of the gastric tube demand frequent mouth care to protect the lips and prevent halitosis and a foul taste in the mouth.

PEPTIC ULCER

A peptic ulcer is a loss of tissues lining the lower esophagus, the stomach, or the duodenum (Fig. 23–10). The most common site is in the first few centimeters of the duodenum, just beyond the pyloric muscle. Acute lesions that do not extend through the muscular mucosae are simply called *lesions*. Chronic lesions, which are almost always called *ulcers*, involve the muscular coat, destroying the musculature and replacing it with permanent scar tissue at the site of healing.

For some unknown reason the incidence of peptic ulcer has been gradually decreasing in the past few decades. It is more common in males than in females.

CAUSATIVE FACTORS

The usual cause of peptic ulcer is the presence of too much gastric juice *in relation to the degree of protection* normally afforded by the gastroin-

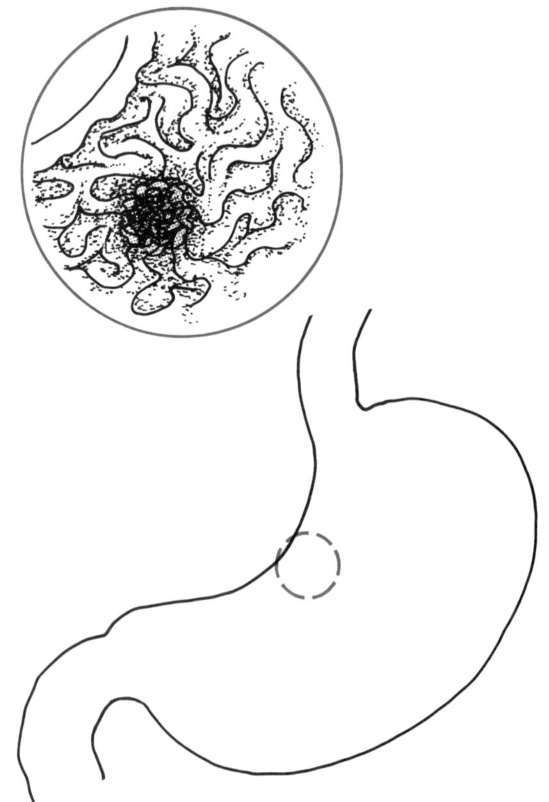

Figure 23–10 Ulcer of the gastric mucosa. The ulcer has penetrated deeply into the stomach wall.

testinal mucosa and the small intestine, which secrete mucus and other substances that neutralize gastric acid. Normally, all areas exposed to the hydrochloric acid and pepsin in gastric juice have an ample supply of mucous glands that secrete a protective alkaline mucus.

Although it is known that gastric acid and pepsin are responsible for ulcer formation, it is not known why mucosal resistance to them should become impaired. Duodenal ulcers and some prepyloric ulcers are associated with an increased amount or hyperacidity of the gastric juice. Gastric ulcers, on the other hand, are characterized by normal or abnormally low levels of hydrochloric acid. It is likely that gastric ulcers develop because there is reduced resistance of the gastric mucosa to digestion by gastric juice.

Theories about genetic and environmental causes of peptic ulcer abound. Both gastric and duodenal ulcers tend to occur in families. Relatives of persons with gastric or duodenal ulcers have three times the expected rate for ulcer formation. One might suspect that because people in the same family share the same environment and tend to eat the same kinds of foods, it is these factors that cause ulcers to run in families. However, there is no evidence that gastric and duodenal ulcers can be attributed to a shared environment alone.

Hot spicy foods once were thought to be a possible cause of ulcers, but there is no evidence to support this belief. It is true, however, that gastric ulcer is more likely to occur in those who are poorly nourished, whether from poverty and the unavailability of nourishing foods or from poor eating habits. Despite the stereotype of the hard-driving executive suffering from an ulcer and gulping antacid tablets, there is a greater incidence of ulcers in blue collar workers and laborers.

This is not to say that stress does not have a bearing on the development of peptic ulcer, however. Tension, anxiety, and prolonged stress do alter gastric function. Prolonged psychological or physiologic stress produces what is known as a *stress ulcer*, which is believed to be the result of unrelieved stimulation of the vagus nerves. A stress ulcer is pathologically and clinically different from a chronic peptic ulcer. It is more acute and more likely to produce hemorrhage; perforation occurs occasionally, and pain is rare. Stress ulcers are an "occupational hazard" of patients who are in intensive care units for prolonged periods. Such patients often receive medication to prevent stress ulcers.

Drug-induced ulcers are most often caused by unbuffered aspirin and nonsteroidal antiinflammatory drugs (NSAIDs), with alcohol running a close second. The glucocorticoids also can be ulcer-producing.

Cigarette smoking is known to be a causative factor in peptic ulcer. Studies have shown that smokers are several times more likely to develop an ulcer than nonsmokers.

DIAGNOSTIC TESTS AND PROCEDURES

The technique most commonly used to diagnose peptic ulcer is an upper GI series *(barium swallow)*. Endoscopy can help locate the site of ulceration and bleeding and in differentiating between benign and malignant ulcerations and between esophageal ulcer and diverticulum (pouching of the intestinal wall).

A gastric analysis to measure the level of hydrochloric acid in gastric juice may be helpful in some cases, but there is a good bit of variation in gastric acid levels among patients with peptic ulcer.

NURSING ASSESSMENT

Significant data the nurse should be looking for when gathering the history of a patient with a suspected ulcer include (1) the presence of peptic ulcer in relatives; (2) the patient's eating habits and how eating affects his symptoms; (3) whether the patient smokes or drinks and to what extent; (4) any history of stressful injuries or diseases such as severe trauma, extensive surgery, severe burns, advanced malignancy, and brain injury, any of which can produce a stress ulcer; and (5) any drugs the patient is currently taking.

The nurse might also gather information about possible psychological sources of stress in the patient's life and how he usually copes with stressful situations. That is, does he "blow off steam" when he is angry and how does he do this? Does he keep his fears, anxieties, and anger to himself? How does he relax? Is he a "workaholic"?

Subjective symptoms of uncomplicated ulcer include epigastric pain that might be described as burning, gnawing, cramping, or aching, and usually comes in waves that last several minutes. The daily pattern of pain is associated with the secretion of gastric juice in relation to the presence of food, which can act as a buffer. For example, the pain is diminished in the morning when secretion is low and after meals when food is in the stomach, and most severe before meals and at bedtime. Discomfort often appears for several days or weeks and then subsides, only to reappear weeks or months later.

Other subjective symptoms include nausea, loss of appetite, and sometimes weight loss. Spontaneous vomiting usually accompanies duodenal ulcer more often than gastric ulcer.

NURSING DIAGNOSIS

The patient with a peptic ulcer may have the following nursing diagnoses:

- Pain related to gastric ulceration.
- Nausea and vomiting related to food intolerance from gastric irritation.
- Alteration in nutrition, less than body requirements, related to abdominal pain and nausea.
- Knowledge deficit related to causative factors and to medication side effects.
- Noncompliance related to refusal to follow recommended lifestyle changes.

COMPLICATIONS

The three major complications of peptic ulcer are hemorrhage, perforation, and obstruction. Hemorrhage has been discussed earlier in this chapter under "Gastrointestinal Bleeding." Perforation is erosion of the ulcer through all walls of the intestine and a spilling of the contents of the GI tract into the peritoneal cavity. It constitutes a surgical emergency because of the danger of hemorrhage and peritonitis.

Peforation is characterized by a sudden and severe pain in the upper abdomen that persists and increases in intensity and sometimes is referred to the shoulders. The abdomen is rigid and boardlike and extremely tender. In a short time the patient shows signs of shock.

Obstruction occurs as a result of scarring and loss of musculature at the pylorus. It is manifested chiefly by persistent vomiting.

MEDICAL TREATMENT AND NURSING INTERVENTION

Peptic ulcer is treated conservatively at first in the hope of avoiding surgery. The goals of treatment are to alleviate symptoms, promote healing, prevent complications, and educate the patient in self-care so that recurrence can be avoided.

Relief of Symptoms

Medications to relieve pain from local irritation of the intestinal mucosa include the antacids, which reduce the pain of ulcer by neutralizing gastric acid. Examples of antacids include aluminum hydroxide (Amphojel), aluminum hydroxide–magnesium trisilicate (Gaviscon), and aluminum hydroxide–magnesium hydroxide–simethicone (Gelusil). Antacids effective for antiflatulence include aluminum hydroxide–magnesium hydroxide–simethicone (Gelusil-M, Maalox Plus, and Mylanta).

Sucralfate (Carafate) tablets may be used for short-term (up to 8 weeks) treatment of duodenal ulcer. It has negligible acid-neutralizing capacity. The action of this drug is local, and its benefits probably derive from its adherence to the ulcer site and protection from further damage by gastric juices.

Sedatives are sometimes prescribed for the peptic ulcer patient to help reduce anxiety and relieve tension.

Cimetidine (Tagamet) is specific for the treatment of peptic ulcer. It inhibits the effect of histamine on H_2-receptors, blocking the secretion of gastric acid. Cimetidine relieves pain, reduces the need for antacids, and promotes healing. Ranitidine (Zantac) is also a histamine inhibitor. It is used for short-term treatment, usually 4 weeks, of peptic ulcers. It does not have to be given at a particular time in relation to food and does not interact with as many other medications as does cimetidine. It should be given 1 hour before an antacid.

Diet

In the past, diet was a major part of treatment of ulcers. Today, most authorities believe that it is best to restrict only those foods that the patient identifies with the onset of symptoms. Exceptions are alcohol and caffeine, both of which can induce gastritis and aggravate erosion of the gastric mucosa.

It is generally agreed that the kind of food eaten by an ulcer patient is not as important as when the food is eaten. He should eat at frequent and regular intervals throughout the day, rather than two or three large meals. He should not skip meals and should try to have some food that agrees with him in his stomach at all times.

Education of the Patient

Before a peptic ulcer can be successfully controlled, the patient must understand how and why he probably developed an ulcer in the first place. Once he has understood the predisposing factors, he must be helped to avoid them as much as possible. Unless he can cooperate fully with the physician and nurses, there is a strong possibility that he will continue to develop ulcers despite medical or even surgical treatment. Nursing interventions for selected problems in a patient with a bleeding peptic ulcer are summarized in Nursing Care Plan 23–1.

TEACHING A PATIENT WITH A PEPTIC ULCER

- He must learn to regulate the types of foods he eats and the manner in which he eats them. Mealtimes should be unhurried, relaxed, and spaced at regular intervals.
- His emotional health, ability to cope with distressing situations, and his occupation and

NURSING CARE PLAN 23–1

Selected nursing diagnoses, goals/outcome criteria, nursing interventions, and evaluations for a patient with a bleeding peptic ulcer

Situation: Mr. Lee is a 47-year-old long-distance truck driver who is admitted to the hospital with a tentative diagnosis of bleeding peptic ulcer. He has had recurrent bouts of epigastric pain that is more pronounced before meals and at bedtime. Mr. Lee states that he eats "whenever I can grab a bite." He eats mostly fried and spicy foods and he smokes two packs of cigarettes a day. He went to the doctor because of fatigue and discomfort that seemed to be getting progressively worse in spite of antacid use. He also admits to having some vomiting episodes with blood in the secretions. Mr. Lee is the sole support of his wife and four children and is very concerned about the expense of hospitalization and the time away from work. He is scheduled for an endoscopic exam of the esophagus, stomach, and duodenum.

Nursing Diagnosis	Goals/Outcome Criteria*	Nursing Intervention	Evaluation
Anxiety related to expenses, time off work, and worry about what is wrong with him. SUPPORTING DATA Sole support of family; expresses worry over hospital expenses; worried about blood in vomitus.	Patient will verbalize reduction in anxiety before discharge. Patient will devise plan to cover hospital expenses so as to decrease anxiety. Patient will verbalize understanding of diagnosis and treatment of his condition.	Encourage verbalization of concerns and fears. Ask for financial consultant collaboration regarding handling of hospital expenses. Explain all diagnostic procedures and medications. Assess usual coping techniques and teach new ways to cope as necessary. Reinforce wife's assurances that they can manage expenses at home. Encourage relaxation techniques.	Appt. with social worker; taught relaxation exercise and encouraged to practice it; wife says he tends to be a "worry wart"; encouraged him to talk about fears; is afraid of being off work; continue plan.
Pain related to irritation and possible ulceration of gastric mucosa. SUPPORTING DATA Recurrent bouts of epigastric pain more pronounced before meals; blood-tinged vomitus; stressful occupation.	Patient will verbalize relief of pain. Patient will verbalize ways to prevent gastric pain.	Assess location and severity of pain q shift. Administer ordered antacids, antispasmodics, and H_2 inhibitors. Give caffeine-free diet. Encourage him to quit smoking. Give frequent feedings to neutralize gastric acid. Provide quiet, relaxed environment.	Pain is epigastric, now occurring between meals; taking meds as ordered; no caffeine drinks; encouraged him to quit smoking; said he would think about it; continue plan.
Alteration in tissue perfusion related to loss of blood from gastric mucosa. SUPPORTING DATA Blood-streaked vomitus; history suggestive of peptic ulcer; increasing fatigue; pale conjunctiva.	No signs of intestinal blood loss by discharge. Hemoglobin and hematocrit will be within normal levels within 30 days.	Monitor CBC count for evidence of continued bleeding. Assess vomitus for blood. Check stool for occult blood as ordered. Monitor vital signs and assess for continued or rapid blood loss as ordered. Teach about foods high in iron content to correct anemia.	Stool positive for occult blood × 2; taught him about foods high in iron; continue plan.
Mr. Lee's physician found a duodenal ulcer on endoscopic examination. He has prescribed sulcrafate (Carafate), 1 gm po qid 1 h ac and hs, ranitidine (Zantac), 300 mg hs, and Mylanta II, 30 mL 30 min pc, in hopes of healing the ulcer and preventing surgery.			
Knowledge deficit related to factors that contribute to peptic ulcer and information about medications. SUPPORTING DATA Was unaware that cigarette smoking contributed to ulcers; never has heard of the medications prescribed for him, except for the antacid.	Patient will verbalize factors that contribute to ulcer formation. Patient will attempt to quit smoking within 2 weeks. Patient will verbalize reason for each medication, dosage schedule, and side effects.	Instruct in contributing factors of ulcer formation. Assist him to learn new ways to cope with stress. Instruct him in food substances to avoid, including caffeine and alcohol. Discuss ways to manage proper eating when on the road. Teach action, dosage, and side effects of each medication. Obtain feedback for material taught.	States that he will quit eating foods that cause pain (i.e., spicy foods); has cut smoking down to ½ pack per day, states he will try to quit; verbalizes side effects of medications and proper dosage schedule; will begin exercise program for stress reduction.

* Can be used as outcome criteria to evaluate patient's progress.

home life are all important to his state of physical health. He must either learn to avoid situations of anxiety or strive to develop a more placid and serene outlook on life.

- Most patients who have peptic ulcers drink very little water. Because water dilutes the gastric juices and thereby makes them less corrosive, the patient should develop the habit of taking several swallows of water at least every hour during the day.
- It is known that there is a relationship between the use of tobacco and aggravation of a peptic ulcer. If the patient is unable to discontinue smoking altogether, he might at least use more moderation in his smoking habits.
- The patient is encouraged to cooperate with his physician and remain under medical supervision for as long as the physician deems advisable. He must report regularly for periodic assessment to determine his progress.
- There are certain side effects from antacids that should be reported to the physician should they occur. These include constipation or diarrhea, flatulence, and signs of edema resulting from sodium retention. Because drug interactions can occur, the patient should inform the physician about all the drugs he is taking.
- Unless otherwise ordered, antacids should be taken 1 hour after meals. If antacid tablets are used in preference to liquid preparations, the tablet must be chewed thoroughly and followed by a full glass of water.
- Aspirin and NSAIDs should be avoided. There are more than 300 prescription and nonprescription medications that contain aspirin. The patient should develop the habit of reading carefully the labels of any medications he is taking without a prescription. He also should inform any physician who is treating him for some condition other than his ulcer that he cannot take aspirin.

SURGICAL TREATMENT OF A PEPTIC ULCER

Indications for Surgery

Surgical treatment becomes necessary when a chronic ulcer fails to respond to medical treatment; when complications such as perforation, obstruction, or hemorrhage occur; or when a malignancy is present.

Types of Surgical Procedures

In *pyloroplasty with truncal or proximal gastric vagotomy*, the pylorus, which has been narrowed by scarring, is widened. The branches of the vagus (Xth cranial) nerve that stimulate acid secretion in the stomach are selectively severed (vagotomy) so that the stomach does not receive impulses from the brain and therefore does not secrete hydrochloric acid. A vagotomy is often done at the same time a gastric resection is performed.

Subtotal gastrectomy (gastric resection) consists of removing a part of the stomach and then joining the remaining portion to the small intestine by *anastomosis* (Fig. 23–11*A*). Anastomosis is the joining of two hollow organs by suturing the open ends together so that they become one continuous tube.

An *antrectomy*, in which the gastrin-producing portion of the stomach (the antrum) is removed, may be done in conjunction with a truncal vagotomy. When the fundus of the stomach is anastomosed to the duodenum, the procedure is known as a *Billroth I*. In the *Billroth II* procedure, the duodenum is closed and the fundus of the stomach is anastamosed to the jejunum.

Total gastrectomy is the surgical removal of all of the stomach. The esophagus is anastomosed to the small intestine (Fig. 23–11*B*).

NURSING CARE OF THE PATIENT UNDERGOING GASTRIC SURGERY

PREOPERATIVE CARE

The diet of the patient is restricted to liquids during the 24 hours before surgery. In case of obstruction, a nasogastric tube is inserted and gastric suction is begun to remove all stomach contents before surgery.

The patient receives routine preparations necessary for all major abdominal surgery. These

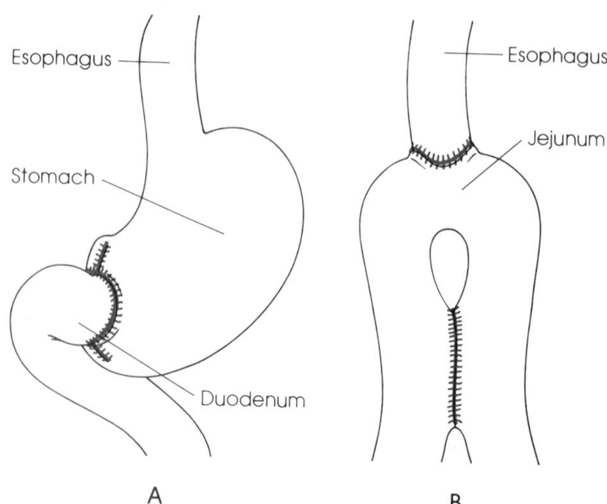

Figure 23–11 Subtotal and total gastrectomy. *A*, One type of subtotal gastrectomy, with the duodenum attached to remaining portion of stomach. *B*, Total gastrectomy. The jejunum is attached directly to the esophagus; the duodenum is closed.

include enemas so that the colon is emptied of fecal material. If the patient has had a barium enema, the nurse should look for and report returns that contain whitish material. This is barium, and it will become hardened if left in the colon, thus presenting the possibility of a fecal impaction later on.

POSTOPERATIVE CARE

Care of the patient having gastric surgery is routine, with the following exceptions. Following surgery in which part of the stomach has been removed, care must be taken in the handling of the nasogastric tube so as to avoid injury to the sutures and introduction of infectious agents. The surgeon will have written specific orders about irrigating fluids allowed and movement of the gastric tube.

After the tubing is removed, the patient is given small amounts of liquid to determine if he can tolerate them. These liquids are gradually increased according to the patient's ability to take them without nausea, vomiting, or abdominal distress. If the liquids are well tolerated, the patient progresses to small, frequent feedings. Within 6 months, most patients are able to take three regular meals a day as the remaining portion of the stomach stretches to accommodate more and more food. Patients who have had a *total* gastrectomy are usually restricted to small, frequent feedings of easily digested semi-solids for the rest of their lives. When the patient is to be dismissed from the hospital, the hospital dietitian usually is called to help the patient and his family learn about the special diet that the patient must follow after undergoing gastric surgery.

"DUMPING SYNDROME"

Some patients who have had a gastrectomy experience a complication known as the "dumping syndrome." The patient has nausea, weakness, abdominal pain, and diarrhea and may feel faint and perspire profusely or experience palpitations when he eats. These sensations probably are caused by the rapid passage of large amounts of food and liquid through the remaining portion of the stomach (if any) and into the jejunum. This occurs because part or all of the stomach and duodenum has been surgically removed and is no longer present to slow down the progress of the intestinal contents through the upper portion of the gastrointestinal tract. When a patient experiences the dumping syndrome, he is instructed to avoid eating large meals and to drink a minimum of fluids during the meal. He may take the fluids in small amounts later, between meals. If sweet foods and liquids seem to aggravate the condition, and they sometimes do, the patient should try to avoid them. It also may be helpful for the patient to lie down flat in bed for 30 minutes after a meal.

CANCER OF THE LARGE INTESTINE

Cancer of the large intestine, also called colorectal cancer, is the third most common malignancy in the United States. The American Cancer Society estimates that 155,000 new cases of colon and rectal cancer will be treated in 1990 (American Cancer Society, 1990). Colorectal cancer is the most curable of all cancers if it is found in the early stages.

The disease mainly occurs in persons over the age of 40 and is slightly more prevalent in females than in males. Persons most at risk include those with disorders of the digestive tract, especially ulcerative colitis and familial polyposis. Other risk factors are lack of dietary fiber and a diet that includes large amounts of red meat, refined carbohydrates, and saturated fat. Hence preventive measures include a diet that is high in fiber and low in simple sugars and animal fat.

The most common sites of colorectal cancer are shown in Figure 23–12.

NURSING INTERVENTION

Nursing intervention is directed at public education. Patients should be taught the following information:

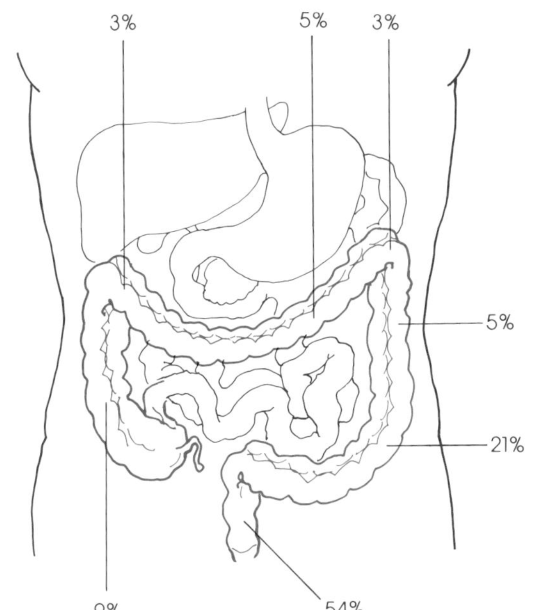

Figure 23–12 Most common sites of colorectal cancer. Rectum, 54%; upper rectum and lower sigmoid, 21%; upper sigmoid and descending colon, 5%; splenic flexure, 3%; transverse colon, 5%; upper ascending colon and hepatic flexure, 3%; cecum and lower ascending colon, 9%.

- A change in bowel patterns or rectal bleeding should be brought to a doctor's attention immediately.
- Everyone over 40 should have a digital rectal examination every year.
- A stool blood test should be done every year after age 50.
- A proctosigmoidoscopy examination should be done every 3 to 5 years after the age of 50, assuming that two consecutive annual examinations have been negative. If the examination locates suspected lesions, biopsy and/or surgery is performed.
- The nurse should listen closely when doing admission interviews and carefully question patients over the age of 40 about changes in bowel patterns and abdominal discomfort or fullness.

SYMPTOMS AND MEDICAL DIAGNOSIS

In the early stages symptoms are typically mild and vague and depend on the location of the tumor and the function of the affected area. Later signs of colorectal cancer are the result of obstruction of the bowel and, eventually, extension of the growth to adjacent structures. Any change in bowel habits, either diarrhea or constipation, could be a sign of cancer of the colon.

Other symptoms include black, tarry stools and anemia resulting from intestinal bleeding. Abdominal pain and a sensation of pressure in the lower abdomen or rectum frequently are present. Digital examination reveals a mass in the anus, rectum, or lower sigmoid when the tumor mass is located in these structures.

Diagnostic tests include a stool guaiac test, endoscopic examinations and barium radiograph, and an intravenous pyelogram to detect any displacement of the kidneys, ureters, or bladder.

SURGICAL TREATMENT

Surgical treatment of colorectal cancer involves removal of the affected portion of the intestine with anastamosis of the remaining portions if the lesion is small and localized. Larger tumors are treated by excision of the colon and provision for elimination of fecal matter via a surgically created opening on the abdomen (colostomy). See Chapter 25 for the care of the ostomy patient.

See Nursing Care Plan 23–2 for postoperative care of the patient who has had abdominal surgery with a colectomy.

INTESTINAL OBSTRUCTION

Intestinal obstruction is a blockage of the intestinal tract that prevents the normal passage of gastrointestinal contents through the intestines. The condition may occur suddenly or progress gradually.

CAUSATIVE FACTORS

Obstruction of the bowel may be *mechanical*, resulting from blockage of the lumen of the bowel, or *nonmechanical*, resulting from the absence of peristalsis.

Mechanical obstructions include tumors, adhesions, strangulated hernia, twisting of the bowel *(volvulus)*, telescoping of one part of the bowel into another *(intussusception)*, gallstones, barium impaction, and intestinal parasites. Abdominal adhesions are a common cause of intestinal obstruction. Adhesions form when inflammation from abdominal trauma or surgery has occurred and fibrous bands of scar tissue hold two segments of bowel together that are normally separated.

Nonmechanical obstructions may occur as a result of paralytic ileus following abdominal surgery or as a consequence of hypokalemia, or they may be secondary to intestinal thrombus. Infections can occur in some pelvic inflammatory diseases or peritonitis, in uremia, and in heavy-metal poisoning. All of these conditions can interfere with normal peristaltic action and produce a nonmechanical obstruction.

ASSESSMENT

The symptoms of intestinal obstruction vary according to the location of the obstruction. Obstructions occurring high in the intestinal tract are characterized by sharp, brief pains in the upper abdomen that are coordinated with increased bowel sounds in the area of peristaltic contractions above the point of obstruction. Other symptoms include vomiting with rapid dehydration and only slight abdominal distention.

Obstructions of the colon are characterized by a more gradual onset with marked abdominal distention as the bowel fills, infrequent vomiting (which occurs late in the process if at all), and pains that last several minutes or longer and correspond to peristaltic waves. Bowel sounds above the point of obstruction are low in pitch.

MEDICAL AND SURGICAL TREATMENT AND NURSING INTERVENTION

Diagnostic radiographs will be ordered to determine where the obstruction is located. Surgery is indicated for obstruction caused by adhesions, volvulus, hernia, or tumor.

The physician may first try to relieve the obstruction with the use of a Cantor tube, which is a long intestinal tube inserted via the nose. It has

NURSING CARE PLAN 23–2

Selected nursing diagnoses, goals/outcome criteria, nursing interventions, and evaluations for a patient undergoing colectomy for colon cancer

Situation: Mrs. Simpson, age 58, just returned from surgery. She had a colectomy because of a malignant lesion in the upper portion of the sigmoid colon. She is very frightened, because her father died with colon cancer. She has a family history of polyposis of the colon. Mrs. Simpson is a loan officer with a national bank, is very busy, and had put off having a physical and sigmoidoscopy until this month, when she noticed some blood in a loose stool. She had had some bouts of loose stools but thought these were a result of the stress she was experiencing on her job.

Nursing Diagnosis	Goals/Outcome Criteria	Nursing Intervention	Evaluation
Pain related to abdominal surgery. SUPPORTING DATA Colectomy; abdominal incision with wound drain.	Pain will be controlled with analgesia. Pain will be controlled by oral medication at discharge. Patient will use relaxation techniques to decrease pain.	Assess for pain q 3 to 4 h and document location and characteristics. Medicate with morphine q 3 h as ordered; assess respirations before giving. Teach relaxation techniques to decrease anxiety and lessen pain. Provide comfort measures to decrease pain.	Requesting pain med q 2 h; resp., 24; attempted to teach relaxation techniques; plan: seek order for PCA pump or increased dosage of analgesic.
Alteration in nutrition related to NPO status and nasogastric tube. SUPPORTING DATA Will be npo for 3 to 5 days with an NG tube in place; IV fluid therapy.	Patient will develop fluid or electrolyte imbalance as evidenced by good skin turgor, moist mucous membranes, and electrolyte studies within normal range. Patient will not develop complications of IV therapy.	Maintain patency of NG tube with irrigations of 30 mL normal saline every 2 h as ordered. Keep tube above level of stomach; loop with tape and pin to gown; maintain on low suction. Assess amount and character of stomach secretions q shift and document. Maintain intake and output. Auscultate for bowel sounds q shift; assess for abdominal distention. Assess IV site q shift for redness, leaking, pain, and patency; document. Check for adequate urine output before hanging IV solution containing potassium. Assess IV site before administering each antibiotic IV piggyback medication. Maintain IV flow at ordered rate; check q 30 min.	IV site without redness or swelling; mucous membranes moist, skin turgor normal; electrolytes within normal limits; NG tube draining well.
Potential for infection related to colectomy and abdominal incision. SUPPORTING DATA Colectomy with abdominal incision and wound drain.	Patient will not experience wound infection as evidenced by temperature and WBC count within normal range at discharge, wound clean and dry without redness, pain, or purulent drainage.	Reinforce dressings prn; change q 24 h or prn when ordered. Use strict aseptic technique for dressing changes. Clean skin around incision with hydrogen peroxide or povidone-iodine (Betadine) as ordered. Maintain patency of drain. Monitor temperature and WBCs. Administer prophylactic antibiotics as ordered.	Incision clean with slight serosanguineous drainage; cleaned with Betadine; drain patent; temp., 99.6°F; WBCs, 12,200. Antibiotics administered as ordered; continue plan.
Potential alteration in tissue perfusion related to possible bleeding at surgical site. SUPPORTING DATA Fresh colectomy.	Patient will maintain adequate tissue perfusion as evidenced by stable vital signs and adequate urine output.	Assess vital signs per postop routine: q ½ h for 2 h; q 1 h for 2 h; q 2 h for 4 h; then q 4 h if stable. Notify physician of tachycardia with increased respirations that is not relieved by pain medication,	Vital signs stable; dressing clean and dry; abdomen soft; urine output > 30 mL/h; continue plan.

Nursing care plan continued on following page

NURSING CARE PLAN 23–2, *Continued*

Nursing Diagnosis	Goals/Outcome Criteria	Nursing Intervention	Evaluation
		or blood pressure 15 to 20 points below preoperative baseline level. Report urine output that falls below 30 mL/h for 2 consecutive hours. Assess dressings for bleeding; check underneath patient. Monitor for internal bleeding with each set of vital signs for first 24 h: assess abdomen for increasing girth or rigidity.	
Potential for ineffective breathing pattern related to anesthesia, analgesia, and postoperative pain. **SUPPORTING DATA** Underwent general anesthesia; requiring morphine q 3 h for pain. Does not wish to cough.	Patient will not develop atelectasis as evidenced by normal breath sounds in all lobes of lungs. Patient will not develop respiratory infection from retained secretions.	Assist patient to turn, cough effectively, and deep breathe (TCDB) at least every 2 h; assist to side of bed for TCDB first postoperative day. Auscultate lungs q shift and document. Encourage use of incentive spirometer if ordered. Monitor temperature; assess characteristics of sputum.	TCDB sitting on side of bed at 8, 10, 12, and 2; bilateral breath sounds clear; using incentive spirometer correctly; no signs of infection; continue plan.
Anxiety related to fear of cancer and treatment and possible death. **SUPPORTING DATA** Father died of colon cancer; expresses fear of cancer and death; dreads chemotherapy.	Patient will openly discuss fears and concerns with nurse, family, and physician. Patient will verbalize positive outlook on chances for survival by discharge.	Establish trusting relationship with patient by active listening and attentive caring. Encourage "labeling" fears; talk through each one. Provide patient with positive statistics regarding colon cancer treated in early stages. Encourage patient to view cancer as a challenge rather than a defeat. Explain that she has a lot of control over her body and immune system and assist her with relaxation and imagery exercises. Help patient to express positive things about herself.	Withdrawn and quiet; doesn't wish to discuss situation until pathology report is back; sat with patient for 15 min; continue plan.

a mercury bag on the distal end that is carried through the intestine by peristalsis. In some patients this treatment can resolve the problem without the trauma of surgery.

The patient with acute intestinal obstruction is very seriously ill. He often has respiratory difficulty because of the pressure of the distended abdomen against the diaphragm. Placing the patient in Fowler's position helps relieve this pressure and also aids in the removal of gas and intestinal contents through the intestinal tube. This tube is inserted before the patient goes to surgery and offers some relief of the symptoms of intestinal obstruction until surgery can be performed.

If the obstruction cannot be resolved, surgical correction must be done. Lysis (breaking apart) of adhesions may be all that is necessary, or a more extensive procedure such as described in the next section may be needed.

NURSING CARE OF THE PATIENT UNDERGOING SURGERY OF THE LOWER INTESTINAL TRACT

TYPES OF SURGICAL PROCEDURES

Colectomy. This is simply the removal of the diseased portion of the colon.

Colostomy. In this procedure, an abdominal incision is made, and the colon is brought to the outside for the purpose of providing a means of draining fecal material. A colostomy is usually done after a colectomy. The colostomy may be permanent or temporary. If it is a temporary colostomy, the patient must return to surgery later for anastomosis of the open ends.

Abdominoperineal Resection. This is a very extensive surgical procedure in which part of the colon and the entire rectum, anus, and regional lymph nodes are removed. Both an abdominal incision and a perineal incision are necessary for this procedure. Because of the nature of the surgery, a permanent colostomy is necessary.

Care of patients with colostomies and ileostomies is discussed in Chapter 25.

PREOPERATIVE CARE

Before surgery of the large intestine, efforts are made to remove as much fecal material from the colon as possible. To accomplish this, the patient is usually placed on a low-residue diet as early as 7 to 10 days before surgery. The last 24 to 72 hours before surgery, his diet is changed to liquids only. Vitamins and minerals may be given to supplement these restricted diets. Antibiotics such as neomycin and sulfasuxidine are given as prophylaxis against infection of the operative site.

In addition to the dietary preparation, laxatives and enemas are administered to cleanse the lower bowel further. Contents of the stomach are removed by inserting a nasogastric tube and connecting it to a suction apparatus the morning of surgery. If it is necessary to remove the contents of the small intestine, a specially designed tube that passes through the stomach and into the duodenum is inserted. This tube is called a Miller-Abbott tube (see Fig. 23–6). It is attached to the suction apparatus and given the same care as a gastric tube. The tube is usually left in place after surgery to remove accumulations of mucus and gas that may cause distention and strain on the sutures.

POSTOPERATIVE CARE

The immediate postoperative care for the intestinal surgery patient is the same as for other patients having major abdominal surgery. Operations on the large intestine are usually of long duration.

The prolonged period of anesthesia and exposure of the body, with loss of essential fluids, leaves the patient susceptible to shock. Therefore the patient must be watched closely for signs of shock during the immediate postoperative period.

Difficulty in voiding after surgery is a common problem with these patients. To avoid the retention of urine in the bladder during the postoperative period, a retention catheter is usually inserted and attached to a drainage apparatus while the patient is in the operating room.

The gastric or intestinal tube is connected to an electrical suction device as soon as the patient is returned to his room. The physician usually does not want the patient to have anything by mouth for the first 48 hours after surgery. Peristalsis usually becomes active after this period of time, and the patient will then be able to take liquids by mouth.

The passing of gas, liquids, or solids through the rectum is an indication of active peristalsis.

In any surgery of the intestine, the surgeon is always concerned with the return of normal peristalsis. It is the nurse's responsibility to observe these patients carefully for evidence of the return of peristalsis and to chart it in the nurse's notes.

ABDOMINAL HERNIA

The internal organs of the body are contained within their respective cavities by the outside walls of the cavity. In the abdomen, the wall is *muscular*. If there is a defect in this muscular wall, the contents of the abdominal cavity may break through the defect. This protrusion is called a *hernia* or simply a *rupture*.

The most common locations for a hernia are in areas where the abdominal wall is normally weaker and more likely to allow protrusion of a segment of intestine (Fig. 23–13). These include the center of the abdomen at the site of the umbilicus, and the lower abdomen at the points where the inguinal ring and the femoral canal begin. The most common contributing factors in the development of a hernia are straining to lift heavy objects, chronic cough, straining to void, straining at stool, and ascites.

Hernias are classified as *reducible*, which means the protruding organ can be returned to its proper place by pressing on the organ, and *irreducible*, which means that the protruding part

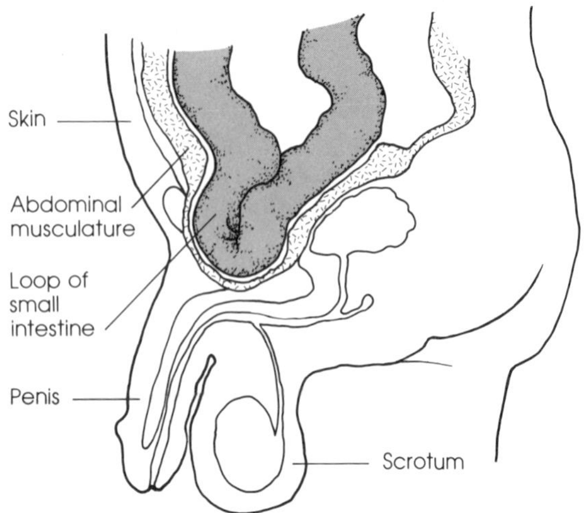

Figure 23-13 Inguinal hernia. A loop of small intestine passes through the inguinal ring, a weak point in the abdominal musculature.

of the organ is tightly wedged outside the cavity and cannot be pushed back through the opening. Another name for an irreducible hernia is *incarcerated* hernia. If the protruding part of the organ is not replaced and its blood supply is cut off, the hernia is said to be *strangulated.*

MEDICAL DIAGNOSIS

There is a "lump" or local swelling at the site of the hernia. The most common sites are the umbilicus, groin, or along a healed abdominal incision. When pressure on the abdominal wall is removed by lying down, the swelling disappears. Lifting of heavy objects, coughing, or any activity that puts a strain on the abdominal muscles may force the organ back through the opening, and the swelling reappears. Pain occurs when the peritoneum becomes irritated or when the hernia is incarcerated or strangulated. The flow of intestinal contents becomes blocked by an incarcerated hernia, and the patient has the symptoms of an intestinal obstruction.

SURGICAL TREATMENT AND NURSING INTERVENTION

Hernias are best treated by surgery. If surgery is not possible because of age or poor surgical risk, the patient may be fitted with an appliance called a *truss.* The truss is put on each morning before the patient gets out of bed, because the hernia is more likely to be reduced at that time. A truss simply reinforces the weakened cavity wall and prevents protrusion of the intestines. It is only a symptomatic measure and does not cure the hernia.

The surgical procedure used in the treatment of a hernia is called a *herniorrhaphy,* which means a surgical repair of a hernia. The defect is closed with sutures. If the area of weakness is very large, a *hernioplasty* is done. In this procedure, some type of strong synthetic material is sewn over the defect to reinforce the area. The procedure is now done on an outpatient basis.

Careful discharge instructions are given to the patient to prevent respiratory problems, because the patient should not cough in the immediate postoperative period. Guidelines as to signs and symptoms of complications are sent home with the patient, along with a written list of activities to avoid until healing is complete.

IRRITABLE BOWEL SYNDROME

This is a group of symptoms that together represent the most common disorder presented by patients who consult a specialist in gastrointestinal disease. The three characteristics that are typical of this disorder are (1) alteration in bowel elimination, either constipation or diarrhea or both; (2) abdominal pain; and (3) the absence of detectable organic disease. Although the pattern of bowel dysfunction varies from case to case, each patient seems to have a pattern unique to him.

Although stress is not thought to be the cause of this disorder, it is definitely a contributing factor, as most patients experience an increase in symptoms during times of stress.

The cause of irritable bowel syndrome is not known. Diagnosis is based on clinical manifestations and ruling out (by barium enema and other tests) the presence of organic bowel disease.

MEDICAL TREATMENT AND NURSING INTERVENTION

Treatment of irritable bowel syndrome is inevitably long and, because of the psychological factors involved, often includes such modes of therapy as psychotherapy, biofeedback training, and instruction in relaxation techniques. It is important to reassure the patient that there is no relationship between his disorder and malignancy of the bowel.

Medications are prescribed according to each patient's need. Drugs that have been used include antidepressants, antispasmodics, and mild analgesics to relieve discomfort. A diet high in bran and fiber also may be prescribed. Metamucil or other bulk stool softeners are very beneficial. Gas-forming foods such as the legumes and those in the cabbage family should be avoided. In some patients the intake of milk is restricted if they have shown evidence of intolerance to it.

The more common nursing diagnoses and interventions for patients with irritable bowel syndrome are essentially the same as for any patient with alteration in bowel elimination, either diarrhea or constipation. Instruction of the patient about the nature of his disease can help diminish unwarranted fears.

Ineffective coping patterns also are likely to be present in these patients. Consultation with a psychiatric nursing specialist can help the staff nurse develop more realistic goals and effective nursing interventions to improve the patient's coping skills.

DIVERTICULA

The term *diverticula* refers to small, blind pouches resulting from a protrusion of the mucous membranes of a hollow organ through weakened areas of the organ's muscular wall. Diverticula occur most often in the intestinal tract, especially in the esophagus and colon. When they are present, the patient is said to have *diverticulosis*. If the diverticula become inflamed or infected, the condition is referred to as *diverticulitis*.

Diverticulitis occurs when food caught in the diverticulum mixes with bacteria. The intestinal wall becomes irritated and infected, and if it is not treated, perforation and peritonitis may occur.

Treatment is with parenteral antibiotics, withholding solid food, and hydration with IV fluids as necessary. If the patient experiences recurrent episodes of diverticulitis, or if perforation and peritonitis occur, surgical removal of that part of the colon is performed.

ASSESSMENT

A person may have diverticulosis and remain unaware of his condition for quite a while because it often presents no symptoms. Eventually, however, the diverticula may fill with some material passing through the intestinal tract and become inflamed or infected, causing symptoms. If the diverticulitis is in the esophagus, the patient may have difficulty in swallowing, foul breath, and emesis of food that was eaten several days prior to the vomiting. Diverticulitis of the intestine produces symptoms of diarrhea or constipation, abdominal pain, fever, and rectal bleeding. The condition may be complicated by intestinal obstruction or by peritonitis if the intestinal wall ruptures.

MEDICAL-SURGICAL TREATMENT

The symptoms of the patient will to some extent govern the treatment necessary. Esophageal diverticulitis, if severe, usually is treated by surgical removal of the sacs and repair of the muscular wall. Intestinal diverticulosis often can be managed conservatively with a high-residue diet and antidiarrheic medications or stool softeners to control constipation.

HEMORRHOIDS

Hemorrhoids are varicosities of the veins of the rectum. They may be *internal* (inside the sphincter muscles of the anus) or *external* (outside the sphincter muscles) (Fig. 23–14).

ASSESSMENT

Local pain and itching are the most common symptoms of hemorrhoids. Bleeding from the rectum at the time of defecation may also be present. External hemorrhoids are less likely to bleed, but they are more evident to the person examining the patient, because they appear as tumorlike projections around the rectum.

Constipation, prolonged standing or sitting, and pregnancy are predisposing causes of hemorrhoids. The habit of sitting on the toilet and straining at the stool for long periods of time is one of the primary factors responsible for many cases of hemorrhoids.

TREATMENT AND NURSING INTERVENTION

The symptoms of hemorrhoids may be relieved by correction of constipation, local applications of heat or cold, sitz baths, and the use of ointments that contain a local anesthetic. The patient should also be instructed to wash the anal region with warm water and soap after each bowel movement.

Hemorrhoids can be treated by scleropathy (injection of a solution that causes the vessel to dry up and disintegrate), cryotherapy (freezing), photocoagulation (burning), or hemorrhoidectomy using a laser or standard surgical procedure. Another treatment method is rubber banding, in which a rubber band is slipped around the hemorrhoidal vessel, cutting off the blood supply.

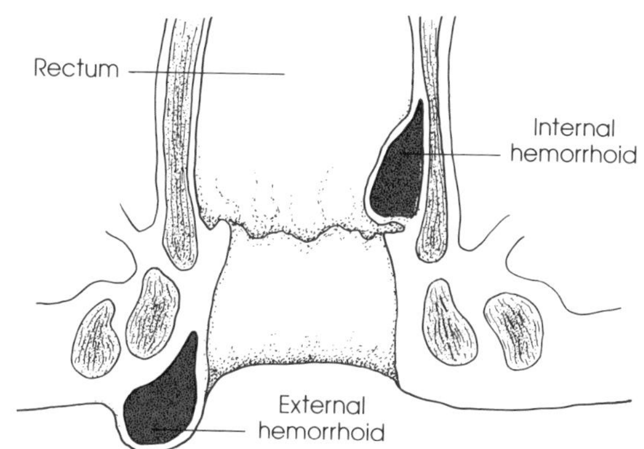

Figure 23–14 Internal and external hemorrhoids.

This causes the hemorrhoid to shrivel and disintegrate. All of these methods except hemorrhoidectomy are usually done as outpatient treatment now.

Thorough discharge teaching is done, and written instructions are sent home with the patient. A prescription for analgesics will be sent home also, as these patients experience quite a bit of pain. Cold or warm compresses and warm sitz baths using a rubber ring to support the buttocks also help relieve pain. Mild, wet dressings that are commercially prepared may also be used on the surgical site. These dressings have a glycerin base and contain a mild astringent that reduces swelling and relieves pain.

The rubber ring may also be used while the patient is lying down to remove pressure from the rectal area. Sitz baths are usually ordered twice a day.

Most patients dread the first bowel movement after a hemorrhoidectomy. There is no doubt that it will cause some pain, and the usual procedure is the administration of a stool softener to make defecation less traumatic. The patient and family should be warned that the patient may become faint, and someone should stay close by.

A high-fiber diet is started right away, as it is best if formed stool is passed regularly. A sitz bath after each bowel movement will offer relief and also cleanses the affected area, keeping it free from irritation.

The patient should continue to make a practice of sitting in a tub of warm water after bowel movements until healing is complete.

MALABSORPTION

Many disorders interfere with the normal absorption of nutrients, water, and vitamins from the intestine. Adult celiac disease, in which the patient cannot properly metabolize gluten (a protein found in all wheat products, barley, and rye) is one cause. Pancreatic disease with interference in secretion of pancreatic digestive enzymes also causes malabsorption. Some patients who have undergone chemotherapy for treatment of cancer experience alteration of the intestinal mucosa that causes malabsorption. Whatever the cause, malabsorption creates a nutritional deficiency.

A key sign of malabsorption is passage of stool that is bulky, frothy, and foul smelling and usually floats in the toilet. Other signs and symptoms include weight loss, weakness, and various signs of vitamin deficiency depending on the type of malabsorption the patient is experiencing.

Treatment is directed at the underlying cause. Pancreatic insufficiency can be treated by administration of pancreatic enzymes with meals. Celiac disease is treated by omitting gluten from the diet.

PILONIDAL SINUS (PILONIDAL CYST)

The word *pilonidal* means "having a nest of hair." A pilonidal sinus is a lesion located in the cleft of the buttocks at the sacrococcygeal region. It is sometimes called a *pilonidal cyst,* but it is believed to be a subcutaneous canal (sinus) with one or more openings into the skin (rather than a true cyst or fluid-filled sac). The condition occurs when the stiff hairs in the sacrococcygeal region irritate and eventually penetrate the soft skin in the cleft of the buttocks. Factors that can lead to development of such a sinus include local injury, improper cleaning of the area, and obesity. People who have more than the usual amount of body hair are particularly susceptible.

ASSESSMENT AND TREATMENT

A pilonidal sinus may cause no trouble until it becomes infected, and then the patient experiences pain in the area, with swelling and a purulent drainage. When this occurs, the area must be incised surgically and the connecting canals opened and drained. Hairs and necrotic tissue must be removed so the area can heal. This is usually done as an outpatient surgical procedure.

Postoperative care includes changing of dressings and measures to avoid contamination of the wound. A lubricating laxative and an oil enema usually are given before the first bowel movement to avoid strain on the sutures. Antibiotics may be given to control infection.

Concerns for the Elderly

After the age of 70, the parietal cells in the stomach decrease their secretion of hydrochloric acid. The pancreas also shows structural alterations that cause a decrease in the secretion of lipase, the enzyme that aids fat digestion. The mucosa of the small intestine is altered, providing a less absorptive surface area. The large intestine may develop diminished motility.

Digestive disorders are common in the elderly population. Hiatal hernia and diverticulosis are very prevalent. Cancer of the colon incidence also rises with each year of age over 70.

The elderly patient who develops a peptic ulcer usually does not display the typical symptoms. Pain is less typical and may be poorly localized, or it may be described as lower chest discomfort or left-sided pain. Anorexia, weight loss, general weakness, anemia, nausea, and painless vomiting may occur, which makes peptic ulcer difficult to diagnose. Nurses who work in long-term-care facilities should keep this possibility in mind if a patient is experiencing these symptoms. Often peptic ulcer in the elderly is not discovered until perforation or obstruction has occurred.

Many older patients live alone and do not go to the trouble to cook adequate, nutritious meals. They may become anemic and develop protein and vitamin deficiencies. When taking a diet history, it is best to ask about specific food intake for each meal of the day and what quantity of food is eaten.

BIBLIOGRAPHY

Alltop, S. A.: Teaching for discharge: Gastrostomy tubes. RN, Nov., 1988, p. 42.

American Cancer Society: Cancer Facts and Figures—1990. Atlanta, 1990.

Andreoli, T. E., et al.: Cecil Essentials of Medicine, 2nd ed. Philadelphia, W. B. Saunders, 1990.

Crocker, K.: GI manifestations of AIDS. Nurs. Clin. North Am., June, 1989, p. 395.

Deters, G. E.: Managing complications after abdominal surgery. RN, March, 1987, p. 27.

Groth, K.: Age-related changes in the gastrointestinal tract. Geriatr. Nurs., Sept., 1988, p. 278.

Guyton, A. C.: Textbook of Medical Physiology, 8th ed. Philadelphia, W. B. Saunders, 1991.

Hannessy, K.: Nutritional support and GI disease. Nurs. Clin. North Am., June, 1989, p. 373.

Harrington, D., and Gogel, H. K.: When the patient suffers from esophageal bleeding. RN, Feb., 1987, p. 24.

Ignatavicius, D. D., and Bayne, M. J.: Medical-Surgical Nursing. Philadelphia, W. B. Saunders, 1991.

Massoni, M.: Nurse's GI Handbook. Nursing 90, Nov., 1990, p. 65.

Matteson, M. A., and McConnell, E. S.: Gerontological Nursing: Concepts and Practice. Philadelphia, W. B. Saunders, 1988.

McConnell, E. A.: Meeting the challenge of intestinal obstruction. Nursing 87, July, 1987, p. 34.

Meize-Grochowski, A. R.: When the Dx is Crohn's disease. RN, Feb., 1991.

Muscari, M. E., and Lobisser, M.: Teaching the eating disordered client. Adv. Clin. Care, Jan./Feb., 1990, p. 20.

Novak, L. T.: Accelerated recovery technique—a new approach to abdominal surgery. Nursing 90, Nov., 1990.

Perkins, S. B., and Kennally, K. M.: The hidden danger of internal hemorrhage. Nursing 89, July, 1989, p. 34.

Price, S., and Wilson, L.: Pathophysiology, 3rd ed. New York, McGraw-Hill, 1986.

Wardell, T. L.: Assessing and managing gastric ulcer. Nursing 91, March, 1991, p. 35.

STUDENT STUDY AIDS

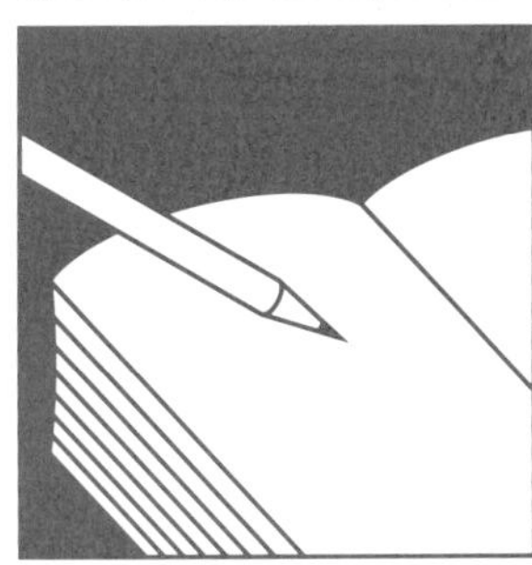

CLINICAL CASE PROBLEMS

Read each clinical case problem and discuss the questions with your classmates.

1. Mr. Post, age 42, is admitted to the hospital because he has epigastric pain, vomiting of blood, and suspected gastric ulcer. The physician prescribes a bland diet for Mr. Post while he is in the hospital and plans to limit Mr. Post's food in the future to items that do not aggravate the patient's condition.

- What tests might be done in order to establish a diagnosis of Mr. Post's illness?
- What kind of information will help Mr. Post to avoid difficulty with his diet after he is discharged?
- What would Mr. Post need to know to keep his ulcer under control and to eventually cure it?

2. Mrs. Penn, age 29, has had frequent bouts of diarrhea associated with physical and emotional stress since her early teens. She is admitted to the hospital with a diagnosis of possible ulcerative colitis. Her admitting physician, a gastroenterologist, feels certain that she has ulcerative colitis and that she will benefit from an ileostomy, as previous efforts on the part of several other physicians have brought no lasting relief from Mrs. Penn's symptoms. She is admitted to the hospital to establish a definitive diagnosis.

Mrs. Penn is 40 pounds underweight and currently is suffering from severe diarrhea and fluid deficit.

- What questions would be relevant when taking Mrs. Penn's nursing history?
- What should be included on Mrs. Penn's nursing care plan regarding observations, measurements, and nursing interventions?
- Discuss some benefits of an ileostomy over the alternative of continued bouts of severe diarrhea.

3. Mr. Horn, age 52, was found to have occult blood in his stool when he underwent a physical examination for a new insurance policy. Fiberoptic flexible sigmoidoscopy revealed a small lesion in the sigmoid colon; the biopsy result was positive for malignancy. He is scheduled for a colectomy.

- What are the probable postoperative nursing diagnoses that should be on Mr. Horn's care plan?
- What are the psychosocial concerns that need to be addressed for this patient? What would be appropriate nursing interventions?
- What further treatment will be necessary for Mr. Horn?

STUDY OUTLINE

I. Introduction

A. Intestinal tract one long tube that serves the functions of ingestion (the intake of food), digestion (physical and chemical changes that foodstuffs undergo), and absorption (passage of nutrients from intestine to blood stream).

B. Accessory organs of digestion: liver, gallbladder, and pancreas.

C. Metabolism is the sum of all physical and chemical processes concerned with the disposition of nutrients.

D. Pathologic conditions of the digestive tract and accessory organs of digestion affect metabolism, the health of the organism, and repair and healing of injury and illness.

II. Causative factors and preventive measures

A. Inflammation and infection.

B. Chemical and physical trauma.

C. Social, economic, and psychological factors.

D. Stress and emotions.

E. Preventive measures concerned with psychological factors and avoidance of irritants and infectious agents.

F. Cautious use of aspirin and nonsteroidal antiinflammatory drugs (NSAIDs).

III. Diagnostic tests and procedures and nursing implications

A. Radiologic examinations: upper and lower GI series (barium swallow and barium enema).

B. Endoscopic examination of the interior of the esophagus (esophagoscopy), stomach (gastroscopy), and small intestine (esophagogastroduodenoscopy).

1. Preparation of patient usually includes NPO, explanation of procedure, and mild sedation.
2. If local anesthetic used, food and liquids withheld after procedure until reflexes return.
3. Patient watched for signs of perforation, bleeding.

C. Proctoscopy, sigmoidoscopy, and colonoscopy: examination of interior of rectum and colon.

D. Gastric analysis to determine level of HCl in stomach contents.

E. Tubeless gastric analysis to find out whether there is any HCl in stomach.

F. Stool examination for infectious organisms, blood, cysts, ova, and parasites.

IV. Specific problems related to ingestion, digestion, and elimination

A. Anorexia: absence of appetite.

1. Assessment to identify cause, if possible
   a. Physical causes: poorly fitting dentures, stomatitis, decaying teeth, halitosis.

b. Psychological factors: unattractive or unfamiliar foods, unpleasant surroundings, company, emotional state.

2. Nursing interventions:
   a. Mouth care.
   b. Cater to patient's preference whenever possible.
   c. Plan meals with variety of foods.
   d. Feed patient slowly and as nurse would eat the meal.
   e. Provide companionship.
   f. Allow foods from home to supplement meals.

B. Eating disorders; have a negative impact on health.
   1. Anorexia nervosa: preoccupation with food coupled with fear of being fat; patient often exercises excessively.
   2. Bulimia: bingeing and induced vomiting; use of laxatives.
   3. Obesity: more than 20% over ideal body weight.
   4. Treatment for eating disorders focuses on behavior modification and psychological counseling along with appropriate diet.

C. Nausea and vomiting: interfere with nutrition (see Chapter 8).

D. Dysphagia: difficult swallowing. Most common symptom of disorders of the esophagus.
   1. Nursing intervention:
      a. Observe patient for foods he cannot tolerate and conditions under which he experiences difficulty.
      b. Instruct patient to chew food thoroughly, eat semisolid foods, drink liquids throughout meal, assume more erect posture when eating.
      c. Provide pleasant surroundings.
      d. Tube feeding may be necessary for severe dysphagia.
      e. Inability to swallow might require gastrostomy feeding.

E. Accumulation of fluid and gas.
   1. Medical intervention:
      a. Insertion of rectal tube or suppository, enemas.
      b. Gastrointestinal intubation using short tube to stomach or longer tube to reach small intestine. Tube is attached to an electric suction apparatus.
   2. Nursing assessment and intervention:
      a. Monitor for nausea, vomiting, complaint of feeling full or bloated, increasing shortness of breath, and increase in girth of abdomen—signs decompression is not taking place.
      b. Hazards of decompression with electric suction: damage to gastric or intestinal mucosa, excessive removal of electrolytes, acid-base imbalance.
      c. Tubes must be kept open and draining freely. Irrigation to remove clots or mucus plugs done by order.
      d. Record amount, characteristics of drainage. Some bloody drainage may be expected following gastric surgery.
      e. Frequent mouth care, lubrication of nares where tube inserted, ice if allowed by surgeon, chewing gum, anesthetic spray and lozenges.
      f. After tube removed, observe for signs of distention, absence of peristalsis.

F. GI bleeding.
   1. Common causes: gastric and duodenal ulcer, esophageal varices, gastritis, tumors and polyps in lower GI tract, ulcerative colitis, diverticula.
   2. Nursing assessment:
      a. Obtain history to identify patients likely to have GI bleeding:

history of anemia, weakness, reported change in color of stools or in pattern of elimination, nausea, chronic indigestion or heartburn.

b. Subjective data: feeling faint, nausea and vomiting of old or new blood, restlessness, thirst, confusion.

c. Objective data: maroon or bright red blood in emesis or stools; black stools; change in vital signs, central venous pressure readings; hematocrit and hemoglobin levels; white cell count.

3. Medical and nursing intervention:

a. Replacement of blood by transfusion of whole blood, packed cells, or fresh frozen plasma; normal saline, Plasmanate, or Ringer's lactate if blood not available.

b. Measure and record intake and output.

c. Oxygen often administered.

d. After condition is stabilized, diagnostic procedures to locate source of bleeding.

e. Surgery when indicated.

f. Injections of vasopressin directly into bleeding artery; insertion of Sengstaken-Blakemore tube to apply pressure and cold; injection of embolus; electric cauterization of bleeding vessels.

g. Reassurance of patient to allay fears and anxiety; continuous monitoring for signs of continued bleeding, hypovolemic shock; daily weighings; measure intake and output, note characteristics of body fluids excreted or aspirated.

G. Hiatal hernia: esophagus passes through defect in diaphragm.

1. Signs and symptoms: indigestion; substernal pain, especially after eating.

2. Treatment: elevation of head of bed, antacids, weight loss; surgery occasionally necessary.

H. Long-term and severe nutritional deficit.

1. Total parenteral nutrition (TPN), also called *hyperalimentation.* A form of intravenous feeding. Must be a coordinated effort on part of all health team members.

a. Staff nurses responsible for monitoring vital signs and fluid and electrolyte balance and other routine interventions, changing dressings, and observing insertion site.

b. Never speed up or slow down prescribed flow rate.

V. Inflammatory disorders of the intestinal tract

A. Stomatitis: inflammation of the oral mucosa.

1. Causes: ill-fitting dentures or malocclusions of the teeth, poor oral hygiene; excessive smoking or drinking; physical trauma, nutritional deficiencies, radiation, and drugs.

2. Assessment: pain and swelling of oral mucosa, bleeding gums, alteration in salivation, halitosis, small, craterlike ulcers.

3. Intervention: frequent mouth care (see Chapter 13), correction of nutritional deficiency, avoidance of irritants.

B. Gastritis: inflammation of gastric mucosa.

1. Causes: overeating, alcohol abuse, contaminated food, ingested poisons, aspirin, NSAIDs.

2. Assessment: nausea, vomiting, heartburn, diarrhea. Nursing diagnoses commonly found: pain, sleep pattern disturbance, self-care deficit, alterations in nutrition, fluid volume deficit, knowledge deficit.

3. Medical treatment and nursing intervention: restriction of foods

followed by bland diet, soothing and antacid medications, antispasmodics, H_2 inhibitors.

C. Ulcerative colitis: inflammation with ulceration of intestinal mucosa.
   1. Similar in symptoms to regional ileitis (Crohn's disease). Tendency is to include both under name of *inflammatory bowel disease*. Major difference is that ulcerative colitis is more likely to develop into malignancy of intestine.
   2. Cause unknown. Immunologic response and emotions play some role.
   3. Medical diagnosis based on medical history and presenting symptoms.
      a. Chief symptoms are attacks of bloody, mucoid diarrhea and cramping pain, usually precipitated by physical or emotional stress.
      b. Endoscopic and x-ray examination helps confirm diagnosis.
   4. Nursing assessment:
      a. Nursing diagnoses common to inflammatory bowel disease include potential or actual fluid volume deficit, diarrhea, sleep pattern disturbance, pain, ineffective individual coping, potential for impairment of skin integrity in anal region.
      b. Long-term problems include anxiety, disturbance in self-concept, and fear of malignancy.
   5. Medical treatment and nursing intervention: inflammatory bowel disease.
      a. Conservative approach: antidiarrheics, long-term sulfasalazine therapy; analgesics; low-residue, bland, high-protein, high-calorie diet.
      b. Surgical intervention: colectomy, colostomy, ileostomy.
      c. Nursing interventions include monitoring bowel elimination and bowel sounds, measurement of intake and output and daily weight, watching for signs of intestinal bleeding, and encouraging stress reduction techniques.
      d. Long-term goals related to patient education and psychological support.

D. Appendicitis: inflammation of vermiform appendix.
   1. Assessment: pain in lower right quadrant, elevated fever with white cell count, nausea and vomiting.
   2. Treatment: appendectomy.
   3. Prior to surgery, patient should not be given laxative or have heat applied to abdomen.

E. Peritonitis: inflammation of peritoneum.
   1. Common causes: ruptured appendix, perforated ulcer, ruptured ectopic pregnancy, infection of peritoneum, any condition in which contents of intestinal tract spill into peritoneal cavity.
   2. Assessment: vomiting, severe abdominal pain, fever, tachycardia, symptoms of shock, paralytic ileus.
   3. Treatment: massive doses of antibiotics, intravenous fluid and electrolytes, intestinal decompression.
   4. Nursing intervention: monitor vital signs, observe for signs of intestinal obstruction, check bowel sounds and other evidence of return of peristalsis, place patient in semi-Fowler's position.

VI. Peptic ulcer

A. Loss of gastric mucosal tissue, ulceration involves loss of muscular coat. Incidence has decreased in recent decades.

B. Causative factors: the presence of too much acid in relation to degree of protection. Reason why mucosal resistance is impaired is unknown.

1. Duodenal ulcers usually characterized by hyperacidity, gastric ulcers by normal or low level of HCl.
2. Genetic predisposition: relatives of persons with peptic ulcers have three times expected rate for development of ulcers.
3. Tension, anxiety, prolonged physical or emotional stress.
4. Diet not thought to be a cause, but ulceration is more prevalent in the undernourished.
5. Drugs: unbuffered aspirin, NSAIDs, alcohol, glucocorticoids.
6. Excessive smoking.

C. Diagnostic tests and procedures:
1. Barium swallow.
2. Esophagogastroduodenoscopy (endoscopy).
3. Gastric analysis.

D. Nursing assessment:
1. Family history of peptic ulcer.
2. Patient's eating habits.
3. History of smoking and extent of alcohol use.
4. History of injuries or other stresses that could cause stress ulcer.
5. Subjective data: epigastric pain and pattern of discomfort in relation of presence of food in stomach, pattern of recurrence of pain; nausea, loss of appetite, weight loss; spontaneous vomiting.

E. Complications: GI hemorrhage, perforation, obstruction.

F. Medical management and nursing intervention:
1. Relief of symptoms: antacids and mild sedatives; cimetidine (Tagamet), ranitidine (Zantac), and sulcrafate (Carafate) relieve pain, reduce the need for antacids, promote healing.
2. Diet: when patient eats is more important than what he eats. Patient instructed to avoid those foods he knows to cause symptoms, to restrict alcohol and caffeine, and to avoid skipping meals.
3. Patient education: see list on pages 572 and 574.

VII. Care of patients having gastric surgery

A. Indications for surgery: complicated peptic ulcer and malignancy.

B. Surgical procedures:
1. Pyloroplasty
2. Total gastrectomy and subtotal gastrectomy: antrectomy; Billroth I or Billroth II.
3. Vagotomy.

C. Preoperative care: routine with exception of intubation and decompression.

D. Postoperative care: after decompression is discontinued, patient is given small amounts of liquid by mouth, diet gradually increased.
1. "Dumping syndrome" may occur after gastrectomy.

VIII. Cancer of large intestine (colorectal cancer)

A. Relatively common; occurs mainly in persons over 40.

B. Persons most at risk are those with other disorders of the digestive tract, especially ulcerative colitis and familial polyposis. Diet low in fiber, high in refined carbohydrate and red meat is a contributing factor.

C. Symptoms and medical diagnosis.
1. In early stages mild symptoms. Later symptoms result of intestinal obstruction and spread to adjacent structures.
2. Diagnostic tests include endoscopy, barium studies, and stool guaiac.

D. Surgical treatment: colectomy and colostomy.

IX. Intestinal obstruction

A. Causes: strangulated hernia, twisting or telescoping of the bowel, or interference with conduction of nerve impulses.

B. Symptoms vary according to the site of obstruction.

1. High obstruction characterized by sharp pain, vomiting, slight abdominal distention.
2. Low bowel obstruction symptoms include marked distention, longer-lasting pain.

C. Treatment: intestinal decompression and surgical correction of obstruction.

X. Nursing care of patient undergoing surgery of the lower intestine

A. Types of surgical procedures:

1. Colectomy (removal of the diseased portion of colon).
2. Colostomy (creation of an artificial anus with bowel opening on the abdominal surface).
3. Abdominoperineal resection: removal of the affected portion of colon, the entire rectum, the anus, and regional lymph nodes; usually done for cancer.

B. Preoperative care: low-residue diet, cleansing of the lower bowel, and intestinal decompression.

C. Postoperative care: observation for signs of shock, care of retention catheter, care of gastrointestinal tube, and observation of drainage (watch for signs of returning peristalsis).

XI. Abdominal hernia: protrusion of the intestines through a weakened area in the abdominal wall

A. Most common sites are umbilical area and beginning of inguinal canal and femoral canal.

B. Reducible hernia: protruding organ can be replaced by pressing on the organ.

C. Incarcerated hernia: cannot be reduced.

D. Strangulated hernia: blood supply to organ has been obstructed.

E. Surgery most effective means for treating hernia (herniorrhaphy); often an outpatient procedure.

XII. Irritable bowel syndrome

A. Characterized by alteration in bowel elimination: constipation or diarrhea, abdominal pain, and absence of detectable organic disease.

B. Cause is not known. Diagnosis established after ruling out organic bowel disease.

C. Medical treatment and nursing intervention:

1. Therapy long-term and focused on psychological factors as well as medications to relieve discomfort and reduce spasms.
2. Nursing intervention essentially the same as for patients with diarrhea and constipation from other causes. Additionally, patient will need help learning effective coping skills.

XIII. Diverticula

A. Small, blind pouches of mucous membrane that have protruded through a weakened wall of a hollow organ.

B. Symptoms not apparent until inflammation (diverticulitis) or infection occurs.

1. Esophageal diverticulitis may produce difficulty in swallowing, foul breath, and emesis.
2. Intestinal diverticulitis produces abdominal pain, fever, diarrhea or constipation, and rectal bleeding.

C. Treatment for diverticulitis may be surgical removal of affected portion of organ or liquid diet, antibiotics, and bulk stool softeners.

D. Treatment for diverticulosis: high-fiber diet, increased fluids, bulk stool softeners.

XIV. Hemorrhoids: varicose veins of the rectum

A. Symptoms: local pain, itching, and bleeding at time of defecation.
B. Treatment by hemorrhoidectomy.
C. Postoperative care concerned with prevention of infection and relief of pain.

XV. Malabsorption: interferes with nutritional status

A. Has many causes: adult celiac disease, pancreatic disease, effects of chemotherapy.
B. Treatment: correct underlying cause, give pancreatic enzymes.

XVI. Pilonidal sinus

A. Subcutaneous canal located in the cleft of the buttocks in the sacrococcygeal area.
B. Produces pain and purulent drainage.
C. Treatment: surgical incision of canal, drainage of purulent material, and removal of hairs and necrotic tissue; antibiotics given to control infection; often an outpatient surgical procedure.

XVII. Concerns for the elderly

A. After age 70, secretion of gastric HCl and pancreatic lipase decreases.
B. Peptic ulcer presents with atypical symptoms.
C. Anemia and vitamin deficiencies common as a result of poor eating habits.

CHAPTER 24

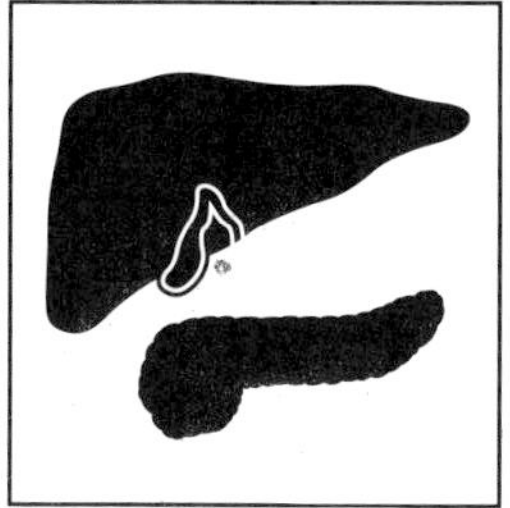

Care of Patients With Disorders of the Gallbladder, Liver, and Pancreas

VOCABULARY

ascites
biliary
cholecystitis
cholelithiasis
encephalopathy
hemolytic
icterus
lithotripsy
pancreatitis
prodromal
pruritus
varices

Upon completion of this chapter the student should be able to:

1. Specify the nursing interventions for pre- and posttest care of patients undergoing tests of the liver, gallbladder, and pancreas.
2. Describe the assessment factors and care of the patient with cholecystitis and cholelithiasis.
3. Describe the pre- and postoperative care for the patient undergoing cholecystectomy.
4. Compare the available methods of treating cholelithiasis.
5. State the care needed for the patient who is having a liver biopsy.
6. Specify the assessment factors to be considered for the patient with possible liver disease.
7. Create a nursing care plan, including psychosocial concerns, for the patient who is jaundiced.
8. List the ways in which the various types of hepatitis can be transmitted.
9. Write a nursing care plan for the patient with viral hepatitis A.
10. Devise appropriate nursing interventions for the patient with cirrhosis.
11. Make a discharge teaching plan for the patient who has been in the hospital with a flare-up of chronic pancreatitis.

The gallbladder, liver, and pancreas are considered the accessory organs of the digestive system. They lie outside the alimentary tract but are directly concerned with digestion.

The gallbladder is a small sac that attaches to the lower portion of the liver. It stores bile produced in the liver and delivers it via the common bile duct to the small intestine. Bile flow from the gallbladder is stimulated by the arrival of fatty food in the duodenum. Fat digestion requires the presence of bile.

The liver performs many life-sustaining functions. It plays a major role in the metabolism of protein, carbohydrate, and fat and performs phagocytosis (destruction of foreign substances) on the blood as it is filtered through the liver. This organ transforms most drugs, hormones, and bilirubin into excretable forms. Bile is manufactured in the liver, and many enzymes are produced here. The liver stores many vitamins and minerals. The body cannot live without a functioning liver.

The pancreas sits behind the stomach. It produces and excretes not only the digestive juices necessary for protein, fat, and carbohydrate metabolism, but also insulin, which is necessary for glucose metabolism. The pancreatic juices empty into the duodenum.

DIAGNOSTIC TESTS

Sonography, radiographs, laboratory tests, nuclear medicine scans, magnetic resonance imaging, and biopsy are used to diagnose problems of the gallbladder, liver, and pancreas. The nurse is responsible for teaching the patient about each of these tests. She also always checks to see if the patient has an allergy that makes a particular contrast medium or injectable marker contraindicated. Psychological care of the patient should not be overlooked. What seems to be a routine test to the nurse can have very different meaning to the patient. It is best to assess what fears the patient might have before beginning teaching about the test.

The purpose, description, and nursing implications for the tests of the gallbladder, liver, and pancreas are listed in Table 24-1.

DISORDERS OF THE GALLBLADDER

CHOLELITHIASIS

Cholelithiasis is the presence of gallstones within the gallbladder itself or in the biliary tract. The stones may vary in size from very small "gravel" to stones as large as an orange. It is usually the smaller ones that cause the most trouble, because they pass into the bile ducts, where they become lodged and cause an obstruction to the flow of bile (Fig. 24-1).

Gallstones are relatively common in persons over the age of 40 and affect women four times more often than men. They do not always cause symptoms and go undetected in anywhere from 60% to 80% of the population.

The use of oral contraceptives by young adults has brought about an increase in gallstones in 20- to 30-year-old women.

TABLE 24-1 **DIAGNOSTIC TESTS FOR GALLBLADDER, LIVER, AND PANCREAS PROBLEMS**

Test Purpose	Description	Nursing Implications
Ultrasonography Obtains images of soft tissue that indicate density changes. Commonly used for the liver, biliary system, gallbladder, pancreas, and spleen.	Sonograms are produced with high-frequency sound waves that pass through the body. Echoes vary with tissue density. Used to diagnose gallstones, tumor, cysts, abscess, etc.	Patient NPO after midnight. Explain procedure: will be supine on table, lubricant will be applied to the skin surface, and a hand-held metal probe is passed back and forth with light pressure. It takes about 30 minutes. Patient needs to remain still.
X-ray studies Cholecystography/Cholangiography Locates obstructions and structural defects in the gallbladder and biliary ducts.	Radiopaque contrast medium is given orally or IV. Serial radiographs are taken at intervals to visualize the gallbladder and the biliary and common ducts. For the cholecystogram, the patient may be asked to drink a substance that contains fat after the first series to cause the gallbladder to contract; more radiographs are then taken to see if the gallbladder functions properly.	For oral cholecystogram, administer the required tablets at 8 P.M. the evening prior to the test. A low-fat dinner is best, and no fats are to be eaten for breakfast. Requirements vary per x-ray department and contrast medium used. There should be no barium in the intestinal tract.

TABLE 24–1 **DIAGNOSTIC TESTS FOR GALLBLADDER, LIVER, AND PANCREAS PROBLEMS** *Continued*

Test Purpose	Description	Nursing Implications
Computed tomography Visualizes soft tissue and density changes when sonography is inconclusive.	Radiographs combined with computer techniques to provide a series of sectional pictures of the gallbladder.	Patient NPO for 3 to 4 hours. May require a consent form. Assess for allergy to iodine or shellfish. Explain to patient that he will be in a supine position on a special narrow table with his body in the circular opening of the scanner. He will have a strap over his waist to secure him to the table. Clicking noises will be heard from the scanner. The test takes about 1½ hours. A contrast agent, which causes a transitory warm feeling, may be given IV to enhance images. He will be asked to hold his breath at certain points in the test. The machine uses narrow x-ray beams.
Endoscopy (ERCP) Performed when common radiologic studies do not reveal the cause of the problem. Used to identify obstruction and other pathologic conditions in the biliary and common ducts.	An endoscope is passed through the mouth into the duodenum with the use of fluoroscopy. A cannula is positioned in the common bile duct, and a contrast medium is injected.	Obtain a signed consent for procedure. Patient NPO after midnight. Explain the procedure to the patient (same as for esophagogastroendoscopy). A pretest sedative may be ordered. Posttest care is same as for esophagogastroendoscopy.
Liver Biopsy Removal of a tissue sample for microscopic exam and diagnosis of various liver disorders.	Under local or general anesthesia, a biopsy needle is inserted into the desired area of the liver, and a tissue sample is aspirated.	Explain the procedure to the patient and obtain signed consent. He will have to remain very still during biopsy if local anesthetic is used. He will feel pain similar to a punch in the shoulder, lasting only a minute or so. Keep patient NPO for 4 to 6 hours prior to biopsy. Assess for allergy to local anesthetics. Have patient empty bladder right before procedure. Take baseline vital signs. Check coagulation studies for abnormalities that contraindicate procedure. Following test, position patient on right side with support to provide pressure over biopsy site. Observe for bleeding: monitor vital signs q 15 min for 1 h; then q 30 min for 4 h; then q 4 h for 24 h; assess for tenderness at biopsy site. Observe for respiratory problems indicative of pneumothorax.
Liver-spleen scan Determines size, shape, and location of abnormal tissue in the liver.	A radioactive isotope is given by IV infusion. The liver is scanned for areas of concentrated radioactivity.	Explain the procedure to the patient. An IV catheter will be inserted for administration of the radioisotope. The small amount of radioactivity is not harmful to the patient or others. He will need to hold very still while the scanner is crossing back and forth over his body. The machine makes a soft clicking noise.

Table continued on following page

TABLE 24-1 **DIAGNOSTIC TESTS FOR GALLBLADDER, LIVER, AND PANCREAS PROBLEMS** *Continued*

Test	Implication	Reference Range
Laboratory tests for liver disorders		
Serum bilirubin	Elevated in all types of jaundice; aids in determining cause.	Total: 0.1-1.2 mg/dL Conjugated: up to 0.3 mg/dL Unconjugated: 0.1-1 mg/dL
Alanine aminotransferase (ALT; formerly SGPT)	Elevated 30 to 50 times normal in toxic hepatitis; 20 times normal in infectious mononucleosis.	1-21 U/L
Aspartate aminotransferase (AST; formerly SGOT)	Elevated within 8 to 12 hours of damage to parenchymal cells; aids in determining degree of problem.	7-27 U/L
Alkaline phosphatase (ALP)	Elevated with metastatic lesions, abscess, cirrhosis, active liver cell damage.	13-39 U/L
Plasma ammonia	Elevated in presence of severe liver damage, as it cannot be detoxified.	12-55 μmol/L
Prothrombin time (PT) Partial thromboplastin time (PTT)	Elevated with liver dysfunction that interferes with production of coagulation factors that are vitamin K-dependent. Prolonged PT is associated with abnormal bleeding.	PT: 25-38 seconds PTT: 11-12.5 seconds
Protein Albumin	Total protein and albumin are decreased in liver failure, as albumin-rich fluid seeps into the peritoneal cavity. Altered protein metabolism also lowers these values.	6.8-8.0 gm/dL 3.5-5.0 gm/dL
Laboratory tests for pancreatic disorders		
Serum amylase	Elevated with acute pancreatitis	4-25 U/mL
Serum lipase	Elevated with acute pancreatitis	2 U/mL or less
Urine amylase	Elevated with acute pancreatitis	24-76 U/mL

Causative Factors

Scientists do not know why gallstones are formed in some persons and not in others. It is known, however, that when bile is saturated with cholesterol, a precipitate settles out and the nucleus of a stone is formed. The stone grows as layers of cholesterol, calcium, or pigment accumulate over the nucleus.

Persons at risk for the development of gallstones are those who have hemolytic disease, have had extensive resection of the bowel as treatment for Crohn's disease, are obese, or have diabetes mellitus. Multiple pregnancies and oral contraceptives increase the chance for gallstone formation.

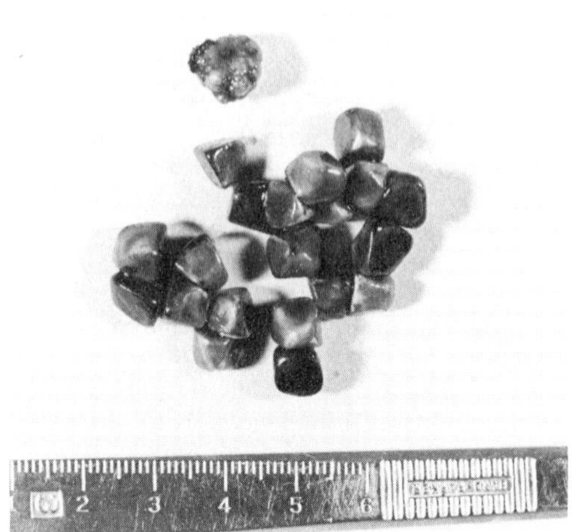

Figure 24-1 Gallstones.

Symptoms and Medical Diagnosis

Symptoms of gallstones vary from none at all to severe and unbearable pain (biliary colic), depending on the degree of obstruction to bile flow and extent of inflammation of the gallbladder. Early signs include indigestion, nausea after eating, and some discomfort in the gallbladder region.

If a stone becomes lodged in the common bile duct, it prevents the flow of bile into the small intestine. The bile accumulates in the blood, causing jaundice. The absence of bile in the intestine results in clay-colored stools that float as a result of undigested fat content. If unrelieved, this condition can cause cholecystitis, which can progress to cirrhosis of the liver.

Gallstones usually can be diagnosed with sonography or computed tomography (CT) of the gallbladder and biliary tract. If the patient is jaundiced, endoscopic retrograde cholangiopancreatography (ERCP) may be done.

Medical and Surgical Treatment

If the patient does not respond to treatment with a low-fat diet and loss of excessive body weight, surgical correction of the obstructed biliary tract is indicated.

The surgical procedure of choice is cholecystectomy. When stones are thought to be in the common bile duct, it is explored during surgery, and a T tube is inserted to drain bile during healing.

CHOLECYSTITIS

Cholecystitis is an inflammation of the gallbladder and is most often associated with gallstones. Other causes include typhoid fever and obstructive tumors of the biliary tract. A systemic streptococcal infection also can cause cholecystitis, but in most cases the infection is secondary to biliary obstruction rather than a primary factor.

Symptoms and Medical Diagnosis

The symptom most often presented in chronic cholecystitis is biliary colic. The pain sometimes is referred to the back at the level of the shoulder blade. Attacks can occur as frequently as daily, or may not appear but once every year or so. Vomiting may accompany acute flareups, and the person may experience chills and fever. If the inflammation is not corrected or if there is an infection, the gallbladder can become filled with pus and will eventually rupture, spilling its contents in the abdominal cavity and causing peritonitis.

The diagnosis of cholecystitis is aided by abdominal sonogram, cholecystogram, intravenous cholangiography, and endoscopic examination. Laboratory tests helpful in the diagnosis of gallbladder and biliary tract disease include evaluation of direct bilirubin and alkaline phosphatase; levels of both are elevated in biliary obstruction.

Medical and Surgical Treatment

The preferred treatment of cholecystitis with gallstones is surgical removal of the gallbladder *(cholecystectomy)*. If surgery is contraindicated, the symptoms might be controlled to some degree by a low-fat diet, restriction of alcohol intake, and spacing of meals so that large amounts of food are not put into the intestinal tract at any one time to stimulate gallbladder activity.

An alternative for patients who are not candidates for surgery, or for elderly patients with mild symptoms, is bile acid therapy. A drug, either chenodiol (CDCA) or ursodiol (UDCA), is given orally that successfully reduces small cholesterol stones. The drug is expensive and may take up to 2 years to dissolve the stones. Often stones appear again after the patient stops the therapy.

Lithotripsy, or "shock wave" therapy, is being done in some major medical centers. This involves the use of sound waves directed through the body to break up the stones. The procedure takes 1 to 1½ hours, and the debris is then carried by the bile into the intestine. There must be no more than three cholesterol gallstones, each smaller than 1½ inches. Only a small percentage of people qualify for this procedure, and the stones tend to recur after treatment. The procedure may be done on an outpatient basis.

A new, less traumatic gallbladder surgical procedure is the laparascopic cholecystectomy. The gallbladder is removed by dissection through an endoscope, often with the use of a laser. This requires only two or three puncture wounds in the abdomen through which the equipment is introduced, rather than the large upper abdominal incision of the standard cholecystectomy. Not all patients are candidates for this procedure, and not all surgeons are willing to perform it, as the view of the operative site is very limited. One advantage is that the hospitalization period is shorter and the patient usually can return to work within 1 to 2 weeks. In some locales this procedure is being done as outpatient surgery.

Nursing Assessment and Intervention

During history taking the nurse should be alert for patients at risk for the development of gallstones and record on the patient's chart those risk factors she has identified. Additionally, she should assess the patient for subjective and objective signs and symptoms of gallbladder disease and liver involvement.

Nursing intervention focuses on problems of discomfort, nausea and vomiting, and acceptance of a low-fat diet. Nursing diagnoses for the patient with gallbladder disease include:

- Pain related to inflammation and contraction of the gallbladder.
- Fluid volume deficit from persistent vomiting and inability to eat.
- Noncompliance with a low-fat diet.

If the patient is scheduled for surgery, his needs will be similar to those of any patient having abdominal surgery. Care of the patient having surgery of the gallbladder is presented below.

NURSING CARE OF PATIENTS HAVING SURGERY OF THE GALLBLADDER

PREOPERATIVE CARE

Preoperatively the patient may have a nasogastric (NG) tube to relieve nausea and vomiting. Meperidine may be ordered to decrease pain, and antiemetics are given for nausea. IV fluids are begun to prevent dehydration if the patient is experiencing symptoms. Coagulation times are monitored if jaundice is present, and vitamin K, if needed, is administered prior to surgery to improve clotting ability of the blood.

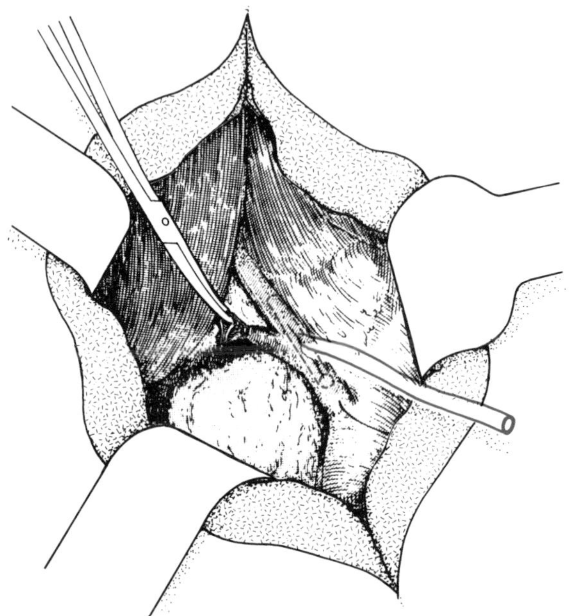

Figure 24-2 T tube inserted into the common bile duct and sutured in place. A hemostat *(left)* holds the end of the cystic duct, which has been cut and tied. The T tube is brought to the outside and attached to a drainage bag.

POSTOPERATIVE CARE

Because the surgical incision is in the upper section of the abdomen, the patient is placed in the semi-Fowler's position after he recovers from anesthesia. Aside from being more comfortable and having less strain on the sutures, the patient will also be able to take deep breaths and cough more easily in this position.

One of the most confusing aspects of nursing a patient who has had gallbladder surgery is proper care of the drains or tubes that may be in place when the patient returns from the operating room.

In many cases, the surgery has been performed to relieve an obstruction to the flow of bile through the bile ducts or to provide a means of draining purulent material to the outside. If the patient has had an infection of the gallbladder, the drainage is absorbed by the dressings over the surgical wound. These must be changed often and should be checked quite frequently for signs of fresh bleeding. The drain is left in as long as necessary and is then removed by the surgeon.

When an obstruction of the common bile duct has occurred because of stones or tumors, the surgeon may insert a small T shaped tube (T tube) directly into the common bile duct (Fig. 24-2). This tube must be kept open at all times and is connected to a bedside drainage bag. The length of time the T tube is left in place depends on the condition of the patient. While the tube is in the common bile duct, no bile will be going to the duodenum as it normally would.

Precautions must be taken so that no tension is put on tubes or drains that have been inserted in the surgical wound (Fig. 24-3).

T tubes are sutured in place, and if they are accidentally pulled out, the patient must be returned to the operating room and the incision reopened to replace the tube.

Dressings must be changed with careful handling of the tube or drain. There is usually so much drainage that the dressings must be changed often, and Montgomery straps are best for holding the dressings in place. The sight of so much greenish-yellow discharge (bile) on the

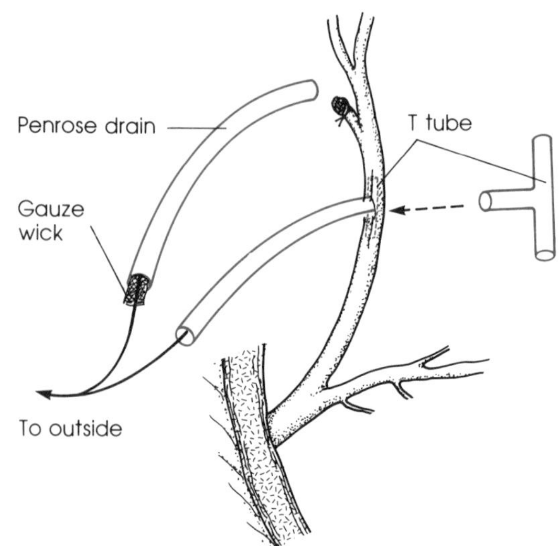

Figure 24-3 After cholecystectomy, the Penrose drain helps to remove exudate from the area formerly occupied by the gallbladder. The T tube diverts bile to the outside.

dressings may upset the patient unless he is told that this is to be expected.

Because the surgeon will be concerned with whether bile is beginning to flow through the duct and into the duodenum as it normally should, the nurse must carefully observe the color of the patient's stools. A return of the characteristic brown color to the stools is an indication that bile is entering the small intestine. If the obstruction remains in the bile duct, the patient will show signs of jaundice.

The cholecystectomy patient is reluctant to deep breathe and cough because of considerable pain in the operative area. He should be assisted with these exercises, and his lung sounds should be auscultated every shift to quickly discover any signs of extra secretions or atelectasis. Administering analgesia regularly, as ordered, will help the patient cooperate with turning, coughing, and ambulating, thus preventing complications.

For the laparoscopic cholecystectomy, the patient will have dressings over the two or three holes on the abdomen. It is especially important to monitor this patient closely for internal bleeding. The nurse should watch for signs of increasing abdominal rigidity and pain and for changes in vital signs. The patient is discharged 1 or 2 days postoperatively and must have careful discharge teaching regarding signs of complications. He should monitor his temperature daily and watch his stool for changes in color. Increasing pain or abdominal distention should be reported to the surgeon.

There is no specific diet recommended for the patient who has had surgery of the gallbladder, although he is usually warned to avoid excessive amounts of fatty foods.

Light-colored stools, dark urine, or the early appearance of a yellowish cast to the skin must be reported as soon any as one of these is noticed.

NURSING ASSESSMENT OF PATIENTS WITH LIVER DISEASE

The liver is subject to infection (abscess) and inflammation (hepatitis), chronic inflammation and degeneration of its cells (cirrhosis), and malignancy.

Because of its many functions, assessment of the patient with liver disease must include all systems of the body. A comprehensive history of illnesses and exposure to toxic agents, both chemical and infectious, is part of a thorough assessment. Some major areas for history taking include:

- Exposure to toxins—(1) Inhalation of agents toxic to the liver (for example, cleaning agents containing carbon tetrachloride or anesthetics, such as halothane). (2) Ingestion of alcohol. How much and how often? (3) Drugs. What medications is the patient taking? How long has patient been on each medication? Does the patient use recreational (illegal) drugs?
- Exposure to infectious organisms—contact with person who has hepatitis; ingestion of contaminated shellfish; blood transfusions.
- Trauma—accidental injury or surgery of the liver, pancreas, or spleen.

Subjective symptoms of liver disease include fatigue, weakness, headache, anorexia, abdominal pain, nausea, and vomiting. Objective symptoms include skin rashes, itching, fever, urine that is darker than normal because of the presence of bile, stools that are gray or clay-colored, thigh and leg edema, palmar erythema (redness of the palms that blanches with pressure), clubbed fingers, and bluish varicose veins radiating from the umbilicus (indicating portal hypertension). Bleeding and bruising also are associated with liver disease because of deficiencies in vitamin K and other substances necessary for clot formation. Jaundice also can be a sign of damage to the liver cells.

JAUNDICE

Jaundice is a symptom, not a disease. It indicates excessively high levels of bile pigment (bilirubin) in the blood. The pigment is deposited in the skin, mucous membranes, and body fluids, causing a change in color ranging from pale yellow to golden-orange. There are three main types of jaundice: obstructive, hepatic, and hemolytic (breakdown of red blood cells [RBCs]).

Obstructive jaundice is caused by a blockage to the flow of bile in the bile ducts. The pigment in the dammed-up bile enters the blood stream and causes the yellowing typical of jaundice. It can occur as a result of inflammation, stones, and tumors in the liver, gallbladder and biliary ducts, or pancreas. If the obstruction is not relieved, congestion eventually will lead to ischemia and destruction of liver cells.

Hepatic jaundice occurs as a result of the inability of the liver either to process bilirubin or to transport it to the bile ducts for excretion via the intestines. It can be caused by inflammation of the liver, cirrhosis, liver congestion, or malignancy of the liver cells.

Jaundice is not always a sign of liver damage. In hemolytic jaundice there may be an increased level of bilirubin as a result of excessive destruction of RBCs, with resultant release of the pigment into the blood stream. Liver function can be normal in hemolytic jaundice, and the liver may actually speed up its function of processing bilirubin.

Some causes of hemolytic jaundice are transfusion reactions, sickle cell and hemolytic anemias, septicemia, and erythroblastosis fetalis caused by Rh-factor incompatibility between fetal and maternal blood.

The patient who is jaundiced experiences a drastic change in body image. He knows his skin color attracts attention and that he looks sick. The nurse needs to provide time for sharing of feelings and affirmation of his self-worth.

DISORDERS OF THE LIVER

VIRAL HEPATITIS

There are four types of viral hepatitis: type A, type B, type C (non-A, non-B), and type D, or delta, hepatitis. Hepatitis A (HAV) is transmitted primarily by the oral-fecal route and is responsible for epidemic forms of viral hepatitis.

Hepatitis B (HBV) is transmitted mainly by parenteral routes and is present in all body fluids and stool of carriers. Sexual partners of patients who are carriers of HBV are at high risk for contracting the virus. Hepatitis D (HDV) coexists with hepatitis B, is transmitted in the same ways, and is present only as long as hepatitis B is in the body.

Hepatitis C is largely transmitted by parenteral routes. It is the main cause of posttransfusion hepatitis, largely because there are no known diagnostic markers for this virus (meaning that donor blood cannot be screened for this type of hepatitis). Hepatitis C also occurs in hemodialysis patients.

The incubation period, clinical manifestations, major route of transmission, and other characteristics differ among the four types of viral hepatitis. A comparison of these characteristics is shown in Table 24–2.

Medical Diagnosis

The clinical signs and symptoms of type A hepatitis and type B hepatitis are similar, except that the onset of type A is acute, whereas in types B, C, and D the onset is slower and more insidious. In these types the patient can be virtually without symptoms and unaware that he is ill. When symptoms do occur they include such vague and nonspecific manifestations as malaise, fever, loss of appetite, nausea, fatigue, and abdominal discomfort. The liver becomes tender and enlarged. The patient might think he has a mild case of influenza because the symptoms are so similar.

Hepatitis D sometimes causes massive death of liver cells, causing liver failure and death of the patient. Hepatitis B and D can become chronic in about 10% of infected patients. The patient is then a constant carrier of the virus.

A more specific group of symptoms are related to jaundice and include gray or clay-colored stools and dark, foamy urine. Viral hepatitis without jaundice is two to three times more common than viral hepatitis with jaundice.

The medical diagnosis is established by serologic testing for immunoglobulins, specifically the presence of IgM-specific anti-HAV antibody in the serum to distinguish current infection from past infection. There are more sophisticated tests for HBV and HDV components, but most laboratories test only for surface antigens and antibody to the surface antigen. There is no laboratory test specific for hepatitis C (non-A, non-B). The majority of patients are treated on an outpatient basis.

Preventive Measures

Both feces and blood of patients with hepatitis A contain virus during the prodromal (infected but without symptoms) stage and early symptomatic stage. Good hygiene, with hand washing after contact and careful handling and disposal of clothing and eating utensils, is necessary. The strict use of universal precautions is essential. Close contacts of patients with hepatitis A should be given immune serum globulin as soon as possible.

The greatest risk for transmission of HBV is from commercially prepared clotting concentrates derived from the plasma of paid donors. Serologic testing for the presence of hepatitis B surface antigen (HBsAg) in whole blood has significantly decreased the incidence of transfusion-related hepatitis B.

Hepatitis B and D are rarely transmitted by the fecal-oral route, but it is best to be very careful when disposing of a patient's stool. Universal precaution guidelines must be carefully followed for handling and disposal of equipment contaminated with blood. These viruses are transmitted by sexual contact, and homosexual men in particular are at risk. About 10% of patients with these forms of hepatitis become carriers. Carriers of HBV are at risk for chronic hepatitis, cirrhosis, and carcinoma of the liver. A carrier of HBV has a 300 times greater risk of liver cancer than someone in the general population.

Hepatitis B carriers are counseled to adhere to strict hygienic principles. They should not share personal items such as razors likely to be contaminated with their blood. Dentists, physicians,

TABLE 24-2 **COMPARISON OF CLINICAL AND EPIDEMIOLOGIC CHARACTERISTICS OF VIRAL HEPATITIS**

Characteristic	Type A Hepatitis	Type B Hepatitis	Type D Hepatitis	Type C (Non-A, Non-B Hepatitis)
Incubation period (days)				
Range	15 to 48	28 to 180	Similar to type B	10 to 180
Usual	25 to 30	70 to 75	Similar to type B	50 to 60
Usual type of onset	Acute	Insidious	Present only with HBV	Insidious
Fever	Common; precedes jaundice	Less common	Less common	Less common
Jaundice	Rare in children, more common in adults	Same as in type A	Same as in type A	Same as in type A
Abnormal AST or ALT	Transient (1 to 3 weeks in duration)	Prolonged (may be elevated 1 to 8+ months)	Prolonged	Prolonged
Age group affected	Usually children and young adults	All age groups	All age groups	All age groups
Virus in feces	2 weeks before jaundice	No direct evidence of presence	Possible	Unknown
Virus in blood (viremia)	Present during late incubation period and *early* acute phase	Present during late incubation period and acute phase; may persist for months or years.	Present during entire clinical course of HBV	Unknown
Virus in urine	Very low level or negative	Low level	Low level	Low level likely but unproved
Virus transmitted by saliva	Unlikely	Yes, but direct transfer probably necessary	Yes, but direct transfer probably necessary	Unknown
Usual mechanism(s) of transmission	Fecal-oral route	Percutaneous; oral-oral route; direct contact and non-percutaneous	Similar to HBV	Percutaneous (especially via transfused blood); body fluids
Carrier state	No	Yes	Yes	Evidence suggests yes

Adapted from Jackson, M. M.: Virus hepatitis. Nurs. Clin. North Am., Dec., 1980, p. 735.

nurses, and other health care workers must be informed of their carrier status.

Hepatitis C is transmitted by blood and body fluids; other modes of transmission are unknown at present. Universal precautions and careful handling of all body fluids are recommended.

Various drugs, toxic agents, and other viruses also occasionally cause hepatitis.

Medical Treatment

Hepatitis A and B are diagnosed by history, physical examination, elevations in liver function tests (LFTs), and laboratory tests for the presence of the serologic markers HAsAg (hepatitis A surface antigen) or HBsAg. Hepatitis D is identified by the presence of the delta antigen or a rise in the anti-HD titer. Hepatitis C is diagnosed by ruling out other possibilities. Liver function tests include bilirubin, alkaline phosphatase, alanine aminotransferase (ALT), and aspartate aminotransferase (AST). Chronic hepatitis is determined by liver biopsy.

No specific treatment or drug can kill the hepatitis viruses. Medical treatment is directed at supportive care to enhance the patient's natural defenses and promote regeneration and healing of the liver. Hydration, sufficient rest, and adequate nutrition are the goals of treatment. Medication for nausea may be prescribed to encourage adequate nutrition. Because the patient tends to be anorexic, small, high-calorie meals several times a day are received better than three normal meals. Sucking on hard candy is recommended and adds to caloric intake.

A vaccine is available to provide active immunity against HBV for persons at high risk for infection. The vaccine produces immunity in about 95% of vaccinated individuals.

Passive immunity to type A hepatitis can be conferred by the administration of immune serum globulin (ISG). There also is a high-titer immune globulin for type B hepatitis (HBIG). Both ISG and HBIG are recommended for those who have been exposed to persons infected with HBV.

Viral hepatitis is an occupational hazard for all persons who have direct contact with patients. The first line of defense is scrupulous hand washing, wearing rubber gloves when handling plasma-containing body fluids from a patient, and extreme care when handling used needles, syringes, and intravenous tubing. One does not have to be stuck with a contaminated needle or have an open wound to contract hepatitis B. The mucous membranes of the eye, nose, and mouth also can serve as ports of entry.

Health care personnel who work in high-risk areas such as emergency departments, hemodialysis units, critical care units, surgery, and clinical laboratories should be immunized by administration of hepatitis vaccine.

Nursing Assessment and Intervention

The nursing assessment of a patient with hepatitis should include a nursing history of previous contacts at home and at work and whether the contacts have been reported and the persons immunized. Viral hepatitis must, by law, be reported to the Department of Public Health. This will necessitate filling out papers for patients being treated at home. When a patient with viral hepatitis has been admitted to the hospital, the infection control officer must be notified as soon as possible and no later than 48 hours after admission. Infection with type A hepatitis in a person who handles food as his occupation must be reported promptly so that a follow-up can be done by the health department.

Because the liver detoxifies many chemicals and metabolizes certain drugs, the nurse must have a complete list of medications the patient has recently taken or is currently receiving. It may be necessary to discontinue some drugs that are particularly toxic to the liver. Examples include acetaminophen, aspirin, chlorpromazine, and tetracycline. Sedatives can have a profound effect on patients with hepatitis and must be given with caution, because a diseased liver cannot detoxify them very well. Alcohol is particularly damaging to the liver and is prohibited for 4 months following recovery from hepatitis.

In her assessment the nurse will look for data to verify need for rest and any potential or actual nutritional deficit or fluid imbalance. The patient and his family probably will need instruction in special precautions to prevent the spread of the infectious agent. This may include properly handling and disinfecting body secretions, proper hand washing, and limiting contact with others.

Assessment of hospitalized patients also should include data that would be helpful in identifying problems related to silent gastrointestinal bleeding, respiratory distress, and neurologic dysfunction, especially mental confusion and coma associated with portal systemic encephalopathy. Nursing interventions include monitoring the patient's progress by reviewing reports of serum enzyme levels and serum bilirubin values.

Prevention of the spread of infection is a major concern in the nursing care of patients with viral hepatitis. In addition to knowledge of the type of hepatitis a patient has, the nurse also should know what stage the disease process has reached. For example, the greatest danger of infection with type A hepatitis is during the incubation period and early prodromal phase of the disease. As the infection progresses and jaundice and other symptoms appear, the shedding of viruses declines rapidly, and there is far less danger of contamination. In hepatitis B the virus lingers in the body and remains a threat for a much longer period of time.

The Centers for Disease Control (CDC) have published guidelines for the care of patients hospitalized with viral hepatitis. These same guidelines can be modified for home care to prevent the spread of the infection.

The convalescence of the hepatitis patient is slow and long. Psychological support from the nurse during this period can help prevent depression. A variety of diversional activities that are not physically taxing should be planned. Perhaps this is the time for the patient to take up a new hobby or learn a new skill.

In a small percentage of cases the patient can develop a massive necrosis of liver cells (fulminant hepatitis). Death occurs in about 75% of these cases. Symptoms of fulminant hepatitis include mental confusion, disorientation, and drowsiness. These symptoms indicate portal systemic encephalopathy. Ascites and edema, which also usually are present, indicate liver failure.

Nursing interventions for selected problems in a patient with viral hepatitis are summarized in Nursing Care Plan 24–1. Nursing assessment and interventions for problems associated with severe liver damage are discussed in the following section on cirrhosis.

CIRRHOSIS OF THE LIVER

In cirrhosis of the liver there is destruction of normal hepatic structures and their replacement with necrotic parenchymal tissue. Fibrous bands of connective tissue develop in the organ and eventually constrict and partition it into irregular

NURSING CARE PLAN 24–1

Selected nursing diagnoses, goals/outcome criteria, nursing interventions, and evaluations for a patient with hepatitis

Situation: JoAnn, age 33, is admitted for hepatitis B infection. She is experiencing nausea and vomiting, muscle weakness and fatigue, and pain in the upper right quadrant of the abdomen. Objective data include an enlarged liver, jaundice, and elevated results on liver function tests (AST, ALT, LDH, ALP, and bilirubin).

Nursing Diagnosis	Goals/Outcome Criteria	Nursing Intervention	Evaluation
Pain/discomfort related to jaundice and bile pigments in skin causing itching. SUPPORTING DATA Constantly scratching; asks, "Can't you stop this itching?"	Pain/itching will be minimized by nursing measures as verbalized by patient.	Assist patient to bathe with tepid water three times a day; apply lotion q 2 h. Provide activities to keep mind off of itching. Teach patient relaxation exercises.	Taught relaxation exercises; bathed ×3; lotion applied q 2 h; states it only helps a little; encouraging handwork while watching television; continue plan.
Fluid volume deficit related to nausea and vomiting. SUPPORTING DATA Dry mucous membranes, decreased skin turgor; states she is very nauseated.	Fluid volume will be restored within 24 hours as evidenced by moist mucous membranes and good skin turgor.	Monitor IV infusion site and fluid rate. Encourage oral fluids as tolerated. Monitor electrolyte levels for imbalances.	Able to tolerate fluids in small amounts; mucous membranes moist; electrolytes within normal limits.
Alteration in nutrition, less than body requirements, related to anorexia, nausea, and vomiting. SUPPORTING DATA States she has eaten very little for past 2 weeks, is nauseated, and vomits frequently.	Patient will ingest 1,200-calorie diet per day within 4 days. Patient will not lose weight.	Initiate IV fluids as ordered if dehydration occurs. Keep room door closed to keep odors out. Offer mouth care before meal time. Provide six small meals a day plus small, high-calorie snacks between meals. Weigh every other day and record. Keep hard candy at bedside for snacking.	States nausea has lessened; eating ⅔ of meal; taking between-meal snacks; continue plan.
Knowledge deficit related to ways in which hepatitis B is transmitted, impact of hepatitis on the body, self-care measures, and measures to prevent transmission to others. SUPPORTING DATA Has not had hepatitis before; states she knows nothing about it.	Patient will verbalize ways hepatitis B is transmitted, impact on body, self-care measures, and measures to prevent transmission to others before discharge.	Teaching ways in which hepatitis B is transmitted: parenteral routes, sexual contact. Give explanation in understandable terms of what hepatitis B does to the body. Reinforce teaching regarding self-care measures: hygiene, diet, rest, follow-up. Teach importance of not sharing personal articles, especially razor, toothbrush, etc., with others. Instruct her to inform health care workers that she has the virus until she tests negative. Inform her that sexual partner(s) will need injection of special immune globulin for protection.	Teaching done on transmission of hepatitis B and self-care measures; will seek feedback tomorrow; continue plan.
Potential for injury related to bleeding tendency from decreased production of vitamin K and decreased synthesis of coagulation factors. SUPPORTING DATA Prolonged PT and PTT; excessive bruising at needle stick sites.	Patient will not experience bleeding episode. PT and PTT will return to normal within 4 weeks.	Administer vitamin K as prescribed. Monitor for signs of bleeding: check gums, urine, and stool, and assess for bruising q shift. Monitor PT and PTT times.	Vitamin K injection administered; slight bleeding of gums after teeth brushing; bruises on arms from lab sticks. PT, 14.2 sec.; continue plan.

Nursing care plan continued on following page

NURSING CARE PLAN 24–1, *Continued*

Nursing Diagnosis	Goals/Outcome Criteria	Nursing Intervention	Evaluation
Body image disturbance related to yellow skin color from jaundice. SUPPORTING DATA Moderately jaundiced; states: "I don't want any of my friends to see me like this."	Patient will accept present body image by allowing visitors within 3 days. Patient will not be jaundiced within 3 weeks.	Assure patient that jaundice is not permanent. Allow her to ventilate feelings about illness and appearance. Encourage verbalization of positive aspects about self. Increase fluid intake to help flush bilirubin from blood during recovery.	Taking fluids in moderate amounts; still does not want to see visitors; is fatigued; continue plan.

nodules. The scarring of liver tissue is generally considered irreversible and often is progressive. The outcome of cirrhosis of the liver is failure of its cells (liver failure) and the development of portal hypertension.

The disease process of cirrhosis is lengthy and ultimately leads to a rather sudden appearance of symptoms. There probably is no one specific cause of cirrhosis. Although its incidence is high among known alcoholics, this does not mean that all those who have cirrhosis have a history of alcohol abuse. From 30% to 60% of all cases of cirrhosis are associated with alcohol abuse.

Cirrhosis that is associated with alcoholism is called *Laennec's cirrhosis* or *portal cirrhosis*. *Postnecrotic* cirrhosis is caused by viral hepatitis, toxic substances, or infection. Biliary disease and some cardiac disorders can also lead to cirrhosis.

Cirrhosis is a common disorder. It is the fifth most frequent cause of death in the United States and the third most common cause of death in persons between 25 and 65 years of age.

Medical Diagnosis

Elevations in ALT and AST levels usually do not occur until 65% of liver function is gone. The disease usually progresses without symptoms until severe liver damage is present. The patient may not seek medical attention until he develops ascites, gastrointestinal bleeding from esophageal varices (dilated, distorted blood veins), or neurologic symptoms associated with hepatic encephalopathy. (Encephalopathy is any dysfunction of the brain.) These complications are directly related to liver failure. Other problems occur because the liver no longer performs its normal functions.

A definitive diagnosis of cirrhosis of the liver is made by liver biopsy. Laboratory testing may show hypoalbuminemia, and elevated prothrombin time as well as elevated AST, ALT, and lactate dehydrogenase (LDH).

Medical Treatment

The major goals of medical treatment are to (1) stop further degeneration of liver tissue, (2) minimize further trauma to liver cells by hepatotoxins, (3) reinforce the body's natural defenses and ability to heal itself, and (4) manage disabling symptoms.

Accomplishment of these goals requires a coordinated effort on the part of the physician, nurse, and patient. The intake of alcohol and administration of hepatotoxic drugs must be restricted completely. Sedatives and opiates are either avoided or given with great caution. Rest may be prescribed to aid healing. The degree of rest and activity is dictated by the patient's stage of illness.

Jaundice occurs either because the liver cannot metabolize bilirubin or because bile flow is obstructed.

The liver normally provides protection against infectious organisms. When the liver cells fail to function as they should, the patient is at great risk for infection. The patient should be protected from exposure to infectious agents and antibiotics should be given quickly when infection occurs.

The management of symptoms usually is focused on the effects of pathologic changes that occur as a result of degeneration of liver cells. When liver cells begin to degenerate, the blood vessels within the liver also fail to function normally. This causes an obstruction to the flow of blood through the portal circulatory system, causing portal systemic hypertension. This in turn leads to altered vessel permeability and fluid leakage into the abdomen, resulting in ascites.

Ascites is an abnormal accumulation of serous (edematous) fluid within the peritoneal cavity. As pressure increases in the hepatic veins, there is a shift of protein-rich plasma filtrate into the lymphatic ducts. Some of the fluid enters the thoracic duct, but if the pressure is high enough, the excess fluid will ooze from the surface of the liver into the peritoneal cavity. Because the fluid has a high colloidal pressure owing to its high protein content, it is not readily reabsorbed and therefore accumulates in the cavity, causing increased abdominal girth.

Medical treatment of ascites includes restriction of fluid and sodium intake and administration of diuretics. Surgical management of ascites was at one time entirely limited to abdominal paracentesis to remove accumulated fluid. This is, however, only a temporary measure that poses problems of rapid fluid shift, loss of protein, and the potential for introducing infectious organisms into the peritoneum. In recent years a procedure involving the shunting of ascitic fluid into the venous system has been used more effectively. The procedure is called a peritoneal-venous shunt (LeVeen or Denver shunt).

Symptoms of bleeding from the upper GI tract may indicate *esophageal varices.* These are engorged veins (similar to varicose veins) that line the esophagus. They, too, are the result of portal congestion and hypertension. In advanced cirrhosis, blood that normally flows from the intestines to the portal vein and on through the liver is shunted to other veins, including the veins of the upper stomach and lower esophagus. The added load of blood causes congestion of these veins and can lead to massive bleeding when the vein walls rupture from the increased pressure or esophageal irritation. Another factor in hemorrhage is that the liver is no longer able to make vitamin K, which is an essential factor in the production of clotting factors in the blood. The patient is given vitamin K by injection. The treatment of hemorrhage of the upper GI tract resulting from esophageal varices was discussed in the previous chapter in the section on gastrointestinal bleeding. Propranolol, a beta blocker that lowers blood pressure, may be prescribed to prevent rebleeding.

A third group of symptoms has to do with damage to the brain cells by abnormally high levels of ammonia in the blood. The liver is responsible for removing ammonia, a product of protein metabolism, from the blood and using it to form urea so it can be excreted by the kidneys. When the liver is diseased and can no longer handle the ammonia, it accumulates in the blood. Excessively high levels of ammonia in the blood are a primary cause of the neurologic changes that constitute portal systemic *encephalopathy* and produce such symptoms as delirium, convulsions, and coma.

An important aspect of treatment of patients with this condition is limitation of dietary protein intake. Dietary protein is limited to 40 to 60 gm per day in an effort to lower ammonia levels. Thiamine and multiple vitamins are given to counteract vitamin deficiency. Neomycin is given orally or by enema to decrease the colonic bacteria that break down protein; this prevents formation of ammonia. The bowel is cleansed by enemas to further decrease ammonia production. Lactulose is given orally or by a feeding tube to prevent diffusion of ammonia out of the intestinal tract. The excessive ammonia levels also can cause persistent itching of the skin.

Kidney failure sometimes accompanies liver failure, further complicating the care of the patient.

Ascites, bleeding esophageal varices, and portal systemic encephalopathy are the most dangerous complications of cirrhosis and the most frequent causes of death. Of these three, esophageal varices can be the most deadly because of massive rapid hemorrhage. About half of the patients suffering from bleeding esophageal varices do not survive.

Liver Transplantation

Liver transplantation is considered for patients with progressive and advanced liver disease that does not respond to treatment. It is most commonly done for nonalcoholic cirrhosis, chronic active hepatitis, sclerosing cholangitis, metabolic disorders, and biliary atresia in children. Seventy to eighty percent of liver transplant patients survive at least 3 years with good quality of life (Andreoli et al., 1990).

Nursing Assessment

The liver performs about 1,500 chemical functions that are essential to health and the maintenance of life. In general, these functions are related to (1) the storage of glycogen and fat and the regulation of energy metabolism from foodstuffs in the diet; (2) the synthesis of proteins that function outside the liver (for example, albumin, which plays a role in osmotic pressure and fluid balance; gamma globulins, which help in antibody formation; and fibrinogen and prothrombin, which are necessary for normal clotting of blood); (3) protection against harmful bacteria that enter the body; (4) detoxification of harmful compounds synthesized within the body (for example, ammonia) or ingested (for example, harmful drugs and alcohol); and (5) the storage of vitamins and minerals.

In view of the many functions of the liver, it is obvious that a patient with cirrhosis will require a thorough assessment to determine his status and identify specific patient care problems related to abnormal liver function. Nursing diagnoses for the care plan of the patient with cirrhosis may include:

- Fluid volume excess related to ascites.
- Potential for alteration in tissue perfusion

related to danger of hemorrhage from esophageal varices and decreased clotting factors.
- Potential for infection related to decreased resistance.
- Alteration in nutrition, less than body requirements, related to nausea, anorexia, and inability of liver to metabolize nutrients.
- Diarrhea related to decreased tolerance to fatty acids because of diminished bile production.
- Altered thought processes related to increased levels of circulating ammonia.
- Potential impairment of skin integrity related to edema and itching from increased levels of ammonia.
- Self-care deficit related to fatigue, ascites, and nausea.
- Potential impaired gas exchange from pressure of ascites on diaphragm.

Nursing Intervention

Nursing measures to help prevent, minimize, or alleviate the many problems associated with cirrhosis of the liver are planned according to the specific conditions presented by the patient. Many of the nursing diagnoses listed above and appropriate nursing interventions have already been discussed earlier in this text. Interventions for selected problems in a patient with cirrhosis of the liver are summarized in Nursing Care Plan 24–2.

PANCREATITIS

Pancreatitis is an inflammation of the pancreas. It may be acute or chronic in nature and frequently accompanies obstruction of the pancreatic duct resulting from gallstones or the backflow of bile into the pancreatic duct.

Most cases of pancreatitis are related to alcoholism or biliary disease. Viral infections, trauma from certain types of surgery, ERCP, penetrating ulcers, drug toxicities, metabolic disorders, and a variety of other things can occasionally cause pancreatitis. Men tend to develop pancreatitis related to alcohol; in women, it is seen more frequently with cholelithiasis.

In some types of pancreatitis, the severe inflammation and damage are caused by escape of pancreatic digestive enzymes, which act directly on the tissue, causing hemorrhage, autodigestion, and necrosis.

ASSESSMENT

Pancreatitis causes abdominal pain that is usually very acute, but this can vary among individuals. The pain is steady and is localized to the epigastrium or left upper quadrant. As it progresses, it spreads and radiates to the back and flank. Eating makes the pain worse. Nausea and vomiting often accompany the pain.

MEDICAL TREATMENT AND NURSING INTERVENTION

Diagnosis is based on the presenting symptoms plus risk factors and results of tests performed to rule out other disorders. An abdominal sonogram, CT scan, and serum and urine amylase studies are usually ordered. Amylase levels are elevated and the pancreas is enlarged in patients with pancreatitis.

Treatment is supportive and consists of pain control, fluid replacement, nasogastric decompression, and treatment of complications such as diabetes mellitus. IV meperidine may be needed to control pain. The patient is allowed nothing by mouth during the acute phase, so as to prevent stimulation of the pancreas and further aggravation of the inflammation. Fluids are given intravenously until the edema of the pancreas and the pancreatic duct has subsided and the digestive juices from the pancreas can once again flow into the duodenum. Most patients with acute pancreatitis recover after receiving this type of treatment.

If the pancreatitis becomes chronic, there is some destruction of the cells of the pancreas and the pancreatic duct becomes fibrotic.

Chronic pancreatitis most frequently is seen in men who have been drinking alcohol for many years. Long-term pain control presents problems. The patient is started on non-narcotic pain medications to try to prevent addiction, but these are often not sufficient for pain control. Pancreatic enzymes are prescribed to be taken with meals, which should be low in fat. No alcohol is to be consumed. Chronic pancreatitis greatly interferes with the patient's usual lifestyle and is often accompanied by depression requiring psychiatric intervention.

CANCER OF THE PANCREAS

Cancer of the pancreas is almost always fatal. It is increasing in incidence and is now the seventh most common malignant tumor in the United States (American Cancer Society, 1990). It is usually in a very advanced state when discovered, as the patient is asymptomatic in the early stages. Epigastric pain and weight loss are the main symptoms. The patient may develop a dislike for red meat.

Diagnosis is made by ultrasonography, imaging techniques, and fine-needle biopsy.

Surgical treatment has not been highly successful and is used mainly to relieve symptoms of obstructive jaundice or other complications. A

NURSING CARE PLAN 24–2

Selected nursing diagnoses, goals/outcome criteria, nursing interventions, and evaluations for a patient with cirrhosis of the liver

Situation: Joe, a 59-year-old male with a 20-year history of alcoholism, is admitted with progressive alcoholic cirrhosis. His complaints include extreme fatigue, a swollen abdomen, edema of the feet and ankles, jaundice, itching, nausea and indigestion, drowsiness, and slight confusion.

Nursing Diagnosis	Goals/Outcome Criteria	Nursing Intervention	Evaluation
Potential for injury related to alteration in thought processes. SUPPORTING DATA Very drowsy; smokes; disoriented as to time and place.	Patient will not experience injury while hospitalized.	Keep long siderails raised and call bell within reach. Monitor mental status q 4 h. Supervise smoking.	Siderails up continuously; call bell in reach; confused; continue plan.
Potential alteration in tissue perfusion related to possible hemorrhage from esophageal varices and decreased clotting factors. SUPPORTING DATA Elevated liver function tests; known cirrhosis; signs of liver failure and portal systemic hypertension; prolonged PT and PTT.	Patient will not experience death from hemorrhage.	Feed only soft foods to decrease mechanical irritation of esophagus. Give vitamin K as ordered. Monitor stool and vomitus for blood. Monitor vital signs every 2 to 4 h as ordered. Observe for increasing restlessness and confusion that might indicate hypoxia from bleeding. Monitor PT and PTT.	Vitamin K injection given; PT and PTT still prolonged; arms bruised from lab sticks; no signs of hemorrhage; continue plan.
Alteration in thought processes related to increased ammonia levels caused by liver failure. SUPPORTING DATA Elevated serum ammonia, confusion and drowsiness.	Serum ammonia levels will not increase further. Serum ammonia levels will return to normal.	Low-protein diet as ordered. Neomycin enemas as ordered. Administer lactulose as ordered to decrease absorption of ammonia; provide protective lubricant for anal region to decrease irritation from diarrhea. Monitor serum ammonia levels.	Lactulose given; profuse diarrhea; serum ammonia unchanged; continue plan.
Fluid volume excess related to ascites and edema from portal systemic hypertension. SUPPORTING DATA Ascites, edema of feet and ankles, 6 lb weight gain in 2 days	Patient will have no further increase in ascites as evidenced by abdominal girth measurement. Patient will return to normal fluid balance as evidenced by normal weight and absence of edema.	Measure abdominal girth q shift and record. Administer diuretics as ordered. Maintain intake and output. Maintain fluid restriction as ordered. Weigh daily and record. Turn at least q 2 h. Provide good skin care.	Abdominal girth down ¼ inch; weight down ½ lb; intake, 500 mL; output, 1,200 mL; turned 8, 10, 12, and 2; continue plan.
Self-care deficit related to fatigue, drowsiness, and ascites. SUPPORTING DATA Cannot perform ADL; very drowsy; ascites.	Patient will be able to assist with ADL within 6 weeks. Patient will be able to perform ADL independently.	Perform ADL for patient while in liver failure. Bathe with tepid water and baking soda q shift to decrease itching. Offer mouth care q 2 h. Apply lotion to skin prn. Offer fluids as permitted. Assist with meals.	ADL done; mouth care 8, 10, 12, and 2; continue plan.
Fear related to possibility of death from liver failure. SUPPORTING DATA States he is afraid he is going to die.	Patient will verbalize fears openly within 3 days. Patient will seek spiritual support.	Establish trusting relationship by attentive, caring attitude. Encourage verbalization of fears; actively listen. Encourage contact with minister or hospital chaplain or use of other spiritual supports.	Does not wish to see minister or chaplain; talks about fear of death; continue plan.

Whipple procedure, or radical pancreaticoduodenectomy, may be done for cancer of the head of the pancreas. The head of the pancreas, gallbladder, duodenum, part of the jejunum, and all or part of the stomach are removed. Remaining structures are anastamosed to the jejunum.

Concerns for the Elderly

Gallbladder action becomes sluggish in the older person, and gallstones increase in incidence. The pancreas decreases secretion of lipase, thereby altering the digestion of fat and contributing to a decreased nutritional state. Pancreatic cancer occurs mostly in the over-70 age group and affects more males than females.

BIBLIOGRAPHY

Adinaro, D.: Liver failure and pancreatitis: Fluid and electrolyte concerns. Nurs. Clin. North Am., Dec., 1987, p. 843.

American Cancer Society: Cancer Facts and Figures. New York, 1990.

Andreoli, T. E., et al.: Cecil Essentials of Medicine, 2nd ed. Philadelphia, W. B. Saunders, 1990.

Bullock, B. L., and Rosendalhl, P. O.: Pathophysiology: Adaptations and Alterations in Function, 2nd ed. Boston, Scott, Foresman, 1988.

Dobberstein, K.: The liver: To know it is to love it. Am. J. Nurs., Jan., 1987, p. 74.

Fain, J. A., and Amato-Vealey, E.: Acute pancreatitis: A gastrointestinal emergency. Crit. Care Nurs., Aug., 1988, p. 47.

Groth, K.: Age-related changes in the gastrointestinal tract. Geriatr. Nurs., Sept., 1988, p. 278.

Guyton, A. C.: Textbook of Medical Physiology, 8th ed. Philadelphia, W. B. Saunders, 1991.

Harrington, D., and Gogel, H. K.: When the patient suffers from esophageal bleeding. RN, Feb., 1987, p. 24.

Ignatavicius, D. D., and Bayne, M. J.: Medical-Surgical Nursing. Philadelphia, W. B. Saunders, 1991.

Jeffres, C.: Complications of acute pancreatitis. Crit. Care Nurs., April, 1989, p. 38.

Jermier, B. J., and Treloar, D. M.: Bringing your patient through gallbladder surgery. RN, Nov., 1986, p. 18.

Matteson, M. A., and McConnell, E. S.: Gerontological Nursing: Concepts and Practice. Philadelphia, W. B. Saunders, 1988.

Quinless, F. W.: Severe liver dysfunction. Focus Crit. Care, Dec., 1985, p. 24.

Ricci, J. A.: Alcohol-induced upper GI hemorrhage: Case studies and management. Crit. Care Nurs., July, 1987, p. 56.

Rowland, G. A., et al.: The new gallstone destroyers and dissolvers. Am. J. Nurs., Nov., 1989, p. 1473.

Wilkinson, M. M.: Your role in needle biopsy of the liver. RN, Aug., 1990, p. 62.

Willis, D. A., et al.: Gallstones: Alternatives to surgery. RN, April, 1990, p. 44.

STUDENT STUDY AIDS

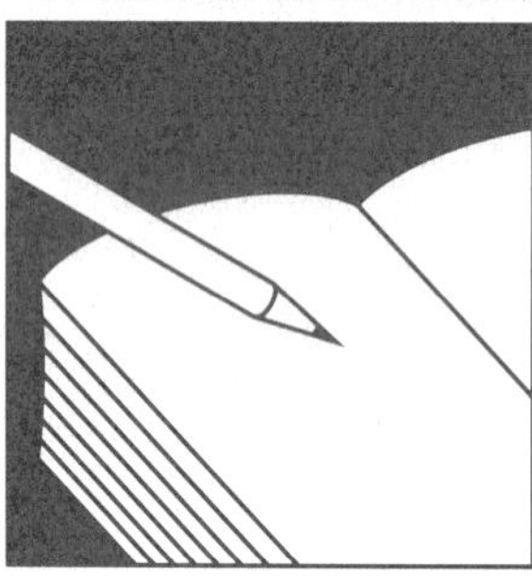

CLINICAL CASE PROBLEMS

Read each clinical situation and discuss the questions with your classmates.

1. Mr. May is admitted to the hospital with a diagnosis of cirrhosis of the liver. He is 59 years of age and has been hospitalized several times for his condition. He suffers from shortness of breath as a result of a swollen and enlarged abdomen, is anemic because of minimal but constant esophageal bleeding, and appears jaundiced. He has severe abrasions on his arms, legs, and abdomen from repeated scratching to relieve his pruritus.

Mr. May is very depressed and will not converse with you when you enter his room with his breakfast tray the first morning you are assigned to his care. He refuses to eat and indicates his attitude by pushing the tray away and turning on his side, face to the wall.

- What nursing measures might help relieve some of Mr. May's problems?
- Why do you think he is mentally depressed?
- How would you go about helping him emotionally?
- What special observations must you make while caring for Mr. May?
- How would you explain a paracentesis to Mr. May if one were ordered for him?

---

2. Mrs. Luke, aged 46, is admitted to the hospital for a cholecystectomy. She is extremely obese and enjoys eating rich, fatty foods even though she knows this will add to her obesity and precipitate attacks of cholecystitis. You are assigned to care for Mrs. Luke when she returns from surgery.

- How will you position this patient?
- If she has a large amount of drainage from the surgical incision, how will you take care of this problem?

- When you get this patient out of bed the next day, how are you going to manage the dressings and prevent strain on the sutures?
- What other problems might you anticipate?

STUDY OUTLINE

I. Diagnostic tests of the gallbladder, liver, and pancreas

A. Purpose, description, and nursing interventions included in Table 24–1.

II. Disorders of the gallbladder

A. Cholelithiasis: gallstones in gallbladder or biliary tract
  1. Relatively common in persons over 40. Do not always cause symptoms.
  2. Causative factors:
     a. Specific cause not known.
     b. Persons at risk are those who have hemolytic disease, who have had extensive bowel resection for treatment of Crohn's disease, or who are obese.
     c. Multiple pregnancies and oral contraceptives also contribute to stone formation.
  3. Medical diagnosis confirmed by sonography. ERCP ordered if patient is jaundiced.
     a. Severity of symptoms depends on location of stone and degree of inflammation.
     b. Obstructive jaundice can be present. Cirrhosis is a possibility if obstruction of bile unrelieved.
  4. Medical and surgical treatment:
     a. Low-fat diet and weight loss.
     b. Cholecystectomy, with or without insertion of T tube.
  5. Nursing assessment and intervention:
     a. Nursing history of persons at risk for gallstones.
     b. Common nursing diagnoses: pain, fluid volume deficit, and noncompliance with low-fat diet.

B. Cholecystitis: inflammation of gallbladder. Most often caused by gallstones. Other causes include tumor, infection, and typhoid fever.
  1. Medical diagnosis:
     a. Clinical signs: indigestion, pain and tenderness in upper right quadrant, malaise, low-grade fever. Indigestion and pain most noticeable after ingestion of fatty meal.
     b. Can lead to rupture of gallbladder, resulting in peritonitis.
     c. Diagnosis confirmed by sonography and x-ray studies.
     d. Laboratory data show elevated levels of direct bilirubin and alkaline phosphatase.
  2. Medical and surgical treatment:
     a. Conservative treatment with low-fat diet, restriction of alcohol intake, spacing of meals.
     b. Cholecystectomy is preferred treatment.
     c. Drug to dissolve the stone (cholelithiasis).
     d. Laparoscopic cholecystectomy.

III. Nursing care of patients having gallbladder surgery, diagnostic procedures, or gastric decompression

A. Preoperative care:
  1. Pre- and posttest care for diagnostic procedures.
  2. Gastric or intestinal decompression.
  3. Pain control.

4. Relief of nausea.
5. Maintenance of hydration.
6. Treatment of infection.

B. Postoperative care:
1. Place in semi-Fowler's position.
2. Monitor tubes for drainage.
3. Frequent dressing changes.
4. Medication for pain.
5. Careful observation of stools for signs of return of bile to intestinal tract.
6. Close attention to respiratory care to prevent complications such as atelectasis or pneumonia.

IV. Disorders of the liver

A. Viral hepatitis: inflammation of the liver:
1. Caused by one of four strains of virus: hepatitis A virus (HAV), hepatitis B virus (HBV), hepatitis C (non-A, non-B), and hepatitis D.
2. Comparison of clinical manifestations of each shown in Table 24–2.
3. Medical diagnosis based on clinical signs and symptoms and serologic testing for immunoglobulins: surface antigens and antibodies to surface antigens.
4. Preventive measures:
   a. Measures to prevent cross-infection and spread of disease; universal precautions.
   b. Vaccination for active immunity against HBV.
   c. Passive immunity: immune serum globulin for hepatitis A and immune globulin for hepatitis B.
   d. Serologic testing on whole blood prior to transfusion.
5. Medical treatment: no cure, treatment is supportive and symptomatic. Majority of patients not hospitalized.
6. Nursing assessment and intervention:
   a. Identify learning needs of patient and family to protect themselves and others.
   b. History of previous contacts.
   c. Prompt reporting of hepatitis to health department.
   d. Seek data to identify needs for rest, adequate nutrition and hydration, potential for cirrhosis and its complications.

B. Cirrhosis of the liver: diffuse fibrosis of liver cells and formation of nodular malfunctioning compartments in liver tissues. Scarring progressive and irreversible.
1. Types:
   a. Laennec's cirrhosis: associated with alcoholism (30% to 60% of all cases).
   b. Posthepatitis or toxin-induced cirrhosis; postnecrotic cirrhosis.
   c. Biliary cirrhosis from obstruction to bile flow.
2. Incidence: fifth most common cause of death in the U.S.; third most common in persons between 25 and 65 years of age.
3. Medical diagnosis:
   a. Often not made until disease has progressed to serious stage.
   b. Definitive diagnosis made by liver biopsy.
   c. Elevated serum enzymes, abnormal liver scan, hypoalbuminemia, and elevated PTT also indicate cirrhosis.
4. Medical treatment:
   a. Major goals are to stop further degeneration of liver tissues,

minimize further hepatotoxic damage, manage disabling symptoms.

b. Restrict alcohol intake.
c. Stop administration of all hepatotoxic drugs.
d. Avoid sedatives and opiates.
e. Prescribe rest to aid healing.
f. Antibiotics as indicated to prevent infection.
g. Manage ascites: restrict sodium and fluids; give diuretics to remove excess fluid in peritoneal cavity; insert peritoneal-venous shunt.
h. Control bleeding from esophageal varices: pitressin infusion; scleropathy; Blakemore-Sengstaken tube with iced saline lavage.
i. Portal-caval shunt to divert blood flow and reduce portal systemic pressure sometimes done.
j. Manage portal systemic encephalopathy: limit protein intake; administer lactulose; neomycin enemas.

V. Nursing assessment of patients with liver disease

A. History to include exposure to hepatotoxins or infectious organisms; physical or surgical trauma; drug abuse.
B. Subjective data: fatigue, anorexia, abdominal pain, nausea, and vomiting.
C. Objective data: skin rashes, itching, fever, dark urine, light stools, thigh and leg edema, palmar erythema, varicose veins radiating from umbilicus; bleeding and bruising easily; jaundice.
D. Jaundice: a group of symptoms caused by excessively high levels of serum bilirubin and the deposition of bile pigment in skin, mucous membranes, and body fluids.
   1. Causes: liver disease, hemolytic jaundice resulting from excessive destruction of red blood cells, and obstructive jaundice caused by blockage of flow of bile to intestines.
   2. Nursing assessment and intervention: see Table 24–2.
E. Nursing diagnoses for patients with liver disease:
   1. Fluid volume excess related to ascites.
   2. Potential for alteration in tissue perfusion related to danger of hemorrhage from esophageal varices and decreased clotting factors.
   3. Potential for infection related to decreased resistance.
   4. Alteration in nutrition related to nausea, anorexia, and inability of liver to metabolize nutrients.
   5. Diarrhea related to decreased tolerance to fatty acids because of diminished bile production and from lactulose therapy.
   6. Altered thought processes related to increased levels of circulating ammonia.
   7. Potential impairment of skin integrity related to edema and itching from increased levels of ammonia.
   8. Self-care deficit related to fatigue, ascites, and nausea.
   9. Potential impaired gas exchange from pressure of ascites on diaphragm.
F. Nursing intervention: see Nursing Care Plan 24–2.

VI. Liver transplantation: for biliary atresia, nonalcoholic cirrhosis, chronic active hepatitis, sclerosing cholangitis, metabolic disorders

A. Seventy to eighty percent of transplant patients survive at least 3 years.

VII. Pancreatitis: inflammation of the pancreas

A. Usually caused by long-term alcoholism or by biliary disease.

B. Symptoms: acute attack similar to acute indigestion; severe pain that radiates to the back.
C. Diagnosis: elevated amylase levels; abnormal abdominal sonogram and CT scan.
D. Treatment and nursing care: medications to relive pain, restriction of foods and fluids, intravenous feedings (TPN).
E. Chronic pancreatitis treated with pain medication, restriction of fat, pancreatic enzymes, and abstinence from alcohol.

VIII. Cancer of the pancreas

A. Insidious disease; discovered when well advanced; usually fatal.
B. Symptoms: epigastric pain and weight loss.
C. Diagnosis by ultrasound, imaging techniques, and fine-needle biopsy.
D. Surgery to decrease tumor bulk: Whipple procedure.

IX. Concerns for the elderly

A. Increased incidence of gallstones; gallbladder sluggish.
B. Decreased lipase secretion; lowers fat metabolism.
C. Higher incidence of pancreatic cancer in men over 70.

CHAPTER 25

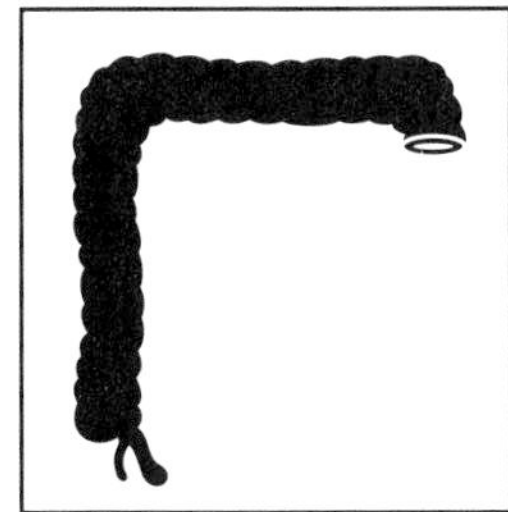

Care of Ostomy Patients

VOCABULARY

anastamosis
conduit
effluent
enterostomal
periostomal
prolapse
stenosis
stoma

Upon completion of this chapter the student should be able to:

1. List four ways the enterostomal therapist can be helpful to the patient with an ostomy.
2. Describe the reasons why each type of ostomy is surgically created.
3. Perform an assessment on a clinical patient with a new ostomy.
4. Formulate a nursing care plan for each type of intestinal ostomy, considering the type of stoma and the effluent it produces.
5. List four interventions for helping the patient psychologically adjust to his ostomy.
6. State the differences in caring for a ureterostomy and a colostomy.
7. Prepare a teaching plan for the following patients: a patient with an ileal conduit; a patient with an ileostomy; and a patient with a permanent sigmoid colostomy and abdominoperineal resection.
8. List six resources and community support services available to ostomy patients.

The term *ostomy* comes from a Greek word that means *mouth* or *opening*. An ostomy is created surgically and can be *internal*, in which a passageway is made between two cavities or organs, or *external*. An external ostomy provides a channel leading from a hollow internal organ to the outside. It is, in effect, a bypass that is needed because the normal passageways for wastes are no longer able to function normally. The surgeon prepares a new opening on the surface of the body so that wastes can be excreted by way of the stoma. Ostomies are necessitated by trauma, disease, or congenital defects. In this chapter, we discuss the ostomy patient who has an external opening surgically created for the purpose of diverting either fecal material or urine to the outside.

ENTEROSTOMAL THERAPY

Although the surgical diversion of fecal material and urine has been done since the 1800s, it is only in the past few decades that new techniques and collection devices have reduced and in some cases completely eliminated many of the inconveniences such procedures could cause the patient. Today, there is no reason why an ostomy operation should prevent a person from leading an active and productive life.

In order to meet the unique needs of ostomates, a specialty has been developed, and a position for this specialist on the health care team has evolved. The field is called *Certified Enterostomal Therapy*. Certification as an enterostomal therapist is not required, but it is encouraged for those who work extensively with patients and clients who have stomas. In order to be certified, one must be a registered nurse, complete a program in an approved school, and pass a qualifying examination.

Many health care agencies employ enterostomal therapists on their staff. These specialists work with ostomates to help them adapt to the many changes in self-care and body image that ostomy surgery can cause. They also serve as consultants to surgeons and members of nursing staffs to help provide more effective care for ostomates. Because they have had special training in skin care, enterostomal therapists also work with patients with draining wounds, decubitus ulcers, and other skin care problems.

The availability of an enterostomal therapist for assistance in special care problems does not relieve staff nurses of the responsibility for the care of those patients assigned to them. The enterostomal therapist is meant to augment nursing care for patients with special needs. She cannot be expected to function as a substitute for the nurse who has resisted learning the special care needed for these patients.

Each year, the number of ostomates increases. Nurses employed in all kinds of health care settings will encounter patients needing physical and psychologic support on a continuing basis as they strive to cope with their ostomies. The nurse who is knowledgeable about such care and has a positive attitude toward the challenges presented by these patients can do much to help them reach the goal of total rehabilitation and adjustment.

There is still much work to be done to prepare health care personnel to meet these challenges and responsibilities. A recent survey in a Florida outpatient clinic indicated that over half the patients who visited the clinic for the first time, in search of help with the management of their ostomies, were sadly lacking in the knowledge and skills they needed to handle their problems. As more nurses become familiar with the types of ostomy surgery and the proper instruction of ostomy patients, it is hoped that there will be fewer and fewer cases of confused and discouraged ostomates.

In this chapter, we discuss the various kinds of stomas, the specialized care of each type, and current equipment used for collection of wastes and control of odor. These are the primary concerns of the patient, who must learn a different way to handle and dispose of body wastes and to adjust emotionally and socially to this change in body image.

LOCATIONS AND TYPES OF STOMAS

As previously explained, the stomas discussed in this chapter are concerned with the diversion of either feces or urine. Stomas are identified according to location and type. If the stoma allows for the passage of fecal material from the colon, it is called a *colostomy*. The stoma leading from the portion of the small intestine called the *ileum* is known as an *ileostomy*. Several techniques are used to permit passage of urine, including *ureterostomy*, which leads from the ureter, and *vesicostomy*, which is a stoma from the bladder.

Table 25–1 summarizes ostomies and the effluent or discharge from each.

COLOSTOMY LOCATIONS

An *ascending colostomy* is one in which either one end or a loop of a portion of the ascending colon is brought to the surface of the abdomen to form a stoma. An ascending colostomy is the least commonly used for passage of fecal material; it involves the portion of the large intestine closest to the small intestine, and therefore the fecal material passing through it has not yet had

TABLE 25-1 **TYPES OF OSTOMIES**

Ostomy	Effluent
Colostomy	
Ascending	Watery and unformed stool.
Transverse	Semiliquid or very soft feces.
Sigmoid	Semisolid to firm feces.
Variations in stomas depend on surgical technique.	
Double-barreled colostomies have two stomas; only the active one discharges feces.	
Single-barreled, or end, colostomies have only one stoma.	
Loop colostomies have one opening, but two tracks: an active (proximal) opening that discharges fecal matter, and an inactive (distal) one that has a mucous discharge.	
Ileostomy	
Continent ileostomy	Continuous discharge of liquid or soft feces. Fecal discharge removed from ileal pouch via catheter several times a day.
Ureterostomy	
Cutaneous	Urine. Output is constant through ureters brought to the surface for excretion of urine.
Ileal conduit	Urine. Output is constant.
Sigmoid conduit	Urine. Output is constant.

much water reabsorbed from it. The stool from an ascending colostomy is thus watery and unformed. Remember that the farther down the intestinal tract waste material travels, the more solid it becomes and the more slowly it moves. It would be expected, then, that the feces expelled would be more liquid and more likely to escape frequently and unpredictably than feces from a stoma nearer the rectum.

An ascending colostomy usually is temporary and is done to allow the bowel distal to the ostomy to rest and heal. This is sometimes necessary for the patient with inflammatory bowel disease, for reconstruction of an intestinal birth defect, or for the patient who has experienced an intestinal tear from trauma. After the rest and healing period, the surgeon will replace the intestine in the abdominal cavity, and fecal material can be defecated normally.

A *transverse colostomy* is situated toward the middle of the abdomen, which is where the transverse colon is located (Fig. 25-1*A*). This kind of colostomy also usually is temporary. The stool from a transverse colostomy is semiliquid and is discharged unpredictably.

Indications for a transverse colostomy are basically the same as for ascending colostomies, the difference being dictated by the location of the condition necessitating diversion of fecal material.

A *sigmoid (descending) colostomy* is located on the surface of the lower quadrant of the abdomen (Fig. 25-1*B*). It is the most common type of permanent colostomy and usually is done as a treatment for cancer of the rectum. The surgical removal of malignant tissues and adjacent structures prevents normal passage of feces. The stoma acts as an artificial anus. The stool from a sigmoid colostomy is more solid and well formed and may be discharged no more often than once a day or every 2 days. It is therefore much easier to establish a pattern of evacuation to control the flow of fecal material through a sigmoid colostomy.

TYPES OF SURGICAL PROCEDURES

There are three basic types of ostomy surgery, and the stomas thus created are called (1) *loop ostomy,* (2) *single-barreled* or *end colostomy,* and (3) *double-barreled ostomy.* The loop ostomy involves pulling a loop of intestine through the incision and securing it to the abdominal wall. In a loop urostomy, the loop of ureter is pulled through an incision in the area of the kidney, which is in the back. In a single-barreled ostomy, there is only one stoma, and in a double-barreled ostomy, there are two.

The loop ostomy is most often seen when a

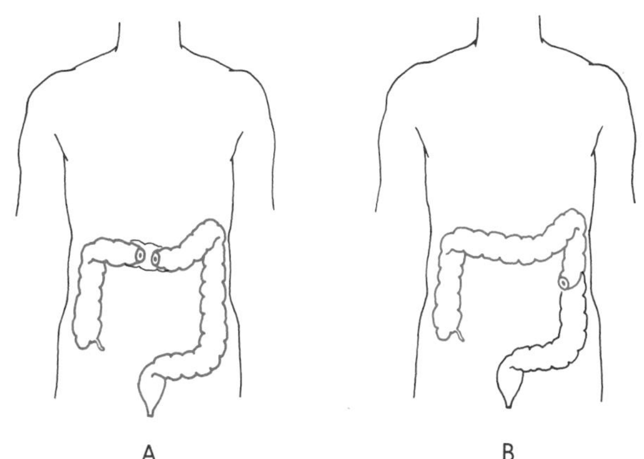

Figure 25-1 Locations for colostomy. *A,* Transverse colostomy. Note two stomas. *B,* Descending colostomy (sigmoid colostomy).

colostomy is performed. For the sake of brevity, we describe each *type of* stoma that is possible when a colostomy is performed, but the reader should bear in mind that these types may be found at locations other than the colon.

Loop Colostomy

As the name implies, a loop of the colon is brought through an abdominal incision and onto the surface of the body. Some kind of supportive device is placed under the loop to prevent it from slipping back into the abdominal cavity (Fig. 25–2). The loop is formed and secured in place while the patient is in the operating room. About 2 days later, the surgeon will open the colostomy at the patient's bedside. This may be done with an electric cauterizing instrument, a scalpel, or surgical scissors and does not require anesthesia because the bowel has no sensory nerve endings.

Once the surgeon has made the opening in the wall of the intestine, fecal material passes through the opening (stoma) in the loop of the intestine. An appliance for collection of fecal material should be on hand before the intestine is opened so that it can be attached immediately after the stoma has been created. The pouch for collection of feces fits over the stoma made by the slit in the loop of intestine. After about 5 to 7 days, the surgeon may remove the rod if the stoma has adhered to the abdominal wall.

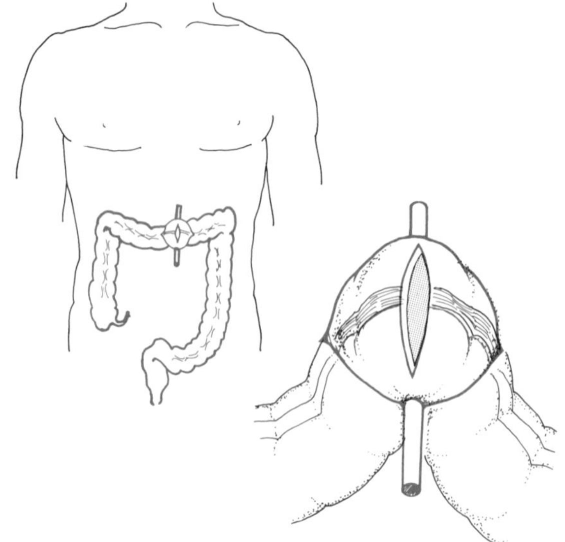

Figure 25–2 A loop transverse colostomy is created from a segment of transverse colon that is brought out through the abdominal wall and supported by a glass rod or temporary support. A slit in the bowel allows feces to drain from proximal colon. Support is removed 5 to 7 days after surgery or when the bowel adheres to the abdominal wall.

Double-Barreled Colostomy

In a double-barreled colostomy, there are two separate stomas. The loop of intestine is completely severed, creating a *proximal stoma* and a *distal stoma*. The proximal stoma is the one closer to the small intestine, and so fecal material passes through it to the outside. The distal stoma leads from the rectum and should discharge only small amounts of mucus. The distance between the stomas varies. It is best if the stomas are widely separated; when they are too close together, it is difficult to get a good seal for the collection device around each one.

Single-Barreled or End Colostomy

There is only one stoma in a single-barreled colostomy. It is located on the lower left quadrant of the abdomen and is the proximal end of the sigmoid colon—that is, the end nearest the small intestine. The end is brought to the abdominal surface, effaced (cuffed over itself), and sutured to the skin, making what is called a *surgically mature stoma*. If the ends are not sutured to the skin, the stoma may be clamped open, allowing the stoma to cuff itself during the healing process. Stomas that mature in this way are more likely to develop strictures. Any type of stoma may be matured surgically.

If the colostomy is temporary, the remaining portion of bowel and rectum are left intact. If the colostomy is permanent, an abdominal perineal resection (APR) is done. This procedure involves removal of the freed bowel, anus, and rectum.

ILEOSTOMY

An ileostomy is performed for the purpose of draining fecal material from the ileum (Fig. 25–3). It is indicated when disease, congenital defects, or trauma require bypassing the entire colon. The most common indications for ileostomy are chronic inflammatory bowel disease (IBD), such as ulcerative colitis and regional ileitis, malignancy, and the presence of many polyps

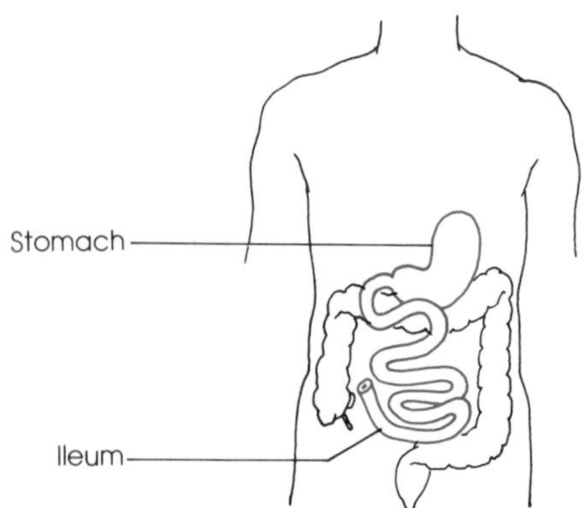

Figure 25–3 Location of ileostomy.

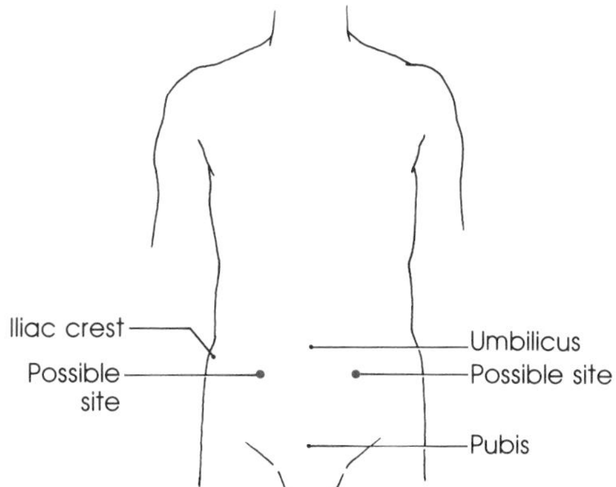

Figure 25-4 Selection of stoma sites.

in the colon *(multiple polyposis)*. The last disease is hereditary, and the polyps have a high potential for malignancy.

The site for the stoma of an ileostomy must be carefully selected so that it is not near any bony prominences, folds of skin, or scars and is in a place where the patient can see it and care for it (Fig. 25-4). The reason for this is apparent when we realize that the stool from an ileostomy is liquid, and even though digestion is completed by the time the fecal material reaches the stoma, it still contains digestive enzymes that are highly irritating to the skin. Bony prominences and scars, folds, and creases in the skin prevent a snug fit of the collection device around the stoma and therefore permit leakage onto the skin.

In recent years, some surgeons have begun using a newer technique for the creation of an ileostomy. The *pouch ileostomy* or *continent ileostomy* frees the ileostomy patient from the need to wear a collection device. A small segment of the ileum is looped back on itself to form a pouch, and a nipple effect is created. Pressure from the accumulating feces closes the nipple valve, preventing constant drainage through the stoma. The patient empties the pouch several times a day by inserting a catheter into the stoma.

Not every patient can be treated by this surgical technique. It has some disadvantages and must be performed by a surgeon skilled in the procedure. Among those who are not good candidates for a continent ileostomy are patients with chronic inflammatory disease that tends to recur. If they develop inflammation within the pouch itself, the pouch must be removed. Another contraindication has to do with the patient's potential for self-care. Because the patient must be able to handle insertion of the catheter for periodic drainage of the pouch, he must be mature enough and sufficiently able to comprehend instructions in self-care and carry them out. The third contraindication is related to previous surgery. Patients who have had a conventional ileostomy cannot have a continent ileostomy done if they have less than 30 mm of terminal ileum remaining. This much is needed to construct the nipple valve.

Although not every patient needing an ileostomy can have a continent ileostomy, it is a safe and effective procedure for many. It eliminates the need for an external appliance, is a more natural way to handle waste, greatly reduces fear of embarrassment from leakage of gas and feces, and minimizes periostomal skin problems.

URINARY DIVERSION

Diversion of urine so that it bypasses the bladder and urethra usually is indicated by (1) malignant disorders of the bladder, (2) congenital structural defects, (3) trauma to the urinary tract, and (4) neurogenic bladder. There are several ways in which urinary diversion can be accomplished (Fig. 25-5), including *ileal conduit* or *ileal loop, sigmoid conduit, cutaneous ureterostomy, vesicotomy,* and *ileal reservoir (Kock's pouch).*

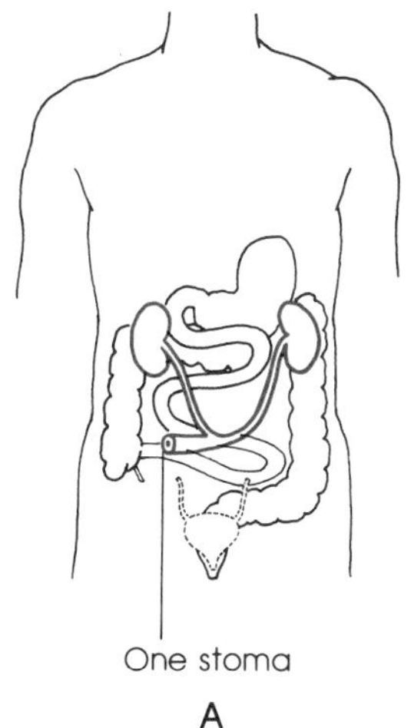

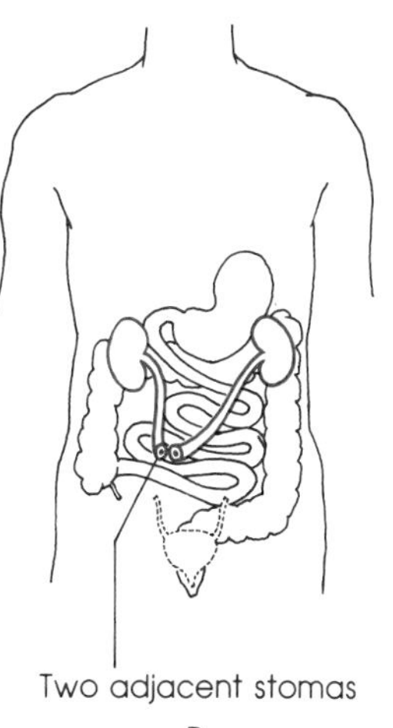

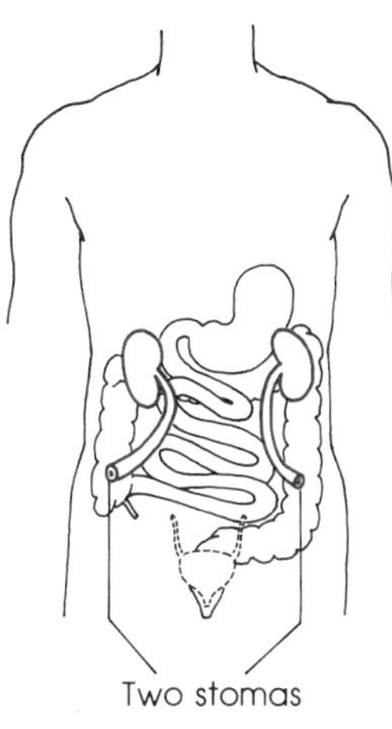

Figure 25-5 Locations for ileal conduit and ureterostomies. *A*, Urinary diversion (ileal loop, ileal conduit). *B*, Ureterostomy. *C*, Bilateral ureterostomy.

Ileal Conduit

This procedure is also called urinary *ileostomy* and *ileal loop*. A portion of the ileum is used as a tube or conduit through which urine flows to the outside. It is important to realize that the section of ileum is removed from the intestinal tract. Urine does *not* flow through it to the intestines, as when the ureters are sutured to the sigmoid.

The surgeon cuts out a portion of the ileum, leaving nerve and blood supply intact so that it remains a viable tissue. The two ends of the intestine from which the section of ileum is removed are rejoined. The "borrowed" section of ileum is sutured together at one end to form a pouch, while the other end is brought outside to form a stoma. The ureters are attached to the ileal conduit so that urine can flow through the conduit to the outside.

Sigmoid Conduit

A sigmoid, or colonic, conduit is similar to an ileal conduit, the difference being that a portion of the sigmoid colon is used to form the conduit.

Cutaneous Ureterostomy and Vesicotomy

In a cutaneous ureterostomy, the surgeon detaches one or both ureters from the bladder and brings them to the surface of the body, usually in the region of the flank. The patient may have one or two stomas.

A vesicotomy is an incision into the bladder just above the pubic area. After incising the bladder, the surgeon moves it forward and sutures the cut edges to the skin, forming a stoma.

Ileal Reservoir (Kock's Pouch)

The surgeon creates an internal pouch, with nipple valves at the entrance and exit, from a portion of ileum (small intestine). The ureters are implanted in the proximal nipple valve, which helps prevent reflux of urine back to the kidney. The distal nipple valve is brought flush to the skin on the right side of the abdomen, forming a stoma. The patient is continent of urine, needing to catheterize the pouch several times a day to empty the urine. An adhesive bandage or gauze pad over the stoma will absorb the mucus it secretes. One daily irrigation of the pouch is performed to empty it of the mucus that has collected there.

POSTOPERATIVE NURSING CARE

Assessment

The postsurgical goals for the patient with a new ostomy include promoting healing, preventing complications, maintaining bowel function, maintaining adequate nutrition, and promoting comfort. The nurse assesses the incision for infection or separation and watches for hemorrhage. Nasogastric and wound drainage are monitored for characteristics and amount. Because paralytic ileus is a potential postoperative problem, bowel sounds are auscultated, and the patient is questioned about the passage of flatus, which usually occurs on about the third postoperative day. The IV site, fluids, and electrolyte levels are monitored very carefully, as the patient is especially prone to fluid and electrolyte imbalances.

Observation of the Stoma

The stoma is inspected for a normal pink or red color, which indicates adequate blood supply. It should look like healthy mucous membrane such as that inside the mouth. Later, the stoma will shrink in size and may be less highly colored. There may be slight bleeding around the stoma and its stem, but any more bleeding than this should be reported. Fortunately, most collection devices are transparent so that checking for color and bleeding does not require removal of the appliance. The skin around the stoma is assessed for irritation or signs of breakdown.

A noticeable lightening or blanching of color in the stoma may indicate inadequate blood flow through the tissues of the stoma itself. A deepening of color to a purplish hue may indicate obstruction to the flow of blood to the stoma.

Prolapse of the stoma is a common occurrence that may result from an opening that is too large or from inadequate securing of the stoma to the abdominal wall. An increase in pressure within the abdominal cavity causes a segment of intestine to protrude several inches beyond its usual position. Sneezing, coughing, and vigorous peristalsis are contributing factors in the occurrence of prolapse. It is most likely to occur in a loop colostomy. If the nurse determines that prolapse has occurred, a note is made on the patient's chart, and the patient is observed for signs of obstruction to the flow of fecal material. The surgeon or enterostomal therapist may be able to gently manipulate the intestine back into place.

Stenosis of the stoma caused by the formation of scar tissue at the point at which the segment of intestine passes through the abdominal wall is a more common complication. If the stenosis is not relieved, obstruction occurs, prohibiting drainage. If stenosis is present, the nurse notes it on the chart and observes for obstruction. Treatment consists of dilation of the stoma by the surgeon.

The stoma is also observed for signs of edema. However, in the early postoperative period, the stoma will be slightly edematous and larger than it will be after complete healing has taken place. Stoma edema can be caused by application of a collection device that has an opening too narrow to accommodate the stoma.

The opening of the collection device should be at least 1/8 inch larger than the circumference of the stoma.

Fecal output from the colostomy stoma does not occur for 7 to 10 days, as the patient is NPO for several days after surgery. IV lines are checked for patency and problems at the cannula site. The patient's fluid status and weight are assessed. Urinary output is assessed. Vital signs are monitored for changes that might indicate beginning shock or, later, signs of infection. Pain assessment is ongoing, and the nurse should be certain to reassess the patient after administering pain medication for effectiveness of analgesia.

If there is a perineal wound, the appearance, amount, and character of drainage are assessed and charted. Careful inspection for signs of infection is done. Such a wound may be left open to heal by secondary intention, in which case it may be 3 months before it is completely healed. A few days of antibiotic therapy is usually given postoperatively to prevent infection.

Additional assessment for the patient with a stoma for urinary diversion includes assessing the amount and characteristics of the urine and mucus it is expelling, and recording accurate output of urine every hour for the first 24 hours and then every 4 to 8 hours. An obstruction to the flow of urine through a ureter causes a backflow of urine into the renal pelvis and eventually a hydronephrosis. If the patient has had a cutaneous ureterostomy with two stomas (one from each ureter), the flow of urine from each stoma must be measured. Any tubing leading from the ureterostomy should be kept open so that urine can flow freely. The tube is checked frequently for signs of obstruction by mucus or blood clots.

Threads of mucus in the urine are to be expected; these are secreted by the mucous membrane of the ileal or colonic segment of the conduit. Whitish crystals or encrustations in or near the stoma indicate an alkaline urine; this should be reported so that treatment can be prescribed to prevent stone formation.

Psychosocial assessment postoperatively focuses on the patient's perception of his altered body image, the meaning of the altered body part, his usual and current coping skills, emotional state, support systems, presurgery lifestyle, and his perception of physical prognosis and its impact on his life.

NURSING DIAGNOSES

Nursing diagnoses appropriate for the patient with an ostomy include the following:

- Bowel incontinence related to loss of portion of colon and anal sphincter.
- Urinary incontinence related to loss of bladder and sphincter muscle.
- Self-care deficit related to surgical pain and knowledge deficit.
- Potential for fluid balance deficit related to excessive water loss through ileostomy.
- Potential impaired skin integrity related to irritation from wastes expelled from ostomy.
- Potential for dysfunctional grieving over loss of normal bowel elimination and altered body image.
- Disturbance in self-esteem related to alteration in intestinal elimination.
- Knowledge deficit related to self-care and care of stoma.
- Potential alteration in patterns of sexuality related to perception of alteration in body image.
- Potential alteration in role performance related to malignancy and therapy and inability to work.

NURSING INTERVENTION

The patient who has undergone surgical creation of an external ostomy will require basic postoperative care as for any patient who has had abdominal surgery. In addition, he will need specific attention to the stoma, the surrounding skin, and the appliance used for collection of wastes discharged through the stoma. The nurse's attitude toward the patient, his stoma, and his care has a major impact on the attitude the patient develops about his new body image and his own self-care. Disposing of body waste is not a pleasant nursing task, but response to the sight and smells can be controlled. A matter-of-fact, efficient approach to caring for the stoma, effluent, and drainage device is best. Nursing Care Plan 25–1 is a sample care plan for a patient with an ostomy.

A surgical dressing is never placed over an ileal stoma. If there is a significant decrease in ileal output accompanied by stomach cramping, the ileum may be obstructed. Such symptoms should be reported to the surgeon immediately. If the condition is not relieved, perforation or rupture of the intestine eventually may occur.

NURSING CARE PLAN 25–1

Selected nursing diagnoses, goals/outcome criteria, nursing interventions, and evaluations for a patient with an ostomy

Situation: A 22-year-old female patient has a long history of ulcerative colitis that has not responded to conservative therapy. A permanent ileostomy was performed 5 days ago.

Nursing Diagnosis	Goals/Outcome Criteria	Nursing Intervention	Evaluation
Potential for alteration in fluid and electrolyte balance; deficit related to loss of fluid and electrolytes via ileostomy. SUPPORTING DATA New ileostomy; recovering from surgery; beginning solid foods.	Fluid and electrolyte balance will be maintained as evidenced by sodium and potassium levels within normal range and normal skin turgor, stable weight, and balanced intake and output.	Monitor for signs of fluid volume deficit; weigh daily; check electrolyte values. Observe for signs of hypokalemia and hyponatremia. Accurately record intake and output and assess pattern. Instruct her to avoid foods that may cause diarrhea: whole milk, raw fruits, iced or hot fluids; administer antidiarrheal agents as ordered.	I, 2,800; O, 2,300; skin turgor normal; electrolytes within normal limits; weight stable; continue plan.
Potential for impaired skin integrity related to irritation of ileostomy drainage. SUPPORTING DATA Ileostomy drainage containing enzymes and bile salts; unfamiliarity with caring for ileostomy stoma and skin.	No evidence of skin irritation or breakdown at discharge. Skin integrity will be maintained.	Inspect skin with each appliance change; document status. Wash skin with mild soap and water; dry very thoroughly; apply skin barrier before applying appliance. Maintain an intact appliance. Treat beginning irritation immediately.	Stoma cherry red and moist; skin intact and without signs of irritation; continue plan.
Anxiety related to self-care of ostomy and impact on lifestyle. SUPPORTING DATA "I'm afraid it will smell." "I'm not sure I can handle this." "How will I work?" "Can I still exercise?"	Anxiety will be decreased by discharge as evidenced by expressed confidence in ability to handle problems of odor, appliance change, application of skin barrier, and work schedule. Within 6 months patient will have adjusted lifestyle and be able to participate in usual activities without problems.	Establish trusting relationship; allow her to verbalize concerns and fears freely. Answer questions honestly. Assist her to identify potential problems and ways to solve them. Encourage learning of self-care; give praise for efforts and accomplishments. Enlist aid of enterostomal therapist for suggestions of how to handle ileostomy during exercise class and at work. Obtain referral to local ostomy support group; have well-adjusted visitor establish contact and answer questions.	Enterostomal therapist in; watched appliance change and asked questions today; ostomate visitor scheduled for tomorrow; continue plan.
Knowledge deficit related to care of ileostomy and self-care. SUPPORTING DATA States she has never seen an ostomy stoma. Doesn't know anything about ostomy care; unaware of diet restrictions and precautions.	Patient will demonstrate ability to empty appliance, clean skin, apply skin barrier, and reattach a clean appliance by discharge. Patient will verbalize ways to prevent odor, protect skin, and prevent problems of fluid and electrolyte imbalance.	Encourage patient to look at stoma; utilize consistent teaching plan for care of stoma, appliance, and skin. Demonstrate care of ileostomy step by step; leave written instructions with patient. Have patient begin by doing one part of care and increasing the tasks each day. Instruct her in dietary precautions, signs and symptoms of fluid and electrolyte imbalance and what to do should they occur. Show various ways to prevent odor; instruct in foods to avoid because they cause offensive odor; have enterostomal therapist work with patient.	First teaching session on ostomy care; able to hold supplies and watch procedure; asked questions; taught dietary restrictions; will obtain feedback in 2 days; continue plan.
Self-esteem disturbance related to altered method of elimination.	Will begin acceptance of ileostomy before discharge as evidenced by looking	Assist her to list reasons the ileostomy was necessary; list the positive benefits of having the	Assisting with ostomy care; will see fellow ostomate tomorrow; continue plan.

NURSING CARE PLAN 25–1, *Continued*

Nursing Diagnosis	Goals/Outcome Criteria	Nursing Intervention	Evaluation
SUPPORTING DATA States she feels that she will not be attractive to any man now that she has an ileostomy.	at stoma, applying own appliance, and cleaning equipment. Within 6 months will be comfortable with new body image.	ileostomy vs. the way things were before the surgery. Encourage discussion of male-female relationships for ostomates with ostomy group visitor and enterostomal therapist. Assist her to look at positive strengths of the person she still is.	

Measurement of Intake and Output

Accurate recording of intake and output is especially important in the care of an ostomy patient. Total output of fecal material is calculated every 8 hours. If the stool is liquid, the accuracy of measurement is very important. When the patient's condition is stable, ostomy output is regular, and the patient's nutrition and hydration status are normal, intake and output recording is discontinued. It is necessary, however, to check occasionally to be sure that the flow of fecal matter has not been impeded. The stools from an ileostomy are mainly liquid, because they have not had time to have water reabsorbed before they are expelled; as a result, the *ileostomy patient must always be watched for signs of dehydration and fluid imbalance.* This is especially important during the immediate postoperative period but remains a concern as long as the patient has the ileostomy. In order to prevent dehydration, fluid intake should be sufficient to compensate for the loss of fluid through the feces.

Evacuation and Irrigation

Once the patient is eating again, ileostomy drainage is usually emptied every 2 or 3 hours. The patient sits on the toilet, unclamps the drainage device, and allows the effluent to drain into the bowl. The clamp is then closed, and the outside of the bag is cleansed of any debris. Ileostomies are not usually irrigated unless there is blockage by large particles of undigested food.

A continent ileostomy has a tube attached to suction in the immediate postoperative period to prevent distention and allow the pouch to heal. After 2 to 3 weeks, a catheter is inserted into the pouch to drain the contents. As the pouch matures and its capacity increases, the time between drainings will lengthen. The pouch is irrigated occasionally to remove fecal residue.

A sigmoid colostomy will usually drain formed stool on a relatively regular schedule. Irrigation of the colostomy gives the patient some control over when elimination takes place. The procedure is done daily or every other day at about the same time and takes close to an hour. A catheter with a cone tip is attached to a bag, which is filled with 500 to 1,000 mL of warm (not hot) tap water. The bag is positioned 18 to 20 inches above the height of the stoma. The colostomy appliance is removed and an irrigating sleeve attached to direct the drainage into the toilet. The cone tip is lubricated and inserted gently into the ostomy stoma, and the water is slowly infused to prevent cramping and distention. The cone tip is removed, and the drainage flows through the sleeve into the toilet. When drainage is complete, the sleeve is removed, skin care is performed, and a clean appliance is secured in place.

If the patient is fortunate enough to have a regular evacuation pattern, irrigation is not necessary.

The major reason for irrigating a colostomy is to establish a pattern of predictable bowel movements at the convenience of the colostomate.

If the patient prefers not to irrigate, suppositories can be used to stimulate evacuation. The patient does need to wear a drainable pouch if he does not irrigate, as evacuation can be unpredictable.

Urinary diversion procedures direct urine drainage immediately. The evacuation of the ostomy depends on which type of procedure was done. If a ureterosigmoidostomy was done, urine will be eliminated via the rectum. There is no external stoma or pouch. The Kock's pouch, or continent urinary conduit, is catheterized at intervals to drain the urine. With other procedures, such as an ileal conduit or Bricker's procedure, urine usually flows into the bag placed over the stoma at the time of surgery and will need to be emptied frequently. If there is considerable edema at the implantation site of the ureters, urine may not flow for 12 to 18 hours.

Periostomal Skin Care

The area of skin around the stoma must be kept clean and protected from fecal material seeping around the opening of the collection device and pooling on the skin. Drainage from an ileostomy contains enzymes and bile salts that are very damaging to the skin. In the immediate postoperative period, the pouch should not be changed any more than is necessary in order to avoid trauma to the skin.

The urostomy patient must be protected from pooling of urine on the skin. The flow of urine across the skin is not as much a cause for concern as are accumulations of stagnant urine.

The two major principles to follow for protection of the skin are cleanliness and provision of a protective barrier to prevent contact between the skin and the discharge from the stoma. If there is a proper seal to prevent seepage of either feces or urine around the stoma, irritation and breakdown of the skin occur much less frequently.

When the appliance is changed, it should be removed carefully and the skin washed gently with soap and water so that it is not damaged by vigorous rubbing and scrubbing. The area should be rinsed thoroughly and dried by patting, not rubbing, the skin. In humid weather, a hair dryer on the low setting may be used to dry the skin. A protective skin barrier paste, which serves to prevent contact between the skin and the waste being discharged through the stoma, is applied after cleansing. This may or may not be used for a sigmoid colostomy stoma.

Protective barriers are available in a number of forms and types. The enterostomal therapist or surgeon will indicate which type of barrier is most effective for the individual patient. Should the skin become highly irritated in spite of efforts to protect it, the physician will prescribe medications to be applied topically.

Causes of skin problems include removing the appliance too roughly or changing faceplates too frequently, an allergic reaction to a particular adhesive or other substance, and yeast infections, particularly around the stoma of a ureterostomy.

Changing the Collection Device

Appliances for the collection of wastes differ according to the type of surgery the patient has had and the specific purposes for which the appliance is designed. There are essentially two kinds of pouches or appliances: the temporary, or disposable, pouch and the permanent, or reusable, pouch. Both types are either drainable or closed-ended (Table 25–2). Drainable pouches are used when regulation of the flow of waste cannot be established and the contents (either urine or feces) must be emptied frequently throughout the day. Closed-end pouches are usually used only for security once bowel movements have been regulated.

The drainable pouches are designed with either wide openings at the bottom for draining fecal discharge or narrow openings to drain urine. In order to avoid the leakage of either urine or feces from around the stoma, a faceplate is attached to the upper end of the pouch. The faceplate is custom-made to fit around the stoma and accommodate the contours of the body.

If the patient does not have a continent ostomy or a colostomy that is irrigated regularly, it is necessary for him to use a drainable pouch at all times. The patient is taught to drain the pouch as necessary. As he adjusts to this new way of handling body waste, he learns the times of day when it is best to empty the pouch or to attach a new one if he is using the disposable type.

Open-ended pouches can be drained rather easily. All that is necessary to drain the pouch is for the patient to sit or stand over a toilet bowl, open the lower end of the pouch, and direct its contents into the bowl.

The manufacturers of appliances for the ostomate provide excellent instructional materials and have representatives who are anxious to be of help to the ostomate and the nurses who care for him. The names and addresses of several sources of information for the nurse and the ostomate are listed at the end of this chapter.

The choice of postoperative collection appliances depends on the individual needs of the patient. In the case of a patient with a loop colostomy, an appliance with an opening large enough to fit around the loop of the bowel should be on hand when the surgeon incises the bowel at the bedside. A patient with an external urinary diversion may already be wearing a collection device when he returns from the operating room. In any event, it is suggested that an enterostomal therapist be consulted on the type of appliance best suited to the patient's need.

At the time an appliance is changed, the used device is removed very gently, the skin is cleansed, the stoma is measured, and, if not done by the manufacturer, an appropriate-sized hole is cut in the faceplate that fits around the stoma. If the patient has a loop ostomy and the supporting device is still in place, the rod may be moved up and down to help position the faceplate securely, but it must *never* be twisted, as this can damage the bowel. The procedure for removal and application of an appliance for collection of discharge from a stoma should be stated in the hospital procedure manual for the nursing department. Before attempting to carry out this procedure, the nurse should seek instruction and guidance.

TABLE 25–2 **TEMPORARY AND PERMANENT POUCHES FOR THE OSTOMY PATIENT**

Type	Use	Basic Designs
Drainable	When regulation cannot be established and contents must be emptied frequently during the day.	Wide opening for draining fecal discharge.
	To collect continuous flow of urine.	Narrow opening for draining urine or liquid drainage. 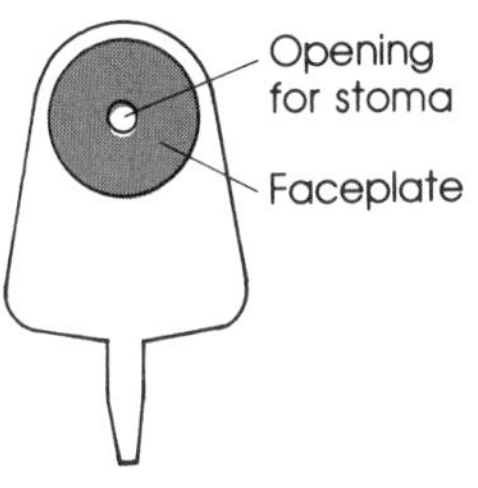
Closed-end	When bowel regulation has been established, either naturally or by irrigations. Usually used for security.	No opening (usually one piece). 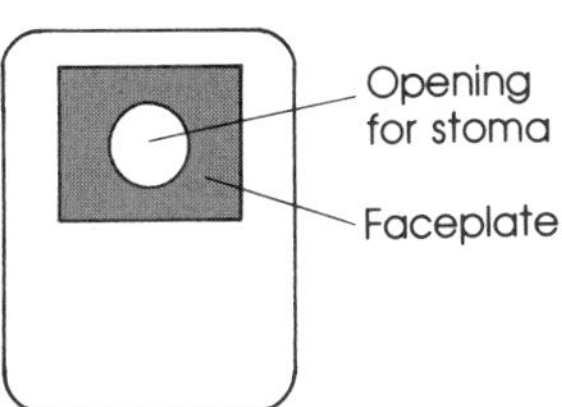

If the drainage device is not disposable, it will need to be cleaned with soap and water, rinsed very well, and allowed to dry.

Perineal Wound Care

When an abdominoperineal resection is performed along with the colostomy, the perineal wound requires considerable care to promote healing and repair. The wound may be packed with gauze, which will need to be changed regularly. To avoid stress on the operative site, the patient should be taught to avoid sitting on an air ring or commode seat. When sitting in a chair, he should be sure his buttocks are pressed together. The patient is taught how to take a sitz bath and administer perineal care for cleanliness as prescribed by the surgeon.

Psychosocial Concerns

The ostomy patient will go through the stages of grief and loss (see Chapter 14). The nurse provides active listening, emotional support, and understanding of the process. It is essential that a trusting nurse-patient relationship be established in order to assist the patient with his psychosocial concerns. Only then will the patient respond to encouragement to share feelings openly.

Social interaction with others is encouraged, and contact with available support groups should be initiated. As soon as postoperative pain is well controlled, it is best if the ostomate can talk with another who has fully adjusted to his ostomy and is living a full and active life. A series of visits is best in order to provide time for formulation and answering of questions. Such visits do require an order by the physician.

The ostomate should be treated warmly and acceptingly by the nurse. The patient should be guided to express his specific concerns about physical, sexual, and social problems he might encounter as a result of his ostomy. Most patients have concerns about odor, leakage, and noise from the passing of flatus. The nurse encourages joint exploration of necessary changes in lifestyle and suggests realistic alternatives.

The nurse should indicate to the patient that he might have some concerns about sexual function, thereby cueing him that it is acceptable to talk about this area of his life. Concerns should be addressed matter-of-factly, and his sexual partner should be included in discussions. The enterostomal therapist is a wonderful resource for specific information and suggestions in this area as well.

The nurse should encourage early participation in care, beginning with simple assistance by holding supplies or other small tasks not directly involved in stoma care. The transition is then made more easily to performing the direct care of the ostomy itself. If the patient is capable of caring for his own ostomy, family member participation and teaching are sometimes best left until later in the recovery process, after the patient has shown acceptance of his ostomy and responsibility for his self-care. Otherwise there may be too much reliance on care given by the spouse or other family member, and the patient may assume a more and more passive role. However, this depends on the personality and psychological status of the patient and the family dynamics.

When the patient continues with dysfunctional grieving too long, becomes clinically depressed, or cannot accept his altered body image, the nurse should seek referral for professional counseling for him. See Nursing Care Plan 25–1 for an example of an individualized care plan for an ostomy patient.

Patient Teaching

After teaching the patient about the physiology of his ostomy and the steps involved in physical care of the stoma and skin, the nurse teaches the patient how to control odor. Good basic hygiene is essential. Another measure used to control odor is to eliminate from the diet certain foods known to cause problems with odor or gas. Such foods include eggs, fish, garlic, raw onions, vegetables in the cabbage family, beans, and spicy foods. Eating too quickly and not chewing food well can cause gas.

Gas entering the pouch from the stoma will accumulate there until the pouch is opened and the gas released. This can be done by opening the lower end of the pouch and gently pressing against its sides to remove the gas. If not released, the gas may cause enough pressure to make the device separate from the stoma. Newer pouches have a filtered valve that allows gas to escape.

The major causes of odor problems in urinary diversion are improper techniques in cleaning and storing appliances, inadequate use of deodorant acidifiers, urinary tract infections, a poor-quality collection pouch that allows leakage, and poor basic hygiene. Dietary factors include asparagus, which causes a peculiar odor in the urine. Urine can be acidified by taking ascorbic acid (vitamin C) tablets four times a day. Another way in which urine may be acidified is by regulating the diet so that it is high in acid-ash foods and low in alkaline foods. The patient may also be instructed to drink cranberry juice daily, as this helps control odor. Some of the newer pouches have built-in odor control.

To help deodorize urine in the collecting bag, a few ounces of white vinegar can be instilled through the lower spout. This is most helpful during the night. There are also commercial deodorants available for ostomy bags.

Urinary tract infections are characterized by a foul odor, encrustation on the skin and drainage apparatus, and pus cells in the urine. The infection should be treated promptly to avoid other problems, as well as those of odor control.

Reusable pouches are washed with soap and water and rinsed with cool vinegar solution.

Dietary guidelines are also taught to prevent problems with diarrhea, constipation, and blockage. Blockage of the ileostomy is fairly common. The major offenders in the case of blockage are foods that absorb water—for example, dried fruits, corn (including popcorn), hard nuts, and those foods that are high in fiber. Particles from these foods are not small enough to pass through the ostomy stoma, thereby causing abdominal cramping, vomiting, and decreased flow from the ileostomy. Treatment for this condition consists of oral administration of enzymes to encourage digestion, gentle lavage, and massage of the abdomen to encourage passage of the obstructing food particles. As a last resort, surgical intervention may be necessary. *Laxatives are never given, as they will only add to the problem.*

Of course there is odor when the drainage pouch is changed or emptied, just as there is with normal urination or bowel movements.

Other pointers that ostomates are taught include the following:

- Ileostomy patients should not take time-release capsules and enteric-coated tablets, as there is not enough time for adequate absorption before the medication is expelled through the stoma.
- Suppositories may be inserted into a colostomy stoma. If it is a double-barreled colostomy, which stoma the suppository is placed into depends on the action of the drug. Glycerin suppositories for stimulation of evacuation are inserted in the proximal stoma; a drug that is to be absorbed from the intestine, as for relief of vomiting, should be inserted into the distal stoma, where it will not be expelled. Adequate intake of fluids is important for all ostomates to prevent dehydration and electrolyte imbalance.

Concerns for the Elderly

Adjustment to an ostomy by an older person depends on the degree to which the person can cope with his own physical and emotional changes. This depends partly on his previous coping style and personality and on the type of support he receives during the adjustment period. Fear of losing independence and curtailment of usual activities are major concerns. The nurse should keep the focus on the fact that the ostomy is done to improve the quality of the patient's life.

The elderly often have vision and hearing problems that need to be considered in teaching and in making self-care as easy as possible. Ostomy pouches that have precut openings are best, and the steps involved in pouch application should be kept to a minimum. Easy-to-read, printed instructions, together with well-labeled equipment, make the whole process of ostomy care smoother. When teaching, the nurse should make certain that the patient can hear her adequately; she should speak clearly and slowly and provide a quiet room for the session.

The decrease in sense of smell that occurs with aging sometimes makes it difficult for the elderly ostomy patient to detect leakage odor. Therefore the patient is taught to check visually for leakage several times a day.

Because the elderly patient's skin is extra fragile, great care must be taken in removing the appliance. Some type of skin barrier should be used at all times.

It is important to encourage high fluid intake, as the older patient often takes in little fluid and is consequently prone to constipation, which can predispose him to problems. A small glass of prune juice at night and a hot drink before irrigation of a colostomy can help regulate elimination.

For those patients who have severe arthritis or debilitating chronic diseases that make ostomy care very difficult, if not impossible, help from a family member or visiting nurse will have to be provided.

OSTOMATES AND THEIR CARE

Ostomates, with sufficient support and encouragement, do adjust to their stomas. Most realize that the surgery was necessary and will improve the quality of or prolong their lives, and they do whatever must be done to go on with their lives. Unless they have other physical limitations, ostomates are able to enjoy social activities, dress more or less as they please, enjoy all kinds of sports (including water sports), and pursue their careers.

There are more than 1 million ostomates in the United States and Canada. Most can manage their self-care and carry on busy, active lives with only minor inconveniences. For the person who has recently undergone an ostomy, a visit from a person who has adjusted to a stoma, when approved by the surgeon, can do much to facilitate the adjustment process.

During the early postoperative period, when care of the stoma and changing the appliance are the responsibility of the nurse, the patient probably will not be able to absorb very much information about stomal care. The nurse still should explain what she is doing and why she is doing it. Later, as the patient begins to participate in the technical aspects of stomal care, he should be given ample opportunity to ask questions. He should not be rushed into accepting total responsibility for his stomal care.

Before the ostomate is discharged from the hospital, he should be able to demonstrate an ability to carry out all procedures that are related to the technical care of his ostomy, or he should work closely at home with an enterostomal therapist. He must know about possible complications and to whom he should report early signs of trouble.

The long-range goals of an ostomy patient are healthy acceptance of the stoma and competence in performing the manual skills needed to take care of it.

AVAILABLE INFORMATION

There are many sources of information available to the ostomate. These include the local branches of the American Cancer Society, ostomate clubs, enterostomal therapists, and other members of the health care team who have expertise in the management of a stoma.

Information about local ostomate clubs and groups can be obtained from the United Ostomy Association, Inc., 36 Executive Park, Suite 120, Irvine, CA 92714.

A directory of enterostomal therapists to contact for local consultation can be obtained from the International Association for Enterostomal Therapy, 2081 Business Circle Dr., Suite 290, Irvine, CA 92715.

Teaching aids and printed material for patient education can be obtained without cost from the following sources:

- Convatech
  Division of Squibb Derm
  Product Plant Manager
  P.O. Box 4000,
  Princeton, NJ 08540
- Hollister, Inc.
  2000 Hollister Limited
  Libertyville, IL 60048
- Hollister Limited
  Dept. N82
  322 Consumens Rd.
  Willowdale, Ontario, Canada M2J IPA
- United Division of Howmedica
  Dept. N82
  11775 Starkey Rd.
  P.O. Box 1970
  Largo, FL 33540

BIBLIOGRAPHY

Alterescu, K. B.: Colostomy. Nurs. Clin. North Am., June, 1987, p. 281.

Broadwell, D. C.: Periostomal skin integrity. Nurs. Clin. North Am., June, 1987, p. 321.

Broadwell, D., and Jackson, B.: Principles of Ostomy Care. St. Louis, C. V. Mosby, 1982.

Erickson, P. J.: Ostomies: The art of pouching. Nurs. Clin. North Am., June, 1987, p. 311.

Kock, M. O.: Bladder substitution with intestine: Past and present. J. Urol. Nurs., Aug., 1989, p. 610.

Motta, G. J.: Life span changes: Implication for ostomy care. Nurs. Clin. North Am., June, 1987, p. 333.

Petillo, M. H.: The patient with a urinary stoma: Nursing management and patient education. Nurs. Clin. North Am., June, 1987, p. 253.

Rideout, B. W.: The patient with an ileostomy. Nurs. Clin. North Am., June, 1987, p. 253.

Shipes, E.: Psychosocial issues: The person with an ostomy. Nurs. Clin. North Am., June, 1987, p. 291.

Shipes, E.: Sexual function following ostomy surgery. Nurs. Clin. North Am., June, 1987, p. 303.

Shipes, E.: Nursing care of the patient with CUR: Continent urinary reservoir. J. Urol. Nurs., Aug., 1989, p. 595.

STUDENT STUDY AIDS

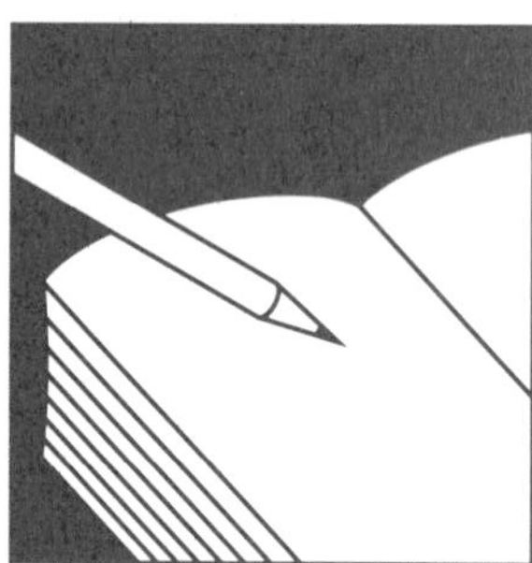

CLINICAL CASE PROBLEMS

Read each clinical case problem and discuss the questions with your classmates.

1. Mr. Jason is a 28-year-old victim of a gunshot wound of the abdomen who has had an emergency transverse double-barreled colostomy. The surgeon plans to repair the damaged intestine and reinstate the continuity of the colon after the wounds have healed sufficiently.

- Describe the care for Mr. Jason's stoma in the early postoperative period.
- What potential complications would you observe for following this type of surgery?
- What type of nursing interventions would you include in your plan of care for the psychological care of Mr. Jason?
- What precautions will be necessary for Mr. Jason when he undergoes barium radiographs next week?

---

2. Terry Santos is a 21-year-old male student who has had chronic ulcerative colitis since childhood. As a treatment for this condition, the surgeon has performed an ileostomy.

- Why would an ileostomy be done as treatment for ulcerative colitis? What type of ileostomy would be done?
- How might an ileostomy affect Terry's social life? How could it affect his future as a clothes designer?
- What specific types of knowledge and skills will your teaching plan need to include to help Terry learn to manage his own ileostomy? Include diet, care of stoma, and care of pouch.

3. Mr. Ivan is a 60-year-old farmer who has undergone a continent ileal conduit procedure (Kock's pouch) for treatment of cancer of the bladder.

- What is an ileal conduit? How does it work?
- How is the care for an ileal conduit different from that for a colostomy? How is it similar?
- What does Mr. Ivan need to know about his diet, fluid intake, and prevention of complications?

STUDY OUTLINE

I. Introduction

A. Ostomy: mouth or opening.
B. Stoma functions as new opening for discharge of waste.
C. Ostomy necessitated by trauma, disease, or congenital defects.
D. No reason why an ostomy should prevent one from leading an active life.

II. Enterostomal therapy

A. Certified enterostomal therapist (ET) specializes in care of ostomates.

III. Locations and types of stomas (see Table 25–1)

A. Colostomy location depends on whether stoma is from ascending, transverse, or sigmoid (descending) colon.
  1. The farther along the length of colon the stoma is made, the less liquid the stool.
  2. Easier to establish control of bowel movements from a sigmoid colostomy.

B. Types of surgical procedures:
  1. Loop: a loop of either intestine or ureter is brought to the outside through an incision.
    a. A support is used to keep loop from sliding back through the incision; removed after 7 to 10 days.
    b. Surgeon slits the intestine or ureter to create stoma.
  2. Double-barreled: two stomas.
    a. In a colostomy of this type, the proximal limb is closest to the small intestine; the distal limb leads from the rectum.
  3. Single-barreled or end: only one stoma on surface of the body.

C. Ileostomy: stoma from the ileum, completely bypasses the colon.
  1. Indications: ulcerative colitis, regional ileitis, and multiple polyposis.
  2. Site for stoma must be carefully selected.
  3. Continent or "pouch" ileostomy frees patient from need to wear external pouch; some patients are not good candidates for this procedure.

D. Urinary diversion.
  1. Indicated by malignancy of bladder, congenital defects, trauma, and neurogenic bladder.
  2. Locations include ileal conduit (stoma or abdomen) and cutaneous ureterostomy (stomas over flanks in kidney region).

IV. Postoperative nursing care

A. Assessment.
  1. Goals include the following:
    a. Promote healing.
    b. Prevent complications.
    c. Maintain bowel function.
    d. Maintain adequate nutrition.
    e. Promote comfort.

2. Observation of the stoma.
   a. Color should be similar to that of mucous membrane inside the mouth.
   b. Will eventually become smaller as it heals.
   c. Check for excessive bleeding.
   d. Watch for increase or decrease in output from stoma.
   e. Prolapse is not necessarily an emergency.
   f. Stenosis is treated by progressive dilatation or surgery.
   g. Edema is usually caused by too narrow an opening on the collection device.
3. Accurate intake and output; monitor for dehydration and electrolyte imbalance.
4. Perineal wound, if present, is assessed.
5. Urinary stoma is assessed for output and condition.
6. Threads of mucus are expected; assess for infection.
7. Psychosocial assessment focuses on patient's perception of altered body image and self-esteem.
8. There are many possible appropriate nursing diagnoses for the patient with an ostomy.

B. Nursing intervention.
1. Postoperative care is essentially the same as for any abdominal surgery patient.
2. Nurse's attitude strongly influences patient's acceptance of stoma.
3. Measurement of intake and output especially important for ostomy patient.
   a. Includes flow of urine as well as feces.
   b. Obstruction can be very dangerous.
   c. Ileostomy patient must always guard against fluid and electrolyte imbalance.
4. Evacuation and irrigation.
   a. Ileostomy drainage is emptied every 2 to 3 hours.
   b. Continent ileostomy is allowed time to heal.
   c. Sigmoid colostomy drains formed stool on a fairly regular schedule.
   d. Irrigation of the colostomy allows control over elimination.
   e. Irrigation is done with bag of 500 to 1,000 mL warm tap water and a cone-tipped catheter.
   f. Suppositories can be used to stimulate evacuation instead of irrigation.
   g. Urine drainage is immediate when urinary diversion procedures are performed.
   h. Continent urinary conduit is catheterized to drain the urine.
5. Periostomal skin care: cleanliness is very important.
   a. Cleanse skin and use protective barrier.
   b. Remove appliance gently.
   c. Possible causes of skin problems are changing the faceplate too frequently, allergic reaction, yeast infections.
6. Changing collection device.
   a. Change faceplate only as often as necessary.
   b. Measure stoma to be sure opening is correct size.
   c. There are disposable and nondisposable types of collection devices.
   d. Reusable devices must be cleansed thoroughly and dried.
   e. Pouches are designed so that drainage can be removed without disturbing the faceplate.

7. Perineal wound care.
   a. Gauze packing is changed regularly.
   b. Prophylactic antibiotics are given to prevent infection.
8. Psychosocial concerns.
   a. Patient will go through stages of grief and loss.
   b. Contact with ostomy support group is desirable.
   c. Encourage verbalization of questions and concerns.
   d. Enterostomal therapist is an excellent resource.
   e. Encourage self-care by slowly increasing participation in care of stoma and collection device.
   f. If clinical depression occurs, refer for counseling.
9. Concerns for the elderly.
   a. Simplify steps in care and provide easy-to-read printed instructions.
   b. Focus on improving the quality of life and ways to remain independent.

C. Patient teaching.
   1. Physiology and care of ostomy.
   2. Odor and gas control.
   3. Dietary guidelines.
   4. Helpful suggestions for ostomates.
   5. Sources of information and support.

CHAPTER 26

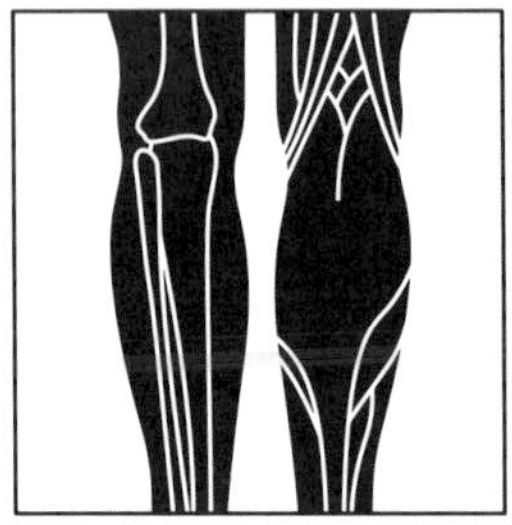

Care of Patients With Disorders of the Musculoskeletal System

VOCABULARY

abduction
adduction
ankylosis
arthroplasty
callus
comminuted
contracture
dislocation
extension
flexion
goniometry
greenstick
intraarticular
isometric
lupus erythematosus
maceration
obliterate
orthopedics
ossification
polyarteritis
prosthesis
sprain
strain
subluxation
synovectomy
tophi
temporomandibular
torsion

Upon completion of this chapter the student should be able to:

1. Devise a teaching plan for the following diagnostic tests: bone scan, arthroscopy, electromyography.
2. Describe the steps included in a nursing assessment of the musculoskeletal system.
3. Describe the steps used in transferring a patient from the bed to a chair.
4. List the steps utilized when moving a patient from a stretcher to the bed.
5. Describe factors to be assessed for the patient who has a cast.
6. Identify the "do's" and "don'ts" of cast care.
7. Describe nursing assessment and intervention for the patient in traction.
8. Identify important postoperative observations and nursing interventions in the care of the patient who has undergone an amputation.
9. Identify the special problems of patients with arthritis and specific nursing interventions that can be helpful.
10. Discuss the preoperative and postoperative care of a patient with a total joint replacement.
11. Demonstrate proper placement of a patient who has had a hip replacement in the lateral and supine positions.
12. Demonstrate range of motion for each joint.

The special branch of medical science concerned with the preservation and restoration of the functions of the skeletal system is called *orthopedics*. We cannot confine a discussion of orthopedic nursing to patients with diseases and deformities of bones and joints, however, because the basic principles of orthopedic nursing are applicable to the nursing care of all patients, and most especially to those with limited mobility.

> ***The three main functions of the musculoskeletal system are* motion, support, *and* protection. *Of these, the preservation of motion is probably the most important consideration as far as prevention of orthopedic disabilities resulting from inactivity is concerned.***

It is the long bones of the limbs that give the body support and provide motion by acting as levers to which the muscles are attached (Fig. 26–1). Joint motion is a result of the shortening and stretching of opposing sets of muscles. For example, when the flexor muscles of the leg contract and shorten, the opposing extensors must relax and lengthen. Disuse or undue strain on these muscles can lead to permanent disabilities and loss of motion.

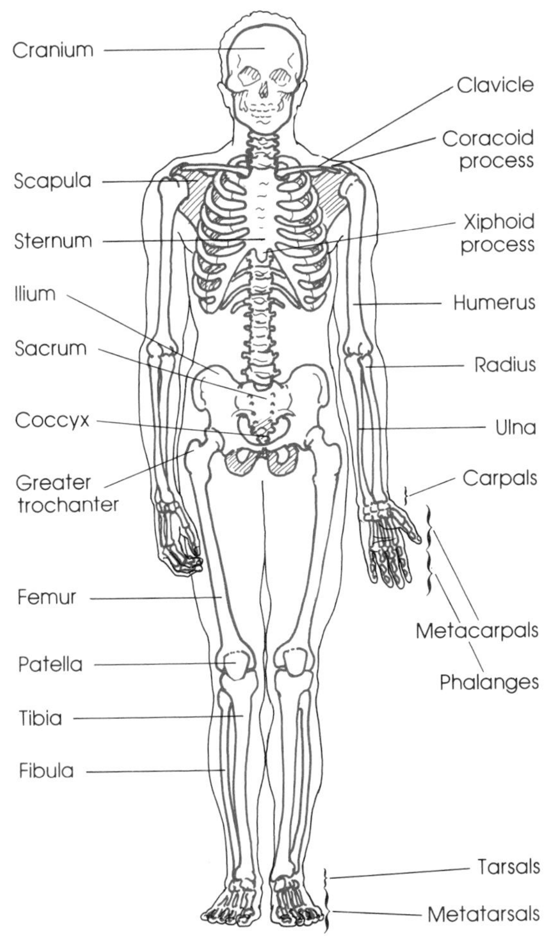

Figure 26–1 Skeletal system.

If we follow the development of bones within a person from conception to old age, we can see that the bony tissues of the infant differ greatly from those of the adult. That is because bone cells do not all follow the same pattern of development from the embryonic stage to full maturity. *There are two distinct groups of bone cells.* The cells in the first group are designed so that they are immediately transformed into mature cells. The normal infant will have this type of firm bone cells in his skull and shoulder bones. In the second group, the bone cells form cartilage first and then are gradually replaced by mature bone cells as the person grows older. Thus most of the bones of an infant are really mainly cartilage. *Ossification*, or replacement of cartilage by more solid bony tissue, is not completed throughout the body until 20 to 25 years of age.

Because the bony structures of infants and young children are softer and more pliable than those of adults, there is less danger of breaking bones during the time of life when they are learning to walk and run and are therefore more likely to have frequent falls. If a fracture does occur, however, it will heal more rapidly in a very young person, because growth is still taking place within the bone.

On the other hand, the bones of elderly people are brittle and less compact; thus they break easily. In addition, they do not heal readily when a fracture is sustained, because the physiologic exchange of minerals has decreased with advancing age, making the process of repair much slower.

In studying the process of bone development and repair, it must be remembered that *bone is a living tissue*, with a complex system of canals through which blood and lymph vessels pass. This system allows for the adequate transportation of nutrients to the bone cells and for the removal of wastes. Certain minerals that are essential to the normal functioning of bones are continually being deposited, stored, and removed from the bony tissues.

Muscles constitute one third to one half of the body's entire bulk. In this chapter, we are concerned only with the skeletal muscles that are instrumental in moving the various parts of the body. Involuntary muscles and cardiac muscle tissues are discussed in appropriate chapters.

DIAGNOSTIC TESTS AND PROCEDURES AND NURSING IMPLICATIONS

Specific diagnostic tests of the musculoskeletal system are listed in Table 26–1. Blood counts,

TABLE 26–1 DIAGNOSTIC TESTS FOR MUSCULOSKELETAL PROBLEMS

Test	Purpose	Description	Nursing Implications
Radiographs of the bones or joints	Detect fracture, avulsion, joint damage.	No preparation necessary. Part to be radiographed is positioned by technician and radiographs are taken.	Explain the purpose, procedure, and possible sensations.
Bone scan	Detects tumor, metastatic growths, bone injury, or degenerative bone disease. Can detect problems earlier than can radiographs.	An IV injection or oral dose of a radioisotope is given, and after an interval time for the substance to be taken up by the bone, the area is scanned by scintillation camera.	Explain the purpose and procedure. Check for allergies and pregnancy. Patient will be asked to lie quietly for 30 to 60 minutes during the scanning. All metal should be removed from the area to be scanned. Explain that the dose of radiation he will receive is lower than usual with radiographs. Assure him he will not be "radioactive." The isotope is eliminated from the body in 6 to 24 hours.
Arthroscopy	Inspects the interior aspect of a joint, usually a knee, with a fiberoptic endoscope to diagnose problems of the patella, meniscus, and synovium. Also used to evaluate the progress of arthritis or effectiveness of treatment.	After injection of local anesthesia, an incision is made, and the arthroscope is introduced into the interior of the joint; instruments for tissue biopsy or surgical procedures may be passed through the arthroscope.	Explain the purpose and procedure. A preprocedure sedative may be administered. When the patient has recovered from any sedation he is allowed to walk but should not overuse or strain the joint for a few days. The area is observed for bleeding or swelling; ice packs may be used in the immediate postprocedure period, especially if biopsy or surgery was performed. Assessment for swelling, circulation, and sensation is done periodically to detect any complications.
Arthrocentesis	Performed to extract synovial fluid for analysis or to reduce swelling.	A needle is inserted into the joint space, and synovial fluid is aspirated. Synovial fluid analysis may detect cells indicating infection, inflammation, rheumatoid arthritis, or lupus erythematosus. Corticosteroid may be injected after aspiration of fluid. If a large amount of fluid is aspirated, the joint is immobilized with an elastic bandage. Ice packs are applied to relieve pain and reduce swelling.	Explain the procedure. Have ice packs ready to apply afterward. Wrap with elastic bandage if ordered and show patient how to do this. It should be worn for 2 to 3 days. Instruct him not to overuse the joint until pain and swelling have subsided. Administer ordered analgesics if needed after corticosterioid injection, as this can be quite painful.

TABLE 26–1 **DIAGNOSTIC TESTS FOR MUSCULOSKELETAL PROBLEMS** *Continued*

Test	Purpose	Description	Nursing Implications
Biopsy	Bone biopsy done to detect tumor cells. Muscle biopsy done to obtain tissue for cellular analysis, which is helpful in differential diagnosis of several muscle disorders	Under local anesthesia, a piece of bone or muscle is excised and sent for pathologic analysis.	Offer emotional support during the procedure. Afterward, medicate for discomfort as needed, apply ice packs to decrease swelling, observe for bleeding; perform circulation and sensation checks distal to the area biopsied.
Culture of synovial fluid	Determine organism responsible for infection.	Explain purpose and procedure. See that specimen of fluid is transported to laboratory immediately.	Synovial fluid is aspirated and sent for culture and sensitivity to determine appropriate antibiotic for therapy. Results take 48 to 72 hours.
Electromyelography (EMG)	Detects abnormal nerve transmission to the muscle and abnormal muscle function. Determines rehabilitation progress.	Needle electrodes are inserted in affected muscles, and as the muscles are stimulated, the electrical impulses generated by the muscle contractions are amplified and displayed on an oscilloscope; tracings are also made on graph paper.	Obtain a signed consent form. Caffeine-containing drinks and smoking are restricted 3 hours prior to the test. Muscle relaxants, anticholinergics, and cholinergic drugs should be withheld prior to the test; check with the physician. Explain that there may be slight discomfort when the electrodes are inserted. Explain that he will be asked to relax and contract the muscles. The test usually takes about an hour. If serum enzyme tests are ordered, draw the blood before the EMG.
Uric acid	Detects abnormally high levels of uric acid in the blood, which is a sign of gout.	Requires 5 to 10 mL of blood in a clot (red-top) tube. Normal range: female: 2.8–6.8 mg/dL; male: 3.5–7.8 mg/dl.	No food or fluid restrictions.
Rheumatoid factor	Detects antibodies, indicating possible rheumatoid arthritis, lupus, or scleroderma.	Requires 5 to 10 mL of blood in a clot (red-top) tube. Normal range: adult: <1:120 titer; >1:80 indicates rheumatoid arthritis.	No food or fluid restrictions.
Antinuclear antibodies (ANA)	Assesses tissue antigen antibodies; useful for diagnosis of rheumatoid arthritis, lupus erythematosus, and other connective tissue disorders.	No food or fluid restrictions. Check drugs patient is receiving for interference with this test. Normal finding: negative.	Requires 2 to 5 mL of blood in a clot (red-top) tube.

blood cultures, and various tests for problems of the immune system may also be performed to detect rheumatoid arthritis, lupus erythematosus, or other connective tissue diseases. These tests include an erythrocyte sedimentation rate (ESR), serum protein electrophoresis, and tests to determine the levels of serum complement and immunoglobulins. Magnetic resonance imaging can also be done to detect tumor or joint problems and provides excellent data, but it is a very expensive procedure.

Range-of-motion testing involves both active and passive maneuvers. In active testing, the part being measured must be moved by the patient himself. In passive testing, the evaluator moves the body part while the patient is relaxed.

The measurement of range of motion in a joint is called *goniometry*. One system of measurement that is commonly used is based on a full circle of 360 degrees. Each joint is evaluated in terms of the number of degrees it can be moved from the zero-degree position.

Muscle strength can be measured on the basis of the ability of a muscle to move the part to which it is attached, working against the force of gravity. A grading system is used, ranging from grade 5 (normal strength) to grade 0 (complete paralysis).

Other techniques used to evaluate musculoskeletal function include inspection, palpation, and tests for stability of a joint under stress.

NURSING ASSESSMENT OF MUSCULOSKELETAL FUNCTION

HISTORY TAKING

When reviewing the patient's past history the nurse should keep in mind the significance of disorders that primarily affect other systems but secondarily affect the bones and muscles. For example, diabetes mellitus can predispose a patient to degenerative joint disease; sickle cell disease and hemophilia can cause bleeding into the joints and muscles, and psoriasis is sometimes the first sign of psoriatic arthritis. Nutritional deficiencies can affect the mineral composition of bone and muscle, making them more susceptible to trauma and loss of function.

Family history also can be significant, as there are some bone and muscle disorders that either are inherited or have a familial tendency. For example, muscular dystrophy is inherited, gout is believed to be inherited, and about 30% of those who have psoriatic arthritis have a family history of psoriasis.

OBSERVATIONS

When gathering information about the patient's present illness or injury, the nurse will need to know whether there is pain, where it is, what seems to make it worse, and what provides relief. She will ask about and observe the patient for signs of joint stiffness, when it is most apparent, and whether it is always present or has a tendency to come and go. In some types of arthritis, pain and stiffness migrate from one joint to another or tend to be worse at certain times of the day, as in morning stiffness in rheumatoid arthritis.

The nurse also will observe her patient for signs of deformity and whether he uses any support equipment such as a cane, elastic bandage, or crutch. She also will look for signs of inflammatory changes and infection, such as fever, malaise, redness, swelling, and limited motion.

Pressure from swelling or deformity can injure adjacent nerve endings and produce sensory changes and loss of feeling. In her assessment the nurse will need to ask whether the patient has experienced any sensory changes, when they were first noticed, and what they feel like to the patient.

If the patient is admitted with a fracture, obtain a history of the precipitating event so that an assessment can be made of other areas that may have been injured.

An assessment of the patient's ability to perform activities of daily living (ADL) should also be made. Does he have any difficulty with eating, bathing, dressing, grooming, toileting, ambulation, or social interaction? A self-care deficit is one of the primary problems for patients who are immobilized.

NURSING INTERVENTION

LIFTING AND TURNING THE PATIENT

Special skills are necessary for the proper care of a patient with musculoskeletal disorders, particularly in regard to moving the patient and changing his linens.

First, the nurse must use good body mechanics herself so that she can safely and correctly use her strength to the greatest advantage. An awkward posture or failure to use the correct methods of lifting and moving the patient will often cause him unnecessary discomfort and apprehension about being moved and will also lead to painful muscle strain for the nurse.

Secondly, all movements must be *gentle* and *firm*. When moving or turning the patient, the nurse should have sufficient help from adequately trained personnel. Each person involved, including the patient, should understand exactly what is going to be done and the steps to be taken in accomplishing the move. If the patient can help without damaging the diseased joint or limb, he should be encouraged to do so. If he is not able to help, the nurse explains the procedure to him and asks him to cooperate by relaxing completely during the procedure.

Many times the patient is afraid that moving and turning will cause him pain. It is then necessary to help him understand the reasons for the frequent changing of position and to gain his confidence and cooperation so that he will not make the task more difficult by resisting all efforts to turn him.

Nurses are sometimes tempted to allow their patient the privilege of assuming any position and remaining in that position as long as he appears comfortable. They believe it is unkind and unnecessary to force the patient to move about when he is apparently resting and does not wish to be disturbed. This is actually not a kindness and could be considered as nothing short of neglect when we know the terrible consequences or poor body posture and inactivity. Unfortunately, the position preferred by the patient often is the very one most likely to cause permanent disability if it is maintained for long periods of time.

The nurse might also take the time to find a reason for the patient's assuming certain postures in bed. It is possible that the patient is curled up in a fetal position because he is trying to keep warm. Older patients and those with poor circulation instinctively huddle their shoulders and tuck their limbs close to their bodies when they are chilly. It is also possible that the patient is flexing his knees, hips, and back because he is attempting to relieve pain in his abdomen or lower legs.

ORTHOPEDIC BED MAKING

When traction is being applied to a patient's lower limb, or when he is in a large body cast, it is not always convenient to arrange the bed linens in the conventional manner. Some institutions in which there are large orthopedic units provide specially made linens designed so that bed making and changing of linen are much easier for the nurse and less disturbing to the orthopedically handicapped patient. If there is such linen available, the inexperienced nurse should seek specific instructions in its use.

In institutions where there is no such linen available, the nurse must improvise with the materials she has at hand. This requires some ingenuity and imagination, but it can be done. For example, two draw sheets may be used for the foundation of the bed in lieu of one large bottom sheet. This would be useful in instances in which the patient's lower limb is in a traction apparatus that uses a frame resting on the mattress, rather than one that hangs from an overhead frame. Obviously, there will be a good bit of disturbance of the frame and the traction if the large bottom sheet must be changed each time it becomes soiled. When two draw sheets are used, however, only the draw sheet under the patient's body need be changed, and the frame will not be disturbed at all. When changing the bottom sheet for the patient in traction, the nurse begins on the side opposite the traction. For example, if traction is on the left leg, she works from right to left and from the foot of the bed toward the head. Top covers may be folded so that the limb in traction is not covered. If extra warmth is needed for the affected limb, it can be covered with a small baby blanket.

One important point to remember in changing the linen is to avoid pulling sheets from under the patient and causing friction against the skin.

It is imperative that the skin of the patient confined to bed for a long time be preserved. He must be gently turned on and off the sheets being changed; sheets are never pulled from under him.

PREVENTION OF DISABILITY

The formation of contractures, loss of muscle tone, and fixation of joints can be prevented in most cases by aggressive and consistent nursing intervention. The major components of the intervention are gradual mobilization, an exercise program, proper positioning, and instruction of the patient and family.

Whenever a patient is immobilized for whatever reason, the time to begin a plan of nursing intervention is immediately after the person is immobilized. It is the responsibility of the nursing staff to initiate the necessary measures and to carry them out consistently. To wait for a physician's order for care that is within the domain of nursing is tantamount to negligence on the part of the nursing staff.

Pathologic Changes

Within a matter of a few days the structures of immobilized muscles and joints begin to undergo changes. If no effort is made to prevent these changes the patient will become permanently disabled. The pathologic changes most commonly associated with lack of motion include (1) contractures, (2) loss of muscle tone, and (3) ankylosis.

Contractures

When skeletal muscles are not regularly stretched and contracted to their normal limits, they attempt to adapt themselves to this limited use by becoming shorter and less elastic. This "adaptive shortening" is called contracture. Contracture formation begins within 3 to 7 days after immobilization of a part, and the process usually is completed in 6 to 8 weeks. This means that there is no time to lose in planning and implementing nursing measures to prevent permanent and crippling disability. The most frequent contractures occurring in patients immobilized for long periods of time are "foot drop," knee and hip flexion contractures, "wrist drop," and contractures of the fingers and arms (Fig. 26–2).

Loss of Muscle Tone

Joint motion is the result of a shortening and stretching of opposing muscles. For example, when the flexor muscles of the leg contract and shorten, the opposing extensor muscles relax and tighten.

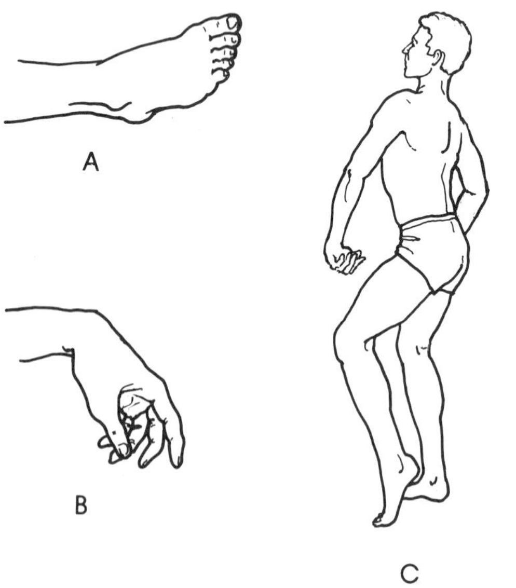

Figure 26–2 *A,* Foot drop resulting from improper support of the feet while patient is confined to bed. A simple footboard could easily prevent this deformity. *B,* Wrist drop resulting from improper support of the hand. *C,* Flexion contracture of knee and hip force this patient to walk on tiptoe on the affected side. If both legs are involved, walking is impossible.

Muscle tone is defined as the readiness of the muscle to go to work—to contract and relax as needed. If a muscle is not regularly stimulated to action or if it is stretched beyond its normal limits for an extended period of time, it will lose its ability to contract and relax. For example, in foot drop, the calf muscles are shortened while the opposing flexor muscles are stretched. The result is loss of muscle tone and inability to produce motion.

Ankylosis

This is permanent fixation of a joint. It is the result of injury or disease in which the tissues of the joint are replaced by a bony overgrowth that completely obliterates the joint. Sometimes it is extremely difficult to prevent this process (as, for example, in some types of arthritis). In these cases the physician may brace the joint in the position that will be most useful to the patient, even though there is no motion in the joint.

To illustrate the importance of properly positioning joints in what are called *positions of optimum use or maximum function,* imagine your wrist locked in a position in which the palm and fingers are at right angles to the lower arm. Try to pick up an object such as a hair brush and bring it to your head. Now imagine that your wrist is slightly flexed and locked in that position. Try to perform the same maneuver as before. If you had your choice of positions, you would choose the one in which your wrist was either straight or slightly flexed, because this would allow you to perform many of your daily activities.

Gradual Mobilization

The first step in nursing intervention to accomplish goals of progressive mobilization is assessment of the patient's ability to move his limbs, turn himself in bed, transfer himself from bed to chair and back again, and stand and walk. These measurable signs of independent movement can represent various stages to which it is hoped the patient will gradually progress.

Setting goals for progressive mobilization must take into account the pathologic condition causing immobility, any contraindications to movement of a body part, and the ability of the patient to understand and take part in carrying out the rehabilitation activities. In some cases passive exercises and positioning may be necessary until the patient is able to carry out exercises and positioning on his own. If the patient is to be cared for by family members once he returns home, it is essential that they may be included in planning and goals of intervention to prevent disability and promote mobilization.

Exercise

Range-of-motion (ROM) exercises, both passive and active, are planned and carried out as soon as feasible after immobilization occurs as a result of disease, injury, or surgery. The exercises are done to maintain functional connective tissue within the joint and thereby ensure that every joint retains its function and mobility. ROM exercises should be done three to four times a day. Other kinds of exercises are planned according to each patient's needs and the amount of motion allowed by the physician.

A sample of exercise programs in which a variety of exercises are used and the rationale for each type of exercise is shown in Table 26–2. *Isometric* exercises involve generating tension between two opposing sets of muscles. For example, trying to flex the lower arm while at the same time using the opposite hand to try to extend it. *Muscle setting* involves contracting a set of muscles such as the gluteal muscles and holding the contraction tightly for a count of eight and then completely relaxing the muscles for a count of two.

Patients suffering from intense joint pain as a result of rheumatoid arthritis will need proper timing of exercises to follow administration of analgesic and antiinflammatory drugs. If at all possible, the schedule for drug administration should be adjusted so that the patient receives his first dose of medication in the morning *before* he begins his daily activities.

Sometimes after joint surgery, especially after a total knee replacement, the surgeon will attach an apparatus to the affected limb that provides continuous passive motion within the limits desired. The apparatus is driven by a motor and requires no effort on the part of the patient or nurse to move the limb. It usually is left on all day and is discontinued at night while the patient sleeps. When this kind of apparatus is used, the nursing care plan should include specific instructions regarding its proper use. Figure 26–3 shows how the apparatus is connected to the patient. Bed supports are mounted on the side of the affected limb. The patient's foot is secured in a running shoe, which is attached to the foot support with a Velcro strap. The foot support moves back and forth along a track, thus providing motion of the knee and hip joints.

TABLE 26–2 EXERCISE PROGRAMS

Exercise Program	Rationale
Dorsiflexion and plantar flexion 10 times, four times daily	Muscle pump; promotes venous flow
Quadriceps femoris muscle setting	Isometric exercises maintain muscle strength, mass and joint stability.
Abdominal muscle setting	
Gluteal muscle setting 10 times, four times daily	Isometric exercise also helps maintain cardiac work capacity.
Active or passive range of joint motion three times daily	Maintains loose latticework of connective tissue
Simulated crutch walking three times daily	Strengthens triceps muscles
Pushing with legs against footboard or use of a bungee cord 10 times, four times daily	Promotes longitudinal stress on long bones to reduce demineralization

From Lentz, M.: Selected aspects of deconditioning secondary to immobilization. Nurs. Clin. North Am., Dec., 1981, p. 729.

Positioning

Even though it is well understood by most nurses that turning a patient, changing his body position, and getting him up in a chair will prevent decubitus ulcers, circulatory stasis, and respiratory and urinary complications, nurses may not realize that *changing body position does not necessarily guarantee freedom from orthopedic deformities. It is also necessary to change joint positions.* Figure 26–4 illustrates this very important point.

Assessment of a patient's need for proper positioning should include watching for early signs of muscle tightness and resistance to joint motion. This can be done during routine ROM exercises and could signal the need for positioning a body part so that the joint is extended and muscles are stretched to their normal capacity.

Patients with flaccid paralysis are not necessarily positioned in the same way as those with spastic paralysis. For example, a footboard is appropriate for proper positioning of the feet to prevent foot drop in a patient with flaccid paralysis. In contrast, putting the soles of the feet of a patient with spastic paralysis in contact with a footboard could trigger muscle contraction and aggravate the spasticity. Using a bed cradle to relieve pressure of the bed clothes can help prevent foot drop in these patients.

Some guiding principles for proper positioning are as follows:

- When the patient is lying on his back, place only one pillow under his head and position it so that it also supports his neck and upper shoulders.
- *Don't* place two or three pillows under his

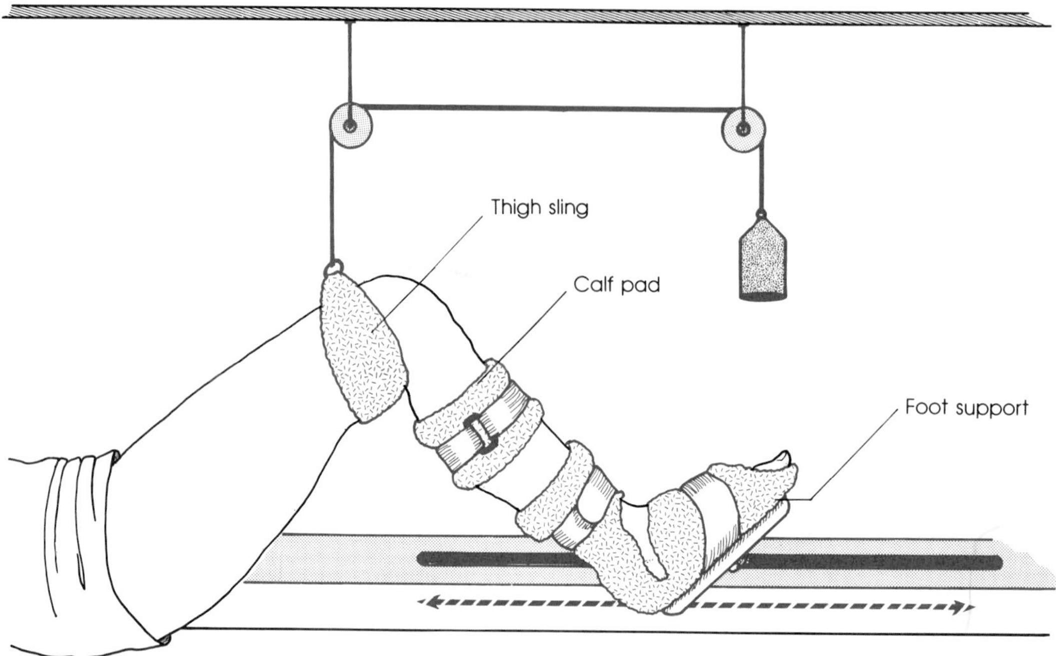

Figure 26-3 A device for providing passive exercise of the knee and hip joints. The thigh sling supports the weight of the upper leg and is attached to pulleys and a weight to allow motion. As the foot support slides back and forth on the track, the knee and hip joints are alternately flexed and extended. Limits of joint motion and length of time for periods of exercise are prescribed by the orthopedic surgeon.

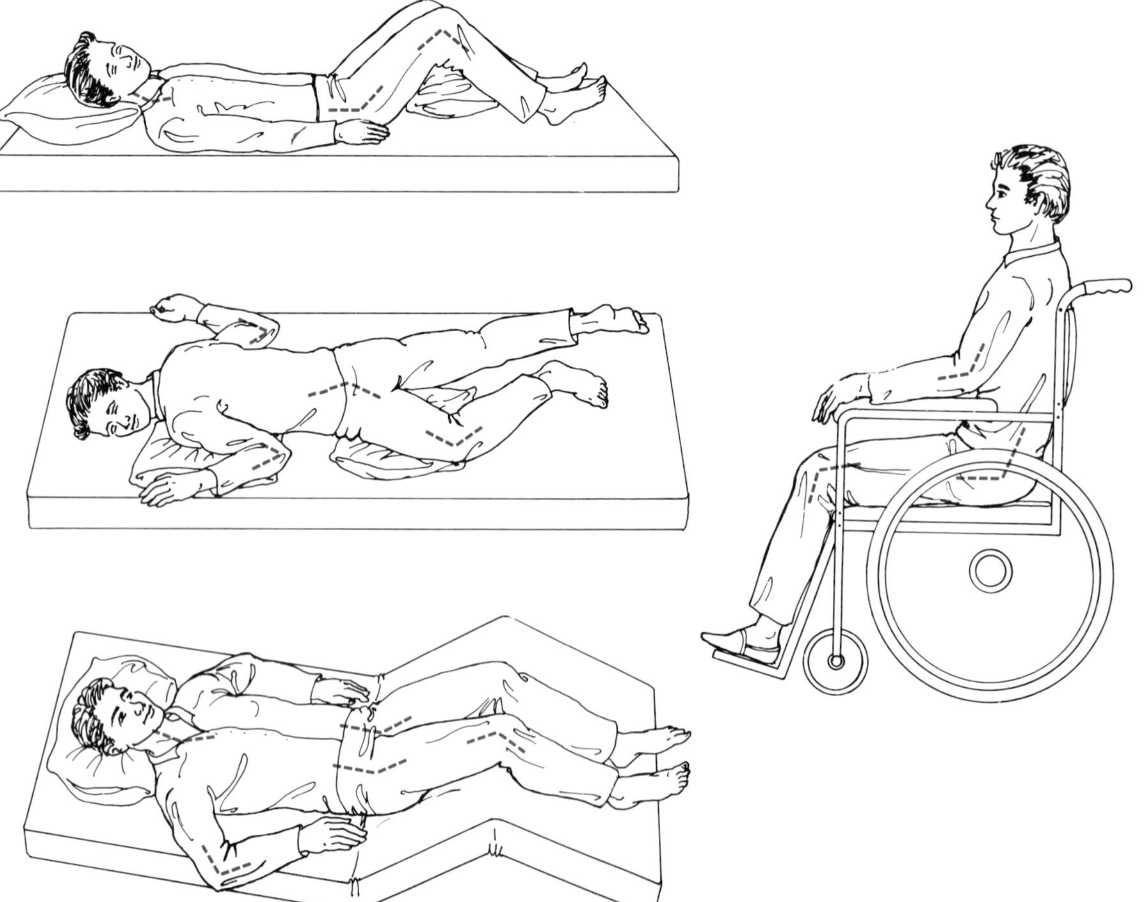

Figure 26-4 In these illustrations, the patient's body position has been changed four times, and yet the positions of the joints at the knees, hips, elbows, and neck have been changed very little or not at all.

head so that his neck is flexed and his chin is close to his chest.

- Place a folded towel under the achilles tendon to relieve pressure on the heels when the patient is lying on his back with his legs extended.
- *Don't* put a pillow under the knees or break the Gatch bed at the knees so that they are flexed.
- Use a trochanter roll and other supports along the leg and ankle to prevent abduction of the leg.
- *Don't* allow the patient to lie on his back with one leg flexed and rotated outward.
- Keep the arms extended and supported and the fingers extended.
- *Don't* allow the patient to keep his arms folded or flexed against his chest and his fingers curled into a fist.

EMOTIONAL ASPECTS OF ORTHOPEDIC DISORDERS

Unfortunately, many orthopedic conditions require prolonged periods of confinement to bed or, at best, immobilization of a part of the body and restricted physical activities. This leads to frustration and a feeling of hopelessness and despair on the part of the patient. When the patient is young and unaccustomed to dependence on others for his personal care, he may react with anger and bitterness toward his plight. If the patient is a wage earner or an active member of the family and one upon whom others are dependent, he has the additional burden of financial and social problems.

Immobilization and some degree of helplessness can greatly affect a patient's personality. Some never cease to rebel against the situation, whereas others become "institutionalized" and do not wish to return to their former lives and responsibilities. The nurse must understand that the long convalescent period filled with tedious hours of waiting for the bone to heal and the surrounding tissues to mend is a very difficult time for the patient. She will need much tact and patience as well as a lively imagination to help the patient spend his time happily and busily. Occupational therapy is available in most institutions and should be used to the fullest for the orthopedic patient.

Involving the patient in setting realistic and measurable goals for self-care and providing him with the guidance and information he needs to accomplish the goals can help him regain some control over what is happening to him. Being able to make some decisions about his care and seeing himself accomplish desired goals can enhance his self-image and improve his mental outlook.

CARE OF THE PATIENT IN A CAST

Casts are used for the purpose of immobilizing a certain part of the body so that it is firmly supported and completely at rest in a specific position.

TYPES OF CASTS

Leg and arm casts may cover all or part of the limb. These are called *long-leg* or *short-leg* casts, depending on how much leg they cover. A *walking cast* is a leg cast with extra material added to the sole for weight bearing. This is most often a metal bar ("walking iron") covered with rubber. A *spica* cast covers the trunk of the body and one or two extremities. There are long-leg and short-leg spicas that cover one or both legs and shoulder spicas that include the trunk and one arm (Fig. 26–5). Each type of cast presents unique problems of mobility and self-care activities.

PLASTER CASTS

The material most commonly used for casts is plaster of Paris. This material is used because it is cheap, durable, fairly easy to apply, and readily available. Plaster of Paris is gypsum from which the water has been removed. Strips of crinoline impregnated with this plaster are available in various widths. When they are to be used, these strips are soaked in water and applied wet. When the cast dries, there is a firm shell of plaster molded to the exact shape of the part of the body to which it has been applied.

Preparation for Application of a Plaster Cast

The mattress and pillows of the patient in a plaster cast should be protected with a waterproof material until the cast is completely dry. Most orthopedic surgeons prefer a cotton mattress with steel or wooden slats underneath to prevent sagging of the mattress. A soft or sagging mattress results in improper support of the cast.

Before a cast is applied, the patient's skin is thoroughly cleansed with soap and water, and any breaks in the skin are reported to the doctor if he is not aware of them. Shaving is not done unless surgery is to be performed before application of the cast. In this case, a special orthopedic surgical preparation according to the hospital procedure is necessary.

In emergencies, a thorough explanation of what is going to be done is not always possible. In all other cases, however, it is best if the patient is prepared for the type of cast that will be applied, the precautions that must be taken while the cast is drying, and any special devices

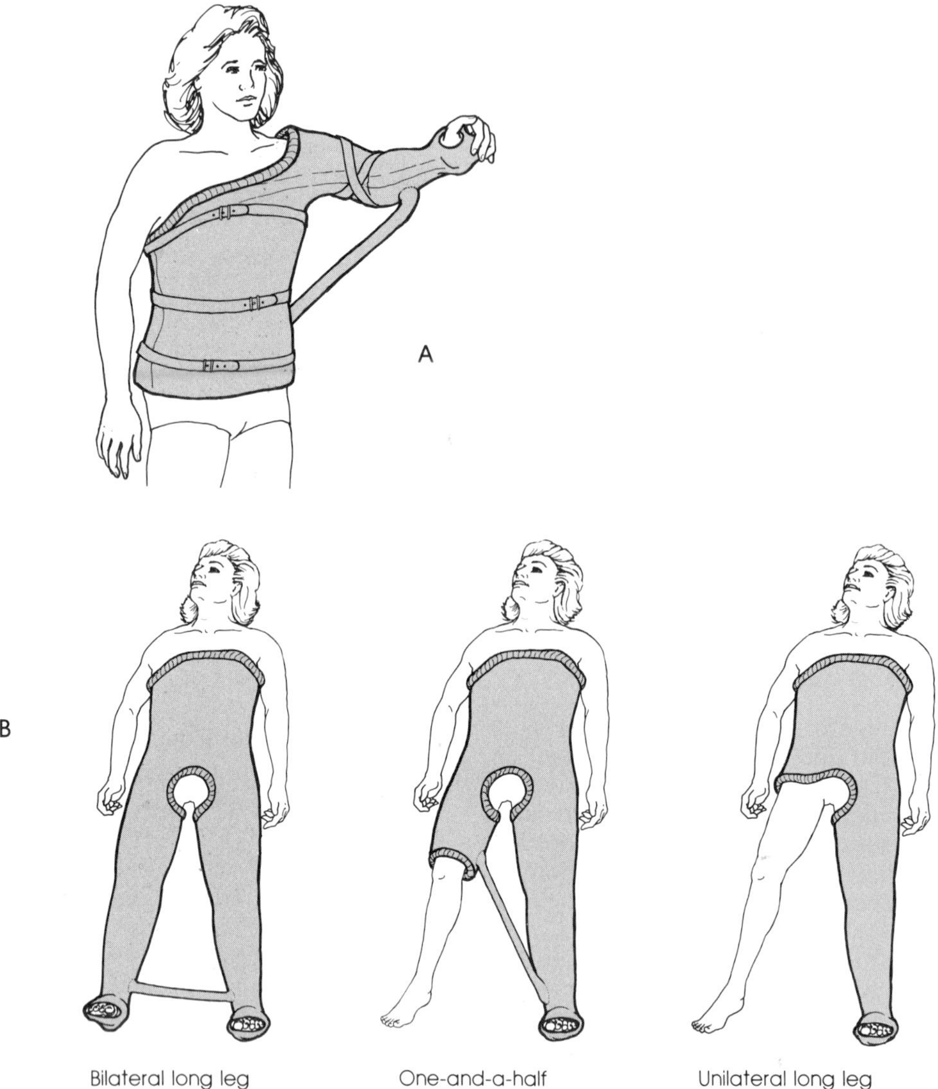

Figure 26–5 Spica casts. *A,* Shoulder spica cast. *B,* Hip spica casts.

that may be put on his bed to help him turn and move about in the bed. An example is the trapeze bar attached to an overhead frame, which allows the patient to lift himself and turn without strain on the affected part.

Care of the Fresh Plaster Cast

The newly applied cast is usually not dry for about 48 hours, depending on the type of cast. While the plaster is damp, its shape can be changed by careless handling or improper support. It follows, therefore, that extreme care must be used in moving the patient or the cast during this time. During the first 24 to 48 hours after a cast has been applied to an extremity, the extremity should be elevated to minimize swelling.

Ice bags also can be used to help control swelling. Because the weight of an ice bag could make an indentation in a wet cast, the ice bags should be only about half full, and they should be laid against the cast and propped in position, rather than set on top of it.

When the patient is transferred from the stretcher to the bed, there must be enough help available so that the patient is not "tumbled" into bed. Pillows for support should be placed on the bed *before* moving the patient onto them. Pillows are used to support the curves of large casts so that there will be no cracking or flattening of the cast by the weight of the body (Fig. 26–6).

The patient in a body cast or spica is more comfortable if pillows are not put under the head and shoulders, because they push the chest and abdomen against the front of the cast, causing an uncomfortable crushing sensation and dyspnea.

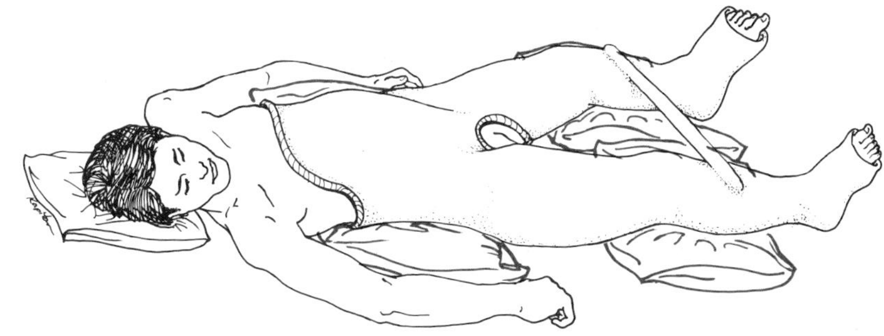

Figure 26-6 Proper support of a cast so that the weight of the body does not flatten curves in the cast.

Turnbuckles or braces such as the one shown between the legs of the cast in Figure 26-6 are never to be used as handles for lifting and turning the patient. Even after the cast is dry, these braces may be dislocated or pulled out of the cast.

While a cast is still damp, it should not be grasped by the fingers in the process of lifting or moving it. An effort should be made to use only the palms of the hands or the flat surface of the extended fingers. The reason for this is that fingertips can sink into the damp plaster and make impressions through the thickness of the cast, thus pressing mounds of plaster against the tissues under the cast. These can harden and in time lead to pressure sores.

After the cast is properly supported and positioned for drying, attention should be given to the patient's skin. Excess plaster on the skin and bits of plaster under the edge of the cast should be removed. A soft cloth dampened with warm water is all that is needed. Reddened areas can be cleansed with alcohol or a mild antiseptic.

Drying the Plaster Cast

The speed with which a plaster cast will dry is directly affected by the (1) humidity of the atmosphere around the cast and (2) circulation of air around the cast.

Thick body casts sometimes take several days to dry out completely. Others, such as the thin casts for club foot or long-leg casts, may dry within a few hours. A cast dryer, similar in principle to a hair dryer, may be used to speed up the evaporation of moisture from the cast.

The advantage of using the dryer is the increased circulation of air around the cast, not ***the application of heat. The use of heat is dangerous, because it may easily lead to burns under the cast.***

It is also possible that heat exhaustion and excessive loss of body fluids from perspiration will occur. A dryer should *not* be used without a written order.

Frequent turning of the patient helps the cast dry evenly and prevents prolonged pressure and flattening of one side of the cast. The patient should always be turned onto his "good side"—that is, with the fractured limb uppermost—while the cast is drying.

Bed cradles are not advisable, as they trap the moisture and increase the humidity around the cast. The patient in a cast may experience chilling from the dampness. He should be covered adequately with blankets, but the cast must remain uncovered until it is thoroughly dry.

It is not possible to determine whether a cast is dry simply by feeling its surface; therefore, it should be handled very carefully for the first few days or until the physician states specifically that the cast is dry. A dry cast is white, has a shiny surface, and will resound when tapped. A wet cast is grayish and dull in appearance and will give a dull thud when tapped.

Nursing Assessment

Any body part encased in a cast is in danger of pressure against nerves and blood vessels and a resultant nerve damage or serious obstruction to blood flow. Periodic assessment of the patient's neurovascular status is an essential part of the nursing care plan for a patient in a cast. Failure to notice the early signs of pressure on nerves or blood vessels and to initiate preventive measures can cause an avoidable paralysis and possibly gangrene.

A thorough assessment of a patient in a cast should include the following:

- *Listen to the patient's complaints.* He may report numbness, a tingling sensation, increased pain with motion of his fingers or toes, or sharp localized pain; any of these symptoms could be caused by pressure from a tight cast. Do not attempt to judge whether his complaints are justified. Assess his sensory response by checking his ability to distinguish between two distinct points on the skin (the *two-point discrimination test*). If elevating the limb does not relieve the patient's complaints, notify the physician.

- *Observe the fingers or toes protruding from a cast for signs of impaired circulation.* These signs include a bluish-gray discoloration to the skin, coldness to the touch, and slow return of color to the skin after applying and then releasing pressure. This latter test, called *blanching* or *capillary refill time,* can be done by sharply compressing the nail of the thumb or great toe. When the pressure is released the capillaries should fill immediately, returning the color to the nail bed.
- A sudden, unexplained elevation of temperature or the presence of a foul or unusual odor from the cast could indicate infection.
- Check frequently to see if the cast is properly supported or if there is undue pressure on any part of the body. A sharp, localized, burning pain could mean the beginning of a pressure sore. This should be reported so that the surgeon or orthopedic technician can cut a "window" in the cast to relieve pressure.

Daily Care

After the cast is thoroughly dry and the initial swelling under the cast has subsided, the nurse must concern herself with the cleanliness of the patient and the cast. The problems involved will vary according to the type of cast and the area it covers. All parts of the body not included in the cast should be bathed daily, using care not to wet the cast. The skin around the edges of the cast should receive special attention, including massage with alcohol or lotion and close observation for signs of pressure or breaks in the skin. The edges of plaster casts tend to crumble, with bits of plaster dropping down inside the cast and causing the patient discomfort and skin irritation. This can be avoided by covering the rims of the cast with stockinette or tape.

Wetting a cast will cause it to disintegrate rapidly. The patient in a long-leg cast or a spica can very easily soil the cast when attempting to use the bedpan. The problem of protecting the cast is even more difficult when the patient is a very young child who is not yet toilet trained, or an older patient who is incontinent. To avoid soiling, the perineal area of the cast can be covered with a waterproof material, such as the waxed paper or plastic wrapping used to keep refrigerated foods airtight. The material should be applied so that it covers the outside edge of the cast and extends down inside the cast for a few inches. This covering may be changed as often as necessary and also gives the added advantage of allowing for thorough cleansing of the buttocks and perineal area without danger of wetting the cast.

When a bedpan is used by the patient in a spica, there is the possibility of a backward flow of urine under the cast unless the head of the bed is slightly elevated. Because the patient cannot bend at the hips to sit up on the pan, the head of the bed should be elevated on shock blocks or some other device and the lumbar area of the cast supported to prevent cracking.

Itching is a common complaint of the patient in a cast. Patients must be instructed not to use sharp objects such as pencils or rulers to scratch under the cast. These can, of course, tear the skin, leaving an open break for the entrance of bacteria. An experienced orthopedic nurse has found that forceful injection of air, using a 50-ml bulb syringe or one with a plunger and directing the air under the cast, can relieve intense itching.

When a cast is removed, the underlying skin is usually dry and scaly. Cleansing of these areas should be done in consultation with the physician, because the type of care to be given will depend on whether another cast is to be applied. In any case, overenthusiastic scrubbing of the area must be avoided to prevent damage to the deeper layers of skin.

Nursing interventions for selected problems of a patient in a cast are summarized in Nursing Care Plan 26–1.

SYNTHETIC CASTS

Casts made from synthetic materials such as fiberglass, plastic, or a combination of cotton and polyester do not require as long a drying period as do those made from plaster of Paris. They set in a matter of minutes, rather than the 48 hours required for plaster casts, and can bear weight almost immediately after application. In addition to their advantage of setting quickly, synthetic casts are not as heavy as plaster casts and therefore allow more freedom of movement. They also are less bulky, do not crumble as easily, and are less likely to be damaged by wetting.

In spite of all the advantages of synthetic casts, they do have limited use. They cost three to seven times more than plaster casts. They are less easily molded to a body part and are not suitable for immobilizing the fragments of severely displaced bones or for stabilizing serious fractures. Their rough exterior surfaces can damage the skin and tend to snag clothing and other soft materials.

Assessment of the status of nerves and blood vessels under a synthetic cast is the same as for a plaster cast. If the patient is allowed to go home after the cast has been applied, he will need to know how to conduct a neurovascular assessment during the first 14 to 48 hours after the cast has been applied. He also will need to know the signs of infection and appreciate the importance of promptly reporting these signs to the physician. A broken or loose cast should be reported immediately.

The synthetic material of the cast will not be

NURSING CARE PLAN 26–1

Selected nursing diagnoses, goals/outcome criteria, nursing interventions, and evaluations for a patient in a cast

Situation: Mark Johnson, age 24, was injured in a motorcycle accident in which he sustained a fracture of the left femur. He is admitted to the orthopedic unit after surgical reduction of the fracture and casting.

Nursing Diagnosis	Goals/Outcome Criteria	Nursing Intervention	Evaluation
Potential alteration in tissue perfusion SUPPORTING DATA Open reduction and casting of fracture of left femur.	Capillary refill within 3 seconds; normal color and sensation of toes.	Assess toes for color, temperature, and capillary refill q 2 hr for 24 h, then q 4 h. Assess sensation in toes with two-point discrimination test. Place half-full ice bags against cast to reduce swelling; elevate leg on two pillows.	Feet warm and pink; capillary refill 10 sec.; sensation equal bilaterally; ice bags in place; left leg elevated; continue plan.
Potential impaired skin integrity related to cast. SUPPORTING DATA Cast on left femur; may cause pressure areas and irritation of skin around edges.	Visible skin clear and intact; no musty odors; no reports of burning pain or pressure from under cast.	Leave cast exposed to air; dry with cool cast dryer if still wet after 24 hours. Turn at least q 2 h to back or right side; handle cast gently with palms of hands. Check q 2 h to be sure cast is well supported and there is no undue pressure on any body part; monitor for sharp, localized, burning pain and report promptly. Circle any blood stain on cast with pen; place ice to area of cast where blood stain noted. Check for further bleeding q 2 h; report if stain continues to enlarge.	Cast with two areas still moist—exposed to air; no complaints of pressure; skin at edges intact; turned 8, 10, 12, and 2; continue plan.
Potential for infection related to pressure of cast on skin, broken bone, and surgical incision. SUPPORTING DATA Fractured femur in motorcycle accident; open reduction and cast; potential for bacterial entry into wound.	Skin under cast remains intact and free of infection.	Check vital signs q 4 h; monitor for temperature elevation. Monitor WBCs. Check for foul or unusual odor from under cast.	VS within normal limits; temp., 98.6°F; WBCs, 8,200; no unusual odor at cast; continue plan.
Knowledge deficit regarding cast care at home. SUPPORTING DATA States he has never had a cast before.	Patient will verbalize basics of cast care correctly.	Teach the following points of cast care: • Do not put any object down cast to try and scratch itching skin. • When leg itches under cast, scratch the opposite leg. • Report signs of infection, pressure sores, and impaired circulation to physician. • If bothered by swelling and throbbing, elevate leg. • Wrap cast in plastic bag and securely tape before showering; do not let water flow directly on casted leg. • If any area of cast becomes soft or broken, make appointment for a new cast.	Teaching regarding cast care complete; will obtain feedback tomorrow.

damaged by water, so in some cases the physician may allow the patient to bathe, shower, and even swim while wearing the cast. Patient education includes warning the patient about getting soap under the cast while bathing, and telling him to dry the cast well each time the cast is wet. This can be done by blotting excess water with a large towel and then using a blow dryer to thoroughly dry the cast and the stockinette under it. Care must be taken *not* to get water inside the cast. He should know that failing to get the cast completely dry can lead to maceration of the skin under the cast. Because it takes more than an hour to get a well-soaked synthetic cast completely dry, the patient may decide that swimming or soaking in a tub for long periods of time is not worth the trouble.

CAST BRACE

In the late 1960s, an appliance called a *cast brace* was introduced as an alternative to the more traditional leg casts. It combines the support and stability offered by a plaster cast with the support and mobility provided by a hinged brace (Fig. 26–7).

The cast brace permits early ambulation and weight bearing in patients who have a fracture in the shaft of the femur. It is applied 2 to 6 weeks after the fracture has been reduced, during which time skeletal traction has been used to hold the fragments in alignment during healing.

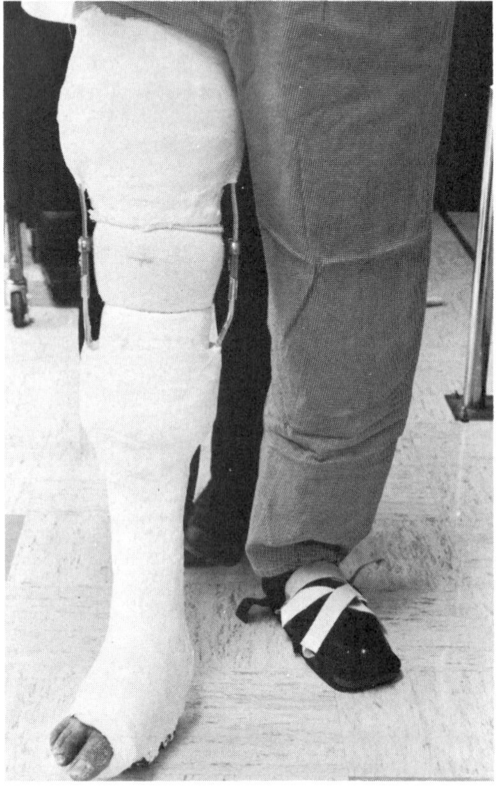

Figure 26–7 Cast brace, anterior view.

The upper end of the cast brace is a *thigh cuff*, which compresses the thigh muscle, thereby immobilizing the fractured fragments. The middle component is a pair of *hinges*, which permit motion of the knee joint. The hinges attach the thigh cuff to a short-leg walking cast, which is the lowest part of the cast brace.

A frequent problem with a cast brace is swelling of the knee. The most effective measure to relieve this condition is elevation of the leg whenever the patient is sitting or lying down. Other nursing care activities and observations are the same as for any patient with a cast.

As soon as the cast brace is dry, the patient is allowed to get out of bed. His gradual progression from standing to partial weight bearing, full weight bearing, and walking is supervised by the physical therapist.

CARE OF THE PATIENT IN TRACTION

TYPES AND USES OF TRACTION

Traction is the application of a mechanical *pull* to a part of the body for the purpose of extending and holding that part in a certain position. Through a system of ropes and pulleys, weights are attached to a fixed point below the area of injury or disease. The apparatus is rigged so that the weights on one end and the weight of the patient's body on the other will pull the affected part in opposite directions, thus straightening and holding that part in the desired position. There are several ways to accomplish this.

The two general types of traction are *skeletal* and *skin*. In skeletal traction, the surgeon inserts pins, wires, or tongs directly through the bone at a point distal to the fracture so that the force of pull from the weights is exerted directly on the bone. With skin traction, a bandage such as moleskin or ace-adherent is applied to the limb below the site of fracture and the pull is exerted on the limb in this manner.

Traction may be continuous, as in the alignment and resultant immobility of fractured bones, or it may be intermittent, as in traction on the spinal column to relieve the symptoms of a slipped disc or muscle spasms.

The system of ropes, pulleys, and weights used to provide the various kinds of traction can be very confusing at first, but the principles on which traction is based are actually quite simple. Some types of traction are named for the orthopedic surgeons who first designed them. Figure 26–8 illustrates some of the different types of traction.

Bryant's traction for small children with frac-

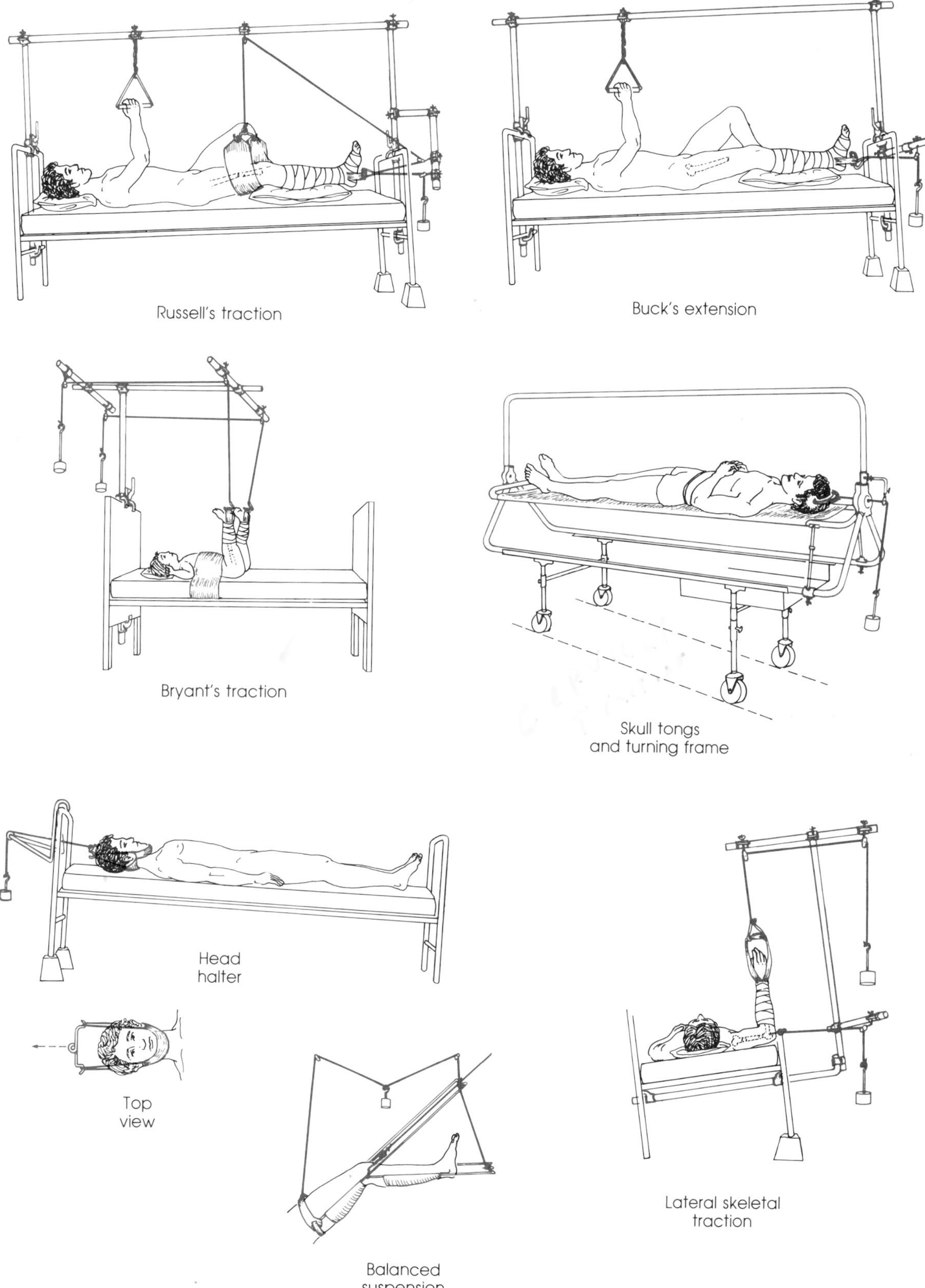

Figure 26-8 Various types of traction and suspension.

ture of the femur uses the weight of the child's lower body to pull the bone fragments of the fracture leg into alignment. In order to accomplish this, the child's buttocks should just clear the mattress and his legs should be at a 90-degree angle to his trunk.

Buck's extension is a simple skin traction that is used to treat muscle spasms and minor fractures of the lower spine.

Russell's traction utilizes a knee sling to provide support of the affected leg. It is commonly used to treat knee injuries and hip fractures.

Balanced suspension with the *Thomas splint* and *Pearson attachment* is used to treat fractures of the leg and to stabilize total hip replacements. The Thomas splint supports the thigh and knee and provides countertraction. The Pearson attachment supports the lower leg.

Cervical traction can be provided through the use of tongs inserted into the skull or by using a head halter (see Chapter 15).

Side traction is indicated when stabilization is needed to treat fractures and dislocations of the arm and shoulder.

NURSING INTERVENTION

Most patients in traction for the treatment of fractures and other orthopedic conditions requiring a continuous pull on a part of the body must lie on their backs, with only a limited amount of turning permitted. This is not an excuse for neglect of the patient's body. He must still be kept clean and comfortable and free of pressure sores.

If the physician will not permit turning the patient far enough to allow for adequate back care, the patient may use a trapeze bar to lift himself so that back care can be given and the bottom sheet changed or tightened. The patient should be instructed to lift himself straight up so that the amount of pull exerted on the limb in traction will not be altered. This same maneuver can be used when the patient is placed on a bedpan. A small, child-size bedpan should be used and the lower back supported by a small pillow or folded blanket.

OBSERVATIONS

Frequent observations of both the patient and the traction apparatus should include the following:

- *Be sure the weights are hanging free.* If the weights are resting on or against any support such as the foot of the bed or the floor, the purpose of the traction is defeated. Be careful not to bump against the weights when walking around the foot of the bed. This can be painful to the patient and may cause damage to the healing bone. It is not necessary to lift the weights when pulling the patient up in bed. The amount of pull on the limb will remain the same as long as the weights are hanging free.
- *Check the position of the patient, making sure his body weight is counteracting the pull of the weights.* Should the patient slip down in bed so that his feet are resting against the footboard, there will be a loss of force exerted on the limb.
- Observe all bony prominences for signs of impaired circulation and tissue necrosis.
- Observe the patient's posture in bed and position of joints for proper alignment.
- To prevent pressure sores, be sure slings and ropes are not pressing against or cutting into an area of the extremity.
- When a patient has skeletal traction, observe the sites of entry of pins, tongs, etc., for signs of infection.
- Devise a systematic routine for observing the patient and the apparatus at specified times during the day so that no aspect of the assessment will be overlooked.

CARE OF THE PATIENT ON A FRAME

There are times when the nursing care of a patient with an orthopedic condition is extremely difficult if the patient is lying on a conventional hospital bed. To solve the nursing problems brought about by these conditions, specially designed frames or orthopedic beds are available, such as the Stryker frame and the Foster bed (Fig. 26–9). They are used (1) to facilitate the nursing care and frequent turning of patients who are helpless, (2) to aid in immobilizing the spine as a means of treating spinal fractures and other diseases of the spine, and (3) to provide a means of keeping those patients clean and dry who cannot be moved for placement of a bedpan or those who are incontinent.

There are several modifications of the frames, but the basic structure consists of two metal frames covered with a heavy duck or canvas material. One of the frames is designed so that there is a perineal opening under the buttocks; this is used when the patient is lying on his back. The second frame is covered so that it matches its mate and is used when the patient is lying in a prone position. The position of the patient may be alternated from back to abdomen by using alternate frames. In the prone position, the head of the patient is supported with a strap across the forehead so that the face is uncovered, allowing for eating, reading, or any simple recreational activity. In addition to the frames, there are detachable supports for the arms and a footboard attachment for proper positioning of the patient's feet.

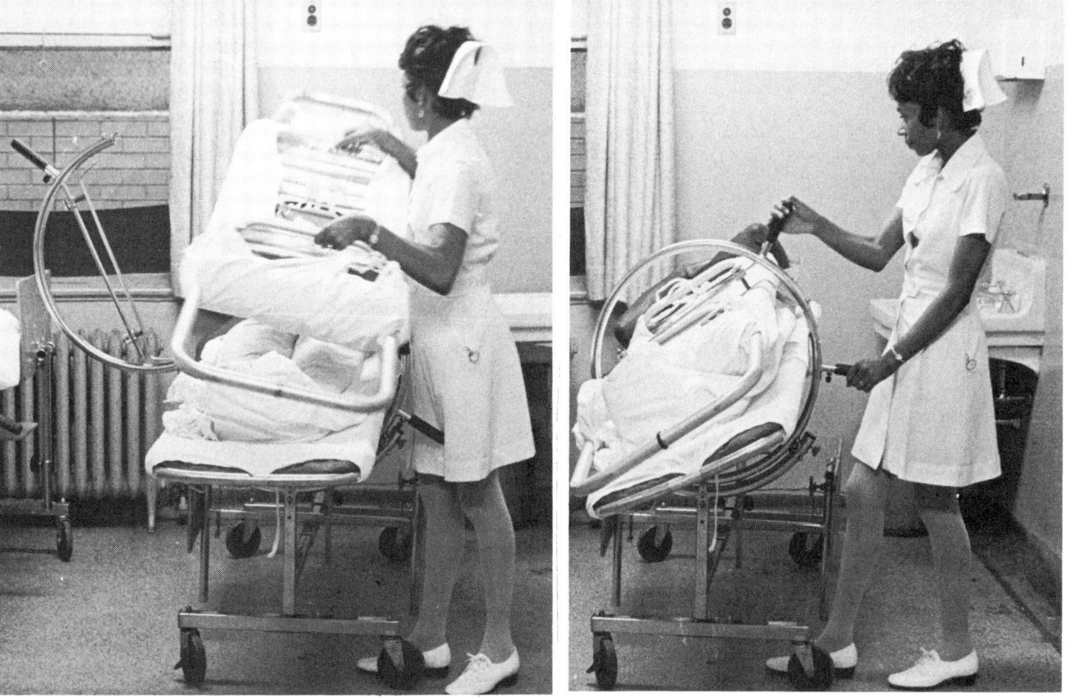

Figure 26-9 The Stryker wedge turning frame. This specially designed frame permits frequent turning of severely injured patients with a minimum of effort on the part of the nurse. *A*, Nurse applying the anterior frame in preparation for turning the patient from supine to prone position. *B*, Nurse turning the patient without assistance.
(Courtesy of Orthopedic Frame Company, Kalamazoo, MI.)

Because turning the patient is a comparatively easy procedure when these frames are used, many complications caused by the patient's lying in one position too long can be avoided. It must be remembered, however, that these patients are *more likely to develop decubitus ulcers* than those in a conventional bed unless they are turned at least every 2 hours.

TURNING THE PATIENT

The nurse caring for a patient on a frame must seek instruction in the use of these frames before accepting any responsibility for a task such as turning the patient.

Unless the patient is turned quickly and smoothly and is adequately strapped onto the frame, there is danger of injury to the patient and disturbance of the body alignment desired by the physician.

It is strongly recommended that the inexperienced nurse observe and assist with the use of the frame before attempting to care for a patient on a frame.

DAILY CARE

The usual procedure for a bed bath must be altered for bathing a patient on an orthopedic frame. The anterior portion of the patient's body is washed while the patient is lying on the posterior frame. He is then turned onto the matching frame while the remaining portions of the body are bathed.

There should be adequate support of the buttocks over the perineal opening of the frame while the patient is on his back, or the alignment of the spine will be disturbed and additional pressure will be placed on the sacral region. When the patient wishes to use the bedpan, the perineal or buttock strap is removed, and the pan is placed on the rack beneath the opening. A piece of waterproof material may be tucked up under the buttocks and the other end placed in the bedpan to direct the flow of urine into the bedpan. Before replacing the supporting strap under the buttocks, the perineum and buttocks are thoroughly cleaned, dried, and powdered.

THE CIRCOLECTRIC BED

The CircOlectric bed (Fig. 26-10) is an electrically operated frame similar in principle to the Stryker frame, except that the patient is turned head-over-heels rather than from side to side. Although this procedure may be somewhat frightening to both patient and nurse who are unfamiliar with the operation of the apparatus, the bed is relatively simple to operate and has several advantages.

The bed can be rotated so that the patient is in a prone position, a supine position, or a sitting

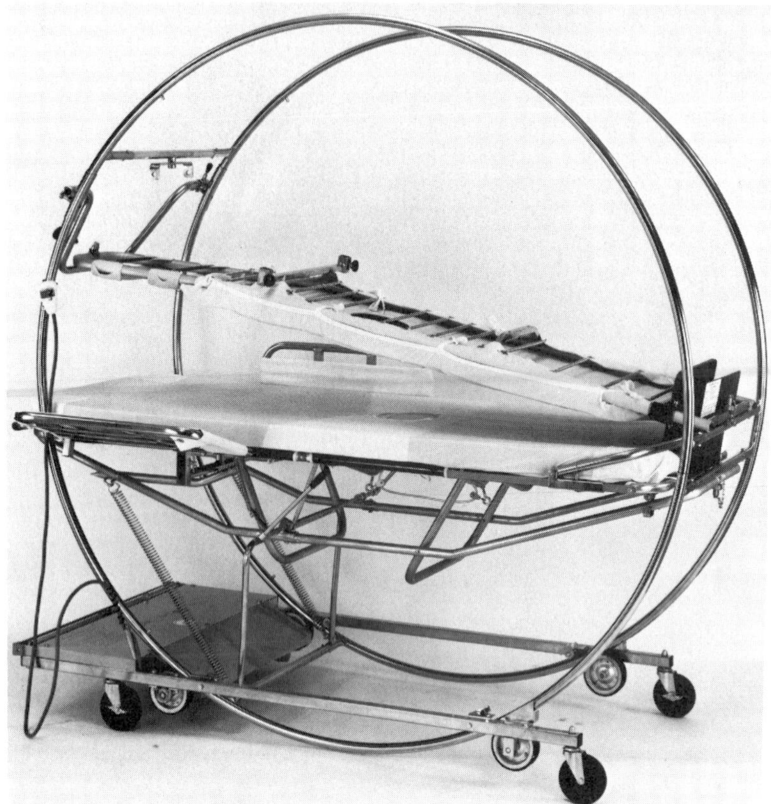

Figure 26-10 The CircOlectric bed. The CircOlectric bed is used to facilitate positioning of severely injured patients and for those with chronic orthopedic or neurologic problems. Like the Stryker turning frame, the CircOlectric bed has an anterior and posterior frame to permit placing the patient in both prone and supine positions. In addition, it has the advantage of preparing a patient for the transition from recumbency to ambulation. When it is used as a tilt table several times a day, the patient can regain standing balance without having to assume a sitting position on the side of the bed. The bed also can be used for controlling weight bearing when sitting is contraindicated.
(Courtesy of Orthopedic Frame Company, Kalamazoo, MI.)

position. If the patient is able to do so and is confident about the operation of the bed, he can manipulate it himself using the hand controls. Use of the CircOlectric bed is not limited to patients in traction. It can also be utilized for burn patients to facilitate turning and applications of medication and for patients with neck injuries.

OTHER BEDS

Another type of bed that is often used for patients in cervical traction is the Rotorest bed. This bed very slowly turns the patient about 300 times a day. It provides passive exercise and stimulates peristalsis without risk of injury to the patient. The bed has many other advantages, including several hatches that provide the nurse access to all of the common pressure points on the patient. There is a hatch for bowel and bladder care so that a bedpan can be placed without moving the patient. The back side of the patient can be bathed through the various hatches also. Once the nurse is familiar with the bed, it greatly simplifies care of the immobilized patient.

The Clinitron therapy bed is also used for various types of immobilized patients. It is an air-fluidized bed and is very helpful in preventing pressure sores.

CRUTCH WALKING

For the convalescent patient or for one who may always need support while walking, crutches can mean the difference between freedom to move about and confinement to one location. Before attempting to walk with crutches, one should have sufficient instruction in their use and manipulation so that they can be handled safely and effectively. The ease with which some people apparently handle themselves on crutches is the result of patience and hard work to learn the proper methods.

The type of crutch to be used will depend on the extent of disability or paralysis and the patient's ability to bear weight and keep his balance on his feet. If the crutches are too short or too long, they can create problems of lifting and moving about for the patient. In regard to this, one must bear in mind that the muscles of the arms, shoulders, back, and chest are all used in the manipulation of crutches. Because this is true, many physical therapists start the patient on special exercises to strengthen these muscles several weeks before the patient begins to use the crutches.

Although the physical therapist supervises preparation and instruction of the patient before he starts to use crutches and then evaluates his ability to use them correctly, the nurse will sometimes be responsible for assisting a patient with crutch walking while he is in the hospital.

The position of the crutches for stability and the gaits used for mobility are the two major components of instruction. The tripod position shown in Figure 26–11 shows how the patient can use his crutches to hold himself steady before starting to move. As shown in the illustration, he can use various gaits to move faster or more slowly. The term *point* as used in Figure 26–11 refers to the number of points of contact with the floor. A three-point gait, for example, uses two crutches and one foot; a four-point gait uses both feet and two crutches.

FRACTURES

A fracture is a break or interruption in the continuity of a bone. The amount of injury to the neighboring tissues varies according to the type of fracture, but there is always some degree of tissue destruction, interference with the blood supply, and disturbance of muscle activity at the site of injury.

TYPES OF FRACTURES

Complete fracture is the breaking of a bone into two parts with complete separation of the two broken ends. An *incomplete fracture* is the breaking of a bone into two parts, without complete separation of the fragments.

A *comminuted fracture* is one in which the bone is broken and shattered into more than two fragments.

A *closed (simple) fracture* is one in which there is no break in the skin.

An *open (compound) fracture* is one in which there is a break in the skin through which the fragments of broken bone protrude.

A *greenstick fracture*, commonly found in children, is one in which the bone is partially bent and partially broken.

Other types of fracture may be classified according to their appearance on the radiograph (Fig. 26–12).

SURGICAL TREATMENT AND RATIONALE

The primary aim in the treatment of fractures is the establishment of a sturdy union between the broken ends of bone so that the bone can be restored to its former state of continuity. The healing and repair of a fracture begins immediately after the bone is broken and goes through four stages:

1. Blood oozing from the torn blood vessels in the area of the fracture clots and begins to form a hematoma between the two broken ends of bone.
2. Other tissue cells enter the clot, and granulation tissue is formed. This tissue is interlaced with capillaries, and it gradually becomes firm and forms a bridge between the two ends of broken bone.
3. Young bone cells enter the area and form a tissue called "woven bone." At this stage, the ends of the broken bone are beginning to "knit" together.
4. The immature bone cells are gradually replaced by mature bone cells, and the tissue takes on the characteristics of typical bone structure.

It is hoped that a thorough understanding of these stages of healing in the process of bone repair will make the nurse more aware of the need for gentle handling of a fractured bone while it is in the process of healing.

To facilitate the process of repair and ensure proper healing of the bone without deformity or loss of function, the surgeon must bring the two broken ends together in proper alignment and then immobilize the affected part until healing is complete. The procedure for bringing the two fragments of bone into proper alignment is called *reduction of the fracture* (Fig. 26–13).

Four methods of reducing a fracture are (1) closed reduction, (2) open reduction, (3) internal fixation, and (4) external fixation.

In *closed reduction* the bone is manipulated into alignment; no surgical incision is made. A general anesthetic may be given before the fracture is reduced.

An *open reduction* is done after a surgical incision is made through the skin and down to the bone at the site of the fracture. In cases of open (compound) fractures and comminuted fractures, an open reduction has always been necessary so that the area can be adequately cleansed and bone fragments removed.

When a fracture cannot be properly reduced by either open or closed reduction and it is impossible to guarantee adequate union of the bone fragments, the physician must perform a procedure called *internal fixation* of the bone. This means that pins, nails, screws, or metal plates must be used to stabilize the position of the two broken ends. Internal fixation is particularly useful in the treatment of fractures in elderly patients whose bones are brittle and may not heal properly (Fig. 26–14).

External fixation of fractures involves the use of a device composed of a sturdy external frame to which are attached pins that have been drilled into the bone fragments. Figure 26–15 shows a fixator that is applied by inserting heavy pins on either side of the fracture and then reducing the fracture by tightening nuts attached to the connecting rods.

External fixation is indicated when (1) there are massive open fractures with extensive soft tissue damage, (2) infected fractures do not heal

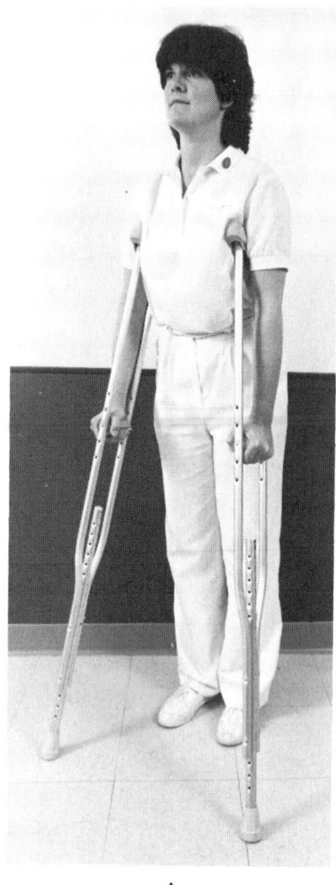

A

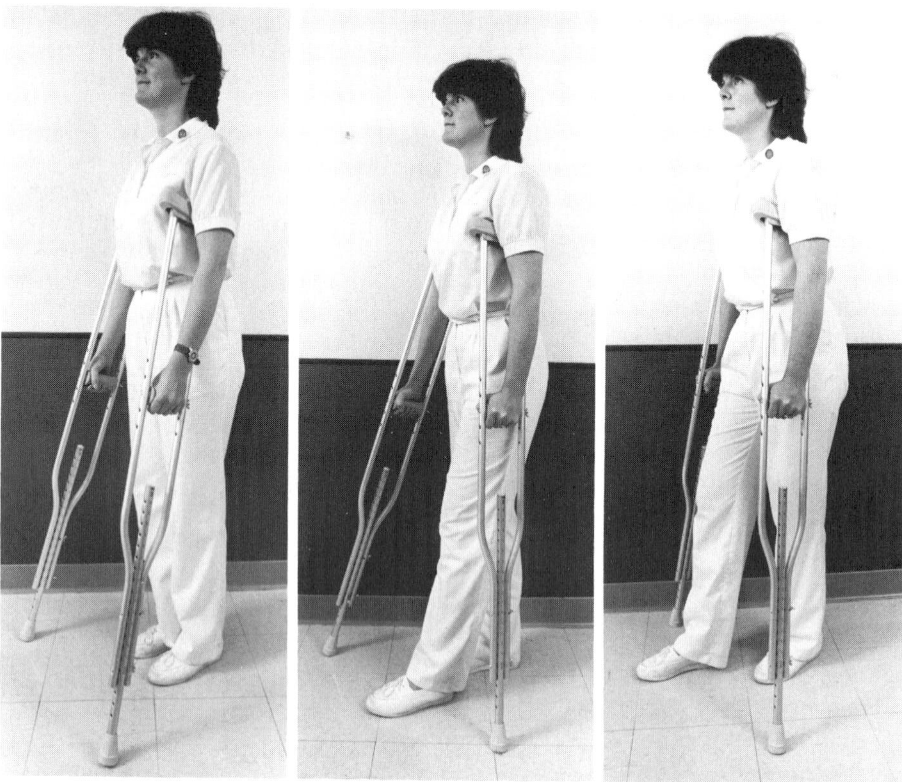

B

Figure 26-11 Crutch-walking gaits. *A,* The tripod position from which all gaits begin. *B,* The four-point gait. There are always three points of contact with the ground to give stability and balance. The right crutch is brought forward, followed by the left foot. The left crutch is then brought forward, followed by the right foot.

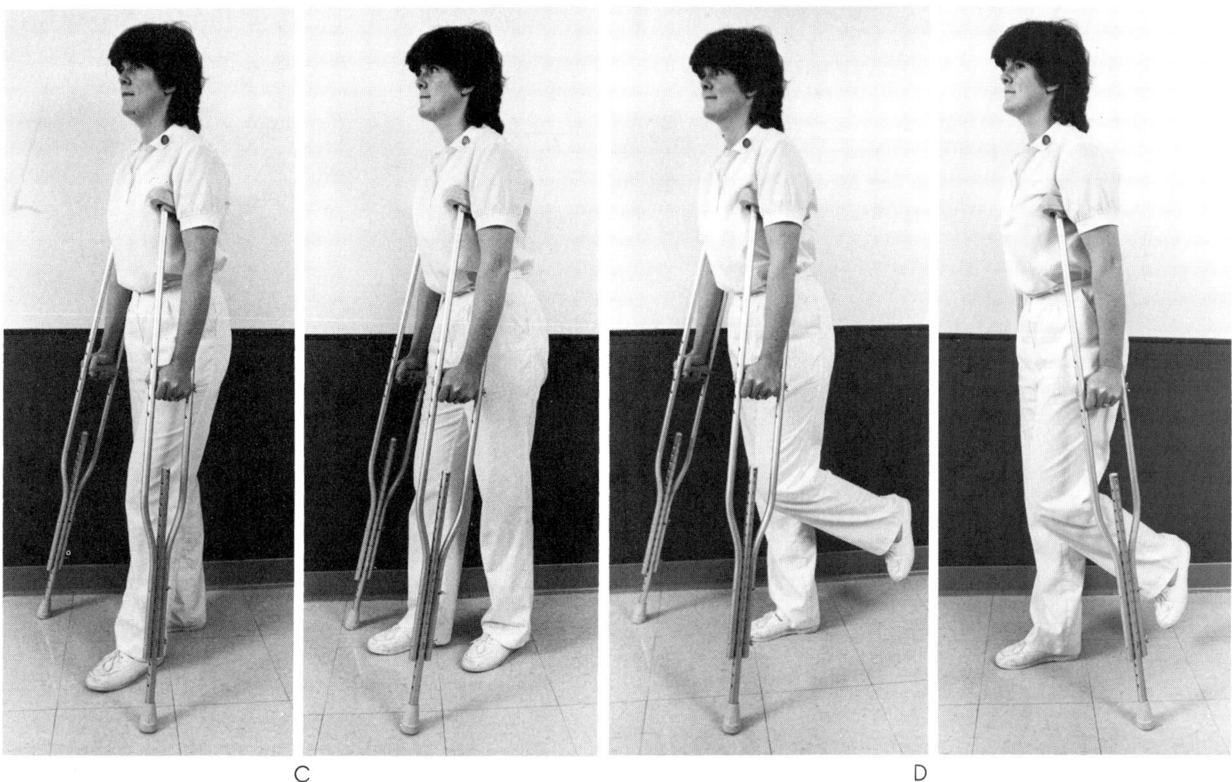

Figure 26-11 *Continued C,* The three-point gait, used when some weight bearing is allowed on the injured part. It begins in the tripod position with both crutches and the affected limb resting on the ground. The unaffected foot is swung forward and supports the body weight while the affected limb and the crutches are brought forward at the same time. Then, while the crutches provide support, the unaffected limb is brought forward. *D,* Alternate three-point gait, used when weight bearing by the affected limb is *not* allowed. It begins with the tripod position. Both crutches are brought forward, and the unaffected limb is swung through the crutches. The affected limb is not allowed to touch the ground.

Illustration continued on following page

properly, and (3) there is multiple trauma with one or more fractures and other injuries such as burns, chest injury, or head injury.

Because the pin sites are left open to the air during convalescence, special daily care is necessary to prevent infection. As soon as it is feasible, the patient is taught to care for the pin sites and to report any signs of infection.

External fixation has the advantage of allowing more freedom of movement than traction or casting, and usually is more comfortable. With good stability there is no need for restricting the patient to bed. In some cases it is possible for the patient to bear weight on his affected limb, but even if this is not allowed, he is free to move about on his own, perform physical therapy exercises, and avoid many of the problems of immobility.

Nonunion of a fracture can be treated by a bone growth-stimulating device, which is an electromagnetic device whose current stimulates osteogenesis (growth of bone cells). The stimulator may be either external or internal. Use of this device can prevent the necessity of further surgery and bone grafting.

In elderly patients who have suffered a fracture of the head of the femur, the surgeon may choose to take out the broken head fragments. He replaces the fragments with a prosthesis that is designed with a ball to replace the head of the femur and is shaped so that it can be fitted into or onto the shaft of the femur in such a way that the patient can bear weight on it. Although a prosthesis is not as good as a normal hip joint, many patients who have such a prosthesis are able to walk again and use the limb effectively. Total hip replacement for osteoarthritis is discussed later in this chapter.

Vertebral Fracture

Care of patients with injury to the spinal column and spinal cord is covered in Chapter 15. The chapter also includes care of the patient with cervical tongs, halo traction, and laminectomy.

Sometimes, when trauma has made the spinal column unstable or it will not heal sufficiently, a spinal fusion is done to provide stability. Bone chips are grafted between the vertebral spaces. *Spinal fusion* is usually done only after traction, bed rest, and other treatments have proven ineffective.

After spinal fusion, the head of the bed is kept

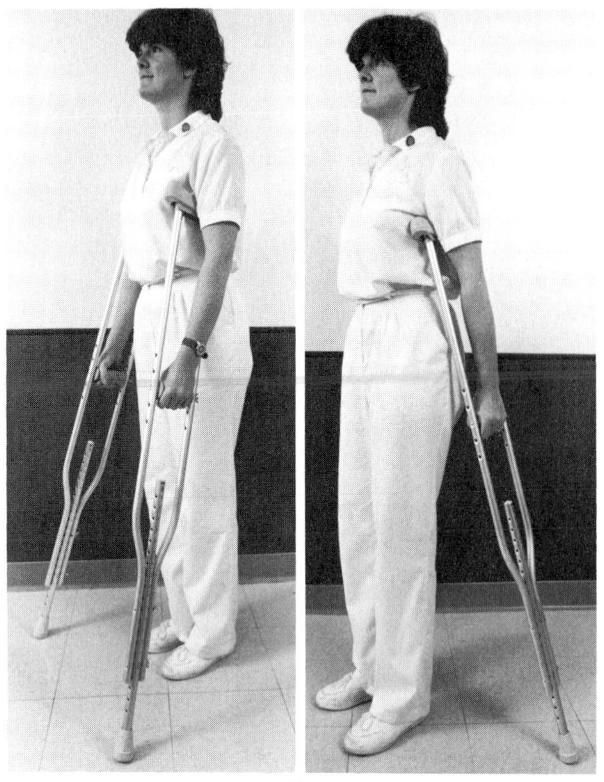

E

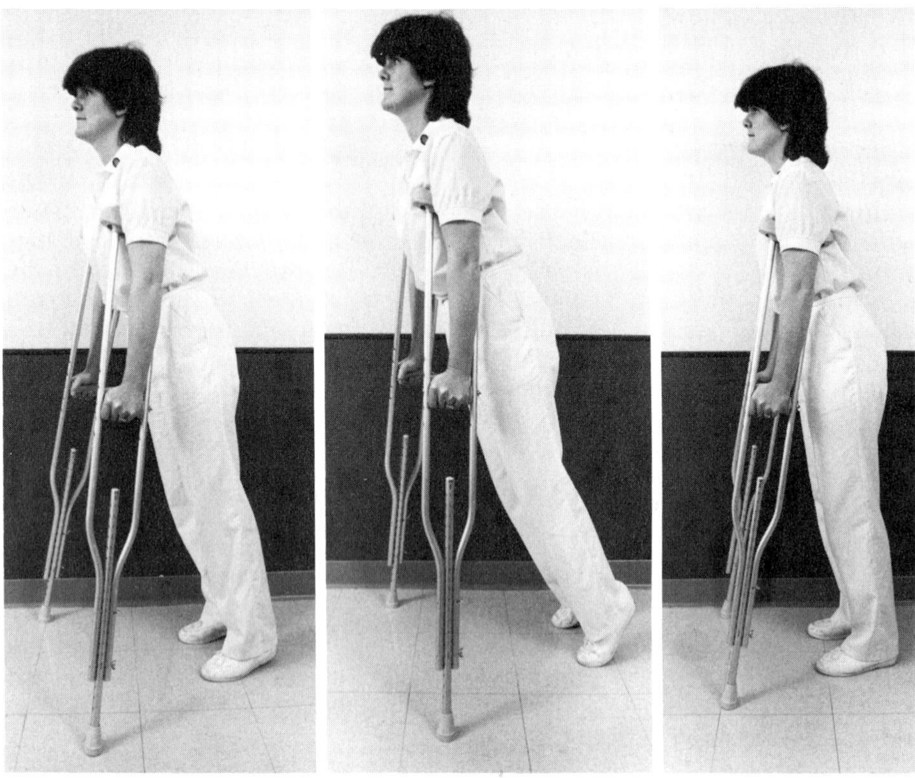

F

Figure 26–11 *Continued E,* Swing-through gait, used when there is adequate balance and muscle power in the arms and legs. The tripod position is attained by two crutches and both feet together as one. The two crutches are moved forward, followed by both feet, which are swung through as the body weight is borne by the hands on the handpieces. The position is then one of a reversed tripod.

F, Swing-to gait, which is similar to but slower than the swing-through gait. From the tripod position, the body is swung forward to the crutches while the feet are brought to the area behind the crutches. The crutches and feet are not ever allowed to be even; to do so would cause loss of balance. The feet and crutches must form a tripod.

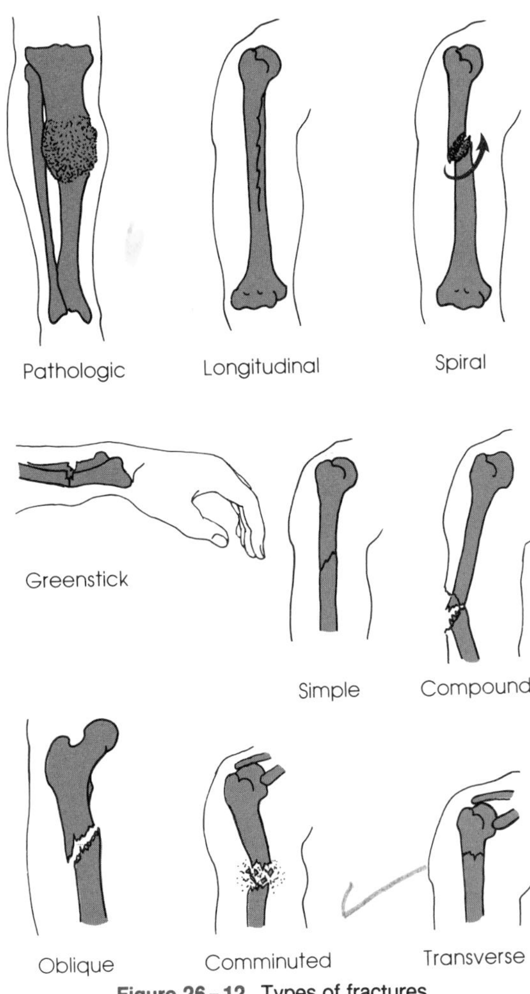

Figure 26-12 Types of fractures.

flat for 24 hours. When the patient is turned to a side-lying position, the spine must be kept straight, with the knees flexed and drawn up toward the chest. The hips are kept abducted by inserting a pillow between the knees. The dressing should be inspected frequently for bleeding or cerebrospinal fluid leak. Signs of either blood or cerebrospinal fluid (CSF) should be reported immediately. An assessment of motor and neurologic function of the trunk and extremities is done every 2 to 4 hours. A circulation check is performed at the same time.

Before discharge, a review of allowed activity and restrictions is given along with printed instructions for wound care. Usually sitting for prolonged periods and bending over are prohibited. Lifting of more than five pounds is forbidden, and long flights of stairs should be avoided. A review of good body mechanics is also pertinent before discharge. A very firm mattress should be used for sleep.

COMPLICATIONS

The healing of a fracture can be impeded by improper alignment and inadequate immobilization of the bone. Malalignment almost inevitably leads to some permanent deformity. Inadequate immobilization of the bone allows continued twisting, shearing, and abnormal stresses that prohibit a strong bony union.

Infection

Infection of the fracture site is probably the most serious impediment to healing. It is of special concern in open comminuted fractures. Systemic infections, inadequate levels of serum calcium and phosphorus, vitamin deficiency, and generalized atherosclerosis—which deprives the healing site of adequate blood supply—also can complicate a fracture by delaying healing. It is important to monitor the patient's temperature and white blood cell (WBC) count for elevations and to carefully monitor the appearance of the area for redness, swelling, heat, or purulent drainage.

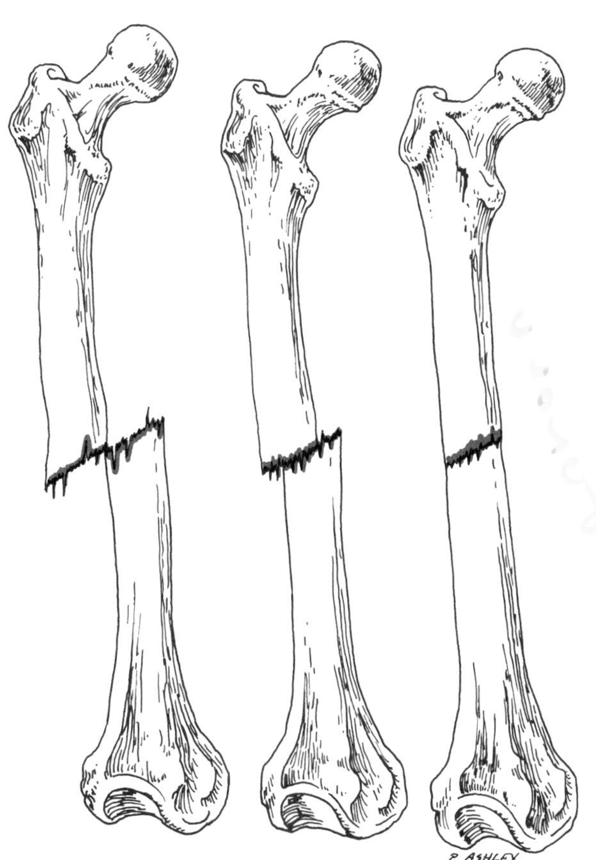

Figure 26-13 Reduction of a fractured bone. A gradual pull is exerted on the distal (lower) fragment of the bone until it is in alignment with the proximal fragment.

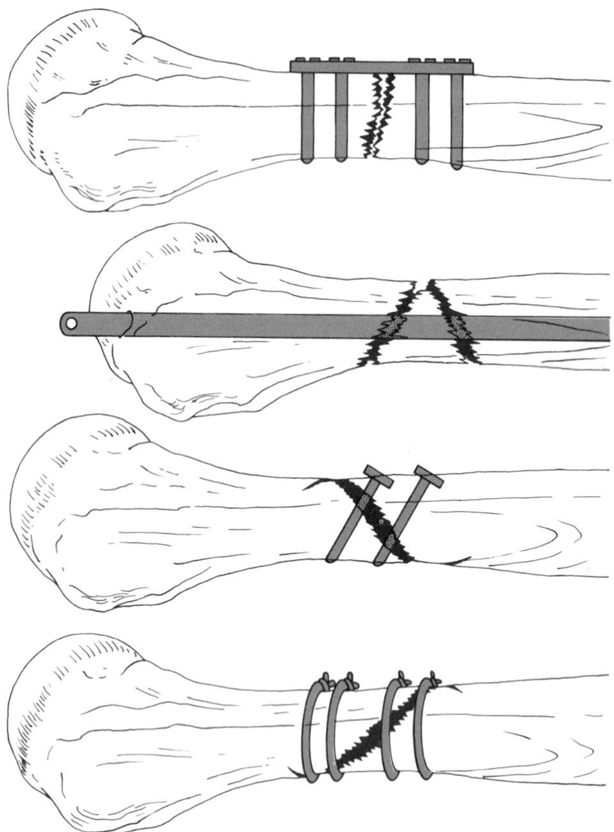

Figure 26-14 Illustrations of various methods of internal fixation, using plates, pins, nails, or screws to hold fragments of bone in place.

Fat Embolism

Fat embolism can be one of the most serious complications of a fracture of bony tissue that has an abundance of marrow fat (e.g., the long bones, pelvis, and ribs). A high percentage of patients with multiple fractures resulting from severe trauma die from this complication. It occurs at any age but is most commonly seen in young men age 20 to 40 and in older persons between 70 and 80 years of age. Not all fat emboli are fatal. To be life-threatening, the fat globules released when a bone is fractured must be large enough or sufficient in number to partially or completely occlude a blood vessel. The fat embolism arises from injury of the fat-bearing bone marrow and rupture of small venules in the area, thus permitting the entrance of fat globules into the circulation. Embolism, if it occurs, happens within 48 hours of fracture.

The first sign of fat embolism is usually respiratory distress accompanied by hypertension, tachypnea, fever, and petechiae (a measles-like rash over the neck, upper arms, chest, or abdomen). Signs must be reported immediately, as there is about an 80% mortality rate from this complication.

The nurse should stay with the patient; put him in a high Fowler's position, if possible, to ease the dyspnea; remain calm; begin oxygen administration at 2 to 3 L/min if it is available; and summon the doctor immediately.

Compartment Syndrome

Compartment syndrome occurs in one or more muscle compartments of the extremities. It is caused by external or internal pressure and seriously restricts circulation to the area. External pressure can occur from dressings or casts that are too tight. Internal pressure occurs from excessive IV fluid infusion, inflammation, and edema (a shifting of fluid from the vascular spaces to the intercellular spaces). The increased fluid puts pressure on the tissues, nerves, and blood vessels, thereby decreasing blood flow. Considerable pain results.

Signs and symptoms of compartment syndrome include edema, pain, pallor, tingling, paresthesia, numbness, weak pulse, cyanosis, paresis, and se-

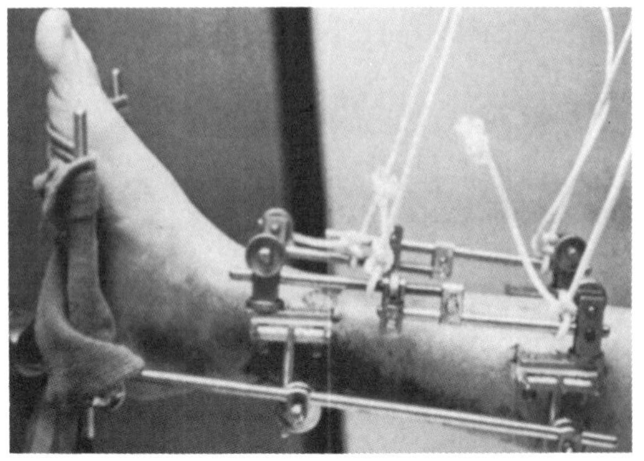

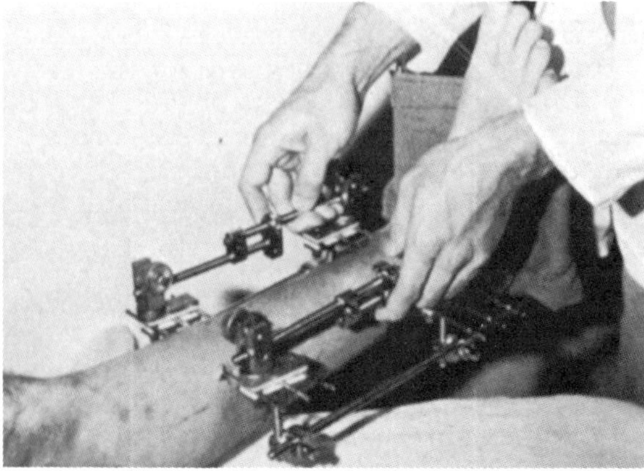

Figure 26-15 External fixator. Heavy pins or wires are inserted through the fractured bone and attached to an external frame that provides stability and immobilization of the bone fragments. Ropes are attached to an overhead frame to elevate the limb during the immediate postoperative period.
(From Kryschysen, P. L., and Fischer, D. A.: External fixation for complicated fractures. Am. J. Nurs., Feb., 1980, p. 258.)

vere pain. The pressure can cause permanent tissue and nerve damage if unrelieved. The physician should be notified immediately if this complication is suspected.

Surgical fasciotomy (linear incisions in the fascia) may be necessary to relieve the pressure on the nerves and blood vessels.

NURSING ASSESSMENT AND INTERVENTION

The emergency treatment and nursing care of fractures consist of preventing shock and hemorrhage and the immediate immobilization of the part to avoid unnecessary damage to the soft tissue adjacent to the fracture.

For the emergency care of a possible fracture, the reader is referred to Chapter 36.

After an x-ray film of the injured part has been made and the type of fracture and extent of damage have been established, the physician will decide which method to use in reducing the fracture and providing immobilization. Assessment and appropriate intervention for problems associated with reduction and immobilization of a fracture are summarized in Table 26–3.

The nurse should assess for signs of infection, sensation, and motor function beyond the fracture and for adequate circulation at least once each shift. When a fracture is fresh, this assessment should be performed every 2 to 4 hours. The cast should be inspected for problems such as flattened areas, soft spots, cracking, and crumbling. Traction devices must be assessed to see that they are in correct position and that the weights are hanging free. The patient's body position should be assessed for proper alignment.

Every immobilized patient should be consciously assessed for the various problems of immobility. The most commonly found problems include skin breakdown, urinary tract infection or stones, and constipation. In the elderly patient, respiratory problems are also common and can be prevented by scheduled coughing and deep breathing or the use of incentive spirometers.

Attention to pain control is important, espe-

TABLE 26–3 PROBLEMS ASSOCIATED WITH REDUCTION AND IMMOBILIZATION OF FRACTURE

Problem	Assessment	Intervention
Increased pressure within a fascial compartment	Increased pain when toes or fingers are passively moved Numbness, loss of sensation, progressive neurovascular deficit	Two-point discrimination test Capillary refill time test
Inadequate immobilization	Patient reports grating sensation, constant, unrelenting pain, especially with motion	Notify physician A change in immobilization device is necessary
Migration of traction pin	Pain at site of insertion Stretching of skin at pin site (tenting)	Pin may need to be replaced
Venous thrombosis	Diffuse pain Swelling of limb Tenderness Engorged veins Increased warmth of affect limb	Elevate affected limb Report to physician
Infection of pin site and fracture site	Dull pain, increasing in severity Tenderness, fever, purulent drainage, foul odor	Initiate skin and wound care routine Culture wound Notify physician for antibiotic and possibly replacement of pin
Fat embolism	Disorientation Elevated pulse rate and temperature Tachypnea, dyspnea, rales and wheezing Petechial rash, lesions do not blanch with pressure	Notify physician promptly; condition can be fatal

cially when the patient is adjusting to traction or a new cast. It is essential to try to keep the patient's mind occupied, as boredom can greatly increase discomfort.

A patient with a fracture is often immobilized for an extended period, which interferes with his usual roles. The patient may be very worried about his usual responsibilities and about his job and finances. Allowing him to ventilate his concerns and fears and then assisting him in solving problems can often bring him some peace of mind.

AMPUTATION

About 80% of all limb amputations involve lower extremities. The most common reasons for amputation of a lower limb are related to peripheral vascular disease and resultant gangrene. Other conditions necessitating lower limb amputation include severe trauma, malignancy, and congenital defects (Fig. 26–16).

About 70% of upper extremity amputations are brought on by crushing blows, thermal and electric burns, and severe lacerations. Vasospastic disease, malignancy, and infection also can necessitate amputation of an upper extremity.

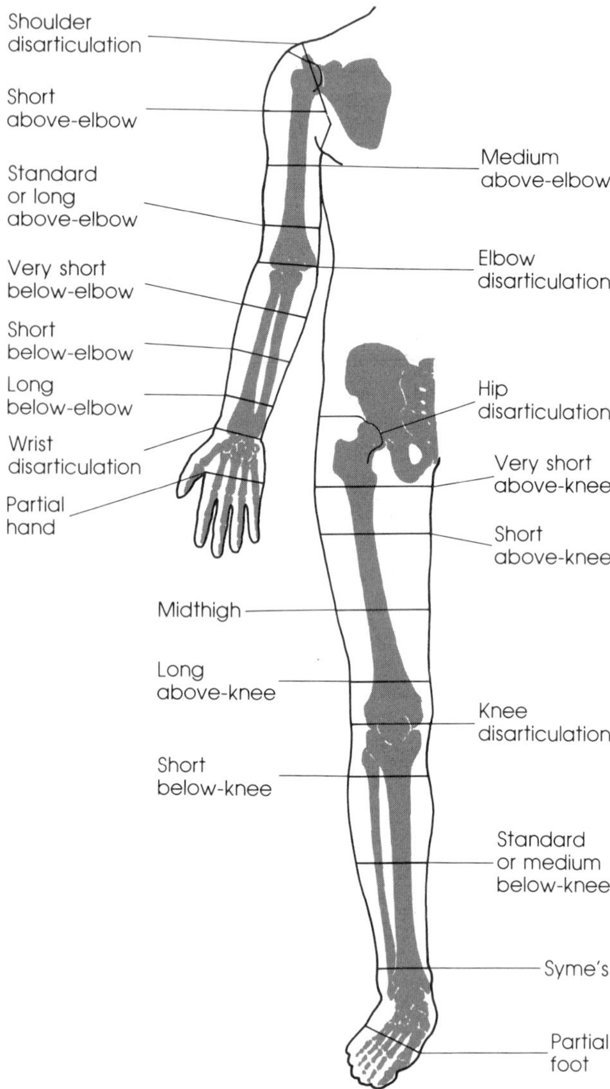

Figure 26–16 Levels of amputation of the upper and lower extremities.

PREOPERATIVE CARE

Unless the amputation of a limb is an emergeny procedure, the patient is prepared physically and psychologically for the removal of all or part of the extremity. If at all possible, the patient should participate in the decision to amputate a limb. He should understand the need for the amputation and have opportunity to discuss realistic goals of rehabilitation with several members of the health care team.

Although the loss of a limb can be very difficult for the patient and his family to accept, they can find some consolation in knowing that the procedure is absolutely necessary and that every effort will be made to take full advantage of the patient's remaining resources. The patient may experience stages of denial, anger, and so on, similar to those of the dying process as discussed in Chapter 14. In a sense, the patient must recognize the death of his former "self," work his way through the grief process, and move toward acceptance of a new body image.

A member of the rehabilitation team should discuss with the patient what he can expect postoperatively in regard to pain, immobility, and readjustment to caring for himself.

"Phantom sensations" in the limb that has been removed are not unusual. There is no scientific explanation for these sensations, but they are nonetheless real to the amputee who experiences them.

If the patient is informed preoperatively that the sensations are not unusual, are not considered a psychiatric problem, and will be dealt with as the reality that they most certainly are, he will be less apprehensive about asking for help should the problem arise.

Physical preparation of the patient includes muscle strengthening exercises if there is any hope that the patient can be active following amputation. These exercises are the first stages of the rehabilitation process, designed to help the patient achieve independence as rapidly as possible.

IMMEDIATE POSTOPERATIVE CARE

When the patient returns to his room from the surgical suite, the two most immediate problems are hemorrhage and edema. To combat these problems, the stump is elevated for 24 to 48 hours. A lower extremity is not elevated for more than 48 hours because of the danger of hip contractures, which would prohibit rehabilitation efforts to achieve ambulation.

The stump is checked at frequent intervals to determine whether bleeding is excessive. A large tourniquet is kept at the bedside in case severe hemorrhage occurs. Fresh bleeding onto the dressing should be reported immediately.

Postoperative wound care is essentially the same as that discussed in Chapter 12. Wound drainage usually is handled with a Hemovac or similar wound drainage system.

Phantom limb sensations, mentioned earlier, may or may not be painful but are quite disconcerting if the patient has not been previously warned that they may occur. There is no satisfactory solution to this problem, but it does help for the patient to know that the sensations are not unusual.

Three alternative modes for the management of the stump after amputation are (1) soft dressing with delayed prosthetic fitting, (2) rigid plaster dressing and early prosthetic fitting, and (3) rigid plaster dressing and immediate prosthetic fitting.

Each method has its particular advantages and disadvantages. If a soft dressing is used, it is important that the stump be wrapped properly to control edema and ensure proper shrinkage of the stump for later fitting of a prosthesis.

Many complications can be avoided if the patient is able to get up and about early in the postoperative period. However, weight bearing before the stump is adequately healed can cause weakening of the suture line and rupturing of the operative wound. Patients with amputations below the knee are better able to begin early walking and weight bearing than are those whose limb has been amputated above the knee.

The bedridden patient who has had a lower extremity amputation should be encouraged to lie on his abdomen several hours each day. This will help prevent joint contractures. He also will require proper positioning to prevent *abduction* contractures. Range-of-motion exercises are carried out with the amputee as with any patient who must be protected from the disabilities of immobility.

When a lower limb has been removed, the patient must learn how to balance himself on one leg, how to stoop and bend over without losing his balance, and how to use his back muscles to maintain good posture while wearing an artificial limb.

REHABILITATION

Most surgeons agree that unless there are complicating factors, the most important factor in successful rehabilitation of the amputee is early ambulation, so that the patient can see for himself that he can eventually become independent once again.

Usually a physical therapist and occupational therapist work with the patient who has suffered an amputation to help him regain mobility, confidence, and the ability to handle tasks of daily living. The nurse then assists with practice at bathing, shaving, dressing, etc. The nurse's attitude and encouragement can make a positive difference in the adjustment the patient makes to his situation.

Elderly and chronically ill amputees can benefit from a positive yet realistic approach to their problems. The nurse must, of course, avoid giving false hopes or unreal assurances that everything is going to be all right. It is insulting to the patient to tell him that he will be "just like new again" when he obviously can't be restored to his former state of health. The focus of attention should be on what the patient can do for himself and on what strengths he has in his favor. By helping her patient find short-range goals that can be accomplished without great difficulty and that indicate progress toward independence, the nurse can be of real help to the amputee. For example, she can guide him toward devising ways in which he can meet his own personal needs, such as bathing and shaving. Later, he can be encouraged to sit up, exercise his other limbs, and assist with changing his dressing. Finally, she can set for him the goal of wearing a prosthesis successfully and walking without assistance. Types of lower-limb and upper-limb prostheses are shown in Figures 26-17 and 26-18.

OVERUSE AND TORSION INJURIES

Sprains, strains, and dislocations are the kinds of injuries likely to occur when ligaments, muscles, and joints are subjected to undue stress, twisting, or a physical blow to the joint. A summary of each type of injury of this kind is presented below.

SPRAIN

A sprain is defined as a partial or complete tearing of the ligaments that hold various bones together to form a joint.

- **Most common sites:** Ankle and knee.
- **Symptoms:** *Grade 1* (mild)—tenderness at site; minimal swelling and loss of function; no abnormal motion.

  Grade 2 (moderate)—more severe pain, especially with weight bearing; swelling and bleeding into joint; some loss of function.

  Grade 3 (severe, complete tearing of fibers)—pain may be less severe, but swelling, loss of function, bleeding into joint, and loss of function more marked.
- **Intervention:** Apply ice immediately after injury and at 20- to 30-minute intervals for

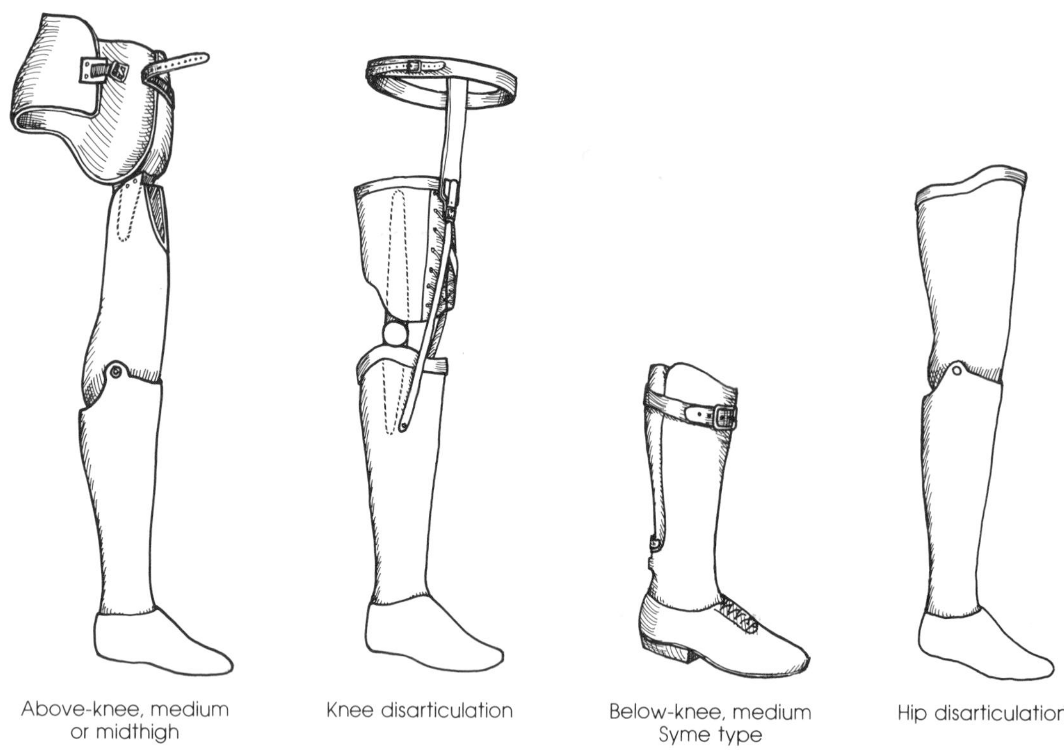

Figure 26-17 Types of lower extremity prostheses.

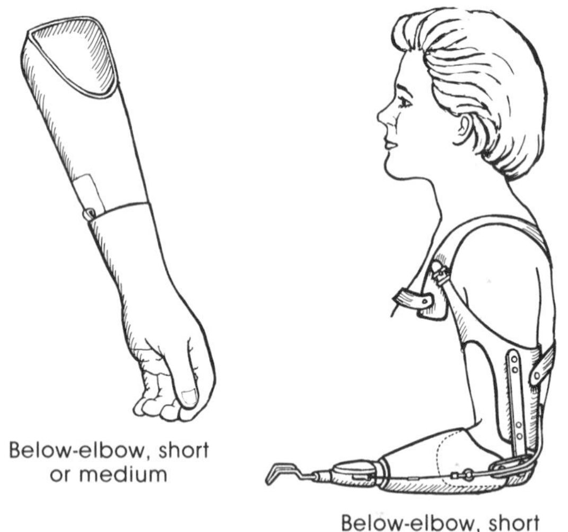

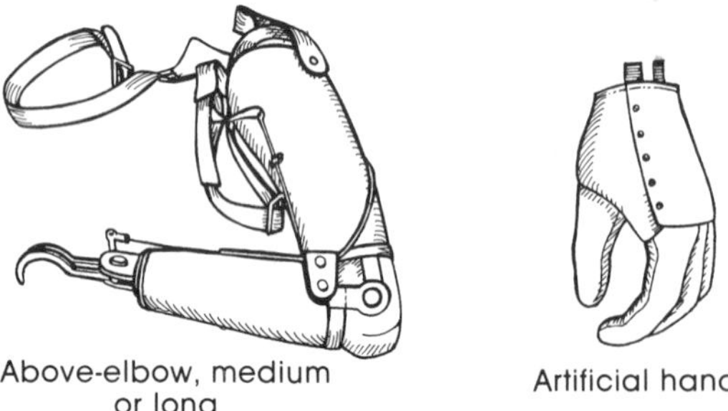

Figure 26-18 Types of upper limb prostheses.

first 24 to 36 hours. Wrap tightly, being careful not to cut off circulation, and elevate the injured part. These measures can help minimize swelling and pain and stabilize the joint in proper alignment. The goal of treatment is to protect the ligament until it heals by scarring. Ligaments do not "grow" back together. Braces or supports are used only until a joint has been strengthened. If a joint is immobilized too long and muscles are not exercised, muscle atrophy, which begins in a matter of days, can cause permanent disability. In some cases surgical repair may be necessary.

STRAIN

A strain is defined as a pulling or tearing of either muscle or tendon or both.

- **Most common sites:** Hamstrings, quadriceps, and calf muscles.
- **Symptoms:** History of overexertion; soft tissue swelling and pain; bleeding (ecchymosis, hemorrhagic spot) present if muscle is torn.
- **Intervention:** Immediately apply ice and compression and rest the part. Surgical repair may be necessary.

DISLOCATION

A dislocation is defined as stretching and tearing of ligaments around a joint with complete displacement of a bone. *Subluxation* is a partial dislocation.

- **Most common sites:** Shoulder, knee, temporomandibular joint.
- **Symptoms:** History of an outside force pushing from certain direction; severe pain aggravated by motion of joint; muscle spasm; abnormal appearance of joint. A radiograph will reveal displacement of bone.
- **Intervention:** Reduction of displacement under anesthesia or manual or spontaneous reduction. Stabilization of joint and rehabilitation to minimize muscular atrophy and strengthen joint.

OSTEOMYELITIS

Osteomyelitis is a bacterial infection of the bone. The causative organism is most often *Staphylococcus aureus*, which enters the blood stream from a distant focus of infection such as a boil or furuncle or from an open wound, as in an open (compound) fracture. It occurs most often in children under the age of 15 and is usually found in the tibia or fibula, but it can also occur in patients at any age.

SYMPTOMS

Osteomyelitis has a sudden onset with severe pain and marked tenderness at the site, high fever with chills, swelling of adjacent soft parts, headache, and malaise.

DIAGNOSIS

Diagnosis of osteomyelitis is made on the basis of (1) laboratory findings indicating an acute infection—for example, high sedimentation rate and white cell count; (2) radiographs, which may show bone destruction 7 to 10 days after onset of the disease; (3) history of injury to the part, open fracture, boils, furuncles, or other infections; and (4) biopsy, in which the bone sample exhibits signs of necrosis.

MEDICAL TREATMENT AND NURSING INTERVENTION

The earlier the condition is diagnosed and treatment is begun, the better the prognosis for the patient with osteomyelitis, as it can be difficult to eradicate. General treatment and nursing care are aimed at improving and maintaining the physical condition of the patient through adequate fluid, mineral, and vitamin intake. Specific treatment includes elimination of the infection through the use of long-term antibiotics and immobilization of the affected limb for complete rest. In some unusually stubborn infections, this treatment is not adequate, and surgical incision for drainage of the abscess and removal of dead bone and debris from the site of infection is necessary. The care of a patient with an infection is presented in Chapter 6.

INFLAMMATORY DISORDERS: ARTHRITIS

The word *arthritis*, translated literally, means inflammation of a joint. Most laypersons use the term to cover any kind of joint disease; however, specialists in the treatment of arthritis limit its meaning to diseases of the joint that are the result of inflammatory changes. There are approximately 100 different types of arthritis, ranging from hereditary disorders such as gouty arthritis and hemophilic arthritis to the more common types in which the exact cause is known (Table 26–4).

In adults, the two most prevalent forms of arthritis are osteoarthritis and rheumatoid arthritis. A comparison of these two types of arthritis is shown in Table 26–5.

All forms of arthritis are capable of producing joint pain and disability. Medical management, surgical procedures, and nursing interventions are intended to minimize the problems associated with inflammatory changes in the joint, deformities and limitation of motion, and the systemic reactions to these pathologic changes.

OSTEOARTHRITIS

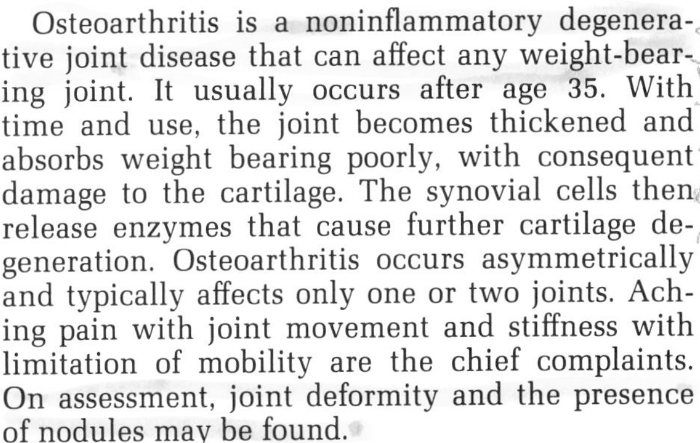

Osteoarthritis is a noninflammatory degenerative joint disease that can affect any weight-bearing joint. It usually occurs after age 35. With time and use, the joint becomes thickened and absorbs weight bearing poorly, with consequent damage to the cartilage. The synovial cells then release enzymes that cause further cartilage degeneration. Osteoarthritis occurs asymmetrically and typically affects only one or two joints. Aching pain with joint movement and stiffness with limitation of mobility are the chief complaints. On assessment, joint deformity and the presence of nodules may be found.

Treatment consists of pain management and maintenance of joint function. Salicylates or nonsteroidal antiinflammatory drugs (NSAIDs) may be used. Corticosteroid injection into the joint is performed if oral medication does not control the problem. Exercises for joint mobility are encouraged. Surgery or joint replacement may be done to relieve severe pain and improve mobility. The hip and knee are the most common sites for joint replacement.

Nursing interventions for osteoarthritis include teaching the patient to balance exercise and rest, moist heat application, the use of imagery and diversion to reduce pain, and encouragement to

TABLE 26-4 ARA NOMENCLATURE AND CLASSIFICATION OF ARTHRITIS AND RHEUMATISM (TENTATIVE)

I. Diffuse connective tissue diseases
  A. Rheumatoid arthritis
  B. Juvenile rheumatoid arthritis
    1. Systemic onset (Still's disease)
    2. Polyarticular onset
    3. Pauciarticular onset
  C. Systemic lupus erythematosus
  D. Systemic sclerosis
  E. Polymyositis/dermatomyositis
  F. Necrotizing vasculitis and other vasculopathies
    1. Polyarteritis nodosa group (includes hepatitis B associated arteritis and Churg-Strauss allergic granulomatosis)
    2. Hypersensitivity vasculitis (includes Henoch-Schönlein purpura, hypocomplementemic cutaneous vasculitis, and others)
    3. Wegener's granulomatosis
    4. Giant cell arteritis
      a. Temporal arteritis
      b. Takayasu's arteritis
    5. Mucocutaneous lymph node syndrome (Kawasaki disease)
    6. Behçet's disease
    7. Cryoglobulinemia
    8. Juvenile dermatomyositis
  G. Sjögren's syndrome
  H. Overlap syndromes (includes undifferentiated and mixed connective tissue disease)
  I. Others (includes polymyalgia rheumatica, panniculitis (Weber-Christian disease), erythema nodosum, relapsing polychondritis, diffuse fasciitis with eosinophilia, adult onset Still's disease)
II. Arthritis associated with spondylitis
  A. Ankylosing spondylitis
  B. Reiter's syndrome
  C. Psoriatic arthritis
  D. Arthritis associated with chronic inflammatory bowel disease
III. Degenerative joint disease (osteoarthritis, osteoarthrosis)
  A. Primary (includes erosive osteoarthritis)
  B. Secondary
IV. Arthritis, tenosynovitis, and bursitis associated with infectious agents
  A. Direct
    1. Bacterial
      a. Gram-positive cocci (staphylococcus and others)
      b. Gram-negative cocci (gonococcus and others)
      c. Gram-negative rods
      d. Mycobacteria
      e. Spirochetes including Lyme disease
      f. Others including leprosy and mycoplasma
    2. Viral including hepatitis
    3. Fungal
    4. Parasitic
    5. Unknown, suspected (Whipple's disease)
  B. Indirect (reactive)
    1. Bacterial (includes acute rheumatic fever, intestinal bypass, postdysenteric—shigella, yersinia, and others)
    2. Viral (hepatitis B)
V. Metabolic and endocrine diseases associated with rheumatic states
  A. Crystal-induced conditions
    1. Monosodium urate (gout)
    2. Calcium pyrophosphate dihydrate (pseudogout, chondrocalcinosis)
    3. Apatite and other basic calcium phosphates
    4. Oxalate
  B. Biochemical abnormalities
    1. Amyloidosis
    2. Vitamin C deficiency (scurvy)
    3. Specific enzyme-deficiency states (includes Fabry's, Farber's, and others)
    4. Hyperlipoproteinemias (types II, IIa, IV, others)

TABLE 26-4 ARA NOMENCLATURE AND CLASSIFICATION OF ARTHRITIS AND RHEUMATISM (TENTATIVE) *Continued*

5. Mucopolysaccharidoses
6. Hemoglobinopathies (SS disease and others)
7. True connective tissue disorders (Ehlers-Danlos, Marfan's, osteogenesis imperfecta, pseudoxanthoma elasticum, and others)
8. Hemochromatosis
9. Wilson's disease (hepatolenticular degeneration)
10. Ochronosis (alkaptonuria)
11. Gaucher's disease
12. Others

C. Endocrine diseases
1. Diabetes mellitus
2. Acromegaly
3. Hyperparathyroidism
4. Thyroid disease (hyperthyroidism, hypothyroidism, thyroiditis)
5. Others

D. Immunodeficiency diseases, primary immunodeficiency, acquired immunodeficiency syndrome (AIDS)

E. Other hereditary disorders
1. Arthrogryposis multiplex congenita
2. Hypermobility syndromes
3. Myositis ossificans progressiva

VI. Neoplasms
A. Primary (e.g., synovioma, synoviosarcoma)
B. Metastatic
C. Multiple myeloma
D. Leukemia and lymphoma
E. Villonodular synovitis
F. Osteochondromatosis
G. Other

VII. Neuropathic disorders
A. Charcot joints
B. Compression neuropathies
1. Peripheral entrapment (carpal tunnel syndrome and others)
2. Radiculopathy
3. Spinal stenosis
C. Reflex sympathetic dystrophy
D. Others

VIII. Bone, periosteal, and cartilage disorders associated with articular manifestations
A. Osteoporosis
1. Generalized
2. Localized (regional and transient)
B. Osteomalacia
C. Hypertrophic osteoarthropathy
D. Diffuse idiopathic skeletal hyperostosis (includes ankylosing vertebral hyperostosis—Forestier's disease)
E. Osteitis
1. Generalized (osteitis deformans—Paget's disease of bone)
2. Localized (osteitis condensans ilii; osteitis pubis)
F. Osteonecrosis
G. Osteochondritis (osteochondritis dissecans)
H. Bone and joint dysplasias
I. Slipped capital femoral epiphysis
J. Costochondritis (includes Tietze's syndrome)
K. Osteolysis and chondrolysis
L. Osteomyelitis

IX. Nonarticular rheumatism
A. Myofascial pain syndromes
1. Generalized (fibrositis, fibromyalgia)
2. Regional
B. Low back pain and intervertebral disc disorders
C. Tendinitis (tenosynovitis) and/or bursitis
1. Subacromial/subdeltoid bursitis
2. Bicipital tendinitis, tenosynovitis
3. Olecranon bursitis

Table continued on following page

TABLE 26–4 **ARA NOMENCLATURE AND CLASSIFICATION OF ARTHRITIS AND RHEUMATISM (TENTATIVE)** *Continued*

4. Epicondylitis, medial or lateral humeral
5. DeQuervain's tenosynovitis
6. Adhesive capsulitis of the shoulder (frozen shoulder)
7. Trigger finger
8. Other

D. Ganglion cysts
E. Fasciitis
F. Chronic ligament and muscle strain
G. Vasomotor disorders
  1. Erythromelalgia
  2. Raynaud's disease or phenomenon
H. Miscellaneous pain syndromes (includes weather sensitivity, psychogenic rheumatism)

X. Miscellaneous disorders
  A. Disorders frequently associated with arthritis
    1. Trauma (the result of direct trauma)
    2. Internal derangement of joints
    3. Pancreatic disease
    4. Sarcoidosis
    5. Palindromic rheumatism
    6. Intermittent hydrarthrosis
    7. Erythema nodosum
    8. Hemophilia
  B. Other conditions
    1. Multicentric reticulohistiocytosis (nodular panniculitis)
    2. Familial Mediterranean fever
    3. Goodpasture's syndrome
    4. Chronic active hepatitis
    5. Drug-induced rheumatic syndromes
    6. Dialysis-associated syndromes
    7. Foreign body synovitis
    8. Acne and hydradenitis suppurative
    9. Pustulosis palmaris et plantaris
    10. Sweet's syndrome
    11. Other

maintain weight within normal limits to decrease joint stress.

RHEUMATOID ARTHRITIS

Rheumatoid arthritis is an inflammatory disease of the joints. It most frequently begins between age 25 and 55. There is a familial tendency. The cause is not known, but it is thought that it is the result of an autoimmune defect or an infectious agent.

The signs and symptoms of rheumatoid arthritis are joint pain, warmth, edema, limitation of motion, and multiple joint stiffness in the morning. The joints of the hands, wrists, and feet are the most commonly affected, and involvement is usually symmetrical. Subcutaneous nodules may appear over bony prominences. Systemic symptoms of low-grade fever, weight loss, and malaise also occur. Considerable joint deformity and consequent dysfunction can occur.

MEDICAL TREATMENT

Treatment is aimed at pain relief, minimization of joint destruction, and the promotion of joint function. Rest and exercise, medication, immobilization with splints and other supportive devices during periods of severe inflammation, and hot and cold treatments are standard. Medications include salicylates, NSAIDs, corticosteroids, antimalarial drugs, methotrexate, gold compounds, and penicillamine. Surgical joint repair or replacement can be done to reduce pain and improve mobility.

Medications

There is a wide selection of drugs from which the physician can choose to treat the various forms of arthritis. There is no drug that will cure the disease, however, and medication is but one part of the overall regimen of treatment. NSAIDs

TABLE 26–5 **COMPARISON OF RHEUMATOID ARTHRITIS AND OSTEOARTHRITIS**

Characteristic	Rheumatoid Arthritis	Osteoarthritis
Definition	A systemic disease, but pathologic changes and disability result from chronic inflammation of the joints.	A progressive degenerative joint disease.
Pathology	Chronic inflammation of synovial membranes and formation of chronic granulation tissue (pannus) in the joint. Pannus capable of eroding cartilage in joints and spreading to bone, ligaments, and tendons.	Microscopic changes in the cartilage in the joint. Eventually there is loss of cartilage, bony enlargement, and malalignment of joints.
Etiology	Unknown. Evidence that the pathologic changes are immunologic.	Unknown. May be caused by "wear and tear" of aging.
Rheumatoid factors (autoantibodies)	Usually present.	Usually absent.
Age at onset	30 to 40 years.	50 to 60 years; rarely before 40.
Weight	Normal or underweight.	Usually overweight.
General state of health	Usually anemic, "chronically ill." Low-grade fever and slight leukocytosis.	Well nourished.
Appearance of joints	Early; soft tissue swelling. Late: ankylosis: extreme deformity.	Early: slight joint enlargement. Late: enlargement more pronounced, slight limitation of motion.
	Joint involvement usually symmetric and generalized.	Joints usually involved are weight bearing; spine, hips, and knees.
Muscles	Pronounced muscular atrophy, particularly in later stages.	Usually not affected.
Other	Morning stiffness, pain on motion, swelling and tenderness of joints. Subcutaneous nodules. Typical rheumatoid changes seen on radiograph.	Stiffness, relieved by moderate motion; joint malalignment. Symptoms increase in cold, wet weather.

are usually the first kind of agents used for arthritis. Of these, aspirin is the drug of choice if the patient can tolerate it. The amount of aspirin prescribed is quite large and ranges from 15 to 25 tablets a day. Other drugs in the NSAID group include salicylates such as sodium salicylate, indomethacin (Indocin), phenylbutazone (Butazolidin), ibuprofen (Motrin), ketoprofen (Orudis), meclofenamate (Meclomen), naproxen (Naprosyn), sulindac (Clinoril), fenoprofen (Nalfon), piroxicam (Feldene), and diclofenac (Voltaren).

The greatest disadvantage of these drugs is that they can cause serious gastrointestinal irritation, ulceration, and bleeding. Some of the NSAIDs are combined with other agents or are specially coated to minimize adverse gastrointestinal side effects. These agents include aspirin compounded with antacids (Ascriptin), enteric-coated aspirin (Ecotrin) and choline salicylate (Trilisate). Although these newer agents are associated with a lower incidence of GI bleeding and heartburn, they are more expensive than plain aspirin.

Although the major difficulty with NSAIDs is gastrointestinal intolerance, all of the agents can be toxic to the liver, kidney, and central nervous system. Blood dyscrasias, tinnitus, and hearing loss also can occur. Only a small percentage of patients suffer toxicity to NSAIDs, but the side effects can be serious and sometimes permanent. If early signs of toxicity appear, they should be reported promptly to the physician.

In selected cases of rheumatoid arthritis that do not respond to other forms of drug therapy, more potent drugs may be prescribed. Although these medications provide periods of remission, they also have some serious side effects in most patients. Remissive agents included in this group of drugs include gold, D-penicillamine (Depen,

Cuprimine), hydroxychloroquine (Plaquenil), and methotrexate.

Systemic corticosteroids have a profound antiinflammatory effect on arthritis. They were once thought to be "miracle drugs" for treatment of arthritis, but their use is now questioned by many authorities. Their antiinflammatory action tends to diminish over a period of time, thus requiring higher doses to obtain the same results. Additionally, long-term steroid therapy exposes the patient to some rather severe side effects. These include diabetes mellitus, osteoporosis, hypertension, acne, and weight gain. Because of these and other problems associated with steriod therapy, long-term oral steroid preparations are reserved for patients who cannot find relief from other drugs.

The injection of steroids directly into a joint (intraarticular administration) has been used successfully in the treatment of painful flare-ups, shortening the period of exacerbation and relieving pain and other symptoms. When intraarticular steroid therapy is used, it is recommended that not more than three or four doses be injected into any joint within 1 year's time.

Immunosuppressive therapy is limited to patients who do not respond to other, less dangerous forms of therapy. Experimental drugs and modalities of therapy continue to be tried in an effort to find some form of treatment in which the benefits far outweigh the risks.

As with many other chronic and incurable diseases, arthritis victims are particularly vulnerable to unproven claims for a cure and to outright quackery. Because rheumatoid arthritis sometimes goes into spontaneous remission, many patients who undergo an unorthodox treatment at the same time their disease is in remission give credit for their improvement to the treatment. Later, when their symptoms return or become worse, they are disappointed and angry and, many times, financially worse off for their experience. Studies have shown that, as a group, arthritics have a stronger positive placebo effect to medications than other people. This probably is one reason that fraudulent claims for cures are so successful in their appeal to many victims of arthritis.

SURGICAL INTERVENTION AND ORTHOPEDIC DEVICES

In the past, surgical intervention was reserved for patients who already had suffered severe joint deformity and loss of motion. There is now a trend toward the use of surgery in the early stages of the disease to prevent or at least modify deformities and mechanical abnormalities.

One such surgical procedure is synovectomy, which is the excision of the synovial membrane of a joint. The goal of synovectomy is to interrupt the destructive inflammatory process that eventually led to ankylosis and invasion of surrounding cartilage and bone tissues.

Surgical repair of a hip joint (arthoplasty) is performed when there is extensive damage and ambulation is not possible. The purpose of joint repair is to restore, improve, or maintain joint function. In cases in which it is not possible to repair the damaged hip joint, total hip replacement may be done. A similar operation can be done on the knee joint.

Braces, splints, and casts sometimes are used to immobilize an affected part so that it can rest during an active phase of the disease (Figs. 26–19 and 26–20). Devices that immobilize the affected joint also should allow for motion of adjacent muscles, thereby improving muscle strength and permitting more independence on the part of the patient. Braces also may be used to prevent deformities by maintaining optimal functional position of the joints.

NURSING ASSESSMENT

The manifestations of arthritis are many and varied, particularly when the diagnosis is rheumatoid arthritis. Pain, limited motion, and the chronic and incurable nature of the illness have some impact on almost every aspect of the patient's life. In order to set realistic goals and plan for their accomplishment, the nurse will need to know about the patient's social history, his personal and family health history, current status of his general health and ability to do the things he wants to do, and his experience of pain and how he has been dealing with it.

Social History

Information about the conditions under which a patient lives and works can help the nurse identify any obstacles that make it difficult or impossible for him to follow instructions and carry out his responsibilities for self-care. For example, if the patient does not have the financial resources to buy the drugs and self-help devices or lives in a crowded apartment in an unsafe neighborhood, it may be very difficult for him to obtain the medications and special apparatus he needs and to get adequate rest and appropriate exercise and maintain his indepen-

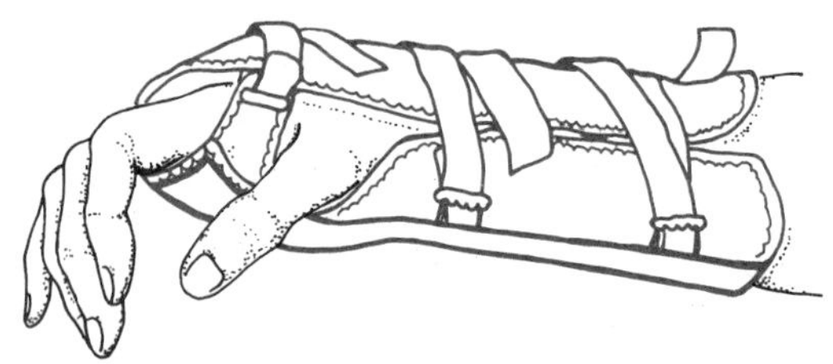

Figure 26–19 Wrist splint.

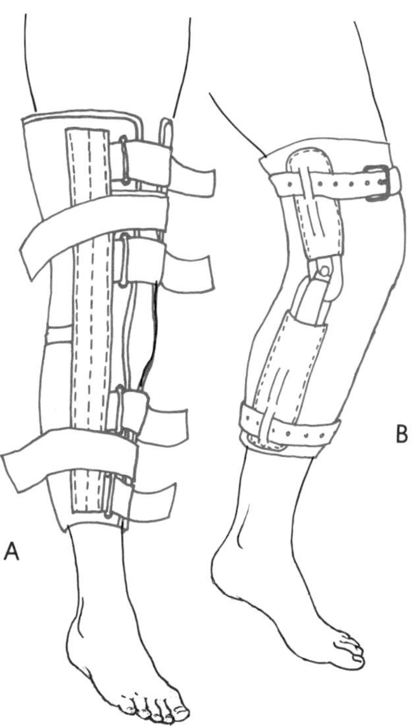

Figure 26-20 *A*, Universal knee splint with laminated canvas, loop lock closures, and rigid aluminum stays. *B*, Knee brace with surgical elastic, jointed steel braces, and leather strap top and bottom.

dence. If he has limited resources for transportation, this could limit his access to health care and discourage him from keeping appointments with the physician and nurse.

Other pertinent social history data include his former or current occupation, exposure to physical and emotional stress, and the usual climatic conditions under which he lives and works. Factors such as heat, cold, and dampness can influence the course of arthritis. Hence whether the patient's home is comfortably warm in the winter and cool in the summer can be significant to management of his symptoms.

Health History and Current State of Health

Among the many kinds of arthritis are those that tend to run in families. These include rheumatoid arthritis, osteoarthritis, and gouty and psoriatic arthritis. Familial diseases in which joint involvement can occur include systemic lupus erythematosus, inflammatory bowel disease, hemophilia, and sickle cell disease. Data related to the occurrence of these diseases in family members can help identify the type of arthritis affecting the patient.

The patient's health history also can help clarify the kind of inflammatory joint disease he has. Past infections, injuries, and such systemic diseases as those mentioned in family history are relevant to the assessment of a patient with arthritis. Perhaps more important is the patient's general health status, sense of well-being, and perception of his ability to carry out a prescribed regimen. For example, fatigue, muscle wasting, and anemia can prevent the patient from enthusiastically accepting plans for his rehabilitation. Patients who have been ill for an extended period of time could have a different attitude toward and be less motivated to participate in efforts to restore joint function than would a patient who sees himself as basically healthy.

Pain

As with any assessment of pain, the nurse is concerned with the time and circumstances surrounding its onset; conditions that aggravate, intensify, or relieve it; and a description of how it feels. Additional subjective data include the duration of the pain, whether it is continuous or intermittent, and its daily pattern (for example, whether it is worse in the morning or evening).

The patient's emotional response to his pain is significant to the development of plans and appropriate interventions to help him deal with it. He may exhibit anger, reticence in talking about it, or refusal to acknowledge it. If he is able to discuss his pain, this could give the nurse an opportunity to identify some nonproductive things he is doing to try to cope with the pain and its effects on his life. Additionally, his self-concept could interfere with his acceptance of the fact that it is no disgrace to admit that he has pain and needs help in managing it.

Objective Data

In addition to reviewing the results of recent laboratory tests such as blood analysis for anemia and leukocytosis, and erythrocyte sedimentation rate to evaluate the status of the inflammatory process, the nurse also can gather objective data by noting radiologic evaluations and the physical findings of the examining physician. In her own inspection and palpation of the affected joints she notes any swelling, warmth, redness, loss of motion, and deformity.

Evaluating the range of motion of various joints and testing for muscle strength can verify whether or not goals for self-care are realistic and attainable. Observation of gait and posture, improper use of a cane or crutches, and inappropriate shoes can reveal specific problems amenable to nursing intervention.

NURSING DIAGNOSES AND INTERVENTIONS

Nursing diagnoses common to patients with arthritis or connective tissue disease include:

- Pain.

- Chronic pain related to inflammation.
- Impaired physical mobility related to inflammation and joint destruction.
- Activity intolerance related to pain and inflammation.
- Impaired home maintenance management related to decreased mobility.
- Potential for injury related to immobility.
- Self-esteem disturbance related to altered body image.
- Self-care deficit.
- Potential impaired skin integrity related to bed rest.

Nursing interventions are aimed at providing a balance of rest and exercise, providing freedom from pain, minimizing emotional stress, preventing or correcting deformities, and maintaining or restoring function so that the patient can enjoy as much independence and mobility as possible.

Rest and Exercise

The amount of rest needed will depend on the extent of inflammation. The more inflamed a joint is, the more rest is needed; this includes rest of the whole body, as well as of the inflamed joint. Fatigue is a common problem and usually requires that the patient change his lifestyle somewhat so that he has rest periods during the day before he becomes too fatigued or exhausted. During periods of acute exacerbation of symptoms, the patient may need continuous bed rest.

During the time the patient is lying down he should maintain good body position and avoid pillows and other devices that support joints in a position of flexion. A firm mattress is recommended, with only one pillow under the head and neck.

The purpose of rest is to allow the body's natural defenses and healing powers to overcome the inflammatory process. It is necessary, however, even in the acute phase, to balance rest with exercise. The exercise program is prescribed on the basis of assessment of each patient's status, the severity of inflammation, the particular joints affected, and the patient's tolerance for activity. Because anemia and other blood dyscrasias can accompany arthritis, the fatigue experienced by a patient may be somewhat alleviated by correction of the underlying blood disorder.

Therapeutic exercise should be just that: a form of treatment that improves the patient's situation. In any exercise program it is necessary to enlist the patient's cooperation or compliance, as the exercises must be continued at home. The patient may need to be taught how to perform specific exercises so that they do not increase his pain. In many instances, doing the exercises in the right way can actually diminish discomfort. If pain persists for hours after exercises have been done, the patient's status should be reassessed and the exercise program revised. Overactivity and physical stress can contribute to the inflammatory process.

When a patient is performing routine physical activities at home, carrying out general exercise, or following a prescribed exercise program at home away from the supervision of the nurse or physical therapist, he should be aware of precautions he should take to avoid injury to his joints. These precautions are as follows:

- Always stop at the point of real pain. Some discomfort can be expected, but it should be minimal. If your joints are still hurting 1 or 2 hours after exercise, you have done too much.
- Always use your biggest muscles and strongest joints. For example, push doors open with your arm instead of your hand; carry a shoulder bag instead of a hand purse.
- Try to do only those jobs that will allow you to stop and rest if you need to when pain develops. Learn to conserve your energy to do the things you really want to do.
- Exercise in a way that doesn't put strain on the joints.
- Slow down and move slowly and smoothly. Avoid rapid, jerky movements.
- Don't lift weights.
- Let swollen, red, hot, and painful joints rest as much as possible. Don't use them any more than absolutely necessary.
- Change your body position frequently, alternating standing, sitting, and lying down.
- Set your own limits and compete with yourself, not with anyone else.

Patients can make adjustments in their exercise performance if they know their own limitations and can identify any changes that indicate consultation with a health care professional. These changes include (1) worsening of either systemic or local joint symptoms, (2) decrease in range of motion, (3) decrease in muscle strength, and (4) involvement of joints not previously affected by arthritis.

Applications of Heat and Cold

There is no hard and fast rule to follow in deciding whether heat or cold is best for treating arthritic joints. Either one may be suitable, depending on the patient's preference and the effectiveness of each. The purpose of either hot or cold applications is to minimize pain, increase joint range of motion, and improve exercise performance. In general, heat is better for subacute or chronic joint inflammation and cold is more effective in the acute phase when joints are hot, red, and obviously inflamed.

Various forms of heat therapy can be used, including moist or dry heat and superficial or deep heat. For dry heat a therapeutic infrared lamp is convenient and inexpensive for home use. For treatment of the hands, paraffin baths are effective. Wet heat can be applied by hot tub baths with the water temperature not exceeding 102°F (39°C) or by means of a towel dipped in hot water, wrung out, and applied to the joint. Whirlpool baths promote relaxation and motion with minimal pain, especially when prolonged treatment is indicated. However, immersing the whole body in warm water can cause physiologic changes in respiration and pulse rate and may be contraindicated in debilitated or elderly patients.

Whatever method of heat or cold application is used at home, the patient will need specific instructions on how to avoid injury to the skin, accidental falls, and other hazards. Information for teaching patients methods and precautions for applications of heat and cold is summarized in Table 26–6.

Diet

There is no special diet that will cure or relieve arthritis, in spite of many fraudulent claims to the contrary. The patient should eat an average, well-balanced diet with no excess or limitations in amount or types of foods. Obesity can contribute to additional stress on the weight-bearing joints and aggravate the arthritic condition. This should be explained to the patient who has a tendency to be overweight so he can be properly motivated and encouraged to lose weight and continue to keep his weight within normal limits.

Resources for Patient and Family Education

It is very easy for the arthritis patient and his family to be overwhelmed with information about the illness and what is best to do to maintain and restore function and achieve some level of independence. The Arthritis Foundation provides some excellent printed material written with the layperson in mind. "Rheumatoid Arthritis—Handbook for Patients" and "Arthritis—The Basic Facts" are available free of charge from the Arthritis Foundation, 1314 Spring St. N.W., Atlanta, GA 30309.

The Self-Help Device Office of the World Rehabilitation Fund, 400 East 34th St., New York, NY 10016, supplies information on specially designed self-help devices for arthritic patients.

Another source of information is the Arthritis Information Clearinghouse, P.O. Box 9782, Arlington, VA 22209.

GOUT

Gout is arthritis of one joint caused by high serum levels of uric acid. Uric acid crystals precipitate from the body fluids and settle in joints and connective tissue. Gout affects men more than women and generally occurs during the middle years. It is more common among populations that consume a high-protein diet. Two factors seem to be implicated: (1) a genetic increase in purine metabolism and (2) consumption of a high-purine diet or excessive alcohol. The big toe is the most common site, but many other joints can be affected.

Typical signs and symptoms are elevated serum uric acid and tight, reddened skin over an inflamed, edematous joint, accompanied by temperature and extreme pain in the joint.

Treatment during acute attacks consists of administration of NSAIDs or colchicine. Allopurinol or probenecid may be prescribed to prevent further attacks. Dietary management includes restriction of high-purine foods, alcohol, and weight control.

SYSTEMIC LUPUS ERYTHEMATOSUS

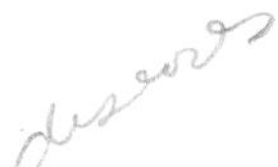

Lupus is a chronic inflammatory disease of the collagen contained in connective tissue. Systemic lupus is an immune complex disorder in which the inflammation and tissue damage occur from the formation of soluble immune complexes that are deposited in tissues and cells.

Signs and symptoms of systemic lupus erythematosus (SLE) include joint inflammation and pain; skin rashes; and involvement of the nervous, vascular, and renal systems. The skin rash characteristically forms a "butterfly" over the cheeks and nose. Vasculitis and Raynaud's phenomenon are vascular manifestations; nephritis may occur; and cardiac, pulmonary, and nervous system manifestations are common.

Diagnosis is made by history, physical examination, and results of multiple diagnostic tests, including lupus erythematosus (LE) cell reaction, erythrocyte sedimentation rate (ESR), and increased serum globulins.

Management is based on the system involved and administration of salicylates, NSAIDs, and corticosteroids. Nursing care is aimed at symptom management, assessment for complications, and psychosocial support.

OSTEOPOROSIS

Osteoporosis is a metabolic bone disorder that causes a decrease in bone mass and makes the person more susceptible to fractures. Causative factors for osteoporosis include long-term calcium deficiency and estrogen deficiency, particularly after menopause. Contributing factors are thought to be cigarette smoking, excessive caffeine ingestion, alcoholism, various medications

TABLE 26-6 METHODS AND PRECAUTIONS FOR APPLICATIONS OF HEAT AND COLD AT HOME

Method	Comments and Precautions
Applications of heat	Generally recommended for chronic and subacute inflammation. Regardless of method, do not apply heat for more than 20 to 30 minutes at a time. Not safe for patient with circulatory stasis, impaired sensitivity to heat.
Tub bath	Use rubber mat, handrails, or bathtub seat to prevent falls and fatigue.
Foot or hand soaks	Exercises can be performed while soaking, but full range of motion not always possible.
Shower	Turn on cold water first, or adjust temperature of water before entering shower. Can provide gentle massage. Use stool in shower if fatigue likely.
Hot water bottle	Cools quickly; temperature difficult to evaluate.
Heating pads:	Patient should not go to sleep with a pad on. Provide heat to relatively small area.
Standard electric heating pad	Do not allow to become wet.
Electric moist heating pad or commercial hot pack	Moist heat more penetrating.
Applications of cold	Generally recommended for acute phase of inflammation. Do not apply to one area for more than 15 to 20 minutes. Discontinue when numbness occurs. Not recommended for patients with hypersensitivity to cold or impaired circulation. Assess skin before and after treatment for signs of injury. Dry skin well after treatment.
Ice water bath	To surround one body area (e.g., hands or feet). Encourage exercise during application.
Ice pack made by partially filling double plastic bag with ice	Wrap bags in *warm* wet towel to help adjustment to cold. Can be applied only to limited area; not entire joint. Exercise not possible during application.
Commercial packs	Can be kept in freezer.
"Slush pack" made with 2 cups water and 1 cup denatured alcohol in double plastic bag which is fastened at top, put in bowl, and placed in freezer	Adding more water will make it pack firmer. Return to freezer after use. Do *not* place ice between hard surface and body part being cooled.
Ice massage	Protect hand holding ice with rubber glove or pad. Rub large cube of ice onto body part until skin feels numb, but no longer than 10 to 15 minutes.

Data from Simpson, C. F.: Adult arthritis: Heat, cold, or both. Am. J. Nurs., Feb., 1983, Vol. 83, No. 2, p. 270.

such as corticosteroids, endocrine disorders, prolonged bed rest, and liver disease, because these factors either have an effect on estrogen production or calcium metabolism.

Signs and symptoms of osteoporosis are height loss, kyphosis, and back pain. Often it is diagnosed after the patient sustains a fracture following little or no known trauma. On radiographs the bone of the patient with osteoporosis appears porous. However, this occurs late in the disease. A screening test known as photon absorptiometry is used to assess loss of bone density in postmenopausal women in order to arrest and possibly correct the problem before it becomes severe.

Treatment is aimed at stopping loss of bone density, increasing bone formation, and preventing fractures. Postmenopausal estrogen replacement therapy and adequate dietary or supplemental calcium are the mainstays of treatment. Calcium supplementation of 1,000 mg is recommended for premenopausal women and 1,500 mg after menopause. Daily weight-bearing exercise is thought to greatly decrease the incidence of osteoporosis. Walking down stairs seems to be especially helpful. Salicylates and NSAIDs are prescribed to control back pain.

BONE TUMORS

Bone is subject to both benign and malignant tumors. They arise from several different types of tissue including cartilage (chondromas), bone (osteomas), and fibrous tissue (fibromas). Benign tumors are often found on radiograph or at the time of fracture.

Malignant bone tumors are either primary or secondary to metastatic disease. Primary malignant bone tumors are most often seen in people 10 to 30 years of age. The most common type is osteosarcoma or osteogenic sarcoma. More than half of the cases affect the distal femur. However, the humerus and proximal tibia are other frequent sites of occurrence. Other types of primary malignant tumors include Ewing's sarcoma, chondrosarcoma, and fibrosarcoma.

Signs and symptoms of malignant bone tumor include pain, warmth, and swelling.

Metastatic bone tumors greatly outnumber primary bone malignancies. Malignancies of the prostate, kidney, thyroid, breast, and lung commonly metastasize to bone. Sites of metastases are usually the vertebrae, pelvis, ribs, and femur.

Treatment for malignant bone tumors includes surgery, radiation, and chemotherapy.

JOINT REPLACEMENT

An arthroplasty (joint replacement) may be done for a knee, shoulder, elbow, finger, ankle, or hip. The hip is the most frequently replaced joint.

TOTAL HIP REPLACEMENT

A hip joint may be replaced with either a low-friction polyurethane socket for the acetabulum with a metallic replacement for the head of the femur or with synthetic materials combined with a porous bone implant (Fig. 26–21). The totally synthetic joint is held in place with surgical bone cement that bonds it firmly to the bone to which it is attached. Partial weight bearing is then permitted very soon after surgery. The porous bone implant requires 6 weeks of healing before weight bearing.

A surgical bacteriostatic scrub solution is usually prescribed for use during the daily shower for several days prior to hip replacement to lessen the chance of infection. The patient is placed in an orthopedic bed with an overhead trapeze bar attached prior to surgery and often is transported to and from the operating room on the bed. The triangular abductor pillow is shown to the patient, and its use between the legs for turning postoperatively is explained. Other care is much the same as for other types of major surgery.

There are several kinds of prostheses to replace the hip, and the surgeon chooses the appropriate one according to an individual patient's needs.

The primary purpose of total hip replacement (THR) is to relieve chronic pain. The greatest dangers to successful replacement are infection, dislocation, and failure to function. Rehabilitation of the patient is a team effort involving the patient himself, the surgeon, nurse, and physical therapist.

Preoperative Care

Preoperatively the patient is given specific instructions about the kind of surgery to be performed, the prosthesis to be used, the procedures

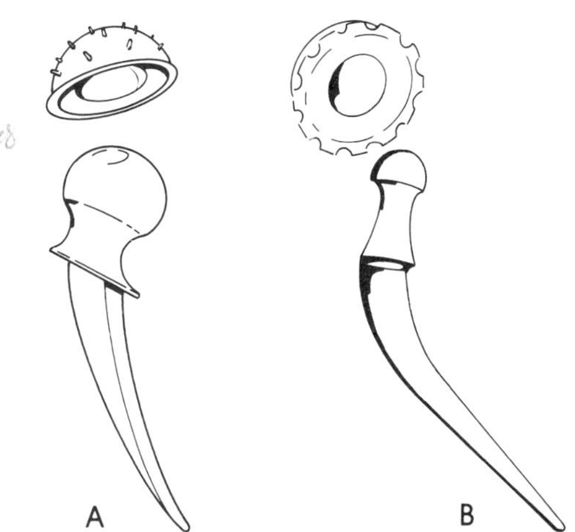

Figure 26–21 Prostheses used in two types of surgical procedure for total hip replacement. The McKee-Farrar procedure involves the replacement of both the femoral head and acetabulum by a metal prosthesis. *(A)*. The Charnley prosthesis *(B)* involves total prosthetic replacement of the hip joint.

NURSING CARE PLAN 26-2

Selected nursing diagnoses, goals/outcome criteria, nursing interventions, and evaluations for a patient undergoing total hip replacement

Situation: Mrs. Thompson, a 62-year-old female, has a history of osteoarthritis of the left hip. She has been in constant pain for months and cannot perform her usual activities of daily living. She is scheduled for a hip replacement.

Nursing Diagnosis	Goals/Outcome Criteria	Nursing Intervention	Evaluation
Impaired physical mobility related to joint pain. SUPPORTING DATA Constant pain in left hip prevents usual mobility.	Range of motion of other joints will be maintained. No signs of joint contractures at discharge.	Supervise active and passive ROM to all other joints at least tid. Be certain body is in correct alignment after turning.	Active and passive ROM at 10 and 2; maintaining good body alignment; continue plan.
Potential for injury related to possible hemorrhage, thrombophlebitis, or dislocation of hip joint. SUPPORTING DATA Total hip replacement; improper positioning or movement can dislocate prosthesis.	Bleeding, should it occur, will be stopped quickly. No evidence of thrombophlebitis. No dislocation of hip joint.	Observe dressing for bleeding; monitor drainage in Hemovac q 1 h for 8 h, then q 2 h for 24 h. Monitor vital signs q 4 h. Assess for signs of thrombophlebitis and possible emboli; apply antiembolic stockings. Use wedge pillow between legs when turning to prevent adduction; turn q 2 h to back or unaffected side. Assess circulatory and nerve function of affected leg q 1 h for 8 h, then q 2 h. Encourage leg and foot exercises q 2 h. Turn q 2 h. Maintain hip abduction at all times. Do not raise head of bed more than 45 degrees. Assess circulatory and nerve function of affected leg q 1 h for 8 h, then q 2 h. When she is up out of bed, do not allow her to sit for long periods of time. Maintain in good body alignment at all times. Monitor for severe pain, external rotation of hip with noticeable shortening of leg, palpable bulge over head of femur.	Hemovac drainage 80 mL this shift; vital signs stable; antiembolic stockings in place; turned with wedge 8, 10, 12, and 2; pedal pulses, 2+; capillary refill, 12 sec; ankle and foot exercises 8, 10, 12, and 2; cautioned again not to raise head of bed >45 degrees; dressing dry and intact; no evidence of external rotation of hip; continue plan.
Potential for infection related to surgical incision. SUPPORTING DATA Incision for implantation of hip prosthesis	No signs of infection as evidenced by normal WBC count and normal temperature; wound clean and dry.	Administer prophylactic antibiotics as ordered. Monitor temperature trends and WBCs. Inspect wound q shift for redness, swelling, and tenderness. Use strict sterile technique for dressing changes.	Antibiotics administered on schedule; temp., 99.2°F.; WBC count, 9,800; incision without redness; slight serosanguinous drainage; no signs of infection; continue plan.

to be followed after surgery, and what is expected of him to help achieve the goals of rehabilitation. He is given instructions in postoperative exercises and in the use of ambulation equipment such as a walker, crutches, or canes.

Postoperative Care

It is imperative that all concerned with the patient's care after surgery understand what is necessary to ensure successful hip replacement and rehabilitation and to prevent dislocation of the prosthesis. Immediately after surgery, nursing intervention includes all the measures required to avoid respiratory and circulatory complications. However, extreme care must be exercised in positioning and repositioning the patient. In order to prevent dislocation, an abduction wedge is secured between the legs (usually in the operating room) and left in place until the surgeon requests its removal.

In most cases the patient is allowed to stand at the bedside on the first postoperative day, supported by a walker and two persons. Weight bearing on the operated joint is sometimes allowed, but there should be a specific written order from the physician saying it is all right to permit weight bearing on the joint. The patient will need instruction in transferring himself from bed to chair, wheelchair, and toilet. Whenever he sits down, the chair seat should be raised so that the hips are never flexed beyond a 90-degree angle.

Patient Teaching

Before he is discharged, the patient who has had hip surgery should be given instructions so he can care for himself at home. These include:

- It is all right to lie on your operated side.
- For 3 months you should not cross your legs. You should put a pillow between your legs when you roll over on your abdomen or lie on your side in bed.
- It is all right to bend your hip, but not beyond a right (90-degree) angle.
- Continue your daily exercise program at home in the same way you did the exercises at the hospital.

In addition to these instructions, the nurse and physical therapist may want to refer the patient and his family to an outside agency, liaison nurse, or social worker if there is evidence of a need for continued support and guidance.

Nursing interventions for selected problems of a patient with a total hip replacement are summarized in Nursing Care Plan 26–2.

KNEE REPLACEMENT

Chronic, uncontrollable pain is the main indication for knee arthroplasty. Either part or all of the knee joint may be replaced. For the best result postoperatively, emphasis is placed on exercise. A continuous passive motion (CPM) machine is used soon after surgery. The patient must be kept well medicated for pain in order to tolerate the exercise. Within 2 to 5 days, quadriceps-strengthening exercises and straight-leg raising are started. Exercises are taught by the physical therapist, and the nurse often assists the patient in performing them. The patient then progresses to ambulation with a walker or crutches. Other pre- and postoperative care is similar to that of the patient undergoing any major surgery.

Concerns for the Elderly

- The elderly person is at risk of sustaining a fracture because of decreased reaction time, failing vision, lessened agility, and decreased muscle tone.
- Many chronic diseases require the use of corticosteroids for treatment. Osteoporosis is a side effect of steroid treatment and makes the older person more susceptible to fractures. Arthritis occurs in at least 50% of the population over age 50 and increases in severity during the later years.
- Kyphosis from compression fractures of the spinal column resulting from osteoporosis can restrict lung expansion and cause decreased respiratory reserve.
- Hip fracture is much more common in the over-60 age group and is a major cause of morbidity and eventual death from complications.
- When the elderly person has to be immobilized because of trauma and fractures, he is much more prone to the complications of immobility than is a younger patient.

Perhaps with the trend in America toward considerable exercise during the middle years, the next generation will have fewer problems of the musculoskeletal system. Also, with the emphasis that has been placed on calcium intake throughout life, the incidence of osteoporosis and fracture in the older age group should decrease.

BIBLIOGRAPHY

Beare, P. G., and Myers, J. L.: Principles and Practices of Adult Health Nursing. St. Louis, C. V. Mosby, 1990.

Bergman, H. D.: Gout: Medical management. J. Pract. Nurs., Sept., 1987, p. 48.

Brassell, M. P.: Pharmacologic management of rheumatic diseases. Orthop. Nurs., March/April, 1988, p. 43.

Ceccio, C. M.: Rx: Home care. Keeping pin sites problem-free. RN, Feb., 1988, p. 70.

Ceccio, C. M., et al.: Teaching the elderly amputee to meet the world. RN, Sept., 1988, p. 70.

Cerrato, P. L.: Nutrition support: Piecing together the osteoporosis puzzle. RN, April, 1990, p. 77.

Chambers, J. K.: Metabolic bone disorders: Imbalances of calcium and phosphorus. Nurs. Clin. North Am., Dec., 1987, p. 861.

Chestnut, C. H. III, et al.: New options in osteoporosis. Patient Care, Jan. 15, 1988, p. 160.

Dunajcik, L. M.: The hip: When the joint must be replaced. RN, April, 1989, p. 62.

Hanell, M. J.: Fractures and the healing process. Orthop. Nurs., Jan./Feb., 1988, p. 43.

Ignatavicius, D. D., and Bayne, M. J.: Medical-Surgical Nursing. Philadelphia, W. B. Saunders, 1991.
Krug, B. M.: The hip: Nursing fracture patients to full recovery. RN, April, 1989, p. 56.
Lavin, R. J.: The high-pressure demands of compartment syndrome. RN, Feb., 1989, p. 22.
Lockskin, M. D., et al.: A better prognosis in lupus. Patient Care, Feb., 29, 1988, p. 75.
Madson, S.: How to reduce the risk of postmenopausal osteoporosis. J. Gerontol. Nurs., Sept., 1989, p. 20.
Milde, F. K.: Impaired physical mobility. J. Gerontol. Nurs., March, 1988, p. 20.
Morris, L., et al.: Nursing the patient in traction. RN, Jan., 1988, p. 26.
Morris, L., et al.: Special care for skeletal traction. RN, Feb., 1988, p. 24.
Perry, G. R.: Living with osteoporosis: Early awareness and attention to life-style can delay or prevent osteoporosis. Geriatr. Nurs., May/June, 1988, p. 174.
Price, S., and Wilson, L.: Pathophysiology, 3rd ed. New York, McGraw-Hill, 1986.
Rakel, R. E., ed.: Conn's Current Therapy 1990. Philadelphia, W. B. Saunders, 1990.
Ranawat, C. S., et al.: What to expect from joint replacement. Patient Care, Sept. 30, 1990, p. 105.
Ruhl, J.: Pelvic trauma. RN, July, 1991.
Schoen, D. C.: Assessment for arthritis. Orthop. Nurs., March/April, 1989, p. 31.
Sica, S., et al.: Immobility syndrome: Use it or lose it. A. D. Nurse, Nov./Dec., 1987, p. 6.

STUDENT STUDY AIDS

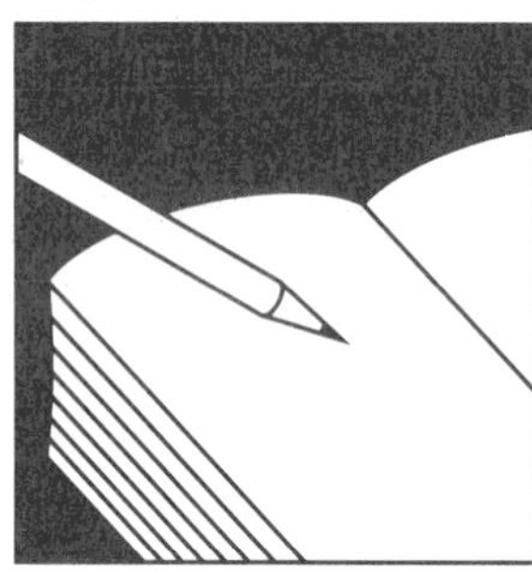

CLINICAL CASE PROBLEMS

Read each clinical case problem and discuss the questions with your classmates.

1. Mrs. Wilkins, aged 38, weighs 210 pounds and has been admitted to the hospital with a diagnosis of fracture of the right femur. You have been told that when the patient returns from the cast room, she will have on a hip spica that will cover the entire right leg and foot except the toes; the left leg will be covered down to the knee. The body section of the cast will stop at the waistline. You have been assigned to assist in the care of Mrs. Wilkins when she returns from the cast room.

- How will you prepare the bed for the patient's return?
- What equipment do you anticipate needing?
- How can you support the cast and reduce swelling while it is drying?
- How is the patient to be transferred from the stretcher to the bed?
- What provision can be made for drying the cast?
- List the observations you must make while the cast is on Mrs. Wilkins's leg?
- If the doctor orders a trapeze bar installed over the patient's bed, how would you plan the procedure for getting Mrs. Wilkins on and off the bedpan?

---

2. Mr. Moss, aged 33, has been injured in a fall from a building on which he was working. When you are assigned to the care of this patient, you are told that the tibia and fibula of the left leg are fractured. These fractures were reduced with the patient under anesthesia, after which pins were inserted for skeletal traction. The accident occurred 3 days ago, and now you are assigned to give morning care to this patient.

- What nursing problems will skeletal traction present?
- What subjective and objective symptoms would you look for when assessing Mr. Moss's condition?

---

3. Mrs. Carter, aged 50, is a very obese woman who comes to the orthopedic clinic for treatment of arthritis of the knees and ankles. She has great difficulty walking and would use a wheelchair if she could afford one. Her daughter states that she is becoming more and more inactive and, though her mother says she does not want to become an invalid, that she refuses to move about and do things for herself. Mrs. Carter lives alone and prefers not to live with her daughter because the grandchildren make her nervous. In fact, she prefers to be left alone because she feels that she cannot be of use to anyone. Her daughter feels that her mother could find many useful things to do in her neighborhood if she would only try.

- How does obesity interact with arthritis in causing immobility?
- What medications might decrease Mrs. Carter's pain?
- What sort of exercise would be best for this patient?
- How could you make Mrs. Carter feel more useful and motivate her to move about and get out of the house more?

---

4. Mrs. Lewis, aged 52, has been told she has osteoarthritis. She is a very nervous individual and extremely apprehensive about her condition. She tells you that she knows she will be helpless and completely useless as a wife and mother within a few months, because she has arthritis and she knows what a crippling disease this is. She is very depressed and has stopped doing the things she normally does around the house, placing the burden of housekeeping on her husband and children.

- How can you help this patient understand the type of arthritis she has and the ways in which she can prevent deformity and crippling?
- How would you approach the psychosocial aspects of her problem?
- What self-help programs are available for Mrs. Lewis? What can she do at home to help herself?

STUDY OUTLINE

I. Introduction

A. Orthopedic nursing is not confined to primary diseases and disorders of the musculoskeletal system.

B. Health of muscle and bones is essential to general well-being and continued mobility.

II. Diagnostic tests and procedures and nursing implications (see Table 26–1).

A. Radiologic studies: most often used. Help diagnose changes in the contour, size, and density of bone. No special preparation or postradiologic care needed.

B. Bone scan: use of radioactive tracer compound to locate areas of abnormal activity in bone.

C. Arthroscopy: endoscopic visualization of interior of a joint. Allows for collection of biopsy specimen; concurrent surgery of joint.

1. Valuable in examining meniscus, patella, condyles, and synovia of knee and internal structures of other joints.
2. Patient watched for signs of infection, bleeding into joint, swelling, thrombophlebitis, and injury to and loss of motion of joint.

D. Arthrocentesis (aspiration of synovial fluid) and analysis of synovial fluid. Also can be therapeutic. Synovial fluid analyzed for abnormalities; for example, white blood cells, bacteria, rheumatoid arthritis cells, and lupus erythematosus cells.

1. After arthroscopy the extremity is supported on pillows. Ice or cold packs used to relieve pain and swelling.
2. Elastic bandage applied to give joint stability after removal of large amount of fluid.
3. Patient cautioned not to overuse joint until after pain and swelling subside.

E. Cultures aid in diagnosing bone infection.

F. Biopsy aids in determining type of tumor present.

G. Electromyography to evaluate intrinsic electrical properties of muscle in response to stimulation.
   1. Helpful in diagnosing neuromuscular disease, location of site of muscle disorder.

H. Blood tests:
   1. Uric acid: high levels indicate presence of gout.
   2. Rheumatoid factor: detects antibodies that possibly indicate rheumatoid arthritis, lupus, or scleroderma.
   3. Antinuclear antibodies (ANA): useful for diagnosis of lupus erythematosus, rheumatoid arthritis, and other connective tissue disorders.

I. Other testing procedures: ROM testing (goniometry), muscle strength, stability of joint under stress.

III. Nursing assessment of musculoskeletal function

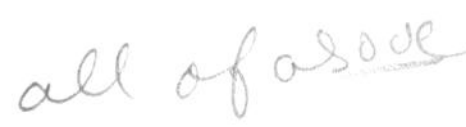

A. History taking: diseases that secondarily affect musculoskeletal system; family history of bone and muscle disease, gout, psoriasis.

B. Observations:
   1. Pain and discomfort: location, description, factors that aggravate or relieve pain. Daily pattern of pain.
   2. Signs of joint stiffness, daily pattern.
   3. Signs of deformity; sensory changes; use of supports such as cane, crutch, elastic bandage.
   4. Signs of inflammatory changes or infection, sensory changes.

C. Assessment of ability to perform activities of daily living also important.

IV. Nursing intervention

A. Lifting, turning, and positioning to avoid injury to patient and self.

B. Orthopedic bedmaking: make bed with minimum of disturbance to limb in traction and damage to skin.

C. Prevention of disability:
   1. Goal is to prevent permanent disability and limitation of motion.
   2. Pathologic changes resulting from immobility and inadequate intervention.
      a. Contractures: adaptive shortening of the muscles when they are not regularly contracted and stretched to their normal limits.
         (1) Process begins 3 to 7 days after immobilization of a part. Completed in 6 to 8 weeks.
         (2) Evident in foot drop, wrist drop, contractures of fingers and arms.
      b. Loss of muscle tone from disuse.
      c. Ankylosis: permanent fixation of a joint; little or no motion possible. If it cannot be avoided, joint is immobilized in position of optimum use or maximum function.
   3. Gradual mobilization: progressive improvement in motion and ability to perform self-care activities.
      a. Must take into account cause of immobility.
      b. Patient involved in goal setting.
      c. Passive exercises and positioning until patient is able to do these on his own.
   4. Exercise:
      a. ROM, both passive and active, should be done at least three to four times daily.
      b. Other exercises summarized in Table 21–1.
      c. Daily exercises scheduled after pain medication given.

d. Continuous passive motion can be accomplished by motor-driven apparatus.

5. Positioning:
    a. Changing body position does not necessarily change joint positions.
    b. Patients with spastic paralysis and those with flaccid paralysis not always positioned in same way.
    c. Follow guidelines to avoid positioning problems.

D. Emotional aspects of orthopedic disorders:
1. Consider impact of prolonged periods of immobility and dependence on others.
2. Involve patient in setting realistic and measurable goals for self-care to improve self-concept and promote better mental outlook.

V. Care of the patient in a cast

A. Cast used to immobilize certain part of the body so that it is firmly supported and completely at rest.

B. Types of casts:
1. Long-leg, short-leg, walking casts.
2. Spica covers trunk and one or two extremities.
3. Shoulder spica covers trunk and one arm.

C. Plaster casts:
1. Applied wet; when dry, cast forms firm shell to immobilize; and protect part.
2. Care of the fresh plaster cast:
    a. Handle patient gently.
    b. Wet cast is picked up only with the palms of the hands.
    c. Supporting pillows should be waterproofed.
    d. Turn patient frequently to avoid misshaping cast.
    e. Ice bags may be used to control swelling.
3. Drying the cast:
    a. Use of heat is dangerous.
    b. Circulating air is best method.
4. Nursing assessment:
    a. Listen to patient.
    b. Check neurovascular status.
        (1) Two-point discrimination test.
        (2) Blanching or capillary refill time.
    c. Watch for signs of infection.
5. Daily care:
    a. Do not wet cast during bath or when patient uses bedpan.
    b. Observe condition of skin at edge of cast.

D. Synthetic casts allow more freedom:
1. Not suitable for serious fractures.
2. If patient allowed to go home with cast on, instructions in proper care must be given.

E. Cast brace:
1. Combines stability of cast with mobility of brace.
2. Used for patients with femoral shaft fracture.
3. Ambulation with cast brace under supervision of physical therapist.

VI. Care of the patient in traction

A. Types and uses of traction:
1. Traction extends and holds part of the body in desired position by mechanical pull.
    a. Skeletal traction exerts pull on bone; skin traction exerts pull on the skin.

2. Types include Bryant's traction, Buck's extension, balanced suspension, and side traction.

B. Nursing intervention:
   1. Special and diligent back care.
   2. Bed is changed so that traction apparatus is disturbed as little as possible.
   3. Weights must be hanging free and patient positioned so that his body weight is counteracting the pull of weights.
   4. Check bony prominences frequently for signs of impaired circulation and pressure.
   5. Patient's body must be kept in good alignment.

VII. Care of the patient on a frame

A. Stryker frame or Foster bed may be used to:
   1. Facilitate nursing care and frequent turning.
   2. Immobilize the spine as a means of treating fractures and other disorders of the spinal column.
   3. Provide a means of keeping clean and dry those patients who cannot move with ease.

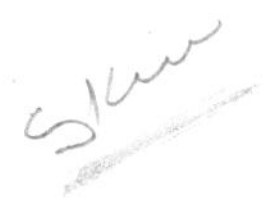

B. CircOlectric bed similar in principle and purpose. Is electrically manipulated.

C. Other beds: Rotorest bed turns patient gently 300 times a day.

D. Clinitron air-fluidized bed is useful for immobilized patients.

VIII. Crutch walking

A. Type of crutch will depend on amount of disability and patient's ability to bear weight and keep his balance on his feet.

B. Muscles of shoulders, arms, and back used to manipulate crutches.

C. Gaits vary according to patient's needs and mobility.

IX. Fractures

A. A break in the continuity of bone.

B. Types (see Figure 26–12).

C. Surgical treatment and rationale:
   1. Purpose is to establish a sturdy union between broken ends of bone.
   2. Closed reduction done by manual manipulation without surgical incision.
   3. Open reduction: surgical incision made over fracture and exposed bone is aligned.
   4. Internal fixation: pins, plates, or screws may be used to stabilize position of the broken ends of bone.
   5. External fixation: pin sites need special care. Patient can be more mobile.

D. Nonunion of bone can be treated with a bone growth–stimulating device.

E. Vertebral fracture: sometimes treated by spinal fusion of the involved vertebrae.
   1. Keep head of bed flat for 24 hours after fusion.
   2. Keep spine straight when turning patient to side: knees flexed and drawn up toward chest.
   3. Check dressing for bleeding and spinal fluid leak.
   4. Assess motor and neurologic function q 2 to 4 hours.
   5. Discharge teaching: no sitting for prolonged periods; no bending from waist; no lifting more than 5 lb; review good body mechanics.

F. Complications:
   1. Infection, especially in open fracture; danger of osteomyelitis.

2. Delayed healing as a result of inadequate levels of serum calcium and phosphorus.
3. Fat embolism: most common to fracture of long bones, pelvis, and ribs.
   a. Occurs within first 48 hours of fracture; high mortality rate.
   b. Signs and symptoms: respiratory distress, hypertension, tachypnea, fever, and petechiae over neck, upper arms, chest, or abdomen.
   c. Place patient in high Fowler's position to ease breathing; remain calm; begin oxygen administration at 2 to 3 L/min if available; summon physician.
4. Compartment syndrome: Occurs in muscle compartments of the extremities.
   a. Caused by external or internal pressure; seriously restricts circulation.
   b. Causes considerable pain; signs and symptoms include edema, pallor, tingling, paresthesia, numbness, weak pulse, cyanosis, paresis, loss of function.
   c. Can cause permanent tissue and nerve damage if unrelieved.
   d. May be treated by surgical fasciotomy to relieve pressure.

G. Nursing assessment and intervention (see Table 26–3)
   1. Assess for infection, sensation, circulation, and motor function each shift.
   2. Inspect casts for flattened areas, soft spots, cracking and crumbling; inspect skin at junction of cast; sniff for signs of infection inside of cast.
   3. Check traction devices for correct positioning and to see that weights are hanging free; check weights each time room is entered.
   4. Assess for problems of immobility: skin breakdown, urinary tract infection, constipation, respiratory problems.
   5. Pain control is important; prevent boredom, offer distraction.
   6. Attend to psychosocial concerns of long-term immobilization and disruption of usual roles.

X. Amputation

A. Surgical removal of part or all of a limb because of severe physical trauma, malignancy, or gangrene. Eighty percent involve a lower extremity.

B. Preoperative care: prepare patient and family emotionally for loss of limb.
   1. Help patient deal with sense of loss.
   2. Prepare for "phantom sensations."
   3. Team effort to plan rehabilitation with patient.

C. Postoperative care:
   1. Observe for signs of hemorrhage.
   2. Encourage lower extremity amputee to lie on his stomach as much as possible, keeping the stump in good alignment to prevent flexion contractures.
   3. Early ambulation to enhance recovery and rehabilitation.
   4. Exercises done to keep joint mobile and prepare a limb for fitting of prosthesis.

D. Emotional aspects and rehabilitation:
   1. Early ambulation and self-care to improve patient's morale and help achieve independence.
   2. Nurse should have positive, hopeful attitude, help patient set short-range goals, and avoid giving false hope.

3. Focus on patient's strengths and what he is able to do.
4. Types of lower-limb prostheses (Fig. 26–17).

XI. Overuse and torsion injuries

A. Sprain: stretching or tearing of ligaments around a joint.
   1. Most common sites are ankle and knee.
   2. Symptoms vary from tenderness and minimal swelling (grade 1) to bleeding into joint and marked loss of function (grade 3).
   3. Intervention: apply ice immediately and at 20- to 30-minute intervals for first 24 to 36 hours. Wrap tightly and elevate part. Surgical repair may be necessary in some cases.

B. Strain: pulling and tearing of either muscle or tendon or both.
   1. Most common sites are hamstring, quadriceps, and calf muscles.
   2. Symptoms: soft tissue swelling and pain. History of overexertion.
   3. Intervention: Apply ice and compression immediately; rest. Surgical repair may be necessary.

C. Dislocation: stretching and tearing of ligaments with complete displacement of bones of the joint.
   1. Most common sites are shoulder, knee, temporomandibular joint.
   2. Symptoms: severe pain, muscle spasm, abnormal appearance of joint. History of outside force pushing against joint.
   3. Intervention: reduction of displacement. Stabilization of joint and rehabilitation to minimize muscle atrophy and strengthen joint.

XII. Osteomyelitis: bacterial infection of bone

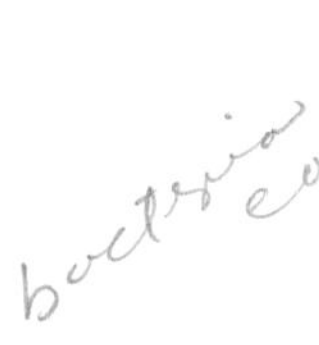

A. Symptoms: sudden onset with severe pain and marked tenderness at site of infection, fever, swelling of adjacent parts.

B. Treatment: rest, antibiotics, and measures to improve general health of patient. Surgical incision for drainage of abscess and débridement of infected bone if necessary.

XIII. Inflammatory disorders

A. Arthritis: literally means inflammation of a joint.
   1. There are more than 100 different forms of arthritis.
      a. All forms produce joint pain and some degree of disability.
      b. Two forms most prevalent in adults are rheumatoid arthritis and osteoarthritis. Comparison of these two disorders in Table 26–5.
   2. Osteoarthritis: noninflammatory degenerative joint disease.
      a. Typically affects only a few joints.
      b. Occurs after age 35.
      c. Chief complaints are aching pain with joint movement and stiffness with limitation of mobility.
      d. Treatment: salicylates or NSAIDs; corticosteroid injection into joint if treatment does not control pain.
      e. Balance exercise and rest; exercise is encouraged.
      f. Nursing interventions: moist heat, imagery, and diversion to reduce pain; encourage weight control.
      g. Surgery may be done to relieve severe pain and improve mobility: joint replacement of hip or knee done frequently.
   3. Rheumatoid arthritis: inflammatory disease of the joints.
      a. Usually begins between age 25 and 55.
      b. Familial tendency, but is thought to be caused by autoimmune defect or an infectious agent.
      c. Signs and symptoms: joint pain, warmth, edema, and limi-

tation of movement and multiple joint stiffness in the morning.
   d. Joints of hands, wrists, and feet are most commonly affected; involvement is usually bilateral and symmetric.
   e. Systemic symptoms include low-grade fever, weight loss, and malaise.
   f. Causes considerable joint deformity and dysfunction.
   g. Treatment aimed at pain relief, minimization of joint destruction, and promotion of joint function.
   h. Rest, exercise, medication, and immobilization with splints and supportive devices during periods of severe inflammation, heat and cold applications are all helpful.
   i. Medications include salicylates, NSAIDs, corticosteroids, antimalarial drugs, methotrexate, gold compounds, and penicillamine.
   j. Surgical joint repair or replacement done to reduce pain and improve mobility.
4. Medications:
   a. Aspirin remains drug of choice. Other NSAIDs include salicylates, ibuprofen, Indocin, Butazolidin, Meclomen, Nalfon, Naprosyn, Voltaren, and Clinoril.
   b. Gastrointestinal irritation and ulceration major adverse side effects.
   c. Newer NSAIDs developed to avoid gastrointestinal problems.
   d. NSAIDs still have potential for toxicity to liver, kidney, and central nervous system, and can cause tinnitus, hearing loss, and blood dyscrasias.
   e. Systemic steroids reserved for patients who cannot find relief from other less dangerous drugs.
   f. Intraarticular injections of steroids useful for relief of painful flare-ups. Number of injections per year should be limited to three or four.
   g. Immunosuppressive therapy largely experimental but proving successful in many cases.
5. Surgical intervention and orthopedic devices:
   a. Synovectomy and arthroplasty to prevent or modify deformities of joints.
   b. Braces, splints, and casts to rest affected part during active flare-ups of symptoms.
6. Nursing assessment:
   a. Social history to identify obstacles to patient compliance, for example, finances, home environment. Also includes occupational, physical, and emotional stresses.
   b. Health history and current state of health:
      (1) Family history of arthritis or of diseases with associated joint pathology.
      (2) Patient's history of past infections, injuries, and systemic diseases with associated arthritis.
      (3) Patient's perception of his health status and ability to follow regimen of exercise and self-care.
   c. Pain:
      (1) Characteristics of pain.
      (2) Patient's emotional response to pain and ways of coping.
   d. Objective data:
      (1) Laboratory tests, radiologic studies, physical examination.

(2) Evaluation of appearance of joints, range of motion, muscle strength, gait, posture.
(3) Note the use of canes, crutches, inappropriate shoes.

7. Nursing diagnoses for patients with arthritis and connective tissue disorders:
   a. Pain.
   b. Chronic pain related to inflammation.
   c. Impaired physical mobility related to inflammation and joint destruction.
   d. Activity intolerance related to pain and inflammation.
   e. Impaired home maintenance management related to decreased mobility.
   f. Potential for injury related to immobility.
   g. Self-esteem disturbance related to altered body image.
   h. Self-care deficit.
   i. Potential impaired skin integrity related to bed rest.
8. Nursing intervention:
   a. Rest and exercise.
      (1) Body in good alignment when patient is in bed.
      (2) Fatigue, muscle weakness, pain can inhibit exercise.
      (3) Patient instructed in proper way to engage in therapeutic exercises. Should take precautions not to injure joints.
   b. Applications of heat and cold.
      (1) Either hot or cold may be suitable, depending on patient's preference and effectiveness of each.
      (2) In general, heat is better for subacute or chronic joint inflammation; cold for acute inflammation.
      (3) Safe methods for hot and cold applications shown in Table 26–6.
   c. Diet: no special diet other than that necessary to maintain normal body weight and avoid obesity.
   d. Resources for patient and family education:
      (1) Information available from local Arthritis Foundation, Arthritis Information Clearinghouse, and Self-Help Device Office of the Institute of Physical Medicine and Rehabilitation.

XIV. Gout: type of arthritis caused by high serum levels of uric acid

A. Uric acid crystals precipitate and settle in joints and connective tissue.

B. Signs and symptoms: elevated serum uric acid; tight, reddened skin over an inflamed, edematous joint; temperature elevation; and extreme pain in the joint.

C. Treatment: analgesics, allopurinol, probenecid or colchicine, NSAIDs; low-purine diet; restriction of alcohol; weight control.

XV. Systemic lupus erythematosus (SLE): immune complex disorder with inflammation and damage of connective tissue throughout the body

A. Signs and symptoms: joint inflammation and pain, butterfly skin rash on face.

B. Vasculitis; Raynaud's phenomenon; nephritis; cardiac, nervous, and pulmonary system problems are also common.

C. Treatment aimed at symptom management, assessment for complications and psychosocial support; no cure.

XVI. Osteoporosis: metabolic bone disorder causing decreased bone mass and susceptibility to fractures

A. Thought to be caused by long-term calcium deficit, estrogen deficiency, and inactivity.
B. Contributing factors: cigarette smoking, excessive caffeine ingestion, and excessive alcohol intake.
C. Signs and symptoms: height loss, kyphosis, collapsed vertebrae and back pain, frequent fractures.
D. Treatment aimed at prevention, with estrogen replacement therapy after menopause, calcium supplementation in midlife, regular weight-bearing exercise.

XVII. Bone tumors: both benign and malignant

A. Primary malignant tumors seen mostly between age 10 and 30; osteogenic sarcoma is the most common.
B. Metastatic bone tumors from cancer of the prostate, breast, kidney, thyroid, and lung are the most common and affect the pelvis, ribs, vertebrae, and femur.
C. Treatment includes surgery, radiation, and chemotherapy.

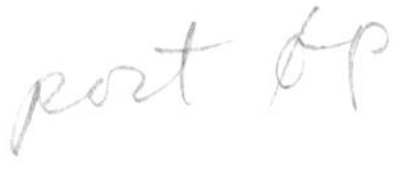

XVIII. Joint replacement: arthroplasty may be done for hip, knee, shoulder, elbow, finger, or ankle

A. Total hip replacement:
   1. Joint replaced with combination of bone and synthetic joint parts or total synthetic joint.
   2. Performed to relieve pain and provide mobility or to replace joint destroyed by trauma.
   3. Preoperatively the patient is taught about the prosthesis and expected goals for rehabilitation after surgery.
   4. Preoperative bacterial skin scrubs are usual for several days before surgery.
   5. Postoperatively, proper positioning and exercise are essential to prevent complications and attain good mobility and joint function.
   6. Discharge planning includes instruction of patient in ways to avoid injury to the artificial joint when he goes home.

B. Knee replacement:
   1. Chronic, uncontrollable pain is indication for knee replacement.
   2. Emphasis on exercise postoperatively for best results; may use CPM machine soon after surgery.
   3. Patient requires good analgesia in order to perform necessary exercises.

XIX. Concerns for the elderly

A. Greater risk of fracture due to decreased reaction time, failing vision, lessened agility, and decreased muscle tone.
B. Many chronic diseases require corticosteroids for treatment; these contribute to osteoporosis and fractures.
C. Arthritis occurs in 50% of population over 50 and increases in severity with aging.
D. Kyphosis from compression fractures of the spinal column can cause restricted lung expansion and predispose the patient to lung problems.
E. Hip fracture is common in people over 60 and is a major cause of morbidity and death from complications of immobility.
F. The elderly are more susceptible to problems of immobility.

CHAPTER 27

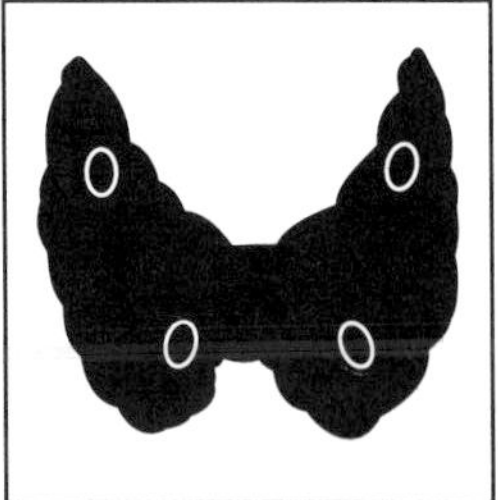

Care of Patients With Endocrine Disorders: Thyroid and Parathyroid Glands

VOCABULARY

cretinism
exocrine
exophthalmia
goiter
hyperplasia
idiopathic
myxedema
radioimmunoassay
resorption
synthesis
tetany
thyroid storm
thyrotoxicosis

Upon completion of this part of the chapter the student should be able to:

1. Describe the diagnostic tests performed on patients who have symptoms of thyroid or parathyroid problems.
2. Describe nursing assessment of patients with hyperactivity of the thyroid gland.
3. Formulate a nursing care plan for a patient with hyperthyroidism.
4. Describe pre- and postoperative assessment and nursing care for a patient who has had a thyroidectomy.
5. List common nursing diagnoses and appropriate nursing interventions for a patient with hypothyroidism.
6. Describe the medical treatment and nursing interventions for patients with hyperparathyroidism.

Pathophysiology

The endocrine system is made up of groups of cells whose primary function is the synthesis and release of hormones directly into the blood stream and body fluids (Fig. 27-1). The endocrine hormones are transported by the blood to various parts of the body, where they act on cells to control their physiologic functions. The cells and tissues that are affected by a specific hormone are called its *target cells* or *target tissues* (Table 27-1).

Some of the endocrine hormones, such as the thyroid hormones, affect practically every cell in the body. Others, such as the sex hormones, exert their special effects on only one kind of organ. Moreover, hormones from one endocrine gland can affect another endocrine gland. The pituitary, for example, secretes several different kinds of hormones that affect other endocrine glands.

The endocrine, or hormonal, system and the nervous system are the two major control systems of the body, and their regulatory functions are interrelated.

However, the primary regulatory activities of the hormonal system are concerned with (1) altering chemical reactions and controlling the rates at which chemical activities take place within the cells, (2) changing the permeability of the cell membrane and thus selecting the substances that can be transported across the membrane, and (3) activating a particular mechanism in the cell (for example, the system that controls cellular growth and reproduction).

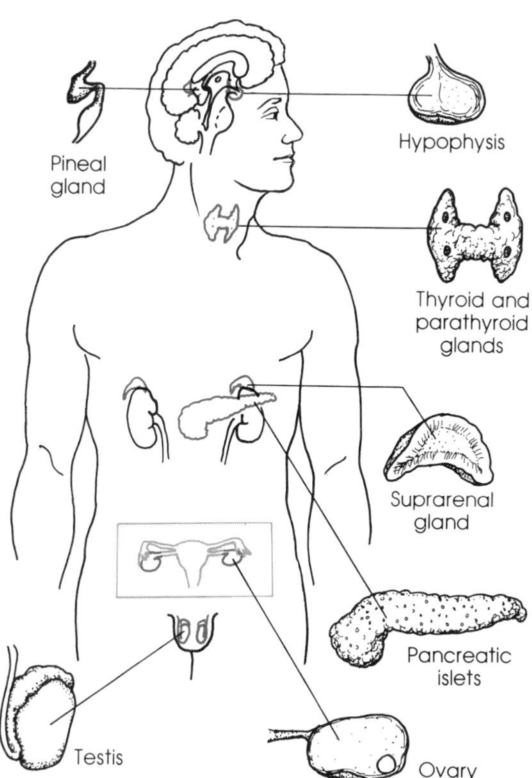

Figure 27-1 Endocrine glands.

The secretion of a particular hormone normally depends on the physiologic need for it at any given moment. Thus if an endocrine gland receives a message that its particular hormone is in short supply, it will synthesize and release more of the hormone. If, on the other hand, the hormonal need of a target tissue is being satisfied, elaboration of the hormone will be inhibited.

Some glands, such as the adrenal medulla and posterior pituitary, receive their information about hormone levels in the body directly and respond only to appropriate stimulation of nerve endings in the glands themselves. However, the adenohypophyseal glands indirectly receive notice either to release or to inhibit their hormones. Their stimulation comes by way of the hypothalamus and the anterior lobe of the pituitary gland (the adenohypophysis). The hypothalamus contains special nerve endings that produce releasing and inhibiting hormones (factors) that are absorbed into the capillaries of a portal system that transports them to the adenohypophysis. Thus the hypothalamus controls the secretion of hormones from the adenohypophysis, which in turn controls the release or inhibition of hormones from other glands. Many of the hormones of the anterior pituitary are "tropic" hormones; that is, they tend to cause a change in the endocrine gland for which the specific corresponding pituitary hormone is produced. An example is corticotropin (adrenocorticotropic hormone, or ACTH), which acts on the adrenal cortex. The various tropic hormones and their target tissues are shown in Table 27-1.

The interrelationships between endocrine glands, the hormones they synthesize and release, and the systems and subsystems that affect and are affected by hormones are complex. There are many steps between recognition of a need for and eventual release of a particular hormone. Thus it is that endocrine disorders cannot be thought of in terms of simply overproduction or underproduction of hormones, even though many disorders (for example, hypothyroidism) are named in this way.

In this chapter, as well as in Chapters 28 and 29, only those endocrine disturbances most frequently encountered in nursing practice will be covered.

The thyroid and parathyroid glands are anatomically very close to one another, but their hormones have quite different physiologic functions. Essentially, the thyroid hormones affect a variety of metabolic activities vital to the life of every cell in the body. The parathyroids,

TABLE 27-1 FUNCTIONS OF ENDOCRINE GLANDS

Gland	Hormone	Action on Target Tissues
Pituitary		
Anterior lobe	Thyroid-stimulating hormone (TSH); also called thyrotropin	Controls all known activities of thyroid glandular cells; influences body's metabolic processes
	Growth hormone (GH); also called somatotropic hormone (SH) and somatotropin	Causes growth of all tissues capable of growing; enhances protein synthesis, increases utilization of fats, and conserves carbohydrate by decreasing utilization of glucose
	Follicle-stimulating hormone (FSH)	Stimulates development of ovarian follicles and estrogen secretion; stimulates production of sperm
	Luteinizing hormone (LH)	Affects maturation of ovarian follicles, ovulation, and progesterone secretion; stimulates Leydig cells of testes and testosterone secretion
	Prolactin (PRL)	Maintains corpus luteum and secretion of progesterone; promotes lactation
	Adrenocorticotropic hormone (ACTH); also called adrenocorticotropin and corticotropin	Controls secretion of some of the hormones of the adrenal cortex; e.g., the glucocorticoids (chiefly cortisol and, to some extent, aldosterone and adrenal sex hormones)
Posterior lobe	Vasopressin (VP); also called antidiuretic hormone (ADH)	Elevates blood pressure in relatively high doses; conserves water by decreasing urinary output
	Oxytocin (OT)	Activates uterine contraction and, in response to sexual stimulation, transports sperm during coitus; increases secretion of milk
Intermediate part	Melanocyte-stimulating hormone (MSH)	Increases pigmentation of skin
Thyroid	Thyroxine (T_4); also called tetraiodothyronine and levothyroxine Triiodothyronine (T_3); also called liothyronine	Stimulates metabolism (catabolic phase); e.g., increases respiratory rate and utilization of oxygen, production of body heat, gluconeogenesis, strength, and force of heart rate; enhances muscle tone
	Calcitonin	Decreases serum calcium
Parathyroid	Parathyroid hormone (PTH); also called parathormone	Maintains constant serum level of calcium
Adrenal		
Cortex	Glucocorticoids (chiefly cortisol)	Increase protein breakdown; impair utilization of glucose; increase hepatic output of glucose; hence are called diabetogenic hormones; essential for survival under stress
	Mineralocorticoids (chiefly aldosterone)	Promote retention of sodium and loss of potassium and hydrogen in urine
	Androgens and estrogens	(See under testes and ovaries)
Medulla	Epinephrine, norepinephrine (to a much smaller extent)	Increase cardiac output; elevate blood glucose and blood lipids; raise blood pressure
Ovaries	Estrogens: β-estradiol, estrone, and estriol	Cause proliferation and growth of sexual organs and other reproductive tissues; induce proliferative phase of the menstrual cycle
	Progesterone	Prepares endometrium for implantation of the fertilized ovum; decreases frequency of uterine contractions; promotes secretory changes in mucosal lining of uterine tubes for nutrition of fertilized ovum; prepares mammary tissue for lactation

TABLE 27-1 **FUNCTIONS OF ENDOCRINE GLANDS** *Continued*

Gland	Hormone	Action on Target Tissues
Placenta	Human chorionic gonadotropin (hCG)	Maintains the corpus luteum and stimulates progesterone secretion
	Human placental lactogen (hPL)	Acts in combination with prolactin to induce lactation; also promotes growth and acts as an insulin antagonist
Testes	Androgens; testosterone, dihydrotestosterone, androstenedione	Promote development of male sex characteristics in fetus; stimulate descent of testes into scrotum; stimulate protein production; responsible for masculinization
Islets of Langerhans of pancreas		
Beta cells	Insulin	Promotes uptake, storage, and use of glucose, particularly by liver, muscles, and fat tissue; increases transport of glucose into cells and their usage of glucose; causes active transport of many amino acids into cells; promotes proteins; depresses rate of gluconeogenesis; and has synergistic effect with GH
Alpha cells	Glucagon	Causes glycogenolysis in liver and release of glucose, which raises blood glucose level; increases rate of gluconeogenesis, which causes continued hyperglycemia
Delta cells	Somatostatin	Inhibits secretion of both insulin and glucagon; also secreted by hypothalamus as growth hormone-inhibiting hormone
Thymus	Thymosin	Induces differentiation of T lymphocytes involved in cell-mediated immunity

From Miller, B, J., and Keane, C. B.: Encyclopedia and Dictionary of Medicine, Nursing, and Allied Health, 4th ed. Philadelphia, W. B. Saunders, 1987.

however, only influence serum calcium levels through the action of a single hormone called *parathormone.*

THE THYROID

The thyroid gland has two lobes, is highly vascularized, and is located below the pharynx in front and on either side of the trachea. The principal hormones secreted by the thyroid gland are thyroxine (T_4), triiodothyronine (T_3), and thyrocalcitonin. The more potent form of thyroid hormone is T_3, but there is about 20 times more T_4 than T_3 in normal circulating blood. When T_3 is needed, it is converted from the abundant supply of T_4. Sufficient quantities of dietary protein and iodine are needed for the synthesis of both of these thyroid hormones.

Thyroid hormones influence many metabolic functions within the cell. They activate the cellular production of heat; stimulate the synthesis of protein and lipids and their mobilization and degradation; stimulate the manufacture of coenzymes from vitamins; regulate many aspects of carbohydrate metabolism; and affect tissue response to epinephrine and norepinephrine.

The secretion or elaboration of thyroid hormones is regulated by the hypothalamic-pituitary-thyroid control system (Fig. 27-2). In other words, all three organs are involved in the closed-loop negative feedback system. Internal conditions such as low thyroid and norepinephrine (NE) serum levels can activate the hypothalamus, as can external conditions such as cold. In response to feedback received by the hypothalamus, thyrotropin-releasing hormone (TRH) is secreted. The TRH acts on the pituitary gland, bringing about its release of thyroid-stimulating hormone (TSH). The TSH then acts on the thyroid cells, causing them to release thyroid hormones. When sufficient heat has been produced by increased metabolic activities (if cold was the stimulus), or when there are sufficient levels of thyroid hormone in the body fluids (if a deficit was the stimulus), feedback to the hypothalamus causes it to stop releasing TRH.

There are three major abnormalities of the

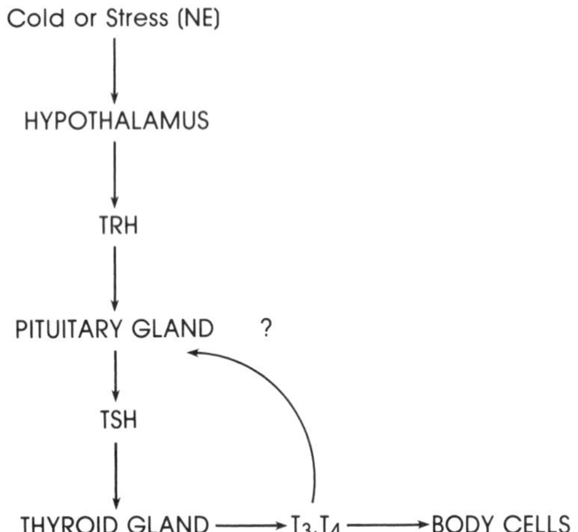

Figure 27-2 Hypothalamus-pituitary-thyroid axis. The cycle for regulation of thyroid hormone (triiodothyronine, T_3; thyroxine, T_4) involves either cold or norepinephrine (NE), which stimulates thyrotropin-releasing hormone (TRH). This hormone, in turn, triggers the release of thyroid-stimulating hormone (TSH), which then stimulates the release of T_3, T_4. Feedback from T_3, T_4 reaches the pituitary gland and probably the hypothalamus.

(From Wake, M. M., and Brensinger, J. F.: The nurse's role in hypothyroidism. Nurs. Clin. North Am., Sept., 1980, p. 454.)

thyroid gland: (1) enlargement of the gland (goiter), (2) overactivity of the gland (hyperthyroidism), and (3) underactivity of the gland (hypothyroidism).

GOITER

The person with goiter has a greatly enlarged thyroid gland. The serum levels of the thyroid hormones may or may not be within normal limits. One type of goiter is caused by a deficiency of iodine in the diet. It can be prevented by providing iodine intake, as in the use of iodized salt. Although the administration of iodine will not cure goiter, it will stop the continued enlargement of the gland. Another type of goiter occurs as a result of unknown causes.

Medical Diagnosis

Because there may be no systemic symptoms or changes in the metabolic rate of a person with simple goiter, the first sign that is usually noticed is an enlargement in the front of the neck. Later, if the gland continues to grow bigger, it presses against the esophagus and causes some degree of dysphagia. The goiter also can press against the trachea and interfere with normal breathing.

Medical Treatment and Nursing Intervention

If goiter resulting from iodine deficiency is treated early, the growth of the gland can be arrested, and in some cases the enlargement will eventually disappear. Medications prescribed include preparations containing elemental iodine (the iodide ion).

Iodine preparations should be given well diluted and administered through a straw, as they can stain the teeth a dark brown. Adverse effects of iodine preparations can include gastrointestinal (GI) upset, metallic taste, skin rashes, allergic reactions, and epigastric pain.

A very large goiter that continues to grow and produce local symptoms of pressure or presents the possibility of developing into a malignant growth or a toxic goiter is surgically removed in a procedure similar to the one sometimes done for hyperthyroidism.

OVERACTIVITY AND UNDERACTIVITY OF THE THYROID

Abnormalities in the activity of the thyroid gland and resultant changes in the levels of thyroid hormones are some of the most common disorders affecting the endocrine system. More than one test is necessary to determine if the thyroid gland is functioning properly. Usually a group of tests, called a *thyroid panel,* is performed. Assessment of serum T_4 and T_3, free T_4 index, serum calcitonin, thyroid antibody, and serum TSH may be included in such a panel.

Diagnostic Tests and Nursing Responsibilities

Tests currently used to evaluate thyroid function involve little more than a venipuncture and collection of blood samples. The nurse should be aware of factors that can distort test results. Contrast media for radiologic tests such as gallbladder studies and intravenous pyelogram contain iodine, Betadine used for skin preparation contains iodine, and so do some drugs taken internally. Moreover, oral contraceptives, aspirin, and other rather commonly used drugs can render thyroid hormone assays useless, because they either increase or decrease the levels of various thyroid hormones. When assessing a patient prior to diagnostic tests for thyroid function that involve radioimmunoassay or competitive binding analysis, the nurse should be sure to ask about any drugs the patient is taking, any previous radiographs, and other possible sources of iodine.

Other diagnostic tests for thyroid disorders include the thyroid scan, which is useful for detecting nodules on the thyroid, and radioactive iodine uptake, done during the scan to evaluate the ability of the thyroid to accumulate iodine. A TSH stimulation test, thyroid suppression test, and TRH stimulation test may be performed, depending on the clinical picture.

Patients with hyperthyroidism usually have high levels of both T_3 and T_4 in their serum and evidence of overactivity of thyroid cells during iodine uptake tests. However, it is possible that only the T_3 level will be above normal if the patient has Graves' disease, toxic adenoma of the thyroid, or toxic nodular goiter. These conditions are discussed below.

High serum levels of T_4 can be caused by either overactivity of the thyroid gland or excessive doses of T_4 given in replacement therapy.

Patients with primary hypothyroidism will have low levels of T_3 and T_4 and high levels of thyroid-stimulating hormone. The latter is the result of the body's attempt to compensate for low thyroid hormone levels by producing more TSH to stimulate the gland to produce more hormones.

Hyperthyroidism

Primary hyperthyroidism is the result of an abnormality of function involving the thyroid gland itself and causes excessive circulation of thyroid T_4 and T_3 hormones. Primary hyperthyroidism is more common in women 30 to 50 years of age. *Secondary* hyperthyroidism usually is the result of an abnormality in another gland, such as the pituitary gland, which could produce too much TSH and therefore overstimulate the thyroid gland.

Primary hyperthyroidism is also known as *Graves' disease, toxic goiter,* and *thyrotoxicosis.* Medications containing iodine such as amiodarone can predispose to thyrotoxicosis.

Symptoms and Medical Diagnosis

The earliest symptoms of hyperthyroidism may be weight loss and nervousness. However, symptoms can vary from mild to severe and also include weakness, insomnia, tremulousness, tachycardia, palpitations, exertional dyspnea, and ankle edema. The condition sometimes is not diagnosed in its early stages because of vagueness of symptoms. In some cases hyperthyroidism is misdiagnosed as a cardiovascular disease because the symptoms are so similar. If the hyperthyroidism is not diagnosed correctly and continues untreated for any length of time, the patient can develop true organic heart disease.

The symptoms manifested by a hyperthyroid patient are the result of an accelerated metabolic rate and a speeding up of all physiologic processes. Emotional upheaval occurs as a result of the action of thyroid hormones on the nervous system. The patient often reports episodes of emotional extremes with uncontrollable crying and depression followed by intense physical activity and euphoria.

The patient with Graves' disease also exhibits an enlarged thyroid gland (toxic goiter) and abnormal protrusion of the eyeballs (*exophthalmia*).

Medical diagnosis is based on clinical manifestations of hyperthyroidism and the results of laboratory tests for thyroid hormone levels. An excellent indicator of thyrotoxicosis is assessment of the heart rate while the patient is sleeping. A rate that is consistently above 80 could signify a toxic state resulting from excessive levels of thyroid hormone.

Medical Treatment

Hyperthyroidism may be treated medically by the administration of radioactive iodine and antithyroid drugs, mild sedatives, and antiadrenergic drugs to control tremor, restlessness, and tachycardia.

Radioactive iodine (131 I) is the drug of choice for middle-aged persons and nonpregnant women. Its main disadvantage is the possibility of hypothyroidism caused by "overeffective" treatment. The hypothyroidism can occur immediately after treatment or long after it is completed; hence the patient must have ongoing follow-up.

Dosage depends on the size of the gland and the thyroid's sensitivity to radiation. Patients receiving small doses can be given the drug orally for several doses and on an outpatient basis. Larger doses require isolation of the patient for 8 days, which is the half-life of 131 I. Because the iodine circulates in the blood and is excreted by the kidneys, precautions must be taken in handling needles, syringes, and other equipment likely to be contaminated with blood and bedpans, urinals, and specimen bottles likely to be contaminated by urine.

All patients receiving radioactive iodine must be observed for signs of thyroid crisis resulting from radiation-induced thyroiditis. (Thyroid crisis is discussed later.) If hyperthyroidism is not controlled within several months of therapy with radioactive iodine alone, the patient will require adjunctive therapy in the form of potassium iodide and antithyroid drugs.

Throughout therapy the patient is checked frequently to be sure thyroid activity is being reduced to normal levels. This is not easily accomplished, as hypothyroidism may be induced by an overly aggressive treatment regimen, whereas persistent hyperthyroidism may result if treatment is ineffective.

Antithyroid drugs are prescribed as the initial treatment of hyperthyroidism in children, young adults, and pregnant women. Iodine preparations such as propylthiouracil and potassium iodide (SSKI) have only a temporary effect. Methimazole (Tapazole) is the main drug utilized. The patient must take the antithyroid drug at the prescribed time and strictly according to schedule. A dangerous side effect is agranulocytosis, which can develop rather quickly.

Iodine preparations also may be given for a period of 10 to 14 days before surgery of the thyroid. This is done to reduce the vascularity of the gland, minimizing the danger of releasing large amounts of thyroid hormone into the blood stream during surgery.

Nursing Assessment

Patients most at risk for hyperthyroidism are adult women between the ages of 30 and 50. Women over 50 years of age often do not show the typical signs of hyperthyroidism but do exhibit shortness of breath, palpitations, and chest pain, which are typically thought of as indicative of angina pectoris and congestive heart failure. Hence their hyperthyroidism might be overlooked and they could be treated for a cardiovascular rather than an endocrine disorder. In her assessment of older women, the nurse should be alert for the possibility of an overactive thyroid gland as the cause of cardiovascular symptoms.

During history taking the nurse is aware of the significance of unexplained weight loss in spite of a voracious appetite and increased intake of food; changes in mental status such as anxiety, nervousness, difficulty concentrating, extreme agitation, and paranoid tendencies; diarrhea; increased thirst and urination; and palpitations. Patients with hyperthyroidism also can experience decreased interest in sexual activity, short and scanty menstrual periods, infertility, and immaturity of sexual organs.

During her history taking the nurse should ask whether any family members have had thyroid disease. There is strong evidence that there is an inherited factor in the development of Graves' disease and myxedema.

In addition to the subjective and objective symptoms listed above, the nurse will look for tremors (for example, when the patient holds an arm out in front of his body for a long period of time), smooth and silky hair, flushing and intolerance to heat, and warm and moist skin. The vital signs are very significant, because they give an indication of the metabolic rate, which would be expected to be elevated in a patient with hyperthyroidism. As mentioned above, an elevated sleeping pulse is typical of an elevated metabolic rate. The objective and subjective signs and symptoms of hyperthyroidism are not always obvious.

Some elderly patients may be lethargic or depressed, experience muscle weakness, and give the impression of hypo- rather than hyperthyroidism. Also they are very likely to show signs of cardiovascular dysfunction.

Nursing Diagnoses

Nursing diagnoses commonly associated with hyperthyroidism include the following:

- Sleep pattern disturbance related to insomnia, fatigue, and excessive physical activity.
- Alteration in nutrition, less than body requirements, related to increased metabolic rate.
- Fluid volume deficit related to increased urine output.
- Ineffective individual coping related to emotional lability.
- Sexual dysfunction related to abnormalities of sexual maturity or function.
- Anxiety related to difficulty in concentrating and agitation.
- Knowledge deficit related to information about illness and treatment.

Nursing Intervention

Because of the effect hyperthyroidism has on physical and mental health status, caring for these patients presents a very real challenge to the nurse. Physical and mental rest are extremely important, because physical stress and emotional upset can stimulate the thyroid gland to become even more active. Adequate rest is essential to conserve the strength of the patient, but it is difficult for a person with hyperthyroidism to relax and get sufficient rest.

The diet of the patient should be sufficiently high in calories to meet his metabolic needs. This will vary from person to person, but continued loss of weight is an indication that more high-calorie foods are needed in the diet. It may be necessary to refer the patient to a dietitian who can work with him to develop a satisfactory diet that helps maintain normal body weight.

Patients who are being treated medically for hyperthyroidism must understand that they have an illness that requires ongoing medication and frequent monitoring to assess the effectiveness of treatment. Sometimes it is difficult for the patient's family to accept and deal with the emotional outbursts and mood changes that are present when the disease is not under control. Once hormone levels return to the normal range, the mental and physical symptoms should subside.

Many patients will be rendered hypothyroidic because of surgery or radiation therapy that alters thyroid function. It is then necessary that their illness be managed with long-term thyroid replacement therapy.

Nursing interventions for selected problems of patients with hyperthyroidism are summarized in Nursing Care Plan 27–1.

Thyroidectomy

Patients who do not respond well to antithyroid drug therapy, are unable to take radioactive iodine, have greatly enlarged thyroid glands, or are likely to or have already developed malignancy of the thyroid are candidates for a subtotal thyroidectomy. In this procedure two thirds of

NURSING CARE PLAN 27–1

Selected nursing diagnoses, goals/outcome criteria, nursing interventions, and evaluations for a patient with hyperthyroidism

Situation: Mrs. Jackson, age 35 years, has been having symptoms of hyperthyroidism. She complains of feeling "hot and soaked with perspiration all the time." She is 25 pounds underweight even though she reports a "ravenous" appetite. Her vital signs are: pulse, 120; bounding respirations, 30; and somewhat irregular blood pressure, 170/90. Her serum calcium level was found to be 11.5 mg/dL when she had a physical examination at her physician's office. She has been admitted for control of hypercalcemia and for more diagnostic tests. Mrs. Jackson is very apprehensive, agitated, and irritable.

Nursing Diagnosis	Goals/Outcome Criteria	Nursing Interventions	Evaluation
Anxiety related to nervousness and agitation. SUPPORTING DATA "I don't understand what is happening to me. I feel so nervous all of the time." Wringing her hands, eyes darting around the room, fidgeting in bed.	Anxiety and agitation will be controlled with medication within 3 days.	Keep environmental stimuli at a minimum. No visitors other than family as requested by patient. Approach in a calm and unhurried manner. Provide 30-minute rest periods before lunch, in afternoon, and after supper. Change sweat-soaked linens and gown as needed. Keep room as cool as possible.	Linens changed × 2; rested after bath and lunch; door to room kept closed; encouraged to play quiet, low music; continue plan.
Knowledge deficit related to lack of information about disease and treatment. SUPPORTING DATA States she does not know anything about hyperthyroidism or its treatment.	Patient will verbalize basic understanding of disease and treatment before discharge.	Explain disease process; teach about diagnostic tests and what to expect for each one. Encourage questions and supply answers. Explain options for treatment.	Teaching for diagnostic tests done; questions answered.
Alteration in nutrition, less than body requirements, related to increased metabolic rate. SUPPORTING DATA Has lost 25 lb over last 6 months although appetite has increased considerably.	Will gain 2 lb/week when thyroid production is under control.	Weigh daily; encourage high-calorie between-meal snacks. Increase caloric intake to 3,000 calories per day. Try to accommodate food preferences.	Eating entire meals; two between-meal snacks taken; weight up ½ lb; continue plan.
Potential for injury related to excess circulating thyroid hormone and excess serum calcium. SUPPORTING DATA Thyroid levels: T_3, 230 mg/dL; T_4, 16 μg/dL; calcium, 16 mg/dL.	No permanent cardiac problems will develop; thyroid production will be controlled with medication within 2 weeks; serum calcium will be within normal levels before discharge.	Check vital signs q 4 h. Assess cardiac function each shift and watch for symptoms of thyrotoxicosis such as increased pulse, dyspnea, edema, and rising blood pressure; report such signs at once. Medicate with calcium channel blocker as ordered; observe for side effects. Give medication to decrease calcium levels (diuretic) and monitor electrolyte levels.	Heart rate, 86; rhythm regular; BP, 132/86; electrolytes within normal limits except for calcium (11.2 mg/dL); continue plan.

Nursing care plan continued on following page

NURSING CARE PLAN 27–1, *Continued*

Nursing Diagnosis	Goals/Outcome Criteria	Nursing Interventions	Evaluation
Ineffective individual coping related to labile moods. SUPPORTING DATA States she has been very moody; family says that she keeps changing her mind about things.	Return to former emotional stability when thyroid production returns to normal.	Assure her that mood swings are manifestations of her thyroid disorder. Stress importance of complying with treatment regimen after discharge and keeping appointments with doctor. Give positive reinforcement for correct behavior; encourage verbalization of feelings. Establish trusting relationship; be accepting of behavior; spend uninterrupted time with her each shift; display acceptance of her and her behavior.	Expressing frustration with being "highly emotional"; discussed mood swings and how to cope; encouraged walking daily to reduce stress; continue plan.

the glandular mass is removed. The remaining portion of the gland is left intact so there can be continued production and release of thyroid hormones.

Preoperative Nursing Care. The preoperative nursing care of the patient having a thyroidectomy is much less difficult than it was before antithyroid drugs became available. Most patients who enter the hospital for this type of surgery are much calmer emotionally and less active physically than formerly, because they have received medications to stabilize the activity of the gland.

The responsibility of the nurse for preparation of the patient who is to have a thyroidectomy is essentially the same as for other types of major surgery. If the patient does appear nervous, tense, and apprehensive, his condition should be reported to the physician. These symptoms may indicate improper control of the activities of the thyroid gland and may predispose the patient to the postoperative complication of "thyroid crisis" (see the following section).

Postoperative Nursing Care. As soon as the thyroidectomy patient returns from the operating room, he is placed in the *Fowler's* position to facilitate breathing and reduce swelling of the operative area. The head may be supported with sandbags on either side to relieve tension on the sutures.

Close observation of the patient is an essential part of immediate postoperative care. The vital signs are checked at frequent intervals, and the patient is watched closely for signs of bleeding and swelling of the operative area. Any rise in temperature, pulse, or respiration rate should be reported when first noticed, because it may indicate a high level of thyroxine in the blood stream. External swelling may cause constriction of the bandage around the neck.

Difficulty in swallowing or breathing should also be reported immediately, as this may indicate internal edema and pressure on the esophagus and trachea.

In many hospitals, a tracheostomy set is kept at the bedside of the postoperative thyroidectomy patient in case severe respiratory embarrassment develops. Other symptoms to be reported are persistent hoarseness or loss of the voice, as they may indicate damage to the vocal cords. *Tetany* and *thyroid crisis* are other complications of a thyroidectomy that may occur. These complications are rare, but when they do occur, the nurse must be alert for the beginning signs and report her observations immediately.

Tetany is actually a symptom and results from injury to, or accidental removal of, the parathyroid glands. These small glands are located on the posterior surface of the thyroid gland. *Parathormone*, or *parathyroid hormone*, is secreted by the parathyroid glands and is important in the regulation of the calcium and phosphorus levels in the body tissues. A deficiency of parathyroid hormone produces muscle cramps, twitching of the muscles, and, in some cases, severe convulsions.

These symptoms represent a medical emergency and must be reported to the physician at once.

This complication is treated by the intravenous administration of calcium gluconate during the emergency stage and subsequent maintenance doses of parathyroid hormone to maintain the proper calcium and phosphorus balance in the body.

Thyroid crisis, sometimes called *thyroid storm*, is another complication to be considered following a thyroidectomy. The condition is caused by a sudden increase in the output of thyroxine caused by manipulation of the thyroid as it is being removed. Another cause may be improper reduction of thyroid secretions before surgery (see "Preoperative Nursing Care").

The symptoms of thyroid crisis are produced by a sudden and extreme elevation of all body processes. The temperature may rise to 106°F or more, the pulse increases to as much as 200 beats per minute, respirations become rapid, and the patient exhibits marked apprehension and restlessness.

Unless the condition is relieved, the patient quickly passes from delirium to coma to death from heart failure.

Treatment of thyroid crisis must be begun immediately after the first symptoms are noticed. Measures are employed to reduce the temperature, cardiac drugs are given to slow the heart beat, and sedatives, such as one of the barbiturates, are given to reduce restlessness and anxiety.

Hypothyroidism

Hypothyroidism can be caused by inflammation of the thyroid gland (thyroiditis) or by treatment of hyperthyroidism that results in destruction of too many thyroid cells and a resultant deficit of thyroid hormone. Genetic defects can cause congenital hypothyroidism (cretinism). Cretinism is caused by a severe lack of thyroid hormone during fetal life and infancy and is characterized by growth failure. Underactivity of the thyroid gland can also be caused by a pituitary or hypothalamus dysfunction that causes inadequate stimulation of the thyroid, inducing secondary hypothyroidism.

Signs, Symptoms, and Nursing Assessment

The child with hypothyroidism will have retarded physical and mental growth and will become very sluggish within a few weeks after birth. Adults who have myxedema (very low thyroid production) have a decrease in appetite but an increase in weight as a result of lowered metabolic rate. Other typical signs are bagginess under the eyes and swelling of the face. In both children and adults there is a tendency to be lethargic and to sleep for abnormally long periods of time during the day and night. The speech may be slurred, and the individual will appear sluggish in both mental and physical activities.

Medical diagnosis is based on clinical signs and symptoms and laboratory testing of serum levels of thyroid hormones and TSH.

During history taking the nurse will need to ask about weight gain; constipation, flatulence, and other symptoms of decreased gastrointestinal motility; anorexia; mental changes such as impaired memory, a slowing of thought processes, and depression; and personality changes.

Subjective data include fatigue, muscle cramps, numbness and tingling, increased sensitivity to cold, and loss of a zest for living. Objective data include evidence of changes in almost all of the major systems of the body. The skin is dry and scaly, sometimes with a yellowish tint. Hair is coarse and the nails are thick and brittle. Nonpitting edema occurs as a result of accumulations of fluid in the interstitial spaces. Edema also can affect hearing and cause the voice to become hoarse and husky. Swelling usually is noticed in the face and around the eyes.

Gastrointestinal symptoms are the result of decreasd peristaltic activity and can lead to paralytic ileus if the hypothyroidism continues untreated.

Geriatric patients who are lethargic, slow in thinking, and unenthusiastic about whatever is going on around them could be showing signs of hypothyroidism rather than senility or some other convenient label.

Nursing diagnoses associated with adult hypothyroidism include the following:

- Sleep pattern disturbance related to somnolence.
- Alteration in nutrition, more than body requirements, related to decreased metabolic rate.
- Potential for injury related to inability to think clearly and mental and physical sluggishness.
- Decreased alteration in cardiac output related to decreased stroke volume and heart rate and increased peripheral resistance.
- Constipation related to decreased intestinal motility.
- Knowledge deficit related to information about illness and treatment.
- Potential impaired skin integrity related to dryness and scaling.

Medical Treatment and Nursing Intervention

Hypothyroidism can be treated effectively with replacement of thyroid hormones. The dosage is gradually increased until a proper level has been reached, and then a delicate balance must be maintained so that the patient does not suffer from either hypothyroidism or hyperthyroidism.

The results of treatment of hypothyroidism are very striking, and most patients show a remarkable abatement of their symptoms. The nurse may not see many cases of hypothyroidism in the hospital, because treatment usually does not require hospitalization. If the patient is admitted for some other condition or illness and is also being treated for hypothyroidism, some special considerations must be made. As stated previously, these patients have very rough and dry skin, and they will need massage with lotions and creams to prevent cracking and peeling of the skin. Provisions for extra warmth must also be made for those patients who have an increased sensitivity to cold as a result of their hypothyroidism.

The nurse must also bear in mind the psychological aspects of hypothyroidism. She must avoid rushing these patients or giving them the impression that she is annoyed and inconvenienced by their sluggishness. Forgetfulness, inability to express themselves verbally, and physical inertia are mannerisms that are a direct result of the thyroid deficiency, and the nurse must recognize them as unavoidable as long as the condition is uncontrolled.

THE PARATHYROIDS

The parathyroid glands, usually four in number, are located on the posterior surface of the thyroid glands. They produce a polypeptide hormone called *parathormone*. Production and secretion of this hormone are regulated by the plasma calcium level, which is part of the feedback mechanism that either stimulates or inhibits the release of parathormone. A low calcium level will stimulate the release of parathormone, which increases the level of calcium in the plasma. Conversely, a high calcium level will inhibit the release of parathormone.

Parathormone raises the calcium level in the plasma by acting on the renal tubules to increase the excretion of phosphorus in the urine and the reabsorption of calcium. It also acts on bone, causing the release of calcium from the bone into the blood stream.

HYPOPARATHYROIDISM

Hypoparathyroidism is caused by atrophy or traumatic injury to the parathyroid glands. This can occur as a result of accidental removal or destruction of parathyroid tissue during a thyroidectomy or irradiation of the thyroids or from idiopathic atrophy of the glands.

Symptoms and Medical Diagnosis

A deficiency of parathormone will result in a drop in serum calcium levels and an increase in phosphorus levels. The chief symptom resulting from a lowered serum calcium level is *tetany*. Muscular twitching and spasms occur because of extreme irritability of neuromuscular tissue. If the calcium level continues to fall, the patient will suffer from convulsions, cardiac arrhythmias, and spasms of the larynx. Other symptoms related to hypocalcemia are discussed in Chapter 8 and summarized in Table 8–2. Medical diagnosis is established by clinical signs and laboratory data.

Medical Treatment

Acute hypoparathyroidism is treated by measures to raise serum calcium levels to normal range. Oral or parenteral administration of calcium salts is used in the acute phase. In chronic hypoparathyroidism, treatment is aimed at restoring and maintaining normal calcium levels in the blood. This can be accomplished by parathormone replacement therapy, administration of vitamin D in massive doses to enhance absorption of calcium from the small intestine, and oral adminstration of calcium salts.

HYPERPARATHYROIDISM (VON RECKLINGHAUSEN'S DISEASE)

Hyperparathyroidism is one of the most common disorders of the endocrine system. In recent years a greater number of cases are being diagnosed because of improved radiologic and laboratory screening procedures. The disorder occurs most often in postmenopausal women.

Excessive synthesis and secretion of parathormone can occur as a result of benign enlargement of the parathyroid glands (adenoma) or hyperplasia of two or more glands.

Signs and Symptoms

Hypercalcemia with a calcium level above 10.5 mg/dL occurs with hyperactivity of the parathyroid glands. Signs and symptoms may be mild or severe and include dehydration, confusion, lethargy, anorexia, nausea, vomiting, weight loss, constipation, thirst, frequent urination, and hypertension. If serum calcium levels are high, indicating hypercalcemia, there may be skeletal changes including thinning of the bone and bone cysts. A fracture is often what causes the patient to seek medical attention.

Medical Diagnosis

Many cases of hyperparathyroidism are now being diagnosed in the earliest stages of the disease before the clinical manifestations of hypercalcemia become apparent. Laboratory testing for

TABLE 27-2 CLINICAL MANIFESTATIONS OF PRIMARY HYPERPARATHYROIDISM AND HYPERCALCEMIA

Renal system
- Tubular calcium deposits
- Kidney stones
- Decreased glomerular filtration rate
- Decreased urine concentration
- Polyuria
- Nephrocalcinosis
- Nephrolithiasis
- Decreased acid excretion
- Renal failure
- Hypertension
- Urinary alkalosis
- Metabolic acidosis

Skeletal system
- Increased osteoclastic activity
- Decalcification
- Fractures
- Punched-out bony lesions
- Bone pain
- Osteitis fibrosa cystica
- Osteopenia

Gastrointestinal tract
- Anorexia
- Constipation
- Peptic ulcer
- Pancreatitis

Myocardium
- Increased contractility
- Decreased automaticity
- Sensitive to effects of digitalis
- Shortened QT interval in electrocardiogram

Neuromuscular system
- Hypotonic muscles
- Lethargy
- Vague weakness
- Depressed reflexes

Psyche
- Decreased mental function
- Mood swings
- Depression
- Personality changes
- Apathy, confusion, coma

Other
- Calcium deposits in palpebral fissure of eyes
- Gout
- Deafness

From Hoffman, J. T., and Newby, T. B.: Hypercalcemia in primary hyperparathyroidism. Nurs. Clin. North Am., Sept., 1980, p. 471.

serum calcium and phosphate levels helps verify the diagnosis.

Excessively high levels of calcium in the blood (hypercalcemia) are manifested in virtually every major system in the body (Table 27-2).

Medical Treatment and Nursing Intervention

The treatment of hyperparathyroidism will depend on the severity of the symptoms produced by hypercalcemia and hypophosphatemia. Methods of therapy include the infusion of isotonic sodium chloride and administration of diuretic agents to promote excretion of excess calcium in the urine; phosphate therapy to correct the deficit; administration of mithramycin to inhibit skeletal resorption (release) of calcium; and administration of calcitonin to decrease the rate of skeletal resorption.

Nursing intervention for patients receiving diuretic therapy includes accurate measuring of intake and output, daily weight, monitoring of serum electrolytes, ongoing assessment of the patient for electrolyte imbalance, and appropriate nursing intervention (see Chapter 8).

Surgical Treatment

Surgical removal of a major portion of the parathyroids (subtotal parathyroidectomy) is recommended for patients who have severe systemic disorders associated with excessively high levels of parathormone. The remaining parathyroid tissue will continue to function and prevent the problem of hypoparathyroidism.

Concerns for the Elderly

Tissue changes of the thyroid gland do occur during aging, and thyroid nodules are not uncommon among the older age group. The only significant change seen in this age group is that the T_3 levels are decreased.

Parathyroid hormone levels vary in some older individuals but overall tend to remain constant. Research in this area regarding phosphorus and calcium metabolism is lacking. Circulating levels of both calcium and phosphorus do decrease with advanced age.

BIBLIOGRAPHY

Andreoli, T. E., et al.: Cecil Essentials of Medicine, 2nd ed. Philadelphia, W. B. Saunders, 1990.

Croce, J.: Parathyroid disorders: Hyperparathyroidism, hypoparathyroidism, and other problems. *In* Nurse Review Series. Goldberg, K. (ed.). Springhouse, PA, Springhouse Corporation, 1986.

Guyton, A. C.: Textbook of Medical Physiology, 8th ed. Philadelphia, W. B. Saunders, 1990.

Ignatavicius, D. D., and Bayne, M. J.: Medical-Surgical Nursing. Philadelphia, W. B. Saunders, 1991.

Jones, S.: Thyroid disorders: Hyperthyroidism, hypothyroidism, and other problems. *In* Nurse Review Series. Goldberg, K. (ed.). Springhouse, PA, Springhouse Corporation, 1986.

Kee, J. L.: Laboratory and Diagnostic Tests with Nursing Implications, 2nd ed. Norwalk, CT, Appleton & Lange, 1987.

Sarsany, S. L.: Thyroid storm. RN, July, 1988, p. 46.

Walpert, N.: An orderly look at calcium metabolism disorders. Nursing 90, July, 1990, p. 60.

STUDENT STUDY AIDS

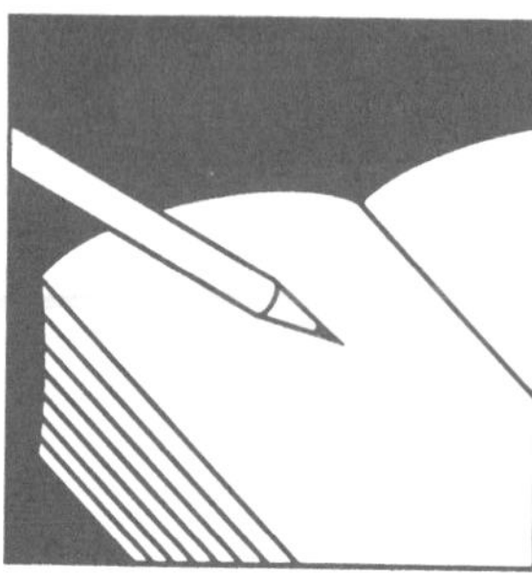

CLINICAL CASE PROBLEMS

Read the following clinical situation and discuss the questions with your classmates.

1. Mrs. Tate has a tentative diagnosis of hyperthyroidism. She is 45 years old, 5 feet 7 inches tall, and weighs 102 pounds.

- What subjective and objective signs and symptoms would you expect Mrs. Tate to present during nursing assessment?
- How would you go about preparing Mrs. Tate for laboratory diagnostic tests for thyroid function?
- If Mrs. Tate's physician decided to treat her condition with large doses of radioactive iodine, what special nursing care will she require?
- What other forms of therapy are used for the treatment of hyperthyroidism?

STUDY OUTLINE

I. Introduction

A. Endocrine glands secrete their hormones directly into blood stream or body fluids.

B. Cells and tissues affected by a specific hormone are called its *target cells* or *tissues.*

C. Hormonal regulation concerned with changing chemical activities within the cells, altering cell membrane permeability, and activating a particular mechanism in the cell.

D. Endocrine glands, their hormones and target cells are summarized in Table 27–1.

E. Regulation of secretion of hormones is a negative feedback system that acts in response to a biologic need.

F. Many endocrine disorders related to overactivity or underactivity of a gland.

II. Thyroids and parathyroids are close anatomically, but have quite different physiologic functions

III. The thyroid

A. Introduction

1. Has two lobes and is highly vascular.
2. Principal hormones are thyroxine (T_4) and triiodothyronine (T_3).
3. These hormones stimulate protein and lipid synthesis, regulate many aspects of CHO metabolism, stimulate synthesis of coenzymes from vitamins.

B. Goiter.

1. Marked enlargement of the thyroid gland; thyroid hormone levels may or may not remain within normal range.
2. May be prevented by adequate intake of iodine for one type.
3. Medical diagnosis based on enlargement of thyroid, local symptoms, absence of systemic changes.
4. Medical treatment and nursing intervention:
   a. Large goiters not responsive to medical treatment are removed surgically. Smaller ones may respond to administration of iodine.

(1) Iodine preparations must be given diluted and through a straw to avoid staining the teeth.

C. Overactivity and underactivity of the thyroid.
1. Diagnostic tests and nursing responsibilities:
a. Involve little more than venipuncture to obtain blood sample.
b. Test results can be altered by presence of iodine in body from previous radiologic studies using contrast media, certain drugs.
c. Thyroid hormones measured include both T_3 and T_4.
d. Other tests include thyroid scan and radioactive iodine uptake.
(1) Patients with hyperthyroidism usually have high levels of both T_3 and T_4.
(2) Patients with hypothyroidism have low levels of T_3 and T_4, and high levels of thyroid-stimulating hormone (TSH).
2. Hyperthyroidism: systemic condition resulting from overactivity of thyroid and overproduction of thyroid hormones.
a. Primary hyperthyroidism also known as Graves' disease, toxic goiter, and thyrotoxicosis.
b. Symptoms and medical diagnosis.
(1) Clinical signs and symptoms indicative of increased metabolic rate.
(2) Sleeping pulse rate elevated.
(3) Serum levels of thyroid hormones elevated.
c. Medical treatment:
(1) Radioactive iodine. Small doses given to outpatients. Large doses require isolation and precautions in handling blood and urine.
(2) Antithyroid drugs include propylthiouracil, SSKI, and Tapazole. Frequently given in preparation for surgery of thyroid.
d. Nursing assessment.
(1) Patients most at risk: women between ages of 30 and 50.
(2) Older women might be misdiagnosed and treated for cardiac disorders.
(3) Family history of thyroid disease significant.
(4) Physical and mental symptoms related to increased metabolism: elevated pulse and blood pressure, palpitations, weight loss and increased appetite, tremors, fatigue, outbursts of physical activity followed by fatigue, emotional instability, possibly exophthalmia.
(5) Patient observed for typical symptoms of hyperthyroidism.
(6) Monitor sleeping pulse.
(7) Problems commonly presented by patients with hyperthyroidism:
(a) Sleep pattern disturbance.
(b) Alteration in nutrition, less than body requirements.
(c) Ineffective individual coping.
(d) Sexual dysfunction.
(e) Knowledge deficit.
(f) Anxiety.
(g) Fluid volume deficit.
e. Nursing interventions:
(1) Provide physical and mental rest.
(2) Diet sufficiently high in calories to meet metabolic needs.
(3) Administer medications and instruct patient about them.
(4) Explain relationship between symptoms and pathology associated with disease.

f. Subtotal thyroidectomy:
(1) For patients who do not respond well to drug or radiation therapy, have greatly enlarged thyroid glands, or actual or potential malignancy of the thyroid.
(2) Two thirds of gland removed.
(3) Preoperative care: observe patient for signs of overactivity or other indications that metabolic rate may be too high for safety during surgery.
(4) Postoperative care:
(a) Patient placed in high Fowler's position.
(b) Vital signs checked frequently and carefully.
(c) Patient watched for signs of bleeding or swelling in operative area.
(d) Two most dangerous complications are thyroid crisis and tetany (from damage to parathyroids).

3. Hypothyroidism: underactivity of the thyroid with insufficiency of thyroid hormones. Can be genetic or acquired.
a. Symptoms and medical diagnosis:
(1) In children, symptoms of cretinism are retarded physical and mental growth.
(2) In adults, condition (myxedema) is characterized by bagginess under the eyes, facial swelling, weight gain, diminished mental acuity, dry and scaly skin, and increased sensitivity to cold.
(3) Diagnosis based on clinical manifestations and serum levels of T_3, T_4, and TSH.
b. Nursing assessment:
(1) Subjective data: fatigue, muscle cramps, numbness and tingling, increased sensitivity to cold, loss of zest for living.
(2) Objective data: changes in almost every body system.
(a) Skin dry and scaly, yellowish in color.
(b) Nonpitting edema.
(c) Hearing loss.
(d) Voice change.
(e) GI symptoms of decreased peristalsis, can lead to paralytic ileus.
(f) Geriatric patients who appear lethargic and disinterested could be suffering from hypothyroidism.
(3) Nursing diagnoses associated with hypothyroidism:
(a) Sleep pattern disturbance.
(b) Alteration in nutrition, more than body requirements.
(c) Potential for injury.
(d) Alteration in cardiac output, decreased.
(e) Constipation.
(f) Knowledge deficit.
(g) Potential impaired skin integrity.
c. Medical treatment and nursing intervention:
(1) Condition usually responds to replacement therapy.
(2) Meticulous skin care necessary.
(3) Provide warmth if patient sensitive to cold.
(4) Avoid rushing patient.
(5) Educate patient of necessity for taking medication daily.

IV. The parathyroids

A. Parathyroids located on the posterior aspect of the thyroid.
B. Parathyroid hormone regulates calcium and phosphorus serum levels. Acts on renal tubules to increase excretion of phosphorus and

reabsorption of calcium. Also acts on bone to release calcium into blood stream.

C. Hypoparathyroidism.
   1. Caused by atrophy or traumatic injury to parathyroids, as in thyroid surgery or radiation.
   2. Medical diagnosis based on abnormal calcium and phosphorus serum levels, symptoms of hypocalcemia, tetany, cardiac arrhythmias.
   3. Signs and symptoms: decreased calcium level with elevated phosphorus level, fatigue, muscular twitching, muscle spasm, possible tetany.
   4. Medical treatment:
      a. Measures to raise serum calcium levels.
      b. Parathormone replacement therapy.

D. Hyperparathyroidism.
   1. One of the most common endocrine disorders. Often diagnosed during routine physical examination and screening techniques.
   2. Results from benign secreting tumors of parathyroid or hyperplasia of the gland.
   3. Signs and symptoms: elevated serum calcium level, GI complaints, dehydration, confusion, weight loss, thirst, and hypertension.
   4. Medical diagnosis based on clinical manifestations and laboratory tests.
   5. Medical treatment and nursing intervention:
      a. Saline infusions, diuretics to remove excess calcium.
      b. Phosphate therapy, mithramycin, and calcitonin to correct skeletal release of calcium.
      c. Nursing measures as for patients receiving diuretic therapy, monitoring serum electrolytes, measuring intake and output.
   6. Surgical treatment: subtotal parathyroidectomy.

V. Concerns for the elderly

A. Thyroid tissue changes include formation of nodules in many patients in this age group.

B. T_3 levels are decreased.

C. Parathyroid levels tend to remain constant.

CHAPTER 28

Breakfast		Lunch		Dinne	
Insulin Dose	Blood Glucose Tests	Insulin Dose	Blood Glucose Tests	Insulin Dose	Bl Glu T
	Time		Time		T
	Result		Result		Re
	Time		Time		T
	Result		Result		Re
	Time		Time		T

Care of Patients With Diabetes Mellitus and Hypoglycemia

VOCABULARY

atrophy
exocrine
exogenous
functional disorder
glucogenesis
hyperglycemia
hypoglycemia
ketoacidosis
ketosis
lipodystrophy
oxidation

Upon completion of this chapter the student should be able to:

1. State significant differences in the two major types of diabetes mellitus.
2. Identify each of the four kinds of factors that influence the development of diabetes mellitus.
3. Describe laboratory tests used in the diagnosis of diabetes mellitus.
4. Describe nursing assessment and intervention for the management of type I and type II diabetes mellitus.
5. Prepare a general teaching plan for the patient with newly diagnosed diabetes.
6. Identify sources of support and information for diabetic patients and their families.
7. Describe the early signs and symptoms that might indicate that your diabetic patient is in early ketoacidosis.
8. List the signs and symptoms of an insulin reaction (hypoglycemia) and describe the appropriate nursing interventions.
9. Describe the acute and long-term complications and sequelae of poorly controlled diabetes mellitus.
10. Identify signs and symptoms of hypoglycemia in nondiabetic patients.
11. Describe nursing assessment and intervention for patients with hypoglycemia.

Diabetes mellitus is not a single disease caused by a deficiency of the hormone insulin, which is produced by the pancreas. It is a complex group of disorders that have in common a disturbance in the oxidation and utilization of glucose that is secondary to a malfunction of the beta cells of the pancreas.

Glucose cannot enter the cells when insulin is absent, and the cells enter a state of starvation even though there is an excess of glucose in the blood.

The pancreas is both an endocrine and exocrine gland. Its endocrine function is production of the hormones *insulin* and *glucagon*. Because insulin is involved in the metabolism of carbohydrates, proteins, and fats, diabetes mellitus is not limited to a disturbance of glucose homeostasis. However, the one disorder that all diabetic persons share is an intolerance to glucose.

TYPES OF DIABETES MELLITUS

There are at least two major types and five subtypes of diabetes mellitus.

The categories of diabetes are not defined by hard and fast rules. Table 28–1 summarizes the major characteristics of various forms of diabetes mellitus. In this section we will be concerned primarily with type I and type II.

Type I, or insulin-dependent, diabetes mellitus (IDDM) accounts for about 5% to 10% of all cases. It occurs twice as frequently in women as men. Black Americans are twice as likely to develop the disease as white Americans, and Hispanic Americans have a five times greater incidence of diabetes mellitus than the rest of the population. As the name implies, persons who have this type

TABLE 28–1 **CLINICAL CATEGORIES OF DIABETES MELLITUS AND THE CHARACTERISTICS OF EACH**

Type	Former names	Characteristics
Type I (IDDM)	Juvenile diabetes Juvenile-onset Ketosis-prone Brittle diabetes	Little or no endogenous insulin produced. New patients can be any age but usually are young. Patient must receive exogenous insulin and follow prescribed diet and exercise program. Renal, cardiovascular, retinal, and neurologic complications likely if disease is not kept under tight control.
Type II (NIDDM)	Adult-onset diabetes Maturity-onset diabetes Ketosis-resistant Stable diabetes	Rarely develop ketosis except during infection or other stress. Patients vary in need for exogenous insulin. New patients usually over 40 and most are obese. Disorder often responds to diet and exercise.
Impaired glucose tolerance	Asymptomatic diabetes Chemical diabetes Subclinical diabetes Borderline diabetes	Glucose levels between those of normal people and those of diabetics. Are at high risk for atherosclerotic disease and cardiovascular problems. Do not seem to be particularly susceptible to renal and retinal complications.
	Gestational diabetes	Occurs only during pregnancy.
	Statistical risk of diabetes	Those who have had impaired glucose tolerance in the past but have normal glucose tolerance now; prediabetes, latent diabetes, subclinical diabetes. Those who are predisposed to diabetes because of family history, age, race, or obesity.

of diabetes require injections of exogenous insulin to maintain life, because they produce little or no endogenous insulin on their own. In general, persons with IDDM are more prone to a serious complication associated with an excess of ketone bodies, leading to metabolic acidosis (ketoacidosis). IDDM also is more likely to appear early in life. In fact, this type of diabetes was formerly called *juvenile diabetes* and *ketosis-prone diabetes* because of its typical early onset and potential for ketoacidosis.

Type II, or non-insulin-dependent diabetes mellitus (NIDDM), affects about 90% of the diabetic population. It is believed to be related to inappropriate insulin production, such as an insufficient amount or a delayed response to a glucose load. NIDDM has a tendency to develop later in life than IDDM, and these patients rarely develop diabetic ketoacidosis.

Gestational diabetes may occur as a result of the stress of pregnancy. It is treated with insulin. After delivery, the condition must be reevaluated; the patient may revert to impaired glucose tolerance, or she may prove to have true IDDM or NIDDM, especially if she is overweight.

CONTRIBUTING FACTORS

There are at least four sets of factors that influence the development of diabetes mellitus: genetic, metabolic, microbiologic, and immunologic.

Genetic factors are included in the etiology of diabetes because diabetes tends to run in families, even though research has not yet pinpointed the responsible genes. It is known that the risk of having some form of diabetes increases in proportion to the number of relatives who are affected, the genetic closeness of the relatives, and the severity of their disease.

Metabolic factors involved in the etiology of diabetes are many and complex. Emotional or physical stress can unmask an inherited predisposition to the disease, probably as a result of glucogenesis induced by increased production of hormones from the adrenal cortex, especially the glucocorticoids.

Perhaps even more significant than metabolic factors and the occurrence of diabetes is the association of NIDDM and obesity. About 80% of these patients are obese, and there is a higher incidence of NIDDM in persons who lead a sedentary life and eat a high-calorie diet. With weight reduction and increased physical activity, blood glucose can be restored to normal levels and maintained there; hence the importance of diet and exercise in the management of NIDDM. In this type of diabetes there also seems to be a relationship to aging and a reduction in the function of the pancreatic beta cells and their synthesis of insulin.

Microbiologic factors have to do with the suspicion that some forms of IDDM are related to viral destruction of the beta cells. The mumps or coxsackievirus is thought to be the trigger. Evidence that supports viruses as causative factors include the following:

- Both IDDM and viral infections tend to have sudden onsets.
- Seasonal fluctuations in the onset of IDDM —late autumn and early spring—correspond with the times of the year when "flu" and other viral illness are most common.
- Viral infections can and often do attack the pancreas; many viral infections are characterized by inflammation of the pancreatic beta cells.

There are known cases in which children developed IDDM after having had a recent viral infection.

Immunologic factors are considered, because research studies have presented strong evidence that some types of IDDM are an autoimmune reaction associated with the HLA-DR3 gene. At the time IDDM is diagnosed, about three fourths of the cases studied have islet cell antibodies circulating in the blood. Such antibodies are not found in normal individuals. Diabetics who continue to produce insulin will eventually stop producing normal amounts of the hormone if islet cell antibodies remain in the blood.

INCIDENCE AND PREVALENCE

For reasons not yet fully understood, the incidence of diabetes mellitus is increasing at an alarming rate. The incidence of diabetes mellitus in the United States is 6%, affecting an estimated 11 million people.

The alarming rate of increase can be explained in part by improved methods of diagnosing and reporting and by more effective management of the disease, which has increased the life span of diabetic persons. Successful management has saved the lives of many diabetic infants who formerly could not survive more than a few months. Moreover, improved methods of control have allowed young diabetic adults to have children safely, and their offspring are more likely to develop diabetes.

DIAGNOSTIC TESTS

The most common diagnostic tests for diabetes mellitus are those that test for glucose in the blood and urine. Glucose normally is excreted by the kidneys in minute amounts, whereas uncontrolled diabetes causes a "spilling" of excess glucose in the blood over the renal threshold and into the urine. Before the invention of the glucometer for blood testing, urine testing was the mainstay of monitoring therapy. However, as a person grows older, urine tests for glucose are less reliable because of the kidneys' inability to rid the blood of excess sugar. The presence of glucose in the urine (glycosuria) may be normal if the specimen is checked immediately after ingestion of a high-carbohydrate meal. Blood testing is much more accurate.

Fasting Blood Glucose

The fasting blood glucose level should show the normal amount of glucose in the blood, which can range from 80 to 120 mg of glucose per 100 mL of blood. A fasting glucose level of 140 mg/dL or more, plus at least two plasma glucose readings of >200 mg/dL, usually accompanied by the presence of ketones in the blood and urine, indicates IDDM. A high blood glucose level is suggestive of diabetes mellitus but can also be found in chronic liver disease and in overactivity of the pituitary and adrenal glands. The test involves the withdrawal of 5 to 7 mL of blood while the patient is in a fasting state.

Two-Hour Postprandial Glucose Test

This test may be done to determine whether a full glucose tolerance test is necessary. A single blood specimen is taken 2 hours after a normal meal. A result above 140 mg/dL is considered abnormal.

Glucose Tolerance Test

This test does not always give a definitive diagnosis of diabetes mellitus, nor can it be depended on to rule out the disease in every case. It is, however, commonly used as one of the criteria for diagnosing diabetes mellitus. The glucose tolerance test is a challenge test, in which the patient is given a large amount of glucose in order to evaluate insulin secretion and the body's ability to metabolize glucose. Testing is done in the morning with the patient in a fasting state. It is a timed test; that is, blood and urine samples are taken before the ingestion of the glucose and then at 30 minutes and 1, 2, and 3 hours after the glucose is consumed. Additional hourly monitoring is sometimes done to aid in the diagnosis of hypoglycemia. Normal plasma glucose levels reach their highest level of 160 to 180 mg per 100 mL within 30 minutes to 1 hour after ingestion of the glucose preparation. The plasma glucose should return to fasting level or lower after 2 to 3 hours. The urine should be negative for glucose throughout the test. Because of confusion over the meaning of glucose tolerance test results, the American Diabetes Association has recommended that physicians use a point system to interpret the values obtained during the test.

Glycosylated Hemoglobin Test

This test is used not to diagnose diabetes but to monitor the progress of a person who is already known to be a diabetic. Commonly called *hemoglobin* A_{1c} (pronounced *A-one-see*), the test measures blood glucose control over a period of many weeks rather than at any one time. No preparation is necessary for the test. It involves only a venipuncture to obtain a small sample of blood and can be done at any time of the day. Hemoglobin A_{1c} is hemoglobin with glucose attached to it. Hemoglobin A, the normal type of adult hemoglobin, is "sticky"; therefore glucose in the blood stream attaches itself to the hemoglobin A molecules and remains there for the life span of the red blood cell. Because red cells live about 120 days, measurement of the amount of glucose attached to the hemoglobin can give an average blood glucose level for the past 3 to 4 months. This test offers advantages for both the patient and the physician who is helping him gain and maintain control over his blood sugar. Patients who monitor their own blood glucose levels at home and follow the prescribed control regimen can determine whether the methods they are using for control are working. Physicians can use test results to change and improve prescribed programs for the management of diabetes. Knowing the test results every 3 to 4 months also can work as a motivator to patients who can see for themselves whether their compliance with the prescribed program is keeping their blood glucose at an acceptable level over a period of time. A normal value for hemoglobin A_{1c} depends on the laboratory method used.

SYMPTOMS AND MEDICAL DIAGNOSIS

In addition to the results of laboratory tests, the physician depends on clinical signs and symptoms of diabetes mellitus to establish a diagnosis. The classic symptoms of the disorder, regardless of type, are related to an elevated blood glucose level. The excess glucose in the blood stream (hyperglycemia) increases the concentration of the intravascular fluid, raising its osmotic pressure and pulling water from the cells and interstitial fluid into the blood. This causes cellular dehydration and the loss of glucose, electrolytes, and water in the urine.

Cellular dehydration causes thirst and a resultant increased intake of water (polydipsia) and diuresis with increased urination (polyuria).

Hunger (polyphagia) is the result of the body's effort to increase its supply of energy foods, even though the intake of more carbohydrates does not meet the energy needs of the cells.

Classic signs and symptoms of diabetes mellitus are polydipsia, polyuria, and polyphagia.

Fatigue and muscular weakness occur because the glucose needed for energy simply is not metabolized properly. Weight loss in patients with IDDM occurs partly because of the loss of body fluid and partly because in the absence of sufficient insulin, the body begins to metabolize its own proteins and stored fat. The oxidation of fats is incomplete, however, and so fatty acids are converted into ketone bodies: beta-hydroxybutyric acid, acetoacetic acid, and acetone. When the kidney is unable to handle all of the ketones accumulated in the blood, the patient has what is called *ketosis*. The overwhelming presence of the strong organic acids in the blood lowers the pH and leads to a severe and potentially fatal acidosis.

Weight gain is common in persons with NIDDM because of a high caloric intake and the availability of endogenous insulin to fully utilize the food that is eaten.

The metabolism of body protein when insulin is not available causes an elevated blood urea nitrogen (BUN) level, because the nitrogen component of protein is discarded when the body metabolizes its own protein to obtain the glucose it needs.

Diabetic persons also are prone to infection, delayed healing, and vascular diseases. The ease with which poorly controlled diabetics develop an infection is thought to be partly a result of decreased chemotaxis of leukocytes and abnormal phagocyte function. Another contributing factor to infection and delayed healing probably is decreased blood supply to the tissues because of atherosclerotic changes in the blood vessels. An impaired blood supply means a deficit in the protective cells brought by the blood to a site of injury.

Moreover, it is believed that the neurologic, vascular, and metabolic complications of diabetes predispose the diabetic person to infections by allowing organisms to enter tissues that are normally better defended and less accessible. For example, a neurogenic bladder predisposes the patient to stagnant urine and accumulations of bacteria, and a leg ulcer resulting from peripheral vascular disease is without the protection of the skin as a barrier to organisms. Chronic neurologic and vascular complications of diabetes are discussed later in this chapter.

MANAGEMENT OF DIABETES

There is no cure for diabetes mellitus; the goal is to maintain blood glucose and lipid levels within normal limits and to control these factors as tightly as possible to prevent complications. Although there is some controversy over the need for rigid control of diabetes, the American Diabetes Association wholeheartedly supports the concept that many of the sequelae of diabetes can be minimized by optimal control.

The controversy over whether keeping blood glucose of a diabetic person at near-normal levels will prevent many long-term complications probably will continue until the effects of insulin pumps, self-monitoring of blood glucose, and other measures for tighter control can be studied over a period of years. Within the next decade studies currently being conducted should give more substantial evidence about the advantages of strict control.

There are some risks associated with perfect control of blood glucose levels. The most serious of these is hypoglycemia or insulin reaction. The long-term risks of tight control have not yet been identified, because in the past few people were able to achieve perfect control with the techniques and modes of management available to them.

In general, "good" or "tight" control is thought to be achieved when fasting blood glucose stays within normal limits, glycosylated hemoglobin tests show that blood glucose has stayed within normal limits from one testing period to the next, the patient's weight is normal, blood lipids remain within normal limits, and the patient has a sense of health and well-being.

The protocol for control of diabetes mellitus is highly individualized and depends on the type of diabetes a person has; his age, general state of health, ability to follow the prescribed regimen, and acceptance of responsibility for managing his illness; and a host of other factors. Both IDDM and NIDDM patients must follow their prescribed diets and carry out some form of regular exercise. These are the cornerstones of management, regardless of the specific problem with glucose intolerance.

Insulin therapy can be prescribed for non–insulin-dependent patients as well as those who are insulin-dependent. In most cases, those who have NIDDM can control their blood glucose by reducing caloric intake and increasing physical exercise. In addition, oral hypoglycemic or antidiabetic agents may be prescribed for NIDDM patients to help keep their blood glucose levels under control.

DIET

The diet of each diabetic patient is calculated on an individual basis. There is no such thing as a "typical" diabetic, and because diabetes is an unstable and changing process, each patient's needs will change from time to time. In general, the diabetic diet is geared toward providing adequate nutrition with sufficient calories to maintain normal body weight and to adjust the intake of food so that blood glucose is kept within safe limits. In recent years, less emphasis has been placed on caloric intake and restriction of carbohydrates and more attention paid to the regulation of body weight and control of cholesterol and blood glucose levels in each patient.

The individual diet is based on the patient's type of diabetes, his height: weight ratio, usual dietary intake, cultural preferences, exercise level, and daily schedule. Meal plans are generally made up of 55% to 65% carbohydrate, 12% to 15% protein, and 20% to 30% fat. Concentrated sweets are avoided, and meals should include an adequate amount of fiber.

The American Diabetes Association and the American Dietetic Association have worked together to devise a simplified method of calculating a diabetic diet and planning a diabetic's meals. The booklet containing this information is entitled "The Exchange List for Meal Planning." The principal foods are divided into six groups, as summarized below.

Each group contains foods that are similar in kind and have equal nutritional value in regard to carbohydrate, protein, and fat. For example, more than 30 fruits from which the diabetic can choose are listed, each providing 10 gm of carbohydrate, a negligible amount of protein and fat, and 40 calories per serving. Other lists contain similar information for a great variety of foods. The booklet also includes instructions for substitutions among the food groups, as well as a table for the conversion of weights and measures. With this simple method of choosing a menu from the exchange lists, a diabetic or a member of his family can calculate caloric and nutritional value with ease.

Other diabetic dietary programs available include the point, constant carbohydrate, and total available glucose (TAG) plans. In the point system, 75 kcal equals 1 point. An assessment of the patient's needed caloric level and lifestyle is done, and a point total is listed for each meal and snack. Recommended daily allowance (RDA) guidelines are also followed so that balanced nutrition is achieved. However, regardless of the type of dietary planning system used, it is essential that the nurse determine whether the patient and family truly understand how to properly use it.

It is important that the diabetic patient not develop a defeatist or negative attitude toward his diet. Emphasis should be placed on the positive aspects of his diet, on the foods he is allowed rather than those that are forbidden. He should not be made to feel guilty about experiencing difficulty with staying on his diet or the times he deliberately "cheats" and helps himself to foods that are not allowed. Each of us has our moments when we are likely to yield to the temptation to do what we know is not in our best interest.

One of the most effective means of helping the diabetic patient follow his diet is by teaching him about food values and how they affect diabetes so that he can understand how food elements affect his health and well-being. In order to help the diabetic and his family learn which foods he should eat and those he should avoid, the physician, the dietitian, and the nurse must all participate in the instruction. Fortunately, many well-written and clearly illustrated booklets and pamphlets are available that are very helpful to the diabetic and his family. Such organizations as the American Diabetes Association (National Service Center, 1660 Duke St., Alexandria, VA 22314. Telephone: 800-232-3472) and the Joslin Diabetes Center (One Joslin Place, Boston, MA 02215. Telephone 617-732-2415) will send instructive material on request. This material not

THE SIX FOOD EXCHANGE LISTS

List I: Milk exchanges	Nonfat, low-fat, and whole milk
List II: Vegetable exchanges	All nonstarchy vegetables
List III: Fruit exchanges	All fruits and fruit juices
List IV: Bread exchanges	Bread, cereal, pasta, starchy vegetables, and prepared foods
List V: Meat exchanges	Lean, medium-fat, and high-fat meat and other protein-rich foods
List VI: Fat exchanges	Polyunsaturated, saturated, and monosaturated fats

only covers diets but also warns the diabetic against misleading or fraudulent information in regard to quick "cures" or special diets that will cure diabetes.

EXERCISE

Physical exercise is an important part of the management of diabetes. Muscular activity improves the utilization of glucose by using it for energy and also improves circulation. In addition to lowering blood glucose levels by "burning up" the glucose, exercise makes the insulin receptors on cells more sensitive to the hormone and thus improves utilization of the available glucose. Because diabetic control also considers blood lipid levels, exercise contributes to that control by reducing triglyceride levels and increasing high-density lipoprotein (HDL) levels.

The exercise program should be designed for the individual patient.

It should consider the age and overall physical condition of the patient, his ability to carry out the exercises regularly, and how well controlled his diabetes is. For some patients a brisk walk of 1 or 2 miles daily is as much exercise as they can tolerate. Others may be able to perform more strenuous exercises, but they must be cautioned against extremes, especially if they are taking insulin. Exercise can rapidly lower blood glucose levels and cause serious hypoglycemia.

All exercise programs should begin with milder forms of exercise and gradually increase until the patient's level of tolerance or the desired therapeutic effect is reached. A program should not be started until the patient's blood glucose is under control. The exercise program should be planned so that the patient performs the exercises at the same time every day, preferably after a meal when the blood glucose is highest. The patient is encouraged to exercise with a friend who knows the signs and symptoms of hypoglycemia and how to treat it.

Recommendations for Increased Food Intake During Exercise

During moderate exercise such as brisk walking, bowling, or vacuuming, 5 grams of simple carbohydrate should be consumed at the end of 30 minutes and at 30-minute intervals during the continued activity. Jogging, swimming, or scrubbing floors should be preceded by consumption of 15 to 20 grams of complex carbohydrate plus protein 15 to 30 minutes prior to beginning the exercise, and then, if the activity continues for more than 30 minutes, 10 grams of simple carbohydrate should be taken every 30 minutes. Vigorous exercise such as fast jogging, skiing, or playing tennis requires intake of 30 to 40 grams of complex carbohydrate plus protein 15 to 30 minutes ahead of time and then 10 to 20 grams of simple carbohydrate intake every 30 minutes after the first half hour.

Performing exercise when insulin or an oral antidiabetic agent is at its peak of action can bring on an acute hypoglycemic reaction. Another precaution for insulin-dependent patients is to avoid injecting insulin into an area that will soon receive extra exercise (for example, the leg). Eating a piece of fruit before even light exercise, if done between meals, also can help prevent hypoglycemia in insulin-dependent diabetics.

Once a patient begins to follow a regular exercise program, his insulin dosage and diet may need revision. In general, he probably willl need to take less insulin and to increase his caloric intake if he exercises regularly. Keeping a daily record of his exercise, along with his weight, insulin dosage, and urine and blood glucose levels can help motivate the patient to continue with his exercises.

ADMINISTRATION OF INSULIN

Insulin is a potent drug that must be treated with respect by the patient and any others involved in its administration. Exogenous insulin is a liquid hormonal preparation obtained from the pancreas of animals. Since the advent of genetic engineering techniques, human insulin (sometimes called *humulin*) is the preferred form, because it is less likely to cause allergies and other problems associated with insulin from an animal source. Human insulin is produced in the laboratory by splicing genetic material into the deoxyribonucleic acid (DNA) of a bacterium. The interjected genetic material contains information for the structure of the insulin protein. The bacteria use this information to produce the insulin over and over again in successive generations.

Exogenous insulin was first developed in 1921 by Sir Frederick Banting and Dr. Charles Best. The plain insulin, known today as *regular insulin*, acts for no longer than 6 to 8 hours after injection. In 1936, Hagedorn, a Danish physician, found that by adding a protein (protamine) to insulin, its action could be prolonged to a period of 12 hours. It was later discovered that by adding zinc to the protamine and insulin, blood glucose levels could be reduced for as long as 24 hours with a single injection. This combination of protamine, zinc, and insulin is known as *protamine zinc insulin*, or *PZI*.

After continued research, scientists developed an intermediate-acting insulin that reaches its peak of action at some time between that of the fast-acting regular insulin and the long-acting PZI. The first to be used was globin insulin. Later, neutral protamine Hagedorn (NPH), lente, and semilente insulin were developed. NPH insulin is one of the most popular types used today.

The variety of rapid-acting, slow-acting, and intermediate-acting insulins provides alternative types from which to choose to find the one best suited for the individual patient. In order to achieve a level of insulin throughout the day that is as near as possible to that of endogenous insulin, some patients may take both regular and a long-lasting insulin once or twice a day (Table 28–2). Humulin 70/30 is a combination of regular and NPH insulin and is often prescribed so that patients do not have to mix insulins. Table 28–3 shows various regimens in which regular (short-acting) and long-acting insulins are used.

TABLE 28–2 MIXING TWO TYPES OF INSULIN

1. Inject air into the long-acting insulin bottle first and then into the short-acting insulin bottle; draw up the correct amount of short-acting insulin.
2. Remove the needle from the bottle and immediately draw up the long-acting insulin from the second bottle, being careful not to inject any of the short-acting insulin into the bottle and drawing up the insulin slowly so that minimal problems occur in obtaining the exact dosage.
3. Follow the remainder of the steps as listed in the text and Table 28–4.

TABLE 28–3 INSULIN REGIMENS

Regimen	Type Insulin Used	Time Administered With Expected Time-Action Curve*	Advantages	Disadvantages
Single-dose	Intermediate insulin (I)	7 A.M. (I); Noon; 6 P.M.; Midnight; 7 A.M.	1 injection should cover noon and P.M. meal; hypoglycemia during sleep is not a problem	No fasting, breakfast, or nighttime coverage of hyperglycemia
Split-mixed dose	Intermediate and regular insulin (I) + (R)	7 A.M. (I)+(R); Noon; 6 P.M.; Midnight; 7 A.M.	2 injections provide coverage over 24-hour period	2 injections required; "locks" patient into set meal pattern
Split-mixed dose	Intermediate and regular insulin (I) + (R)	7 A.M. (I)+(R); Noon; 7 P.M. (R); 9 P.M. (I); Midnight; 7 A.M.	3 injections provide coverage over 24 hours, particularly over early A.M. hours	3 injections required; evening intermediate insulin dose may potentiate early morning hypoglycemia
Multiple dose	Regular insulin and intermediate insulin (I) + (R)	7 A.M. (R); Noon (R); 7 P.M. (R); 9 P.M. (I); Midnight; 7 A.M.	Allows more flexibility in meal times and amount of food intake	4 injections required; requires premeal blood glucose checks; establishing and following individualized algorithm; tighter control may predispose to hypoglycemia
Multiple dose (insulin delivery via the pump is similar to this regimen)	Regular insulin and longest-acting insulin (R) + (LA)	7 A.M. (R)+(LA); Noon (R); 7 P.M. (R); Midnight; 7 A.M.	Provides insulin delivery pattern that more closely simulates normal endogenous insulin pattern; allows for some flexibility in food-intake pattern	Requires 3 or 4 injections plus premeal and blood glucose check on retiring; requires establishing and following individualized algorithm; tight control may predispose to hypoglycemia

* Short-acting insulin ———. Long-acting insulin ---------.
From Price, M. J.: Insulin and oral hypoglycemic agents. Nurs. Clin. North Am., Dec., 1983, p. 695.

PZI, NPH, and lente insulin are all cloudy and milky in appearance and must be thoroughly mixed before they are administered so that the patient will receive the prescribed dose. This is done by gently rolling the bottle between the palms of the hands. The bottle is not shaken, because this produces very fine air bubbles that are almost impossible to see but can alter the dosage given and may contribute to breakdown of the insulin.

The type of insulin prescribed for a patient should not be confused with its strength. Insulin labeled "U100" means that there are 100 units of insulin per milliliter of solution; that is, each milliliter contains 100 units. The syringe used for measuring and administering U100 insulin is calibrated to accommodate insulin of this strength. A "Lo-dose" syringe will accommodate up to 50 units of insulin. If the dose is higher than this amount, the larger 100-unit syringe is needed. If regular insulin and a longer acting insulin are to be mixed in one syringe, the regular insulin is drawn up first to prevent any contamination of the regular bottle of insulin with the longer acting variety.

No matter what the type, insulin must be given by injection. It cannot be taken orally, because it is destroyed by gastric juices. Oral hypoglycemic drugs, which are prescribed for some non-insulin-dependent diabetics, are not an oral form of insulin.

Insulin injections can cause depressions in the fat beneath the skin (lipodystrophy) when the insulin is repeatedly injected in the same place over a period of time. Rotation of sites can help minimize this problem. Patients are given charts showing the places on the arms, legs, buttocks, and abdomen where insulin can be injected (Fig. 28-1). They are then encouraged to keep a daily record of injection sites to help them avoid the

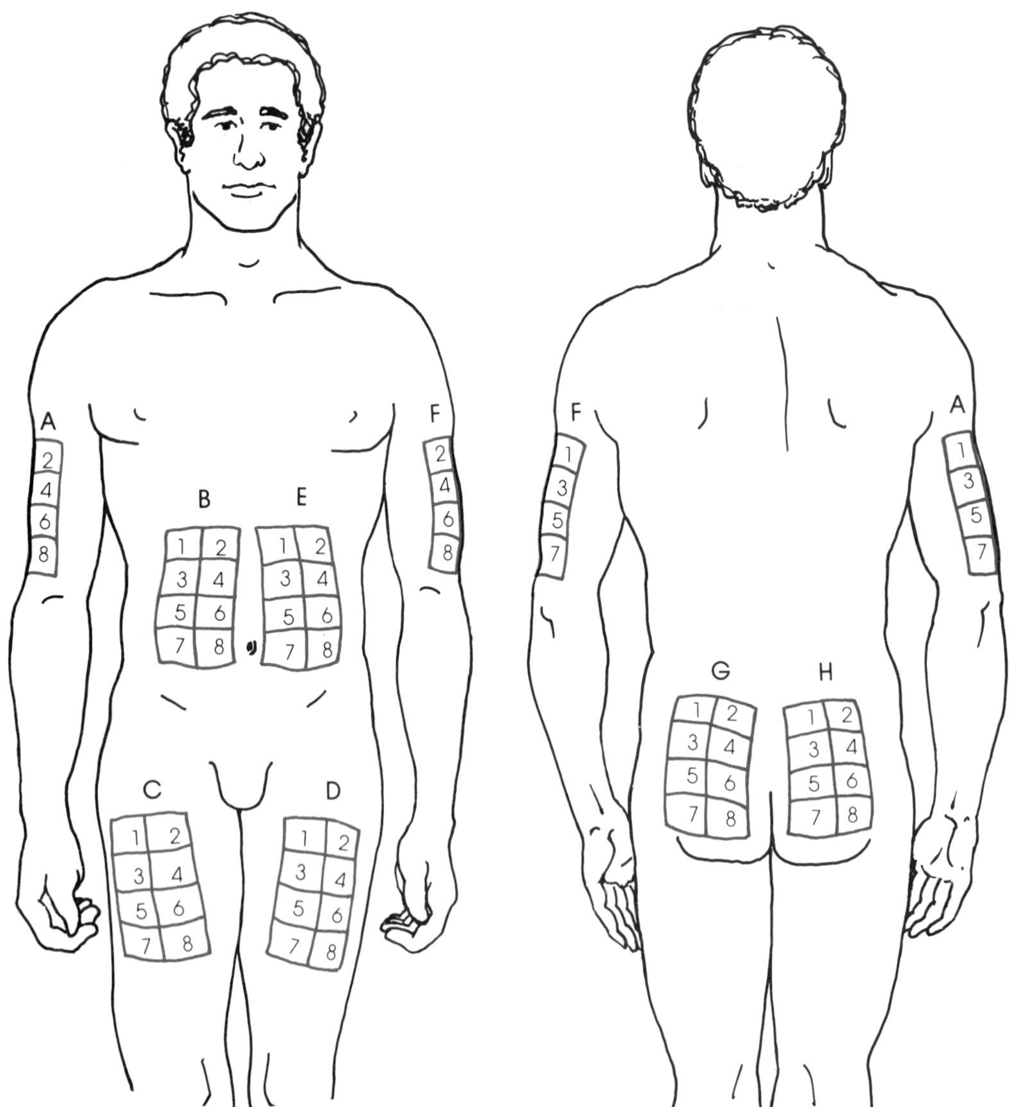

Figure 28-1 Rotation sites for injection of insulin.

TABLE 28-4 **TEACHING GUIDELINES FOR SUBCUTANEOUS INSULIN ADMINISTRATION**

1. Wash hands thoroughly.
2. Check type of insulin and expiration date on bottle label.
3. Check that syringe type is correct (e.g., U100 for U100 insulin).
4. Roll the bottle of insulin between the palms of the hands to gently mix it.
5. Cleanse the top of the rubber stopper with an alcohol swab.
6. Remove the needle cover and pull the plunger back to a point equal to the desired amount of insulin you will draw up; place the needle into the bottle above the surface of the insulin and inject the air (this prevents bubbles).
7. Turn the bottle and syringe upside down, holding them with one hand; with the bevel of the needle well into the insulin, slowly draw up the correct amount of insulin.
8. Remove air bubbles in the syringe by tapping on the barrel of the syringe, reinjecting into the bottle, and then redrawing up the correct dosage of insulin without bubbles.
9. Remove the needle from the bottle; select a site for injection that has not been used in the past month.
10. Clean the site with an alcohol swab; pinch up the area of skin and insert the needle all the way at a 90-degree angle; inject the insulin.
11. Pull the needle straight out quickly.
12. Do not recap the needle; dispose of the syringe and needle in a puncture-proof container.

problem of lipodystrophy. Pain at the injection site may be caused by injecting insulin that has been refrigerated. If insulin is refrigerated, it should be warmed by gently rotating the filled syringe between the hands. Table 28-4 presents guidelines for teaching a patient how to give insulin subcutaneously.

Insulin requirements change as metabolic needs are altered by diet, exercise, age, and even changes in seasons. In the summer, for example, many people are outdoors and exercising more than during the winter months. Also, as a person grows older, his level of physical activity may decrease. Insulin requirements are also altered when the patient has an infection or illness or is under added stress.

If a patient is monitoring his own blood glucose at home and his physician has recommended adjustments of insulin dosage on the basis of daily blood glucose levels, he will need to be taught how to calculate the amount of insulin he should take to achieve the desired blood glucose level.

Research is in progress to determine whether it is possible to effectively deliver insulin dosages by eye drop or nasal inhalation. Someday insulin by injection may be obsolete.

Insulin Pump

An alternative to conventional insulin therapy by daily injections is the insulin pump. These pumps are capable of delivering a continuous infusion of insulin by way of an automated system composed of a battery-driven electronic "brain," an electric motor and drive mechanisms, and a syringe. The syringe is attached to plastic tubing and a subcutaneous needle, which is inserted into the abdomen or thigh. Insulin pumps are especially useful for "brittle" diabetics (those whose blood glucose levels swing widely each day).

The pump partially imitates the action of the beta cells by delivering insulin continuously. Current models do not yet have a mechanism by which the pump can sense the body's ever-changing needs for insulin, as happens in a normal physiologic closed-loop feedback system. In all of the commercially available models, the patient still must check his blood glucose to determine the amount of insulin needed on a day-to-day or moment-to-moment basis.

At the present time insulin pumps are recommended only for a select few patients who are able to discipline themselves to monitor their blood glucose frequently during the day, who can understand the principles of continuous insulin infusion, who are compliant with their diet and self-care, and who have no physiologic and pathologic contraindications.

Soon a programmable implantable medication system may be available to deliver continuous insulin directly into the peritoneal cavity. The device technically would only have to be replaced every 5 years. A small, hand-held external radio transmitter is used by the patient to program insulin release from the pump. The patient will still have to do regular blood glucose monitoring. The advantage of the system is the decreased risk of infection compared with the external pump and needle system.

SYNTHETIC HYPOGLYCEMIC AGENTS

Oral hypoglycemic or antidiabetic agents are sometimes prescribed for patients with NIDDM to help control their blood glucose. These drugs are sulfonylureas, which stimulate the beta cells to release more insulin. They are related to the sulfonamide antibiotics. In addition to their ability to stimulate the beta cells, they also appear to inhibit glucose production and facilitate the transport of glucose into the muscle cells. Recent research indicates that the sulfonylureas also increase the number of receptor sites where insulin is bound and where it initiates the process of breaking down glucose. This action is particularly beneficial to diabetics who produce enough insulin but whose cells resist it.

Because the sulfonylureas are from the same family of drugs as the sulfonamide antibiotics, they must be given with caution to persons known to have an allergy to sulfa drugs.

There are four first-generation oral hypoglycemic agents in use: acetohexamide (Dymelor, Dimelor), chlorpropamide (Diabinese), tolazamide (Tolinase), and tolbutamide (Orinase) (Table 28–5). Side effects occur in less than 5% of patients. Those that do occur are common to all four agents, which belong to the sulfa family and have similar properties. Side effects include hematologic and gastrointestinal disorders, jaundice, skin rash, photosensitivity, and a reaction to alcohol similar to that associated with disulfiram (Antabuse). The symptoms of alcohol intolerance include severe vomiting, throbbing headache, respiratory difficulty, blurred vision, and confusion.

Second-generation sulfonylurea hypoglycemics include glyburide (Micronase and Diabeta) and glipizide (Glucotrol). These hypoglycemics are more potent, meaning that lower dosages can be used to control blood glucose. Their primary side effects include gastrointestinal distress and skin reactions. When used in pregnant women, glyburide is discontinued 2 weeks before delivery to prevent severe hypoglycemia in the newborn. Glipizide has not been released for use during pregnancy.

Among the drugs that enhance or increase the effect of the sulfonylureas are dicumarol, chloramphenicol (Chloromycetin), the salicylates, and the sulfonamides. Drugs that can inhibit or decrease the action of the oral antidiabetic agents include diazoxide, rifampin, and the thiazides.

Patients receiving hypoglycemic agents should know that the drug does not eliminate the need for following their prescribed diet and exercise program. Some may be under the mistaken notion that if they go off their diet and indulge themselves, they can just take more oral hypoglycemic pills to make up for this. Others who have been on a diet and exercise program for a

TABLE 28–5 ORAL HYPOGLYCEMIC AGENTS

Name	Dosage	Metabolism	Duration of Effect
Tolbutamide (Orinase)	500–3,000 mg daily total, taken bid or tid Available in 250- and 500-mg tablets	Metabolized by liver Excreted in urine	6–12 hours
Acetohexamide (Dymelor)	250–1,500 mg daily total, taken once a day or bid Available in 250- and 500-mg tablets	Metabolized by liver Excreted in urine	12–24 hours
Chlorpropamide (Diabinese)	100–500 mg daily total, taken once daily Available in 100- and 250-mg tablets	Very little metabolized by liver 99% excreted in urine	Up to 60 hrs
Tolazamide (Tolinase)	100–1,000 mg daily total, taken once daily or bid Available in 100-, 250-, and 500-mg tablets	Metabolized by liver Excreted in urine	12–24 hours
Glyburide (Diabeta, Micronase)	1.25–20 mg daily with breakfast or in two doses	Metabolized by liver Excreted in urine	12–24 hours
Glipizide (Glucotrol, Minidiab)	5–15 mg daily before breakfast or in two doses	Metabolized by liver Excreted in urine	12–24 hours

while and then have an oral hypoglycemic agent prescribed for them think it is all right to stop planning their meals and exercising regularly.

All hypoglycemic agents are capable of producing gastric irritation, nausea, vomiting, and diarrhea. There also can be liver damage with resultant jaundice, bone marrow depression, and allergic skin reactions in some patients.

An oral hypoglycemic that is not a sulfonylurea is being tested for release in the United States for the use of NIDDM patients who are allergic to the sulfonylureas. Metformin, a biguanide, has been used in Canada and Europe. It is unclear how this medication works, but it is thought to mimic the action of insulin.

Pre- and Postoperative Insulin Management

The emotional and physical stress of surgery can increase the blood glucose level and alter the amounts of medication needed for good control. NIDDM patients may be taken off of oral hypoglycemic medication up to 48 hours prior to surgery and are started on insulin by injection in order to achieve adequate control of their diabetes during this stressful period. The patient should be reassured that this does not indicate that his diabetes is worse and that the insulin injections are only a temporary measure.

For all diabetic patients, intravenous fluids are begun as soon as the patient is NPO and are continued until he is eating again after surgery. Insulin may be added to the IV glucose solution. Blood glucose monitoring is done every 2 to 4 hours, and urine is checked for signs of acetone. The nurse must be especially alert for signs of hypoglycemia in patients who are receiving insulin intravenously. Insulin dosage may be ordered by injection according to a sliding scale in which increments of regular short-acting insulin are used to attempt to keep the blood glucose within a safe range.

NURSING ASSESSMENT AND INTERVENTION

ASSESSMENT

The nurse should always assess each patient, regardless of his complaint, for signs and symptoms of diabetes mellitus. Questions regarding family history of diabetes, weight loss combined with increased hunger, thirst, urination patterns, and fatigue should be included in the general assessment. Other questions to include are: Does the patient seem to have trouble with wound healing? Does he find that even small scratches frequently get infected? Does he have any numbness or tingling in his feet or legs?

For the patient who is a known diabetic, an assessment of neuropathy progression should be included. Has he noticed any new areas of numbness or paresthesia or dysfunction of the bladder or colon? Is constipation becoming a problem? What about sexual function? Are there any problems there?

Can he correctly perform his blood glucose determinations? Can he properly plan his meals, and is he sticking to his dietary plan? Does he take his medication regularly? Are there any problems related to the medication? Do the records he has kept indicate adequate control of blood glucose? Is he having his eyes examined regularly to detect retinopathy?

NURSING DIAGNOSES

The following diagnoses are common for patients with diabetes mellitus:

- Alteration in nutrition, less than (or more than) body requirements, related to food and energy needs.
- Knowledge deficit related to disease process, possible complications, and self-care.
- Potential for infection related to elevated blood glucose level.
- Ineffective individual coping related to denial of need for effective self-care.
- Sensory perceptual alteration related to effect of elevated blood glucose on nervous system.
- Sexual dysfunction related to effect of elevated blood glucose on nervous system.
- Potential for injury related to severe decrease in tissue perfusion in feet and possibility of gangrene requiring amputation.
- Self-esteem disturbance related to diagnosis of chronic disease requiring insulin injections for survival.

There are many other nursing diagnoses related to the various complications that the diabetic patient may develop over the years. Nursing care plans must be carefully individualized to the particular problems and needs of each patient.

NURSING INTERVENTION

Intervention is geared toward assisting the patient with self-care, performing blood glucose determinations and admininstering medication when he is ill and cannot do so for himself, observing for signs and symptoms of complications, assessing learning needs, and carrying out a teaching plan as indicated.

The nurse should monitor the trend of blood glucose readings over time, rather than focus only on the current reading. She should check how well the patient is eating, as well as his fluid intake. Intake and output recordings are appropriate if the patient is ill or is having surgery. Any type of stress can alter the control of his diabetes. Electrolytes should also be monitored, with particular attention to potassium levels, which can shift suddenly when insulin is insufficient.

Every patient on insulin should be monitored for hypoglycemia after his insulin injections. The nurse must know how many hours after injection of each type of insulin this might occur and should then assess her patient at that time. Patients are taught to report signs of hypoglycemia promptly in order to avoid a crisis.

Monitoring for signs of ketoacidosis is also essential. Some of the earliest symptoms may be polyuria, fatigue, anorexia, and abdominal pain. Look for beginning signs of dehydration with decreased tissue turgor, sunken eyeballs, and dry mucous membranes. Report such findings to the physician promptly.

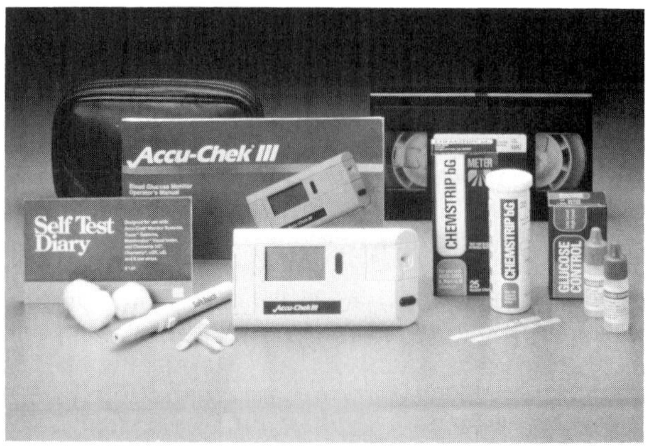

Figure 28-2 Accu-Chek blood glucose reflectance meter and Chemstrip blood glucose reagent strips used for home monitoring of blood glucose levels.
(Courtesy of Boehringer Mannheim Diagnostics, Inc.)

Patient Education

Successful management of diabetes requires that the patient be so well informed about his illness and the protocol for controlling it that he can assume responsibility for changing his former dietary habits, administering his own medication, and monitoring his progress. In addition he probably will need to make some adjustments in his lifestyle, recreational choices, and self-image.

The problem of noncompliance can be devastating to the welfare of the patient and can mean the difference between leading a nearly normal life or becoming an invalid; eventually it may mean the difference between life and death for the diabetic person. Many hospitals and clinics have developed standardized teaching programs for diabetes education, because the task of teaching the diabetic patient is very challenging and complex.

Major topics covered in a standardized program usually include the following:

- Pathophysiology of diabetes mellitus, including functions of the pancreas and potential contributing or precipitating factors in the development of diabetes.
- How to manage a diabetic diet program.
- Blood glucose monitoring at home using either a visually read test or a glucose monitoring meter. (Specific step-by-step instructions come with each individual device; Fig. 28-2.)
- Foot care (Table 28-6).
- Urine testing when blood glucose is over 240 mg/dL to check for acetone. (Dipstick instructions are included with each particular type of testing material.)
- Identification tag, ID card, and medical information (Fig. 28-3).
- Information on what to do on "sick" days, especially when nauseous or vomiting and unable to maintain diet (Table 28-7).

TABLE 28-6 TEACHING GUIDELINES FOR DIABETIC FOOT CARE

1. Each foot should be inspected daily for cuts, cracks, blisters, abrasions, or discoloration of the toes; report any abnormality to your health care provider.
2. The feet should be washed in warm (not hot) water, using mild soap; they should not be soaked, as this can cause cracking of the skin.
3. Thoroughly dry the feet after washing and apply an unscented, unmedicated cream.
4. Cut the nails straight across; have corns, calluses, and ingrown nails managed by a podiatrist.
5. Wear clean cotton socks and properly fitted shoes that do not pinch or bind the foot; never walk barefoot.
6. Use blankets to warm the feet; never use a heating pad or hot water bottle near them.
7. Elevate the feet whenever possible to improve circulation.

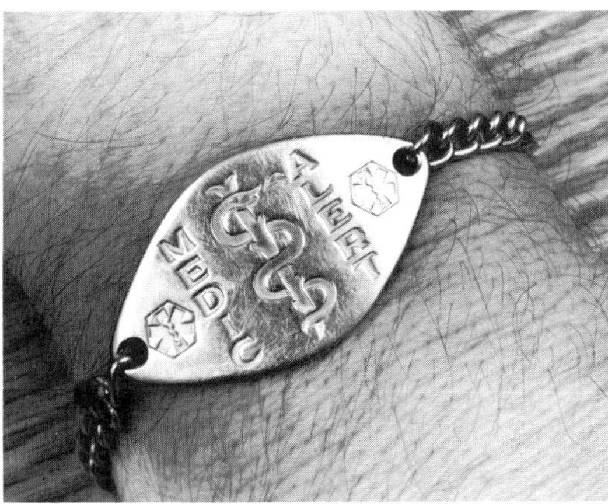

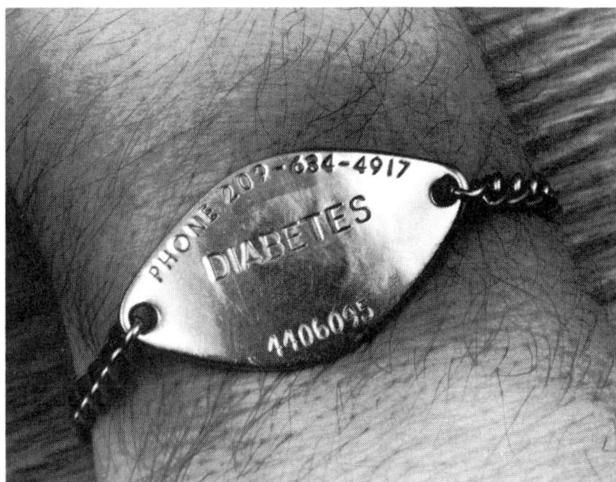

Figure 28-3 The Medic-Alert emblem worn as bracelet (also may be worn as necklace). Reverse side denotes specific medical problem of the wearer.
(Photographs by Ken Kasper.)

TABLE 28-7 SUGGESTIONS AND PRECAUTIONS FOR SELF-CARE WHEN DIABETIC PERSONS HAVE A COLD, FLU, OR MINOR GASTROINTESTINAL UPSETS

Medication

Insulin: Take your insulin as prescribed; it is essential to meeting your metabolic needs. If you check your blood glucose and notice it is higher than usual, you may need to increase the dosage while you are ill. Call your physician.

Oral hypoglycemic agents: Continue taking your usual dose. Do not increase the dose unless told to do so by your physician. He may order insulin *temporarily* if you are vomiting and unable to take medicine by mouth.

Food and drink

If you do not have nausea and vomiting, eat your normal diet and on your usual schedule.

Drink fluids often, using only calorie-free liquids if you are eating normally. Keep fluid intake at about ½ cup per each waking hour for an adult. For a child, ¼ teaspoon per pound of body weight each hour is advised.

If you are not able to eat your usual foods, replace them with carbohydrates in the form of liquids or soft foods. Examples include: ½ cup apple juice, ½ cup of regular 7-Up, 1 cup of chicken noodle soup, ½ cup of sherbet, ½ cup cooked cereal, 6 saltine crackers, or ½ cup fruit-flavored yogurt. Eat (or drink) at least 50 grams of carbohydrates every 3 to 4 hours.

Monitoring

Take your temperature every 4 hours or more often if you think you are running a fever.

Test your urine for glucose and acetone *or* your blood glucose every 4 hours and record results.

Be alert for signs of dehydration (fluid loss) such as dry mouth, thirst, dry skin, decreased urination, and concentrated urine.

If you are alone, call someone to stay with you if you are unable to care for yourself.

Notifying physician

Call your physician right away if (1) you are vomiting or have abdominal pain, (2) you are showing large amounts of glucose and acetone in your urine or your blood glucose levels are above 200 mg/100 mL and do not come down even after extra doses of insulin have been taken, or (3) your temperature rises to 100°F or more.

If you cannot get in touch with your physician right away, go to a hospital emergency room for treatment.

Data from Miller, L., et al.: Sick-Day Guide. Diabetes '83. New York, American Diabetes Association, 1983; and Lind, D., et al.: Managing Well on Sick Days. New York, American Diabetes Association, 1988.

TABLE 28-8 **TIPS FOR TRAVELING FOR DIABETICS**

1. Carry extra medication or insulin in case a bottle gets lost or broken. Keep one set of pills or insulin with 48 hours of syringes in your purse, briefcase, or carry-on luggage, along with your blood glucose-monitoring device.
2. Wear a Medic-Alert bracelet or tag and carry a medical information card in your purse or wallet.
3. Carry an emergency supply of simple sugar at all times in case of a hypoglycemic episode.
4. Plan ahead at least 2 days for replenishing supplies for blood glucose monitoring, insulin, and syringes in case the correct items are hard to find in a foreign city. (It is best to take supplies with you for the entire time you will be gone.)
5. If you become severely ill, seek medical attention immediately before you get into a dangerous condition.
6. Stick to prescribed meal plans as well as possible, substituting available foods according to food group classification.
7. Obtain sufficient rest and avoid stressful situations as much as possible to prevent stress-induced hyperglycemia.
8. If you are a "brittle" diabetic, it is best to travel with someone who is familiar with your condition and treatment.
9. Obtain your usual amount of exercise or adjust food and medication intake accordingly.

- Community resources and help groups available to diabetic and family.
- Devices that make insulin administration easier (especially for the elderly, visually impaired, or arthritic patient).

The health care team helping the diabetic manage his illness should include a diabetologist, nurse practitioner, dietitian, podiatrist, and periodontist and, of course, the patient himself and his significant others. Because of frequent updates and changes in the management of diabetes, all persons responsible for the care of diabetic patients should read and continue to study and learn about the current protocols for management of diabetes mellitus. Table 28-8 provides traveling tips for diabetic patients.

SOURCES OF INFORMATION

There are at least two free publications that are published regularly and made available to diabetics, their families, and others interested in learning more and keeping current with new developments in the management of diabetes. *Diabetes in the News*, published by the Ames Education Corporation, can be obtained by sending name and address to *Diabetes in the News*, Subscription Department, 38135 Benham, Elkhart, IN 46517. The second publication, a newsletter published bimonthly by the American Diabetes Association, can be obtained by writing to that organization at 1660 Duke Street, Alexandria, VA 22314.

A third publication, also published by the American Diabetes Association, is called *Diabetes Forecast*. It is written and edited by health care specialists and is aimed at providing information for diabetics so that they can manage their illness more effectively. There is a charge for this publication, which can be obtained by writing to the American Diabetes Association, National Service Center, at the address given above. Pharmaceutical companies, local chapters of the American Diabetes Association, and the American Dietetic Association are also excellent sources of information for continuing education in the management of diabetes.

COMPLICATIONS

In general, diabetic patients are susceptible to two types of complications: short-term, or acute, problems and long-term sequelae.

SHORT-TERM PROBLEMS

Acute complications arise when the blood glucose suddenly becomes either too high (hyperglycemia) or too low (hypoglycemia). The symptoms, causes, treatment, and prevention of each of these conditions are summarized in Table 28-9. When a patient is admitted to the hospital for treatment of critical hyperglycemia, decisions about the proper modes of therapy are based on whether the patient has type I or type II diabetes and the objective and subjective symptoms presented. Type I diabetes is more likely to be complicated by ketoacidosis than is type II.

Diabetic Ketoacidosis

Diabetic ketoacidosis is a serious condition caused by incomplete metabolism of fats as a result of the absence or insufficient supply of

TABLE 28-9 COMPARISON OF HYPOGLYCEMIC (INSULIN) REACTION AND HYPERGLYCEMIA (DIABETIC KETOACIDOSIS)

Hypoglycemic Reaction	Hyperglycemia
Causes	
Overdosage of insulin	Failure to take insulin
Skipped or delayed meal	Illness or infection
Unplanned strenuous exercise	Overeating or eating sweets
	Severe stress (surgery, trauma, emotional upset)
Symptoms	
Early stage: tremor; dizziness; numbness in mouth; cool, wet skin; fluttering in chest; hunger	Polyuria, polydipsia, polyphagia, blurred vision, dizziness
Middle stage: headache, mental confusion, combative behavior	Loss of appetite, stomach cramps, nausea and vomiting, dehydration, fatigue
	Deep, rapid breathing
	Loss of consciousness
Treatment	
Early stage: If patient can swallow, give orange juice, 6 to 7 Life Saver mints, glucose tablets or gel	Physician may prescribe insulin
Late stage: If patient cannot swallow, give glucagon, 2-mg kit (home or hospital); give IV glucose	Hospital admission for severe cases
Prevention	
Eat meals 4 to 5 hours apart, plus prescribed snack.	Take correct dose of insulin
Take correct dose of insulin. Test urine or blood for glucose, especially during illness	See physician for illness
Eat extra food for extra exercise, (i.e., activity other than regular exercise)	Follow diet; don't overeat or eat sweets

insulin. When insulin is not present in adequate amounts to meet metabolic needs, the body breaks down proteins and fats for energy. This produces an abundance of the by-products of fat metabolism, which are potent organic acids called *ketones*. In an attempt to rid itself of the excess ketones, the body excretes some of them in the lungs. This produces a characteristic fruity odor to the breath. Acetone, a ketone body, is excreted in the urine, causing acetonuria or ketonuria. As the kidney excretes excess glucose and ketones, it also eliminates large quantities of water and electrolytes. These pathologic changes are responsible for metabolic acidosis, dehydration, and electrolyte imbalances.

Signs and symptoms of diabetic ketoacidosis include hyperglycemia; thirst; abdominal pain; nausea and anorexia; vomiting; excessive urine output; alteration in level of consciousness; fruity odor to the breath; flushed face; rapid, thready pulse; hypotension; Kussmaul's respirations; and possibly coma.

Treatment of ketoacidosis is aimed at restoring normal pH of the blood and other body fluids, correcting the fluid and electrolyte imbalance, lowering the blood glucose level gradually, providing life-support measures as necessary if the patient is comatose, and eventually correcting the underlying cause of poor control of insulin-dependent diabetes.

Somogyi Phenomenon

Another acute condition sometimes encountered in patients with IDDM is the Somogyi phenomenon, a rebound hyperglycemia that occurs in response to hypoglycemia from too much insulin being administered. Determination of the correct dosage of insulin for a particular patient is not an exact science. Many variables enter into the situation, including a change in stress level because of surgery, illness, or some other event in the patient's life. At times an insulin-dependent patient may receive a dose of insulin that is too large and may develop hyperglycemia in response to a very low blood glucose level. This phenomenon is corrected by gradually lowering the insulin dose. There may be times when it will be necessary for the nurse to explain to a patient why he is receiving less insulin even though his blood glucose level is well above normal.

Whenever a diabetic person is subjected to additional stress, as in an unrelated medical illness or when surgery is necessary, his metabolic needs change, and thus the delicate balance between hyperglycemia and hypoglycemia is threatened. Selected nursing diagnoses and nursing interventions for a diabetic patient having surgery are summarized in Nursing Care Plan 28-1.

NURSING CARE PLAN 28–1

Selected nursing diagnoses, goals/outcome criteria, nursing interventions, and evaluations for a diabetic patient having a hysterectomy

Situation: Mrs. Sanchez, age 53, has had type I diabetes since age 18 and is scheduled for a hysterectomy. She has been performing blood glucose monitoring at home and has achieved fairly good control of her diabetes. Her blood lipids are within acceptable limits, but she is 10 pounds overweight.

The morning of surgery, an IV infusion of D5W is started, and regular insulin is added to the infusion. On her return from surgery, the surgeon ordered the intravenous infusion continued for 24 hours, blood glucose determinations q 4 h, and sliding scale administration of regular insulin (based on the blood glucose level). The following day the IV is discontinued, and blood glucose determinations are ordered twice a day. Mrs. Sanchez' usual dosage of insulin is resumed, with additional units of regular insulin per sliding scale.

Nursing Diagnosis	Goals/Outcome Criteria	Nursing Intervention	Evaluation
Potential for injury related to wide fluctuations in blood glucose. SUPPORTING DATA Undergoing surgical stress; receiving IV insulin.	Blood glucose will remain within safe limits (60 to 180 mg/dL).	Perform blood glucose determination q 4 h; administer insulin as needed per sliding scale; observe for signs of hypoglycemia. Monitor intake and output. Be alert for signs of insulin reaction as she recovers from the stress of surgery (insulin needs decrease as stress decreases).	Blood glucose of 250 at 7:30 A.M.; insulin per sliding scale given; 11:30, blood glucose 160; intake, 1,050; output, 760; continue plan.
Potential for injury related to possible infection at surgical site. SUPPORTING DATA Hysterectomy; diabetic (high blood glucose levels make tissues more susceptible to bacterial growth.)	No signs of infection: normal vaginal secretions, normal WBC count, no temperature elevation by day 3.	Vital signs q 4 h; monitor WBC count for signs of infection; check vaginal discharge for characteristics of infection and bleeding. Monitor venipuncture sites for signs of infection q shift. Administer prophylactic antibiotics as ordered.	VS stable; temp., 100°F; WBCs, 8,400; vaginal pack in place; no signs of infection; antibiotics administered as scheduled; continue plan.
Knowledge deficit related to self-care after surgery. SUPPORTING DATA Asking questions about activity, resumption of intercourse, required care after surgery.	Patient will verbalize understanding of limitations of activity, need for increased rest, and signs and symptoms of complications.	Explain need for increased rest after surgery; inform her of signs and symptoms of infection to report to physician; teach regarding prophylactic antibiotics, medication schedule; assess knowledge of general diabetic care; assess self-administration of insulin and glucose monitoring.	Teaching for postop and home care done; tomorrow will assess self-care knowledge regarding diabetes and insulin injection.
Potential for self-esteem disturbance related to loss of child bearing ability. SUPPORTING DATA States that although she doesn't want more children, it will seem strange not to be able to have another.	Patient will verbalize feelings regarding new body image by discharge.	Encourage verbalization of feelings regarding hysterectomy and loss of child-bearing ability. Assist her to focus on positive aspects of self. Encourage discussion of feelings with spouse.	States she is glad she won't be bleeding all of the time, but it seems funny that a part of her is gone; continue plan.

Hypoglycemia

The word *hypoglycemia* means low blood glucose. Hypoglycemia is a rather common complication of type I diabetes mellitus. Most often it is a response to either too large a dose of insulin or too much exercise in relation to the amount of food eaten. Signs and symptoms of hypoglycemia include tremulousness, hunger, headache, pallor, sweating, palpitations, blurred vision, and weakness; symptoms may progress to confusion and loss of consciousness. Individual reactions vary considerably. Some patients are alert with a glucose level of 40 mg/dL, and others are comatose.

Treatment depends on the degree of hypoglycemia. Glucose levels of 40 to 60 mg/dL respond to ingestion of food such as milk, crackers, or orange juice. Glucose levels of 20 to 40 mg/dL respond best to simple sugars such as honey, table sugar, or juice. In the hospital, if the person is experiencing seizures or is comatose as a result of severe hypoglycemia, a solution of 50% glucose is given intravenously.

When there is doubt as to whether the patient is suffering from hyperglycemia or hypoglycemia, treatment is begun for hypoglycemia until a blood glucose determination is obtained. This is done in order to prevent brain damage from extremely low cerebral glucose levels. Administration of glucagon is another treatment for the unconscious patient who is hypoglycemic. Its advantage is that it can be given intramuscularly when a vein cannot be found for IV glucose administration.

Diabetic patients must be taught to monitor themselves for beginning signs of hypoglycemia and to always carry a source of simple sugar with them to be taken if the symptoms occur.

LONG-TERM SEQUELAE

The long-term consequences of diabetes mellitus are chiefly the result of damage to the large and small blood vessels. Although the controversy over whether tight control prevents or minimizes the long-term effects of diabetes is still not resolved, there is no doubt that elevated blood glucose levels over a period of years will seriously damage blood vessels and the organs they serve. Diabetes remains among the three leading causes of death in the United States, the other two being cardiovascular disease and cancer. However, cardiovascular disease and other less frequent causes of death often can be attributed to diabetes.

Cardiovascular Disease

Thickening of the vessels occurs when blood glucose is elevated over a long period of time. The basement membrane grows thicker. The vessels of the retina, renal glomeruli, peripheral nerves, muscles, and skin are affected. Larger vessels are also affected, which predisposes the patient to atherosclerosis and vascular occlusion. A person with diabetes has a 50% higher chance of suffering from heart disease or stroke than does a nondiabetic person. About half of all diabetics suffer premature death from myocardial infarction; the survival time for those diabetics whose first heart attack was not fatal is about 50% less than that of nondiabetic heart attack victims.

Nephropathy

Diabetic nephropathy (disease of the kidney) occurs directly from changes in the renal blood circulation. As damage from inadequate blood circulation is done, the patient experiences signs of renal failure. Proteinuria (protein in the urine) and hypertension are early signs of renal failure. A large percentage of those who have chronic renal failure and are on renal dialysis are also diabetic.

Peripheral Vascular Disease

Gangrene, which often necessitates amputation, is 40 to 50 times more common in diabetic persons. Vascular changes frequently cause very poor circulation in the feet and lower extremities. Healing of wounds in these areas is difficult because of the poor blood supply, and also because increased levels of glucose in the blood provide a good medium for bacterial growth, making it harder to eradicate infection. The teaching and practice of excellent foot care is essential to prevent eventual amputation in the diabetic patient.

Retinopathy

Visual impairment and blindness are common sequelae of diabetes mellitus. The three most common problems of this kind are diabetic retinopathy, cataracts, and glaucoma. Retinal damage, which can cause visual impairment and blindness, occurs in most diabetics within 10 years of diagnosis. Changes in the retinal vessels lead to hemorrhages and also to retinal detachment. Recent surgical techniques using photocoagulation of destructive lesions of the retina with laser beams now offer hope for preservation of sight by preventing further progress of diabetic retinopathy. Good glucose control, frequent eye examinations, and treatment can help preserve vision.

Neuropathy

Pathologic changes in the nervous system cause deterioration, with symptoms such as paresthesia, numbness, and loss of function. Diabetic neuropathies primarily affect the peripheral nerves, causing sexual impotence in the male, neurogenic bladder, and pain or anesthesia in the lower extremities. It is for this reason that foot care and daily inspection of the feet is so important. Because the patient often cannot feel cuts, blisters, or abrasions on the foot, there is great danger of a neglected sore becoming infected. The patient typically experiences an anesthesia beginning about 10 years after onset of diabetes. There eventually may be almost total anesthesia of the affected part, bringing with it the potential for serious injury to the patient without his being aware of it. In contrast, some patients experience debilitating pain and hyperesthesia; some lose deep tendon reflexes. Other problems related to diabetic neuropathies are the result of autonomic nervous system involvement. These include orthostatic hypotension, delayed gastric emptying, diarrhea or constipation, and asymptomatic retention of urine in the bladder.

Prevention of the potentially devastating long-term consequences of diabetes is a major goal in the management of the disease. Preventive measures related to heart disease, stroke, and peripheral vascular disease are discussed in Chapter 21. There is some evidence that tight control is espe-

TABLE 28–10 **STAGES OF DIABETES**

Stage I

Fasting blood glucose greater than 110 mg/100 mL, or 2-hour postprandial (after a meal) blood glucose greater than 140 mg/100 mL, and without ketoacidosis or other complications

Stage II

Diabetes with infection in one or more systems (skin, genital tract, urinary tract, etc.)

Diabetes with septicemia

Diabetes with acidosis (diabetic ketoacidosis present, but without coma); serum pH less than 7.35 or CO_2 less than 23 mEq/L, and presence of acetone in serum

Diabetes with retinopathy but *without* loss of vision; glomerulonephrosclerosis (without azotemia), neuropathy (peripheral or autonomic), or gangrene (tissue breakdown)

Stage III

Diabetes mellitus with acidosis and coma (CO_2 less than 10 mEq/L)

Diabetes with retinopathy and loss of vision

Diabetes with necrotizing papillitis (evidenced by papillae in urine or visible on intravenous pyelogram)

Diabetes with azotemia (blood urea nitrogen greater than 30 mg/100 mL or creatinine greater than 2 mg/100 mL)

Adapted from Grimaldi, P. L., and Micheletti, J. A.: Diagnosis Related Groups: A Practitioner's Guide. Chicago, Pluribus Press, Inc., 1983, p. 43.

cially beneficial in preventing pathologic changes in the small blood vessels serving the kidneys, thereby preventing renal failure. Care of patients with urologic disorders is discussed in Chapter 22.

STAGES OF DIABETES IN RELATION TO COMPLICATIONS

Although not every diabetic person will suffer from long-term complications such as those just described, many will for one reason or another be hospitalized in some later stage of the disease. Criteria for determining the three stages of diabetes mellitus are presented in Table 28–10. This table indicates the kinds of medical problems long-term diabetes is likely to cause and shows the various states in which the nurse might find diabetic patients who are hospitalized.

HYPOGLYCEMIA

A low blood glucose state can exist whenever the homeostatic mechanisms designed to maintain blood glucose within a rather narrow range fail to function as they should. The organs involved in meeting the challenge of carbohydrate ingestion include the intestines, liver, and pancreas (specifically, the beta cells that produce insulin). Thus any condition affecting these organs and their systems can lead to hypoglycemia. Examples, other than diabetes mellitus, include gastrectomy and surgical bypass procedures. These types of surgery provide more rapid access of glucose to the absorptive sites in the small bowel. Tumors of the pancreas, liver disease, and disorders of the adrenal cortex and pituitary gland can produce abnormally low blood glucose levels. Alcoholics and drug addicts also are prone to hypoglycemia.

Functional hypoglycemia, for which there is no known cause, may be a very early indicator of diabetes mellitus. In fact, studies have shown that almost one third of the people who have functional hypoglycemia may eventually develop diabetes if the hypoglycemia is not effectively controlled.

REACTIVE AND SPONTANEOUS HYPOGLYCEMIA

The pathophysiology of hypoglycemia and its attendant symptoms are quite different after eating than in a fasting state. These differences are the basis for classification of the disorder into *hypoglycemia in the fed state* (also called *reactive hypoglycemia)* and *hypoglycemia in the fasting state (spontaneous hypoglycemia).* Reactive hypoglycemia has been the subject of the most debate as to its cause, effect, and treatment. The term *hypoglycemia* is often mistakenly used to explain symptoms that may or may not be indicative of reactive hypoglycemia. These symptoms include rapid heart beat, tremulousness, weakness, anxiety, nervousness, and hunger, and they occur rather suddenly several hours after carbohydrates are eaten. The diagnosis of reactive hypoglycemia is very difficult to confirm, as abnormally low blood glucose levels often cannot be demonstrated.

TREATMENT

Treatment of hypoglycemia is modification of eating patterns. Smaller and more frequent meals that are relatively free of simple sugars are recommended. The diet should include a balance of proteins, fats, and the complex carbohydrates found in fruits, vegetables, and whole grains. Refined sugar and white flour are omitted. Cases in which gastric surgery and intestinal bypass are believed to be the cause of hypoglycemia may also be treated with drugs that reduce intestinal motility.

NURSING ASSESSMENT AND INTERVENTION

One of the most tragic consequences of hypoglycemia from any cause involves mistaking the physiologic symptoms for indication of a psychiatric illness. These symptoms include irritability, personality change, temper tantrums, and other psychoneurotic manifestations.

Nurses are in an excellent position to observe and help identify patients who might be hypoglycemic. In addition to information about his physical and mental symptoms, assessment should include a rather detailed history of the person's eating habits. Does he eat regularly? How often during each day? What kinds of foods constitute a typical meal for him? Does he crave sweets? Has he had episodes of weakness, sweating, visual disturbances, and confusion or inability to concentrate? If these symptoms have occurred, when are they most noticeable (that is, in a fed or fasting state)?

Nursing interventions for patients with hypoglycemia include explanations of the nature of the disorder and the need for diagnostic testing to confirm or rule out reactive hypoglycemia, objective and nonjudgmental observation and reporting of symptoms, and reinforcement of dietary instruction and restrictions.

Concerns for the Elderly

Type II diabetes has its onset in adulthood and can occur at any time after age 30. Very often it is not discovered until the sixth or seventh decade. Many patients in these age groups have difficulty adjusting to the new diet, medication, and required exercise. Income is generally reduced, and some patients have difficulty obtaining the necessary foods or medicine because of financial constraints.

Diabetics often have developed many of the complications of the disease by the sixth, seventh, or eighth decade. Hypertension and renal failure are common problems. Failing vision from retinopathy is very common and causes problems with insulin administration as well as self-care. Total blindness occurs in many patients. Cardiovascular problems occur in the normal population in these age groups and are compounded for those with diabetes mellitus. There is a much larger incidence of stroke and myocardial infarction in those with diabetes. Peripheral vascular disease and infection lead to amputation of the toes or foot in approximately 50,000 diabetics per year. Neuropathy is yet another complication, leading to bladder and bowel problems as well as limb numbness and paralysis, especially of the legs.

Older NIDDM patients are particularly prone to develop hyperglycemic hyperosmolar nonketotic HHNK syndrome. This disorder is similar to diabetic ketoacidosis, except that the level of ketones does not become excessive. It most frequently occurs after a febrile illness or gastrointestinal flu in which the patient has stopped eating properly and possibly discontinued his oral hypoglycemic agent. As his blood glucose level rises, he experiences thirst and polyuria but, because of his illness, does not recognize these danger signs. As the blood glucose level continues to rise, he experiences lethargy, a decreased level of consciousness, and further dehydration. The blood glucose level may rise to between 600 and 2,000 mg/dL. Blood osmolality is considerably elevated (> 350 mOsm/kg). HHNK is treated with IV normal saline, plus IV glucose and regular insulin. Like blood glucose, intake and output must be monitored closely. HHNK can be fatal, and mortality is directly correlated with higher elevations of blood glucose.

There is a great need for home care and monitoring of the diabetic elderly population. If nurses could follow the progress of these patients over the years with good assessments, the incidence of complications could probably be decreased. As the national trend shifts toward preventive medicine and health care, perhaps the funds for such a program will be forthcoming.

BIBLIOGRAPHY

Andreoli, T. E., et al.: Cecil Essentials of Medicine, 2nd ed. Philadelphia, W. B. Saunders, 1990.

Armstrong, N.: Coping with diabetes mellitus. Nurs. Clin. North Am., Sept., 1987, p. 559.

Bell, D. S. H., and Clements, R. S.: Diabetes and the digestive system. Diabetes Forecast, Dec., 1987, p. 43.

Christman, C., and Bennett, J.: Diabetes: New names, new test, new diet. Nursing 87, Jan., 1987, p. 34.

Donohue, P. O.: Diabetes now: Patient education makes all the difference. RN, Nov., 1989, p. 56.

Dunning, D.: Diabetes now—safe travel tips for the diabetic patient. RN, April, 1989, p. 51.

Freinkel, R. K.: Caring for your skin. Diabetes Forecast, July, 1988, p. 76.

Galuk, D.: The nurse (as) diabetic educator. Adv. Clin. Care, Sept./Oct., 1990, p. 27.

Galuk, D.: Classes for the diabetic patient: A 5 day format. Adv. Clin. Care, Nov./Dec., 1990, p. 29.

Galuk, D.: Diabetes mellitus types I and II. Adv. Clin. Care, March/April, 1991, p. 5.

Guthrie, D. W., and Guthrie, R. A.: Nursing Management of Diabetes Mellitus, 3rd ed. New York, Springer, 1991.

Guyton, A. C.: Textbook of Medical Physiology, 8th ed. Philadelphia, W. B. Saunders, 1991.

Hull, M.: How to set up a diabetes education program. RN, Nov., 1989, p. 61.

Huzar, J. G.: Diabetes now: Preventing acute complications. RN, Aug., 1989, p. 34.
Huzar, J. G., and Cerrato, P. L.: The role of diet and drugs. RN, April, 1989, p. 46.
Ignatavicius, D. D., and Bayne, M. J.: Medical-Surgical Nursing. Philadelphia, W. B. Saunders, 1991.
Lumly, W.: Hypoglycemia and hyperglycemia. Nursing 88, October, 1988, p. 36.
Nath, C., et al.: Lessons in living with type II diabetes mellitus. Nursing 88, Aug., 1988, p. 45.
Peterson, A., and Drass, J.: Managing acute complications of diabetes. Nursing 91, Feb., 1991, p. 34.
Ramsey, R. W.: Hyperglycemia at dawn. Am. J. Nurs., Nov., 1987, p. 1424.
Robertson, C.: Diabetes now: Coping with chronic complications. RN, Sept., 1989. p. 34.
Sabo, C. E.: Managing DKA and preventing a recurrence. Nursing 89, Feb., 1989, p. 50.
Steil, C. F., and Deakins, D. A.: Today's insulins: What you and your patient need to know. Nursing 90, Aug., 1990, p. 34.
Tomky, D.: Diabetes now: A 3-pronged approach to monitoring. RN, March, 1989, p. 24.
Whitehead, E. D.: Diabetes-related impotence: Putting new knowledge to use. Geriatrics, Feb., 1988, p. 114.
Wozniak, L.: Your teaching plan: The key to controlling type II diabetes. RN, Aug. 1988, p. 29.

STUDENT STUDY AIDS

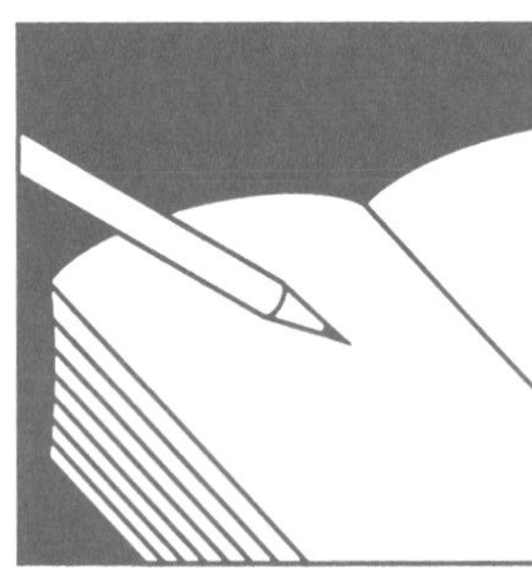

CLINICAL CASE PROBLEMS

Read each clinical situation and discuss the questions with your classmates.

1. Mrs. Loomis is 42 years old and has had non–insulin-dependent diabetes mellitus (NIDDM) for the past 10 years. She is admitted to the hospital for treatment of an infection of the great toe on her left foot, which is the result of improper care of an ingrown toenail. She is 45 pounds overweight and admits to frequent binges of eating foods not on her diet. She does not exercise regularly because she says the housework she does gives her enough exercise. When asked about the oral antidiabetic agent that has been prescribed for her, she tells you that she only takes it "when I feel like my blood sugar is high or when I eat too much."

- Devise a specific teaching plan for Mrs. Loomis in order to help her manage her illness better.
- What could you suggest to Mrs. Loomis to help her lose weight?
- What do you think might motivate Mrs. Loomis to accept more responsibility for managing her illness?

---

2. Mr. Tower is a 22-year-old construction worker who has recently experienced fatigue, excessive thirst and urination, and weight loss. A routine urinalysis revealed glycosuria and a trace of acetone. His physician has arranged for Mr. Tower to have an oral glucose tolerance test to determine whether he has diabetes mellitus.

- What is the significance of the findings of the routine urinalysis?
- What is involved in an oral glucose tolerance test?
- If Mr. Tower is found to have insulin-dependent diabetes mellitus, what kinds of information will he need to manage his illness?
- How would you explain the importance of "good" or "tight" control of his blood glucose levels to Mr. Tower?
- What criteria could be used to determine whether his diabetes is under control?

STUDY OUTLINE

I. Diabetes mellitus

A. Diabetes defined as a complex group of disorders that have in common a disturbance in the oxidation and utilization of glucose.

B. Types of diabetes summarized in Table 28–1.

C. Contributing factors

1. Genetic: tends to run in families (genetic predisposition).
2. Metabolic: obesity, emotional and physical stress.
3. Microbiologic: some cases of IDDM related to viral infections.

4. Immunologic: IDDM thought to be an autoimmune disorder because of islet cell antibodies found in the blood of about 75% of diabetics.

D. Incidence and prevalence:
1. Incidence increasing at an alarming rate; currently there are about 11 million diabetics in the United States.
2. Increasing incidence can be explained in part by improved methods of case finding and reporting.

E. Diagnostic tests:
1. Fasting blood glucose above normal is suggestive of diabetes.
2. Fasting blood and urine samples taken, then patient given large amount of glucose. Samples taken after 30 minutes and then at hourly intervals for up to 4 hours. Point system used to avoid misinterpretation of blood and urine values.
3. 2-hour postprandial blood glucose test can indicate need for glucose tolerance test.
4. Glycosylated hemoglobin (hemoglobin A_{1c}) not a diagnostic test. Gives information about average blood glucose levels over period of 2 to 3 months. Useful in determining effectiveness of prescribed protocol for management of diabetes.

F. Symptoms and medical diagnosis:
1. Classic symptoms: polydipsia, polyuria, polyphagia.
2. Fatigue, muscle weakness, weight loss, ketoacidosis found in IDDM.
3. Weight gain common in NIDDM.
4. Frequent and slow-healing infections, proneness to vascular disease.

G. Management of diabetes:
1. Continued controversy over advantages and disadvantages of strict control of blood glucose. With better methods of control it is believed that fewer complications will be seen in the future.
2. In general, good control indicated by:
   a. Fasting blood sugars within normal limits.
   b. Hemoglobin A_{1c} indicating average blood glucose within normal range.
   c. Weight staying within normal range.
   d. Serum lipids within acceptable range.
   e. Patient having sense of health and well-being.
3. Diet: prescribed for individual patient.
   a. Intended to provide adequate nutrition from each of major food groups.
   b. Patient must learn to use food exchange list or other dietary planning system.
   c. Patient encouraged to avoid concentrated sweets, excess fats in diet.
4. Exercise: patient encouraged to follow a program of regular exercise daily.
   a. Helps metabolize glucose.
   b. Makes insulin receptors more sensitive to insulin.
   c. Helps lower serum lipid levels.
   d. Patient will need instruction in precautions to take during exercise, especially if he has IDDM.
5. Insulin: types shown in Table 28–3.
   a. Type of insulin not to be confused with strength, which usually is 100 units of insulin per milliliter (U100).
   b. Insulin must be given by injection.

c. Dosage varies according to patient need. Some may require two or more daily injections of two types.
d. Patient or family member will need instruction in how to administer insulin.
(1) Insulin pump: a system for delivering continuous infusion of insulin. Recommended only for selected patients.

6. Synthetic hypoglycemic agents (oral antidiabetic drugs) sometimes prescribed for NIDDM patients.
a. Not an oral form of insulin.
b. Examples: Dymelor, Diabinase, Tolinase, Orinase, Diabeta, Micronase, and Glucotrol.
c. Sulfonylureas, akin to sulfa antibiotics.
(1) Lower blood glucose by stimulating beta cells to produce insulin.
(2) Inhibit glucose production.
(3) Facilitate transport of glucose into cell.
(4) Increase number of receptor sites.
d. Certain drugs enhance the action of oral antidiabetic agents, whereas others inhibit their action.
e. Patient receiving oral antidiabetic drugs will require instruction in how to take the drug and how to avoid drug-drug interactions.

H. Nursing assessment and interventions
1. Every patient should be assessed for signs of diabetes mellitus.
2. General assessment should include questions about family history of diabetes, weight loss, increased hunger, thirst, excessive urination, poor wound healing, and fatigue.
3. Patients known to be diabetic should be assessed for signs of complications.
4. Assessment of performance on blood glucose monitoring and of technique for insulin injection should be done.
5. Common nursing diagnoses for diabetic patients include:
a. Alteration in nutrition, less than (or more than) body requirements.
b. Knowledge deficit.
c. Potential for infection.
d. Ineffective individual coping.
e. Sensory perceptual alteration.
f. Sexual dysfunction.
g. Potential for injury related to severe decrease in tissue perfusion in feet.
h. Self-esteem disturbance.
6. Many other nursing diagnoses become appropriate as the patient experiences the many complications of the disease.
7. Nursing interventions are geared toward assisting the patient with self-care, monitoring blood glucose, administering medication, observing for signs and symptoms of complications, assessing learning needs, and carrying out a teaching plan.
a. The trend of blood glucose readings over time should be monitored.
b. Food and fluid intake should be checked.
c. Electrolytes, especially potassium, should be checked to see that they are within normal limits.
d. The patient should be monitored for hypoglycemia after insulin injections.
e. Monitoring for early signs of ketoacidosis is also essential:

polyuria, fatigue, anorexia, abdominal pain, dehydration, irritability.

8. Patient education: an extremely important component of management.
9. The patient must learn enough about his disease and treatment to take charge of his own care. Topics to be covered include:
   a. Blood glucose monitoring.
   b. Urine testing for acetone when blood glucose is >240 mg/dL.
   c. Pathophysiology of diabetes mellitus.
   d. Type of medication, side effects, and method of administration (insulin injections).
   e. Signs and symptoms of hyperglycemia and hypoglycemia and treatment.
   f. Skin and foot care.
   g. Diet planning and adherence.
   h. Balance of diet, exercise, and medication.
   i. Need for ID tag.
   j. What to do on "sick" days.
   k. Pointers for traveling.
   l. Community resources and help groups available.
   m. Devices that make insulin preparation and administration easier.
   n. Need for close medical follow-up.
10. American Diabetes Association and American Dietetic Association and their local chapters and pharmaceutical companies are excellent sources of information for patient education.

I. Complications:
   1. Short-term problems:
      a. Hyperglycemia and hypoglycemia: symptoms, causes, prevention, and treatment summarized in Table 28–9.
      b. Diabetic ketoacidosis: caused by incomplete oxidation of fats with resultant accumulation of organic acids (ketones) in the urine.
         (1) Symptoms include fruity odor to breath, acetonuria, and signs and symptoms of acidosis and fluid and electrolyte imbalances.
         (2) Treatment aimed at restoring normal blood pH, correcting fluid and electrolyte imbalances, and treating underlying cause.
      c. Somogyi phenomenon: a rebound hyperglycemia caused by administration of too much insulin.
      d. Hypoglycemia: response to too much insulin (insulin reaction) or too much exercise in relation to food intake.
         (1) Signs and symptoms: tremulousness, hunger, headache, pallor, sweating, palpitations, weakness, and blurred vision.
         (2) May progress to confusion and unconsciousness.
         (3) Treated with a form of glucose.
         (4) Glucagon is an alternative treatment.
   2. Long-term consequences chiefly the result of atherosclerotic changes and damage to large and small blood vessels.
      a. Diabetes among the three most common causes of death in the United States.
      b. Cardiovascular disease: a person with diabetes has a 50% higher chance of suffering from heart disease or stroke than does a nondiabetic person.

(1) About half of all diabetic persons die from heart attack, and those who survive live about half as long as others after heart attack.

c. Nephropathy: large percentage of patients on renal dialysis are diabetic.
d. Peripheral vascular disease: gangrene is 40 to 50 times more prevalent among diabetics.
e. Neuropathy: can lead to impotence, neurogenic bladder, and pain or loss of feeling in the lower extremities.
f. Retinopathy: can cause visual impairment and blindness.

3. Stages of diabetes mellitus vary in relation to complications.
   a. Stage I: no ketoacidosis or other complications, but blood glucose is above normal.
   b. Stage II: diabetes with infection, acetone in serum, retinopathy, and other complications.
   c. Stage III: diabetes with acidosis and coma, retinopathy and loss of vision, or azotemia.

II. Hypoglycemia

A. Disturbance of glucose metabolism resulting in abnormally low blood glucose levels.
B. Failure to meet the challenge of carbohydrate ingestion can occur:
   1. Following intestinal surgery.
   2. In tumors of the pancreas.
   3. In liver disease.
   4. In disorders of the adrenal cortex and pituitary.
C. Alcoholics and drug addicts also prone to hypoglycemia.
D. Functional hypoglycemia: no known cause.
E. Fasting hypoglycemia: result of insufficient intake of glucose.
F. Reactive hypoglycemia (person in a fed state): the most controversial type.
   1. Diagnosed only when symptoms are correlated with abnormally low blood glucose levels as determined by extended glucose tolerance test.
   2. Treatment:
      a. Patient placed on diet of complex sugars, high-protein foods; refined sugar and starches restricted or omitted.
      b. Persons with abnormally rapid passage of food through the bowel may also be given medications to decrease motility.
   3. Nursing assessment and intervention:
      a. Recognize physiologic, psychological, and emotional symptoms of hypoglycemia.
      b. Assess patient's eating habits thoroughly.
      c. Explain nature of illness and need for testing to confirm a diagnosis.
      d. Reinforce dietary instruction and restrictions.

III. Concerns for the elderly

A. Type II diabetes has its onset in adulthood and often is not discovered until the sixth or seventh decade.
B. Older patients have difficulty adjusting to the diet, medication, and exercise routine.
C. Financial constraints sometimes make it difficult to obtain needed food and medicine.
D. By the sixth, seventh, and eighth decades, many diabetics have developed the complications of the disease: kidney failure, visual impairment, neuropathy, and severe cardiovascular and peripheral vascular disease.

E. Older NIDDM patients are prone to develop hyperglycemic hyperosmolar nonketotic (HHNK) syndrome.
   1. Similar to ketoacidosis except level of ketones not excessive.
   2. Often occurs during or after a febrile illness or gastrointestinal flu during which the patient has stopped eating normally and possibly discontinued his oral medication.
   3. Signs and symptoms include lethargy, thirst, polyuria, dehydration, and change in level of consciousness.
   4. Blood glucose often rises to 600 to 2,000 mg/dL.
   5. HHNK can be fatal.
   6. Treated with rehydration, IV glucose, and insulin, plus close monitoring of vital signs.
F. Better monitoring and home care of the diabetic elderly population could prevent many of the complications of the disease.

CHAPTER 29

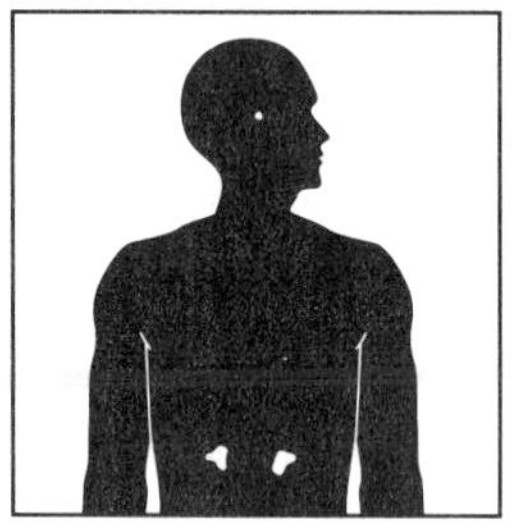

Care of Patients With Disorders of the Adrenal and Pituitary Glands

VOCABULARY

amenorrhea
catabolism
diabetogenic
diurnal
ectopic
endogenous
exogenous
hirsutism
hypophysectomy
impotence
libido

Upon completion of this part of the chapter the student should be able to:

1. List six signs and symptoms of adrenocortical insufficiency (Addison's disease).
2. State four nursing diagnoses and appropriate interventions for patients with Addison's disease.
3. List four major possible causes of Cushing's syndrome.
4. Describe eight signs and symptoms of Cushing's syndrome.
5. Formulate a nursing care plan for the patient with Cushing's syndrome.
6. List four major problems associated with hyposecretion of pituitary hormones and give at least three nursing interventions appropriate for each of them.
7. Identify nursing diagnoses and appropriate interventions for patients with diabetes insipidus.

THE ADRENAL GLANDS

The adrenal glands are composed of two distinct parts that have no direct functional relationship. The *adrenal medulla* (middle portion) secretes two hormones, *epinephrine* and *norepinephrine*. These substances are secreted in response to stimulation from the sympathetic nervous system, and their effects are, in turn, almost the same as direct stimulation of the sympathetic nerves. Epinephrine prepares the body to meet stress or emergency situations and prevents hypoglycemia. Norepinephrine functions as a pressor hormone to maintain blood pressure.

The hormones secreted by the *adrenal cortex* (outer covering) are called *adrenal corticosteroids*. The word *steroid* is sometimes used as an abbreviated form to designate an adrenal corticosteroid or a synthetic compound with similar properties. The two major types of hormones secreted by the adrenal cortex are the *mineralocorticoids* and the *glucocorticoids*. It also secretes small amounts of *androgenic hormones*, which have effects similar to the male and female sex hormones. Normally, the androgenic hormones have very little effect in comparison with the sex hormones secreted by the gonads, but in some abnormalities of the adrenal cortex, such large amounts of androgenic hormones are poured into the blood stream that they can present symptoms of sexual changes in the patient.

The mineralocorticoids and glucocorticoids are so named because of the effects they have on the body. The mineralocorticoids affect the electrolytes, particularly sodium, potassium, and chloride. Without the mineralocorticoids, a person would die within 3 to 7 days, because these hormones directly control fluid balance, blood volume, cardiac output, exchange of nutrients and wastes in each cell, and, in effect, all chemical processes and glandular functions within the body. Little wonder that they are said to be "lifesaving hormones." The glucocorticoids are almost equally important, because they are essential to the metabolic systems for proper utilization of carbohydrates, proteins, and fats.

ADRENOCORTICAL INSUFFICIENCY (ADDISON'S DISEASE)

In this condition, overall decreased function of the adrenal cortex leads to a deficit in all three hormones secreted by the adrenal cortex. The major problems presented by this disorder are, however, related to insufficiencies of the mineralocorticoids and the glucocorticoids. Insufficiency of the androgenic hormones can be compensated for by the ovaries and testes.

Insufficient production of the adrenocortical hormones can result from a disorder affecting the adrenal cortex itself *(primary insufficiency)*, or from a disorder affecting the pituitary gland that stimulates adrenal secretion *(secondary insufficiency)*.

Disorders causing a primary insufficiency include idiopathic atrophy, inflammation, infection, and nonsecreting tumors of the adrenal cortex. Secondary insufficiency is the direct result of failure of the pituitary gland to secrete corticotropin (also known as adrenocorticotropic hormone, or ACTH). This can occur as a result of underfunctioning of the pituitary, surgical removal of the gland *(hypophysectomy)*, and certain pituitary tumors.

Symptoms and Medical Diagnosis

In the early stages of Addison's disease the clinical manifestations may be so vague as to be annoying to the patient but not serious enough to consult a physician. Hence it is easily missed altogether or misdiagnosed. Later, as the hormone insufficiency becomes more pronounced, the patient will begin to exhibit more severe symptoms associated with fluid and electrolyte imbalance and hypoglycemia. Considering the functions of the mineralocorticoids, a major problem is depletion of sodium (hyponatremia), which in turn causes depletion of extracellular fluid and potassium retention (hyperkalemia). The patient experiences generalized malaise and muscle weakness, muscle pain, orthostatic hypotension, and vulnerability to cardiac arrhythmias. The problems of hyponatremia, fluid volume deficit, and hyperkalemia are discussed in Chapter 8.

Insufficiency of the glucocorticoids affects blood glucose levels and causes symptoms of hypoglycemia. There also is decreased secretion of gastrointestinal enzymes, which results in anorexia, nausea and vomiting, flatulence, and diarrhea. These symptoms, as well as anxiety, depression, and loss of mental acuity, are thought to be related to absence of the peaks of cortisol output that normally occur every 24 hours. In fact, abnormal serum electrolyte levels, decreased glucose tolerance, and abnormally low levels of free cortisol are among the criteria used to diagnose Addison's disease.

Medical Treatment and Nursing Intervention

Replacement therapy to provide the missing adrenocorticoid hormones is the major component of treatment. Replacement therapy usually brings about a rapid recovery, but the patient must continue taking the hormones for the rest of his life.

Nursing intervention is concerned with:

- Intensive care and support during *addisonian crisis* when the patient is in a critical condition and in danger of death from fluid vol-

ume depletion, hypotension and shock, and impairment of cardiac function.
- Prevention of problems related to fatigue and orthostatic hypotension.
- Alleviation of GI problems.
- Instruction of the patient in self-care.

Two important nursing measures are providing regular feedings throughout the day and providing adequate rest. The patient may feel well in the morning but becomes progressively weaker and more fatigued as the day goes on. If fasting is necessary for diagnostic studies or surgery, the patient with Addison's disease probably will need intravenous feedings of glucose to avoid profound hypoglycemia. Maintenance doses of exogenous (originating outside) glucocorticoids are especially important whenever fasting is required.

Gastrointestinal problems bring on the possibility of altered nutritional status related to anorexia, nausea and vomiting, and diarrhea. Specific fluid and electrolyte imbalances have already been discussed and are covered in more depth in Chapter 8.

Stress, even relatively mild physical or emotional stress, can quickly bring on an addisonian crisis. The patient should be cautioned to avoid undue stress whenever possible and to learn effective coping mechanisms to deal with the emotional stresses everyone faces.

Addisonian Crisis

Physical stress from the flu or other minor infection can tip the scales for the patient with Addison's disease and send him into crisis. The stress of surgery also presents problems. The nurse must be especially watchful and closely monitor vital signs in these patients.

Addisonian crisis requires immediate fluid replacement therapy, or the patient will go into irreversible shock. Intravenous hydrocortisone is given along with sodium, fluids, and dextrose until blood pressure becomes stable. The hydrocortisone is then tapered off slowly.

Nursing Diagnoses

Nursing diagnoses common to patients with Addison's disease include:

- Fluid volume depletion related to hormone and electrolyte imbalance.
- Alteration in cardiac output related to fluid depletion.
- Potential for injury related to the possibility of stress inducing a crisis.
- Ineffective individual coping related to the inability to decrease and control stress levels.
- Knowledge deficit related to disease process, medication, and necessary lifestyle changes.

Patient Education

Teaching the patient how to manage his illness is as important in Addison's disease as it is in diabetes mellitus. In both insulin-dependent diabetes mellitus (IDDM) and adrenocortical insufficiency, the inadequate supply of endogenous (originating inside an organ or port) hormone must be supplemented with exogenous hormone. Patient education for Addison's disease includes instruction in the signs and symptoms of either inadequate or excessive steroid levels and the importance of reporting these symptoms promptly.

Other points to be covered in patient teaching include:

- The nature of the illness and what can be done to control it.
- The purpose of each medication and the side effects to be reported.
- The importance of never suddenly stopping corticosteroids; they need to be tapered off slowly.
- Methods of adjusting medication dosage to combat the effects of stress.
- Signs and symptoms to report to the doctor immediately (worsening weakness, hypotension, confusion, infection).
- Diet adjustments to provide food throughout the day and a bedtime snack.
- Planned rest periods during the day and sufficient sleep at night.
- The need for a Medic-Alert tag or bracelet.

Additionally, the patient will need to understand the nature of his illness and the reasons for taking his medication every day, following his prescribed diet to avoid gastrointestinal problems, and getting enough rest so as to avoid unnecessary physical stress. The patient also should be instructed to wear some form of identification stating that he has Addison's disease and is receiving steroid therapy.

Nursing interventions for selected problems of patients with Addison's disease are summarized in Nursing Care Plan 29–1.

EXCESS ADRENOCORTICAL HORMONE (CUSHING'S SYNDROME)

The group of symptoms typical of Cushing's syndrome are manifestations of excess levels of the hormones from the adrenal cortex. The condition can be caused by:

- Excessive secretion of corticotropin (ACTH) by the pituitary gland, which may actually result from faulty release of corticotropin-releasing factor (CRF) from the hypothalamus.
- A secreting tumor of the adrenal cortex.
- Ectopic production of corticotropin by tumors outside the pituitary, most commonly lung

NURSING CARE PLAN 29–1

Selected nursing diagnoses, goals/outcome criteria, nursing interventions, and evaluations for a patient with adrenocortical insufficiency (Addison's disease)

Situation: Mr Cox, age 49, is admitted with a tentative diagnosis of adrenocortical insufficiency (Addison's disease). He has recently experienced weight loss, weakness and poor coordination, vomiting, changes in skin coloration, and loss of body hair. During initial assessment, Mr Cox is found to be very irritable and easily upset by the questions. His blood pressure is 90/50; pulse, 70 and slightly irregular; respirations, 16 and deep. He reports that he feels pretty good when he awakens in the morning but quickly becomes tired and his muscles begin to ache. He is concerned about his weight loss and change in appearance and also has noticed that he has been unable to "think straight." Admission laboratory data: blood glucose, 50 mg/dL; sodium, 90 mEq/L; and potassium, 5.6 mEq/L.

Nursing Diagnosis	Goals/Outcome Criteria	Nursing Interventions	Evaluation
Activity intolerance related to weakness and electrolyte imbalance. SUPPORTING DATA States that with the least little exertion, he tires and has muscle aching.	Serum sodium will return to normal within 24 hours.	Administer glucocorticoids and mineralocorticoids as prescribed; observe for side effects. Weigh daily; measure and compare intake and output. Monitor electrolyte levels. Force fluids until steroid therapy takes effect. Encourage him to eat to maintain adequate blood glucose and sodium levels.	Cortisone and fludrocortisone administered as ordered; weight unchanged; I, 2,860; O, 2,320; continue plan.
Potential for injury related to possible severe drop in blood glucose. SUPPORTING DATA Blood glucose on admission, 50 mg/dL.	Blood glucose will be maintained within normal limits. Crisis will not develop.	Observe for signs of hypoglycemia and report promptly. Check to see that meals are served on time; provide snacks as needed. Teach signs of hypoglycemia and instruct him in what to do when this occurs.	Blood glucose, 95; no signs of hypoglycemia; Continue plan.
Ineffective individual coping related to excess cortisol and mood swings. SUPPORTING DATA Very irritable and impatient; states he is unable to "think straight"; tentative diagnosis of Addison's disease; serum cortisol results pending.	Patient will develop effective coping mechanisms; relaxation techniques will be used before discharge. Patient will not be subjected to infection during hospitalization.	Protect him from exposure to infection. Monitor vital signs, WBC count, and lung fields each shift. Observe for signs of infection. Teach relaxation techniques and supervise practice; work with patient on other ways to decrease stress in daily life. Teach him how to handle anticipated stress by adjusting dosage of medications. Encourage verbalization of concerns and fears; answer questions. Discuss alterations in body image and changes that can be expected with therapy.	Lung fields clear; WBC count, 6,800; taught relaxation exercises and encouraged to practice; began survey of usual coping mechanisms and ways to decrease daily stress; continue plan.
Knowledge deficit related to illness, medications, and necessary changes in lifestyle. SUPPORTING DATA States that he knows nothing about Addison's disease, its diagnosis, or treatment. Unfamiliar with corticosteroid therapy.	Patient will simply describe problems of Addison's disease. Patient will verbalize understanding of medications and dosage schedule before discharge. Patient will verbalize plans for obtaining adequate rest before discharge.	Help to identify stressors in his life and assist in determining ways to avoid them. Answer questions and discuss expected effect of continued therapy on his ability to resume pre-illness activities. Help him develop a schedule that allows for periods of rest, work, social interaction, and recreation. Stress importance of balancing rest and activity. Provide written instructions that give warning signs and symptoms of insufficient corticosteroid medication and those of excess medication (Cushing's syndrome). Instruct him to report either set of symptoms to the physician promptly so medication can be adjusted.	First teaching session complete; written guidelines regarding medications given; continue plan.

Nursing care plan continued on following page

NURSING CARE PLAN 29–1, *Continued*

Nursing Diagnosis	Goals/Outcome Criteria	Nursing Interventions	Evaluation
		Discuss how to adjust medication for periods of extra stress (minor illness, such as a cold, an emotional upset, or unusual physiologic or psychological stress). Instruct him to wear a form of Medic-Alert identification with data concerning steroid therapy.	

carcinoma, medullary thyroid carcinoma, and thymoma.
- *Iatrogenic* Cushing's syndrome due to overzealous use of exogenous steroid therapy.

Symptoms and Medical Diagnosis

Diagnosis of Cushing's syndrome is established by laboratory findings indicating consistently high levels of free plasma cortisol rather than the usual 24-hour (diurnal) fluctuations. The symptoms and signs presented by the patient are the outcome of excessive levels of this hormone. They include painful fatty swellings in the intrascapular space (buffalo hump) and in the facial area (moon face), an enlarged abdomen with thin extremities, bruising following even minor traumas, impotence, amenorrhea, hypertension, and general weakness due to abnormal protein catabolism with loss of muscle mass.

Unusual growth of body hair (hirsutism) can occur in women, and streaked purple markings in the abdominal area can occur, owing to collections of body fat. Patients with Cushing's syndrome who have a familial predisposition to diabetes mellitus frequently develop IDDM as a result of the anti-insulin, diabetogenic properties of cortisol.

Medical Treatment

Treatment of Cushing's syndrome is becoming more successful as new modes of therapy become available. Pituitary Cushing's syndrome can be treated by surgical procedures involving the pituitary gland and utilizing microsurgical techniques. In some instances *prevention* of the disorder can be accomplished by the cautious use of steroids and restriction of their administration to patients who do not respond to other forms of therapy.

Nursing Intervention

The nursing care of patients with Cushing's syndrome is primarily concerned with helping each patient cope with the many problems presented by the disorder.

Nursing Diagnoses

Appropriate nursing diagnoses for the patient with Cushing's syndrome may include:

- Potential for infection related to glucose metabolism abnormality.
- Sleep pattern disturbance related to excess cortisol secretion.
- Activity intolerance related to electrolyte imbalance and decreased muscle strength.
- Potential for injury related to muscle weakness, fatigue, and thinning bone.
- Potential alteration in nutrition, more than body requirements, related to increased appetite.
- Ineffective individual coping related to hormone-induced mood swings.
- Knowledge deficit related to illness and treatment.

The more common problems and suggested nursing interventions are summarized in Table 29–1.

THE PITUITARY GLAND

The pituitary gland (hypophysis) lies at the base of the brain and is connected to the hypothalamus by the hypophyseal stalk. The pituitary gland is only 1 cm in diameter, but it plays a key role in many different functions of organs throughout the body. The gland is divided into two distinct portions that secrete different kinds of hormones. The anterior pituitary is called the adenohypophysis, and the posterior pituitary is known as the neurohypophysis.

In view of the many and varied functions of the pituitary gland one can readily understand that dysfunction of the hypophysis can produce a variety of symptoms and syndromes. It is therefore difficult to classify the many syndromes that can occur as a result of a pituitary disorder. Among the more common disorders are tumors of the pituitary, which account for about 10% of all intracranial tumors, and diabetes insipidus.

TABLE 29–1 COMMON NURSING DIAGNOSES AND INTERVENTIONS FOR PATIENTS WITH CUSHING'S SYNDROME

Nursing Diagnosis	Nursing Intervention
Potential for infection related to antiinflammatory effect of excess cortisol.	Monitor carefully for signs of beginning infection. Protect from exposure to infectious agents (see Chapter 6). Teach scrupulous hygiene.
Alteration in nutrition, more than body requirements, related to altered glucose metabolism.	Teach signs and symptoms of hyperglycemia and how to administer insulin; teach diabetic diet exchange system. Assist in designing diet according to food preferences.
Activity intolerance related to muscle weakness and fatigue.	Assist with ADL as needed. Provide rest periods throughout the day; teach to balance rest and activity. Monitor electrolyte levels.
Potential for injury related to alterations in metabolism.	Remove hazards from environment; pad sharp corners. Encourage adequate intake of dietary protein.
Ineffective individual coping related to excess cortisol and mood swings.	Encourage verbalization of feelings and concerns. Assure patient that as disease is controlled, moods will be more stable. Help patient identify strengths and focus on them. Teach relaxation techniques to handle stressful times. Explain physiologic causes of changes in moods.

PITUITARY TUMORS

Tumors of the pituitary gland can produce local and systemic symptoms. Local symptoms are more likely to occur when the tumor is large and creates pressure within the brain. Smaller tumors, as well as the larger ones, can cause various endocrine dysfunctions, depending on whether they stimulate or inhibit the secretion of particular hormones.

Local symptoms include headache and visual disturbances, the latter being due to pressure within the optic chiasm. If the pressure is not released, continued pressure will destroy the optic nerve and produce blindness. Systemic symptoms may be vague and, like the local symptoms, are very slow in their progression. Personality changes, weakness, fatigue, and vague abdominal pain can be present for years before the condition is diagnosed correctly.

Diagnosis is established by immunoassay tests for anterior and posterior pituitary hormones. Other diagnostic tests for pituitary dysfunction include a computed tomographic (CT) scan of the skull and a pneumoencephalogram.

Medical and Surgical Treatment and Nursing Intervention

In some cases the physician may choose to treat the pituitary tumor conservatively with hormone replacement therapy and periodic monitoring of the patient's progress. If the tumor continues to grow or presents serious hormonal imbalances, it may be treated surgically or by irradiation. Some specialists prefer to remove the tumor surgically and then apply radiation to the site to be sure that all tumor cells have been destroyed.

Some of the more common problems presented by patients with pituitary tumor and *hypopituitary* syndromes and recommended nursing interventions are summarized in Table 29–2.

DIABETES INSIPIDUS

This condition is characterized by the production of copious amounts of dilute urine, often as much as 15 to 20 liters in every 24-hour period. Diabetes insipidus occurs as a result of decreased production of the antidiuretic hormone (ADH), which regulates reabsorption of water in the kidney tubules. When ADH is not present in sufficient amounts, the water remains in the tubules and is excreted as urine. Restriction of fluid intake does not control the excessive flow of urine.

Diabetes insipidus is treated by the injections of vasopressin tannate (Pitressin Tannate in Oil) every 2 to 3 days. The drug also can be taken by nasal spray four to six times a day. Nursing care

TABLE 29-2 **SELECTED NURSING DIAGNOSES AND NURSING INTERVENTIONS FOR PATIENTS WITH PITUITARY TUMOR AND HYPOPITUITARY SYNDROME**

Nursing Diagnosis	Nursing Intervention
Self-esteem disturbance related to changes in physical appearance	Provide opportunities for verbalization of feelings Help patient identify strengths and positive aspects of his life and self. Focus on strengths and positive aspects Give sincere compliments
Sexual dysfunction related to decreased libido, amenorrhea, and impotence	Help patient recognize and maintain his personal worth as an individual Assist patient to maintain family role as mother, father, etc. Help family understand patient's illness
Alteration in nutrition, less than body requirements, related to anorexia, constipation	Measure fluid intake and output Weigh daily Alter diet as needed to increase fiber and carbohydrate content Give stool softener as needed Teach patient not to ignore urge to defecate Provide smaller and more frequent meals of preferred foods
Activity intolerance related to fatigue, lethargy, weakness, somnolence	Provide periods of rest Assist with activities of daily living as needed Set slower pace for activities Give patient more time to respond to verbal communications Encourage physical activity to highest level of tolerance
Potential for injury related to possible increased intracranial pressure	Continue steroid replacement therapy Conduct regular checks of neurologic status Assess for vomiting, hypotension, changes in headache, and seizures
Knowledge deficit about management of illness after surgery or irradiation	Teach patient and family about need for ID card and tag Provide written instructions for taking replacement hormones Provide instruction for "sick days" Describe symptoms of too much or too little medication Emphasize importance of follow-up care

TABLE 29-3 **NURSING CARE FOR PATIENTS WITH PITUITARY DIABETES INSIPIDUS**

Nursing Diagnosis	Nursing Intervention
Fluid volume depletion related to insufficient ADH.	Measure and record intake and output every 2 hours; maintain ordered IV fluid rate; encourage oral fluid intake. Compare intake and output; weigh daily; assess for signs of dehydration. Institute measures to prevent skin breakdown (bath oil, lotion, mobilization).
Constipation related to dehydration.	Provide high-bulk diet; encourage fluid intake. Administer stool softener as ordered.
Knowledge deficit related to disorder and treatment.	Emphasize need for Medic-Alert tag or bracelet and wallet card. Teach correct administration of vasopressin preparation. Teach signs and symptoms that indicate need for extra dose of medication and what to report to doctor (e.g., thirst, change in urination patterns). Stress need for regular follow-up visits with doctor.

for patients with pituitary diabetes insipidus is summarized in Table 29–3.

Concerns for the Elderly

From middle age on, there is a decrease in cell mass of the pituitary gland. However, hormonal secretion seems to remain adequate to meet the body's needs. Thus although there are aging-related changes in the mass of the adrenal glands, hormone levels remain constant, because as decreased secretion occurs, the body adjusts and slows metabolism of the adrenal hormones.

BIBLIOGRAPHY

Andreoli, T. E., et al.: Cecil Essentials of Medicine, 2nd ed. Philadelphia, W. B. Saunders, 1990.

Germon, K.: Fluid and electrolyte problems associated with diabetes insipidus and syndrome of inappropriate antidiuretic hormone. Nurs. Clin. North Am., Dec., 1987, p. 785.

Guyton, A. C.: Textbook of Medical Physiology, 8th ed. Philadelphia, W. B. Saunders, 1990.

Ignatavicius, D. D., and Bayne, M. J.: Medical-Surgical Nursing. Philadelphia, W. B. Saunders, 1991.

Kee, J. L.: Laboratory and Diagnostic Tests with Nursing Implications, 2nd ed. Norwalk, CT, Appleton & Lange, 1987.

Price, S. A., and Wilson, L. M.: Pathophysiology: Clinical Concepts of Disease Processes, 3rd ed. New York, McGraw-Hill, 1986.

STUDENT STUDY AIDS

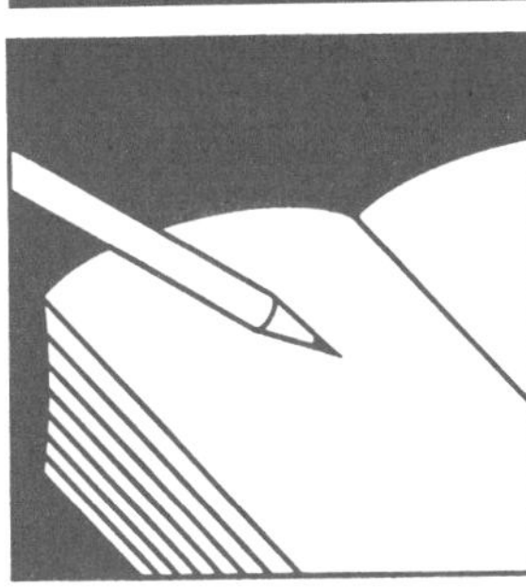

CLINICAL CASE PROBLEMS

Read the clinical situation and discuss the questions with your classmates.

1. Mr. Lake, age 37, is receiving adrenocorticoid hormones as replacement therapy for Addison's disease.

- What kinds of problems does insufficiency of the adrenal cortex hormones bring about?
- What should be included in your instructions to Mr. Lake to help him manage his illness?

2. Mrs. Johnston, age 48, is hospitalized for a cholecystectomy. She has Cushing's syndrome as well as gallbladder disease. She is 35 pounds over-weight and depressed.

- What kinds of problems is Mrs. Johnston likely to have as a result of her Cushing's syndrome?
- What would be your concerns in the immediate postoperative period?
- What would you want to include in your discharge teaching plan?

STUDY OUTLINE

I. Adrenal glands

A. Adrenal medulla secretes epinephrine and norepinephrine; adrenal cortex secretes mineralocorticoids, glucocorticoids, and androgenic hormones.

B. Dysfunction of adrenal cortex more likely to be related to abnormal levels of cortical hormones other than androgenic ones because testes or ovaries can compensate for insufficiency of sex hormones.

C. Adrenocortical insufficiency (Addison's disease).

1. Primary insufficiency due to malfunction of adrenal gland; secondary related to disorders of pituitary.
2. Primary insufficiency can be caused by idiopathic atrophy of gland, inflammation, infection, and nonsecreting tumors of adrenals.
3. Symptoms and medical diagnosis:
   a. In the early stages of Addison's disease clinical manifestations can be very vague.
   b. Eventually patient will show signs of fluid and electrolyte imbalance: hyponatremia and fluid water deficit, hyperkalemia, low blood pressure, and hypoglycemia.
4. Medical treatment and nursing intervention:
   a. Replacement therapy usually brings about rapid recovery.

b. Nursing intervention:
   (1) Intensive care during addisonian crisis.
   (2) Problem of fatigue and orthostatic hypotension.
   (3) Alleviation of anorexia, nausea and vomiting, diarrhea.
   (4) Preventive and coping mechanisms for stress.
   (5) Patient education.
      (a) Medications.
      (b) Signs and symptoms of insufficient or excess adrenocorticoid hormones.
      (c) Prescribed diet.
      (d) Need for extra rest.
      (e) ID card and tag.

D. Excess adrenocortical hormone (Cushing's syndrome).
   1. Can be caused by excess corticotropin, secreting tumor of adrenal cortex, overzealous administration of steroids.
   2. Symptoms and medical diagnosis:
      a. Laboratory testing of 24-hour levels of cortisol. Constantly high level indicative of Cushing's syndrome.
      b. Clinical manifestations include painful fatty swellings, large body with thin extremities, bruising after mild trauma, impotence, amenorrhea, hypertension, and general weakness.
      c. Patients with family history of diabetes can develop IDDM.
   3. Medical treatment and nursing intervention:
      a. Surgical removal and radiation or destruction of pituitary gland when pituitary disorder is primary cause.
      b. Nursing diagnoses common to patient with nursing interventions summarized in Table 22–9.

II. Pituitary gland

A. Pituitary is a pea-sized gland located at the base of the brain and connected to the hypothalamus.

B. Anterior pituitary (adenohypophysis) and posterior pituitary lobe (neurohypophysis) secrete completely different hormones.

C. Among more common disorders of the pituitary are tumors and diabetes insipidus.

D. Pituitary tumors.
   1. Large tumors can create pressure within the brain, causing local symptoms of headache, visual disturbances.
   2. Small tumors may present vague symptoms such as personality change, weakness, fatigue, and abdominal discomfort.
   3. Symptoms can be present years before diagnosis is made.
   4. Medical diagnosis established by immunoassay for hormone levels, CAT scan of skull, and pneumoencephalogram.
   5. Medical and surgical treatment and nursing intervention:
      a. Conservative treatment: administration of pituitary hormones.
      b. Surgical procedure involves removal of tumor or radiation or both.
      c. Common problems and nursing intervention for patients with hypopituitarism summarized in Table 29–2.

E. Diabetes insipidus results from decreased production of ADH; characterized by production of copious amounts of dilute urine.
   1. Treatment consists of injections of vasopressin every 2 to 3 days, or nasal spray of vasopressin several times daily.

III. Concerns for the elderly

A. Adrenal hormone levels remain constant.

B. Pituitary hormone secretion is sufficient to meet the body's needs.

CHAPTER 30

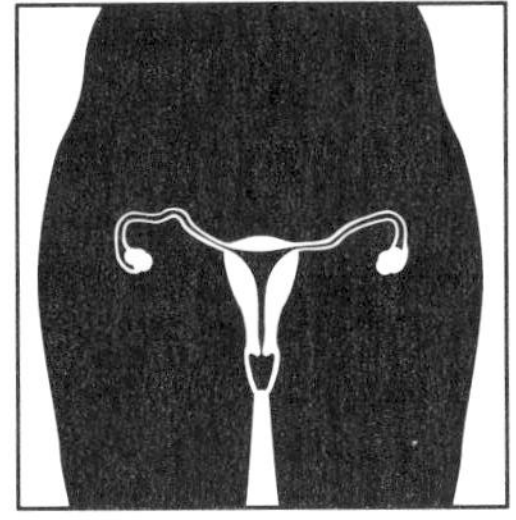

Care of Patients With Disorders of the Female Reproductive System

VOCABULARY

climacteric
coitus
curettage
dilatation
ectopic pregnancy
fibroid tumor
fulguration
gynecology
menopause
perineum
uterine tubes
vulva

Upon completion of this part of the chapter the student should be able to:

1. Discuss the role of normally functioning reproductive organs in the total sexual health of an individual.
2. List nursing responsibilities for the periods before, during, and after gynecologic tests and examinations.
3. Describe points and areas to be included in nursing assessment of the gynecologic status of patients.
4. Describe the procedure for breast self-examination (BSE).
5. Describe the nursing care plan, including instructions for self-care, for patients with common gynecologic problems such as dysmenorrhea, menopause, premenstrual syndrome, endometriosis, vaginitis, and pelvic inflammatory disease.
6. State the risk factors for development of cervical, uterine, and endometrial cancer.
7. List specific nursing interventions to be included in the nursing care plan for the patient with endometrial cancer undergoing intracavitary radiation and hysterectomy.
8. Devise nursing interventions for the patient who has had a vaginal hysterectomy.
9. Prepare a teaching plan for the patient with fibrocystic disease of the breast.
10. Present possible nursing interventions for the psychological care of the patient undergoing a simple mastectomy for breast cancer.

The normal development and proper functioning of the reproductive organs in both male and female depend to a great extent on a properly functioning endocrine system. The glands of the female reproductive system are the ovaries, which lie on either side of the pelvis and are attached to the uterus. The ovaries are both endocrine and exocrine glands, because they secrete hormones directly into the blood stream (estrogen and progesterone) and also have external secretions that contain an ovum, or egg (Fig. 30–1).

A second group of organs are the tubes. In the female, these tubes are the uterine tubes, which conduct the egg from the ovary to the uterus, and the vagina, or birth canal, which serves as a passageway for either the menstrual flow or the products of conception, depending on whether the ovum has been fertilized.

A third group of organs consists of the reservoirs. In the female, the ovary contains and allows for maturation of the egg, or ovum; the uterus serves as a reservoir for the fertilized egg and assists in its maturation and development until the birth of the infant.

The reproductive organs are but one factor in total human sexuality. They represent the biologic aspects of what it means to be male or female and contribute to identification with and acceptance of the role of man or woman. Other factors include social, cultural, psychological, and emotional influences and expectations for feminine and masculine behaviors.

In this chapter we will primarily consider the biologic aspects of reproduction, realizing that whatever affects a part or subsystem of the total human system also has an impact on the whole person. Hence any abnormal function, disease, or surgery of a reproductive organ has ramifications beyond those of physiology that are different from dysfunctions affecting some other body system. All humans are sexual beings, and each person expresses his or her sexuality in many different ways. Any reproductive disorder will in some way create concern in a person about his or her own masculinity or femininity. Dysfunction or loss of a reproductive organ through surgery can cause serious psychological problems related to sexuality, body image, and a sense of wholeness.

DIAGNOSTIC TESTS AND PROCEDURES AND NURSING RESPONSIBILITIES

PELVIC EXAMINATION

The external and internal female genital organs are examined mainly by inspection and palpation. Nurses who are qualified to perform a pelvic examination have learned special skills and techniques and should have a high degree of sensitivity to the patient's feelings and concerns about such an intimate procedure. The specific knowledge and skills required to perform a complete gynecologic examination are not within the scope of this text. The information presented is related to the duties and responsibilities of the nurse when assisting with a pelvic examination. It is expected that in the role of assistant to the examiner the nurse will display a genuine respect for the privacy and feelings of the patient and concern for her needs.

Physical and mental preparation of the patient who is to have a pelvic examination is of utmost importance. The success of the examination will depend to a great extent on the ability of the

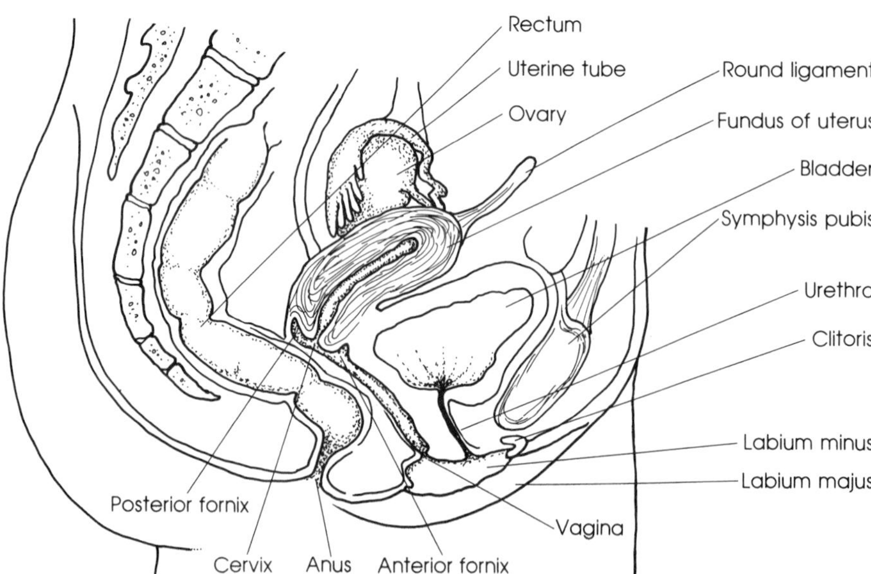

Figure 30–1 Female reproductive system.

patient to relax and cooperate with the examiner. Proper draping of the patient and privacy for the examination are essential.

The necessary equipment, such as a vaginal speculum, gloves, and lubricant, must be assembled and conveniently arranged before the examination begins. The assisting nurse may be asked to remain with the patient during the examination and to assist her in dressing after the examination is completed. She should avoid all signs of haste or lack of interest in the patient's feelings and attitudes toward the examination. A few moments should be taken to explain the procedure if the patient does not know what to expect and to relieve her anxieties and fears by answering her questions simply and honestly.

While preparing the patient for a gynecologic examination, the nurse must be sure to have the patient empty her bladder completely. Otherwise, the distended bladder will interfere with the examination.

The best time for a pelvic examination is between menstrual periods. This is sometimes taken to mean that a pelvic examination is dangerous and undesirable if the patient has any vaginal bleeding. Actually, the presence of persistent vaginal bleeding for several weeks or months may indicate a serious disease that should be investigated *immediately*, rather than delaying the examination in the hope that the bleeding will stop. There is no reason that a pelvic examination should not be done when the patient is bleeding.

Sometimes patients who have an abnormal amount of vaginal discharge will give themselves a vaginal douche before a pelvic examination, unaware that this procedure washes away secretions that may help in diagnosing the cause of the discharge. The nurse may need to explain this to her patients so that they will understand why douching is not advisable immediately before a gynecologic examination.

SMEARS AND CULTURES

In both smears and cultures, samples of cells and fluid from the vagina, cervix, and endometrium can be taken and sent to the clinical laboratory for examination. Cultures are used to identify specific infectious organisms. A Papanicolaou (Pap) smear is useful for cytologic evaluations in screening for cancer of the cervix.

Pap smears are reported as "negative" or in the following terms of cervical intraepithelial neoplasia (CIN) stages:

- CIN I indicates mild dysplasia.
- CIN II indicates moderate dysplasia.
- CIN III indicates severe dysplasia to carcinoma in situ (CIS).

CIN I, II and III results indicate a need for a more complete evaluation of the lesion from which the cells were taken.

An alternative technique is the Gravlee method, in which cells are collected for examination by washing the uterine cavity with normal saline and collecting the returned material in a reservoir that is part of the apparatus. Advocates of this technique claim that it provides more accurate testing for malignancy, particularly for endometrial cancers.

ENDOMETRIAL BIOPSY

Endometrial biopsy often is part of a workup for patients with problems of infertility. It is also done for women with menstrual problems or postmenopausal bleeding and is now recommended yearly for all women who are taking estrogen and progestin after menopause. The test is an office procedure that involves removal of a sample of endometrial cells for microscopic examination. It is often done at the onset of or just before menstruation in order to determine whether the endometrium is responding to the ovarian hormones, estrogen and progesterone. If normal ovulation has occurred, the endometrium should have a thickened secretory lining in preparation for implantation by a fertilized ovum. The biopsy procedure causes some cramping, and the nurse must help the patient relax to minimize the discomfort.

After biopsy the patient is instructed to refrain from sexual intercourse and to avoid using vaginal creams or inserting anything into the vagina until the biopsied area has healed and bleeding has stopped. Tampons are not to be used until complete healing has occurred.

COLPOSCOPY

Colposcopy is an inspection of the vagina and cervix by means of an endoscopic instrument placed at the vaginal opening. Colposcopy is done in the office, and the preparation is similar to that for a pelvic exam. Its purpose is to evaluate abnormal cells and lesions and to examine the vagina and cervix more closely after a positive Pap test. Attachments for the colposcope allow removal of tissue for biopsy and photographs of lesions that need further study.

Preparation of the patient for colposcopy is minimal and requires a simple explanation of the purpose of the test, allowing time for any questions the patient might have. The procedure takes from 10 to 15 minutes in all and, if biopsy is done, causes only a small amount of bleeding and some minor cramping. No tampons are to be used until healing has occurred.

LAPAROSCOPY

Laparoscopy is a surgical procedure that requires a very small abdominal incision for the insertion of a fiber-optic instrument into the peritoneal cavity. It permits inspection of the cavity to detect such abnormalities as cysts, infections, fibroids, and adhesions. Laparoscopy can also be done for such therapeutic procedures as tubal sterilization and removal of adhesions, foreign bodies, and implants of endometrial tissue outside the uterus.

Laparoscopy is done in the outpatient surgery department with the patient under regional or general anesthesia. Therefore the patient's preoperative and postoperative care is similar to that of any patient with abdominal surgery. The major difference is the relatively small incision and minimum trauma to organs in the peritoneal cavity. The patient usually goes home the same day, and the recuperative period is much shorter than that following major abdominal surgery. The patient is told to rest for 1 to 3 days following the surgery. Shoulder pain may be experienced if air or gas was injected into the abdomen during the procedure to aid visualization. The patient should be able to resume normal activity within a week after surgery.

DILATATION AND CURETTAGE (D AND C)

Dilatation of the cervix and curettage, or scraping of the inside of the uterus, is a minor surgical procedure that is performed in the outpatient surgery department. It can be accomplished under regional or general anesthesia.

Postoperatively the nurse monitors the patient for excessive uterine bleeding and for severe abdominal pain, which could indicate uterine perforation.

Discharge teaching includes instructions to rest for 1 to 3 days, to report excessive bleeding and passage of large clots, and to watch for signs of infection. It is done to treat certain diseases of the reproductive system. However, the endometrial tissue removed during the operation is often sent to the laboratory for microscopic examination to aid in the diagnosis of the patient's condition.

MAMMOGRAPHY

Mammography is an x-ray examination of the soft tissues of the breast without the injection of a contrast medium. It can be used in diagnosing lesions of the breast such as tumors and abscesses, but it requires a skilled and experienced radiologist to read the films properly. One of the most difficult tasks is distinguishing between benign and malignant lesions, and therefore mammography cannot take the place of biopsy, palpation, and other examinations of the breast. It should be accepted as one more means of detecting breast disorders rather than as a specific examination that eliminates the need for further study. However, mammography identifies far more malignancies than can be felt by a doctor's examination or self-examination of the breast.

The American Cancer Society recommends a baseline mammogram for all women at 35 to 40 years of age. For women without significant risk factors for breast cancer, mammograms are to be done at least every 2 years between the ages of 40 and 49. Mammograms are recommended yearly for all women over 50 and for women over 40 who have significant risk factors.

BREAST SELF-EXAMINATION

Monthly self-examination of the breast has been widely publicized in an effort to encourage women to look for any lump or thickening in their own breasts. The examination should be done each month 1 week after menstruation begins. Women who have passed menopause are advised to choose a date on which they will examine their breasts each month. The steps for performing the procedure are shown in Figure 30–2.

THE NURSE'S ROLE IN BREAST SELF-EXAMINATION

The nurse can and does play an important role in health teaching. With breast cancer, hers is a dual role—personal as well as professional.

Most nurses are in contact with many people in their 24-hour day; thus their opportunities to teach breast self-examination are limitless. Patients, friends, and relatives all need to know the importance of regular self-examination of the breasts. A nurse should be constantly alert herself and encourage others to be on the lookout for any lump or thickening in the breast. The important factor to be stressed is that each woman takes an unnecessary risk if she gives "lip service" to the breast examination rather than performing an actual examination.

Millions of women have seen the American Cancer Society's film on "Breast Self-Examination," and every nurse should see it herself and encourage all women to see it. This film may be obtained through the local unit or division of the American Cancer Society.

The concerned nurse will ask each female patient during the admission assessment if she performs BSE. If the answer is "no," appropriate teaching should be incorporated into the patient's care plan.

WHY DO THE BREAST SELF-EXAM?

THERE ARE MANY GOOD REASONS FOR DOING THE BREAST SELF-EXAM (BSE) EACH MONTH. ONE REASON IS THAT BREAST CANCER IS MOST EASILY TREATED AND CURED WHEN IT IS FOUND EARLY. ANOTHER IS THAT IF YOU DO BSE EVERY MONTH, IT WILL INCREASE YOUR SKILL AND CONFIDENCE WHEN DOING THE EXAM. WHEN YOU GET TO KNOW HOW YOUR BREASTS NORMALLY FEEL, YOU WILL QUICKLY BE ABLE TO FEEL ANY CHANGE. ANOTHER REASON, IT IS EASY TO DO.

REMEMBER: *BSE COULD SAVE YOUR BREAST—AND SAVE YOUR LIFE. MOST BREAST LUMPS ARE FOUND BY WOMEN THEMSELVES, BUT, IN FACT, MOST LUMPS IN THE BREAST ARE NOT CANCER. BE SAFE, BE SURE.*

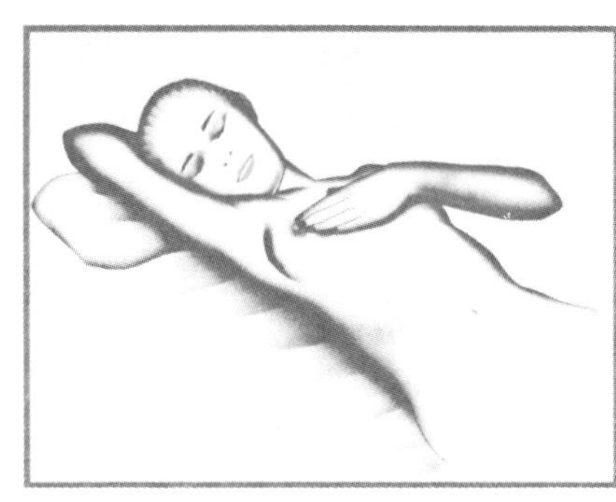

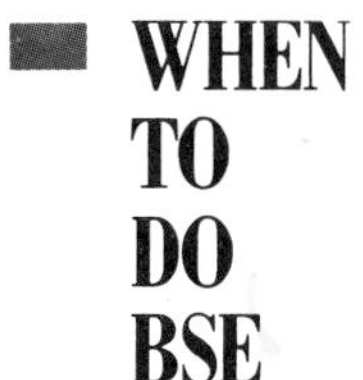

WHEN TO DO BSE

THE BEST TIME TO DO BSE IS ABOUT A WEEK AFTER YOUR PERIOD, WHEN BREASTS ARE NOT TENDER OR SWOLLEN. IF YOU DO NOT HAVE REGULAR PERIODS OR SOMETIMES SKIP A MONTH, DO BSE ON THE SAME DAY EVERY MONTH.

NOW, HOW TO DO BSE

1. *LIE DOWN AND PUT A PILLOW UNDER YOUR RIGHT SHOULDER. PLACE YOUR RIGHT ARM BEHIND YOUR HEAD.*

2. *USE THE FINGER PADS OF YOUR THREE MIDDLE FINGERS ON YOUR LEFT HAND TO FEEL FOR LUMPS OR THICKENING. YOUR FINGER PADS ARE THE TOP THIRD OF EACH FINGER.*

3. *PRESS FIRMLY ENOUGH TO KNOW HOW YOUR BREAST FEELS. IF YOU'RE NOT SURE HOW HARD TO PRESS, ASK YOUR HEALTH CARE PROVIDER. OR TRY TO COPY THE WAY YOUR HEALTH CARE PROVIDER USES THE FINGER PADS DURING A BREAST EXAM. LEARN WHAT YOUR BREAST FEELS LIKE MOST OF THE TIME. A FIRM RIDGE IN THE LOWER CURVE OF EACH BREAST IS NORMAL.*

4. *MOVE AROUND THE BREAST IN A SET WAY. YOU CAN CHOOSE EITHER THE CIRCLE (A), THE UP AND DOWN LINE (B), OR THE WEDGE (C). DO IT THE SAME WAY EVERY TIME. IT WILL HELP YOU TO MAKE SURE THAT YOU'VE GONE OVER THE ENTIRE BREAST AREA, AND TO REMEMBER HOW YOUR BREAST FEELS EACH MONTH.*

5. *NOW EXAMINE YOUR LEFT BREAST USING RIGHT HAND FINGER PADS.*

6. *IF YOU FIND ANY CHANGES, SEE YOUR DOCTOR RIGHT AWAY.*

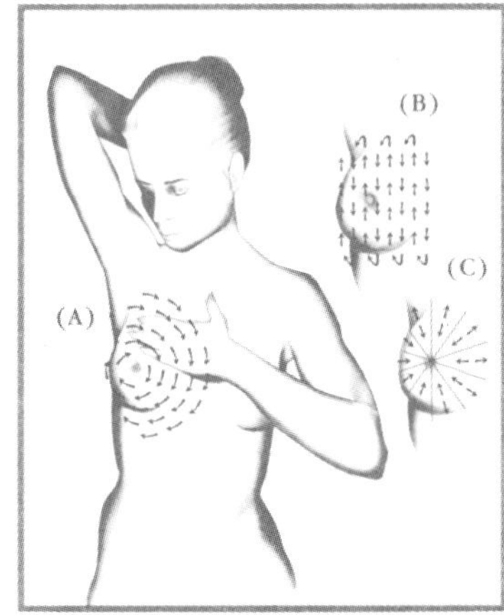

FOR ADDED SAFETY:

YOU MIGHT WANT TO CHECK YOUR BREASTS WHILE STANDING IN FRONT OF A MIRROR RIGHT AFTER YOU DO YOUR BSE EACH MONTH. SEE IF THERE ARE ANY CHANGES IN THE WAY YOUR BREASTS LOOK: DIMPLING OF THE SKIN, OR CHANGES IN THE NIPPLE, REDNESS OR SWELLING. YOU MIGHT ALSO WANT TO DO AN EXTRA BSE WHILE YOU'RE IN THE SHOWER. YOUR SOAPY HANDS WILL GLIDE OVER THE WET SKIN MAKING IT EASY TO CHECK HOW YOUR BREASTS FEEL.

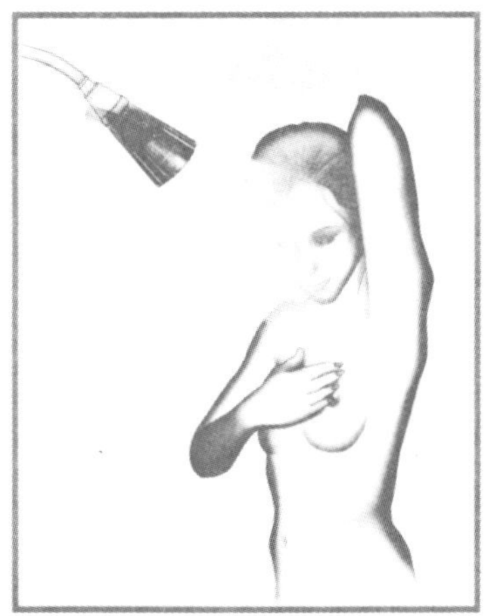

Figure 30-2 Breast self-examination. (Courtesy of the American Cancer Society.)

NURSING ASSESSMENT OF GYNECOLOGIC HEALTH STATUS

HISTORY TAKING

Approaches to women's health care are substantially different from the typically paternalistic and controlling attitudes that once were acceptable or at least tolerated by women patients. Today's female patient usually is more open in expressing her concerns and asking questions about her reproductive organs and their functions. She, in turn, is more likely to be comfortable answering questions about her personal and reproductive health history, especially if the nurse is able to establish a sense of mutual trust and respect.

Because the developmental stages in the reproductive life of a female are unique to her sex, the age of the patient is always relevant to her gynecologic history. Breast cancer and endometrial malignancies are more common in postmenopausal women. Sexually transmitted diseases are more prevalent in sexually active women who are in their teens and twenties.

Questions about a patient's sexual activity should be handled matter-of-factly and tactfully but with appreciation for the patient's right not to answer if she so chooses. It is helpful in the diagnosis of several kinds of vaginal and cervical disorders if one knows at what age the woman became sexually active and how many partners she has had. As pointed out elsewhere, the woman who has had frequent sex in her early teens or sex with many partners is at higher than usual risk for uterine and cervical cancer. Women who are sexually active also are more likely to develop sexually transmitted diseases.

The patient's personal history should include information about the onset of menses (menarche), length of menstrual periods each month, any irregularity in periods, episodes of irregular bleeding, vaginal discharge other than normal menses, history of birth control use, previous pregnancies, sexually transmitted diseases, frequency of BSE, and mammograms.

Symptoms of premenstrual syndrome and discomfort during menstruation also should be recorded. As with other types of pain and discomfort, assessment should include description of location, how it feels and its degree of severity, whether it radiates to another part of the body, and measures that relieve or conditions that aggravate the pain.

Pain and discomfort are among the more common chief complaints presented by a patient with a gynecologic disorder. Other common symptoms include vaginal discharge, pruritus, detectable lumps and masses, and abnormal uterine bleeding.

If the patient has had children and either is experiencing or has been through the climacteric, she should be asked about postpartum blues, irritability or depression during menses, and other emotional disturbances related to birth and menstruation and accompanying hormonal changes. Women who have a history of problems such as these are more likely to experience depression and other emotional difficulties during menopause.

The history should also include medications that the patient takes routinely, because there are several kinds of drugs that affect the female reproductive system. Among these are the more obvious ones such as oral contraceptives and progestogens. Some of the less obvious are antihypertensive agents, cytotoxics for the treatment of cancer, and other endocrine hormones such as thyroid hormones.

Family history is an important part of the overall nursing history because breast cancer on the female patient's maternal side of the family greatly increases her chances of developing a similar malignancy. Another important piece of information is whether the patient's mother received diethylstilbestrol to prevent miscarriage while she was pregnant with her. Women who have this kind of prenatal history are at much greater risk for developing a malignancy of the vagina and cervix.

Other family diseases that could be significant in the history of a patient with a gynecologic disorder include endocrine disorders, such as diabetes mellitus and thyroid disease, and either sickle cell trait or sickle cell disease.

SUBJECTIVE AND OBJECTIVE DATA

Subjective data that could be relevant to a gynecologic disorder include back pain, pain during intercourse, cramping, headache, irritability, emotional instability, feeling of fullness in the pelvis, and itching in and around the vagina.

Objective data might include amount and character of vaginal discharge, evidence of irritation around the vagina and perineum, and blisters, growths, or ulcerations on the external genitalia. If the patient has uterine bleeding, it is helpful to know the amount and character. Amount can be estimated by recording the number of peripads or tampons needed in a 24-hour period. Clots, pieces of tissue, and color of the discharge (bright red, dark brown, etc.) should also be noted and recorded.

Assessment of the patient with a breast disorder should include information about the contour and development of each breast. It is also important to note whether there is any swelling or dimpling, whether the breasts are symmetric, and if there is any discharge from either nipple.

Evaluation of ovarian function can be helped by noting secondary sex characteristics. These would include distribution of body hair, development of breasts, pitch of voice, and texture of the skin.

NURSING DIAGNOSES

Nursing diagnoses commonly associated with gynecologic disorders include the following:

- Activity intolerance related to anemia from excessive blood loss, weakness, or disabling discomfort.
- Ineffective individual coping related to unhealthy attitude about human sexuality or menstruation.
- Fear of mutilating surgery, loss of femininity.
- Fluid volume excess related to premenstrual fluid retention.
- Knowledge deficit about practices of personal feminine hygiene, normal anatomy and physiology of the female reproductive organs, or safe methods of contraception.
- Sexual dysfunction related to dyspareunia or emotional block.
- Disturbance in self-concept related to sterility, menopause, and surgery of a reproductive organ.
- Impairment of skin integrity related to pruritus, genital lesions, and vaginal discharge.
- Pain related to menstruation, decreased vaginal lubrication, or vaginal irritation.

MENSTRUATION

Menstruation is a normal monthly process and certainly should be considered as such in spite of age-old negative attitudes toward it. In the event pregnancy does not take place, the uterine lining is sloughed off and, together with mucus and blood, constitutes the menstrual flow.

The onset of menstruation is called the *menarche*. It usually occurs between the ages of 9 and 16 years; earlier and later onsets are not necessarily abnormal. During the first year after onset, menstruation may be irregular, but by the second year a cycle of about every 28 days should be established. Table 30–1 reviews the phases of the 28-day menstrual cycle.

Attitudes toward menstruation are formed early in a young girl's life and may directly affect the degree of physical discomfort and emotional uneasiness she experiences during each of her menstrual periods. Every young girl should be told about menstruation *before* she begins her periods so that she can be prepared and ready to accept it as a wholesome sign of her maturing process.

Nurses frequently are in a position to inform young children of both sexes about the many physiologic changes that take place in their bodies during puberty. Before attempting to in-

TABLE 30–1 **STAGES OF THE MENSTRUAL CYCLE**

First to Fifth Day	Sixth to Fourteenth Day	Fifteenth to Twenty-eighth Day
*Menstrual stage (dismantling stage)**	*Stage of growth and repair (estrogen or proliferative stage)*	*Secretory stage (postovulatory or progesterone stage)*
1. Endometrium sloughs away as menstrual flow begins.	1. Follicle grows and egg matures.	1. Corpus luteum secretes progesterone.
2. Progesterone and estrogen no longer secreted.	2. Endometrium returns to normal state and then begins to thicken in response to estrogen.	2. Endometrium continues to thicken in response to estrogen and progesterone. Prepares to receive fertilized ovum.
3. New follicle starts to mature.	3. Ovulation occurs 14 days before menses, regardless of length of menstrual cycle. Takes place when follicle ruptures and releases egg.	

* *Note:* In order for menstruation to occur, two organs are essential: (1) the uterus, because menstruation is the sloughing away of about three fourths of the lining of the uterus; and (2) at least part of one ovary, because the ovary secretes the hormones that cause the endometrium to thicken.

struct these young people, the nurse should explore her own attitudes and feelings about discussing the topic of sexuality. She should strive to develop a positive, healthy attitude toward her own body and the process of menstruation. Once she is comfortable with her own self-image and aspects of her femininity, she can communicate to others the concept of menstruation as a normal process, a "rite of passage" to be celebrated by the young girl entering womanhood.

MENOPAUSE

Sometime between the ages of 45 and 50, the *climacteric* usually begins. The word *climacteric* is taken from a Greek word meaning *a rung of a ladder*. Thus a man or woman who enters the climacteric period is taking another step in life. In fact, the common term for menopause in women is *the change of life.*

The climacteric in women is characterized by gradual changes in the menstrual cycle with a decrease in menstrual flow and irregularity in the cycle. When the menstrual flow is completely absent for a full year, menopause, which is the complete cessation of menstruation, is said to have occurred.

Menopause marks the end of the woman's reproductive period. Prior to actual menopause, it is possible for a woman to become pregnant. Women wishing to avoid a "change of life baby" should use some form of contraception for one full year after menstrual flow has stopped.

During the climacteric, which sometimes extends for more than a year, there is a gradual change in ovarian function. Hormonal changes taking place present some physical and emotional disturbances that may or may not interfere with the woman's daily activities. Not all women are aware of problems during the climacteric. About 15% experience no symptoms at all, and of the remaining 85%, only about one fourth are uncomfortable enough to seek relief and consult a physician.

Menopause can actually take place at any time between the ages of 35 and 58 with an average age at onset of 50. Menopause that occurs before the age of 35 is called *premature menopause;* after the age of 58 it is called *delayed menopause.* Either of these conditions may be inherited, or they may be indicative of a primary disorder affecting the endocrine glands or the reproductive organs. In either case, medical attention is advised. Paradoxically, a woman who began menstruating at a relatively early age will experience menopause later than average.

Artificial menopause may be induced by surgical removal or radiation of the *ovaries*. The symptoms usually are more severe than those of natural menopause because of the sudden, rather than gradual, elimination of hormonal secretion. It should be noted that surgical removal of the *uterus only* (simple hysterectomy) causes a cessation of menstrual flow but does *not* produce symptoms of the climacteric. If, however, both ovaries are removed or rendered dysfunctional by radiation, the patient will experience an artificial menopause.

Symptoms

Just as the entire subject of menstruation is clouded by misinformation, so, too, is the subject of menopause. Fortunately, women today are more willing to discuss their gynecologic problems and are interested in finding out more about their bodies and what is happening to them. The informed nurse is in an excellent position to provide women with the information they need to adjust to life's changes and develop healthy coping skills.

The symptoms experienced by women during the climacteric are the result of at least three groups of factors: (1) decreased ovarian function and a resultant deficiency of hormones, (2) sociocultural factors that influence a woman's attitude toward growing older and moving beyond her child-bearing and child-rearing years, and (3) psychological factors related to each woman's inner resources, the support that is available to her from her family and significant others, and the personal coping skills she has developed.

The first sign of the onset of the climacteric is usually menstrual irregularity in which the flow of blood alternates between being very scanty and being profuse. Patchy flushing of the skin, an uncomfortable feeling of warmth in the face, neck, and chest (sometimes called *hot flashes*), and excessive perspiration also are relatively common and can last from a few months to 10 years or more. These symptoms are due to estrogen deficiency, which is the result of decreased ovarian activity. In general, the more abrupt the decline in ovarian function, the more severe the symptoms.

Other symptoms are not as clearly identified with lack of estrogen. They include fatigue, insomnia, emotional instability, and depression. Some women also experience back pain, headache, irritability, and decreased libido. These latter symptoms may be related to psychological factors and ineffective coping skills. A woman who is actively engaged in projects that are meaningful to her and provide her with a sense of productivity and accomplishment is less likely to suffer serious emotional upheavals during menopause than is the woman who sees herself as useless and unattractive. There is no truth to the belief that a postmenopausal woman is less attractive sexually or that she herself loses interest in sexual activities. In fact, many women report that they find sexual intercourse more enjoyable after menopause, because they are free from the fear of pregnancy.

Medical Treatment

Replacement of the estrogen that is no longer produced after menopause is a controversial form of therapy. It has the advantage of helping prevent postmenopausal osteoporosis and atrophic urethritis, as well as providing relief from some of the symptoms experienced during menopause. The major disadvantage is increased risk for endometrial cancer. Most gynecologists agree that estrogen replacement therapy can be used safely during the climacteric, but the period of treatment should be as brief as possible and the dosage only as high as needed to provide relief. Additionally, it is recommended that the patient on estrogen replacement therapy be checked at least every 6 months by a Pap smear and be evaluated for the effectiveness of the drug in relieving menopausal symptoms.

Current therapy calls for the addition of medroxyprogesterone (Provera) during the second half of the month in order to decrease the chance of uterine cancer. New research on osteoporosis indicates that perhaps long-term therapy with estrogen and progestin can decrease the rapid bone demineralization that occurs after menopause.

Nursing Intervention

A nurse can do several things to help patients deal with the problems of menopause. She can encourage the patient to eat a well-balanced diet and to strive to maintain normal body weight. The nurse can also discuss exercise as an important part of physical fitness and of achieving a sense of health and well-being.

When a patient does have hot flashes, she can be taught to lessen their impact by initiating some form of relaxation and mental imagery as soon as a hot flash begins. For example, she can take deep breaths, relax her skeletal muscles from head to toe, and imagine herself as calm and cool until the sensation is gone.

Postmenopausal women should be cautioned to report immediately any spotting or bleeding between periods before complete cessation of the monthly flow or after their periods have stopped. Spotting or bleeding during or after menopause can be the first sign of cancer of the uterus or cervix. Patients receiving progestin need to have an annual endometrial biopsy performed.

Patients who have been using some form of birth control should continue their contraceptive practices for at least a year after they have been through 12 consecutive months with no menstrual flow. Some authorities extend this time to 2 full years. The form of contraception used will depend on the individual patient. However, women over 40 years of age should not take any oral contraceptive ("the pill").

Patients who complain of dyspareunia (painful intercourse) because of vaginal dryness can use an estrogen vaginal cream to decrease thinning of the vaginal mucosa or a water-soluble jelly to provide lubrication. Normal sexual activity benefits the female by keeping the vaginal mucous membranes more flexible and also helps prevent problems of the prostate in the middle-aged male partner.

MENSTRUAL DYSFUNCTIONS

AMENORRHEA

The word *amenorrhea* means absence of menstruation. The term is applied to absence of regular monthly menstrual periods at any time between the onset of puberty and the climacteric. Primary amenorrhea refers to a condition in which menses have never occurred. Secondary amenorrhea refers to the absence of menstruation in women who have formerly had normal menstrual periods. In the context of this discussion, amenorrhea is an abnormal condition.

The causes of amenorrhea are varied and complex. They include (1) anatomic defects, such as imperforate (closed) hymen or some other vaginal defect, that prevent normal flow of menstrual fluids; uterine malformations; and developmental defects of the ovaries; (2) endocrine dysfunction affecting the hypothalamus, pituitary, ovaries, or thyroid; (3) chronic disease and obesity; (4) emotional disturbances; (5) side effects of some drugs; (6) poor nutrition; (7) excessive vigorous exercise causing weight to decrease below 95 lb; and (8) abrupt discontinuation of birth control pills. Malnutrition related to eating disorders such as anorexia nervosa or bulemia affects endocrine function and can cause amenorrhea.

Cessation of menstruation as a probable sign of pregnancy is not an abnormal event and is not considered among the disorders included under amenorrhea.

Medical Diagnosis

The onset of menstruation usually is at about the age of 12; however, there is no cause for alarm if menstruation does not begin at precisely the expected time. Most gynecologists recommend a complete physical workup to determine the cause of amenorrhea only if the woman has not menstruated by her seventeenth or eighteenth birthday.

Mature women who have an unexplained cessation of menstruation should consult a gynecologist because absence of menstrual flow can be symptomatic of many different illnesses other than those affecting the endocrine and reproductive systems.

Once pathologic amenorrhea is suspected, the physician will evaluate it on the basis of a complete physical examination and medical history, hormonal assays, and urine and blood analyses.

Medical Treatment

Treatment of amenorrhea is based on the cause of the condition. Surgical intervention may be necessary to correct anatomic defects. In cases of hormonal deficits, replacement therapy is usually indicated.

Nursing Intervention

An important aspect of nursing intervention in cases of amenorrhea is adequate health education, so that women of all ages become aware of the possible causes of the condition and the importance of consulting a gynecologist when either primary or secondary amenorrhea is present.

The patient may need help in learning to cope with either emotional or physical stress, which may cause menstrual problems. Relaxation techniques, an exercise program balanced with adequate rest, and improvements in dietary intake to restore and maintain normal nutrition and body weight are nursing interventions that could be helpful to the patient with amenorrhea.

DYSMENORRHEA

The word *dysmenorrhea* literally means difficult menstruation. The term is most often used to denote pain and discomfort that occurs either with the menstrual period or immediately before it (premenstrual syndrome). The pain is described in many different ways, ranging from a dull, steady ache in the lower back and pelvis to sharp, cramping pains in the suprapubic region. Symptoms other than pain include nausea and vomiting, diarrhea, headache, dizziness, fatigue, and emotional instability.

Primary dysmenorrhea is not accompanied by any demonstrable pathology. Secondary dysmenorrhea is related to an infection or inflammation of the pelvic organs, endometriosis, or the presence of an intrauterine contraceptive device.

Premenstrual syndrome (PMS) is a group of symptoms, both physical and emotional, that occurs before each menstrual period.

Etiology

Possible causes of primary dysmenorrhea range from hormonal imbalances to obstruction of the cervix. Recently, scientists have found that women with dysmenorrhea have two to four times more prostaglandins in their menstrual fluid than do women who do not have this problem. Prostaglandins are produced by the body from unsaturated fatty acids consumed in the diet. They are present in almost all body tissues and affect many physiologic processes. Among their physiologic effects is stimulation of smooth muscle contraction.

Discovery of the role of prostaglandins in the contraction of smooth muscle cells in the uterus and other organs such as the intestines and blood vessels does help explain the symptoms of dysmenorrhea. However, prostaglandins are not the only factor. Psychosocial factors associated with menstrual pain include lack of knowledge about normal anatomy and physiology of the female reproductive system, suggestion, imitation of the mother or other significant female, and anxiety and fear of recurring monthly pain. The use of tampons early in the menstrual period seems to increase the cramping in young girls and in some women.

The woman's general physical and emotional status and attitude toward menstruation can have some effect on the severity of dysmenorrhea. Although those who are physically fit and emotionally stable often escape severe menstrual pain, one should be careful when making judgments about dysmenorrhea. It is difficult to determine whether the monthly pain has rendered the patient psychologically and emotionally unstable or whether the psychological condition contributes to expectation of pain. In the latter case, the expectation of pain becomes a self-fulfilling prophecy, and the woman experiences dysmenorrhea.

Medical Treatment and Nursing Intervention

Pharmacologic and surgical approaches to the problem of dysmenorrhea have met with limited success in the past. Medications that have been prescribed include analgesics, stimulants and mood elevators, spasmolytic drugs to relax the uterine muscles and improve blood flow, and hormonal therapy to suppress ovulation and the proliferation of endometrial tissue. Diuretics have been tried in an effort to control fluid retention during both the premenstrual and menstrual periods.

All of the above approaches to the problem of dysmenorrhea have not been fully validated by research studies. Recently, prostaglandin synthetase inhibitors (PGSIs) have been used to provide relief. These agents are antiinflammatory compounds that act to inhibit the production of prostaglandins by the uterus. Examples include ibuprofen (Motrin), naproxen sodium (Anaprox), and mefenamic acid (Ponstel), available by prescription, and ibuprofen pills (Nuprin, Advil) that can be purchased over the counter.

Nursing intervention is more likely to be effective if the patient is encouraged to talk about her problem and how she has coped with it each month. Support groups and individuals who allow women to talk about their experience with dysmenorrhea provide significant relief for many women. If nothing else, taking the problem seriously as a legitimate concern of health care professionals and recognizing that the woman is not complaining because she is imagining pain or is neurotic helps her realize that she will no longer be left alone to cope with her problem. Just knowing that she is not maladjusted, lazy, dishonest, or psychologically unbalanced can have a very positive effect on the patient's symptoms and outlook.

Among the self-care measures traditionally used by women to help ease the pain and discomforts of dysmenorrhea are nonprescription analgesics such as aspirin, applications of heat to the back and abdomen, exercise, rest, and relaxation techniques. These measures do provide some measure of relief for many women. Restriction of salt and monosodium glutamate (MSG) to reduce fluid retention during the premenstrual and menstrual periods is also helpful. Women who are overweight should be encouraged to lose weight and strive to maintain normal body weight once it is reached. Diet modifications directed toward an increase in vitamin B_6, calcium, protein, and magnesium are also recommended.

Health teaching should also include information about the role of prostaglandins in dysmenorrhea and the PGSIs currently available, if the woman is not aware of them.

PREMENSTRUAL SYNDROME

Premenstrual syndrome is a group of symptoms that many women experience for several days before the onset of their menstrual periods. Symptoms include accumulation of body fluid, which causes weight gain; acnelike skin eruptions; cravings for special foods; crying spells; severe headaches; and depression.

It is now acknowledged that these symptoms are not simply a matter of emotional instability but represent a pathologic state, even though its exact nature and cause are not known. Increased interest in the phenomenon has led to the opening of several premenstrual syndrome clinics throughout the United States. Clients are given opportunities to discuss their problem and learn about others who have the same kinds of problems and how they have dealt with them. For some women it is a great comfort to know that others have experiences similar to theirs and to be assured that their physical and emotional symptoms are not just a matter of lack of will power or being overly concerned about minor ills. Most of these clinics also prescribe progesterone therapy based on the assumption that the symptoms of premenstrual syndrome are the result of a hormonal imbalance between estrogen and progesterone.

Regular physical exercise, relaxation exercises to decrease tension, and a diet that is lower in sugar, red meats, caffeine, salt, and alcohol also seem to lessen the symptoms of PMS.

DYSFUNCTIONAL UTERINE BLEEDING

Bleeding at times other than during the normal menstrual period is a common problem among women. It can be relatively insignificant, or it can be the first sign of a serious disorder such as a malignancy in the reproductive tract. The term *metrorrhagia* is frequently used to indicate uterine bleeding or spotting that occurs at times other than the regular menstrual flow. *Menorrhagia* refers to an excessive loss of blood during the monthly period. There can be an increased amount of menstrual bleeding, or the menses can continue beyond the usual period of time.

Etiology

Causes of irregular bleeding vary according to the age of the woman. In young teens it can simply be a sign of inadequate progesterone levels or lack of cyclic ovulation, which is not uncommon until the menstrual cycle has been firmly established. Hormonal imbalances also can cause irregular bleeding in women who are menopausal.

When a woman has an intrauterine contraceptive device in place, heavier than usual bleeding is to be expected. When oral contraceptive pills are discontinued, it is not unusual for women who have taken the drug for years to have heavier bleeding than they previously had.

Infections of the endometrium can cause excessive bleeding, because the infection interferes with the normal clotting properties of the endometrium. In addition to the heavy blood loss there is usually a foul-smelling vaginal discharge, fever, and other signs of infection.

Women in their child-bearing years can have irregular uterine bleeding associated with spontaneous abortion, ectopic pregnancy, benign fibroids, and endometriosis.

As previously mentioned, malignancy of the cervix, adenocarcinoma of the vagina, and uterine cancer are all possible causes of irregular bleeding.

Nursing Assessment

Assessment of the patient with irregular bleeding should include information about the onset, duration, and frequency of the vaginal bleeding and the intervals between episodes of bleeding. It also is helpful to have a close estimate of the amount of blood lost. This can be determined by finding out how many tampons or pads are needed each day and the kind used (that is, regular, super, or maxi). The degree of saturation also should be determined.

Other assessment data should include an obstetric history, use of contraceptives in the past and present, menstrual history, and general health history. Obesity, use of legal and illegal drugs (including alcohol), stressful life changes, and thyroid disease are examples of factors that could be relevant to the development of irregular bleeding.

Treatment

Metrorrhagia, or excessive vaginal bleeding, is treated conservatively with hormone therapy. A dilatation and curettage (D and C) is performed if the condition persists. A new laser procedure known as *endometrial ablation* can be performed on an outpatient basis and is an option for childbearing-age women who haven't responded to a D and C and do not wish to have a hysterectomy.

INFLAMMATORY DISORDERS OF THE GENITAL TRACT

PELVIC INFLAMMATORY DISEASE

Pelvic inflammatory diseases (PIDs) include any inflammation in the pelvis *outside the uterus.* If the inflammation is located in the uterine tubes, it is called *salpingitis;* if the ovaries are affected, the term used is *oophoritis;* and involvement of the pelvic peritoneum is called *pelvic peritonitis.*

The organisms causing the infection are usually introduced from the outside and then spread upward through the uterus without affecting the endometrium. Sometimes, however, in an infection following delivery, the inflammatory process may extend outward from the uterus and involve adjoining connective tissues of the pelvis. When this happens, the patient has *pelvic cellulitis.*

Any organism capable of producing an infection can cause pelvic inflammatory disease. However, the majority of cases of PID are caused by *Neisseria gonorrhoeae* or *Chlamydia trachomatis,* both of which are sexually transmitted.

Symptoms

The patient with acute pelvic inflammatory disease is very ill and appears to be in acute distress. She experiences severe abdominal and pelvic pain, elevated temperature, and nausea and vomiting and frequently has a purulent, foul-smelling vaginal discharge.

If the disease progresses to the chronic stage, there are usually disturbances of menstruation, backache, and a feeling of heaviness in the pelvis.

Medical Treatment and Nursing Intervention

Ideally, the condition should be treated in its earliest stages so that further spread of the infection and complications from scarring of the tissues may be avoided. Antibiotics are administered for control of the infection, and hygienic measures to improve the general health of the patient are also employed.

The patient is usually placed on bed rest and positioned in a semi-Fowler's position so that any abscess that may form will be low in the pelvis, where drainage is most easily established. Heat is usually applied to the lower abdomen, and hot sitz baths are ordered to facilitate drainage of the exudate from the site of the inflammation. Analgesics are given for pain. After recovery, any change in the amount, color, or odor of the vaginal discharge should be reported immediately.

Nursing interventions for selected problems in a patient with pelvic inflammatory disease are summarized in Nursing Care Plan 30–1.

The most common complication of pelvic inflammatory disease is infertility. This is a result of the narrowing or complete closure of the uterine tubes, which prevents passage of the sperm through the tube. Sometimes, even if the sperm can pass through and fertilize the egg, there is not room for the enlarged fertilized egg to pass back through the tube into the uterus, and it becomes lodged in the tube, thus leading to a *tubal* or *ectopic* pregnancy.

VAGINITIS

Inflammation of the vagina and accompanying vaginal discharge and itching are among the most common gynecologic problems. About one third of all vaginal discharges are caused by an organism called *Gardnerella vaginalis.* The organism does not invade the vaginal wall and therefore produces only vaginal discharge and odor. There is no itching, burning, or soreness associated with

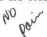

NURSING CARE PLAN 30–1

Selected nursing diagnoses, goals/outcome criteria, nursing interventions, and evaluations for a patient with pelvic inflammatory disease

Situation: Ann Gordon, age 26, is an unmarried secretary who is admitted to the hospital for treatment of severe abdominal and pelvic pain that suddenly appeared the day of admission. A pelvic examination revealed extreme tenderness in the lower abdomen, purulent vaginal discharge, and a red and swollen uterine cervix.

During her assessment the nurse found that Miss Gordon has had recurrent episodes of abdominopelvic pain that she attributed to constipation or some other digestive disorder. Her present complaints, in addition to pain, include malaise, feeling "feverish," and a troublesome vaginal discharge that she has tried to treat at home with daily vaginal douches. She has never had any tests for gonorrhea, syphilis, or any other sexually transmitted disease.

Nursing Diagnosis	Goals/Outcome Criteria	Nursing Intervention	Evaluation
Pain related to pelvic inflammation SUPPORTING DATA Severe abdominal and pelvic pain, tenderness in lower abdomen, purulent vaginal discharge, red and swollen cervix; recurrent episodes of abdominopelvic pain.	Pain is controlled by analgesia as verbalized by patient. Pain is resolved within 3 weeks.	Assess location, type, and degree of pain at least once each shift. Administer analgesics as ordered; monitor for side effects and effectiveness. Provide quiet environment; promote rest. Apply heating pad to lower abdomen as needed. Assist with hot sitz baths tid as ordered.	Using heating pad on lower abdomen; analgesics given q 4 h with relief for 3½ hours; hot sitz bath at 9 and 1 P.M.; states pain is improving; continue plan.
Anxiety related diagnostic tests and possibility of sexually transmitted disease. SUPPORTING DATA Is sexually active; persistent vaginal discharge, abdominopelvic pain.	Patient will verbalize understanding of diagnostic tests and their necessity to determine presence of STDs. Patient will verbalize fears concerning STDs.	Explain purpose, procedure, and tests for possible causative organisms. Assist with pelvic exam to obtain secretion samples for testing. Explain necessity of blood test for syphilis and advantages of prompt discovery of the disease. Use a matter-of-fact approach when discussing STDs. Spend time with her and encourage verbalization of questions and concerns.	Diagnostic tests and purposes explained; beginning to ask questions about her illness and ramifications for future health; continue plan.
Potential for infection and spread of disease related to vaginal discharge. SUPPORTING DATA Persistent vaginal discharge, abdominopelvic pain, sexually active.	No evidence of spread of disease outside of pelvic reproductive organs. No signs and symptoms of pelvic inflammation and infection will remain at 21 days.	Administer antibiotics as prescribed; stress importance of correctly taking entire prescription. Explain importance of follow-up exam after treatment. Monitor for signs of peritonitis: rigid abdomen, absent bowel sounds, increased pain, nausea and vomiting. Assist with perineal care, using universal precautions, after each voiding (at least qid). Monitor vital signs q 4 h. Encourage good hand washing. Handle contaminated linens or pads using universal precautions.	Taking antibiotics correctly; no signs of peritonitis: abdomen soft; temp., 99.2°F; universal precautions used; performing perineal self-care correctly; demonstrating good hand washing; continue plan.
Knowledge deficit related to signs and symptoms of STDs, how to prevent infection and transmission of STDs, and necessity of treatment. SUPPORTING DATA Thought she couldn't get	Patient will correctly verbalize signs and symptoms of STDs. Patient will verbalize usual treatment for STDs. Patient will verbalize ways in which STDs are transmitted.	Explain signs and symptoms of gonorrhea, syphilis, chlamydia, and condyloma. Explain ways in which each disease is transmitted. Instruct her in ways to pre-	First teaching session on STDs finished; reinforced use of condoms with any partner and wisdom of restricting number of partners; verbalizes signs and symptoms of herpes and gonorrhea; continue plan.

Nursing care plan continued on following page

NURSING CARE PLAN 30–1, *Continued*

Nursing Diagnosis	Goals/Outcome Criteria	Nursing Intervention	Evaluation
STDs because she takes "the pill." Unaware of signs and symptoms of STDs other than herpes.		vent the transmission of each STD. Reinforce importance of immediately seeking medical attention if signs and symptoms of STDs occur. Explain need for treatment for her sexual partner(s).	

this kind of vaginitis, and it can produce no symptoms at all.

The other organisms responsible for vaginitis and accompanying symptoms are *Trichomonas vaginalis* and *Candida*, formerly called *Monilia*, or yeast infection.

The characteristics of these three major types of vaginitis are shown in Table 30–2.

Health Teaching

Many kinds of vaginal infections can be prevented by some rather simple hygienic measures. Some do's and don'ts that can be taught to the person uninformed about personal feminine hygiene are listed below:

- Bathe or shower daily, using mild soap and

TABLE 30–2 TYPES OF VAGINITIS

	Gardnerella vaginalis	*Trichomonas*	*Candida*
Onset	May note odor only after sexual intercourse	May appear or worsen immediately after menstruation	Abrupt; before menstruation
Odor	Fishy odor; particularly after sexual intercourse	Foul discharge with acute infection	Absent
Itching	Absent, since does not invade vaginal wall	Occasionally present, but varies according to degree of inflammation	Severe; the most prominent symptom
Discharge	Thin, gray, homogeneous; frothy in 7%	Amount varies, often gray; green in 20%, frothy in 33%	Unusual, except in pregnancy
pH of discharge	5.0–5.5	7.45	4.5
Associated factors	None	Often acute during pregnancy	Often associated with pregnancy, glycosuria, diabetes, antibiotic use
Sexual transmission	Yes	Yes	Possible
Vulvar signs	Absent	Usually absent; erythema or edema can be present if discharge is profuse	Excoriation from scratching; erythema; possible edema of labia
Vaginal signs	Little or no erythema; discharge adherent to vaginal wall; cervix normal	Diffuse erythema; vaginal/cervical petechiae or "strawberry" appearance on 10%; cervix may bleed easily, otherwise normal	Discharge adherent to vaginal wall; "cottage cheese" appearance or "curds" present only in heavy colonization; cervix normal
Treatment and nursing intervention	Oral metronidazole (Flagyl) 500 mg bid × 7 days. Sexual partner should be treated concurrently only if problem is recurrent.	Oral Flagyl (2 gm as a single dose) except during pregnancy. Betadine douche (2 tbsp/liter of water) twice daily for 1 week. Treat sexual contacts concurrently.	Miconazole (Monistat) or clotrimazole (Gyne-Lotrimin) cream or suppositories each night for 1 week.

Adapted from Andreoli, T. E., et al.: Cecil Essentials of Medicine, 2nd ed. Philadelphia, W. B. Saunders, 1990.

water. Separate the folds around the vagina and clean gently but thoroughly. Rinse the area well and dry completely. If the problem is chronic, taking showers rather than tub baths seems to lessen the incidence.

- Avoid strong deodorant soaps and vaginal deodorants. They not only can mask the symptoms of an infection but can themselves be irritating and harmful to the vaginal mucosa and external genitalia.
- Always wipe from front to back after a bowel movement or urination. Bacteria from the bowel can be spread to the urinary and reproductive tracts by improper wiping.
- Try to keep the vulva dry and well ventilated. Cotton underwear traps less moisture than synthetic materials. Tight-fitting panty hose and pants or jeans can be irritating to the external genitalia.
- Replace tampons or pads every 2 to 3 hours; use pads rather than tampons overnight. Wash your hands thoroughly before and after inserting a tampon. Failure to replace tampons frequently can trap blood in the vagina and encourage the growth of bacteria, which sometimes causes toxic shock syndrome.
- Routine douching is not recommended. If douching is done too frequently, it can actually increase vaginal discharge.
- It is normal to have a small increase in vaginal secretions during ovulation. This is related to hormonal changes and an increase in estrogen levels.

DISORDERS OF THE CERVIX, UTERUS, AND ENDOMETRIUM

TUMORS OF THE CERVIX

Cervical polyps are the most common benign growth on the cervix. They occur most frequently in multiparous women 40 to 60 years of age.

Malignant tumors of the cervix are the sixth most common cancer in women. There is an increased incidence of cervical cancer in women who have had multiple sexual partners, those who were sexually active in their teens, and those who have given birth more than once. Some forms of the human papilloma virus that cause genital warts also can predispose a patient to cervical cancer.

Symptoms and Medical Diagnosis

Slight bleeding between menstrual periods, after coitus, and after vaginal examination is the only symptom of cervical polyp. This closely parallels the symptoms of early cervical cancer. Diagnosis is made by direct examination of the cervix during a pelvic examination, at which time the polyp is removed and sent for tissue examination.

Early cervical malignancy is usually asymptomatic, but vaginal discharge and slight vaginal bleeding or spotting can occur. Diagnosis is by Pap smear. Further evaluation by colposcopy, endocervical curettage, and biopsy and x-ray studies of abdominal organs is done before choice of treatment is made.

Surgical Treatment

Carcinoma in situ of the cervix in women who wish to bear further children is treated by conization, in which a wedge-shaped section of the cervix is removed. Hysterectomy or radioactive implant is the treatment for patients who do not wish to have further children.

If the malignancy is invasive, intracavity radiation or radical hysterectomy may be performed. Radical hysterectomy includes removal of the uterus, adjoining vaginal area, and regional lymph nodes. If metastasis has already occurred, irradiation may be used alone. Chemotherapy has had poor success in patients with cervical cancer.

TUMORS OF THE UTERUS

Tumors within the uterus are very common in women between the ages of 25 and 40. Most often, they are benign *uterine myomas* or fibroids, which frequently are asymptomatic.

Endometrial cancer, or tumor of the uterus, is the most common reproductive cancer. It is a slow-growing tumor and usually occurs after menopause. It is asymptomatic in the early stages.

Symptoms and Medical Diagnosis

Bleeding is the most common symptom of all uterine tumors in their early stages. Uterine fibroids sometimes cause very heavy menstrual periods. The hallmark sign of endometrial cancer is postmenopausal bleeding. A watery, serosanguinous vaginal discharge may also occur. Later, as the tumor becomes larger, it causes symptoms of pressure within the abdominopelvic cavity. Diagnosis is made on the basis of clinical manifestations, history, and physical examination.

Surgical Treatment

The treatment of a nonmalignant tumor of the uterus is entirely different from that of a malignant tumor. It is well known that a malignant disease requires immediate surgical removal of the affected part and possibly additional radiation therapy to destroy any remaining malignant cells. A benign uterine tumor, however, may subside spontaneously, especially at the time of menopause, because it is at this time that ovarian hormones that stimulate the growth of these tumors are no longer secreted.

If uterine myoma is asymptomatic, treatment may consist of follow-up examination every 3 to 6 months.

For fibroids that are causing considerable bleeding in childbearing-age women, a myomectomy may be done. This procedure removes the tumors, but not the uterus. In older women who are experiencing excessive bleeding, a hysterectomy may be performed. A new option is laser ablation of the tumor.

The treatment for endometrial cancer varies depending on the stage of the cancer. Often a combination of radiation therapy plus hysterectomy is recommended. A radioactive implant is placed in the uterus 6 weeks prior to surgery. The patient is placed in an isolation room before the procedure, and the implant is left in place for 1 to 3 days. Total bed rest and minimal movement are required during the treatment period. Radiation precautions are used; these can be found in Chapter 13.

A total abdominal hysterectomy and bilateral salpingo-oophorectomy is performed for stage I cancer. Stage II cancer is treated by radical hysterectomy (discussed earlier). External radiation, chemotherapy, and hormonal therapy may also be used for treatment following surgery.

Risk factors for the development of cervical and uterine cancers are shown in Table 30–3.

ENDOMETRIOSIS

Endometriosis is a rather common disorder in which endometrial tissue (that of the inner lining of the uterus) is found outside the uterus, especially in the ovaries, rectovaginal septum, and other areas of the pelvis and abdomen. The misplaced tissue usually undergoes changes during the menstrual cycle in the same way normal endometrium does, and it may bleed at the time of menstruation.

The cause of endometriosis is not known. There is a familial susceptibility, and in some cases uterine surgery may have allowed the escape of endometrial cells and their relocation outside the uterus. While this might explain why endometriosis occurs in some instances, it does not provide an etiologic agent for every case. One theory holds that abnormal implantation is due to a combination of at least two factors: (1) an excessive production of endometrial tissue, which is probably related to estrogen secretion, and (2) a reflux or backflow of menstrual blood and tissue through the uterine tubes at the time of menstruation. The first factor is probably valid, because many women with endometriosis do not ovulate. Hence estrogen secretion continues through the entire monthly cycle rather than decreasing when progesterone secretion should predominate. This causes an overabundance of endometrial tissue inside the uterus as well as in abnormal locations elsewhere in the abdominopelvic region.

Symptoms

Because the aberrant endometrial tissue can cause bleeding into spaces that have no outlet and are likely to be irritated by the blood, the patient experiences pain and often has adhesions in the area of bleeding. Other symptoms may include excessive menstrual flow, bleeding between menstrual periods, and pain on defecation or during sexual intercourse. Some patients have dysmenorrhea that is so severe it is almost incapacitating. Ibuprofen is used for pain relief.

Medical and Surgical Treatment

A relatively conservative treatment of endometriosis involves administration of birth control pills. The objective is to produce extreme sloughing of the misplaced endometrial tissue and thus remove it from the sites of implant. An androgen, danazol (Danocrine), also might be prescribed in the hope it will help shrink the implanted tissue.

Surgical procedures usually are more effective, but they also involve major surgery in which a laparotomy is done and the endometrial implants are excised or fulgurated. The most efficient method of eliminating the symptoms of endometriosis is hysterectomy with removal of both ovaries because they are necessary for continued growth of endometrial tissue. This is not always a viable alternative, however, because endometriosis is a disease of young women in their childbearing years. The latest treatment is the use of laparoscopy with carbon dioxide laser to vaporize adhesions and implant areas. For some women, birth control pills may be the treatment of choice. Of course, if the woman wants to have children and is unable to do so because of endometriosis, she will need to understand that the pills will help get rid of unwanted endometrial implants and increase her chances of becoming pregnant once she stops taking them.

OVARIAN TUMORS

Benign and malignant tumors of the ovary can arise from misplaced endometrial tissue (endometriosis), or they can develop from tissues of the ovary itself. Some tumors are cystic (that is, saclike structures), whereas others are solid. *Dermoid cysts* are neoplasms of the ovary that are believed to be the result of spontaneous growth

TABLE 30–3 RISK FACTORS IN CERVICAL, ENDOMETRIAL, AND OVARIAN CANCERS

Cervical Cancer	Endometrial Cancer	Ovarian Cancer
Multiparity	Nulliparity	Nulliparity
Early and frequent coitus with multiple partners	Infertility	Low parity
Poor medical attention post partum	Annovulatory cycles associated with ovarian pathology	Infertility
History of venereal disease	Hyperplasia	Delayed childbearing
Inadequate personal hygiene	Abnormal uterine bleeding	Older primipara
Low socioeconomic status	Late menopause	Breast cancer
	Prolonged, sustained use of estrogen (especially postmenopausal estrogen replacement therapy)	Familial history of ovarian cancer
	Familial history of endometrial cancer	History of endometrial cancer
	Obesity	
	Diabetes	
	Hypertension	

From Edlund, B. J.: The needs of women with gynecologic malignancies. Nurs. Clin. North Am., March, 1982, p. 167.

of an unfertilized ovum. Seventy percent of ovarian tumors are benign.

Benign ovarian tumors can become very large, weighing as much as 15 pounds, and thus interfere with normal motion of adjacent organs. Malignant ovarian tumors present different and far more serious problems.

Symptoms

Ovarian tumors, either benign or malignant, do not as a rule present specific symptoms until they are fairly well advanced. Ovarian cancer presents very vague symptoms that can be mistaken for indigestion or some other gastrointestinal disorder. The patient may report chronic discomfort in the lower abdomen, enlarging abdominal girth, indigestion, abdominal distention with gas, and constipation. Some symptoms such as low back pain, dysuria, and pressure within the pelvis can be mistaken for urinary disease.

Unfortunately, by the time the above symptoms are noted there usually has been widespread dissemination of malignant cells throughout the peritoneal cavity. Less than one third of ovarian cancers are diagnosed while the tumor is still localized and can be treated by surgical removal.

Risk factors in the development of ovarian cancer are shown in Table 30–3.

Surgical Treatment

If the tumor is benign and involves only one ovary and the patient is relatively young, the surgeon may treat it conservatively by removing the affected ovary and a section of the uterine tube, leaving the other tube and ovary intact. Patients with malignant tumors receive more radical treatment. A *panhysterectomy* is usually performed, in which both ovaries, both uterine tubes, and the uterus are removed. Some patients have responded well to radiation and intraperitoneal chemotherapy.

UTERINE PROLAPSE, CYSTOCELE, AND RECTOCELE

The lower abdominal reproductive organs are supported by the pelvic muscles. These muscles often atrophy with age or weaken with childbearing and no longer provide adequate support. The uterus may then protrude into the vagina (uterine prolapse). Often this is accompanied by cystocele, (protrusion of the bladder into the vagina) and by rectocele (bulging of the rectum into the vagina). The symptoms of these problems are backache, urinary incontinence or retention, and constipation. Stress incontinence of urine is common.

Correction of uterine prolapse is by hysterectomy. Cystocele and rectocele are treated by tightening the pelvic muscles. The procedure is known as an *anteroposterior repair* (AP repair) or *anteroposterior colporrhaphy*.

If the patient is elderly and has health problems that prevent surgery, a pessary, which is a hard rubber ring, can be inserted to help keep the abdominal organs in place.

CARE OF THE PATIENT HAVING GYNECOLOGIC SURGERY

Gynecologic surgery may be classified into three major types: (1) sterilization procedures, (2) reparative and reconstructive procedures, and (3) removal of the internal female organs of reproduction—the uterus, the uterine tubes, and the ovaries.

STERILIZATION PROCEDURES

Sterilization in women, which is done for the purpose of preventing conception permanently, usually involves the tying, cutting, occlusion, or removal of a portion of the uterine (fallopian) tubes. These procedures should *not* be considered reversible. However, pregnancy has occurred in some cases after this surgery, particularly when clips are used to close off the uterine tubes. Tubal ligation can be accomplished with a variety of abdominal and vaginal procedures. It can be done after abortion, with casarean delivery, after vaginal delivery, or at any time a woman desires the surgery.

Three techniques for sterilization in women are the vaginal approach, the abdominal approach, and the newer endoscopic methods. The method used most frequently during the postpartum period (after childbirth) is the *Pomeroy procedure.* As shown in Figure 30–3, this involves removal of a portion of both uterine tubes. The procedure requires a small abdominal incision and can be performed in less than 30 minutes.

A vaginal tubal ligation requires an incision in the vaginal wall with entry into the cul-de-sac at the back of the vaginal vault. However, in order to perform this procedure, the surgeon must undergo special gynecologic training. Vaginal tubal ligation also presents problems of postoperative infection, because surgical asepsis of the vagina is difficult to achieve. Infections also occur because many patients fail to abstain from sexual intercourse until the surgical wound is completely healed.

Endoscopic methods include laparoscopy, culdoscopy, and hysteroscopy. During *laparoscopy* (Fig. 30–4), the fiber-optic instrument is inserted through a small incision in the abdominal wall. Before the procedure is begun, the peritoneal cavity is inflated with carbon dioxide. The patient is placed in the Trendelenburg position so that the bowel falls away from the pelvis, allowing for visualization of the uterine tubes and surrounding structures. A second incision is made for insertion of a cauterizing instrument, which is used to section and electrocoagulate each tube. The procedure can be done on an outpatient basis with regional or general anesthesia.

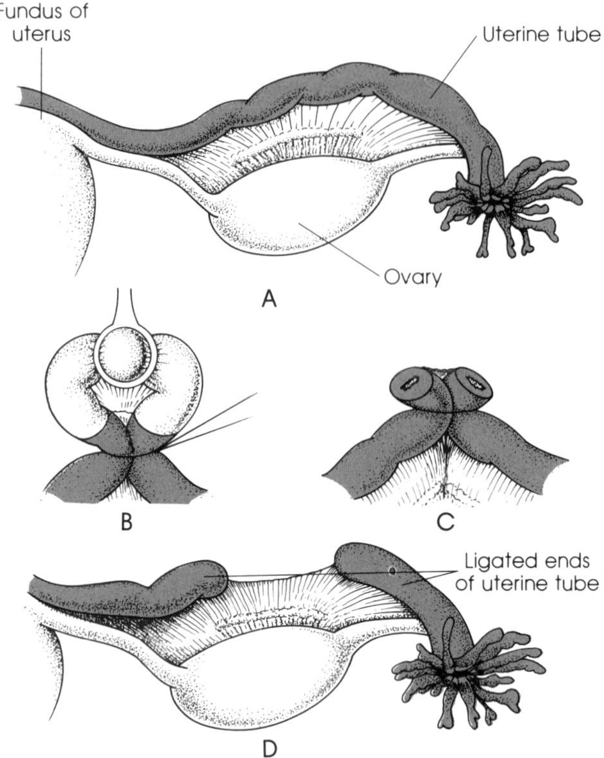

Figure 30–3 Pomeroy procedure for sterilization. *A*, Intact uterine tube and adjacent ovary. *B*, Portion of uterine tube has been pulled through a ring to form a tight loop. Tube is severed. *C*, Severed tube and destruction of its continuity so that ova can no longer pass through to the uterus. *D*, Severed uterine tube.

Sometimes the tubes are closed off with plugs rather than by cauterization. The advantage to using clips or plugs is that the tubes may be reopened at a later time if the patient decides that she wishes to become pregnant. This does not always work, however, and there is also the possibility that the clips or plugs may not completely occlude the tubes, making conception possible at any time.

The *culdoscopic* procedure involves a transvaginal approach and thus eliminates the need for an abdominal incision. The patient is placed in knee-chest position and air is injected into the abdominal cavity, forcing the bowels upward, away from the pelvic organs. The culdoscope is inserted through the cul-de-sac and the tubes are drawn down into the vagina (Fig. 30–5). After the tubes are either cauterized or occluded by clamps, they are returned to their normal position.

A serious drawback of the culdoscopic approach is the incidence of postoperative infection. However, culdoscopy is advantageous because it can be done as an outpatient procedure or with minimal hospitalization.

Discharge instructions for tubal ligation include instructing the patient (1) to keep the dressing dry (for an abdominal procedure) and not to shower for 24 hours, (2) to watch for

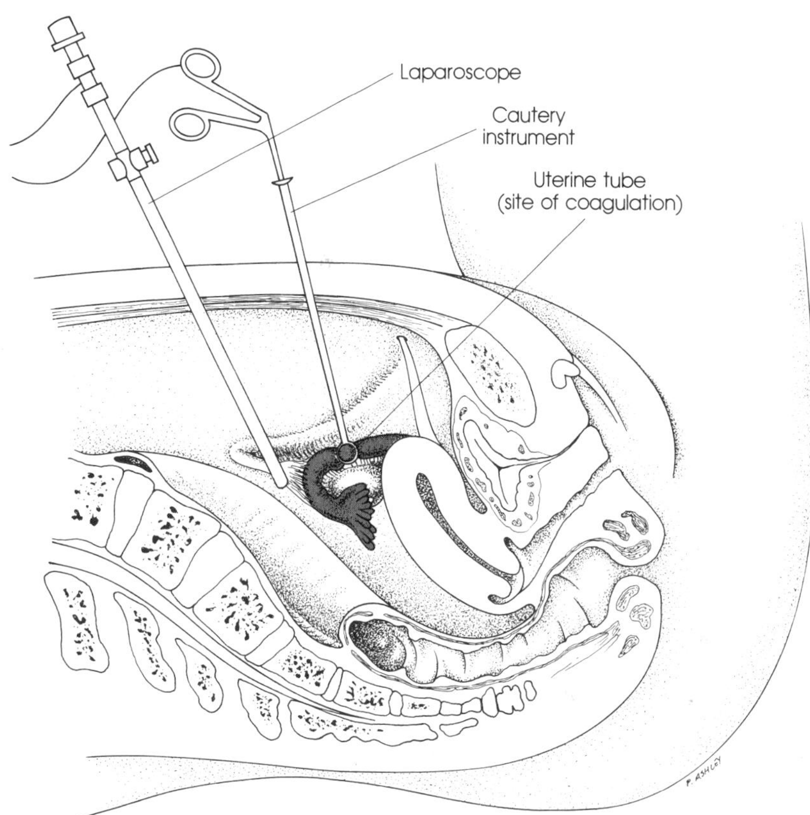

Figure 30-4 Laparoscopic procedure. The laparoscope (visualizing instrument) has been inserted through one small incision in the lower abdomen after inflation of the peritoneal cavity. The cautery instrument has been inserted through a second small incision and is used to cauterize and thus destroy the continuity of the uterine tube.

increased temperature and inflammation at the surgical site that might indicate infection, (3) to take aspirin or acetaminophen for discomfort, and (4) to report any severe abdominal pain to the physician.

VAGINAL AND ABDOMINAL GYNECOLOGIC SURGERY

Terms commonly used to describe various kinds of gynecologic surgery are shown in Table 30-4. Other procedures involve surgical repair

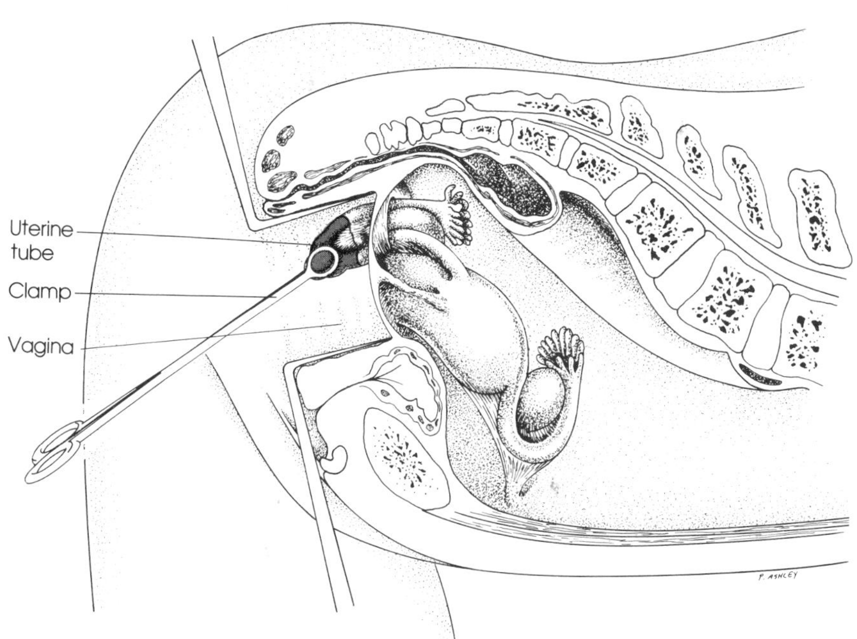

Figure 30-5 Culdoscopic procedure. The culdoscope is introduced vaginally. The tubes are drawn into the vagina with a clamp, cut and tied, and then returned to their normal position.

TABLE 30–4 TYPES OF GYNECOLOGIC SURGERY

Surgical Procedure	Explanation
Dilatation and curettage	Widening the cervix and scraping away the inner lining of the uterus (endometrium).
Conization, or conical excision	Removal of a cone of inflamed tissues of the cervix. Conization is done with an electric cutting wire. Conical excision is done with a surgical knife.
Hysterectomy	Removal of the entire uterus, vaginally or abdominally
Panhysterectomy	Removal of the entire uterus, tubes, and ovaries.
Radical hysterectomy	Removal of uterus, tubes, ovaries, upper third of vagina, and lymph nodes.
Anterior and posterior colporrhaphy	Repair of the anterior and posterior wall of the vagina.
Salpingectomy	Removal of a uterine tube.
Oophorectomy	Removal of an ovary.

and reconstruction of the vagina and adjacent structures.

Fistulas are a common indication for vaginal repair (*colporrhaphy*). A fistula is an abnormal tubelike passage between tissues and organs. Damage to the vagina, rectum, and urethra occurs less frequently during childbirth when women receive adequate prenatal care and skilled assistance during delivery. Pressure against and tearing of the structures in the pelvic floor can produce rectovaginal fistula (between the rectum and vagina), urethrovaginal fistula (between the urethra and vagina), and vesicovaginal fistula (between the bladder and vagina). These fistulas can cause leakage of either feces or urine into the vaginal tract.

Sometimes these fistulas heal spontaneously, but more often they require surgical excision and repair. After surgical repair, measures must be taken to avoid stress on the area and to prevent infection. An indwelling catheter may be inserted to keep the bladder empty and prevent passage of urine through the urethra. Perineal care, irrigations, and scrupulous care of the surgical site are essential measures to prevent infection.

Other vaginal procedures include repair of cystocele and rectocele, correction of prolapsed uterus, and vulvectomy. These procedures should not be confused with a vaginal hysterectomy, which is removal of the uterus by way of the vagina.

Vulvectomy

A radical vulvectomy involves surgical excision of the labia, clitoris, and perineal structures and removal of the lymphatic tissues in the femoral and inguinal areas to control malignancy. Two surgical sites are involved, one in the perineal area and one in the groin.

In most cases, the surgery is necessitated by malignancy of the tissues. As with surgery involving vaginal repair, two major areas of concern are prevention of stress on the operative site and prevention of infection of the wounds.

Preoperative and postoperative care of a patient having a vulvectomy require specialized training, because the patient will have many unique physiologic and psychosocial needs.

Hysterectomy

About 700,000 hysterectomies are performed each year in the United States, more than in any other country in the world. Surgical removal of the uterus ranks second only to tonsillectomies in the list of surgical procedures done. Since the feminist movement and other social changes that have occurred in the past few decades, there has been much controversy over whether many hysterectomies are actually necessary.

The basic factors that should enter into a decision for or against hysterectomy are (1) whether the hysterectomy is clinically justified, (2) whether childbearing is desired by the patient, and (3) the complex psychosocial factors related to the woman's self-image and the value she places on her uterus. The gynecologist and the patient (and her spouse, if she is married) should be involved in the decision-making process. This assumes that communication between the various parties has taken place and that the patient is well-informed about the surgical procedure and its expected consequences.

Clinical indications for hysterectomy include the following: (1) pelvic relaxation with prolapse of pelvic organs; (2) pain associated with pelvic congestion, pelvic inflammatory disease, endometriosis, recurrent ovarian cysts, or possible fibroids; (3) excessive and debilitating uterine bleeding; and (4) cervical and uterine malignancies, premalignancy, and other high-risk conditions.

The mental health of a woman following hysterectomy is profoundly affected by many personal and social factors. Her ability to adjust to the loss of a reproductive organ will be influenced by her sense of self as a woman and her age at the time of the hysterectomy. If she has had a history of uterine pain and excessive bleeding, she may look forward to a more healthy and active life. Her attitude will also be influenced by her perception of the attitudes and expectations of her spouse and significant others and her beliefs about how the surgery will affect her own sexual expression and function and her vocational or avocational involvement and enjoyment of life. A woman who experiences negative attitudes toward the hysterectomy—either within herself or in those significant to her—is likely to have serious psychological upheavals anywhere from 3 months to 3 years after hysterectomy. However, hysterectomy should not precipitate psychological disorders in a woman who is psychologically mature and healthy.

Preoperative Nursing Care

The physical aspects of preoperative preparation for gynecologic surgery and hysterectomy are fairly routine. However, it is usually not the physical aspects of preoperative care that are neglected but rather the psychological preparation of the patient and her significant others. Time must be set aside to talk with the patient, allowing her to express her fears and concerns and answering her questions in a factual and straightforward manner.

Although each patient will react to hysterectomy in an individual way, the uterus can be symbolic of femininity. For some patients, loss of the uterus can mean becoming less female, less attractive, and essentially useless to the male partner, family, and society in general.

Recent research has shown that hysterectomy does have some impact on a woman's sexual response and causes alteration in the quality and frequency of orgasm. Women who have been culturally influenced to accept a highly "feminine" role and who view the uterus as a symbol of femininity are at a greater risk for sexual dysfunction after hysterectomy.

Traditionally, the feminine role encompasses maternal behaviors, duties as homemaker, and an attitude of submission to the spouse or male partner. If a woman is accustomed to working outside the home or has vocational and avocational interests and is comfortable with having both "feminine" and "masculine" traits, she is far less likely to be psychologically impaired by hysterectomy.

The nurse should be prepared to participate in preoperative assessment of the hysterectomy patient in order to determine a lack of specific knowledge about the impending surgery and the reasons why it is indicated. It also is important for effective postoperative care to gather information about the patient's self-concept, social and cultural attitudes toward the role of women in society, and personal fears and anxieties about the loss of her uterus.

Postoperative Nursing Care

During the immediate postoperative period, the patient who has had an abdominal hysterectomy requires essentially the same care as any patient having abdominal surgery. The patient's intake and output are measured and recorded, and she is helped to turn, cough, and deep breathe every 2 hours after recovery from anesthesia.

In order to decrease pelvic congestion, the patient should *not* be placed in the high Fowler's position. There should be no pressure under the knees because of the danger of slowing down venous circulation and of formation of a clot (thrombus). Antiembolic stockings are applied as ordered, and early ambulation is encouraged. Dressings are checked periodically for drainage or hemorrhage. Vaginal bleeding is also monitored.

Nursing care for the patient undergoing an abdominal hysterectomy is summarized in Nursing Care Plan 30–2.

Prior to discharge from the hospital, the patient is given instruction, preferably in writing for reference at home, regarding self-care. Discharge planning should include information on undergoing estrogen and progestin therapy (if this is expected), restricting douching and sexual intercourse, avoiding constipation, caring for the incision, and experiencing and reporting such signs of infection as redness, pain, swelling and drainage, and body temperature over 100°F. Abdominal cramps and changes in bowel habits also should be reported. If the patient is not on hormone therapy, she should be told to report any signs of abrupt climacteric changes unless, of course, she has already been through menopause.

In addition, ample time for discussion of the more personal concerns of the patient regarding sexual activity and new body image is important. Although these topics should have been introduced during the preoperative period, the patient may be in a better frame of mind and more receptive to discussion as she prepares to return home. An excellent resource for instruction of the patient is the pamphlet "After Hysterectomy What?" It can be given to the patient before surgery and used as a basis for continued instruction during hospitalization and prior to discharge. The booklet is available from Semed

NURSING CARE PLAN 30–2

Selected nursing diagnoses, goals/outcome criteria, nursing interventions, and evaluations for a patient who has had an abdominal hysterectomy

Situation: Marilyn Blair, age 52, has just returned to the unit after abdominal hysterectomy for multiple fibroids, metrorrhagia, and greatly increased uterine size that caused abdominal pain. She has an IV of 1,000 mL normal saline in the left forearm, an indwelling urinary catheter, an abdominal dressing, and a patient analgesic control (PAC) device containing morphine. Her vital signs are BP, 138/82; pulse, 86; respirations, 16; temperature, 98.2°F.

Nursing Diagnosis	Goals/Outcome Criteria	Nursing Intervention	Evaluation
Pain related to surgical incision. **SUPPORTING DATA** Abdominal hysterectomy; moaning and grimacing.	Pain will be controlled by analgesia. Pain will be controlled by oral analgesia at time of discharge.	Instruct her in use of PCA pump. Give booster medication as ordered if needed. Assess location, type, and quality of pain q 3 to 4 h. Assist with repositioning and support with pillows to attain comfort. Provide quiet, darkened atmosphere for sleep and rest. Monitor for side effects of morphine, especially respiratory rate; administer antiemetic as ordered at first signs of nausea to prevent vomiting and further pain. Check catheter and tubing for patency frequently to prevent bladder distention and further pain.	Using PCA pump; sleeping at long intervals; resp., 14; bladder not distended; Foley draining; continue plan.
Potential fluid volume deficit related to possible hemorrhage from surgery. **SUPPORTING DATA** Abdominal hysterectomy.	Vital signs will remain stable; no signs of shock. No hemorrhage as evidenced by lack of signs of excessive bleeding.	Monitor vital signs frequently per postoperative routine. Check abdominal dressing and beneath patient for signs of bleeding with each set of vital signs; assess for bleeding from vaginal cuff. Assess for signs of intra-abdominal bleeding; increasing abdominal girth, decreasing bowel sounds, increasing abdominal pain and rigidity.	Abdominal dressing clean and dry; no visible vaginal drainage; VS: BP, 118/68; P, 84; R, 16; abdomen soft; no bowel sounds, continue plan.
Potential ineffective breathing pattern related to pain, anesthesia, and analgesia. **SUPPORTING DATA** Shallow respirations; groggy; sleeping for long periods; states "It hurts too much to cough."	Patient will perform deep breathing and coughing exercises. No signs of atelectasis or pneumonia as evidenced by clear breath sounds in all areas and normal temperature.	Assist patient to sit up to deep breathe and cough q 2 h; give small pillow to splint incision before coughing. Encourage her to take four deep breaths each time a commercial comes on the television while it is on. Enlist aid of family or significant others in reminding patient to deep breathe. Auscultate lung sounds q shift, report diminished or absent breath sounds or crackles. Ambulate as soon as ordered.	Deep breathing and coughing at 8, 10, 12, and 2 sitting on side of bed; lung sounds clear bilaterally; temp., 98.8°F; continue plan.
Potential for infection related to surgery. **SUPPORTING DATA** Abdominal hysterectomy.	Patient will be without signs of infection at discharge.	Administer prophylactic antibiotics as ordered. Monitor incision for signs of redness, swelling, purulent drainage, hardness.	Taking antibiotics; dressing clean and dry; vaginal drainage without change in character; abdomen soft; no signs of infection; continue plan.

NURSING CARE PLAN 30–2, *Continued*

Nursing Diagnosis	Goals/Outcome Criteria	Nursing Intervention	Evaluation
		Keep dressing clean and dry. Use careful aseptic technique when changing dressings. Monitor WBC count and temperature. Assess vaginal drainage for signs of odor or change in character. Assess abdomen for signs of abscess or peritonitis: increasing pain, localized tenderness, swelling, decreased bowel sounds.	
Potential for injury related to possibility of thrombophlebitis from bed rest and abdominopelvic surgery. SUPPORTING DATA Abdominal hysterectomy; reluctant to ambulate.	Patient will not exhibit signs of thrombophlebitis.	Encourage ambulation as soon as it is ordered; explain benefits. Encourage added fluid intake as soon as diet order allows. Assist with leg and ankle exercises q 2 h; encourage her to do them during commercials while watching television. Inspect lower legs q shift; check for positive Homans' sign beginning third postoperative day.	Leg and ankle exercises at 8, 10, 12, and 2; will ambulate this P.M.; continue plan.
Body image disturbance related to removal of uterus. SUPPORTING DATA States "I wonder if my sex life will be different now; it seems strange to be missing a part."	Patient will express her concerns over loss of uterus. Patient will accept new body image within 3 months as evidenced by lack of depression and reinvestment in usual activities.	Provide openings for conversation regarding patient concerns over loss of uterus and its meaning to her. Explore her feelings regarding sexuality after hysterectomy. Encourage expression of positive aspects of having the hysterectomy and how she as a person is unchanged.	Patient still groggy; begin discussion of concerns tomorrow; continue plan.

Pharmaceuticals, S. E. Massengill Co., Bristol, Tennessee.

DISORDERS OF THE BREAST

The breast plays a significant and unique role in the life of a female in every stage of her adult life. Pathologic changes in the breast can produce stress and anxiety in both the patient and her significant others. Although the breast is not a reproductive organ, it is affected by hormonal changes related to the menstrual cycle and pregnancy and is part of a woman's total concept of herself as a female.

FIBROCYSTIC BREAST DISEASE

Fibrocystic breast disease (FBD), also called *chronic cystic mastitis,* is the most common disorder of the female breast, affecting more than 30% of all women. In fact, it is so prevalent in premenopausal women that some authorities question whether it is a disease. It tends to run in families and usually disappears after menopause.

True fibrocystic breast disease is characterized by single or multiple benign tumors in the breast. The tumors can be fluid-filled sacs or cysts that arise from glandular elements or solid fibrous growths containing connective tissue elements (fibroadenomas).

FBD occurs most often in the reproductive

years, beginning in the late teens and early 20s. The symptoms seem to subside after menopause. It is thought that FBD is linked to normal increases and decreases of estrogen and progesterone.

The most outstanding symptom of FBD is, of course, the presence of one or more lumps in the breast. There also is a feeling of fullness and tenderness of the breast, which is more noticeable during the premenstrual period. The presence of cysts and lumps in the breast make self-examination difficult and produces anxiety for many patients. Additionally, the frequent examinations necessary to determine whether malignant changes have occurred add to physical discomfort and psychological stress. However, repeated examinations, radiographs, and biopsies are essential.

Medical Treatment and Nursing Intervention

Medical treatment of FBD usually consists of either vitamin or hormonal therapy. Vitamin B complex seems to be helpful, and trial studies using 600 international units of vitamin E daily for 8 weeks have shown dramatic improvement in 80% to 90% of patients. A daily dose of this much vitamin E should be taken only under the supervision of a physician or nurse clinician.

Administration of a synthetic androgen (danazol [Danocrine]) also produces a significant decrease in the symptoms of women with severe FBD. However, side effects such as menstrual irregularities, weight gain, edema, and acne do occur. Hormonal therapy is usually reserved for women who cannot find relief through more conservative, noninvasive means.

Among the self-help measures that have been successful for many women with FBD are reduction of stressors in their lives and restriction of all forms of methylxanthines (particularly caffeine), which are found in coffee, tea, and chocolate. Drugs that contain caffeine include many over-the-counter remedies for the common cold, headache, and indigestion.

Patients interested in trying the dietary approach to FBD will need to practice self-discipline and learn less harmful substitutes for caffeinated coffee, tea, and chocolate. Sweet and dark chocolate and baking chocolate contain from three to seven times more caffeine than milk chocolate. Carob is caffeine free and is an ideal substitute for chocolate. It also has the advantage of containing far less fat and fewer calories than chocolate.

Before purchasing over-the-counter drugs, the patient should read the label carefully and avoid those containing caffeine and theobromine. The success of the dietary approach depends on the patient's ability to totally eliminate the intake of any of these substances. It usually takes at least 2 months for the results of dietary restriction to become apparent.

Other measures that some patients have used with varying degrees of success include limiting salt and taking a mild diuretic during the week before menstruation begins, applying warm compresses to the breast, wearing a brassiere that gives good support, and taking a mild nonprescription analgesic to relieve discomfort.

Patient education should also include teaching the patient how to perform self-examination of the breast, emphasizing the importance of faithfully carrying out the examination. Once the woman becomes accustomed to the location and size of her breast lumps, she should be able to determine any change that might occur. Because the tenderness and swelling are at a minimum 5 to 7 days after menstruation, this is the ideal time for a woman with FBD to do her self-examination.

Changes that should be reported to the physician include the following: appearance of a new lump; change in the size of a preexisting lesion; change in the contour of the breast; noticeable increase in the prominence of breast veins; increase in pain; and changes in the nipple such as inversion or flattening, discharge or scales, and the direction in which the nipple usually points.

BREAST CANCER

Cancer of the breast is the most common type of malignancy in women in the United States, with 140,000 new cases diagnosed in 1989 (American Cancer Society, 1990). For reasons not fully understood, the incidence of breast cancer is increasing in this country. However, the number of women surviving the disease also is increasing. Recent studies show a 5-year survival rate of 90% for women with localized malignancy and 60% for those with regional metastasis (American Cancer Society, 1990).

Those at highest risk for cancer of the breast are women (1) who are over 40, unmarried, and childless; (2) who have not nursed an infant; (3) whose first pregnancy occurred after they were 25 years of age; (4) who had early menarche and late menopause; (5) who have a positive family history of mothers or sisters with breast cancer; and (6) who have a history of fibrocystic breast disease.

Symptoms

A lump in the breast is one of the prime symptoms of breast tumor. Although pain and tenderness are symptomatic of cystic breast disease, they usually are not associated with a malignant growth until it is in an advanced stage. Abnormal discharge from the nipple can be symptomatic of almost any breast disorder, but it should be considered significant and should receive prompt medical attention.

Dimpling of the breast tissue and overlying skin can occur when a tumor located near the surface adheres to underlying structures. Other symptoms, which may involve one or both breasts, include swelling or enlargement, a change in firmness, and the appearance of a reddened area. A definite diagnosis of malignancy is made by biopsy.

Medical and Surgical Treatment

Traditionally, the choice of treatment for breast cancer has been radical mastectomy with lymph node resection. Today, there is some controversy over the need for such drastic procedures as treatment for all forms of breast cancer. Because of the unpredictability of the disease, however, many physicians still advocate extensive surgery to avoid, insofar as possible, a recurrence of the malignancy. However, conservative surgery with radiation or chemotherapy is another option. The use of carbon dioxide laser for mastectomy has decreased blood loss and shortened healing time.

Figure 30-6 shows the lymphatic drainage of the breast. Because these lymphatic vessels filter drainage from the breast tissues, cancer cells can metastasize along the route.

The various methods of surgical treatment of breast cancer that apply to the tumor itself are as follows:

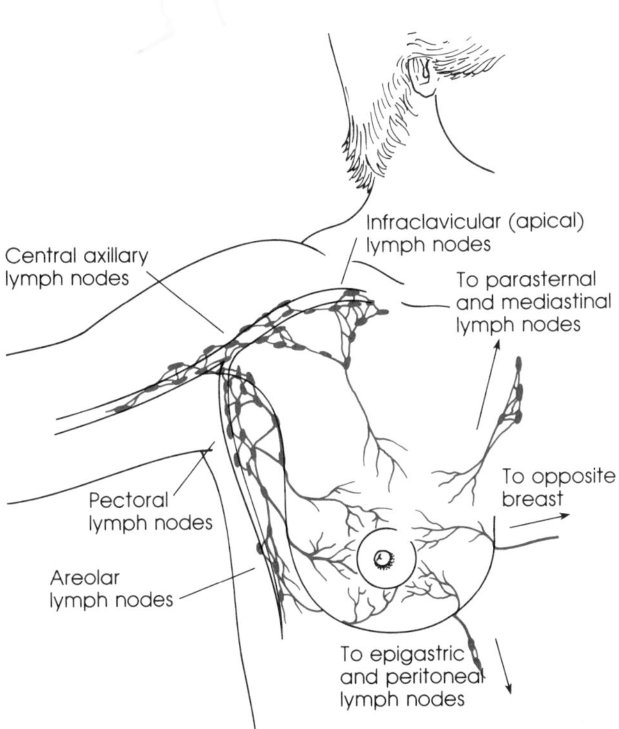

Figure 30-6 Lymph drainage of the breast.

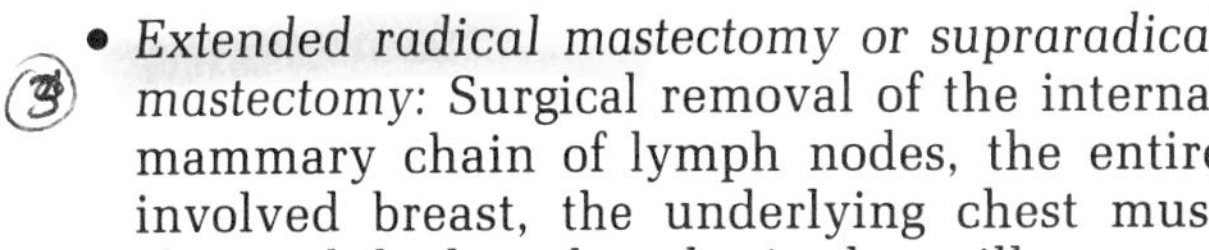

- *Extended radical mastectomy or supraradical mastectomy:* Surgical removal of the internal mammary chain of lymph nodes, the entire involved breast, the underlying chest muscles, and the lymph nodes in the axilla.
- *Halsted radical mastectomy:* Surgical en bloc removal of the entire involved breast, the underlying chest muscles, and the lymph nodes in the axilla.
- *Modified radical mastectomy:* Surgical removal of the entire involved breast and many lymph nodes in the axilla. The underlying chest muscles are removed in part or are left in place after removal of the nodes in the axilla.

Conservative surgeries include:

- *Simple mastectomy* (more recently called *total mastectomy*): Surgical removal of the entire involved breast. The underlying chest muscles and lymph nodes in the axilla are not removed.

  (*Note:* All the above procedures remove the involved breast completely.)

- *Limited Procedures:* These include a variety of techniques—lumpectomy, local excision, partial mastectomy, tylectomy (comparable to lumpectomy). In each instance, the tumor is removed along with a varying amount of surrounding tissue.

Figure 30-7 shows the effects of a radical mastectomy.

Surgical procedures are not the only modes of treatment for malignancy of the breast. The tumor tissue is sent for hormone receptor assay testing after surgery to see if hormone therapy will be helpful. Radiation therapy may be employed before or after surgical excision. Another form of adjuvant therapy is the use of antineoplastic drugs. Among these are the alkylating

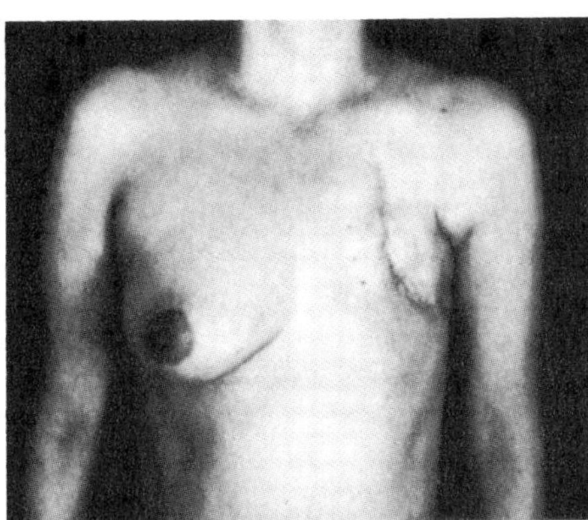

Figure 30-7 Patient after radical mastectomy of left breast.
(From Cohen, B. E., and Cronin, E. D.: Breast reconstruction with the latissimus dorsi musculocutaneous flap. Clin. Plast. Surg., April, 1984, p. 296.)

agents that interfere with the structure of DNA, thus inhibiting rapid cell growth; antibiotic derivatives; steroids; hormones; and nitrogen mustard derivatives.

The choice of adjuvant therapy is based on the stage of the disease, patient age and menopausal status, results of hormone assay tests, and patient preference. The purpose of adjuvant therapy is to decrease the risk of recurrence in patients who have no evidence of metastases or to prolong life in patients who have metastatic disease.

The three adjuvant therapies used are chemotherapy employing multiple-agent combinations; hormonal therapy with tamoxifen, an estrogen antagonist; and radiation.

A common combination of chemotherapy recommended for every woman undergoing mastectomy or lumpectomy is cyclophosphamide (Cytoxan), methotrexate, 5-fluorouracil, and doxorubicin (Adriamycin). Hormone therapy is also recommended for patients with estrogen- or progesterone-dependent cancer.

Radiation is necessary for the woman who has evidence of tumor cells in lymph nodes. Radiation may be used in conjunction with a more conservative surgery, even if the tumor appears localized. Treatment modes vary but are usually given over a 3- to 6-week period.

Many women are choosing to have reconstructive surgery done after mastectomy. This can be done at the time of the mastectomy, but many women wait until after chemotherapy or radiation treatment is complete.

Care of the Patient Having a Mastectomy

Preoperative Nursing Care

The physical preparation of the patient about to undergo a mastectomy differs very little from the routine preoperative care of any patient having major surgery. The emotional preparation, however, demands additional explanation of the type of surgery to be done and the formulation of plans for rehabilitation and prosthesis after surgery. These tasks are the responsibility of the surgeon, but the nurse must be aware of the emotional upheaval that most patients experience when they realize that the breast must be removed. The same fears and anxieties associated with surgery of the genital organs are frequently seen in the mastectomy patient. Because the breasts are secondary sex organs, and as such are closely related to femininity and motherhood, it is only natural that removal of a breast will cause an emotional reaction. The nurse must try to understand her patient's problems in adjusting to this type of surgery and give her as much support and comfort as possible.

Postoperative Nursing Care

A radical mastectomy is an extensive surgical procedure, one that may take 4 to 6 hours and may involve the loss of more than a pint (500 mL) of blood. The patient may have family members bank blood for her prior to the surgery if they are of a compatible blood type. Since the discovery of the acquired immunodeficiency syndrome (AIDS), transfusions with blood from a blood bank are given only if absolutely essential.

Because so much blood is lost, the surgeon usually applies a pressure dressing over the wound to prevent further bleeding after surgery. This dressing must be watched carefully for signs of hemorrhage during the first few postoperative days. In observing for bleeding, the nurse must remember to turn her patient and check the back of the chest as well as the front, because the blood may have seeped downward by gravity flow and collected on the bottom sheet. The pressure dressing may be reinforced but is *never* changed without specific orders to do so.

During the first 24 hours after surgery, there may be some swelling under the dressing, causing it to become tighter and to constrict the blood vessels leading to the arm. When this happens, the patient will complain of numbness of the lower arm, inability to move the fingers, or swelling of the lower arm. Such symptoms should be reported immediately. To minimize edema, the arm on the affected side should be elevated with pillows so that the elbow is at the level of the right atrium and the hand higher than the elbow.

In order to provide adequate drainage of serosanguineous fluid from the surgical site, the surgeon may insert tubes that are connected to a spring-loaded portable suction apparatus (Hemovac). The drainage tubes are usually removed after the third or fourth postoperative day if the drainage has subsided. (Directions for using the Hemovac are printed on the apparatus.) The drainage obtained should be measured and recorded at least every 8 hours. Large amounts of bright red blood may indicate hemorrhage and should be reported immediately. Deep breathing and coughing should be encouraged, even though they will most certainly cause some discomfort in the affected area. The patient is usually allowed out of bed the first postoperative day. When helping the patient get up from bed, the nurse should be aware that the patient will have some difficulty in balancing herself as long as she cannot use one arm, and she will be very likely to fall if she does not have adequate support from those helping her.

Blood pressure must not be taken on the affected arm, and no needle punctures for lab work are allowed. This is also true for the lumpectomy patient, as lymph node dissection is done of one or more nodes with this procedure also, putting this patient at risk for lymphedema. The patient is asked to remind everyone that the arm is not to be used for any procedure.

Although the patient who has more conservative surgery does not require as much physical care, the nurse needs to remember that the psychological impact of cancer is just as severe. Although the patient may seem very self-sufficient and did not lose a breast, the nurse should spend time with her to allow verbalization of fears and concerns.

Special exercises of the arm and shoulder on the affected side are begun as soon as the physician feels the patient may safely do them (Fig. 30–8). Most patients are very cooperative and anxious to do these exercises regularly if they understand how these exercises will prevent deformities and disabilities. The most commonly used exercises are wall hand climbing, hair brushing, elbow pull-in, and paddle swinging. These exercises are fully described and illustrated in the booklet "Help Yourself to Recovery," published by the American Cancer Society and available at any local Cancer Society office. This booklet also contains some excellent information on the selection and fitting of breast forms and specially designed brassieres for the patient who has had a mastectomy (Fig. 30–9).

Rehabilitation of the mastectomy patient is the function of all available members of the health care team. In some communities, volunteers from the American Cancer Society, who are women who have undergone mastectomy, are available for visits with postmastectomy patients. The attending physician may want to make arrangements for such a volunteer to visit and give psychological reassurance to the patient during convalescence from surgery.

Discharge Teaching

Before discharge from the hospital, the postmastectomy patient needs special instructions to help her minimize the possibility of infection and swelling of the arm on the affected side. Special precautions that help prevent such complications are:

- Do not carry a handbag or heavy articles with the affected arm.
- Do not wear a wristwatch or other jewelry on the affected arm.
- Apply hand or body cream daily to the affected hand and arm.
- Never pick or cut cuticles on the affected hand. After bathing, use a towel to push cuticles back.
- Do not immerse affected arm or hand in water for long periods. Use rubber gloves when washing dishes.
- Do not reach into a hot oven with the affected arm.
- Do not move or carry heavy objects.
- Use reliable insect repellent when exposure to insects is expected.
- Do not expose affected limb to sun for long periods.
- Consult your doctor before having any vaccinations or injections.
- Have your blood pressure taken on your *unaffected* arm.
- If any cuts or abrasions are sustained on the affected limb, wash them immediately and apply a protective covering.

RECONSTRUCTIVE BREAST SURGERY

Plastic surgery of the breast may be done to enlarge the breasts, to reduce their size, or to reconstruct one or both breasts so that they are equal in size and contour. Reconstructive breast surgery is an elective procedure that has a psychological as well as physiologic impact. With the advent of less radical surgery for breast malignancies, postmastectomy plastic surgery of the breast is becoming more commonplace.

Reduction Mammoplasty

The purpose of this kind of surgery is to reduce the size of breasts when hypertrophy of breast tissue causes physical and psychological problems. The weight of abnormally large breasts can cause fatigue and a dragging sensation on the shoulders, breast tenderness and pain that are more pronounced during the menstrual period, and difficulties obtaining adequate support even with a sturdy brassiere.

Psychological stress can be created by embarrassment over the deep grooves that shoulder straps of brassieres eventually produce and the fear of ridicule that is often associated with a very large bust size. Hypertrophied breasts also can affect a woman's ability to find suitable clothing and to wear her clothes with confidence.

Surgical correction of breast hypertrophy involves removal of the excess breast tissue by way of a curved incision under the breast. The skin is tightened, and the nipple is transplanted to its normal location in the center of the newly formed breast.

Postoperative nursing care is routine except for attention to psychological acceptance of a new body image and realization that normal lactation is no longer possible. The latter will be signifi-

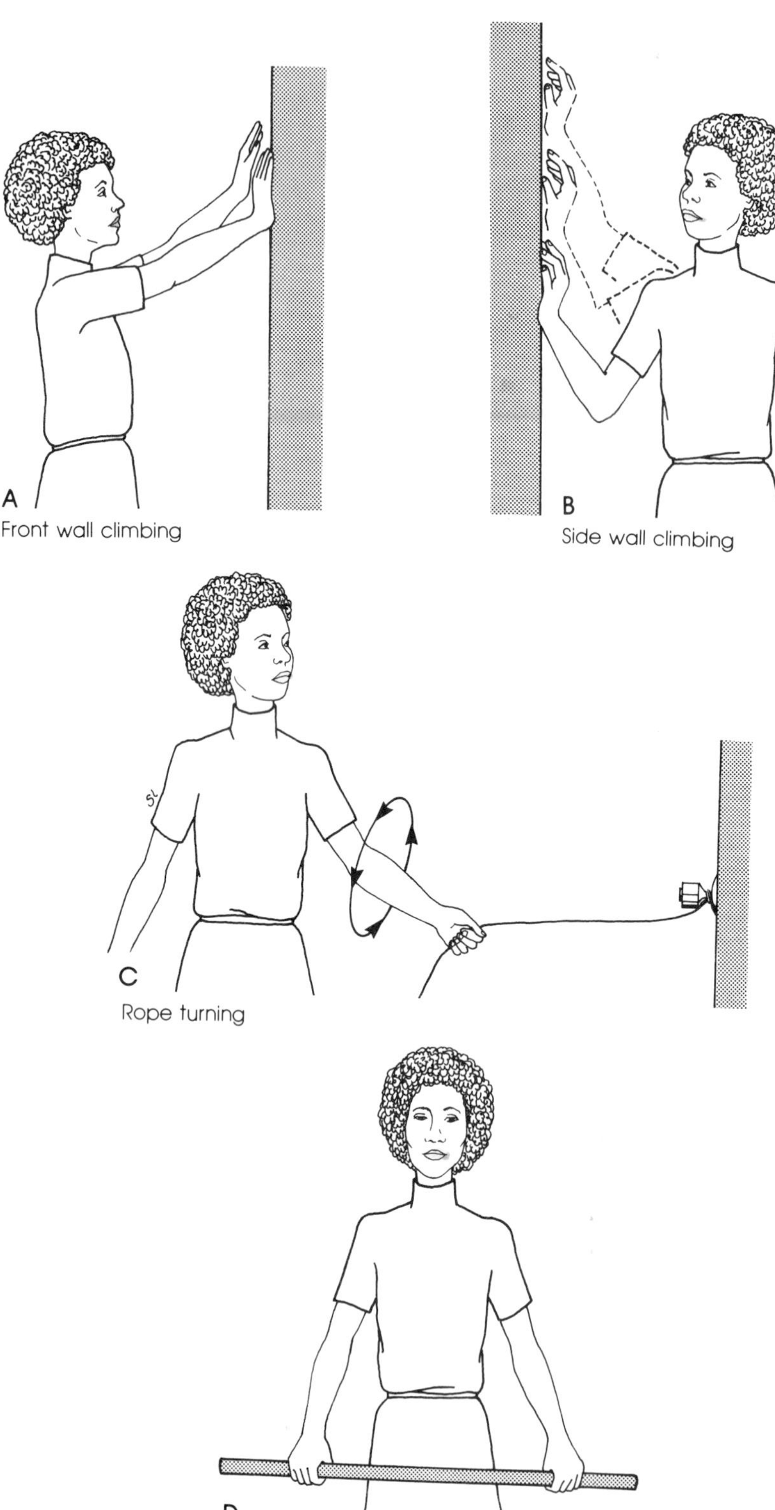

Figure 30–8 Postmastectomy exercises. *A*, Front wall climbing. Patient stands facing the wall, elbows slightly bent. Palms are placed at shoulder level and fingers are flexed and unflexed as hands "walk" up the wall as high as possible. Hands are then walked back down to shoulder level. Patient moves toward wall as fingers climb higher and then away from wall as fingers move downward. *B*, Side wall climbing. With operative side to wall, arm is extended until fingers touch wall. Patient moves toward the wall as fingers climb higher until body touches it. Maneuver is reversed as fingers climb back down wall. *C*, Rope turning. One end of rope is tied to door knob. Patient holds other end of rope and swings it in a circular motion, being sure entire arm and not the wrist is in motion. *D*, Yardstick or broom lift. Holding a yardstick or broom handle with both hands, the back is placed against a wall. Arms are extended straight downward and, with elbows straight, the stick is raised by the straightened arms until knuckles touch the wall over the head.

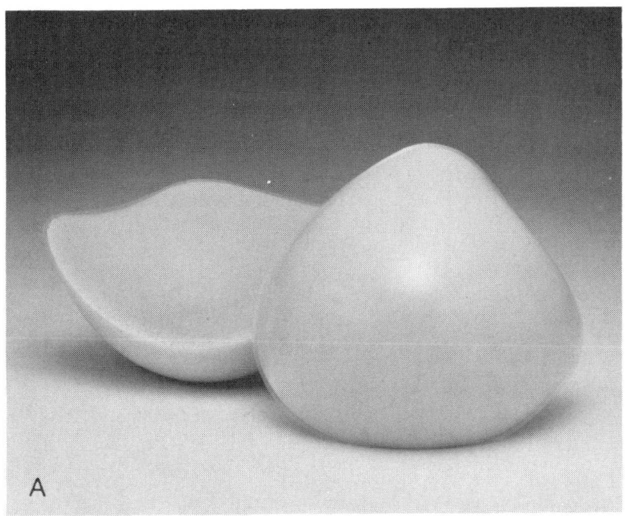
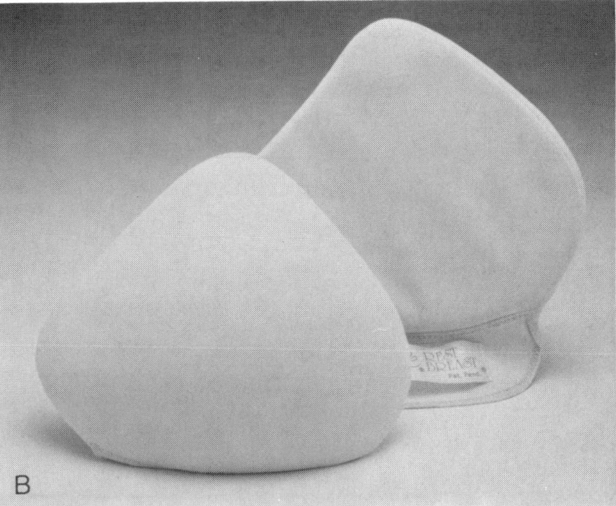

Figure 30-9 Breast prostheses for postmastectomy patients. *A*, "Nearly Me" prosthesis made of silicone gel, with hollowed sculpted foam back, and covered with outer "skin" of smooth polyurethane. Designed to be worn in regular brassieres. *B*, "Nearly Me Rest Breast" that is nonweighted and fabric-covered over foam. Recommended as a leisure-time prosthesis.
(Both photos courtesy of Spenco Medical Corporation, Waco, TX.)

cant only to women of childbearing age who might have planned to breast-feed their infants.

Augmentation Mammoplasty

The purpose of procedures of this type is to enlarge and possibly lift the breasts. It may be done for purely cosmetic reasons, as when a woman wants larger breasts, or following mastectomy to replace the surgically removed tissue (Fig. 30-10). Breast reconstruction after mastectomy sometimes is considered to be but one stage in the total plan for treatment of breast cancer. However, not every mastectomy patient is a candidate for reconstructive surgery.

The criteria used to decide whether postmastectomy breast reconstruction is desirable include (1) the amount of tissue remaining after mastectomy, such as in pectoral muscles, skin, and nipple; (2) the probability of recurrent metastatic disease; (3) appearance and size of the unoperated breast; and (4) the size and angle of the mastectomy scar. Radiation therapy usually does not preclude additional surgery on the breast.

Other considerations are the woman's motivation and psychological stability and available financial resources. The patient must be aware of the additional time and physical stress imposed by plastic surgery. She should also take into account the possibility of surgery on the unaffected breast, so that a match in size and contour of both breasts results. Because reconstructive surgery has become more popular, many insurance companies will cover the expense incurred.

Nursing care of patients having postmastectomy reconstructive surgery depends in large part on the type of surgery performed and its expected outcome. Accomplishment of the goals of plastic surgery of the breast requires a cooperative effort on the part of all members of the health care team, especially the surgeon, nurse, and physical therapist. The patient will need detailed instruction in the amount of physical activity allowed and measures to be taken so that infection and stress on the suture lines do not occur.

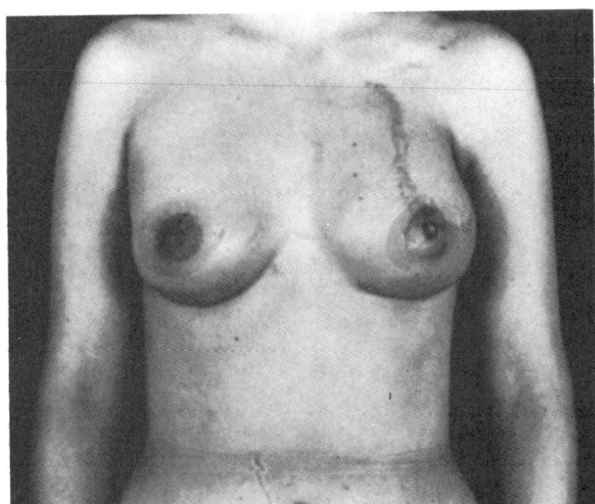

Figure 30-10 Reconstruction of left breast of patient shown in Figure 30-7. A subcutaneous mastectomy was performed on right breast.
(From Cohen, B. E., and Cronin, E. D.: Breast reconstruction with the latissimus dorsi musculocutaneous flap. Clin. Plast. Surg., April, 1984, p. 296.)

Concerns for the Elderly

After menopause, estrogen levels diminish to about 20% of premenopausal levels. Estrogen deficiency causes some atrophy in all of the female sexual organs, as well as loss of elasticity of the pelvic and supportive ligaments. Vaginal dryness can lead to fungal or bacterial infection.

A large number of women are now on long-term hormone replacement therapy to prevent osteoporosis. However, this increases the risk of endometrial cancer. The nurse should encourage female patients to have a pelvic examination every year.

Sexual response in older women is characterized by a decrease in intensity and duration of the response. The diminished amount of vaginal lubrication can interfere with sexual pleasure. This is easily corrected with estrogen cream or lubricants. The degree of sexual desire and pleasure derived appears to be directly related to whether the woman has continued to be sexually active through the years.

Cancer of the breast and endometrium are the main reproductive health problems in older women. Annual mammograms and regular Pap smears need to be encouraged. Patients in long-term-care facilities should not be exempted from these screening procedures.

BIBLIOGRAPHY

American Cancer Society: Cancer Facts and Figures: 1990. New York, 1990.

Andreoli, T. E., et al.: Cecil Essentials of Medicine, 2nd ed. Philadelphia, W. B. Saunders, 1990.

Brown, M. A.: Primary dysmenorrhea. Nurs. Clin. North Am., March, 1982, p. 145.

Caldwell, L. R.: Questions and answers about menopause. Am. J. Nurs., July, 1982, p. 1100.

Clark, E. E., and Sandler, L. S.: Factors involved in nurses' teaching breast self-examination. Cancer Nurs., Dec., 1989, p. 42.

Edlund, B. J.: The needs of women with gynecologic malignancies. Nurs. Clin. North Am., March, 1982, p. 165.

Ellenhorst-Ryan, J. M., et al.: Evaluating benign breast disease. Nurse Pract., Sept., 1988, p. 13.

Ignatavicius, D. D., and Bayne, M. J.: Medical-Surgical Nursing. Philadelphia, W. B. Saunders, 1991.

Khoiny, F. E.: Pelvic inflammatory disease in the adolescent. J. Pediatr. Health Care., Sept./Oct., 1989, p. 230.

King, J.: Vaginitis. J. Obstet. Gynecol. Neonatal Nurs., Jan., 1984, p. 41.

Lauver, D.: Irregular bleeding in women: Causes and nursing intervention. Am. J. Nurs., March, 1983, p. 396.

Mack, E.: Most breast lumps aren't cancer. RN, Dec., 1990, p. 20.

Madson, S.: How to reduce the risk of postmenopausal osteoporosis. J. Gerontol. Nurs., Sept., 1989, p. 20.

National Cancer Institute: Breast cancer: Understanding treatment options, Bethesda, MD, U.S. Department of Health and Human Services, 1988, 86–2675.

Nettles-Carlson, B.: Early detection of breast cancer . . . mammography, clinical breast examination (CBE), and breast self-examination. J. Obstet. Gynecol. Neonatal Nurs., Sept./Oct., 1989, p. 373.

Norwood, S. L.: Fibrocystic breast disease: An update and review. J. Obstet. Gynecol. Neonatal Nurs., March/April, 1990, p. 116.

Olds, S. B., et al.: Maternal Newborn Nursing: A Family-Centered Approach, 3rd ed. Menlo Park, CA, Addison-Wesley, 1988.

Rubin, D.: Gynecologic cancer: Uterine and ovarian malignancies. RN, June, 1987, p. 52.

Rust, D. L., and Kloppenborg, E. M.: Don't underestimate the lumpectomy patient's needs. RN, March, 1990, p. 59.

Springhouse Corporation: Diseases, 2nd ed. Springhouse, PA, 1987.

Thompson, J. M., et al.: Clinical Nursing, 2nd ed. St. Louis, C. V. Mosby, 1989.

STUDENT STUDY AIDS

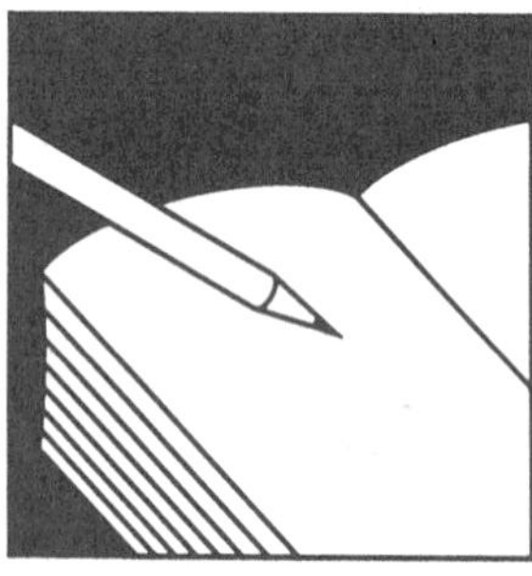

CLINICAL CASE PROBLEMS

Read each clinical situation and discuss the questions with your classmates.

1. Your brother, whose wife is dead, has asked you to explain menstruation to his daughter, who is reaching the age of puberty. You know that the child has some idea of what to expect, but most of her information has come from her friends who are no better informed than she.

- How would you go about explaining menstruation to her?

2. Mrs. Lawrence is a 45-year-old professional woman who is married and has two teen-age sons. She found a lump in her breast, which was diagnosed as malignant. Mrs. Lawrence does not want to have the radical mastectomy recommended by her physician.

- What are some possible reasons for Mrs. Lawrence's hesitation about having a radical mastectomy?
- What alternative surgical procedures are available to Mrs. Lawrence?
- What other kinds of therapy are used for breast malignancy?
- If Mrs. Lawrence chooses to have a lumpectomy, what adjuvant therapy will probably be recommended?

3. A neighbor, age 35, has had fibrocystic breast disease for several years. Her physician has suggested a mastectomy, which she does not want to have done unless it is absolutely necessary. Your neighbor has not tried any approach to relieve her FBD other than taking a mild analgesic when she cannot tolerate the pain.

■ What might you suggest to this person to help her cope with her disease?

STUDY OUTLINE

I. Introduction

A. Female glands (ovaries) secrete estrogen and progesterone and release ova.

B. Uterine tubes of female conduct ova from ovary to uterus; vagina conducts menstrual flow or infant.

C. Reservoirs in female are ovary and uterus.

D. Reproductive organs are but one biologic factor in total human sexuality.

E. Any disorder affecting the reproductive organs of a person will create some degree of concern about his or her own masculinity or femininity.

II. Diagnostic tests and procedures and nursing responsibilities

A. Pelvic examination:

1. Physical and mental preparation of patient will affect success of examination.
2. Explain procedure to patient if this is first pelvic examination or if it will be different from that to which she is accustomed.
3. Warn patient not to take douche before examination.

B. Smears and cultures: samples of fluid and cells are taken from cervix or vagina or both for laboratory examination.

1. Pap smear of sample cells taken from cervix and vagina. Three designations used for abnormal findings: CIN I, which indicates mild dysplasia; CIN II for moderate dysplasia; and CIN III for severe dysplasia or carcinoma in situ. Any of the three designations is indication for further evaluation.

C. Endometrial biopsy: evaluates response to ovarian hormones.

D. Colposcopy: allows better direct visualization of vagina and cervix. Biopsy may be taken at time of examination. Patient should have only minimal bleeding after biopsy; should be cautioned not to have sexual intercourse and to avoid inserting anything into vagina (except tampons) until biopsied site has healed and there is no more bleeding.

E. Laparoscopy: minor surgical procedure for exploration of peritoneal cavity by endoscopy.

F. Dilatation and curettage (D and C): dilatation of the cervix and curettage (scraping) of the endometrium. Can be therapeutic and diagnostic.

G. Mammography: x-ray examination of soft tissue of the breast without injection of contrast medium.

H. Breast self-examination (BSE): Monthly, usually 1 week after onset of menstrual period.

III. Nursing assessment of gynecologic health status

A. History taking:

1. Age relevant to development of a variety of gynecologic disorders.

2. Questions about sexual activities handled with tact and sensitivity.
3. Menstrual history includes onset of menses, average length of menstrual periods, irregularity of periods, excessive or scant bleeding, vaginal discharge, and sexually transmitted diseases or other infections.
4. History of premenstrual syndrome, dysmenorrhea, and character and location of pain.
5. History of depression, anxiety, and other emotional states related to birth and menstrual periods.
6. Drugs the patient is taking or has taken, including contraceptive agents.
7. Family history, especially if mother took diethylstilbestrol (DES) while pregnant with patient. Other significant family diseases include endocrine disorders and sickle cell disease. Obstetric history: number of pregnancies and births.
8. Subjective and objective data:
   a. Back pain, cramping, headache, irritability, feeling of fullness in pelvis, itching or burning of vulva.
   b. Characteristics of vaginal discharge, vaginal bleeding.
   c. Contour of breasts, condition of nipples.
   d. Secondary sex characteristics.
9. Nursing diagnoses commonly related to gynecologic disorders:
   a. Activity intolerance.
   b. Ineffective individual coping.
   c. Fear of mutilating surgery, loss of femininity.
   d. Fluid volume excess.
   e. Knowledge deficit.
   f. Sexual dysfunction.
   g. Disturbance in self-concept.
   h. Impaired skin integrity.
   i. Pain.

IV. Menstruation

A. Normal physiologic process.

B. Health education prior to menarche prepares young girl for monthly periods. Emphasis should be on positive aspects.

C. Menopause (climacteric): a process beginning sometime between ages 45 and 50 years. Usually takes about 1 year, during which there is gradual change in ovarian function and decrease in production of hormones.

1. Symptoms:
   a. Not always severe enough to need medical attention.
   b. Those that do occur are the result of several different physiologic, sociocultural, and psychological factors.
   c. First sign of onset is menstrual irregularity.
   d. Fatigue, insomnia, emotional instability, back pain, headache, decreased libido may be related to sociocultural factors and ineffective coping skills.
   e. In general, the more abrupt the decline in ovarian function, the more severe the symptoms.
2. Medical treatment:
   a. Estrogen and progestin replacement therapy effective in relieving some symptoms. Also helps prevent postmenopausal osteoporosis and atrophic urethritis. Disadvantage is increased risk for endometrial cancer. Estrogen and progestin are given in as small a dose and for as brief a period of time as needed to relieve symptoms.

3. Nursing intervention:
   a. Encourage patient to eat well and exercise.
   b. Relaxation techniques to cope with symptoms.
   c. Patient cautioned to report any spotting or bleeding after menses has completely stopped.
   d. Contraceptive practices continued until after 12 consecutive months of no menses. Women over 40 should not use oral contraceptives.
   e. Dyspareunia because of vaginal dryness alleviated with water-soluble lubricant or estrogen cream.

V. Menstrual dysfunctions

A. Amenorrhea—absence of menstruation:
   1. Causes: hormonal imbalance, malformation of reproductive tract, chronic disease, emotional disturbance.
   2. Medical diagnosis: complete physical workup recommended only if woman has not menstruated by her 17th or 18th birthday.
   3. Treatment medical and surgical, depending on cause.
   4. Nursing intervention: instruction about normal menstruation; assist patient to develop healthful coping mechanisms.

B. Dysmenorrhea: painful or difficult menstruation; other symptoms: nausea and vomiting, headache, dizziness, fatigue, irritability, emotional instability.
   1. Etiology: prostaglandins known to play a role by stimulating contractions of uterine smooth muscle tissue. Woman's attitude, general physical health, and emotional state can also affect symptoms of dysmenorrhea. Expectation of pain can become a self-fulfilling prophecy.
   2. Medical treatment: mild analgesics, uterine relaxants, prostaglandin synthesis inhibitors (PGSIs).
   3. Nursing intervention:
      a. Encourage patient to be open and discuss her problem. This alone often brings relief.
      b. Exercise and rest, applications of heat, relaxation techniques.
      c. Health teaching should include information about role of prostaglandins.

C. Premenstrual syndrome: a group of symptoms experienced for several days before menstrual period begins.
   1. Symptoms include fluid accumulation and weight gain, skin eruptions, cravings for special foods, crying spells, severe headaches, and depression.
   2. Special clinics help women obtain support and treatment, which sometimes includes progesterone therapy.

D. Dysfunctional uterine bleeding:
   1. Metrorrhagia: uterine bleeding or spotting at times other than menses.
   2. Menorrhagia: excessive bleeding.
      a. Causes include:
         (1) Inadequate hormonal level in young women just beginning to menstruate, or in menopausal women.
         (2) Presence of intrauterine device (IUD); infections of the endometrium.
         (3) Women in childbearing years could have irregular bleeding as sign of spontaneous abortion, ectopic pregnancy, benign fibroids, or endometriosis.
      b. Nursing assessment:
         (1) Information about onset, duration, frequency of irregular bleeding, and intervals between episodes.

(2) Estimate of blood loss.
(3) Obstetric history, menstrual history, general health history.
(4) Body weight, use of drugs and alcohol, stressful life changes, thyroid disease.

VI. Inflammatory disorders of the genital tract

A. Pelvic inflammatory disease (PID): any inflammation or infection in the pelvis outside the uterus.
  1. Caused by organisms spreading upward through the uterus and uterine tubes.
  2. Symptoms: severe abdominal pain; foul-smelling, purulent vaginal discharge; fever.
  3. Medical treatment and nursing care: antibacterials and measures to localize infection and prevent complications.

B. Vaginitis: inflammation of vaginal mucosa and possibly vaginal walls. Among the most common gynecologic problems.
  1. Major types and characteristics: see Table 30–2.
  2. Health teaching should include personal feminine hygiene do's and don'ts.

VII. Disorders of the uterus and endometrium

A. Tumors of the cervix
  1. Cervical polyp, usually benign; may exhibit spotting or bleeding between menses or after coitus.
  2. Malignant tumor diagnosed by Pap smear; treated by conization or hysterectomy.

B. Tumors within uterus often benign.
  1. Symptoms and medical diagnosis: abnormal bleeding usually the first sign; if tumor grows, can cause symptoms of pressure.
  2. Risk factors: see Table 30–3.
  3. Treatment:
    a. Benign tumors may subside after menopause or may require simple hysterectomy.
    b. Malignant tumors demand prompt and aggressive therapy: hysterectomy, radiation.

C. Endometriosis: endometrial tissue outside the uterus.
  1. Cause unknown; probably a combination of excessive production of endometrial tissue due to continued estrogen secretion throughout monthly cycle, and reflux of menstrual blood and tissue through uterine tubes.
  2. Symptoms: severe pain in lower abdomen or pelvis, excessive menstrual flow, metrorrhagia, and pain on defecation and during coitus.
  3. Medical and surgical treatment varies with location of misplaced tissue, age of patient, desire to have children, and severity of symptoms. Surgical removal of implants or total hysterectomy.

D. Ovarian tumors:
  1. Symptoms vague and slow to develop; ovarian tumor sometimes mistaken for gastrointestinal or urologic disorder.
  2. By the time symptoms are noted there is often widespread metastasis of malignant cells throughout peritoneal cavity.
  3. Risk factors for ovarian cancer in Table 30–3.
  4. Treatment: combination of surgery, radiation, multiagent chemotherapy, and intraperitoneal chemotherapy have improved prognosis for some patients.

VIII. Care of patients having gynecologic surgery

A. Sterilization procedures for contraception.

1. Vaginal approach for tubal ligation. The most common problem is infection.
2. Abdominal approach: removal of portion of both uterine tubes.
3. Endoscopic procedures can be done on outpatient basis. Include laparoscopy and tubal ligation, culdoscopy, and cauterization or occlusion of uterine tubes.

B. Vaginal and abdominal surgery:
   1. Vaginal repair of fistulas, other structural defects.
   2. Vulvectomy: surgical excision of labia, clitoris, perineal structures, and removal of lymphatic tissues in the femoral and inguinal areas.
   3. Hysterectomy: surgical removal of uterus.
      a. Decision to remove uterus should be based on clinical justification, whether childbearing is desired, and psychosocial factors. Patient should be well informed about need for and consequences of surgery.
      b. Clinical indications include pelvic relaxation, severe recurrent pain, excessive uterine bleeding, and cervical and uterine malignancies.
      c. A woman who experiences negative attitudes (her own and those of others) is likely to have psychological aftereffects months to years after hysterectomy.
      d. Hysterectomy should not precipitate psychological disorders in women who are psychologically stable and mature.
      e. Preoperative care:
         (1) Patient is prepared psychologically.
         (2) Given time to express concerns and receive factual answers.
      f. Postoperative care:
         (1) Do not place in high Fowler's position.
         (2) Take measures to prevent pulmonary and circulatory complications.
         (3) Discharge planning to include instruction in self-care.

IX. Disorders of the breast

A. Breast is part of woman's total concept of herself as a female.

B. Fibrocystic breast disease.
   1. Characterized by small single or multiple tumors or cysts.
   2. Occurs most often in women in their 20s.
   3. Many cases subside after menopause, which indicates some relationship to estrogen and progesterone levels.
   4. Medical treatment and nursing intervention.
      a. Vitamin and hormone therapy.
      b. Self-help measures include restriction of all forms of methylxanthines, especially caffeine; limitation of salt and fluid intake to relieve feeling of fullness, swelling; application of warm compresses; wearing brassiere that gives good support; mild analgesics.
      c. Patient education: how to perform self-examination of breast 1 week after onset of menstrual period. Changes that should be reported promptly.

C. Breast cancer.
   1. Symptoms: lump in breast, dimpling, retraction of nipple, discharge from nipple, swelling, changes in contour or firmness, redness.
   2. Medical and surgical treatment: some type of mastectomy or lumpectomy, radiation, possibly chemotherapy.

D. Nursing care of patients having mastectomy:
   1. Preoperative care: physical and emotional preparation.
   2. Postoperative care: Monitor for bleeding, swelling under dressing or in arm and hand on surgical side, numbness and inability to move fingers must be reported.
      a. Elevate affected arm; do not take blood pressure on that side; no needle sticks.
      b. Deep breathing, coughing exercises to prevent pulmonary complications.
      c. Assist patient from bed until she has adjusted to changes in distribution of body weight.
      d. Teach and supervise arm exercises.
      e. Prepare for self-care at home.

E. Reconstructive breast surgery.
   1. Reduction mammoplasty: done to reduce size of hypertrophied breasts.
      a. Greatly enlarged breasts can create physiologic and psychological problems.
      b. Procedure involves surgical removal of excess tissue, tightening of skin, and replacement of nipple.
      c. Nursing care fairly routine. Patient should be helped with acceptance of new body image and nonfunctioning mammary glands.
   2. Augmentation mammoplasty: done to enlarge breasts or replace tissue removed during mastectomy.
      a. Criteria for postmastectomy mammoplasty:
         (1) Amount of tissue remaining.
         (2) Probability of recurrent malignancy.
         (3) Appearance and size of unoperated breast.
         (4) Size and angle of mastectomy scar.
      b. Other considerations include woman's motivation and psychological stability. Financial resources also must be taken into account.
      c. Postoperative care depends on type of surgery done. Requires cooperative effort on part of surgeon, nurse, and physical therapist.

X. Concerns for the elderly

A. Estrogen levels decrease after menopause to about 20% of premenopausal levels.
B. Postmenopausal dryness of the vagina tends to occur.
C. Postmenopausal hormone replacement is thought to help prevent osteoporosis.
D. Sexual response in older women is decreased in intensity and duration of response.
E. Cancer of the breast and endometrium are the main reproductive problems of the older woman.
F. Annual mammograms and regular Pap smears are to be encouraged.

CHAPTER 31

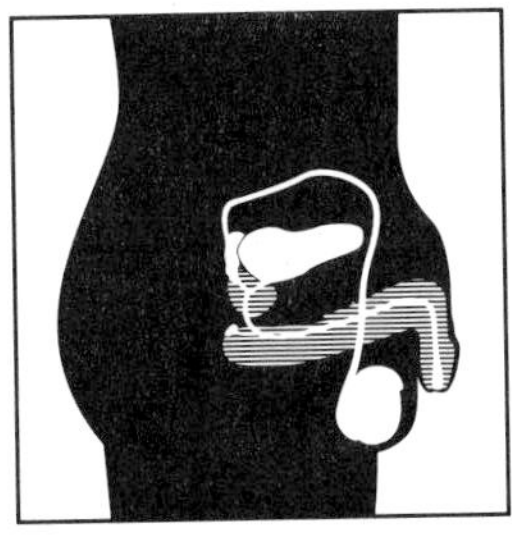

Care of Patients With Disorders of the Male Reproductive System

VOCABULARY

ejaculation
epididymis
impotence
macule
prepuce
seminal
spermatozoa
testis
vesicle

Upon completion of this part of the chapter the student should be able to:

1. List the most common diagnostic tests and examinations of the male reproductive system and significant nursing responsibilities in the care of the patients undergoing each of them.
2. Describe areas and points included during assessment of the male reproductive system.
3. Describe nursing interventions for patients experiencing infection or inflammation of the reproductive organs.
4. Identify the patient teaching involved for early detection of testicular tumors.
5. Explain the nursing care for the patient who has a three-way catheter and continuous bladder irrigation system in the postoperative period.
6. Write a nursing care plan for the patient who has had a perineal transurethral prostatic resection.

The glands of the male reproductive system are called the *testes*. These have both internal hormonal secretions (testosterone) and external secretions, which contain the spermatozoa. The testes, like the ovaries, are oval; however, they are located outside the abdominal cavity in the scrotal sac. The prostate gland, which is located just below the bladder and completely surrounds the urethra, is one of several auxiliary glands that secrete a lubricant for the urethra (see Fig. 31–1).

The system of tubes in the male includes the epididymis, the ductus deferens, the ejaculatory duct, and the urethra; these are all responsible for transporting the spermatozoa from the testes to the outside (Fig. 31–1).

DIAGNOSTIC TESTS AND PROCEDURES AND NURSING IMPLICATIONS

EXAMINATION OF GENITALIA

Because most of the structures that comprise the male reproductive system are located outside the body, they are more easily inspected and palpated than the female reproductive organs.

The penis and foreskin are inspected for signs of macules and papules, vesicles and pustules, erosions and ulcers, and abnormal growths. The foreskin is retracted (pulled back) to examine the surface of the penis under it. The skin enclosing the scrotal sac is similarly examined for abnormalities.

The contents of the scrotal sac include the testis, the epididymis, and the spermatic cord. Each testis and scrotal sac is palpated for abnormal masses, localized and generalized swelling, and tenderness. The perineum is inspected for discoloration, lesions, swelling, growths, and masses.

Palpation of the prostate and seminal vesicles requires insertion of a gloved finger into the rectum. The examiner evaluates the consistency and size of the prostate and determines whether there are any nodules or tenderness.

The examination is performed with the patient standing with his upper body bent over the examining table or with him lying on his left side with the hips and knees slightly flexed. Each step of the procedure is explained, and privacy is provided.

TRANSRECTAL ULTRASONOGRAPHY OF THE PROSTATE

Cancer of the prostate is the second most common malignancy in men over 55. It is very difficult to detect in the early stages. A new tool utilizing a transrectal probe with an ultrasound transducer at its tip can detect differences in tissue densities in the prostate gland, thereby picturing tumor location and size.

The procedure takes 15 to 20 minutes to perform and can be done on an outpatient basis without anesthesia.

BIOPSY OF THE PROSTATE

The purpose of this test is to determine the cause of prostatic enlargement and rule out or confirm a diagnosis of malignancy. The prostate gland can be approached through the perineum, the rectum, or the urethra. A biopsy needle is inserted into several locations of the suspicious area in the prostate, and cells are aspirated and sent for histologic examination.

During the procedure the patient may feel

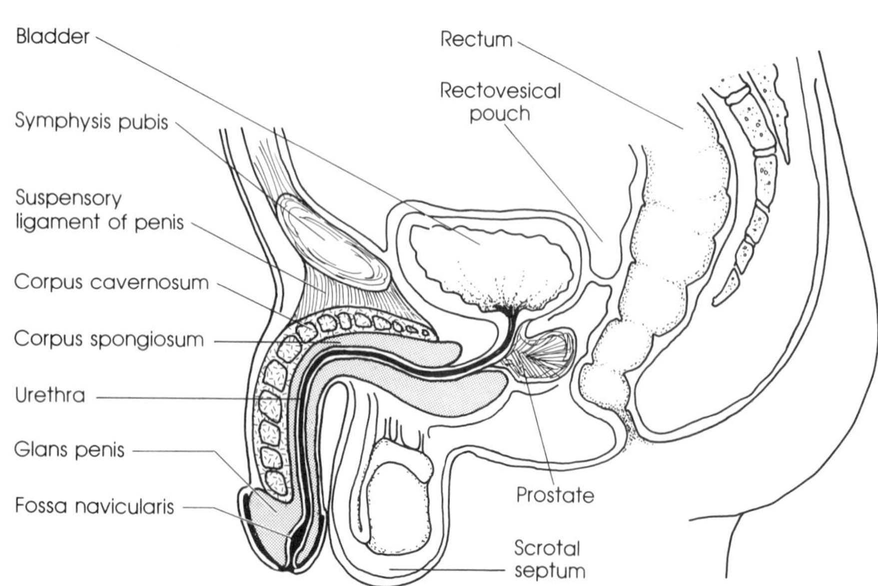

Figure 31–1 Male reproductive system.

some discomfort, even though a local anesthetic is used. After the needle is withdrawn, slight pressure is applied to the insertion site to control bleeding and prevent hematoma. There are few, if any, complications expected from the procedure. Bleeding into the urethra can produce a small amount of blood in the urine.

The biopsy is often done on an outpatient basis, and the patient should be instructed to watch for signs of infection and hematoma and to report these promptly if they occur. The patient also should watch for gross hematuria and a change in urinary flow such as frequency or inability to empty the bladder. If the patient is in the hospital at the time of the biopsy, the nurse monitors him for these signs of complications.

SEMEN ANALYSIS

This test is most often done as part of a total evaluation for fertility. The specimen is analyzed for total volume of seminal fluid, and motility and number of sperm. A microscopic examination of the sperm and fluid is also done to identify infectious organisms. Semen analysis is done for medicolegal purposes, for example, to verify the blood type in a case of alleged rape or to verify sterility as a defense in a paternity suit.

TESTICULAR SELF-EXAMINATION

Testicular cancer is the third leading cause of death in young men between the ages of 20 and 35. In its concern for early detection and treatment of cancer of the testis the American Cancer Society encourages monthly self-examination of the testes by males just as it encourages breast self-examination in the female. If testicular cancer is treated in the early stages, it is one of the most curable forms of cancer.

There are several sources of information for teaching testicular self-examination (TSE). The American Cancer Society publishes a pamphlet written for laypersons that is titled "For Men Only." It also will provide a free film on TSE. Both give some basic facts about testicular cancer and explains the "how to's" of TSE.

It is recommended that TSE be done immediately after a warm shower or bath when the examiner's hands are warm and the scrotal sac is relaxed and the testicles are readily accessible. Each testicle is rolled between the thumb and fingers of both hands to detect any nodules in the testis or abnormalities in the epididymis and spermatic cord (Fig. 31–2). The patient is instructed to contact his physician right away if any abnormality is found.

OTHER TESTS

Tests for general state of health such as complete blood cell (CBC) count, urinalysis, chemistry profile, and thyroid tests are done initially for problems of the male reproductive tract. Serum acid phosphatase is usually elevated in the patient with prostate cancer. Serum alkaline phosphatase is elevated if malignancy of the prostate has metastasized to the bone. A new test, PSA (prostate specific antigen), is able to detect cancer of the prostate. Kidney, urinary, and bladder

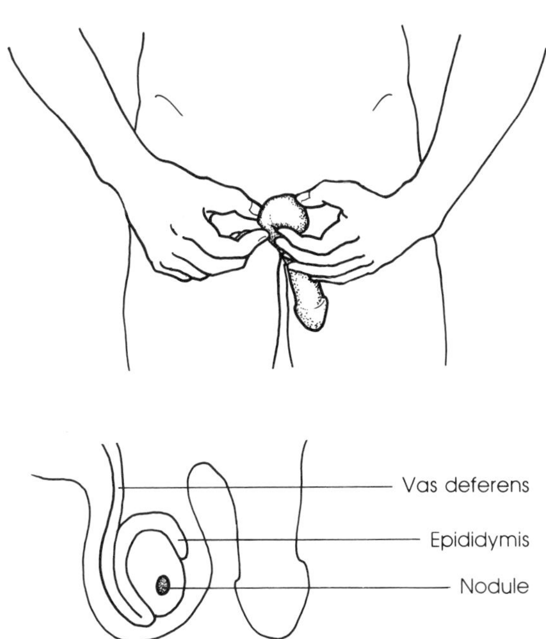

Your best hope for early detection of testicular cancer is a simple three-minute monthly self-examination. The best time is after a warm bath or shower, when the scrotal skin is most relaxed.

Roll each testicle gently between the thumb and fingers of both hands. If you find any hard lumps or nodules, you should see your doctor promptly. They may not be malignant, but only your doctor can make the diagnosis.

Following a thorough physical examination, your doctor may perform certain x-ray studies to make the most accurate diagnosis possible.

Figure 31–2 Testicular self-examination.
(Redrawn from For Men Only. New York, American Cancer Society.)

(KUB) tests; an intravenous pyelogram (IVP); and cystoscopy with urodynamic studies may also be done.

Smears of urethral discharge and serum tests are done to detect sexually transmitted diseases. Tumor protein marker studies are performed for patients with testicular masses for both diagnostic purposes and for follow-up to determine success of treatment. The primary tumor markers are alpha-fetoprotein (AFP) and the beta subunit of human chorionic gonadotropin (β-hCG).

NURSING ASSESSMENT

Because of the predominance of certain kinds of reproductive disorders in males in certain age groups, the age of the patient is relevant to nursing assessment. In males over the age of 50, the assessment is directed more toward detection of prostate problems, whereas younger males are assessed for sexually transmitted disease and testicular cancer.

HISTORY TAKING

It may be awkward for the new nurse to obtain a sexual and reproductive history, but with experience in interviewing male patients of all ages, she will soon become more comfortable and adept at obtaining necessary data. Because questions about urinary problems are usually less sensitive than those dealing with sexual dysfunction, it is best to begin with questions of this kind and then lead into more sensitive ones.

Open-ended questions that start out with "tell me about . . . " or "when did you first notice . . . " give the patient room to discuss only those things he is comfortable talking about. It also is helpful to relate his problem to the inconvenience it has caused in his daily life. For example, tenderness and discomfort in the scrotal area could make sitting at a desk or walking very difficult and interfere with getting assigned work done. Frequent urination can cause distracting and sometimes embarrassing interruptions in his work schedule or recreational activities.

Good communication depends on the sender and receiver of messages using mutually understood language. Many people do not know the medical names of their sex organs. If the nurse suspects that the patient does not understand what particular part of the body she is talking about or if the nurse herself is not familiar with the term the patient is using, it is important to phrase questions differently or ask for clarification from the patient.

Some of the questions to be included in an assessment of the male reproductive system are related to difficulties or changes in patterns of urination, discharge from the penis, tumors or masses noted in the scrotum or inguinal region, tenderness or pain that is located in the external genitalia or perineum, rectal pain, impotence, and infertility.

Questions directly related to sexual activities might include patterns of sexual activity, such as number of partners, frequency of genital contact or oral-genital contact, and the sex of his partners.

The nurse also will need to know about past infections affecting the urinary system and the reproductive organs. Drugs taken by the patient also are relevant because there are many drugs, including alcohol, that can affect the male reproductive system and cause impotence, loss of libido, and sterility.

Metabolic and endocrine disorders such as diabetes mellitus and hypothyroidism also can cause impotence in male patients. Those who have heart disease can have problems of sexual dysfunction because of fear of precipitating a heart attack by sexual activity. Some medications for hypertension occasionally interfere with sexual function.

INFLAMMATIONS AND INFECTIONS OF THE MALE REPRODUCTIVE ORGANS

Many of the inflammations and infections affecting the male reproductive system are similar to those of the female reproductive system in cause and effect. For example, urethritis in the male and female can be caused by common pyogenic and colonic bacteria and by *Neisseria gonorrhoeae*. The male also can be infected with *Trichomonas vaginalis*, which is transmitted by sexual contact. There is always the possibility that the sexual partners will reinfect one another until both are treated simultaneously.

Nonspecific genitourinary infections in the male, including nongonococcal urethritis (NGU), are not caused by any particular organism, but they present substantially the same clinical picture. Among the symptoms of nonspecific urethritis are mucopurulent discharge from the urethra, painful urination of varying degrees of severity, and occasionally the appearance of blood in the urine. A microscopic examination of a smear from urethral secretions usually does not show any specific organisms, but there may be an excessive number of white cells.

Epididymitis is an inflammation of the epididymis and may result from infection of the prostate. The patient with epididymitis complains of groin pain plus swelling and pain in the scrotum. In men below the age of 35, the major cause of epididymitis is *Chlamydia trachomatis*, a sexually transmitted organism. Sometimes an inflammatory epididymitis occurs after vigorous exercise.

Orchitis is inflammation of the testicle and may affect one or both testes. It may be caused by local or systemic infection or by trauma. *Mumps orchitis* occurs in about 20% of adult males who contract mumps. Gamma globulin is usually given to lessen the severity of the orchitis. Bilateral orchitis is serious, as it very often causes sterility.

Prostatitis is inflammation that occurs from virus, bacteria, or congestion in the prostate gland. It can occur from a sudden decrease in sexual activity. *Acute prostatitis* is characterized by fever, chills, burning on urination, and urethral discharge containing many WBCs. Patients with chronic prostatitis complain of backache, perineal pain, urinary frequency and burning, and possibly blood in the urine.

MEDICAL TREATMENT AND NURSING INTERVENTION

Treatment of nonspecific or nongonorrheal urethritis usually consists of oral administration of an antibiotic such as tetracycline, possibly followed by a sulfonamide. Because the infection typically is spread by sexual intercourse, it is possible that both partners will have the disease and should be treated concurrently. Untreated urethritis in the male can lead to acute infection of the epididymis.

Appropriate antibacterial drugs are prescribed to control other urogenital infections once the disorder has been diagnosed. In some cases surgical intervention may be necessary to correct structural defects that help harbor infectious organisms.

Epididymitis is treated by bed rest and elevation of the scrotum on a towel to increase venous drainage and ease pain. Specific antibiotics are administered to combat infection, and analgesics are given for pain. Ice packs or warm sitz baths may also be used to lessen pain. If epididymitis is from a sexually transmitted disease, the patient's sexual partner must be treated also. The nurse instructs the patient to avoid lifting, straining, or sexual activity until the infection is under control (which can take up to 4 weeks). A scrotal support should be worn when the patient is out of bed.

Orchitis is treated in the same way as epididymitis.

Treatment of prostatitis is vigorous in order to prevent abscess of the prostate and to eliminate urinary tract infection. Antimicrobials such as carbenicillin indanyl sodium (Geocillin) or fluoroquinolones (e.g., norfloxacin) are the drugs of choice for acute infection. Long-term therapy (30 days) with trimethoprim and sulfamethoxazole (Bactrim, Septra) is preferred for the patient with chronic prostatitis, because it diffuses into the prostatic fluid. Frequent prostatic massage may be performed to regularly "milk" the prostate for those clients who have recurrent episodes of prostatitis.

HYDROCELE

There is normally a small quantity of fluid in the space between the testis and tunica vaginalis within the scrotum. When a larger than normal amount of fluid accumulates in this space, it is known as *hydrocele.* The fluid accumulation may be caused by infection such as epididymitis or orchitis, or it may occur after trauma. Many times the cause is unknown. Hydrocele causes enlargement of the scrotum and is usually painless, but the weight and added bulk can cause discomfort.

Treatment, when indicated, is surgical excision of the sac. A pressure dressing and a drain are in place postoperatively. The patient will need to wear an athletic support for several weeks.

VARICOCELE

Dilation and clumping of the tributary vessels of the spermatic vein cause this somewhat painful swelling. It usually occurs on the left side of the scrotum. The discomfort is rarely enough to warrant surgery. If infertility has been a problem, surgical correction will sometimes improve the sperm count.

NURSING INTERVENTION

Nursing measures to help the patient cope with fatigue, weakness, and fever are appropriate, because these problems often are associated with urogenital infections. Fluid intake should be increased to help prevent fluid deficit, reduce fever, increase urinary flow, and remove debris and bacteria.

TESTICULAR CANCER

Testicular cancer most commonly occurs in men age 15 to 40 and is the leading cause of death in men 25 to 34 years of age (American Cancer Society, 1990). It is most frequently found in whites and is quite rare in blacks.

Men most at risk for testicular cancer are those who have an undescended or partially descended testicle. This condition, called *cryptorchidism*, occurs during fetal development. As the unborn male child matures, the testes first appear in the abdomen at about the level of the kidneys. They develop at this site until approximately the seventh month of fetal life, when they start to move downward to the upper part of the groin. From there they move into the inguinal canal and then into the scrotum. If the descent of a testis is halted in its progress, it remains at that site as an undescended testis. Sometimes the undescended testicle will drop into the scrotum when the boy starts walking. If it remains undescended, surgical correction is done at 1½ to 3 years of age.

Treatment of cryptorchidism consists of surgical correction in a procedure called *orchiopexy.*

MEDICAL DIAGNOSIS

Assessment for testicular cancer includes questioning about any history of an undescended testicle and the incidence of the disease in relatives. Testicular examination is performed by the physician or nurse practitioner. Any testicular mass that will not transilluminate (allow light to shine through it) is assumed to be malignant until proved otherwise. If a mass is found, diagnostic tests for tumor marker proteins are obtained. Lymphangiography is performed to determine lymph node involvement.

When testicular cancer is suspected, orchiectomy (unilateral removal of the testicle) is performed. Biopsy of a testicular mass is never done, as it can spread malignant cells.

There are three stages for classifying the malignancy. In Stage I, the tumor is confined to the affected testis. In Stage II, malignant cells have spread to the regional lymph nodes, usually on the same side as the affected testis. In Stage III, there is metastasis to other organs such as the lungs and liver. Figure 31–3 shows lymphatic drainage of the penis, testis, and scrotal wall.

SURGICAL TREATMENT

If the testicular tumor is limited to the scrotal sac and there is no metastasis, surgical removal of the testis *(orchiectomy)* may be all that is necessary to cure the patient of his disease. At the time of the orchiectomy a prosthesis is inserted into the scrotal sac to cosmetically simulate the removed testis. Removal of only one testis will not affect the patient's ability to produce the male hormone testosterone or render him impotent, as there remains another testis to carry on normal testicular function.

Further treatment for metastatic testicular cancer includes radical dissection of the lymph nodes and possibly radiation or chemotherapy. This extensive surgery can damage nerves necessary for normal intercourse and ejaculation. The patient could remain potent (that is, capable of having sexual intercourse), but there will be no ejaculation of seminal fluid and so he will be sterile. A young man who is looking forward to fathering children might consider banking his sperm before surgery so that he could father children by artificial insemination of his spouse.

NURSING INTERVENTION

In addition to routine preoperative and postoperative nursing care and attention to the special needs of a cancer patient, the nurse helps the patient with testicular cancer deal with problems related to his masculinity and sexual activity. He will need time to think about and discuss the effects of surgery that have been explained to him by the surgeon.

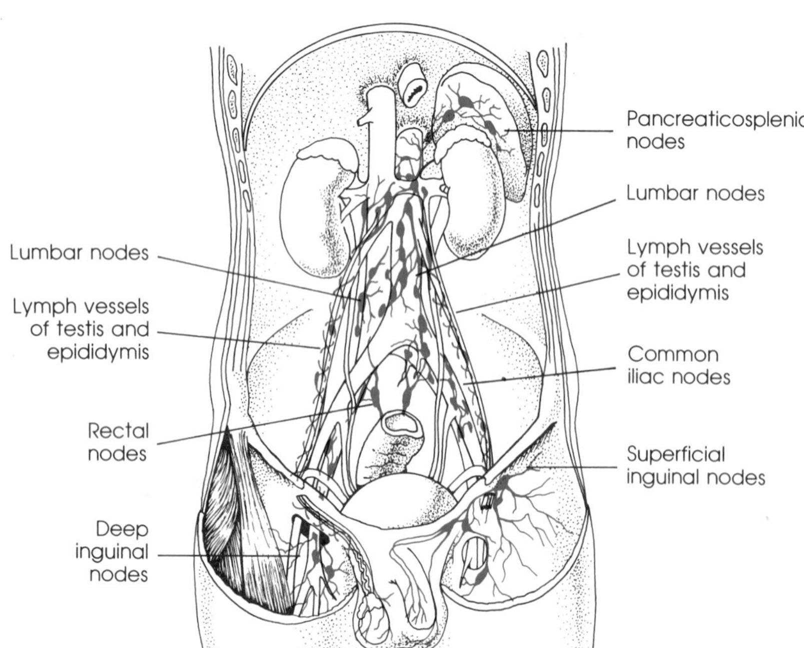

Figure 31–3 Lymph drainage of the penis, testes, and scrotal wall. The lymphatics of the external genitals provide pathways by which gonorrheal and other infections of the urethra and epididymis, as well as malignancies of the testis, can spread.

The lymph vessels of the skin of the scrotum and of the penis and prepuce drain into the superficial inguinal nodes. The lymphatics of the testes and spermatic cord follow testicular vessels through the inguinal canal toward the deeper lumbar nodes.

Many men refuse to undergo orchiectomy because they view it as loss of manhood. The nurse is very instrumental in assisting the patient to accept the procedure. Repeated explanation that removal of one testicle will not cause sterility and assurance that a prosthesis is implanted for normal appearance can overcome the patient's reluctance. Time for questions and discussion of concerns should be provided for the patient and his sexual partner.

TUMORS OF THE PROSTATE

The prostate gland encircles the neck of the bladder and the urethra. It is an exocrine gland, secreting a mucuslike fluid through ducts opening into the prostatic portion of the urethra. The prostate does *not* produce hormones. Prostatic fluid is the fluid in which sperm are transported during sexual intercourse.

As the male ages, the glandular cells in the prostate undergo an abnormal increase in number (tissue hyperplasia), resulting in benign enlargement, or hypertrophy, of the gland. This hyperplasia occurs in all men over 40 to some degree. As the prostate gland enlarges, it extends inward, narrowing the urethral channel, and upward, narrowing the bladder opening and obstructing the outflow of urine. These problems usually occur after age 60. Urinary retention and stasis can result in urinary tract infection. Obstruction to urine outflow can cause backup of urine into the ureters and kidney, causing hydronephrosis and eventual kidney damage.

Malignant neoplasm of the prostate rarely occurs in men under 50 years of age and increases in incidence with each decade of life. It is the most common cancer in American men and occurs twice as frequently in blacks as in whites. Dietary fat is thought to be a factor in the development of prostatic malignancy, and tumor growth is associated with the presence of androgen, a male sex hormone.

SYMPTOMS AND MEDICAL DIAGNOSIS

Benign prostatic hypertrophy (BPH) produces no symptoms until the growth becomes large enough to press against the urethra. Then the patient begins to experience difficulty in urinating, and in the later stages there is complete obstruction of the urinary flow.

Carcinoma of the prostate is usually not discovered until the later stages of development. This type of carcinoma is the slowest growing of all cancers. When palpated, a malignant nodule feels hard and immovable. Needle biopsy and tests to determine whether metastatic spread has occurred are performed to determine the best treatment.

Not all men with benign prostatic hypertrophy need surgery, but those who are experiencing recurrent urinary tract infection or hydronephrosis from bladder neck obstruction or are unable to obtain sufficient sleep because of frequency and nocturia are candidates for prostatic surgery. The type of surgical procedure depends on the size of the gland, the age and physical condition of the patient, and the preference of the patient and surgeon. All the surgical procedures for BPH remove the hyperplastic tissue and leave the prostate capsule.

SURGICAL TREATMENT AND NURSING INTERVENTION

Surgical removal of all or part of the prostate gland is the treatment of choice for tumors of the prostate. Whenever a biopsy shows the tumor to be malignant, the entire prostate and its capsule must be removed.

The location of the incision and the amount of tissue to be removed will depend on the individual patient, his general physical condition, and the type of tumor present.

- *Transurethral prostatic resection (TURP).* This is the most common procedure. There is no surgical incision, as the tissue of the prostate gland is removed by way of the urethra.
- *Suprapubic prostatectomy.* A low abdominal incision is made, with another through the bladder wall. The prostate tissue is removed through the bladder cavity and Gelfoam or some form of hemostatic packing is placed in the cavity to control bleeding. A urethral catheter and a drain for urine are brought out through the incision. This procedure is done when the patient has bladder disease that also needs treatment.
- *Retropubic prostatectomy.* A low abdominal incision is made, and the prostate gland is exposed. A small incision is made in the prostate capsule, and the tissue is extracted. This procedure is done when the gland is too large to resect by the transureteral approach. There should be no urine drainage on the abdominal dressing.
- *Perineal prostatectomy.* This is used to remove enlarged prostate glands that are full of stones. An exaggerated lithotomy position is used, and the incision is U shaped, extending between the ischial tuberosities. A urethral catheter and a perineal drain are placed. Because the pudendal nerve is cut in this procedure, the patient is impotent afterward. Infection is more of a problem because of the closeness of the incision to the rectum.
- *Radical prostatectomy.* This is performed via a suprapubic, retropubic, or perineal ap-

proach. The prostate gland and the capsule are removed along with the cuff at the bladder neck, the seminal vesicles, and the regional lymph nodes. The bladder neck is reconnected to the urethra. This is the procedure of choice for patients with stage I or II prostatic malignancy. The patient undergoing a suprapubic or retropubic procedure will be able to have an erection and orgasm, but the spermatic fluid will travel into the bladder. The perineal approach may cause sexual dysfunction. The patient may also experience urinary incontinence after a radical prostatectomy. If this becomes a continuing problem, an artificial urinary sphincter can be surgically implanted.

Localized prostatic cancer is treated with surgery and radiation therapy. For metastatic disease, hormonal therapy with diethylstilbestrol (DES), progestational agents, and androgen inhibitors; bilateral simple orchiectomy to remove testosterone; and chemotherapy are added to the treatment. Treatment management is based on the stage of the disease and the physical condition of the patient.

Nursing interventions for selected problems in a patient having a transurethral resection are summarized in Nursing Care Plan 31–1.

Preoperative Nursing Care

The preoperative care is the same as for any patient having abdominal surgery. An enema is given the night before to prevent postoperative straining at stool, which can cause bleeding.

The patient with BPH admitted for a prostatectomy will inevitably have some difficulty in voiding. An indwelling catheter may be necessary to drain the bladder. An accurate record of intake and output is essential.

The average age for prostatectomy is 73. Nursing care for this age group requires close attention to assistance with ambulation if a sedative has been given and the appropriate use of siderails.

Preoperative teaching includes deep breathing exercises, leg exercises, the preoperative and postoperative routine, and explanation of the care of the incision, catheters, irrigation system, and drains.

Table 31–1 lists some common preoperative procedures and their purposes.

Postoperative Nursing Care

The postoperative nursing care of the patient varies according to the type of prostate surgery performed. The general principles of postoperative nursing care that apply to all patients having major surgery are necessary for the patient undergoing a prostatectomy.

TURP and suprapubic prostatectomy patients will return from surgery with a three-way urethral catheter connected to continuous bladder irrigation (CBI) with sterile normal saline. Bloody urine is usual for the first few days following the surgery. To decrease clot formation, the flow rate is adjusted to keep the urine diluted to a reddish-pink, clearing to a pink tinge within 48 hours. Some pieces of tissue and small clots will be seen in the drainage. Additional intermittent irrigation with 20 to 30 mL of normal saline may be needed to clear the catheter of obstruction. Hemorrhage is a possible complication and occurs most frequently in the first 24 hours. Vital signs are monitored every 2 hours. An elevated pulse combined with a drop in blood pressure indicates hemorrhage and shock. Persistent bleeding turning the urine darker than cherry red or bright red, viscous drainage with many clots should be reported to the surgeon. Traction may be applied to the catheter to supply pressure to prevent excessive bleeding. The surgeon does this by taping the catheter to the thigh or abdomen. The nurse checks frequently to see that the catheter and tubing are not kinked and that outflow is appropriate. Irrigation is continued for 2 to 3 days. The patient may have some frequency and burning after the catheter is discontinued. Some blood in the urine is not unusual for several more days.

The patient who has had a suprapubic prostatectomy will have a suprapubic catheter in addition to a urethral catheter. Each catheter is attached to a separate sterile drainage system. After the urethral catheter is removed (sometime after the third day), the suprapubic catheter is clamped, and the patient attempts to void. Residual urine is measured afterward by unclamping the suprapubic catheter. When there is no more than 75 mL of residual urine after voiding, the suprapubic catheter is removed. Dribbling of urine often occurs after prostatectomy but usually stops within about 6 months.

The nurse monitors the incisional dressings and changes them as often as necessary to keep the patient dry and comfortable. Urine is very irritating to the skin, and any area that is exposed to drainage is thoroughly cleansed before a new dressing is applied.

Prophylactic antimicrobials and analgesics are administered in the early postoperative period. Bladder spasms are often a problem for the post-TURP and post–suprapubic prostatectomy patient. Before giving medication, the nurse checks to see that the catheter is draining well, as obstruction can cause bladder spasm. Belladonna and opium (B and O) rectal suppositories are effective if they are given when the spasms first begin.

The patient who has had a radical prostatectomy needs good psychological care in addition

NURSING CARE PLAN 31-1

Selected nursing diagnoses, goals/outcome criteria, nursing interventions, and evaluations for a patient having a transurethral resection for benign prostatic hypertrophy

Situation: Mr. Dodge, a 78-year-old diabetic, is admitted for a transurethral resection. He has had difficulty starting and maintaining urination, dribbling of urine after voiding, nocturia, a small amount of hematuria, and burning on urination. He was scheduled for a transurethral prostatic resection.

He returned from the recovery room with an indwelling three-way catheter with continuous bladder irrigation. His blood pressure was 110/86; pulse, 74; and respirations, 16; his color was good and he was fully oriented.

Nursing Diagnosis	Goals/Outcome Criteria	Nursing Intervention	Evaluation
Potential alteration in tissue perfusion related to possible hemorrhage at surgical site. SUPPORTING DATA Had TURP, cherry red drainage in Foley bag; hemorrhage is a potential complication.	Blood loss will be minimal as evidenced by lightened color of urine. No signs of shock as evidenced by vital signs within normal limits.	Assess color and characteristics of urine drainage q 15 minutes for first 2 h, then q 2 h for 24 h, then q 4 h. Report change to dark red, viscous drainage with clots or drainage that is considerably darker in color for an extended period of time. Assess vital signs q 2 h for 24 h. Maintain traction on catheter if present for 6 to 8 h. Give stool softener daily and instruct him not to strain at stool. Caution not to cough vigorously.	Foley with Murphy drip in place draining light red urine with a few clots; VS stable; no signs of shock; stool softener given; continue plan.
Potential fluid imbalance (excess), related to possible absorption of irrigation fluid. SUPPORTING DATA TURP with fluid in contact with open vessels, continuous bladder irrigation.	Fluid balance is maintained as evidenced by balanced intake and output. Absence of signs and symptoms of fluid overload: pulmonary crackles, increased BP, confusion, weight gain, hyponatremia.	Accurately record I & O. Ascultate lungs q shift, assess level of consciousness, check lab values for hyponatremia. Monitor BP and assess for increase. Weigh daily and compare with previous weight.	Lungs clear to auscultation; Na^+, 110 mEq/L; BP, 128/82; no weight change; I = 5600, O = 5050; continue plan.
Pain related to presence of catheter, bladder spasms, and possible obstruction of catheter. SUPPORTING DATA Complains of bladder spasms; keeps asking for the catheter to be removed.	Bladder spasms will be controlled by medication as evidenced by patient's statement.	Catheter and tubing will be checked for patency frequently to prevent obstruction and bladder spasm. Keep continuous bladder irrigation flowing to flush the bladder and prevent clot formation. Remind patient not to try to void around catheter, as this can cause spasm. Administer analgesics and antispasmodics as ordered; assess for side effects and effectiveness. Provide comfort measures and quiet environment.	B and O suppository given at 8 and 1 for bladder spasms; effective; Murphy drip functioning; draining light red urine with scant clots; continue plan.
Potential for infection related to possible invasion of infectious organisms at surgical site. SUPPORTING DATA TURP; history of UTI; diabetic.	Patient will remain free of infection as evidenced by normal urinalysis, WBC count, and temperature.	Maintain strict aseptic technique when handling catheter and drainage system. Encourage 10 to 14 glasses of water during the day after catheter is removed to flush bladder. Monitor temperature, WBC count, and urine for signs of infection. Provide catheter care q shift.	Drinking a glass of water an hour; temp., 98.8°F.; WBC count, 6,800; urine clear with normal odor; no sign of infection; catheter care given; continue plan.

Nursing care plan continued on following page

NURSING CARE PLAN 31-1, *Continued*

Nursing Diagnosis	Goals/Outcome Criteria	Nursing Intervention	Evaluation
Knowledge deficit related to lack of knowledge regarding self-care after discharge. SUPPORTING DATA Asking questions about activity and work.	Patient will verbalize need for increased fluid intake and signs of infection. Patient will state activity that is not permitted. Patient will state what medication is for and when it is to be taken.	Instruct him to increase fluid intake to 10 to 14 glasses of water during the day. Tell him to avoid heavy lifting, driving, and sexual activity until permitted by the urologist. Instruct him to report new onset of burning on urination or cloudy urine. Explain what each medication is for and when it is to be taken. Provide written information about signs and symptoms of urethral stricture or infection and instruct him to report these symptoms to the urologist.	Teaching regarding medications and self-care complete; obtain feedback tomorrow.
Fear of alteration in sexual function related to TURP. SUPPORTING DATA States "Guess that ends my love life."	Patient will verbalize understanding that surgery should not interfere with intercourse once healing is complete.	Encourage verbalization of specific concerns. Explain that TURP does not interfere with ability to have an erection and orgasm, but that the spermatic fluid flows into the bladder rather than out the urethra.	Discussed specific concerns regarding intercourse; answered questions; states he is feeling more confident about resuming his "love life."

to attention for his physical needs. If he is faced with orchiectomy as part of his treatment, he may become very depressed and angry. Fear of what awaits him in both treatment and the progression of the disease is a major concern. The nurse provides emotional support, acceptance of his moods, and an ear to listen to his concerns.

Patients and their wives often worry about sexual activity after prostatectomy. Interference with sexual function depends on the type of

TABLE 31-1 PREOPERATIVE PROCEDURES FOR PROSTATECTOMY PATIENTS

Procedure	Purpose
Rectal examination	Digital examination of the prostate to determine site and presence of tumors.
Intravenous pyelogram (excretory urogram)	To rule out hydronephrosis and hydroureter and to demonstrate benign prostatic hypertrophy.
Urinalysis and midstream cultures	To detect possible pyuria, microscopic hematuria, and bacterial infections.
A 12- or 24-hour urine collection for creatinine clearance	To evaluate kidney function.
Coagulation studies	To rule out potential bleeding tendency.
Blood type and cross-match	To have blood available for replacement during and after surgery.
Urodynamic studies	To determine bladder's ability to empty completely.
Urethrogram	To detect strictures at various levels of the urethra.
Cystoscopy	To visualize bladder and to perform biopsy to rule out cancer of the prostate.

surgical procedure performed and the general health and mental outlook of the patient. The nurse encourages questions and exploration of these concerns and suggests resources for information on issues of sexual function.

Discharge Teaching

The prostatectomy patient is taught to drink 12 to 14 glasses of water during the day to keep urine flowing freely. Strenuous activities such as driving, walking more than a few blocks, lifting more than 8 lb, having sexual intercourse, playing at sports, or riding in a car for more than 25 minutes at a time are to be avoided for the first 2 to 3 weeks after discharge. If blood is noticed in the urine, the patient is instructed to lie down and rest, drink more fluids, and call the surgeon if the bleeding persists. Depending on his type of employment, the patient may return to work in 2 to 4 weeks after surgery, except after a radical procedure, when healing takes much longer.

VASECTOMY

Sterilization of the male by vasectomy is a popular method of permanent contraception. The term *vasectomy* refers to a surgical procedure performed on the vas deferens for the purpose of interrupting the continuity of this duct, which conveys the sperm at the time of ejaculation (Fig. 31–4). Some vasectomies can be successfully reversed by vasovasotomy at a later time if a man's life circumstances change.

The procedure is done on an outpatient basis in a clinic or physician's office with a local anesthetic. An incision is made into the scrotal sac on each side, and the vas is lifted out. A segment of the vas is cut out, the ends are bound, and the incision is closed.

The nurse instructs the patient to use ice applications and aspirin or acetaminophen for scrotal pain and swelling the first 12 to 24 hours postoperatively. It is recommended that the patient wear jockey shorts or a scrotal support for comfort. The patient is told to use another method of birth control until sperm counts are negative, because active sperm are still present in the vas.

IMPOTENCE

Impotence is the inability to achieve or maintain an erection that is firm enough for sexual intercourse more than 25% of the time. The problem is caused by a variety of psychological and physical disorders. Diabetes mellitus is one of the most common causes of impotence, which occurs in about 55% of diabetic men.

If, after extensive testing, the problem is determined to be physiologic, a penile prosthesis may be implanted surgically. There are various types of implants, including a semirigid type, a self-contained type activated by a pump device, and an inflatable prosthesis.

Preoperative care is the same as for other types of general surgery. Postoperatively the patient is monitored for urinary retention, infection, atelectasis, deep vein thrombosis, and other complications of anesthesia and general surgery.

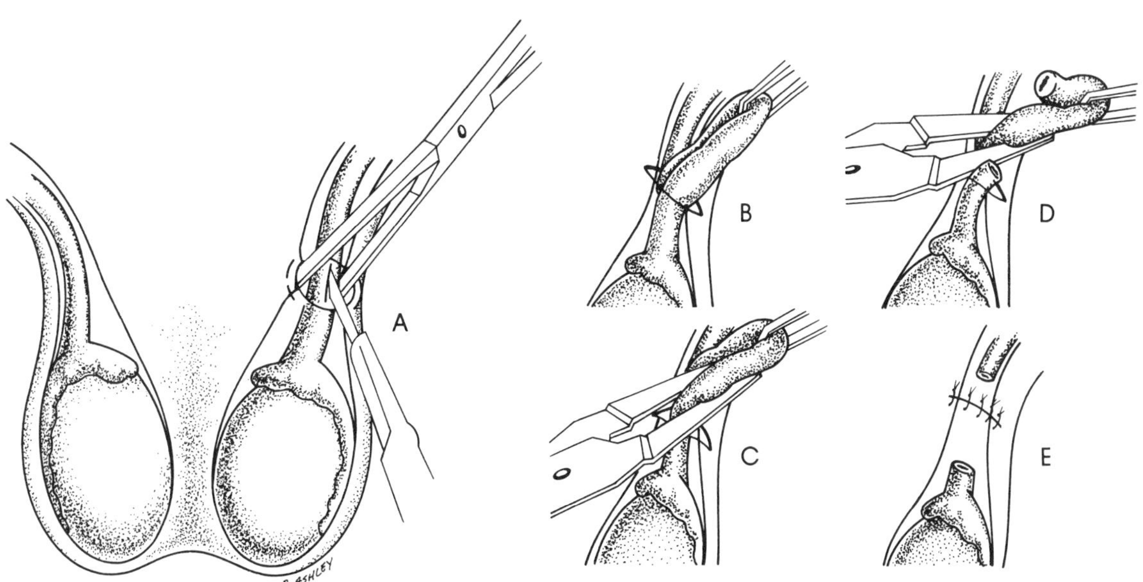

Figure 31–4 Vasectomy. *A*, Incision exposes sheath, which is then opened. Vas is exposed *(B)* and occluded with two clips *(C)*. *D*, Segment of about one-half inch is excised. *E*, Vas is replaced in sheath, and skin is sutured.

Concerns for the Elderly

Testosterone levels remain stable into old age. Impotence, if it occurs, is usually caused by factors other than low testosterone levels. There is a decrease in sperm production, but reproduction can take place. Sexual desire does not cease. The degree of sexual activity in the later years greatly depends on the general health of the patient, his energy level, the degree of sexual activity during his middle years, and the availability of a willing partner. Sexual stimulation is slower to take place and is not as intense as it is in the younger man.

BIBLIOGRAPHY

American Cancer Society: Cancer Facts and Figures—1990. Atlanta, 1990.

Andreoli, T. E., et al.: Cecil's Essentials of Medicine, 2nd ed. Philadelphia, W. B. Saunders, 1990.

Blackmore, C.: The impact of orchidectomy upon the sexuality of the man with testicular cancer. Cancer Nurs., Nov., 1988, p. 33.

Etchells, J. L.: Photodynamic laser therapy: A bladder cancer protocol. AORN J., Aug., 1988, p. 221.

Henrick-Rynning, T.: Prostatic cancer treatments and their effects on sexual functioning. Oncol. Nurs. Forum, June, 1987, p. 37.

Ignatavicius, D. D., and Bayne, M. J.: Medical-Surgical Nursing. Philadelphia, W. B. Saunders, 1991.

LaFollette, S. S.: Radical retropubic prostatectomy: Campbell and Walsh techniques . . . home study program. AORN J., Jan., 1987, p. 57.

McConnell, E. A.: Discovering a post T.U.R.P. complication. Nursing 89, Sept., 1989, p. 96.

Reno, D. R.: Men's knowledge and health beliefs about testicular cancer and testicular self-examination. Cancer Nurs., Nov., 1988, p. 112.

Schaufele, B.: Teaching testicular self-examination. Professional Nurse, March, 1988, p. 409.

Smith, D. B.: Sexual rehabilitation of the cancer patient. Cancer Nurs., Dec., 1989, p. 10.

Thompson, J. M., et al.: Clinical Nursing, 2nd ed. St. Louis, C. V. Mosby, 1989.

Walsh, P. C., et al.: Campbell's Urology. Philadelphia, W. B. Saunders, 1986.

STUDENT STUDY AIDS

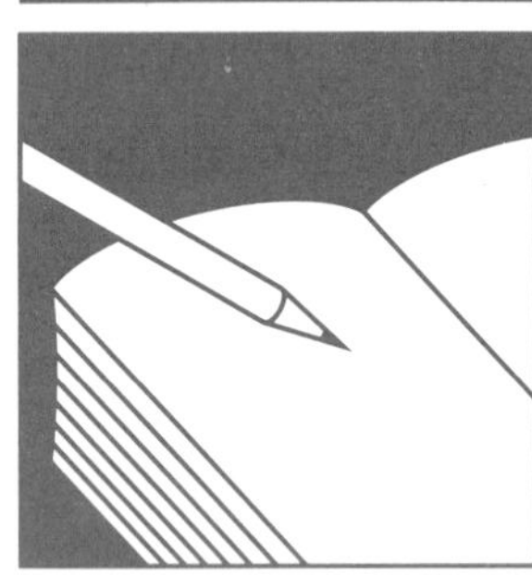

CLINICAL CASE PROBLEMS

Read each clinical situation and discuss the questions with your classmates.

1. Your brother, who is 20 years old, tells you of a friend who has just learned that he has testicular cancer and is scheduled for surgery tomorrow. Your brother is concerned about the effect the surgery will have on his friend's "manhood." He also says that if ever he has that kind of cancer, he doesn't want to know about it, and he certainly wouldn't allow surgery.

- What information could you give your brother about testicular cancer and self-examination of the testes?
- How could you explain that removal of a testis does not render a man less masculine?

2. Mr. Williams, age 67, has been admitted to the hospital to undergo a transurethral resection of the prostate. He is assigned to your care on his second postoperative day. Mr. Williams seems disoriented and restless, and when you begin to give him his bath, he tells you that his bladder is full and he needs to urinate. You check the catheter and find that it apparently is not draining as it should.

- What would you tell Mr. Williams about his need to void?
- What would you do about the catheter, which seems obstructed?
- What observations should you make while caring for this patient?
- What special precautions should be taken for his safety?

STUDY OUTLINE

I. Diagnostic tests and procedures and nursing implications

A. Examination of genitalia: by inspection and palpation.

1. Palpation of prostate and seminal vesicles by gloved finger inserted into rectum. Size, consistency, and presence of nodules evaluated.
2. Provide privacy during examination; explain steps and purposes of examination.

B. Biopsy of the prostate: to rule out or confirm malignancy, determine cause of enlarged prostate.
   1. May experience pain or discomfort during procedure.
   2. After biopsy, pressure applied to needle insertion site to prevent hematoma.
   3. Instruct patient to watch for signs of hematoma, infection, and gross bleeding or urinary retention.

C. Semen analysis: to determine volume of fluid and motility and number of sperm. Also to detect organisms causing infection, and for medicolegal reasons.

D. Testicular self-examination (TSE): to be done monthly for early detection of testicular tumors.

II. Nursing assessment

A. Age is relevant.

B. History taking: do not assume male patient is reluctant to discuss problems related to reproductive organs and sexual activity.
   1. Begin with less sensitive questions about urinary function; then progress to questions about reproductive organs and sexual activity.
   2. Ask open-ended questions; relate symptoms to activities of daily living.
   3. Be sure you and patient are talking about the same things. Patient may not use terms understood by the nurse and vice versa.
   4. Gather information about patterns of urination, penile discharge, tumors or masses noted by patient or someone else, tenderness or pain, impotence, sterility.
   5. Personal and family history of endocrine disorders and prostate and testicular cancer.

III. Inflammations and infections of the male reproductive organs

A. Causative organisms include common pyogenic and colonic organisms and *Neisseria gonorrhoeae*, also organisms that cause vaginitis in women.

B. Nonspecific urethritis (also called nongonococcal urethritis [NGU]) not caused by any specific organism.
   1. Symptoms include mucopurulent urethral discharge, dysuria, occasionally hematuria.
   2. Treatment: oral antibiotics and sulfonamides.

C. Epididymitis: inflammation caused by strenuous exercise or infection; often caused by *Chlamydia trachomatis* in men under 35.

D. Orchitis: inflammation of the testis, usually caused by infection.

E. Prostatitis: inflammation of the prostate. Can be acute or chronic; can be difficult to eradicate.

F. Medical treatment and nursing intervention:
   1. Antibacterials.
   2. Surgical correction of existing structural defect.
   3. Active and passive immunity to prevent effects of mumps.
   4. Instruction of patient in personal hygiene and avoidance of factors that predispose to infections.
   5. Encourage both sexual partners to be treated simultaneously to avoid reinfecting one another.
   6. Warm sitz baths. Extreme heat to be avoided because of possibility of destroying spermatozoa.
   7. Elevation of scrotum and application of ice bag. Athletic scrotal support when patient is ambulatory.
   8. Other measures to deal with fatigue, weakness, and fever.

IV. Testicular cancer

A. One of the most common cancers in men between ages 15 and 34 years.

B. Cryptorchidism places person at greater risk.

C. Biopsy never performed, as it tends to spread malignant cells.

D. Surgical treatment: surgical removal of testis; more extensive surgery and radiation if metastasis has occurred.

1. Effects of surgery and radiation on potence and ability to have children depends on type and amount of tissue damage.

E. Nursing intervention must include helping patient deal with perceived effects on his masculinity.

V. Tumors of the prostate

A. Prostate encircles urethra; enlargement of gland can cause urinary retention.

B. Benign prostatic hypertrophy (BPH) more common in older males.

C. Cancer of the prostate treated by surgery and possibly radiation.

D. Symptoms: usually none until growth obstructs urinary flow through urethra. Enlargement can be felt on rectal examination.

E. Surgical treatment: surgical removal of all or part of prostate.

1. Transurethral prostatic resection (TURP): part or all of the gland removed by way of the urethra, using an endoscope.
2. Suprapubic prostatectomy: gland removed by incision into bladder.
3. Retropubic prostatectomy: gland removed by low abdominal incision.
4. Perineal prostatectomy: U-shaped incision in perineum, through which gland is removed.
5. Radical prostatectomy: done by any of the above methods, but gland, capsule, neck of the bladder, and the regional lymph nodes are removed; performed for malignancy.
6. Preoperative nursing care: maintain urinary flow, protect patient from injury from falls, explain all procedures.
7. Postoperative nursing care: guard against hemorrhage, but realize that bleeding is expected, maintain urinary flow, change dressing (if any) to keep patient dry and comfortable.
   a. Patient education should include information about sexual activity.

VI. Vasectomy

A. Removal of a section from each vas deferens for the purpose of preventing impregnation.

VII. Impotence has many physical and psychological causes.

A. Physical cause may be treated with penile implant.

VIII. Concerns for the elderly

A. Slower and less intense response to sexual stimulation.

B. Generally capable of reproduction into old age.

CHAPTER 32

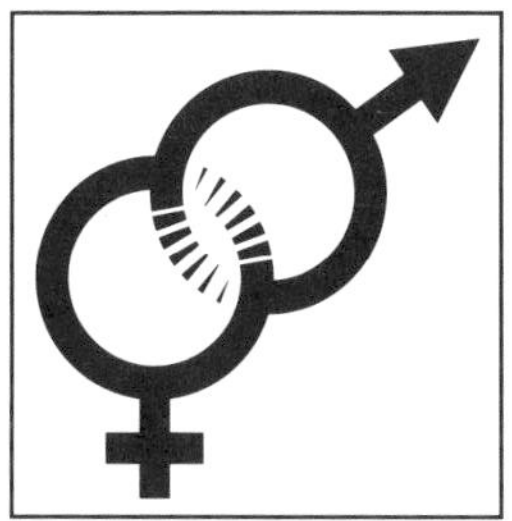

Care of Patients With Sexually Transmitted Diseases

VOCABULARY

chancroid
genital
heterosexual
HIV
recurrent
retinitis
spirochete
tertiary
venereal

Upon completion of this part of the chapter the student should be able to:

1. Identify the signs and symptoms of the following commonly transmitted sexual diseases: syphilis, gonorrhea, genital herpes, venereal warts (condylomata), and AIDS.
2. Compare the symptoms of gonorrhea in the male and in the female.
3. Describe the treatment of gonorrhea and the potential consequences of failure to treat this disease.
4. Specify nursing responsibilities in the diagnosis and treatment of syphilis and prevention of its progression to the secondary and tertiary stages.
5. Describe the characteristics of genital herpes, its treatment, and the resources available to those needing information about it.
6. List the ways in which the AIDS virus is transmitted.
7. Identify specific things people can do to try to prevent contracting the AIDS virus.

Throughout the world the incidence of infections transmitted through sexual contact is rising. The term *sexually transmitted diseases* (STDs) is used for those particular diseases that are spread from one person to another by means of sexual intercourse, either between heterosexual or homosexual partners or by intimate contact with the genitals, mouth, or rectum. These diseases can also be transmitted to the fetus or newborn through the blood or during the birth process. The human immunodeficiency virus (HIV) can be transmitted by contact with blood containing the virus. People who had blood transfusions in the decade before the tests for detection of the virus were available may be carriers of the virus.

Any sexually active person may be at risk for an STD. Persons who have sexual contact with multiple partners are at very high risk. Many of these infections can lie dormant for years; thus even those in monogamous relationships are at some risk if either partner was sexually active with someone else prior to the relationship.

Although the appearance of acquired immunodeficiency syndrome (AIDS) has captured the most attention, the five "classic" STDs still present problems. These include the well-known syphilis and gonorrhea infections and the less familiar diseases of chancroid, lymphogranuloma venereum, and granuloma inguinale. The Centers for Disease Control (CDC) estimate that there are 3 million new cases of gonorrhea and about 35,000 new cases of syphilis each year in the United States. There are no reliable statistics for the "new generation" of STDs—chlamydia, genital herpes, venereal warts (condylomata acuminata), and other infections that are very commonly transmitted sexually—but they are probably contracted in even greater numbers. Hepatitis B and various types of vaginitis are also in this group of disorders.

GONORRHEA

Of the various types of sexually transmitted diseases, gonorrhea is the most reported. In spite of intensive efforts to eradicate the disease, it is still a menace to public health. The infection is caused by *Neisseria gonorrhoeae*, which is easily transferred from one person to another by sexual contact.

SYMPTOMS AND MEDICAL DIAGNOSIS

The symptoms of gonorrhea usually appear in the male within a week after exposure to the organism, but they can take as long as 3 weeks to develop. Not everyone who is infected has noticeable symptoms. About 10% to 40% of all males and 90% of females with gonorrhea are asymptomatic.

In the male the infection and resultant inflammation usually cause dysuria and the discharge of a whitish fluid or yellowish pus from the penis. If the condition remains untreated, the discharge increases in amount and continues for months. As the infection spreads to other tissues, complications such as inflammation of the prostate and testes can occur and can eventually cause sterility.

The female infected with gonorrhea may feel no pain and notice no early symptoms, or she might have a vaginal discharge, pain in the lower abdomen, and burning during urination. If the infection continues to spread, it will eventually involve the uterine tubes and ovaries and cause sterility. The infection may involve the kidneys, bladder, rectum, and eyes. An infant can become infected as he passes through the birth canal of his mother if she has an active case of gonorrhea. Gonorrheal conjunctivitis can cause blindness. To avoid this, it is a law that immediately after birth every newborn infant must be given eyedrops of either silver nitrate or an antibiotic such as penicillin, erythromycin, or tetracycline.

Sometimes gonorrheal infection attacks the joints, causing a painful arthritis. As the infection spreads, it can cause meningitis or peritonitis and may be fatal if the gonococci enter the blood stream and lodge in the valves of the heart.

Diagnosis of gonorrhea is confirmed by the presence of the organism in smears and cultures taken from the discharge.

MEDICAL TREATMENT AND NURSING INTERVENTION

Most types of gonorrhea can be cured with comparative speed if the infection is treated in its earlier stages. Penicillin and other antibacterials such as ampicillin, erythromycin, and tetracyclines in combination are effective in overcoming the infection. The treatment for gonorrhea recommended by the CDC is a 250-mg injection of ceftriaxone (Rocephin) plus oral doxycycline (100 mg bid for 1 week). In case of allergy, spectinomycin or a combination of other antibiotics is used. All sexual partners must be treated at the same time, and there must be no sexual contact during treatment.

Every patient under treatment is encouraged to return for follow-up evaluation, because gonorrhea cannot be considered cured until cultures taken from the discharge are negative for 3 to 4 weeks. The patient also should understand that having a case of gonorrhea does not render a person immune; therefore reinfection is possible.

Although patients are often reluctant to divulge the name or names of their sexual partners, it is not possible to eradicate the disease without effective treatment of all infected persons. The cooperation of the patient with an active case is important to adequate treatment of those who have infected him or are likely to have been infected by him.

Nurses who have contact with the vaginal or penile discharge of a patient with gonorrhea must be careful to follow universal precautions and wear gloves when in contact with body secretions or linens and pads that are contaminated. Gloves must be changed between patients, and hands are washed as soon as gloves are removed. Gown, mask, and goggles or a face guard must be worn when any procedure is done on the patient that might expose the nurse to secretions. Any accidental contamination of the mucous membranes or of an open skin lesion of the nurse should immediately be reported to the infection control officer, a staff member of employee health, or her private physician. Her condition can then be monitored and treatment started as indicated.

The nurse's role is mainly that of teacher and counselor for the general public and the patient with an STD. Safe sexual practices, the need for examinations for STDs in sexually active people, and information on the signs and symptoms of STDs are the areas of information most needed by the general public.

Patients who have STDs need emotional support, information about the treatment of the disease, and teaching regarding safe sexual practices. Universal precautions and thorough, frequent hand washing are essential when caring for a patient with any STD.

Nursing diagnoses for the patient who has an STD may include:

- Knowledge deficit related to ways of transmission, signs and symptoms, and treatment.
- Pain related to inflammation.
- Anxiety related to need to contact partners.
- Fear of becoming HIV positive.
- Noncompliance related to repeated infection with STDs and refusal to use condoms.

SYPHILIS

Syphilis is also a sexually transmitted disease, but it is a more generalized disease affecting the entire body and not limited to the genital organs only. It is caused by a spirochete, *Treponema pallidum*. The causative organism of syphilis cannot survive without moisture, and it can be destroyed with plain soap. Because the spirochete must be wet and warm to survive, syphilis is nearly always transmitted by direct bodily contact; it is extremely rare for the disease to be transmitted by inanimate objects such as toilet seats or eating utensils.

It is possible for an infant to be born with an active case of syphilis, because the spirochete can pass the placental barrier once the fetus has reached the fourth month of development. About 50% of expectant mothers who have an active case of syphilis that is not treated will bear an infant with congenital syphilis. The disease can be fatal to the infant, or it can lead to physical deformities and mental disorders.

MEDICAL DIAGNOSIS

The common tests used for diagnosis of primary and secondary syphilis are the venereal disease research laboratory (VDRL) and rapid plasma reagin (RPR) tests. However, false-positive reactions can occur if the person has a viral or bacterial infection, a chronic systemic illness, or nonsyphilitic treponemal disease.

The VDRL or RPR test usually requires only a small sample of blood, but it can also be performed on a sample of cerebrospinal fluid obtained by lumbar puncture to determine the presence of neurosyphilis in the tertiary stage of the illness.

The patient should be advised not to drink alcohol for 24 hours before the test, as this can produce a transient false-positive reaction. There is no need, however, for any limiting of fluid or food intake.

The fluorescent treponemal antibody absorption (FTA-ABS) test is more sensitive than the VDRL in identifying all stages of untreated syphilis, and can be used to verify or rule out false-positive reactions to the VDRL. It also requires a sample of blood that should be handled gently to prevent hemolysis. No special preparation is needed; a negative result (no fluorescence) indicates the absence of syphilis.

SYMPTOMS

The symptoms of syphilis are not very severe in the early stage of the disease. Some symptoms have a way of subsiding and then reappearing, and the patient unfortunately may not be aware of the serious and permanent damage being done to vital organs of his body until it is too late. This is doubly tragic, because the disease can be cured and serious complications avoided if it is treated in its earliest stages.

There are three stages of syphilis: *primary*, *secondary*, and *tertiary* (late). In the primary stage, a chancre or hard sore appears on the mucous membrane of the mouth or the genitalia. It often goes unnoticed in women. The chancre is teeming with spirochetes, and therefore the individual is highly infectious at this stage. Within 3 to 7 days after infection, the spirochetes enter the blood stream, where they begin to multiply rapidly. Other symptoms of the first stage may include headache and some enlargement of the lymph glands near the chancre, but generally, the infected person does not feel very sick. The chancre and other symptoms disappear within 3 to 8 weeks, and if the patient has used some salve or patent medicine with the mistaken idea that the chancre was a minor infection, he may falsely conclude that the medicine had cured him. Nothing could be farther from the truth, because the disease has now entered the second stage, and spirochetes have invaded his blood stream.

Symptoms of the secondary stage of syphilis vary in individuals. Some may feel basically all right, with only slight malaise or headache. Others may develop a skin rash or sore throat, or they may lose patches of hair from the scalp. There also may be some arthritis, neuritis, or retinitis. Eventually these symptoms subside (though they may reappear), and the disease enters a latent (noninfectious) period.

The tertiary stage of syphilis can begin 1 year after infection, but more often it is 4 or 5 years before the serious effects of the infection are first noticed. In some people, the disease may lie dormant for 20 years before symptoms of the third stage appear. Because the spirochetes have had free access to all tissues of the body, the damage they have caused can present a wide variety of symptoms. The nervous system, blood vessels, and eyes are most often affected.

MEDICAL TREATMENT AND NURSING INTERVENTION

Penicillin is the drug of choice in treating syphilis. Other drugs that can be used as alternatives in case of sensitivity to penicillin include tetracycline and erythromycin. Usually the patient receives 2.4 million units given intramuscularly. The patient must be closely watched for signs of allergic reaction, usually anaphylaxis. He is instructed to return for periodic check-ups. There is no immunity conferred by an attack of the disease, and a person can become infected with syphilis again and again.

One of the most important aspects of treating and controlling syphilis and other sexually transmitted diseases is proper education of the public so that their cooperation can be gained.

One person with many sexual partners can be responsible for infecting several others, who in turn become sources of infection for still others, and the chain reaction can be almost endless. Locating those who have been in contact with an infected person can be a time-consuming and often thankless job, because it necessarily involves asking personal questions and requires convincing the people involved that a simple treatment can prevent very serious complications in later life. The nurse should realize that many of those infected are teenagers who fear being found out by their families and friends and who do not fully appreciate the seriousness of the disease. She must use tact and understanding with these patients, avoid treating them with disgust or censuring them, and encourage them to cooperate with Public Health officials and other members of the health team who are striving to locate and treat infected people.

GENITAL HERPES

Genital herpes (HSV 2) is rapidly approaching gonorrhea as the most prevalent sexually transmitted disease in the United States. It is estimated that almost one-half million new cases occur each year. The rapid increase in incidence is due in part to the fact that the disease currently is incurable and symptoms tend to recur throughout a person's lifetime. Another contributing factor is believed to be the sexual freedom and consequent increased sexual activity of young adults.

The word *herpes* refers to a class of over 50 viruses that share many of the same characteristics. Herpes simplex virus (HSV) types 1 and 2 cause genital herpes. Herpes viruses invade healthy human tissues and rely on their host to provide the materials needed to produce the RNA and DNA necessary for their replication.

Once HSV gains access to the body it enters the nervous system and invades nerve cells located near the site of infection, usually in the sacral ganglia. The virus lies dormant in nerve cells and can remain there indefinitely, predisposing the person to periodic flare-ups of symptoms.

Factors related to recurrent appearances of the symptoms of genital herpes are not well understood. Some infected persons experience no recurrences, while others are plagued with frequent and severe outbreaks. Many patients have reported a correlation between the appearance of lesions and such precipitating factors as exposure to sunlight, local trauma, fever, emotional stress, and hormonal changes during the menstrual cycle.

Genital herpes is highly contagious and is spread by direct person-to-person contact. Its transmission is not limited to sexual contact. Self-inoculation is possible; for example, transferring the virus from a lip ulcer to the genitals. Viral shedding may occur when the disease is active, even if there are no outward symptoms.

SYMPTOMS AND MEDICAL DIAGNOSIS

Genital HSV is diagnosed on the basis of the patient's history and the symptoms presented, which are easily recognized by an experienced clinician. Clinical and serologic tests can help establish whether the patient has a primary infection or is in the initial phase of a recurrent episode.

A diagnostic blood test called the Simplex-2 is specific for HSV 2 and can detect primary or secondary herpes infection even when the patient is without symptoms. It is especially valuable for screening pregnant women whose infants are at risk for herpes during vaginal delivery. Diagnosis by culture is most accurate. A new test called *Herp-Check* can detect the presence of HSV within 4 hours.

Herpes initially causes a tingling or burning sensation in the genital area, which is followed by a rash and itching. Eventually small blisters form on the surface of the skin. These lesions enlarge, break open, and ulcerate. The lesions are painful, especially during coitus, and can cause urinary retention if they involve the urethra.

In the male, the lesions are found on the glans penis, shaft of the penis, and prepuce and can extend to the scrotal sac and inner thighs. In the female, the eruptions usually are located on the vulva, vaginal surface, and buttocks. Lesions on the cervix can vary from small superficial ulcers with diffuse inflammation to a single, large, necrotic ulcer. It is known that genital herpes in the female considerably increases the risk of cervical cancer. There also is danger to the infant born of a mother with genital herpes. The newborn is infected as it passes through the vaginal canal. Hence the general practice is to deliver infants of mothers with active genital herpes by cesarean section.

MEDICAL TREATMENT

At the present time there is no cure for genital herpes. In 1982 the Federal Drug Administration approved the first antiviral drug for the treatment of HSV in the United States. The drug, acyclovir, prevents the virus from making the RNA and DNA necessary for its continued life and thereby shortens healing time during the initial phase. However, the drug cannot be used during pregnancy. It is given orally for 7 to 10 days for initial infection.

NURSING INTERVENTION

The external genitalia and perineum should be examined for lesions. The patient is taught to use scrupulous hand-washing techniques after any contact with the infected area. Herpes lesions must be kept clean and dry to prevent secondary infection. Sitz baths decrease discomfort, and Burow's solution soaks can also be ordered to reduce pain. Ice packs are sometimes helpful.

Increased fluids are advised to dilute urine. Voiding while sitting in a tub of water or standing in the shower or while pouring water over the perineum will decrease pain.

Topical steroids can be applied to the lesions to hasten healing, and local anesthetic sprays or ointments may be prescribed. Oral analgesics are administered as needed.

The nurse educates the patient about the role of poor nutrition, stress, and insufficient rest in recurrent outbreaks. It is very important for a patient, if she becomes pregnant, to tell her physician about her herpes infection, as it can cause a major threat to her baby. The relationship of genital herpes and cervical cancer is addressed, and the patient is encouraged to have yearly Pap tests done.

The nurse should counsel the patient about the possibility of spreading herpes through intimate contact, even when symptoms are not apparent, and recommend the use of condoms for all sexual exposure.

Universal precautions must be followed when dealing with secretions, including saliva, from the patient who has herpes type 1 or 2 lesions anywhere on the body. Double gloving or sturdy rubber gloves provide the most protection.

Because of the widespread incidence of genital herpes and the emotional trauma suffered by its victims, the American Social Health Association has established the Herpes Resource Center (formerly called HELP). Information about the national organization and its local chapters can be obtained by writing to Herpes Resource Center, Box 100, Palo Alto, CA 94302.

CHLAMYDIA TRACHOMATIS

According to the CDC, chlamydia was the most commonly transmitted bacteria in America in 1988, and there are an estimated 4 million acute cases annually (Centers for Disease Control, 1989a). This organism causes about half of the cases of epididymitis and nongonococcal urethritis in men. In women, 30% to 50% of pelvic inflammatory disease (PID) is caused by chlamydia. The disease can be transmitted during vaginal delivery, with resultant eye infection and pneumonia in the newborn.

SYMPTOMS AND MEDICAL DIAGNOSIS

In men, the primary symptom of chlamydia is dysuria, frequency of urination, and a watery, mucuslike discharge. About 75% of infected women have no symptoms. Symptoms of cervicitis may occur with vaginal discharge, urinary frequency, and soreness, itching, or pulling in the vaginal area. Often a woman will simply notice an odor that she had not noticed before. After intercourse, the odor is often "fishy."

Diagnosis is usually made by smear and Gram stain of secretions to identify polymorphonuclear leukocytes (WBCs) and rule out the presence of the gram-negative organism of gonorrhea. Cultures can absolutely identify the bacteria but are expensive. A new test, the fluorescein-labeled monoclonal antibody test, provides results within 30 minutes and is less expensive.

The drug of choice for treatment of chlamydia is doxycycline, a tetracycline. If the patient is allergic to tetracycline or is pregnant, erythromycin can be substituted.

NURSING INTERVENTION

Nursing intervention is directed at educating women regarding the need for examination and treatment any time an unusual vaginal discharge is discovered. Pelvic inflammatory disease resulting from chlamydia infection is becoming a frequent cause of infertility.

VENEREAL WARTS (CONDYLOMATA ACUMINATA)

The human papilloma viruses cause venereal warts, which can be flat or raised, rough, cauliflower-like growths on the vulva, penis, perianal area, vaginal or rectal walls, or cervix. The incubation period is 1 to 3 months. These warts are common among sexually active people, as they are highly contagious.

There are several different types of virus that cause the growths. The flat variety are more likely to contribute to tissue changes that lead to cervical cancer. The papilloma viruses can be transmitted to infants during birth.

SYMPTOMS AND MEDICAL TREATMENT

The warts may cause itching or become excoriated from scratching. Dysuria, vaginal discharge, and bleeding after intercourse may occur. Diagnosis is made on the appearance of external growths. Vaginal and cervical areas require culposcopy and biopsy for accurate identification.

Treatment is by freezing, laser therapy, surgical removal, or topical chemotherapy. Podophyllin resin is an alternative treatment for external warts. All sexual partners must be treated concurrently. No therapy has been shown to eradicate the papilloma virus, and patients are told that they may have recurrent lesions at any time.

NURSING INTERVENTION

Patient education about the mode of transmission, treatment, and complications is the focus of nursing care. Patients are encouraged to use condoms to reduce spreading the disease.

Any woman who has had condylomata acuminata is encouraged to have frequent Pap smears because of the increased incidence of cervical cancer.

AIDS AND ARC

AIDS and AIDS-related complex (ARC) are the most serious of the STDs, because AIDS is ultimately fatal. AIDS results from a chronic retroviral infection that destroys the cell-mediated immune system. ARC is similar to AIDS, but the patient is not as ill. Both AIDS and ARC patients test positive for the human immunodeficiency virus. This virus is transmitted in three ways: (1) by unprotected sexual contact; (2) by blood or blood products, including equipment contaminated with infected blood (IV and injection needles), and (3) from infected mother to fetus in utero or to baby by breast milk. Although most of the people with AIDS are homosexual men or IV drug abusers, there is now an increase of infection in heterosexuals.

Rubber condoms are the only protection against sexual transmission and should be used for each sexual encounter in order to slow the spread of this disease.

AIDS is covered more thoroughly in Chapter 7.

SAFE SEXUAL PRACTICES

For protection against STDs, the CDC recommends having sex with only one monogamous person and avoiding sexual contact with people who have had multiple partners. The sexual partner should be well known; persons at high risk for STDs should be avoided. Rubber condoms lubricated with a substance containing nonoxynol-9 are to be used as a barrier, unless the couple is in a long-term monogamous relationship and neither is in a high-risk category. Anal intercourse should be avoided. Vaginal spermicides also help prevent spread of some STDs. Thorough washing of the hands and of the genital/rectal area before and after intercourse will reduce the number of germs and secretions. Gargling with an antiseptic mouthwash or with a solution of hydrogen peroxide (one part to three parts water) may slightly reduce the risk of oropharyngeal STD infection. The genital area should be examined for sores, pus, or rashes before sexual contact, and contact should be avoided if such signs are present. Water-soluble, rather than oil-based, lubricants will reduce the spread of germs. Vaginal spermicidal contraceptives that are germicidal and virucidal are helpful. Excessive douching should be avoided so that a normal vaginal flora can be maintained.

Voiding after intercourse, especially for men, may reduce the incidence of some types of STDs.

The nurse should encourage any patient who has multiple sexual partners to have at least biannual examinations for STDs.

BIBLIOGRAPHY

Andreoli, T. E., et al.: Cecil Essentials of Medicine, 2nd ed. Philadelphia, W. B. Saunders, 1990.

Andrist, L. C.: Taking a sexual history and educating clients about safe sex. Nurs. Clin. North Am., Dec., 1988, p. 959.

Betolli, E. J.: Herpes: Facts and fallacies. Am. J. Nurs., June, 1982, p. 924.

Bourcier, K. M., and Seidler, A. J.: Chlamydia and condylomata acuminata: An update for the nurse practitioner. J. Obstet. Gynecol. Neonatal Nurs. Jan./Feb., 1987, p. 17.

Breslin, E.: Genital herpes simplex. Nurs. Clin. North Am., Dec., 1988, p. 907.

Centers for Disease Control: 1989 sexually transmitted diseases treatment guidelines (special issue). Morbidity and Mortality Weekly Report, 38 (suppl. 8), 1989, p. 1.

Centers for Disease Control: Sexually transmitted disease statistics 1990, issue 139. Atlanta, 1990.

Deitch, K. V., and Smith, J. E.: Symptoms of chronic vaginal infection and microscopic condyloma in women. J. Obstet. Gynecol. Neonatal Nurs., March/April, 1990, p. 19.

Dirubbo, N.: The condom barrier. Am. J. Nurs., Oct., 1987, p. 1306.

Fogel, C. I.: Gonorrhea: Not a new problem but a serious one. Nurs. Clin. North Am., Dec., 1988, p. 885.

Kee, J. L.: Laboratory and Diagnostic Tests With Nursing Implications, 2nd ed. Norwalk, CT, Appleton-Century-Crofts, 1987.

Loucks, A.: Chlamydia: An unheralded epidemic. Am. J. Nurs., July, 1987, p. 920.

Lovejoy, M. C.: Precancerous lesions of the cervix: Personal risk factors. Cancer Nurs., Feb., 1987, p. 2.

Lucas, V. A.: Human papilloma virus infection: A potentially carcinogenic sexually transmitted disease (condylomata acuminata, genital warts). Nurs. Clin. North Am., Dec., 1988, p. 917.

Lynch, J. M.: Helping patients through the recurring nightmare of herpes. Nursing 82, Oct., 1982, p. 52.

McElrose, P.: The "other" STDs: As dangerous as ever. RN, June, 1988, p. 51.

McMahon, K. M.: The integration of HIV testing and counseling into nursing practice. Nurs. Clin. North Am., Dec., 1988, p. 803.

Nettina, S. M.: When the patients with genital herpes turn to you for answers. Nursing 89, Aug., 1989, p. 61.

Secor, R. M.: Bacterial vaginosis: A comprehensive review. Nurs. Clin. North Am., Dec., 1988, p. 865.

Talashek, M. C., et al.: Sexually transmitted diseases in the elderly: Issues and recommendations. J. Gerontol. Nurs., April, 1990, p. 33.

Warmbrodt, L.: Herpes: the shock, the stigma, the ways you can help. RN, May, 1983, p. 47.

Whelan, M.: Nursing management of the patient with *Chlamydia trachomatis* infection. Nurs. Clin. North Am., Dec., 1988, p. 877.

Wyngaarden, J. B., and Smith, L. H., Jr.: Cecil Textbook of Medicine, 17th ed. Philadelphia, W. B. Saunders Co., 1985.

STUDENT STUDY AIDS

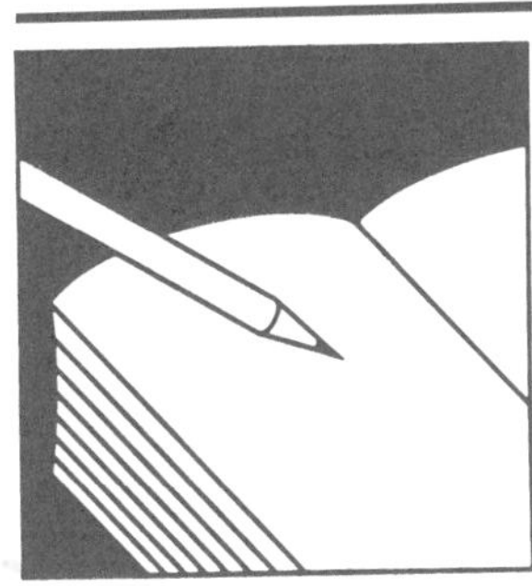

CLINICAL CASE PROBLEMS

Read the following clinical situation and discuss the questions with your classmates.

1. A friend of yours whom you have not seen since graduation from high school calls you unexpectedly on the phone, saying that she knows you are a student nurse and she has a question to ask about her health. She admits to having been sexually active with several partners and recently noticed some "blisters" on her lips and genitalia. She asks if they could be "syphilis sores" or perhaps herpes.

- What might you say to convince your friend that she needs to see an experienced clinician who can diagnose her disease?
- Where might she find such a person if she is not willing to go to her own physician?
- How would you explain the differences between the manifestations and complications of syphilis and herpes?
- What would you tell her about the difference in treatment of syphilis and genital herpes?

2. While at a party at a local club, a small group of friends in their early 20s are gathered in the restroom and the talk has turned to their sex life. It becomes apparent that several of them are active with more than one partner. You know that some of the people at the party use illegal drugs. You wonder about the danger of AIDS, as well as other STDs, for these people.

- How might you introduce the problem of AIDS into the conversation?
- How would you convince them that heterosexuals are also at risk for AIDS?

- What exactly would you tell them about protecting themselves against this disease?

STUDY OUTLINE

I. Introduction

A. Sexually transmitted diseases include the classic venereal diseases plus chlamydia, genital herpes, nonspecific urethritis, trichomoniasis, crab lice, and genital warts.

B. Sexually transmitted diseases include all diseases spread by sexual intercourse between heterosexual and homosexual partners or by any intimate contact with the genitals, mouth, and rectum.

II. Gonorrhea

A. The most common STD.

B. Symptoms and medical diagnosis:

1. Symptoms usually appear in the male within a week of exposure. Not all infected persons have symptoms.
2. Males can have dysuria, whitish or purulent discharge from the penis.
3. In the female, symptoms include vaginal discharge, lower abdominal pain, dysuria.
4. If untreated, infection can spread to bladder and kidney and to uterine tubes, causing infertility. Also can affect the joints and produce arthritis. If valves of the heart become involved, the infection can be fatal.
5. Gonococcal conjunctivitis can lead to blindness. All newborns must have eyedrops to prevent this.

C. Medical treatment and nursing intervention:

1. Ceftriaxone (Rocephin) given by injection, is the drug of choice; doxycycline is given orally for 1 week as well.
2. Patients must have follow-up evaluation; gonorrhea is not considered cured until cultures are negative for 3 to 4 weeks.
3. Teach patient that reinfection is possible; immunity is not established by having the disease.
4. Encourage reporting of sexual partners so they can be treated and will not reinfect patient.
5. Universal precautions are used to prevent spread of organisms.
6. A nurse who suspects that her eyes or skin may have been infected while caring for a patient should report the incident to the infection control officer or her private physician.

III. Syphilis

A. Spread by direct body contact. Can be spread from mother to unborn child.

B. Medical diagnosis: positive VDRL, RPR, or FTA-ABS test result.

C. Symptoms:

1. Primary stage: chancre, headache, enlarged lymph glands. Tends to be self-limiting; very infectious in this stage.
2. Secondary stage: usually asymptomatic but patient might have rash, loss of hair in patches, sore throat, arthritis, or neuritis.
3. Tertiary stage: symptoms will depend on organs infected; do not appear until damage has been done. Organs most often affected are blood vessels, heart, nerves, and eyes.

D. Medical treatment and nursing intervention:

1. Penicillin or other antibacterial will cure the disease and prevent progress to second and third stages.
2. Management of later stages is with combination of antibiotics.

IV. Genital herpes

A. Caused by herpes simplex virus, type 1 and 2 (HSV 1 and HSV 2).

B. Virus lies dormant in nerve tissue, usually in sacral ganglia.

C. Factors leading to recurrence of symptoms not well understood. Some patients report unusual physical or emotional stress just before outbreak.

D. Diagnosis made from symptoms. Culture of lesions is most accurate test. "Herp-Check" newest quick test.

1. Symptoms in male include lesions on glans and shaft of penis, scrotal sac, and inner thighs. In female, lesions are on vulva, vaginal surface, cervix, and buttocks. The lesions are blisters that erupt and become encrusted.
2. Genital herpes in the female greatly increases risk for cervical malignancy. Infant can get herpes from its mother when it is born. Mothers with active herpes usually must have cesarean section.

E. Treatment: there is no cure for the disease. Acyclovir holds the most promise for alleviating symptoms and hastening recovery.

F. Information and help for victims available from Herpes Resource Center.

G. Special precautions: Nurses should wear gloves on both hands when suctioning, giving mouth care, shaving, bathing, and changing the linen of patients with open lesions. Immunosuppressed patients are very susceptible to herpes.

V. *Chlamydia trachomatis* is the most commonly transmitted organism.

A. 75% of infected women have no symptoms.

B. May cause cervicitis.

C. Very frequent cause of PID and epididymitis.

D. In males, causes dysuria, discharge, and frequency of urination.

E. Diagnosis made by smear and Gram stain to rule out gonorrhea; fluorescein-labeled monoclonal antibody test is newest.

F. Treatment is with doxycycline; erythromycin can be substituted during pregnancy.

G. Nurse teaches patients to seek treatment for any different vaginal discharge to prevent incidence of PID.

VI. Venereal warts (condylomata acuminata) caused by human papilloma viruses

A. Highly contagious disease found very commonly in sexually active people.

B. Flat variety can cause tissue dysplasia, leading to cervical cancer.

C. Cauliflower-like growths appear on vulva, penis, perianal area.

D. May cause itching, dysuria, vaginal discharge, and bleeding after intercourse in the female.

E. Treatment: freezing, laser therapy, surgical removal or topical chemotherapy; podophyllin resin is an alternative for external warts.

F. Virus is never completely destroyed, just latent; can recur at any time.

G. Condoms are used as barrier to prevent the spread of condylomata acuminata.

H. Infected women need Pap smear at least semiannually.

VII. AIDS and ARC

A. AIDS: most serious of all STDs, because it is ultimately fatal.

B. Virus is transmitted in three ways:

1. Unprotected sexual contact.
2. Exposure to blood or blood products (IV and injection needles).

3. Infected mother to fetus in utero or to baby by breast milk.

C. Although most cases of AIDS are in homosexual men or IV drug abusers, there now is an increase among heterosexuals.

D. Abstinence from sexual contact is only known prevention.

E. Safe sex practices may lower incidence of the disease.

1. One sexual partner only.
2. Use rubber condoms for barrier protection.

VIII. Safe sex practices

A. There are practices that can decrease the spread of STDs.

B. Sexually active people should be examined at least twice a year for STDs.

CHAPTER 33

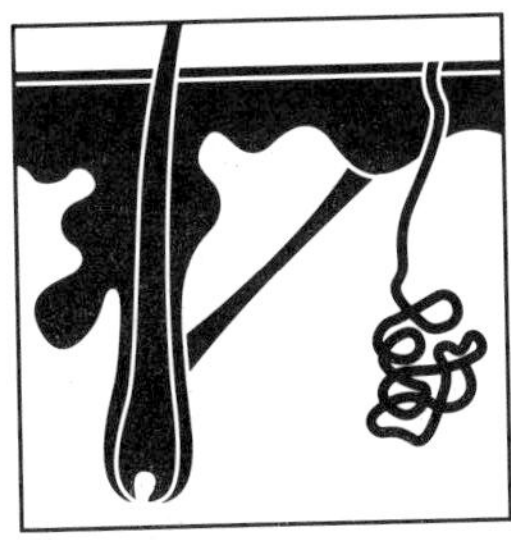

Care of Patients With Disorders of the Skin

VOCABULARY

comedo
débridement
erythrasma
eschar
exfoliate
fissure
fungated
lesion
lichenification
nodular
scaling
sebaceous
thermal

Upon completion of this chapter the student should be able to:

1. List etiologic factors in the development of primary and secondary skin disease.
2. State nursing responsibilities in the diagnosis of skin disorders, including self-examination of the skin.
3. List important factors in the prevention of skin disease.
4. List significant subjective and objective data in the nursing assessment of skin disease.
5. Describe the nursing care plan for the patient with a nursing diagnosis of impaired skin integrity.
6. List the main points of nursing care for patients with herpesvirus infections, impetigo, fungal infections, pediculosis, and scabies.
7. State important characteristics of the various types of skin cancer.
8. Describe five major points specific to the nursing care of patients with major burns.

The skin that covers our bodies is actually an organ and, like the liver or heart, is essential for the maintenance of life and good health. The skin functions very much like a built-in suit of armor; it is our first line of defense against invasion by the hordes of pathogenic bacteria living in our environment. The skin also protects us against loss of body heat by acting as a layer of insulation against changes in the temperature of our environment and as a cooling system that reduces the body temperature through the process of evaporation of moisture from the skin's surface. In addition, the skin functions as a container for body fluids and helps in the disposal of some of the body's waste products. Therefore intact skin is essential to the body's ability to maintain homeostasis.

When an area of the skin is destroyed by disease or trauma, its protective functions are immediately impaired, and the body is susceptible to infection. If very large areas of skin are destroyed, as in an extensive burn, fluid and electrolyte balance is disturbed, and body heat is lost.

Skin diseases are among the most common afflictions in humans. They are also extremely exasperating, because they often are difficult to diagnose and cure and they tend to recur. Although the physical effects of skin diseases usually are not extremely serious, it is difficult to measure the psychological impact of a disorder that renders one unattractive and threatens one's wholesome self-image and damages self-esteem.

Disorders that primarily affect the skin are legion, but the skin also reflects systemic diseases. In this chapter we are mainly concerned with diseases that are primary skin disorders; however, a knowledge of the patient's health history greatly improves the chances of making an accurate diagnosis of any abnormality of the skin.

There are over 3,000 disorders of the skin that have been officially named, and probably many more not included in any official nomenclature. The majority of the recognized and named skin disorders arise from some pathology in the skin itself; the remainder are manifestations of some systemic disease. The etiologic factors responsible for skin disorders, both primary and secondary, are shown in Figure 33–1.

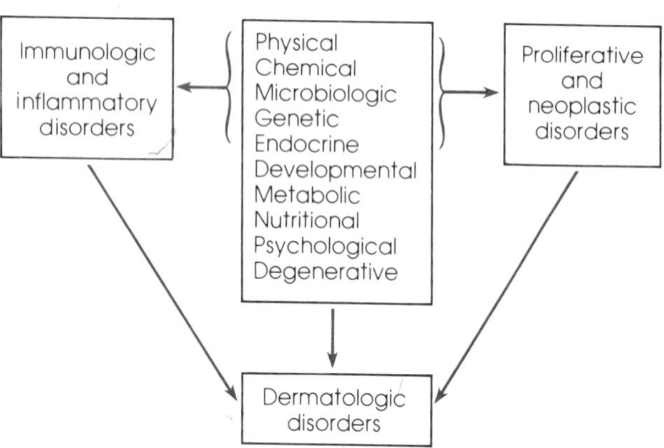

Figure 33–1 Etiologic factors in dermatologic disorders. (Adapted from Smith, L. H., Jr., and Thier, S. O.: Pathophysiology. The Biological Principles of Disease. Philadelphia, W. B. Saunders, 1981.)

Many patients with dermatologic disease are not hospitalized and are seen only in physicians' offices and outpatient clinics. Others do not seek medical attention but treat their skin disorder themselves with home remedies and over-the-counter drugs. In some cases self-care measures are successful, but they also have the potential for either aggravating the condition or temporarily relieving its more severe symptoms. This can lead to delay in treatment and allows the disease to progress to a chronic and sometimes untreatable state.

Caring for those who have a skin disorder can be particularly challenging to the nurse because of the recurrent nature of many skin disorders, the potential they have for disfigurement, and the added burden they can place on the patient when his skin disease can be spread to others.

DIAGNOSTIC TESTS AND PROCEDURES AND NURSING RESPONSIBILITIES

SKIN BIOPSY

Removal of a sample of tissue from a skin lesion usually is done with use of local anesthetic. It can be done by shaving a top layer off a lesion that raises above the skin line *(shave biopsy)*, by removing a core from the center of the lesion *(punch biopsy)*, or by excising the entire lesion *(excisional biopsy)*.

Skin biopsy is used to differentiate benign from malignant lesions and to help in the identification of the causative organism in bacterial and fungal infections.

No special preparation of the patient is necessary beyond giving him a simple explanation of the procedure and its purpose. If a local anesthetic is to be used, the patient should be asked about any personal or family history of allergies.

CULTURE AND SENSITIVITY TESTS

When a bacterial or fungal infection of the skin is suspected, the dermatologist may wish to know the causative organism and the drug most appropriate for treating a specific kind of infection. A sampling of exudate is taken from the lesion and sent to the laboratory for culturing. Once the organism has been cultured, colonies can be tested for sensitivity to certain antiinfective agents. These tests take the guesswork out of treating infectious skin disease and very quickly determine the drug that will be most effective in treating it.

As with the collection of any specimen for culture, care must be taken in handling the specimen and its container so as to avoid contamination of the person collecting and handling the specimen, the outside of the container, and the inside.

INSPECTION UNDER SPECIAL LIGHT

Inspection of the skin is one of the principal means by which skin lesions are diagnosed. To facilitate diagnosis of certain kinds of skin disorders, special lights may be used by the examiner.

A *cold light* is one in which the light is transmitted through a quartz or plastic structure to dissipate the heat. Because there is no danger of burning the skin, the cold light can be applied directly to the skin to illuminate its layers for visualization of malignant changes.

Wood's light is a specially designed ultraviolet light. The nickel-oxide filter holds back all but a few violet rays of the visible spectrum. This special light is especially useful in diagnosing fungal infections of the scalp and chronic bacterial infection of the major folds of the skin (*erythrasma*). Under Wood's light, fungal lesions and erythrasma are fluorescent. Erythrasma usually is seen on the inner thighs, the scrotum, the axilla, and the area between the toes.

SELF-EXAMINATION OF THE SKIN

All persons who have warts, moles, scars, or birthmarks should be taught how to do monthly evaluations of the lesions in order to detect malignant changes in their earliest stages.

Examination can be done by the patient himself or by someone in the family if the patient cannot see well or has difficulty inspecting the area of his body where the lesions are located. The changes the examiner is looking for include the following:

- A darkening or spreading of color.
- An increase in size.
- A change in shape; that is, the lesion becomes elevated, or its formerly regular edges become irregular.
- Redness or swelling of surrounding skin, or any other noticeable change around the lesion.
- Itching, tenderness, or other change in sensation.
- Crusting, scaling, oozing, ulcerating, or other change in the surface of the lesion.

NURSING ASSESSMENT OF SKIN LESIONS

HISTORY TAKING

The diagnosis of skin disorders often requires diligent detective work to identify factors that predispose a patient to or actually cause some type of skin disease. Each of the twelve etiologic factors shown in Figure 33–1 is significant in the history of a patient with a skin disorder.

In regard to the patient's presenting dermatologic disorder, it is important to find out when the lesion or rash first appeared or was first noticed, any particular event or events that took place prior to its appearance, and factors that seem to make it worse or better.

Some environmental factors that could contribute to the development of a skin disorder include exposure to chemicals and other irritants used by the person in performing his job doing household maintenance, or enjoying a hobby. Scabies, lice, and other parasites can be transmitted through close personal contact with infected persons at work, recreation, home, or school. Travel to a different geographic area and climate also is significant because some parasites and infectious organisms are more prevalent in warmer climates and tropical areas. If the patient has recently been exposed to severe cold, his skin may be drier than usual and he may complain of severe itching (*winter itch*).

It is particularly important that the nurse be alert to the possibility of a drug reaction. Almost all drugs can produce skin eruptions in certain individuals. Drug allergy or reaction can produce lesions and rashes that imitate any of a long list of diseases including measles, chickenpox, fungus infections, skin cancers, and psoriasis.

Family history of skin disease is relevant because many disorders such as psoriasis, acne vulgaris, and atopic allergic dermatitis tend to run in families.

SUBJECTIVE AND OBJECTIVE DATA

Itching and pain are the complaints most often presented by the patient with a skin disorder. If the disorder is due to an allergy, the patient also may complain of shortness of breath or cough, or some gastrointestinal symptoms.

The patient also may be able to tell the nurse what other factors, such as stress or excitement, could be related to the appearance of his skin lesions.

Significant objective data include the following:

- Type of lesion (Table 33–1) and distribution, size, and appearance.
- Appearance of skin adjacent to lesions, noting whether reddened areas blanch when mild pressure is applied.

TABLE 33–1 TYPES OF SKIN LESIONS, EXAMPLE, AND DESCRIPTION OF EACH

Name of Lesion	Example	Description
Bulla	Second-degree burn	A blister; a circumscribed, fluid-filled, elevated lesion of the skin, usually more than 5 mm in diameter.
Burrow	Scabies	A linear or zigzag, slightly raised lesion, caused by parasite burrowing under the skin.
Comedo	Blackhead or Whitehead	Plugged duct, formed from sebum and keratin.
Excoriation	Friction or chemical burn	Injury caused by scraping, scratching, or rubbing away layers of skin.
Macule	Freckle, purpura	A discolored spot or patch on the skin. Usually is not elevated nor depressed, and cannot be palpated.
Nodule	Intradermal nevus	Firm, raised lesion; deeper than a papule.
Papule	Measles rash	A solid elevation of skin. Can vary from the size of a pinhead to that of a pea. Usually red, resembling a pimple without pus.
Plaque	Psoriasis	Circumscribed, solid, elevated lesion greater than 1 cm in diameter.
Pustule	Acne, Smallpox	A small elevation of the skin or pimple filled with pus.

TABLE 33-1 TYPES OF SKIN LESIONS, EXAMPLE, AND DESCRIPTION OF EACH *Continued*

Name of Lesion	Example	Description
Vesicle	Blister	A small sac containing serous fluid.
Wheal	Insect sting, hives, nettle rash	An area of local swelling, usually accompanied by itching.

- Localized or generalized edema of skin.
- Characteristics of secretions; that is, color, viscosity, amount.
- Odor: description of odor; strong or faint; source—local or generalized.
- General appearance of skin surface: texture, elasticity, thickness.
- Observation of patient scratching, rubbing, or picking at lesions.
- Temperature changes: location of "hot spots" or cold areas of the skin.

NURSING DIAGNOSES

Nursing diagnoses commonly associated with skin disorders include the following:

- Impaired skin integrity related to autoimmune dysfunction.
- Impaired skin integrity related to infection.
- Potential impaired skin integrity related to inflammatory reaction.
- Pain related to itching, soreness, or tenderness of lesions; exposure of denuded skin to air; or involvement of nerve tissue.
- Disturbance of self-esteem related to disfiguring skin lesions, scarring.
- Anxiety related to chronic, recurring nature of skin disorder and slow healing or potential for malignancy.
- Potential for infection related to loss of intact skin barrier.
- Knowledge deficit related to causative factors of skin lesions, appropriate therapy, and self-care.
- Sleep pattern disturbance related to itching or pain of skin disorder.
- Social isolation related to withdrawal from others because of unsightly appearance of skin.

PREVENTION OF SKIN DISEASE

CLEANLINESS

The ritual of the daily bath is almost an obsession with the average American, and nurses are perhaps guiltier than most in their insistence on using good, strong soap and plenty of hot water. No one will quarrel with the value of cleanliness, but it can be overdone, and the method of cleansing the skin deserves some consideration.

First, we must recognize that there are various skin types. Blondes and redheads usually have very delicate skin that requires special care to prevent drying and irritation. On the other hand, brunettes usually have skin that is more oily and less susceptible to excessive drying and irritation.

If the skin appears dry and scaly, frequent bathing with strong soaps and hot water only aggravates the condition. Oils and creams are available that cleanse the skin quite effectively and help replace the natural oils at the same time. The person with oily skin will need to clean the skin frequently, using a liberal amount of soap and water and avoiding the application of additional oils to the skin.

DIET

Adequate intake of vitamins and minerals is essential to the maintenance of healthy skin. Even borderline deficiencies in these nutrients will cause the skin to take on a sallow and dull appearance. Severe nutritional deficiencies lead to a breakdown of the skin and the development of sores and ulcers. Many teenagers who are so concerned with their physical appearance that they refuse to eat properly for fear of gaining weight fail to realize that they are robbing themselves of one of the sources of real beauty—a healthy and radiant complexion.

AGE

Young people are not the only ones who should be concerned with the care of their skin. As we grow older, our skin undergoes certain changes that easily lead to irritation and breakdown of the skin if proper care is not given. The oil and sweat glands become less active, and the skin has a tendency to become dry and scaly. It also loses some of its tone, making it less elastic and more fragile. Frequent cleansing of the skin becomes unnecessary as the skin ages, and alcohol and other drying agents must be used sparingly if at all. As we grow older, we should establish a regular routine of massaging oils, creams, or oily lotions into the skin, if not for the sake of vanity, at least for the sake of preserving a very important organ of our bodies.

ENVIRONMENT

Several environmental factors can have a direct effect on the health of the skin (Fig. 33–2). These include prolonged exposure to chemicals, excessive drying from repeated immersions in water, and excessive burning by strong sunlight. Some of these are occupational hazards and may necessitate a change of jobs in order to eliminate contact with the causative factor. Also see the discussion of contact dermatitis in Chapter 7.

Overexposure to the ultraviolet rays of the sun can seriously and permanently damage the superficial and deeper layers of the skin, causing severe wrinkling and furrowing, loss of elasticity, and a "tissue paper" transparency of the skin. In addition to the potential for premature aging and degenerative changes, solar damage also can result in malignant changes. Ultraviolet rays from the sun have long been known to be carcinogenic, especially in fair-skinned persons who have subjected their skin to prolonged exposure to sunshine.

Health teaching to apprise the public of the dangers of solar ultraviolet radiation should include the following information:

- Although fair-skinned people who freckle easily are more likely to suffer sun-damaged skin, persons of all complexions and races can and do burn if exposed to sufficient sunlight.
- While a "good tan" might be considered a sign of health, not everyone can acquire such a tan without serious damage to the skin. If one insists on lying out in the sun, the initial exposure should be slow and gradual, and an adequate sunscreen of at least an spf of 15 should always be used. Too much sun too soon will only lead to blistering and peeling.
- Select a sunscreen preparation on the basis

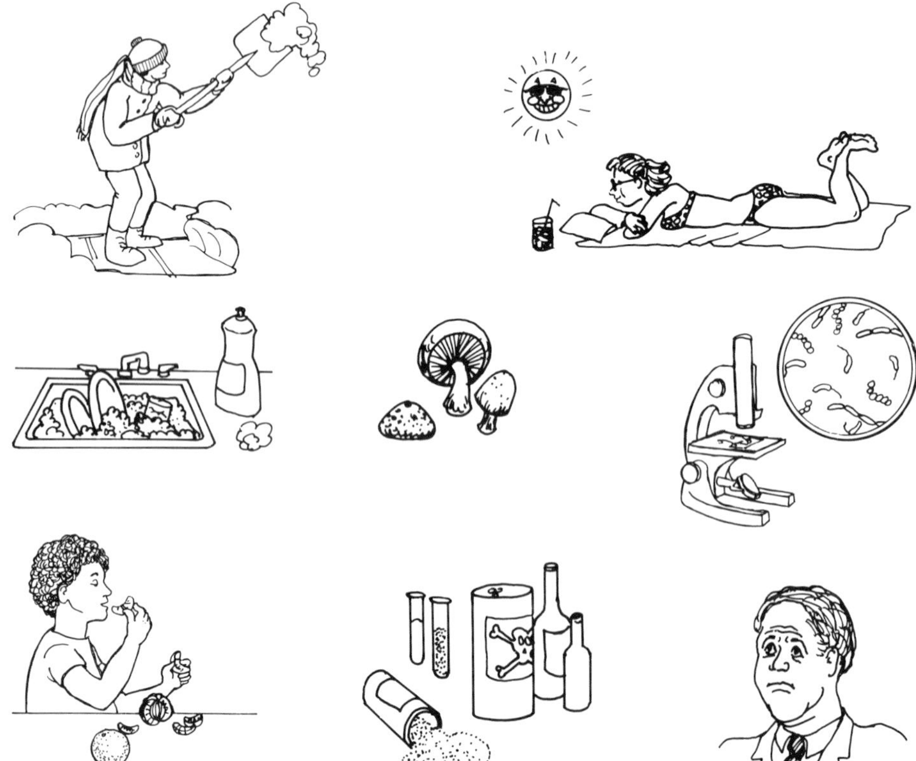

Figure 33–2 Factors that cause or complicate dermatitis include cold; solar radiation; detergents and other chemicals in contact with skin; fungi and molds; microorganisms; foods, drugs, and other chemicals taken internally; and emotional stress.

of your skin type and ability to tan, as well as its active ingredients and the amount of time you plan to spend in the sun. Remember that the sunscreen can be washed off by water or perspiration or rubbed off on sand and towels.

- Avoid long exposure to the sun during the time its rays are most hazardous; that is, between 11 A.M. and 3 P.M. Local radio and television stations often give information about current weather conditions and the chances for being burned by the sun at particular times during each day.
- You can be sunburned on a cloudy or overcast day.
- Light, loosely worn clothing will not give adequate protection from the sun's rays.
- Remember that snow, water, and sand can reflect the sun's rays and increase your chances of being burned.
- Do not try to gauge how much you are being burned while in the sun. It may be 6 to 8 hours before a painful burn becomes obvious.

GENERAL NURSING CARE

The word *dermatology* refers to the study of diseases of the skin. A *dermatologist* is one who specializes in the treatment of disorders of the skin. Many dermatologists have some standing orders or written instructions they wish followed in the care of their patients who have been admitted to the hospital.

Some general rules in the care of the patient with skin disease may be helpful as a guide until specific orders are obtained:

- Bathing with soap is usually contraindicated in all inflammatory conditions of the skin.
- Dressings covering the skin lesions that have been applied by a physician should not be removed when the patient is admitted unless there are specific orders to do so.
- Do not attempt to remove scales, crusts, or other exudates on the skin lesions until the physician has had an opportunity to examine the patient.
- Observe the skin very carefully at the time of the patient's admission and record your observations on the chart or report them to the nurse in charge.
- Avoid excessive handling or rubbing of the skin against the sheets and bedclothes when changing the bed.
- Lotions and alcohol generally used in the hospital for backrubs are never applied to the skin of patients with dermatologic disorders without the permission of their dermatologist.
- If you are not sure about any part of the nursing routine, ask before you act.

Once the physician has determined the type of lesions present, he will order specific treatments to relieve the patient's symptoms and promote healing. The two most commonly used treatments are special dermatologic baths and wet compresses or dressings. In addition, lotions, salves, or ointments may be applied locally at frequent intervals.

Although the vast majority of skin diseases are *not* contagious, nurses should be careful to observe rules of cleanliness and self-protection and universal precautions when caring for any patient with a skin eruption. Special care is needed to avoid spreading infection from the fluid in all pustules and in the vesicles of fever blisters and cold sores.

MEDICATED BATHS

Among the agents that may be added to the bath water are sodium bicarbonate, sodium chloride, cornstarch, oatmeal, medicated tars, oils, and potassium permanganate.

During the bath, the patient must be protected from chilling, because the bath usually lasts from 30 minutes to an hour, and most patients with skin diseases have a lowered resistance to cold. When the patient is removed from the tub, the skin is dried by patting rather than by rubbing. If medication is to be applied locally, it should be put on as soon as the bath is completed, in order to keep pruritus at a minimum.

The medicated bath has a very soothing and relaxing effect on the patient and also helps relieve the itching and burning commonly associated with skin diseases. The nurse should encourage her patient to rest in bed and perhaps to take a short nap after each bath.

LAUNDERING

The bed linens and gowns used for patients with severe skin diseases may need special laundering to eliminate all traces of soap. In the hospital, this requires that specific instructions be given to the personnel in the laundry room and that the patient's linens be carefully labeled. If the patient is to be cared for at home, vinegar may be added to the rinse water to neutralize the soap. One tablespoon of vinegar is used for each quart of water.

WET COMPRESSES OR DRESSINGS

There are various ways in which wet dressings may be applied to the skin. The two general types used are *open dressings* and *closed dressings*. Open compresses must be changed constantly and are never allowed to dry. They are used when the dermatologist wishes to have air circulating to the skin lesions. Closed dressings are thoroughly soaked with the prescribed solution and wrapped in an airtight, waterproof material. It is recommended that the nurse obtain specific instructions from the dermatologist before applying wet dressings to any lesions of the skin.

TOPICAL THERAPY

Many skin lesions are treated by the direct application of medications to the surface of the affected area. This method is called *topical therapy*. Lotion, cream, ointment, powder, or gel may be used.

The physician prescribes the kind of medication to be used and the way in which the drug is to be applied. There are times, however, when a physician is not consulted and the nurse is asked for advice on the use of nonprescription medications. Patients with skin conditions do not always consult a physician and sometimes choose to treat themselves at home. *All patients should be instructed in the proper application of topical medications* (Table 33-2).

INFECTIOUS AND PARASITIC SKIN DISEASES

There are many skin diseases resulting from infection by bacteria, viruses, or fungi or by infestation with parasites. Diseases of this kind require special precautions to avoid spreading the infectious organism or the parasite. The Center for Infectious Diseases, Centers for Disease Control, recommends that *contact isolation* be implemented for a number of these diseases. Specifications for *contact isolation* are as follows:

- A private room is indicated. In general, patients infected with the same type organism may share a room.
- Masks are indicated for those who come in close contact with the patient.
- Gowns are indicated if soiling is likely.
- Gloves are indicated for touching infective material.
- Hands must be washed after touching the patient or potentially contaminated articles and before taking care of another patient.
- Articles contaminated with infective material should be discarded or bagged and labeled before being sent for decontamination and reprocessing.

Skin diseases requiring contact isolation include:

- Diphtheria, cutaneous.
- Furunculosis, group A *Streptococcus*.
- Herpes simplex, disseminated, severe primary, or neonatal.
- Herpes zoster (varicella-zoster).
- Impetigo.
- Infection or colonization by bacteria with multiple drug resistance (any site).
- Pediculosis.
- Scabies.

TABLE 33-2 GUIDELINES FOR USING TOPICAL MEDICATIONS

Powders: Dry the area thoroughly before applying powder, to prevent caking. Do not apply to raw and denuded areas. Some powders such as cornstarch can actually serve as glucose-rich culture media for the growth of bacteria.

Ointments: Use only a small amount and gently massage into the skin until a thin film covers the area. Exception is when ointment is used as an occlusive dressing, as for a burn. Ointments tend to leave a greasy feeling to the skin. They are best for chronic lesions, because they help the skin retain moisture and natural oils. Avoid putting ointment on areas where the skin is creased and overlaps itself.

Gels: A gel is a semisolid mixture that tends to liquefy when applied to the skin. It is absorbed into the skin and dries quickly, leaving a thin nonocclusive film. If applied to abraded or sensitive areas, alcohol in the base can cause a burning or stinging sensation.

Lotions: These are actually powders suspended in water; they will leave a residue once the liquid evaporates from the skin. This residue should be washed off before a fresh dose is applied. Be sure powder is uniformly dispersed in solution before applying, then use a firm stroke to distribute the medication evenly. Do not "dab" on lotions, as this can be irritating to the skin.

All types: Always apply topical medications sparingly and in a thin film that extends beyond the affected area about ¼ inch. Thick layers of topicals are wasteful, and some of these drugs such as corticosteroids are very expensive. Too much of some topicals (for example, antifungal agents) can chemically irritate the skin and delay healing. Thick layers also tend to soften the skin too much.

If the skin condition appears to be getting worse after a topical agent is applied, or if the patient develops eczema, suspect an allergic contact dermatitis caused by the drug.

- Skin wound or burn infection, major (draining and not covered by dressing, or dressing does not adequately contain purulent material), including those infected with *Staphylococcus aureus*.
- Vaccinia (generalized and progressive eczema vaccinatum).

HERPESVIRUS INFECTIONS

The herpesviruses are an extensive family of viruses, many of which are capable of infecting and causing disease in humans. Their nomenclature is complex and does not follow a consistent pattern. For example, some are named for the disease they cause (e.g., herpes simplex and herpes zoster–varicella), and some for the persons who discovered them.

Herpes Simplex

Herpes simplex virus type 2 (HSV 2) is most often associated with genital herpes, whereas herpes simplex virus type 1 (HSV 1) lesions are primarily nongenital. It should be understood, however, that either type can cause lesions in the genital area as well as other regions of the body. Autoinoculation of the virus is possible by direct contact; for example, lips to fingers to genitals or lips to fingers to eyes.

Symptoms

An infection with HSV 1 is manifested by lesions on the lips and nares that are commonly called "cold sores" or "fever blisters." As with other types of herpesvirus infections, there is no drug that will completely cure the infection.

Treatment and Nursing Intervention

The symptoms of itching and burning that accompany oral herpes infection sometimes can be minimized by warm compresses to the sores, followed by local application of tincture of benzoin or spirits of camphor to aid drying and facilitate healing. Sometimes topical and oral acyclovir is beneficial in hastening healing. The disease usually is self-limiting, which means that it does not progress and will subside on its own, but it can recur.

Patients should be cautioned to use good personal hygiene to avoid spreading the virus to the eyes and genital area and other body parts. Hand washing is a very simple but essential part of the prevention of autoinoculation. Canker sores, which are shallow white ulcerations of the tongue and gums, often are mistaken for herpes simplex infection; however, they are not the same and are not known to be caused by any infectious organism.

Herpes Zoster

The causative organism for this skin disorder is herpes varicella–zoster. The virus causes chickenpox (varicella), mostly in young children, and shingles (herpes zoster).

In herpes zoster the herpesviruses replicate in the peripheral nerve ganglia, where they lie dormant until reactivated by trauma, malignancy, or local radiation.

Symptoms

Herpes zoster begins with vague symptoms of chills and low-grade fever and possibly some gastrointestinal disturbance. About 3 to 5 days after onset, small groups of vesicles appear on the skin. They usually are found on the trunk and spread around the body, following the nerve pathways leading from the spinal nerve to the skin.

The vesicles eventually change from small blisters to scaly lesions and are accompanied by pain and itching. The lesions usually affect only one side of the body or face. The pain of shingles often is quite severe and can persist for several days after the skin lesions are completely healed.

Medical Treatment and Nursing Intervention

There is no cure for herpes zoster. The condition can persist for months, especially in older and debilitated patients. One herpes infection does not provide immunity from future attacks.

Symptomatic treatment usually involves the administration of an analgesic to relieve the pain. Antibiotics may be prescribed prophylactically against secondary bacterial infection of the lesions. Most physicians prescribe oral acyclovir to diminish the extent or duration of the lesions.

Narcotic analgesics are avoided, because they can lead to addiction when used for an extended period of time. If the pain persists and is intractable, the physician prescribes a corticosteroid to reduce inflammation. Vidarabine, administered intravenously, is sometimes given to patients who have an immune deficiency. It is usually effective in reducing if not completely relieving the pain.

Fortunately, even though shingles may be difficult to live with while it is running its course, there rarely are any serious complications from the disease. However, the prognosis is obviously less favorable in patients who have an underlying malignancy of the skin.

Nursing intervention is aimed at providing emotional support and symptomatic relief from the pain and itching and preventing a secondary bacterial infection. Cold compresses, calamine lotion, and diversional activities are sometimes helpful. Rest and adequate nutrition can promote healing and shorten the acute phase of shingles.

IMPETIGO CONTAGIOSA

Impetigo is a streptococcal or staphylococcal infection marked by vesicles and bullae that become pustular, rupture, and form yellow crusts. Impetigo can be mistaken for ringworm because of the round patches it forms (Fig. 33–3).

Medical Treatment and Nursing Intervention

The itching that accompanies impetigo brings on scratching of the lesions and contamination of the hands and fingernails. Exudate from the lesions is highly contagious; thus the disease can be spread rather easily to other parts of the body and to other persons.

Treatment consists of cleansing the lesions with soap and water and then wiping the surrounding skin with alcohol. Contact isolation is recommended. The lesions should be kept dry and as open to the air as possible. Local applications of an antibiotic ointment may clear up the lesions; however, systemic antibiotics are recommended in some cases.

It is important that impetigo be recognized early and treated promptly, especially in newborn infants, in whom the infection can be fatal.

FUNGAL INFECTIONS

Fungal infections are called *mycoses;* systemic fungal infections involving the lungs and other internal organs are called *systemic mycoses.* There are actually two groups of fungi: (1) those that are truly pathogenic to humans, and (2) those that are opportunistic infections and can cause an infection when the host has an altered immune system.

True pathogenic fungi can cause infection in an otherwise healthy person, but there are relatively few fungi that are able to do this. Fungal infections are rarely fatal if they involve only the superficial tissues of the body. Nevertheless, mycotic skin infections can be exasperating, because they progress slowly, are difficult to diagnose, and are often resistant to treatment.

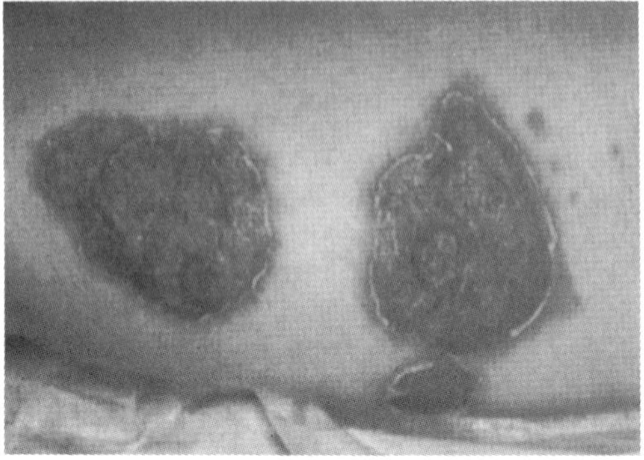

Figure 33–3 Large lesions of impetigo, with smooth red weeping surfaces.
(From Hurwitz, S.: Clinical Pediatric Dermatology. Philadelphia, W. B. Saunders, 1981.)

The most common types of fungal infections involving the skin are *tinea pedis* (athlete's foot or dermophytosis), *tinea of the scalp* (commonly known as ringworm), and *tinea barbae* (barber's itch). *Moniliasis* (thrush) is a fungal infection that can attack the mucous membranes of the mouth, rectum, and vagina (this condition is discussed more fully in Chapter 30).

All surface fungal infections produce itching, some swelling, and a breakdown of tissue. Because fungi thrive in warm, moist places, a tropical climate or other environmental factors that produce prolonged heat and moisture can encourage the development of fungal infections.

Diagnosis of fungal infections is confirmed by microscopic examination of skin scrapings that have been treated with potassium hydroxide solution (KOH). Fungal specimens generally show the typical filaments of fungal organisms.

Instructions to patients for prevention of common fungal infections are provided in Table 33–3.

Tinea Pedis (Athlete's Foot)

Tinea pedis affects the feet, particularly between the toes. The infection may spread to the entire foot and cause blistering, peeling, cracking, and itching. If it continues unchecked, it can spread to other parts of the body. The condition can be complicated by a severe bacterial infection.

Treatment of tinea pedis consists of keeping the area dry, clean, and exposed to the air and sunlight as much as possible. Clean cotton stockings should be worn every day, and the affected areas between the toes should be separated by gauze or cotton. Various topical antifungals can be prescribed, including ciclopirox (Loprox), miconazole, clotrimazole (Mycelex), econazole (Spectazole), ketoconazole (Nizoral), and naftifine (Naftin). Some medicated powders such as undecylenic acid–zinc undecylate (Desenex) work to keep the feet dry and also help control growth of the fungi.

Because most cases are contracted and spread in swimming pools, showers, and other public facilities of this type, one should be careful to wash one's feet and dry them thoroughly after using such facilities. It is difficult to destroy the fungi in public facilities by any method other than by boiling contaminated articles or by use of a strong disinfectant such as 0.1% bichloride of mercury or 0.2% creosol.

Ringworm

The term *ringworm* is often used to designate tinea of the scalp and beard. Actually, the term is incorrect and confusing. The skin lesions do

TABLE 33-3 PREVENTION OF RECURRENT FUNGAL INFECTIONS

Wear shoes that provide ventilation for the feet. Wear cotton socks when rubber-soled shoes or sneakers must be worn.

Wash and dry the feet at least daily, being careful to dry completely the skin between the toes.

Sprinkle an antifungal powder on the feet and between the toes if there is a tendency to have athlete's foot.

Change hose or socks daily; do not wear them more than one day without washing.

Use only clean towels, changing them at least every other day.

Change bed linens at least once a week.

Do not use the toilet articles of others and do not allow them to use yours.

Inspect pets regularly for ringworm. Have veterinarian check the animal if an infection is suspected.

not necessarily appear in rings, and they very definitely are not caused by a worm. If the infection is located on the scalp *(tinea capitis)*, the hair falls out in patches, and there are small, reddish lesions of the skin. Tinea capitis primarily affects children. Because it is highly infectious, any child with this condition should be kept out of school until he is no longer a source of infection. His contaminated clothing should be boiled or destroyed to prevent the spread of the infection, and he should wear a stocking cap or surgical cap to protect his scalp during treatment.

Ringworm of the body may affect the genital area, producing a raw area, particularly where the skin rubs together. The patient should be instructed to dry the area completely after washing and to avoid tight clothing, nylon underwear, or other factors that prevent airing and drying of the area.

Tinea barbae is also called "barber's itch" because it affects the area of the face where the beard grows and is most often spread by unsanitary conditions in a barber shop. The lesions produce a boggy swelling of the skin, soften the hairs of the beard, and involve the lymph glands.

Griseofulvin (Fulvicin or Grifulvin) is the fungistatic antibiotic most often used in the control of ringworm of the scalp and face.

PARASITIC INFESTATIONS: PEDICULOSIS AND SCABIES

The parasites that cause pediculosis and scabies are found throughout the world in all types of climates, and they can infest anyone. The parasites are particularly troublesome, however, wherever people live under crowded conditions and are negligent in their personal hygiene. The occurrence of pediculosis and scabies in the United States has recently increased significantly because of communal living and other "more natural" lifestyles chosen by some people.

Three basic types of lice that infest human beings are (1) the head louse, *Pediculus capitis* (Fig. 33-4*A*); (2) the body louse, *Pediculus corporis;* and (3) the pubic or "crab" louse, *Phthirus pubis* (Fig. 33-4*C*). In addition, human beings may also be infested by the *Sarcoptes scabiei*, the mange mite that produces scabies (Fig. 33-4*B*). All types are acquired by contact with infested people or their clothing, bed linen, and bedding. Dogs have also been known to carry lice and the scabies mite.

Symptoms

The most prevalent symptom of louse infestation is severe itching. The resultant scratching can lead to excoriation of the skin and secondary infection causing impetigo, furunculosis, and cellulitis. Systemic infections are not commonly associated with louse infestation, but they can and do occur in the forms of glomerulonephritis, septicemia, pneumonia, and cystic abscesses. If the lice infest the eyelids and eyelashes, the eyelids become red and swollen. Swelling may also occur in the lymph glands of the neck of a person heavily infested with head lice. The body louse can transmit typhus fever, trench fever, and some other diseases. Other types of lice are not known to be transmitters of disease.

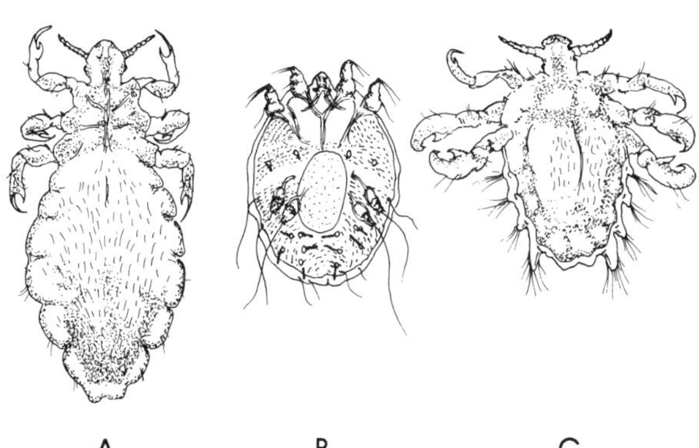

Figure 33-4 Types of lice that infest human beings. *A*, Head louse, dorsal view (2 to 3 mm long). *B*, Scab mite, ventral surface (0.4 mm long). *C*, Pubic louse, dorsal view (1 mm long).

The scabies mites burrow under the top layers of the skin and live their entire life there. They are more likely to be found in the skin between the fingers and toes, in the groin, and in other areas where there may be folds of skin. Excretions from the mites produce irritation with intense itching and blistering. Secondary infection is not uncommon with scabies, and some deaths have occurred when the scabies infestation has led to pneumonia or septicemia.

Medical Treatment and Nursing Intervention

The prescription drugs most commonly used and considered most effective against lice and scabies are 1% lindane (Kwell, Gamene) and 10% crotamiton (Eurax). They are available as creams, lotions, and shampoos. A-200 Pyrinate and Cuprex are nonprescription drugs used to treat louse infestations. The medication is left on the affected ares for 12 to 24 hours and then removed completely with soap and water. If needed, the treatment may be repeated once more 24 hours later.

Lindane is also available as a shampoo for head lice. The shampoo lather is rubbed on the hair and scalp for at least 4 minutes and then removed by thorough rinsing with water. A fine-toothed comb is then used to remove the nits (eggs) that may have remained on the hair.

Contact isolation is recommended. In addition, clothing, bedding, and other infested articles must be decontaminated to prevent reinfection. Laundering and dry cleaning can be effective for decontamination of clothing and bed covering. Mattresses, upholstered furniture, and other articles should be sprayed with a disinfectant specific for destruction of the parasites not located on the infected person's body.

ACNE

Acne is a disorder of the skin characterized by papules and pustules over the face, back, and shoulders. There are many kinds of acne, but the two major types are *acne vulgaris* and *acne rosacea*. Of the two, acne vulgaris is the most common. It typically begins in early puberty, continues through the teens, and then begins to subside. Occasionally it persists, or it can recur several years later.

Some types of acne are related to cosmetics (*acne cosmetica*) or to chemicals in the environment; for example, occupational acne due to prolonged contact with oils and tars.

Acne occurs when the ducts leading from the sebaceous glands become plugged with sebum, the oily secretion of the glands.

The onset of acne vulgaris in adolescents is related to increased release of sex hormones, which stimulate activity of the sebaceous glands, causing increased production of sebum. It is not known why in some persons the ducts from these glands become plugged, but the increased production of sebum triggers the formation of blackheads and whiteheads. These lesions are not a sign of uncleanliness. The color of blackheads is due to the result of particles of melanin, the skin's own pigment.

Accumulations of sebum, skin particles, and dead skin cells can cause an inflammatory reaction. Bacterial infection leads to the formation of pustules. An extensive inflammation can lead to the formation of cysts, with swelling above and below the surface of the skin (Fig. 33–5).

Medical Treatment

Mild, noninflammatory cases of acne respond well to efforts to remove blackheads and whiteheads by promoting dryness and peeling of the top layer of skin. The medication is applied directly on the skin. Nonprescription drugs such as lotions, creams, and gels that contain sulfur, benzoyl peroxide, and sulfur combined with resorcinol usually are effective for noninflammatory acne.

Among the topical medications, tretinoin (Retin-A) is the best agent for papular and pustular acne problems. It should be used once or twice a day. Benzoyl peroxide is the most fre-

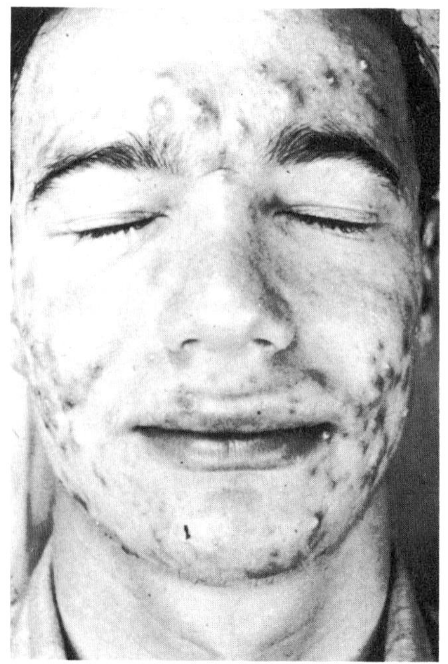

Figure 33–5 Typical appearance of acne. (Courtesy of Medichrome-Clay-Adams, Inc., New York.)

quently used topical agent for acne and is available both by prescription and over the counter.

Antibiotics such as tetracycline and erythromycin also are sometimes prescribed for inflammatory acne to inhibit the growth of bacteria in the plugged ducts.

The antibiotic can be given safely for months or years. Tetracycline should not be given to children under the age of 8 (or before eruption of all permanent teeth) or to pregnant women, because it can lead to weakness of the bones and discoloration of the teeth.

A relatively new drug approved by the FDA for treatment of cystic acne has been especially effective in controlling cases that are resistant to other forms of treatment. The drug is 13-*cis*-retinoic acid and is marketed under the trade name Accutane. Almost all patients experience some adverse reaction to this drug, and it is not recommended for pregnant women. Accutane is taken by mouth daily for 2 to 4 months and inhibits activity of the sebaceous glands. Its effects are sustained for months to years after it has been discontinued. Accutane is only used for severe cystic acne that is resistant to all other treatment.

The appearance of the patient with deep scarring and pitting as a result of cystic acne can be improved by *dermabrasion*. This procedure involves mechanically scraping away the outer layers of skin and smoothing out its surface by applying motor-driven wire brushes or diamond wheels. Chemical dermabrasion is done by applying phenol or trichloroacetic acid to remove the scars.

Nursing Intervention

Nursing intervention is primarily concerned with teaching the patient about the nature of his particular skin disease and giving support while he is trying to cope with its physiologic and psychosocial effects. He should feel that his problems are being taken seriously, even though they are certainly not life threatening. Acne can be particularly distressing to adolescents, who are often deeply concerned about their appearance and acceptance by their peers.

There are many misconceptions about acne and its treatment. It is not a contagious disease. It is not due to uncleanliness or poor personal hygiene. It is not caused or made worse by lack of sleep, constipation, masturbation, venereal disease, or anger and hostility. Diet can contribute to the formation of lesions, but this is true of relatively few people who usually can find a relationship between the intake of certain foods and the appearance of the lesions of acne. In general, however, chocolate, colas, and the fried foods of which most adolescents are so fond need not be restricted or eliminated from the diet in an effort to prevent or cure acne. A well-balanced diet is all that is recommended in the management of acne.

The face should be washed gently and with a mild soap. Scrubbing the skin and using a harsh soap is damaging to the skin and contributes to inflammation. Special medicated soaps do not seem to be any better than a mild face soap. If the hair is oily, it should be shampooed frequently and kept off the face.

It is not a good idea to squeeze pimples and pustules. This can press the sebum and accumulated material more firmly in the clogged duct, increase the chance of inflammation, and spread an infection to other parts of the skin and body. Blackheads and whiteheads are best removed by applying a prescription medication that causes peeling of the skin.

Because the management of acne can go on for years and require periodic evaluation by a dermatologist, patients and their families will need continued support and encouragement to follow the prescribed regimen. They will need to know the expected results of prescribed medications, any adverse reactions that might occur, and symptoms that should be reported immediately.

PSORIASIS

Psoriasis is a chronic and recurring skin disorder that typically appears as patches or "plaques" that are covered with adherent silvery scales. These scales are the result of an abnormally rapid rate of proliferation of skin cells. The skin under the plaques is reddened, and when the scales are removed there is pinpoint bleeding. The plaques most often appear on the skin of the elbows, knees, and base of the spine. It also may affect the scalp, in which case it can be confused with seborrheic dermatitis. When the fingernails are involved there can be pitting of the surface of the nails. The palms and soles also can be affected, making it difficult for the patient to carry out activities of daily living. In some cases the skin eruptions are accompanied by inflammation of the joints, especially those of the fingers and toes. This is called psoriatic arthritis (Fig. 33–6).

The cause of psoriasis is not known. It is not contagious, and tends to run in families, although the precise pattern of inheritance has not been defined. A parent with psoriasis has a 50% chance of passing the presumed gene along to each child. However, since any individual with the gene has only a 50% chance of developing psoriasis, the offspring of a person with the disease has a 25% chance of developing it.

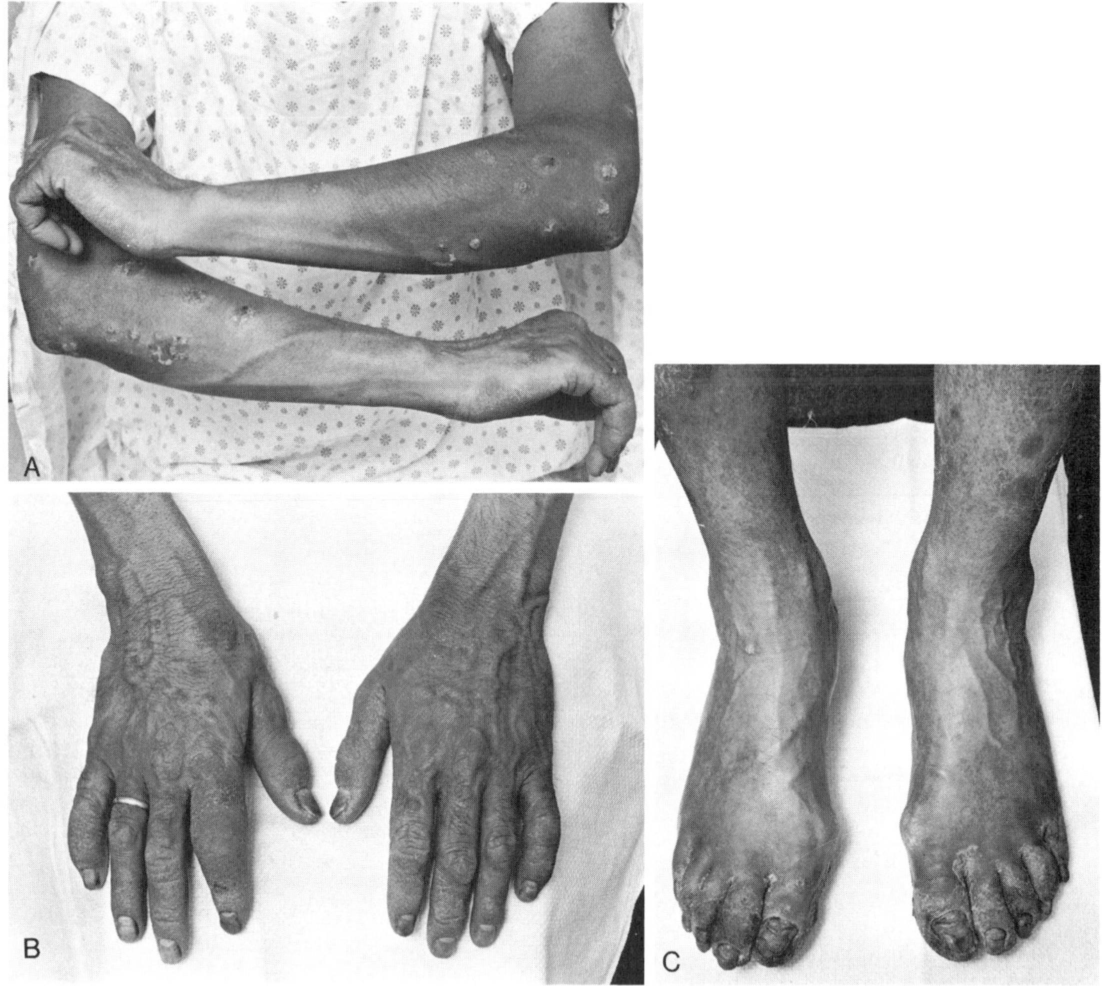

Figure 33-6 Classic lesions in psoriasis. Note arthritic changes in joints. (Photos by Ken Kasper.)

MEDICAL TREATMENT AND NURSING INTERVENTION

Each case of psoriasis is treated individually. The disease is unpredictable, tends to go into remission spontaneously, and sometimes will clear up temporarily with or without treatment.

Mild cases usually respond to steroid creams, but there is a possibility that eventually the disease will become resistant to steroids. Sunlight in moderate doses can help, because the ultraviolet rays slow down the rate at which epithelial cells are produced. Extremes of ultraviolet radiation can have the opposite effect, resulting in an aggravation of the condition.

Tar preparations also act to impede the proliferation of skin cells and have long been used to heal psoriasis lesions. They may be administered in the form of baths, topical applications, or shampoos. Combinations of artificial ultraviolet radiation and a coal tar product often are prescribed for severe cases. This usually requires hospitalization so that the dosage of each component of therapy can be measured precisely. A recently approved form of therapy called PUVA combines application of the drug psoralen, which penetrates the skin, and exposure to ultraviolet light type A (UVA). Oral retinoids can also be added to this therapy.

The Goeckerman technique, named after the physician who developed it, combines ultraviolet light B (UVB) and a crude coal tar ointment for the treatment of psoriasis.

Antimetabolites have more recently been used in the treatment of severe psoriasis, helping to control the disorder by their antiproliferative action. Methotrexate is the most commonly used antimetabolite for this purpose.

Patients with psoriasis will need instruction about the nature of their disease, the purpose of the prescribed treatment, and information about ways to avoid aggravating it. The skin should be kept as moist and pliable as possible. Humidifiers to increase moisture in the environment are sometimes helpful. Lubricating lotions and creams should be approved by the dermatologist before they are applied, but they usually can be used to maintain the integrity of the skin areas not affected by psoriasis.

Minor scratches and abrasions and bacterial infections can trigger the formation of lesions at a new site. Because any irritation or break in the skin seems to stimulate the growth of psoriatic plaques in a person susceptible to psoriasis, the patient should be cautioned to avoid injury of any kind. This includes hangnails, damaged cuticles, blisters from poorly fitting shoes, and potentially harmful agents in the environment such as radiation and chemicals.

CANCER OF THE SKIN

Skin cancer is often neglected, because there is no pain associated with it, and patients fear that treatment will involve extensive or mutilating surgery. It has been estimated that each year, 32,000 people discover they have skin cancer and 8,800 of these cases are fatal because of inadequate treatment. Almost all these deaths could have been averted through early diagnosis and treatment.

CAUSES AND SUSCEPTIBILITY

Several factors predispose an individual to the development of skin cancer. Among these are internal changes in the cells that may be due to hereditary factors, and external influences such as chronic exposure to chemicals or other irritants in the environment. Because children tend to inherit their skin characteristics from their parents, susceptibility to skin cancer tends to run in families. Blue-eyed blondes seem to be most susceptible, probably because they lack sufficient pigment to protect the skin cells from outside irritants. The incidence of skin cancer in blacks is very low.

A major cause of skin cancer today is the alteration in the ozone layer of the earth's atmosphere causing more UV radiation to reach the earth's surface. This type of radiation is causing much quicker damage to skin with much less sun exposure than in years past. Another problem is that the quickly proliferating skin cells of the younger generation are even more susceptible to this type of damage, and it is mostly the young who spend large amounts of time in the sun. It is appropriate for every nurse to instruct all people about the dangers of sunning without an appropriate protective sunscreen.

Another danger is the tanning salon. Many use tanning beds that deliver dangerous UV radiation to the skin. Most dermatologists adamantly state that no one should use artificial tanning equipment.

TYPES OF SKIN CANCER

The three main types of skin malignancy are basal cell epithelioma, squamous cell epithelioma, and melanocarcinoma.

Basal cell epithelioma usually appears first as a small, scaly area and tends to become larger as the disease progresses. It occurs most often on the face and trunk. As the scales shed, there will be a small amount of bleeding and a scab will form. When the scab is shed, the affected area becomes wider, and it is bordered by a waxy, translucent, raised area. This spreading may continue very gradually during several months or years. Even though these malignancies do not metastasize, they can invade underlying tissues, and death can result from complications such as infection, hemorrhage, or exhaustion. Small lesions can be removed under local anesthesia in a doctor's office. Larger lesions respond well to x-ray or radiation therapy.

Squamous cell carcinoma usually begins on the mucous membranes and can metastasize to other areas of the body. The tumor begins as a small nodule, which rapidly becomes ulcerated. Treatment must begin early if the condition is to be relieved before the skin cells sustain extensive damage. Surgical procedures involve total removal or destruction of the lesions and the surrounding tissues that have been invaded. Radiation therapy is advised for patients who are poor surgical risks or who are fearful of surgery.

Malignant melanoma is the least common form of skin cancer. It arises from pigment-producing cells and varies in its course and prognosis according to its type. There are three kinds of malignant melanoma: superficial spreading, nodular, and lentigo malignant melanoma. In general, the superficial lesions can be cured, while the deeper lesions tend to metastasize more readily through the lymphatic and circulatory systems.

Characteristics of the three types of melanoma are shown in Table 33–4.

Malignant melanoma always requires surgical removal of the tumor and excision of adjacent tissues and possibly nearby lymphatic structures. Chemotherapy may be employed to destroy tumor cells believed to have migrated beyond the tumor site. Radiation therapy usually is not indicated unless there is extensive metastasis. The radiation does not eliminate the disease, but it can relieve symptoms by reducing tumor size.

MEDICAL TREATMENT AND NURSING INTERVENTION

Removal of cancerous skin tissue will depend on the type of malignant growth present. In all but the most extensive growths, treatment is

TABLE 33-4 COMPARISON OF THREE MAJOR TYPES OF SKIN CANCER

Type	Characteristics
Basal cell epithelioma	Slowly enlarging, firm, scaly papule. Crusted or ulcerated center that may be depressed; has pearly (semitranslucent) raised border. Dilated capillaries around lesion. Accounts for 70% of all skin cancers. Rarely spreads and is easily treated.
Squamous cell epithelioma	Appearance variable. Frequently seen as well-defined, irregularly shaped nodule or plaque. May be elevated, nodular mass or fungated mass. Varying amounts of scale and crusting. May have ulcerated center. Predominantly on sun-exposed areas: head, neck, hands; 75% occur on the head. Spreads rapidly.
Malignant melanoma Superficial spreading melanoma (SSM)	Appears in a variety of colors: white, red, gray, black, blue over a brown or black background. Has irregular surface and notched border. Small tumor nodules may ulcerate and bleed. Horizontal growth can continue for years. Vertical growth worsens prognosis.
Nodular malignant melanoma (NMM)	Nodule with uniformly grayish-black color, resembles a blackberry. May be flesh-colored with specks of pigment around base of nodule. Itching, oozing, and bleeding may occur. Prognosis less favorable than superficial type.
Lentigo maligna melanoma (LMM)	Relatively rare. Arises from a lesion that resembles a large flat freckle that is of variable color from tan to black. Has irregularly spaced black nodules on the surface. Often located on the back of the hand, on the face, and under fingernails. Develops very slowly; may ulcerate. Tends to metastasize; prognosis poor.

relatively simple and completely successful. Although benign precancerous lesions do not inevitably develop into malignant lesions, the most advisable course of action is to remove them when they are first diagnosed. The nurse often is in a position to notice these lesions in their early stages and should do her best to persuade the person with such a lesion to seek prompt medical attention.

Because victims of skin cancer run a high risk of eventually developing another malignancy, either at the former site or elsewhere in the body, they should visit a physician at least once a year after the skin cancer has been cured. Although most skin cancers are easily curable, they should not be considered harmless and something to forget about after treatment. *Skin cancer may be a warning that another form of cancer will develop later.*

BURNS

Burns are injuries to the skin caused by exposure to extreme heat, electrical agents, strong chemicals, or radiation.

CLASSIFICATION OF BURNS

The classification of burns is based on the amount of the body surface that has been burned and the depth of the burn.

The extent of a burn is calculated according to the "rule of nines" and is expressed as a percentage of total body surface (Table 33-5). The figures used in this method are fairly accurate for gross assessment in adults; however, the rule of nines does not make allowances for the proportionate differences in children at various ages. The Lund and Browder system computes the depth of the burn as well as the extent of the injury according to relative age.

The depth of a burn is more difficult to determine, because various graduations of injury are sustained in a major burn. Some small patches may be more deeply burned than the areas adjacent to them. Burn depth has traditionally been classified according to degrees, a first-degree burn being the most superficial and a fourth-degree burn being the deepest (Fig. 33-7).

A more current method for evaluation of the depth of burns is based on the layers of skin that have been damaged. *Partial-thickness wounds* are

TABLE 33-5 RULE OF NINES

Area of Body	Percentage of Body Surface
Head and neck	9
Anterior trunk	18
Posterior trunk	18
Upper limbs	18
Lower limbs	36
Genitalia and perineum	1

those in which the epidermal appendages (sweat and oil glands and hair follicles) are not destroyed, and the wound will heal by itself if no further injury is done by either infection or inappropriate treatment. Partial-thickness burns are comparable to either first- or second-degree burns. A *deep-dermal* wound is a deep partial-thickness wound that can resurface itself if infection does not destroy the epidermal appendages. *Full-thickness wounds* involve all layers of skin and the destruction of the epidermal appendages. Wounds of this type will require grafting if optimal function is to be restored. Table 33-6 provides a guide for estimating the depth of a burn.

The *crust* is the dry, scab-like covering that forms over a superficial burn. *Eschar* is a hard leathery layer of dead tissue that results when there has been a full-thickness injury. The eschar can act as a protective covering over the wound, serving as a barrier against infectious agents; however, removal of eschar and skin grafting are usually done within a week after the burn. *Slough* is the moist necrotic tissue of a burn.

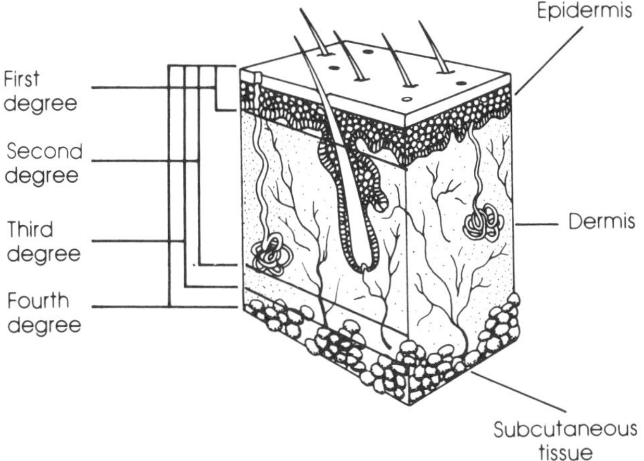

Figure 33-7 Skin cross section with depths of burns.

EMERGENCY TREATMENT

All burns should be considered potentially dangerous until they are thoroughly assessed. The recommended treatment for minor burns is submersion in cool water and applications of cool compresses as soon as possible after the injury. This helps relieve pain and edema and reduces the chances for a deeper burn.

Under no circumstances should salves or ointments or any greasy substance be applied to a burned area. Because the removal of greasy substances is very painful, inappropriate treatment can cause unnecessary suffering and increase the possibility of infection. First aid for the treatment of burns is discussed in Chapter 36.

IMMEDIATE CARE

Most major burn cases are transferred to a major burn unit for specialized care. However, many burn victims are initially treated and stabilized at the community hospital nearest the scene of the accident before being moved to a burn unit. The first hour of treatment, from the time of burn, can be crucial to the eventual outcome of a serious burn.

If possible, details of the nature of the accident should be obtained so that a more thorough assessment can be made. The cause of the burn and whether there is any possibility of thermal damage to the respiratory tract can help identify more closely the specific needs of the patient. Once the depth and extent of the burn has been estimated, efforts are made to establish an intravenous line and infuse an isotonic balanced solution such as Finger's lactate to maintain fluid balance. Oxygen is administered if blood gases indicate a problem with respiratory function.

Care of the wound may involve nothing more than covering the burned area with a clean sheet to protect it from air, which can be very painful to partial-thickness wounds. Moist, cool towels also are sometimes applied to help relieve pain. Analgesics usually are withheld until the patient's vital signs are stable.

Preventing Shock and Infection

A major concern in the care of a burn victim is prevention of shock due to circulatory collapse. The two most important measures used to relieve profound shock in a burn patient are (1) replacement of lost fluids and electrolytes and (2) relief of pain and anxiety. The loss of fluids and electrolytes results from the sudden shifting of the blood plasma and tissue fluids from their normal site to the area of the burn. The fluids are then lost by seepage through the open wounds where the skin has been destroyed.

Unless these fluids are replaced immediately, the blood vessels will collapse and the resultant

TABLE 33-6 DEPTH OF BURN WOUNDS

Depth or Degree	Likely Cause	Characteristics	Pain Level
First degree—Epidermal layers only	Sunshine, moderate heat	Dry, red skin	Painful
Second degree or partial-thickness—superficial to deep dermis	Hot liquids, flashes, flames	Color mottled, whitish to pink, red to a deeper cherry red; skin is moist, with or without blisters.	Very painful
Third degree or full-thickness—all layers of dermis; extends into subcutaneous tissues	Flames, electricity, chemicals	Whitish, leathery appearance or possibly charred; skin is dry and lacks elasticity	Little or no pain
Fourth degree—includes muscle and bone	Usually electrical injury	Skin charred or dead white	No pain

profound shock may be fatal to the patient. Plasma, fluids, and electrolytes are given intravenously, through multiple lines, and sometimes through an incision into a vein, for continuous replacement of fluids until a normal fluid and electrolyte balance is established. In a severely burned patient, intravenous therapy may be necessary for several days or longer. The patient may receive additional nourishment by total parenteral nutrition through a central line.

Managing Pain

Measures to relieve pain include the administration of morphine or meperidine (Demerol IV) as soon as possible after the burn has been sustained.

The nurse must use gentleness and care in handling the patient as she turns him or administers treatments. Not only does this reduce the amount of pain the patient must suffer, but the less the patient is handled, the less danger there is of contaminating the wounds.

Even though there is not usually much pain associated with full-thickness burns during the first few days, most burn patients sustain burns in varying depths and eventually suffer a great deal of pain. Also, burn victims do not lose consciousness. Added to the physical discomfort is the patient's realization that he has been badly injured. He no doubt thinks of all the horrifying sights and smells associated with burned flesh, and he can suffer much emotional shock from such a traumatic experience.

Preventing Other Complications

In addition to the dangers of shock and infection, there is a potential for respiratory failure if upper airway passages have been burned. Dyspnea may or may not be present at first, but if the burn victim inhaled smoke or superheated air at the time of injury, an inflammatory response could obstruct the air passages completely within 24 hours.

Patients who should be watched closely for signs of developing respiratory problems include those who have (1) burns of the face and neck, (2) singed nasal hair, (3) darkened membranes in the nose and mouth, and (4) a history of having been burned in an enclosed space.

Hemorrhage does not occur with burns. If a burned patient shows signs of bleeding, he must be checked for some other type of injury such as a penetrating wound, fracture, or laceration that occurred at the same time that he was burned.

Although the physician chooses the type of medication to be applied topically or administered systemically, the nursing staff is responsible for continued assessment of the burn wounds to determine the effectiveness of the prescribed treatments.

The patient's vital signs must be checked at regular intervals and recorded accurately. The condition of the wounds also should be checked systematically to determine whether healing is taking place as it should and infection is being avoided. Three common conditions that the nurse should guard against and report immediately if signs appear are decreased urine output (indicating dehydration), infection, and cellulitis.

Dehydration may be indicated by an elevated body temperature and a dryness in the wound, with loss of skin turgor in the unaffected areas. A very wet wound that has a foul odor indicates *infection*. A greenish-gray exudate from the wound is a sign of Pseudomonas infection. A bluish-black discoloration at the edges of the wound and other signs of a generalized infection may indicate that the patient is developing septicemia. Signs of inflammation such as redness and swelling of the tissues adjacent to the wound may indicate *cellulitis.*

Healthy granulation tissue does not emit exudate. During the granulation stage of repair, the wound should look slightly pink and somewhat shiny. If there are any deviations from this description, such as those mentioned above, the nurse should notify the physician.

TREATMENT OF THE WOUND

In general, two methods may be used in the treatment of a burn wound: *open* and *closed.* In the open method, the burned area is left uncovered and exposed to the air. In the closed method, the area is covered with multi-layered, bulky dressings and is then wrapped snugly with elastic bandages (Fig. 33–8). An alternative to these two methods is a semi-open method, in which the wound is covered with a topical ointment and cleansed once or twice a day. If dressings are used, they are composed of a few layers of sterile gauze saturated with a topical medication. Cleansing of the wound may be done at the bedside or in the physical therapy department in a whirlpool bath.

There is no one "best" way to treat burns. Each patient must be evaluated according to his age, physical makeup, and type of burn and then treated on an individual basis.

Open Method

When the wound is exposed to the air, the nurse must guard constantly against infection. Usually, the serous fluid that exudes from the burns will harden and cover most of the burned area, but bacteria may enter through the cracks in the dried exudate.

The bed linen is sterile, and a bed cradle or some other device is used to support the weight of the top covers in order to keep them off the burned areas. Those in attendance usually wear sterile caps, gowns, and gloves while caring for the patient.

Aside from preventing infection, the nurse must also provide additional warmth when the open method of treatment is used. Much body heat is lost through the parts of the body where the skin has been destroyed, and the patient is chilled easily. Heat lamps or radiant heat shields will usually provide the extra warmth needed.

Wet compresses or soaks to cleanse the burned area and remove excess exudate and drainage must be used with extreme care and under sterile conditions in order to minimize the danger of infecting the wound.

In recent years, some hospitals have set up special units, staffed with specially trained personnel, in which burn patients are treated by the open method.

Closed Method

This method of treating burns presents fewer problems for the nursing staff because there is less danger of infection. Also, the burned areas are covered; therefore the patient does not have a constant visual reminder of his injuries. It is also true that patients who have pressure dressings are freer to move about and do things for themselves than those who do not have their wounds covered. The main disadvantage of the closed method is the need for frequent changing of the dressings, which may require administration of a general anesthetic and also involves

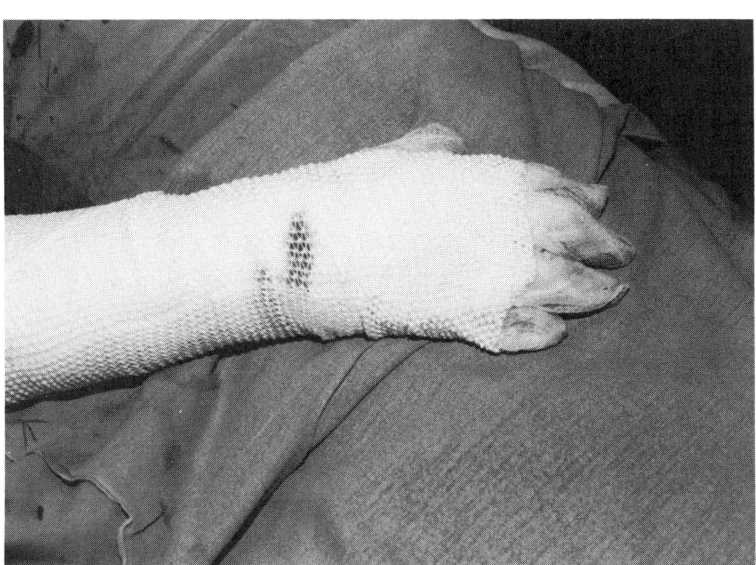

Figure 33–8 Occlusive dressing applied to a burned hand.
(Courtesy of the Burn Center at Saint Agnes Medical Center, Philadelphia, PA.)

some trauma to the regenerating tissue. Other disadvantages of bulky dressings are that they (1) provide a culture medium for the growth of bacteria, (2) are difficult to apply properly to areas such as the face and perineum, (3) may increase fluid loss and heat retention, and (4) can mask bleeding. It is also much more difficult to assess the status of the wound when the closed method is used.

Débridement and Grafting

Débridement involves removal of the eschar and necrotic material from underlying tissues. This must be done with great care so that bleeding is kept at a minimum and healthy tissues are disturbed as little as possible. Some physicians prefer the method of soaking off eschar by placing the patient in a tub containing a temperature-controlled, balanced salt solution. The bath water is gently agitated to facilitate the débridement process. Patients do not object to the bath as they do to other methods of débridement, because the bath is soothing, relaxing, and less painful, and they can exercise more freely in the water. Débridement can also be done with a scrub brush and hand-held shower instrument followed by the use of tweezers and scissors to remove loosened dead tissue.

Surgical removal of eschar and grafting of skin usually are done within the first week after the burn injury. It is most desirable to graft the patient's own skin, but when this is not possible, the skin of another person, porcine grafts, or artificial skin can be used.

Control of Infection

Wound infection remains the major cause of death in burn victims. The necrotic tissue serves as an excellent breeding ground for microorganisms, which multiply rapidly in the burn wound. The past decade has seen a gradual revolution in the treatment of burns. In the early 1960's, most patients with full-thickness burns over 50% of the body did not survive. Today, because of improved care to prevent infection and promote healing, many patients survive such extensive burns.

Some major reasons for the improved prognosis for extensive burns are (1) quicker, more aggressive fluid and electrolyte replacement; (2) better monitoring techniques for physiologic parameters; (3) more adequate nutritional support with total parenteral nutrition or high-calorie, high-protein supplements and other measures to bolster the patient's defense system and meet metabolic needs; (4) establishment of contained burn units that can truly provide an aseptic environment; (5) specially trained nurses who understand and are competent in all aspects of burn care; and (6) better skin grafting techniques, both temporary and permanent.

NURSING INTERVENTION

Prevention of infection in the wound is important throughout the healing process. Applications of topical medications should be done under aseptic conditions, even if the burn is a minor one. When the patient is ready to accept some responsibility for his care, and in preparation for his release from the hospital, the nurse begins teaching him how to apply topicals without contaminating the wound and how to change dressings if these are used.

She also will systematically assess scar tissue formation and help the patient adjust to the fact that burn scars may take as long as 6 months to 2 years to mature completely. Maturing scars usually appear red, hard, and raised before they eventually begin to fade and soften. Pressure garments and masks help prevent thick and disfiguring scars but are uncomfortable. The patient may resist wearing them unless he understands their intended purpose.

Pain and itching often continue beyond the point at which the wound appears to have healed completely. Exercises to prevent contractures can cause pain, because they stretch the skin at a time when it is very tender. Splints to prevent musculoskeletal complications also can be uncomfortable for the burn patient. Analgesics prescribed for management of pain will allow the patient to get sufficient rest, but they should be administered judiciously. If a patient begins to depend too much on one kind of analgesic, alternative drugs can be given. Itching can be controlled by giving regular doses of medication to prevent the problems, rather than waiting until the itching becomes intense and interferes with rest.

Contractures are always a threat to a patient with major burns and sometimes to one with minor burns. Proper positioning and regular exercise are essential to the prevention of musculoskeletal deformities following a burn. Painful as the motion of physical therapy exercises may be, the muscles and skin must be exercised and stretched every day if normal motion is to be maintained. Sometimes it is necessary for the patient to continue visiting the physical therapist for several months after discharge from the hospital.

Fluid intake and output are measured as long as there is a threat to fluid and electrolyte balance. Laboratory data are checked frequently for evidence of either a deficit or surplus of specific electrolytes.

The diet of the burn patient is an essential component of his therapy. Protein and calorie content is increased to several times that of a regular diet in order to assist the body in healing itself and rebuilding lost tissue. Dietary supplements include vitamins, especially vitamin C; minerals such as iron and calcium; and electrolytes.

The odor of the burn and the patient's despondency over his predicament can adversely affect his appetite. Perseverance and ingenuity in making meals and supplemental foods appealing are needed to help the patient meet his metabolic needs and promote healing and repair.

The emotional shock of a burn can be quite serious and long-lasting, especially if there is some loss of mobility and independence, or disfigurement involving the face or other parts of the body usually visible to others. The nurse should strive to develop an attitude of acceptance of the patient, a calm approach to dressing changes and discussions of scar formation, and an optimistic emphasis on what the patient can do and will be able to do in the future. As is true in most long-term and slowly progressing disorders, the severely burned patient can become bored and apathetic and might even lose the will to live. Diversional and occupational therapy and a coordinated effort on the part of all members of the health team are needed to help the burn patient recover and adjust to the effects of his injury.

When a patient has difficulty coping with the physical and psychosocial effects of a severe burn, effective nursing intervention can help him deal with his fears, anxieties, and sense of loss. In order to be most helpful, the nurse should encourage the patient to tell her what he is experiencing and how he feels about what has happened or is happening to him. She might ask him how she and others who care for him can be most helpful and what changes in his environment he would like to see take place. It may be possible to change some elements of the environment. For example, noise, lights, or certain people—visitors or staff—may be very irritating to the patient; these factors usually can be adjusted. If the patient is unhappy about being isolated, bringing in a radio or magazines and books may help him keep in touch with the outside world. Regardless of whether every change desired by the patient can be made, at the very least he is assured that there is someone who will listen to and empathize with him.

The patient's self-esteem can be reinforced by emphasizing the strengths the nurse has noticed when he is coping with pain, inconvenience, or some other unpleasant situation. She can involve him in caring for himself as much as he is able and give him some sense of control over his condition. And she can communicate by words and actions her concern and care.

Nursing interventions for selected problems in a burned patient are summarized in Nursing Care Plan 33-1.

Concerns for the Elderly

It is easy to see that there are many changes in the skin as we grow older. Wrinkled, sagging, and dry skin are universal with age. However, genetic makeup and amount of sun exposure has a great impact on just how much and how quickly the skin shows such changes.

The epidermis thins with advancing age, giving a pale translucent appearance. Collagen decreases through the years, causing a decrease in skin strength and elasticity. Greater vascular fragility in the skin and loss of subcutaneous tissue is the reason for easy bruising. This is evidenced in the extremities in the form of "senile purpura" from even minor trauma. More than 70% of older women have areas of senile purpura, compared with 40% of men. Healing is slower because of the decreased vascularity of the dermal layer.

This decreased vascularity extends to the subcutaneous tissue also and affects the absorption of drugs given subcutaneously.

Sweat glands decrease with age, and in the very old, the capacity to produce sweat is greatly reduced. The skin also loses some of its ability to maintain body temperature. For these reasons, the elderly are at greater risk of hypothermia and heat exhaustion. Sebaceous glands slow their output, resulting in drier, coarser skin. This seems to be more pronounced in fair-skinned people.

Changes in hair growth and distribution are evident with age. The degree of change is determined by racial, genetic, and sex-linked factors. After age 40, there is some progressive loss and thinning of the hair. After age 60, women tend to lose more hair on the trunk and extremities, whereas men lose more from the head.

Nails become dull, brittle, hard, and thick with aging as a result of changes in the vascular supply to the nailbed. This is more evident in the nails of the toes than in those of the fingers. There is an increase in longitudinal striations, which often leads to splitting of the nails.

The main pathologic skin change seen in elderly individuals is development of actinic keratoses caused by sun exposure through the years. Skin cancers also occur, and fungal infections are frequent. Lentigos, or "age spots," are very common. Skin tags are also seen more often after the sixth decade. Senile papillomata (yellow, brown, or black warts) appear on the trunk, extremities or face in more than 60% of the elderly. These are normal occurrences with age and only cause concern because of their appearance. However, they are so commonplace that vigilance is necessary in looking for skin changes that indicate malignant lesions.

NURSING CARE PLAN 33–1

Selected nursing diagnoses, goals/outcome criteria, nursing interventions, and evaluations for a burned patient

Situation: Mr. Young, age 33, sustained second- and third-degree burns over both arms when a container of gasoline he was carrying ignited. He also suffered first-degree burns on his hands and face. In the emergency department his wounds were cleaned, and a topical agent was applied; no dressings were applied. An intravenous line was established, and fluids were administered to avoid potential fluid and electrolyte imbalance. He received meperidine for pain and on admission to his room was fairly comfortable, conscious, and oriented.

Nursing Diagnosis	Goals/Outcome Criteria	Nursing Intervention	Evaluation
Fluid volume deficit related to loss of fluids via open wounds. SUPPORTING DATA Second- and third-degree burns over both arms; weeping.	Adequate circulating blood volume as evidenced by BP, pulse, and urine output.	Monitor VS q 2 h. Monitor urine output, report drop below 50 mL/h. Monitor lab values for electrolyte imbalances. Maintain IV fluids on schedule. Encourage fluid intake of 3,000 mL q 24 h when bowel sounds are present.	BP maintaining 108/62; P, 92; urine output, 45 mL/h; continue plan.
Potential for infection related to damage to skin. SUPPORTING DATA Skin on both arms damaged by burns.	Burn wound will be free of infection as evidenced by normal VS and negative wound cultures.	Use strict aseptic technique when working with patient. Apply silver sulfadiazadine as ordered to wounds tid. Monitor WBC count for signs of infection; observe wounds tid. Encourage good nutrition.	Sulfadiazadine applied, 9 and 1; WBC count, 7,800; temp., 99.6°F.; wounds moist and clean; no purulent material evident; continue plan.
Pain related to open burn wounds. SUPPORTING DATA Is constantly asking for pain medication; grimacing and holding body rigid.	Patient will verbalize that pain control is adequate.	Administer pain medication as ordered before débridement procedures and prn. Teach relaxation and imagery techniques to assist with pain control. Utilize diversionary activities such as television, card games, board games, etc., to help diminish awareness of pain.	Demerol, 100 mg., 9, 12, and 3; relaxation and imagery techniques taught; encouraged to practice; states pain only controlled for 2½ hours; encourage diversional activities; continue plan.
Self-care deficit—bathing, feeding, toileting, grooming—related to inability to use arms and hands. SUPPORTING DATA Unable to perform self-care because of burns on arms and hands.	Patient will resume own self-care activities within 3 months.	Assist with toileting, bathing, grooming, and feeding. Allow him to make decisions as much as possible to lessen feelings of helplessness. Allow him to do as much as he is able to do.	Not ready to resume self-care activities; making decisions about time for bath, diversional activity, etc.; continue plan.
Self-esteem disturbance related to helplessness and fear of losing ability to work as a mechanic. SUPPORTING DATA "With my hands burned, I won't be able to work anymore."	Patient will verbalize improved sense of self-worth within 3 months; able to return to work as mechanic.	Establish trusting relationship; actively listen to concerns and frustrations. Help him establish his active role in recovery of use of hands and arms. Allow him to do whatever tasks of ADL are possible for him. Praise him for his efforts with physical therapy exercises. Help him establish small, accomplishable goals on a weekly basis. Offer emotional support and encouragement that is realistic.	Verbalizing fears about the future and employment; working with physical therapist; established two small goals for the week; continue plan.

BIBLIOGRAPHY

Andreoli, T. E., et al.: Cecil's Essentials of Medicine, 2nd ed. Philadelphia, W. B. Saunders, 1990.

Bayley, E., and Smith, G.: The three degrees of burn care. Nursing 87, March, 1987, p. 34.

Bush, A.: What to look for when the patient suffers an electrical injury. RN, Sept., 1987, p. 39.

Coleman, D., et al.: A worst-case guide for any case of psoriasis. RN, March, 1988, p. 39.

Curtis, M.: Psoriasis: A persistent problem. Nurs. Times, May 9–15, 1990, p. 44.

Cuzzell, J. Z.: Clues: Recurrent, punched-out lesions. Am. J. Nurs., May, 1990, p. 21.

Dunn, M. D., et al.: Treatment options for psoriasis. Am. J. Nurs., Aug., 1988, p. 1082.

Kinney, R. M., et al.: AACN's Clinical Reference for Critical-Care Nursing, 2nd ed. New York, McGraw-Hill, 1988.

Rakel, R. E., ed.: Conn's Current Therapy, 1990. Philadelphia, W. B. Saunders, 1990.

Stern, C.: Melanoma: The most lethal skin cancer. RN, July, 1987, p. 53.

Thompson, J. M., et al.: Mosby's Manual of Clinical Nursing, 2nd. ed. St. Louis, C. V. Mosby, 1989.

Vargo, N. L.: The skin cancer success story. RN, July, 1987, p. 50.

STUDENT STUDY AIDS

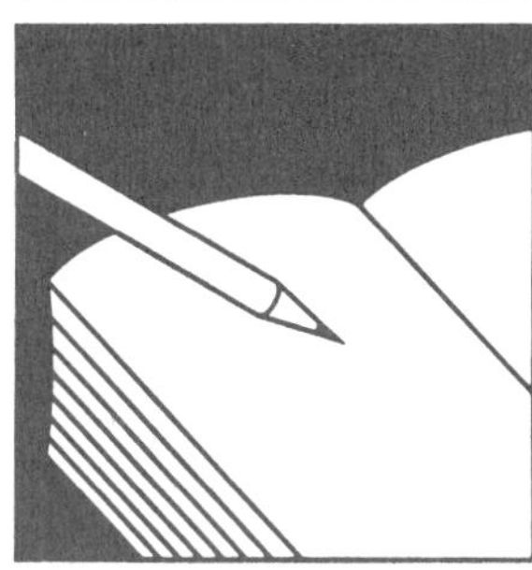

CLINICAL CASE PROBLEMS

Read each clinical situation and discuss the questions with your classmates.

1. You have been asked to give a presentation to your younger sister's ninth-grade class on the subject of skin care and the prevention of skin disease.

- What specific information would you include on the subject of general care of the skin?
- Which skin disorders would you choose to talk about?
- What information would you plan to include about each of these disorders?

---

2. Mrs. Nation, age 32, has been assigned as your patient on the evening shift. She has a severe dermatitis, probably allergic. Her physician has ordered a topical lotion, dermatologic baths twice a day, and an antihistamine to relieve itching.

- What kinds of data would you include in your ongoing assessment of Mrs. Nation's skin disorder?
- What nursing care problems is Mrs. Nation likely to present?
- What objectives and the nursing measures to meet them would you include in Mrs. Nation's nursing care plan?
- What would you teach Mrs. Nation about the application of topicals when she returns home?

---

3. Martha Moore, age 19 years, was badly burned when her clothing caught fire while she was grilling hamburgers on her patio. She has partial-thickness and full-thickness burns over her abdomen and down the front of both upper legs.

- What is the priority of care after assessment when Martha reaches the emergency room?
- What *nursing* measure should be taken to prevent infection of Martha's burns?
- What nursing measures would be included in her nursing care plan to ensure that Martha did not suffer from an undetected fluid and electrolyte imbalance?
- How is Martha's pain treated? Why?
- List some specific things you and the other nurses could do to help Martha handle her sense of loss and altered self-image as a result of the appearance of the burns and scars.

STUDY OUTLINE

I. Introduction

A. Skin protects against invasion of bacteria in the environment.
B. Helps regulate body temperature.
C. Holds in body fluids.
D. Diseases of the skin often difficult to heal; have a tendency to recur.
E. People often try to treat skin diseases themselves.

II. Diagnostic tests and procedures and nursing responsibilities

A. Skin biopsy: shave, punch, or excision. Done to differentiate benign from malignant lesions, and to identify infectious organisms.
B. Culture and sensitivity tests.
C. Inspection under special lights:
   1. Cold light to illuminate layers of skin.
   2. Wood's light to diagnose fungal infections.
D. Self-examination of skin to recognize changes in warts, moles, birthmarks, and other lesions.

III. Nursing assessment of skin lesions

A. History taking:
   1. Potential etiologic factors (see Fig. 33–1).
   2. Present illness: when rash first appeared; precipitating or aggravating factors noticed by patient.
   3. Exposure to infectious or irritating agents.
   4. Drugs currently being taken or taken in recent past.
   5. Family history of skin disease.
B. Subjective and objective data:
   1. Subjective: pain, itching, shortness of breath, gastrointestinal problems.
   2. Objective data: type of lesion (see Table 33–1).
      a. Appearance of adjacent skin.
      b. Edema.
      c. Characteristics of secretions.
      d. Odor.
      e. General appearance of skin surface.
      f. Observations: scratching, rubbing, picking at lesions.
      g. Local changes in temperature of skin.
C. Categories of nursing diagnoses commonly related to skin disorders:
   1. Impaired skin integrity.
   2. Potential impaired skin integrity.
   3. Pain.
   4. Disturbance of self-esteem.
   5. Anxiety.
   6. Potential for infection.
   7. Knowledge deficit.
   8. Sleep pattern disturbance.
   9. Social isolation.

IV. Prevention of skin disease

A. Cleanliness; gentle cleaning with mild soap and water; lotions to combat dryness.
B. Well-balanced, nutritious diet.
C. Age: older persons experience dryness, loss of elasticity, and sometimes poor circulation to the skin.
D. Environment: avoiding irritants such as chemicals and ultraviolet radiation from the sun. Health teaching to warn general public of the hazards of overexposure to the sun.

V. General nursing care

A. Intelligent observation; careful handling of the skin; avoidance of alcohol, lotions, and other skin applications not specifically ordered by the dermatologist.

B. Dermatologic baths:
   1. Prepared by adding soothing agents or disinfectants to bath water.
   2. Avoid chilling patient.
   3. Pat, do not rub, the skin dry after bath.

C. Laundering: bed linens and clothing may require special laundering to remove all traces of soap.

D. Wet compresses and dressings often used.

E. Topical therapy—administration of medication directly to surface of skin (see Table 33–2).

VI. Infectious and parasitic skin diseases

A. Contact isolation measures recommended for certain skin disorders that can be transmitted to others by personal contact or contact with infective material.
   1. Private room, masks, gowns if soiling is likely, gloves for handling infective material, hand washing, and decontamination of articles.

B. Herpesvirus infections: those caused by an extensive family of viruses.
   1. Herpes simplex: acute viral disease:
      a. Symptoms: lesions (blisters, ulcers) on lips and nares, also called cold sores and fever blisters.
      b. Treatment and nursing intervention:
         (1) Disease usually self-limiting. Treatment is symptomatic, as there is no cure.
         (2) Oral acyclovir may be beneficial.
   2. Herpes zoster ("shingles"): caused by herpes varicella–zoster, which causes chickenpox (varicella) in children and shingles in older adults.
      a. Viruses replicate in the peripheral nerve ganglia, where they lie dormant until activated by trauma, malignancy, or local radiation.
      b. Symptoms begin with low-grade fever and possibly GI upset. Lesions appear 3 to 5 days later, along the course of affected nerve. Pain and itching are chief complaints.
      c. Medical treatment and nursing intervention:
         (1) Non-narcotic analgesics.
         (2) Corticosteroids to reduce inflammation and pain.
         (3) Vidarabine intravenously for immune-deficient patients.
         (4) Acyclovir may diminish severity; corticosteroids used to relieve severe pain.
         (5) Emotional support and measures to relieve symptoms and prevent secondary bacterial infection.

C. Impetigo: streptococcal or staphylococcal infection of skin.
   1. Symptoms: vesicles and bullae that become pustular, rupture, and form crusts.
   2. Medical treatment and nursing intervention:
      a. Patient placed on contact isolation.
      b. Lesions cleaned with soap and water.
      c. Local applications of antibiotic ointment.

D. Fungal infections (mycoses).
   1. Two groups: those that are truly pathogenic and those that are opportunistic.
   2. Examples: tinea pedis (athlete's foot), tinea of the scalp (ringworm), and moniliasis (thrush).

3. Symptoms: itching and some breakdown of skin.
4. Treatment: fungistatic medicines.
5. Patient teaching to avoid recurrent fungal infections (see Table 33–3).

E. Parasitic infestations: pediculosis and scabies.

1. Three kinds of lice: head, body, and pubic or "crab" lice.
   a. Most prevalent symptom of lice is severe itching. Scratching causes lesions and entry points for bacterial infection.
   b. Scabies mites burrow under skin and produce irritation with intense itching and blistering. Secondary infection not uncommon.
   c. Lice and scabies treated with lindane (Kwell and Gamene) and 10% crotamiton (Eurax). A-200 Pyrinate and Cuprex do not require prescription.

VII. Acne: characterized by papules and pustules over the face, back, and shoulders

A. Begins when ducts from sebaceous glands become plugged with sebum and cellular debris. Can cause inflammation and formation of cysts.

B. Acne vulgaris most common type. Typically begins in early puberty.

C. Medical treatment:

1. Mild noninflammatory type usually responds well to topicals that peel top layer of skin and remove blackheads and whiteheads.
2. Retin-A best for papular and pustular acne.
3. Benzoyl peroxide most used topical for acne.
4. Antibiotics, especially tetracycline, prescribed to inhibit bacterial infection.
5. 13-*cis*-retinoic acid (Accutane) effective in controlling most cases of treatment-resistant acne. Its effects are sustained for months or years after the drug is discontinued.
6. Scarring and pitting treated by dermabrasion.

D. Nursing intervention: health education and patient teaching.

1. Cleanliness, diet, exercise recommended. No special diet needed unless patient notes relationship between certain foods and appearance of lesions.
2. Patient needs support and encouragement to continue treatment, which can last for months or years.

VIII. Psoriasis: chronic, recurring skin disorder. Patches of skin covered with adherent silvery scales (plaques).

A. Tends to run in families; cause unknown.

B. Comes and goes, often with or without treatment.

C. Medical treatment and nursing intervention:

1. Mild cases respond to steroid creams, moderate doses of sunlight.
2. Resistant cases treated with ultraviolet radiation and tar preparations.
3. Antimetabolites used in severe cases.
4. Patient education includes information about nature of disease, purpose of prescribed treatment, avoidance of factors that aggravate the condition or cause a flare-up.
5. Skin should be kept moist and pliable; scratches and abrasions avoided because they can trigger appearance of plaques at new site.

IX. Cancer of the skin

A. Almost all cases can be treated successfully if caught early.

B. Cause unknown, but skin type, heredity, and exposure to environmental carcinogens—including sunlight—can increase susceptibility.

C. Types and characteristics (see Table 33–4).

D. Treatment: surgical removal, occasionally chemotherapy and radiation therapy once metastasis has occurred.

X. Burns

A. Caused by exposure to heat, electrical agents, strong chemicals, and radiation.

B. Classified according to extent and depth of injury (Tables 33–5 and 33–6).

C. Emergency treatment:

1. All burns should be considered potentially dangerous until they are thoroughly assessed.
   a. Minor burns treated by submersion in cool water, applications of cool compresses. Do not apply any ointment or greasy substance.

D. Immediate care (major burns):

1. First hour can be crucial to successful outcome; fluid replacement essential.
2. Obtain details of nature of accident; cause of burn, possibility of internal burns.
3. Determine depth and extent; establish intravenous lines.
4. Administer oxygen as needed.
5. Cover wound with clean sheet to protect from air.
6. Prevent or relieve profound shock by:
   a. Replacing fluids and electrolytes.
   b. Relieving pain.
7. Management of pain:
   a. Administer morphine or meperidine IV as ordered.
   b. Handle gently.
   c. Consider emotional impact of burn.
8. Other immediate complications:
   a. Damage to respiratory tract.
   b. Hemorrhage not typical of burn. Check for other types of injuries.

E. Nursing assessment:

1. Monitor vital signs frequently and regularly.
2. Check condition of wound for signs of infection, cellulitis. Note color, dryness, appearance of wound, swelling and other signs of inflammation in adjacent tissues.
3. Monitor patient for fluid imbalance: urine output, vital signs.

F. Treatment of the wound:

1. Two general methods: open and closed.
   a. In open there is no dressing. Wound is left open to the air.
      (1) Sterile bed linens, some form of reverse isolation.
      (2) Provide additional warmth.
      (3) Compresses and soaks done under sterile conditions.
   b. In closed method, wound is covered with bulky dressing.
      (1) Advantages are that wound is not so obvious to patient, infection is less likely, patient able to move more freely.
      (2) Disadvantages are pain involved in frequent dressing changes, bacteria can grow on dressing, difficult to apply on certain body parts, can increase fluid loss, and can mask bleeding from healing wound.
2. Alternative method: combination open and closed, using occlusive topical to cover wound.

3. Débridement and grafting to promote healing and cover wound.
4. Control of infection:
   a. Wound infection the major cause of death from burns.
   b. Major reasons for improved prognosis are aggressive fluid replacement, more sophisticated physiologic monitoring, better nutritional support, use of specialized burn units with highly skilled nurses, and better skin grafting techniques.

G. Nursing intervention:
1. Use aseptic technique to avoid infecting patient while administering care.
2. Systematically assess scar tissue formation. Help patient adjust to possibility that scars will get worse before they begin to fade.
3. Measures to relieve pain and itching.
4. Exercises to prevent contractures.
5. Measure intake and output; check laboratory data for electrolyte imbalance.
6. Encourage adequate dietary intake of high-protein foods.
7. Help patient cope with emotional shock and sense of loss, altered self-image.

XI. Concerns for the elderly

A. Epidermis thins with advancing age, giving a translucent appearance to the skin.
B. Collagen decreases through the years, causing a decrease in skin strength and elasticity.
C. Elderly skin is more easily damaged and slower to repair as a result of decreased vascularity of dermal layer.
D. Skin loses some of its ability to maintain body temperature.
E. Sebaceous gland secretion decreases, leading to dry, coarser skin.
F. Hair becomes thinner and more sparse, although baldness is related to genetic factors, rather than to aging alone.
G. Nails become dull, brittle, hard, and thick with aging.
H. Sun exposure over the years causes formation of actinic keratoses, which are premalignant lesions.
I. "Age spots," skin tags, and senile papilloma common among the elderly.
J. Skin cancers and fungal infections also common problems among the elderly.

CHAPTER 34

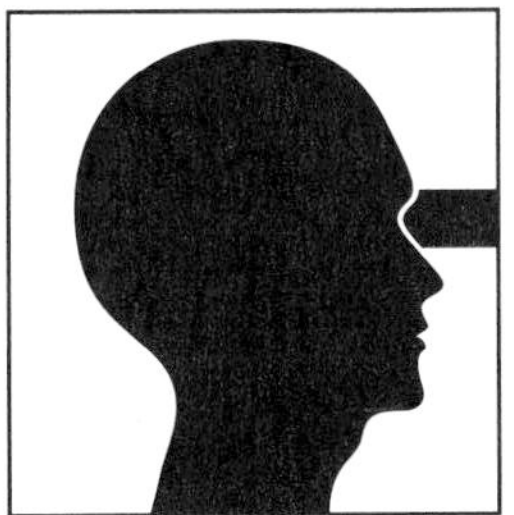

Care of Patients With Disorders of the Eyes

VOCABULARY

aphakia
enucleation
intraocular
miotic
mydriatic
nystagmus
ophthalmologist
optician
optometrist
periorbital
phacoemulsification
photocoagulation
presbyopia
retinopathy
vitrectomy

Upon completion of this part of the chapter the student should be able to:

1. Describe ways in which nurses can contribute to the preservation of sight and prevention of blindness.
2. Discuss tests and examinations used in the diagnosis of eye disorders and visual impairment.
3. Describe nursing activities in assessment of the eye and nursing diagnoses commonly associated with patients experiencing impaired vision.
4. Describe the clinical manifestations of selected inflammations of the eye and appropriate medical treatment and nursing interventions for each.
5. Discuss nursing interventions for care of the visually impaired patient.
6. Describe the nursing care plan for a patient with glaucoma, including education for self-care.
7. Describe the nursing care plan for a patient having eye surgery.

Vision loss is one of the most profound and dreaded of physical disabilities. When a sighted person is no longer able to see, his world changes, and he is required to make many adjustments. There are two general kinds of patients with impaired vision: those who were born blind or unable to see well enough to care for themselves, and those who develop some degree of visual impairment later in life. In this chapter we will focus on the latter type of visually handicapped patient.

The nursing care of patients with severe visual handicaps demands a special awareness of the unique problems encountered by someone who has either partial or total loss of vision. The nurse must be sensitive to these patients' special needs, demonstrating gentleness in her approach, and she must be creative in devising ways to help them accept responsibility for their personal care and enjoyment of life without the benefit of good sight. Patient education is especially important to these patients' acceptance of their visual disorder, their participation in diagnostic and therapeutic measures, and their adjustment to their new surroundings when they are hospitalized or admitted to a long-term-care facility.

Within the past few decades there have been many new developments in the treatment of a number of potentially blinding diseases of the eye. These new surgical techniques and medical treatments offer hope for the preservation of sight in increasing numbers of people. There also have been efforts made to educate the public about eye care, prevention of eye disease, and periodic examinations to detect eye disorders in their earliest and treatable stages.

PREVENTION OF EYE DISORDERS AND IMPAIRED VISION

As health care providers, nurses share responsibility for the maintenance of good eyesight in normal eyes and the preservation of vision throughout the patient's life span. Although some visual problems are related to diseases that occur later in life, management of such chronic diseases as diabetes mellitus and early detection of glaucoma can help prevent blindness.

Two major goals of the maintenance of good vision are (1) health education to inform the general public about basic eye care and (2) prevention of accidental injury to the eye.

BASIC EYE CARE

Teaching people to take care of their eyes sometimes involves dispelling misconceptions they might have and providing them with factual information about the eyes and their care. Following are some facts that should be included in this area of health education.

The term *eyestrain* has often been used as a catchall to explain various visual defects and diseases of the eye. It is actually very difficult to strain the eye. Inadequate lighting or prolonged use of the eyes for close work can overwork the eye muscles, but this will not damage the eyes any more than straining to hear a distant sound can damage the ears. One should rest the eye muscles periodically when watching television, doing needlework, or performing any activity that demands intensive visual effort. If the eyes tire easily or if there is headache or burning, itching, or redness of the eyes, this is not eyestrain. These are symptoms of a visual problem and are an indication that the person's eyes should be examined.

Adequate diet and good nutrition are important to the conservation of sight, but eating large amounts of carrots and other yellow vegetables will not improve eyesight. A lack of vitamin A found in these foods often results in inflammation of the lids and conjunctiva and an increased sensitivity to light. A serious deficiency of vitamin B can cause irreparable damage to the retina and permanent visual defects.

Normal eyes do not require irrigations or periodic "washing out" with over-the-counter eye solutions. Normal secretions of the conjunctiva and tear glands should be sufficient to lubricate the eye and wash away small particles of dust that may collect in the eye. Accumulations of purulent material or excessive tearing usually indicates the need for an eye examination.

Older persons sometimes have what lay persons call "dry eyes." This is due to decreased production of tears and is treated by the instillation of "replacement tears," which are commercial preparations of solutions similar in composition to real tears. If dry eye syndrome occurs in persons younger than 60 years of age, it could be symptomatic of an underlying disease.

Children do not outgrow crossed eyes (strabismus). Until a baby reaches the age of 6 to 9 months, he may have some difficulty focusing his eyes, but this problem should not persist. Neglect of strabismus can result in serious loss of vision. It is generally agreed by ophthalmologists that the sooner treatment is begun, the better the chance of correcting the condition and preserving the child's eyesight.

A more common visual defect in children is amblyopia, or "lazy eye," which is caused by poorer vision in one eye than in the other eye. The child tends to avoid using the weaker eye because of difficulties in focusing both eyes on an object. The result can be permanent damage to vision if the condition is not corrected by the age of 6 or 7.

Every person over the age of 40 should have eye examinations every 2 years. It is particularly important that a test for glaucoma be made at the time of the examination, because this disease usually is asymptomatic until damage to vision has occurred. Persons with a family history of glaucoma should be especially careful to have their eyes tested for increased pressure within the eyeball, as this is the basic pathology of glaucoma and the disorder tends to be familial.

Accidental injury to the eye is a major cause of diminished or total loss of vision, especially in young children. Parents and teachers should be encouraged to teach children the danger of sharp pencils, paper wads, small stones, lawn darts, fireworks, and other small objects children may be tempted to hurl at one another while playing. Older children and adults should be cautioned to wear protective eyewear when engaging in sports such as raquetball and squash where small balls travel at high speeds.

Occupational accidents have been reduced since the establishment and enforcement of rules regarding the wearing of goggles and other protective devices when working in a hazardous environment. The National Institute of Occupational Safety and Health (NIOSH) in Rockville, Maryland, provides information about eye safety and hazards in the work place.

The incidence of injuries to the eye and surrounding structures can be reduced by encouraging people to wear special headgear and devices to protect the head and eyes when participating in sports, doing yardwork, or working in home workshops.

Cosmetics for the eyelids, eyelashes, and eyebrows can be a source of infection and allergy. Most dyes used for hair on the scalp are not intended for use on the eyelashes and eyebrows. Sometimes it is not the cosmetic but the way in which it is applied that causes eye disease. Saliva should not be used to moisten pencils, eye shadow, or mascara, as it may contain organisms that can cause eye infection. When eye cosmetics are being applied, it is important to have a steady hand to avoid accidentally scratching the cornea and eyelids. Cosmetics should never be shared, as this can transmit organisms.

In an effort to promote prompt treatment of eye disease in its earliest stages, the National Society for the Prevention of Blindness lists the following danger signals.

DANGER SIGNALS OF EYE DISEASE

- *Persistent redness of the eye.* Infections and inflammations of the structures of the eye that are not treated may leave scars that can produce loss of vision.
- *Continuing pain or discomfort about the eye, especially following injury.*
- *Disturbances of vision.* Although these symptoms may simply indicate a need for eyeglasses, blurred vision, loss of side vision, double vision, and sudden development of many floating spots in the field of vision may be symptomatic of more serious systemic diseases.
- *Crossing of the eyes, especially in children.*
- *Growths on the eye or eyelids or opacities visible in the normally transparent portion of the eye.*
- *Continuing discharge, crusting, or tearing of the eyes.*
- *Pupil irregularities,* either unequal size of the two pupils or distorted shape.

DIAGNOSTIC TESTS AND EXAMINATIONS

VISUAL ACUITY

The Snellen chart is one of the simpler tools for testing visual acuity. The chart is quite familiar to most of us, even though we may not know it by name. It is usually designed so that there is one large letter at the top and subsequent rows of letters under it, each row in smaller print than the one above it. The Snellen chart is read from a distance of exactly 20 feet, and the letters are scaled according to normal vision. A person with normal visual acuity can read the top letter from a distance of 100 feet, the second row of letters from 70 feet, the third at 50 feet, and so on, down to 10 feet for the last row of letters.

The visual acuity of the person being tested is expressed as a fraction; the *numerator* indicates the distance between the patient and the chart (20 feet), and the *denominator* indicates the distance at which a person with normal vision can read at least half of the letters correctly. For example, 20/50 vision means that the person being tested can read the letters of the specific row at a distance of 20 feet, whereas a person with normal visual acuity could easily read these letters from a distance of 50 feet. Visual acuity of 20/20 is considered normal; vision of 20/200 is legally defined as blindness. Legal blindness is defined as a corrected vision of less than 20/200 in the better eye or a visual field of less than 20 degrees.

NEAR VISION TEST

In order to test an individual's ability to see objects close at hand, the examiner uses a test known as *Jaeger's Test Types*. The patient is given a card that is printed with different sizes of ordinary printer's type. A piece of cardboard is placed over one eye while the other eye reads the print. In this way, each eye is tested separately.

REFRACTION

When light rays enter the eye, they are "refracted," or bent, so that they focus on the retina. The lens, aqueous humor, and vitreous humor are responsible for bending these light rays. Disorders of the lens that prevent the proper focusing of light rays upon the retina are diagnosed by a *refraction*. This eye examination makes use of several glass lenses of different shapes through which the patient reads the Snellen chart. When the patient chooses the lens through which he can best read the chart, the ophthalmologist or optometrist prescribes the same kind of lens to be ground by the optician and fitted as glasses for the patient.

INTRAOCULAR PRESSURE TEST

The chambers of the eyeballs in front of the lens are filled with a watery substance called the *aqueous humor*. This fluid is constantly being produced and drained off in equal proportions so that there is a normal amount of pressure within the chambers. The amount of pressure being exerted by the aqueous humor within the chambers of the eye can be measured with an instrument called a *tonometer*. The testing of intraocular pressure is extremely important in the diagnosis of glaucoma, a condition in which intraocular pressure is increased.

Normal intraocular pressure is approximately 15 to 21 mm Hg. This number is not absolute, however, because the pressure varies from 3 to 5 mm Hg during the day. It is highest in the morning before arising and lowest late in the evening. Moreover, some eyes seem to tolerate higher pressure better than others, and some patients can have a pressure reading of more than 30 mm Hg for long periods of time without suffering damage to their vision. In general, however, intraocular pressure readings in the low 20s should be watched carefully and checked frequently to establish an early diagnosis of glaucoma. If intraocular pressures remain in the high 20s, further testing is recommended. Testing for glaucoma is discussed later in this chapter.

SLIT LAMP OR BIOMICROSCOPIC EXAMINATION

A special instrument called the biomicroscope, or slit lamp, is used to examine the surface of the eye through a microscopic lens (Fig. 34–1). The advantage of the slit lamp is that it reduces the beam of light to a narrow slit that illuminates only a small section of the eye. Because the slit lamp beam can be angled from one side or the other, the examiner can assess one thin section (or slit) of the cornea or the lens at a time.

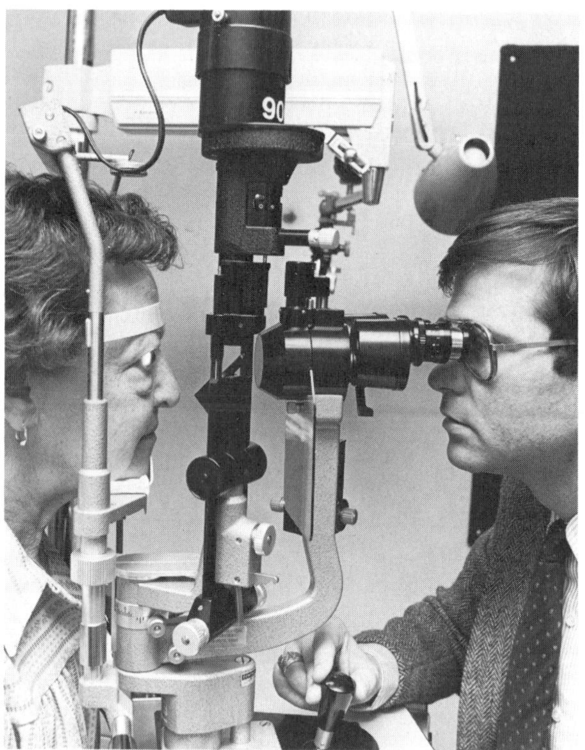

Figure 34–1 Slit lamp examination. (Courtesy of Wills Eye Hospital, Philadelphia, PA.)

The slit lamp technique for examining fluid within the eyeball can be compared to the ability to see sediment floating in a lighted aquarium. Hence cells floating in the aqueous (the fluid in the anterior and posterior chambers of the eye) can be seen and their quantity evaluated. The number of cells is increased in proportion to the degree of inflammation.

TOPICAL DYES

A topical dye can also be used to detect abrasions and tears of the cornea with the naked eye. The dye, which is usually fluorescein, is applied to the eye and the excess washed away with water or saline. The dye will remain on the injured tissue, making it more easily seen without magnification.

OPHTHALMOSCOPY

The direct ophthalmoscope (Fig. 34–2) is an instrument used to inspect the fundus; that is, the back portion of the interior of the eyeball, which is visible through the pupil when the ophthalmoscope is used. Examination is best carried out in a darkened room after the pupils have been dilated.

During *direct ophthalmoscopy* the examiner is

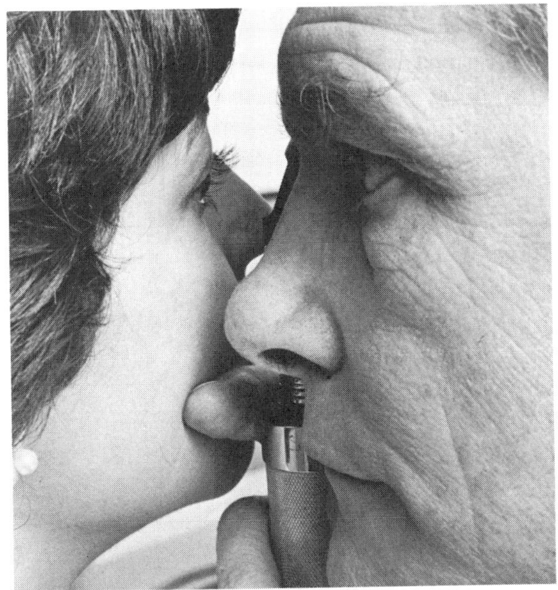

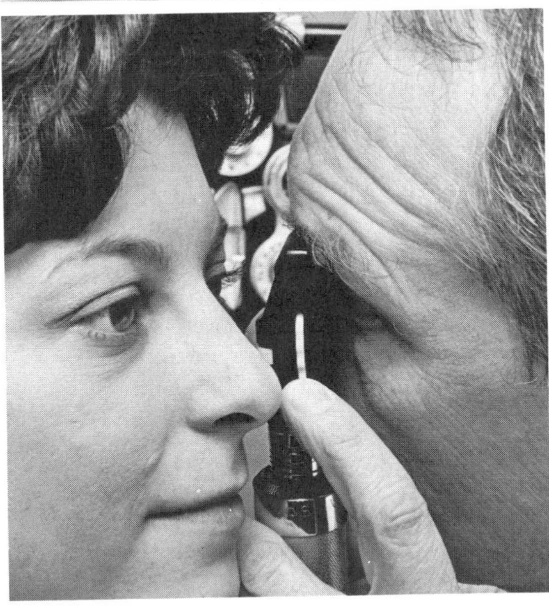

Figure 34–2 Examination of patient with direct ophthalmoscope. Note that examiner views the patient's right eye with his right eye and the patient's left eye with his left eye.
(Photos by Ken Kasper; courtesy of Wills Eye Hospital, Philadelphia, PA.)

looking for discoloration or changes in the color or pigmentation of the fundus, changes in the caliber and shape of retinal blood vessels, increased pressure caused by lesions, areas of hemorrhage, and any abnormalities in the macula. The macula lutea (which means "yellow spot") is the portion of the retina that receives and analyzes light only from the very center of the visual field. It is a very small area directly behind the center of the lens and is densely packed with light detectors. Macular degeneration, which occurs in persons over 50 or 60 years of age, can be seen by direct ophthalmoscopy. Opacities of the lens also can be noted during direct examination with an ophthalmoscope. Figure 34–3 shows a cross section of the eye.

An *indirect ophthalmoscope* provides a stronger light source, a specially designed hand-held lens, and opportunity for stereoscopic observation of the interior of the eye. It is invaluable in the diagnosis and treatment of retinal holes, tears, and detachment. The pupils must be fully dilated for satisfactory indirect ophthalmoscopy.

FLUORESCEIN ANGIOGRAPHY

In fluorescein angiography, an intravenous injection of sodium fluorescein, a contrast medium, is given, and photographs of the fundus of the eye are taken using a special camera. The procedure is used to detect tumors and retinopathy (disorder of the retina).

NURSING ASSESSMENT

Nurses who have had special training in ophthalmic nursing are qualified to conduct a complete assessment of the eye. A detailed explanation of the various diagnostic procedures and techniques used in such an assessment is beyond the scope of this text. However, there are some significant data that can be obtained by nurses without such specialized education.

HISTORY TAKING

Visual defects and eye disease are not always the direct result of infection, injury, or degeneration within the eye itself. Many systemic diseases, including the acquired immunodeficiency syndrome (AIDS), hypertension, and diabetes mellitus, secondarily affect the eye and its functions. In her general assessment of any patient the nurse should be aware of the more obvious indications of an ophthalmic pathology, whether it be primary or secondary.

Normal vision depends in part on (1) adequately functioning nerve cells, including those in the retina as well as the optic nerve; (2) adequate circulation of blood to the retinal cells; and (3) intact and functioning structures of the eyeball itself.

A history of neurologic disorders should be noted. Neuromuscular diseases are especially likely to cause diplopia, blurred vision, or inability to move the eyes. Endocrine disorders that secondarily affect the eyes include thyroid disease and diabetes mellitus. An acute hyperglycemia can alter the shape of the lens and temporarily cause blurred vision. Prolonged hyperglycemia can adversely affect the blood vessels of the retina, causing bleeding and leading to loss of vision. Liver and kidney failure can produce pathologic changes in both neural and

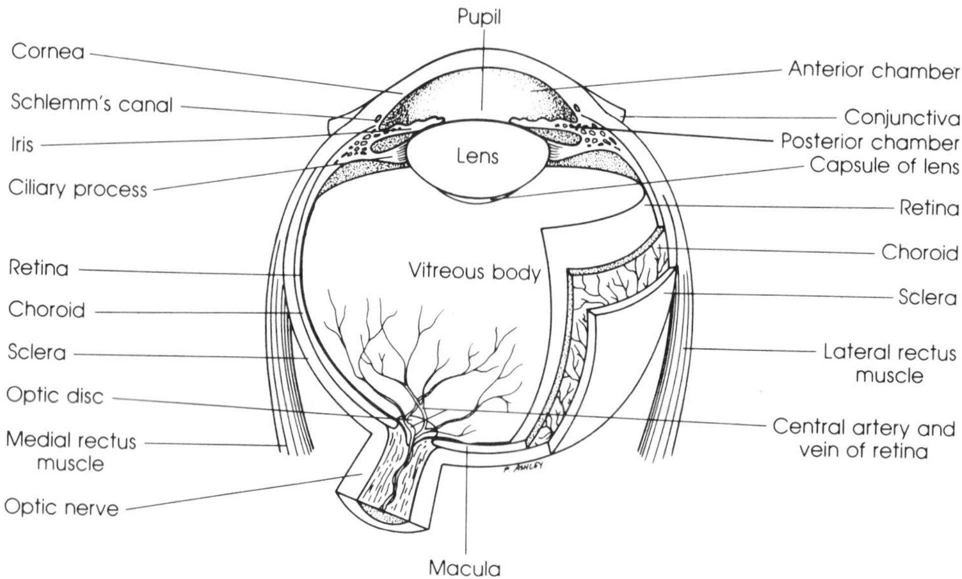

Figure 34-3 Structures of the eye.

vascular structures within the eye. Retinal changes also can be caused by hypertension and atherosclerosis.

Some drugs are capable of producing either transient or permanent ocular changes that lead to disturbances in color vision and visual acuity and the formation of cataracts, retinopathy, and glaucoma. Among common drugs that have possible ocular side effects are digitalis leaf, corticosteroids, indomethacin (Indocin), and sulfisoxazole (Gantrisin).

A family history of eye disorders also can be significant because disorders such as strabismus, retinitis pigmentosa, glaucoma, and cataracts tend to run in families or follow a pattern of inheritance.

Questions about the patient's recent history and present illness should pertain to recent injuries, infections, and changes in activities of daily living brought about by visual impairment. Sometimes patients are not aware of gradual changes in vision but have noticed that they have had more minor accidents lately, seem to be more easily fatigued, or are less interested in doing things that once gave them pleasure, such as sewing or some other hobby.

SUBJECTIVE AND OBJECTIVE DATA

Subjective symptoms of eye disorders include mild discomfort or pain, itching, burning or stinging, abnormal tearing, change in visual acuity, blurred vision, diplopia, and loss of visual field.

Objective data may include redness of the conjunctiva, swelling of the eyelids or in the periorbital space, excessive tearing, change in visual acuity, secretions and encrustations on the eyelids, abnormal position of the eyelid, and exophthalmia. The relationship between certain kinds of subjective and objective data and specific infections and inflammations of the eye and eyelid are shown in Table 34-1. Abnormalities of lid position are summarized in Table 34-2.

In addition to the more obvious signs of eye disease, visual impairment also can be assessed by noting the patient's head, hand, and eye movements. Tilting the head to one side to improve vision could mean that the patient has double vision or that one eye is much stronger than the other. Squinting could mean poor vision. Shading the eyes with the hands may indicate an increased sensitivity to light (photophobia).

Observation of the patient's ability to move his eyebrows and eyes can be helpful in diagnosing nerve damage. Inability to raise the eyebrows indicates damage to the facial nerve. Movement of the eyeball to direct the gaze is controlled by no less than six muscles, which are themselves under the control of three cranial nerves: the oculomotor (third cranial) nerve, the trochlear (fourth cranial) nerve, and the abducens (sixth cranial) nerve.

NURSING DIAGNOSES

Some of the nursing diagnoses most frequently encountered in the care of patients with eye disease include:

- Visual sensory perceptual alteration related to decreased visual acuity.
- Pain related to increased intraocular pressure.
- Potential for injury related to decreased visual field.

TABLE 34–1 CLINICAL MANIFESTATIONS OF SELECTED EYE DISEASES AND MEDICAL TREATMENT AND NURSING INTERVENTION

Disease	Manifestations	Medical Treatment and Nursing Intervention
Blepharitis Infection of glands and lash follicles along lid margin.	Itching, burning, sensitivity to light. Mucus discharge and scaling; eyelids crusted, glued shut, especially on awakening. Loss of eyelashes.	Warm compresses to soften secretions. Scrub eyelids with baby shampoo. Stroke sideways to remove exudate and scales. Antibiotic eyedrops. Systemic and topical antibiotics if skin is infected.
Chalazion Internal style; infection of meibomian gland.	Astigmatism or distorted vision, depending on size and location of chalazion. Small, hard tumor on eyelid.	Chalazion may require surgical excision and antibiotics to avoid chronic state and cyst formation.
Hordeolum External style. Infected swelling near the lid margin on inside.	Sharp pain that becomes dull and throbbing. Rupture and drainage of pus bring relief. Localized redness and swelling of lid.	Hordoleum usually resolves spontaneously. Warm compresses qid for 10 to 15 min to bring stye to a head and hasten rupture. Caution patient never to squeeze swelling, as this could spread infection. Poor health status can predispose a person to recurrence of styes.
Conjunctivitis Inflammation of the conjunctiva. "Pink eye" is a specific type caused by chemical irritants, bacteria, or virus.	Varying degrees of pain and discomfort. Increased tearing and mucus production. Itching; sensation of a foreign body in the eye.	Depends on type of infecting organism. Antibiotic eyedrops and ointments. Special care when handling infective material.
Keratitis Inflammation of the cornea.	Varying degrees of pain and discomfort. Photophobia; blurred vision if center of cornea is affected.	Depends on specific causes. Could be allergy, microbes, ischemia, or decreased lacrimation. Most superficial lesions are self-healing. Antibiotic eyedrops or ointment used for bacterial infections. Steroids can reduce inflammation and discomfort; however, herpes infection can rapidly worsen keratitis unless an antiviral agent is given simultaneously. Patient is encouraged to use good personal hygiene, frequent handwashing.
Corneal abrasion or ulceration	Moderate to severe pain and discomfort aggravated by blinking. History of trauma, contact lens wear.	Change or discontinue use of contact lens. Teach patient proper way to insert, remove, and care for contact lens. Caution not to moisten lens with saliva.

- Fear of blindness related to consequences of diabetic retinopathy.
- Impaired home maintenance management related to impaired vision.
- Anxiety related to an impending surgical procedure on the eye.
- Ineffective coping patterns related to excessive dependence on others.
- Knowledge deficit related to proper method and schedule of instillation of eye drops.
- Noncompliance with prescribed treatment for glaucoma.
- Self-care deficit related to inability to see.
- Social isolation related to reluctance to seek company of others because of visual impairment.

NURSING INTERVENTION FOR THE VISUALLY IMPAIRED

EMOTIONAL ASPECTS OF LOSS OF VISION

Those of us who are fortunate enough to have adequate vision cannot fully realize the tremendous adjustments to be made by those who are deprived of optimum sight. If we were to put on a blindfold and stumble through one day of our usual activities, we might have some slight comprehension of the obstacles to be overcome, but we still would not experience the same sense of hopelessness and despair that besets those who

TABLE 34-2 ABNORMALITIES OF LID POSITION

Abnormality	Causes	Symptoms	Treatment
Entropion: inversion of lid margin; eyelids are turned inward toward eyeball so that lashes rub against it.	Scarring and contraction of skin near eyelid (*cicatricial entropion*); or aging of skin with laxness of tissues supporting the lid and contraction of obicularis muscle (*spastic entropion*).	Pain, tearing, redness, and corneal ulceration due to margin and eyelashes rubbing against cornea.	Splinting the lid, using a pressure patch, or taping lid into everted position. Surgical correction by tightening musculature and everting lid margin.
Ectropion: eversion or outward turning of the lower lid.	Aging and laxness of skin and muscle tissues, facial paralysis, edema of conjunctiva lining the lid, or contraction of scar tissue.	Irritation of palpebral conjunctiva, spilling of tears down the cheeks due to blocked outlet, irritation of skin of cheeks, symptoms of conjunctivitis.	Usually responds to patching of the eye. Surgical correction necessary if paralysis of orbicularis muscle is permanent or if there is severe scarring and contraction of skin near the lid.
Ptosis: drooping of the eyelid so that it partially or completely covers the cornea.	Congenital weakness of the levator superioris muscle or long-term presence of foreign body. One of first signs of myasthenia gravis.	Obvious drooping of eyelid. If not corrected in infants, can lead to blindness because light rays cannot enter and stimulate development of the eye. Patient may be observed tilting head back or raising eyebrows in an effort to see from under eyelids.	Surgical correction. Removal of foreign body, if that is the cause.

have lost their sight. We would have the security of knowing that we could regain our sight by simply removing the blindfold. The blind person has no such promise.

The patient who has lost his sight goes through stages of denial, anger, and bargaining before reaching final acceptance of his condition in much the same way the dying person does. He gradually learns that he can lead a full life despite his visual impairment and the changes it brings about. He is a different person and he must learn to lead a *different kind* of life, but not necessarily one that is less meaningful. In fact, as the blind patient moves out of his preoccupation with himself, he may find that he has much to offer and much to receive from those with whom he associates.

GUIDELINES FOR HELPING A BLIND PERSON

Remember that the person is blind, not deaf. There is no reason to shout at him or address him as though he were deaf or a child. Speak normally, and do not try to avoid using the words "I see." Blind people use this phrase themselves without hesitation.

Speak to the blind person as you enter the room, and do not touch him until after you have spoken to him. This prevents startling or frightening him when he may not have heard you enter the room.

The prevention of accidents is an important part of the care of the blind. Aside from the physical effects of bumping into objects or falling over them, the blind person also suffers from a loss of self-confidence and security if he cannot move about safely and independently. Doors should be kept closed or completely open. They must never be left ajar. If it is necessary to move any object in the patient's room, ask his consent and tell him about its new location.

When you leave the room, tell the blind person that you are going. This will prevent him from becoming frustrated by resuming a conversation only to find that no one is there.

Pity is neither expected nor appreciated by the blind. They only want to be treated as normal people and would prefer to ask for your help when they need it rather than have you do everything for them. It is also important to remember that there are no such things as "extra senses" that many people mistakenly believe blind people have to compensate for the loss of sight. Whatever the blind person has learned about living with his blindness, he has accomplished through hard work and determination.

If you are assigned to the care of a blind person in a general hospital, determine the amount of assistance the patient needs and wants. Do not embarrass him by assuming that he is helpless, but avoid neglecting him when he needs your help.

When a blind or visually handicapped patient is admitted, *he will require special orientation to his room and surroundings.* If he is totally blind, describe the size of his room and the placement of furniture, using his bed as the focal point. An ambulatory patient can be walked around the room and to the bathroom to familiarize him with the location of the commode, bath, and sink. As with any patient, show him how to locate and use the call system, the radio, and the telephone if there is one at his bedside.

Most patients prefer to feed themselves if at all possible. However, it usually is necessary for the nurse to set up the meal tray of the visually handicapped patient, using the "clock" method for placement of food on the plate (Fig. 34–4). Setting up the meal tray includes opening containers of milk and juice, pouring coffee or tea, and cutting meat into bite sizes, unless the patient is accustomed to doing these things for himself.

Do not give a blind person a straw or drinking tube unless you are asked to, because it may be awkward for him to use. If you must feed him all of a meal, work slowly and calmly. Tell him about hot and cold foods on his tray, and alternate dishes rather than feeding him all of one thing before offering another. Avoid talking too much, thus forcing the patient to either stop eating or answer you with a mouth full of food. Whenever possible, help the patient select finger foods such as sandwiches and raw fruit or vegetables from the menu. *Your goal is to help the patient maintain dignity and self-respect while meeting his personal needs.*

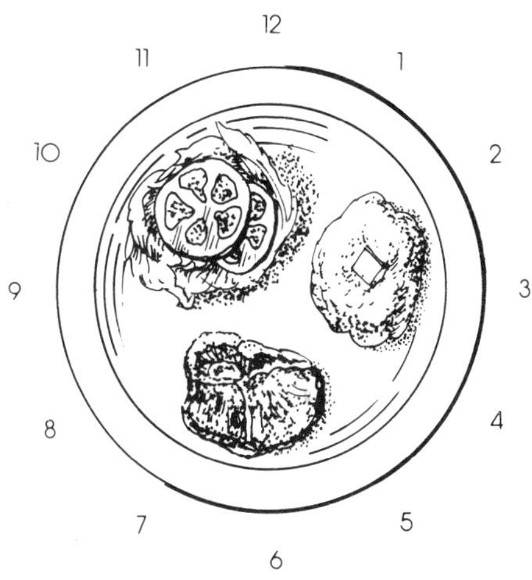

Figure 34–4 Telling the patient that his meat is at 6 o'clock, potato at 2 o'clock, and vegetable at 10 o'clock helps him to locate them on his plate.

NURSING CARE OF THE PATIENT HAVING EYE SURGERY

Preoperative Care

Most eye surgery procedures are done on an outpatient basis unless the patient has other serious disorders such as cardiac arrhythmias, severe diabetes, or a chronic disability that would prevent self-care at home or present greater risk of infection or intraoperative complications. Therefore a large part of nursing care is directed at discharge teaching for home care.

During the preoperative period, the individual needs of each patient anticipating surgery of the eye must be determined and his nursing care and teaching planned accordingly. Some patients will have nearly normal vision, whereas others may be almost totally blind. Each patient is oriented to the outpatient surgery area. Instructions regarding preoperative medications and the times they are to be instilled are given when the surgery is scheduled. The patient or significant other is taught to wash the hands thoroughly, pull the lower lid of the eye downward while the patient is looking up (with the head tilted slightly upward), and squeeze the correct number of drops into the conjunctival sac without touching the tip of the medication container on the eye or lashes. The eye is to be closed gently so as not to squeeze all the medication out of it.

Stool softeners may be started a day or two before surgery to prevent constipation and the Valsalva maneuver postoperatively. Some physicians direct the patient to wash his face with surgical soap several times the evening and morning before surgery.

If the nurse notices any symptoms of a respiratory infection or an allergy that will bring about coughing and sneezing during the postoperative period, she should notify the surgeon. Because such violent motions can bring about hemorrhage within the eye or rupture the surgical incision, the physician may postpone surgery until a later date.

Postoperative Care

In caring for a patient undergoing any type of eye surgery, the key word is *gentleness*. The patient's head should not be jarred when he is transferred from the operating table or stretcher to his bed. Remember to speak before touching a patient who is blind or wearing bandages over his eyes. He could be startled and move suddenly and violently when someone touches him if he is not aware of their presence.

Children or older patients who are unable to cooperate may need someone in constant attendance during the recovery period to prevent their pulling at the bandages.

Nausea and subsequent vomiting can wreak havoc with delicate suture lines in the eye. If the patient becomes nauseated, antiemetic medication should be administered immediately and all food and liquids withheld.

A sudden pain in the eye may indicate hemorrhage and should be brought to the attention of the physician immediately.

Irrigations of the eye and cold or wet compresses sometimes are ordered to remove exudate and reduce swelling of the eyelids and surrounding tissues. These procedures must be carried out with the utmost care, cleansing only the lids and avoiding any contact with the eyeball.

Should the patient need to stay in the hospital because of other problems, the nurse must be thoroughly familiar with his individual care needs. She should know whether the patient can be turned on one or both sides or must remain flat on his back, whether pillows are allowed under the head, and how high the head of the bed may be raised. If the patient is allowed out of bed, he must take care not to jar his head or move too suddenly; all straining and lifting must be avoided. The patient and his family should be encouraged to follow the physician's directions faithfully during the healing period at home so that nothing will jeopardize the success of the surgery.

Discharge planning for the patient having surgery from the outpatient department or the hospital is of utmost importance. The patient and/or significant other is taught the following points for home care:

- The need for asepsis when caring for the eyes. Always wash the hands before instilling medication. Be careful to check the label of the container of the medication to be certain it is the right medication. Do not contaminate the applicator tip of the medication.
- The proper method of instilling eye medications. Instill only the number of drops ordered; apply pressure at the inner canthus to prevent systemic absorption; close the eye gently (do not squeeze the eye shut).
- How to apply cold compresses; how to clean the eye.
- The proper way to change the eye patch dressing(s).
- Adherence to the medication schedule prescribed by the physician. The nurse should send home a written schedule.
- The signs and symptoms of side effects of medications to report to the physician.
- Acceptable positions for sleeping.
- The signs of complications: sudden, increasing pain in the eye, which can indicate hemorrhage; purulent drainage; decreasing vision; signs of increased intraocular pressure.
- The date, time, and importance of the follow-up visit with the surgeon.
- Activity restrictions, especially those pertaining to exercise, reading, and close vision work.
- Caution about getting water in the eye when showering or washing the hair.
- The need to wear eyeglasses to protect the eye during the day, sunglasses for outside wear, and a protective eye shield at night.

COMMON ERRORS OF REFRACTION

The most common visual defects are those of refraction.

This means that light rays entering the eye are not "refracted," or bent, at the correct angle and therefore do not focus on the retina. Errors of refraction may be caused by a number of structural defects within the eyeball itself. For example, if the eyeball is constructed so that the distance between the lens and retina is too short, the light rays focus behind the retina. This causes difficulty in seeing objects close at hand and is called farsightedness *(hyperopia)* (Fig. 34–5).

If the opposite is true, and the eyeball is too elongated, the light rays will converge and focus in front of the retina. The individual then has difficulty seeing objects at a distance and is re-

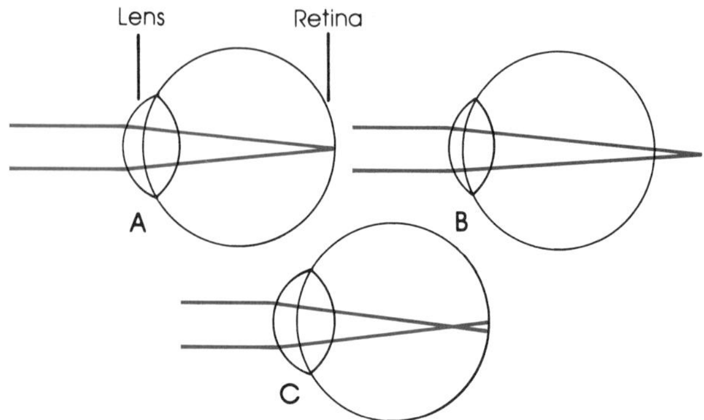

Figure 34–5 *A,* Normal vision. The lens bends light rays so that they focus directly on the retina. *B,* Hyperopia. The lens is too close to the retina; light rays converge at a point beyond the retina. *C,* Myopia. The lens is too far away from the retina; light rays converge before they reach the retina.

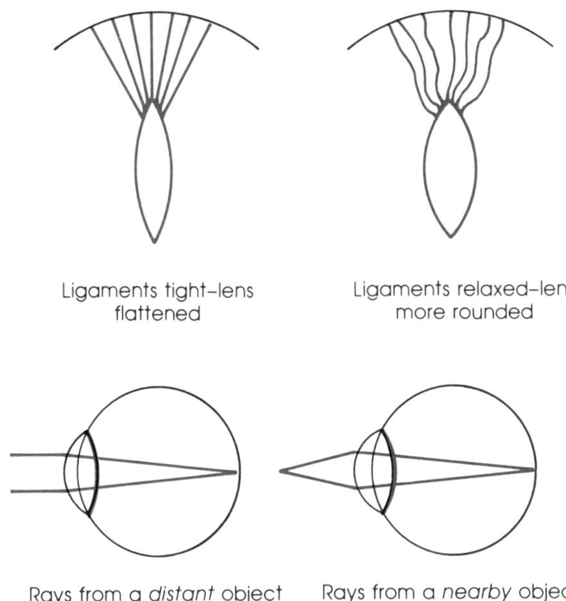

Ligaments tight–lens flattened
Ligaments relaxed–lens more rounded
Rays from a *distant* object are focused on the retina by a flattened lens
Rays from a *nearby* object are focused on the retina by a more rounded lens

Figure 34–6 Flattening and rounding of the lens during accommodation.

ferred to as being nearsighted. Nearsightedness is called *myopia.*

Light rays from distant objects do not enter the eye at the same angle as light rays from near objects. When we look off into the distance and then quickly look down at a book in our hands, our eyes must make an adjustment to the difference in the light rays entering the eye. This adjustment, which is called *accommodation,* is accomplished by ciliary muscles and ligaments that change the shape of the lens, making it more rounded or flatter, thereby allowing light rays to fall on the retina (Fig. 34–6).

As we grow older, our ciliary muscles become less elastic and cannot readily accommodate the needs of distant and near vision. Hardening of the ciliary muscles occurs in many people over 40 years of age and is known as *presbyopia.* Bifocal glasses are usually prescribed for this condition, because they allow for two sets of lenses in one pair of glasses, one for viewing distant objects and one for seeing close objects.

Astigmatism is a visual defect resulting from a warped lens or an irregular curvature of the cornea, either of which will prevent the horizontal and vertical rays from focusing at the same point on the retina. Actually, there are very few people who have perfectly shaped eyeballs, and thus there are very few who do not have some degree of astigmatism. If the astigmatism is very slight, the eye can accommodate for its imperfection by changing the shape of the lens. If there is a serious error of refraction, the eyes will tire very easily or the person will have defective vision because the eyes cannot change the shape of the lens enough to compensate for the abnormality.

The treatment for serious errors of refraction is the prescription of artificial lenses and the fitting of either eyeglasses or contact lenses so that the light rays are brought into proper focus on the retina. In recent years, advances have been made in refractive surgery that permit correction of refraction problems for some people.

FOREIGN BODIES IN THE EYE

The human eye is situated within the eye socket of the skull so that it is partially protected from direct blows. The quick-acting lids, the eyelashes, and the eyebrows also serve to protect the eye from injury. Despite nature's attempts to protect the eye, there are still many instances in which foreign bodies become lodged in the eye.

If the foreign body is not deeply embedded in the tissues of the eye, it can easily be removed by touching it with a moist cotton swab. To evert the lower lid, pull down the skin over the lower rim of the bony orbit, being careful not to place pressure on the eyeball (Fig. 34–7). Have the patient look up, down, to the left, and to the right. To evert the upper eyelid, tell the patient to look downward. Gently holding the eyelashes, and avoiding pressure on the eyeball, place a cotton swab on the eyelid. Roll the eyelid over the cotton swab, and hold the lash border up against the upper lid (Fig. 34–8). However, it is far better to use irrigation with clear, lukewarm water or sterile water or saline to remove a foreign body sticking to the cornea. Continuous

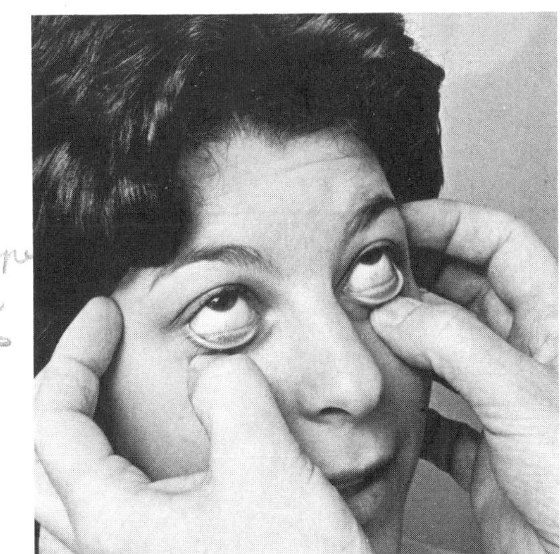

Figure 34–7 Eversion of the lower eyelid.
(Photo by Ken Kasper; courtesy of Wills Eye Hospital, Philadelphia, PA.)

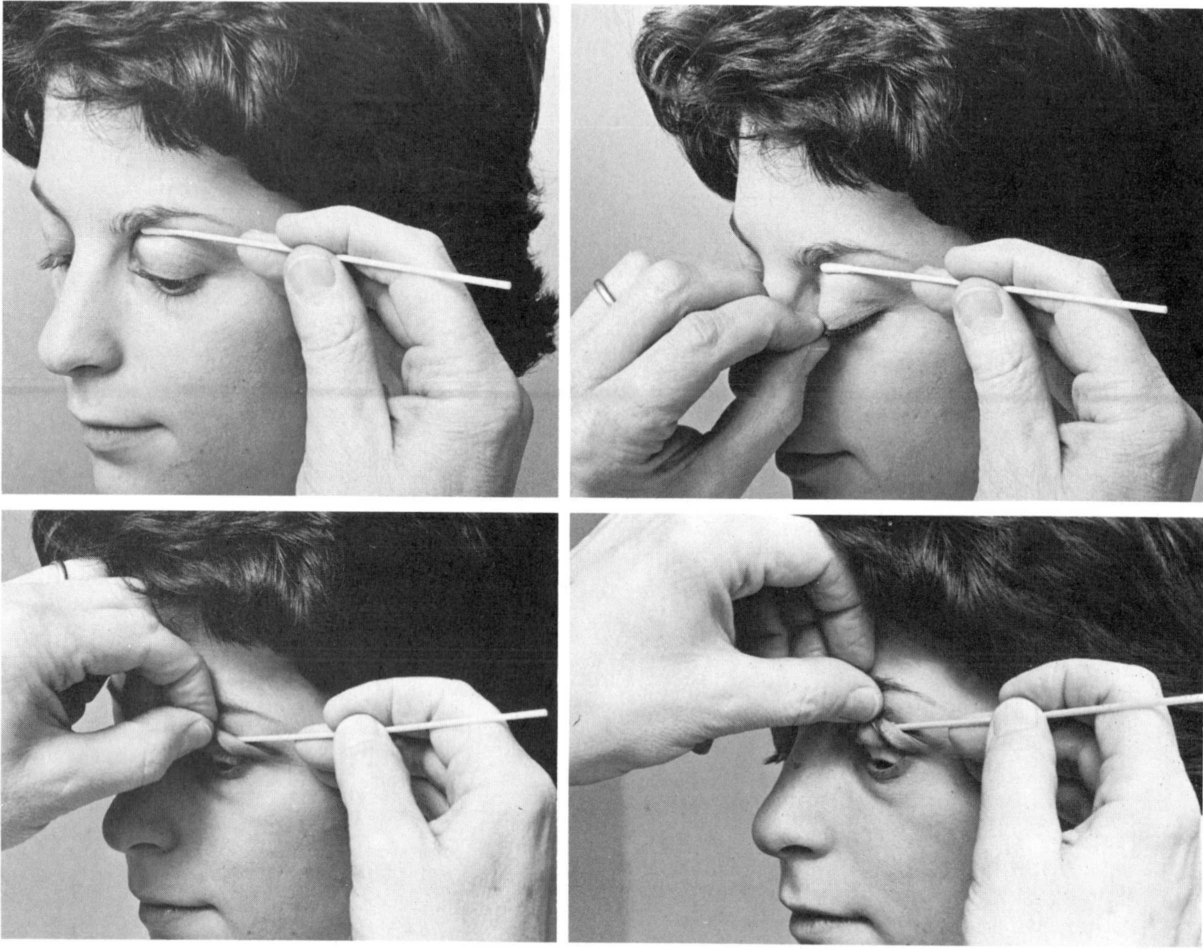

Figure 34–8 Four steps in everting the upper eyelid.
(Photos by Ken Kasper; courtesy of Wills Eye Hospital, Philadelphia, PA.)

irrigation can be done with small tubing, and a bottle of solution or an irrigating syringe can be used. The nurse must be very careful not to touch the eye with the tip of the irrigating device used.

If a foreign body is sticking out of the eye, no attempt to remove it should be made. Both eyes should be patched to prevent further eye movement, and the patient should be transported to the emergency department or to an ophthalmologist.

If the patient continues to complain of the sensation that a foreign body is still in the eye after it appears to have been removed by irrigation or swab, refer him to a physician immediately, as he may have a corneal abrasion.

CATARACT

The word *cataract* literally means waterfall. It is used to designate an opacity of the lens that produces an effect similar to one a person would get when looking through a sheet of falling water. A cataract causes a blurring of vision, because the lens, which is normally transparent, becomes cloudy and opaque.

Cataracts are sometimes present at birth *(congenital cataracts),* but they most often occur as a result of the aging process and are found in people over the age of 50 *(adult-onset cataracts).*

Traumatic cataracts may occur as a result of injury from a physical blow or exposure to radiation, heat, or chemical toxins.

SYMPTOMS AND MEDICAL DIAGNOSIS

In addition to the blurred vision that is typical of opacity of the lens, there may be distortion of vision when looking at distant objects. Uncomplicated cataracts are usually painless, but the patient may have photophobia.

The loss of vision associated with cataracts is progressive and sometimes is partially due to secondary glaucoma. If the patient was formerly farsighted, he may begin to notice improvement in his ability to see objects close at hand. As an untreated cataract progresses, the lens of the eye becomes cloudy or milky white, then may turn yellow, and eventually become brown or black. The patient may have difficulty with color discrimination.

Diagnosis of a cataract is confirmed by examination of the dilated pupil using a slit lamp, which enables the examiner to see opacities more clearly. Glaucoma should first be ruled out as a possible cause of the symptoms.

SURGICAL TREATMENT

The only effective method of treating cataracts is surgical removal of the affected lens. Two surgical techniques are (1) *extracapsular extraction*, in which the lens capsule is excised and the lens removed, and (2) the more radical *intracapsular extraction*, in which both the capsule and the lens are removed. Adult-onset cataracts are sometimes removed by intracapsular extraction.

Historically, the affected tissue was removed by surgical knife. Techniques for intracapsular cataract extraction (ICCE) utilize *cryosurgery*, in which the lens is frozen by a super-cooled probe and then removed. *Phacoemulsification*, in which the tissue is pulverized and the debris is removed by suction, is often used for extracapsular cataract extraction (ECCE) (Fig. 34-9).

After surgery, there is no recurrence of the cataract unless part of the opaque lens had to be left in the eye. This tissue may thicken and block

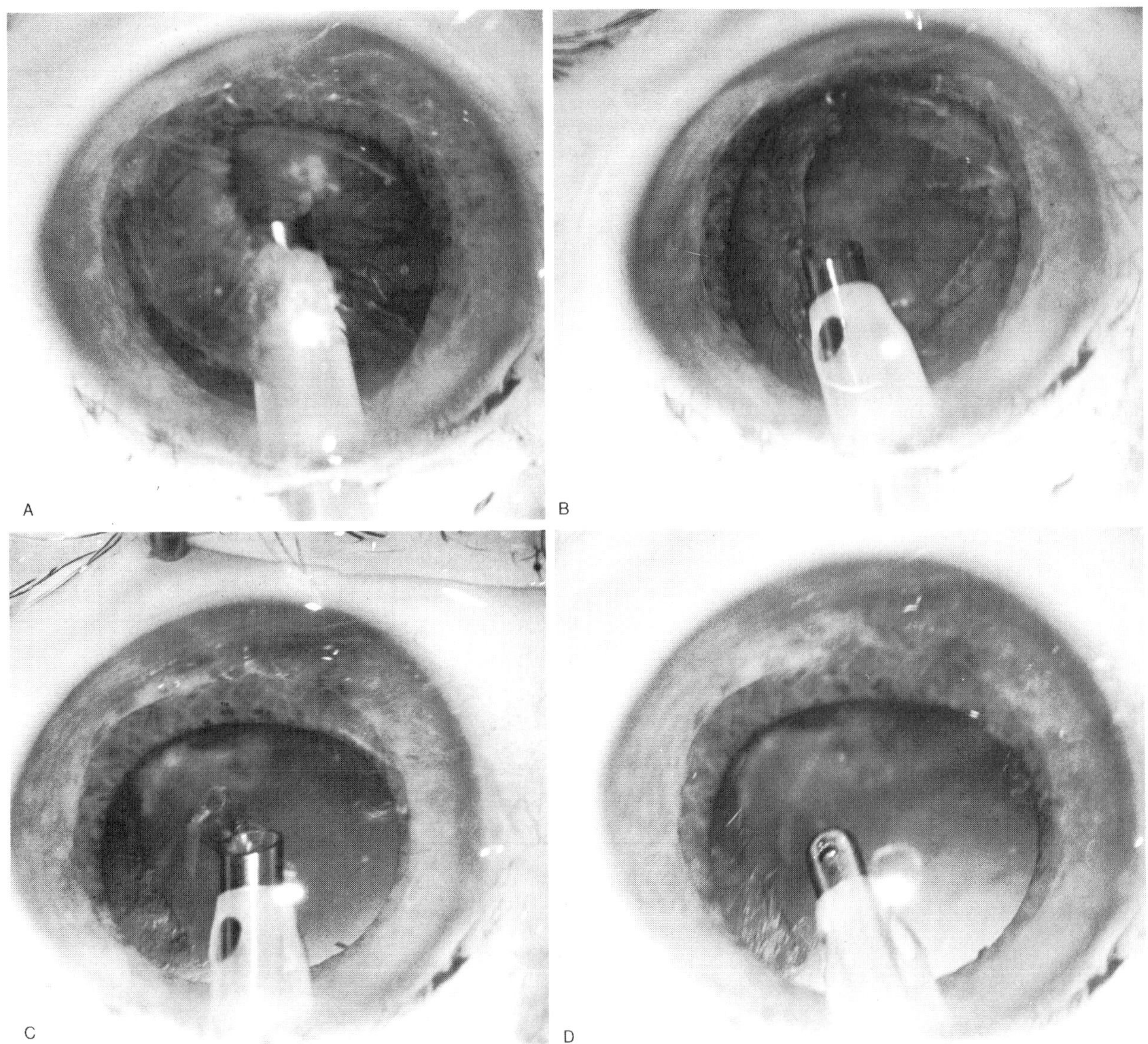

Figure 34-9 Phacoemulsification. *A* to *C*, Ultrasonic emulsifying tip in operation. The instrument has been inserted at the limbus under the cornea through a 3-mm incision and is ultrasonically emulsifying the nucleus. *A*, Early stage. *B*, Middle stage. *C*, Late stage. *D*, Irrigation/aspiration tip is aspirating the cortex of the lens.
(Courtesy of Wills Eye Hospital, Philadelphia, PA.)

off light rays, necessitating further surgery to cut through the tissue so that the light rays may pass through to the retina.

It should be understood that although cataract extraction does *improve* vision, it does not restore the eye to a perfectly normal condition. After cataract surgery, the eye is *aphakic* (without lens). The aphakic eye cannot accommodate to distances, and most of its ability to refract light rays is lost. The visual impairment must be corrected by eyeglasses, contact lenses, or an intraocular lens (Fig. 34–10).

NURSING INTERVENTION

Preoperative Care

Because the great majority of patients undergoing cataract operations are elderly and therefore are most likely to be suffering from some additional chronic disease, the nurse must remember to apply the principles of geriatric nursing in administering care. Fear, anxiety over surgery, and confusion about the expected results of the surgery are all factors to be considered in the preparation of the patient for the operation. Patients sometimes do not fully understand the information given to them about the surgical procedure, what they can and cannot do in the immediate postoperative period, and how surgery might affect the unoperated eye.

Cataract extraction is usually done as an outpatient surgery procedure. The patient is admitted to the outpatient surgery unit and given instructions regarding the layout of the room and area and the ways in which he can call for the nurse. Siderails are usually necessary to prevent falls, and the patient should be cautioned against getting up without assistance. The patient will have had instruction concerning the medications he is to use at home the night and morning before surgery. These usually consist of an antibiotic ointment to prevent infection and the administration of *mydriatic* eyedrops to dilate the pupil.

Drugs must be given with extreme care and accuracy, especially if only one eye is affected. When the abbreviations "o.d." and "o.s." are used to designate the right eye and the left eye, the nurse must be sure that the medication is applied to the correct eye. The term o.u. means both eyes.

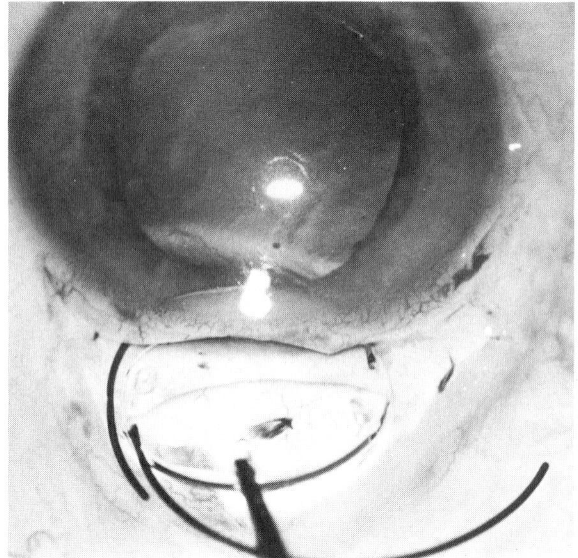

Figure 34–10 Implanting a posterior chamber intraocular lens. The lens is being slid underneath the cornea. Haptics *(dark half-circles)* hold the intraocular lens in place within the eye. (Courtesy of Wills Eye Hospital, Philadelphia, PA.)

Postoperative Care

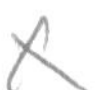

The patient is warned to avoid coughing, sneezing, rubbing the eyelids, or suddenly moving the head. The purpose of restrictions on movement is to prevent hemorrhage and increased intraocular pressure.

Policies regarding the amount of physical activity allowed the patient vary according to the surgeon's preference; some patients are permitted more freedom than others. In recent years, there has been a trend toward allowing the patient more activity.

Patients are usually kept in the recovery area of the Outpatient Surgery department for 2 to 3 hours postoperatively. The patient and a significant other is instructed on how and when to instill the prescribed postoperative eye medications. The use of analgesics such as acetaminophen is suggested for eye discomfort. Instruction on how to gently cleanse the eye using sterile cotton balls and water directed from the inner canthus outward is given, and the patient is told not to rub or place pressure on the eyes. Glasses should be worn to protect the eye during daytime hours, dark glasses should be used when outside, and an eye shield should be worn at night for as long as the surgeon feels is necessary, usually 2 to 6 weeks. The patient is cautioned against doing anything during the healing period that might increase intraocular pressure such as lifting objects weighing 20 lb or more, bending, straining at stool, or coughing. Bathing and hair shampooing is to be accomplished without getting any water in the eye. The patient is advised to immediately report any pain in the eye, decrease in vision, or increased discharge. Sexual activity can usually be resumed 6 to 8 weeks postoperatively. The nurse makes certain that the patient understands when he is to see his ophthalmologist.

Nursing interventions for selected problems in a patient having a cataract extraction are summarized in Nursing Care Plan 34–1.

NURSING CARE PLAN 34-1

Selected nursing diagnoses, goals/outcome criteria, nursing interventions, and evaluations for a patient having a cataract extraction

Situation: Mrs. Fort, age 79, is admitted to the outpatient surgery unit for extracapsular extraction of a senile cataract of the left eye with lens implant. The vision in her right eye also is affected by a cataract, but the visual loss is not as severe in that eye. Mrs. Fort suffers from a crippling osteoarthritis of the hands, but her general health is good. She is well-oriented, outgoing, and physically active. She lives alone in an apartment building for retired senior citizens. Her daughter and son-in-law live nearby and are in daily contact with her.

Mrs. Fort has only been in the hospital once in her life for pneumonia and is concerned about what to expect pre- and postoperatively.

Nursing Diagnosis	Goals/Outcome Criteria	Nursing Interventions	Evaluation
Knowledge deficit regarding pre- and postoperative procedures and care. **SUPPORTING DATA** "I have never had surgery before."	Patient will verbalize preoperative routine activities and postoperative procedures and expectations.	Teach patient and daughter about eye medications to be used at home and how to instill them; how to dress and shield eye properly, how to remove bandage without contaminating eye.	Patient and daughter demonstrate proper way to instill eyedrops and apply eye patch and shield; patient states she understands pre- and postop routine and activities.
Potential for injury related to postoperative complications such as hemorrhage and increased intraocular pressure. **SUPPORTING DATA** Undergoing cataract extraction; hemorrhage and increased intraocular pressure are potential complications.	Intraocular hemorrhage will not occur, and there will not be an increase in intraocular pressure.	Question patient regarding eye pain when taking each set of vital signs. Wash hands thoroughly before instilling eye medications or changing dressing; teach patient and daughter to wash hands before approaching eye area. Demonstrate how to put on eye shield for sleep. Instruct her to avoid rapid or sudden movements and bending from the waist. Medicate immediately for nausea and vomiting. Remind patient not to lie on affected side. Encourage her to seek assistance with ambulation while vision is blurred.	No complaints of increased eye pain; dressing dry and intact; no sign of complication; continue plan.
Self-care deficit related to disabilities imposed by osteoarthritis. **SUPPORTING DATA** Has severe osteoarthritis of the hands with limited dexterity.	Assistance with administration of postoperative eye medications and eye care will be given by daughter.	Explain pre- and postoperative routine to patient. Include daughter in all teaching regarding postoperative care; send home dosage chart and schedule for all postoperative medications. Teach signs and symptoms of complications that are to be reported to physician immediately: increasing eye pain, purulent discharge, decreasing vision, fever or chills. Teach patient and daughter about eye medications to be used at home and how to instill them; how to dress and shield eye properly; how to remove bandage without pressing on eye; importance of hand washing and not rubbing the eye and the importance of follow-up with physician.	Daughter verbalizes correct schedule for medications; lists signs of complications to report to doctor; states she understands postop and home care.

Artificial Lenses

The patient with an aphakic eye has several options for replacement of the lens for improvement of his vision. Cataract eyeglasses have many disadvantages, but they may be the only suitable alternative for patients who cannot wear a contact lens or have an intraocular lens implanted.

Adjusting to cataract eyeglasses can be very frustrating and even frightening for the patient and will require much patience and understanding from those trying to help him during this difficult period. The lenses of cataract glasses are very thick, and the edges tend to cause straight lines to appear curved. Depth perception becomes greatly distorted, and the patient has great difficulty judging distances. If he turns his head suddenly, the curved lines are set in motion, and his only clear vision is directly through the center of the glasses. Also, he has the unnerving experience of seeing someone approach him, disappear into a blind spot, and then reappear much closer to him. In time, the patient will adjust to this and will barely notice the blind spot, but at first it can be very frightening and discouraging.

The nurse can help the patient in his adjustment by reassuring him that such difficulties are to be expected at first and that eventually he can become accustomed to his glasses. He should be instructed to move slowly at first, feeling his way through doorways and other close quarters where he may feel uneasy. The patient should make a special effort to get into the habit of moving his head from side to side rather than shifting his eyes, and he must always try to look directly through the center of his glasses. Adjustment can be more rapid if the patient is able to use his hands and eyes for fine work such as knitting, cooking, carving, whittling, or sewing. This type of precision work trains the eyes to focus through the cataract glasses properly and also serves as a form of occupational therapy that can do wonders for the morale of a person who could barely distinguish between light and dark shadows before surgery.

Contact lenses have many advantages over cataract eyeglasses, but they are not always completely trouble free. They require a certain degree of manual dexterity to remove and reinsert, and they can be irritating to the cornea. Although the adjustment period varies depending on the type of lens used, patients do need to be aware that some adjustment is necessary before the full effect of surgery can be evaluated.

An intraocular lens usually is implanted during surgery, but the surgeon may choose to implant the lens months after the original lens has been removed. Postoperative care of the patient following implantation of an intraocular lens does not differ greatly from that of a patient with simple cataract extraction. The surgeon may prescribe miotic eyedrops after surgery to constrict the pupil and lessen the danger of lens dislocation.

The intraocular lens has many advantages over the removable contact lenses. It is always present in the eye, which can be a safety factor, it does not cause any discomfort or inconvenience, and manual dexterity is not required to care for it, because it is left in place.

There are, however, some risks involved in the implantation of an intraocular lens. Complications such as corneal edema, secondary glaucoma, lens displacement, retinal detachment, and other eye disorders require the removal of the lens in about 5% of those who have an intraocular lens. Additionally, some patients are poor candidates for lens implantation because of retinopathy, chronic iritis, or severe myopia.

GLAUCOMA

The term *glaucoma* comprises a complex group of disorders that involve many different pathologic changes and symptoms but have in common an increased intraocular pressure (IOP) that damages the optic disc and causes loss of vision. Glaucoma may come on slowly and cause irreversible visual loss without presenting any other noticeable symptoms, or it may appear abruptly and produce blindness in a matter of hours.

The normal eyeball is filled with aqueous humor in an amount carefully regulated to maintain the shape of the eyeball. The aqueous fluid is formed by the epithelial cells of the ciliary body. It flows into the posterior chamber of the eye between the front of the lens and the back surface of the iris, through the pupil, and into the anterior chamber. It then flows through angled structures where a network of channels collects and conducts the fluid into the canal of Schlemm and from there to the venous system. As long as production of aqueous is equal to the amount returned to the venous system, the balance is maintained and there is no problem. However, if too much aqueous is produced or it cannot pass through to the venous system, the balance is upset and fluid begins to build up within the eye. As the fluid begins to exert pressure on the optic disc, cells are damaged, and blind spots appear in the visual field.

Glaucoma can be present at birth or can develop at any age. It can result from trauma or from another disorder of the eye, or it can occur without any known etiology. Glaucoma frequently is a manifestation of diseases and pathologies in other systems of the body.

There are two major types of glaucoma: angle-closure (acute) glaucoma, and open-angle (chronic) glaucoma. These two major types differ in their clinical manifestations, treatment, and effects on vision.

ANGLE-CLOSURE GLAUCOMA

Angle-closure, or acute, glaucoma is a medical emergency in which there is severe pain in the eye accompanied by the appearance of colored halos around lights, blurred vision, and regional headache. The problem in angle-closure glaucoma is that the iris lies too close to the drainage canal and bulges forward against the cornea, blocking the drainage area of the trabecular meshwork. Thus there is mechanical blockage of the aqueous humor, and the intraocular pressure rises suddenly, sometimes reaching a pressure of 50 to 70 mm Hg. Symptoms can develop slowly and appear intermittently for short periods, particularly in the evenings when the pupils dilate in the dimmer light. Nausea, vomiting, and abdominal pain may also be present. If the attack is acute with a rapid rise to very high IOP, the patient will experience excruciating eye pain, tearing (lacrimation), nausea, and vomiting. He will seek a dark place and turn away from any light source. His vision will decrease rapidly. Treatment in this situation must be prompt, or damage to the optic nerve will cause blindness in the affected eye.

Because angle-closure is relatively uncommon and its symptoms are nonspecific, the condition may be misdiagnosed. As a result, needed treatment is delayed, and vision is permanently lost.

Medical and Surgical Treatment

Emergency treatment in angle-closure glaucoma consists of measures to reduce intraocular pressure as quickly as possible. During the attack, such drugs as pilocarpine, topical epinephrine, and acetazolamide may be given intravenously. Surgery is performed as soon as inflammation subsides to relieve pressure against the optic nerve endings. In most cases, a *peripheral iridectomy* is done under local anesthesia. This provides an opening in the iris through which the aqueous humor can flow from the posterior chamber into the anterior chamber. The iris falls away from the angle wall, thus preventing another buildup of pressure.

OPEN-ANGLE GLAUCOMA

Open-angle, or chronic, glaucoma, in which there is no angle closure, is much more insidious and more common. It usually is bilateral and can progress to complete blindness without ever producing an acute attack. Its symptoms are relatively mild, and many patients are not aware that anything is wrong until vision has been seriously impaired.

The National Society for the Prevention of Blindness lists the following symptoms as danger signals of chronic glaucoma:

- Glasses, even new ones, don't seem to clarify vision.
- Blurred or hazy vision that clears up after a while.
- Trouble in getting used to darkened rooms, such as in movie theaters.
- Seeing rainbow-colored rings around lights.
- Narrowing of vision at the sides of one or both eyes.

Symptoms and Medical Diagnosis

People at high risk for glaucoma are (1) diabetics, (2) patients with recently controlled hypertension, (3) blacks (eight times as many blacks as nonblacks have glaucoma-related blindness), (4) individuals with a family history of glaucoma, (5) patients with facial hemangioma or other nevi, (6) children with large eyes, and (7) victims of eye injuries.

A commonly used screening technique for early detection of glaucoma is the measurement of intraocular pressure using an air tonometer. A puff of air is directed at the cornea, which causes a momentary indentation while a pressure reading is taken. The test is painless, and nothing but the air touches the eye. Verification of the diagnosis of glaucoma may require the use of a more complex instrument called an *applanation tonometer* (Fig. 34–11). The cornea is flattened and measured with a slit lamp biomicroscope.

Medical and Surgical Treatment

The initial treatment of choice for chronic (open-angle) glaucoma is medication rather than surgery. If drugs are not effective or if they produce worrisome side effects, there are several surgical techniques, including the use of a laser beam, that can facilitate the outflow of aqueous and reduce pressure within the eye.

Drugs prescribed are intended to enhance aqueous outflow or decrease its production or both. Pilocarpine acts to stretch the collecting network and enlarge the channels through which the aqueous flows. However, the drug also causes constriction of the pupil, and can reduce visual acuity. Newer drugs, known as *beta-adrenergic receptor blocking agents*, are used for many patients with glaucoma. It is believed that these beta blockers reduce intraocular pressure by diminishing the production of aqueous humor and increasing the outflow. Because they do not affect pupil size and have fewer side effects, they are gradually replacing pilocarpine. Examples of such agents include timolol maleate (Timoptic), betaxolol hydrochloride (Betoptic), and levobunolol hydrochloride (Betagan).

Diuretics also may be prescribed to reduce production of aqueous fluid. Not all diuretics

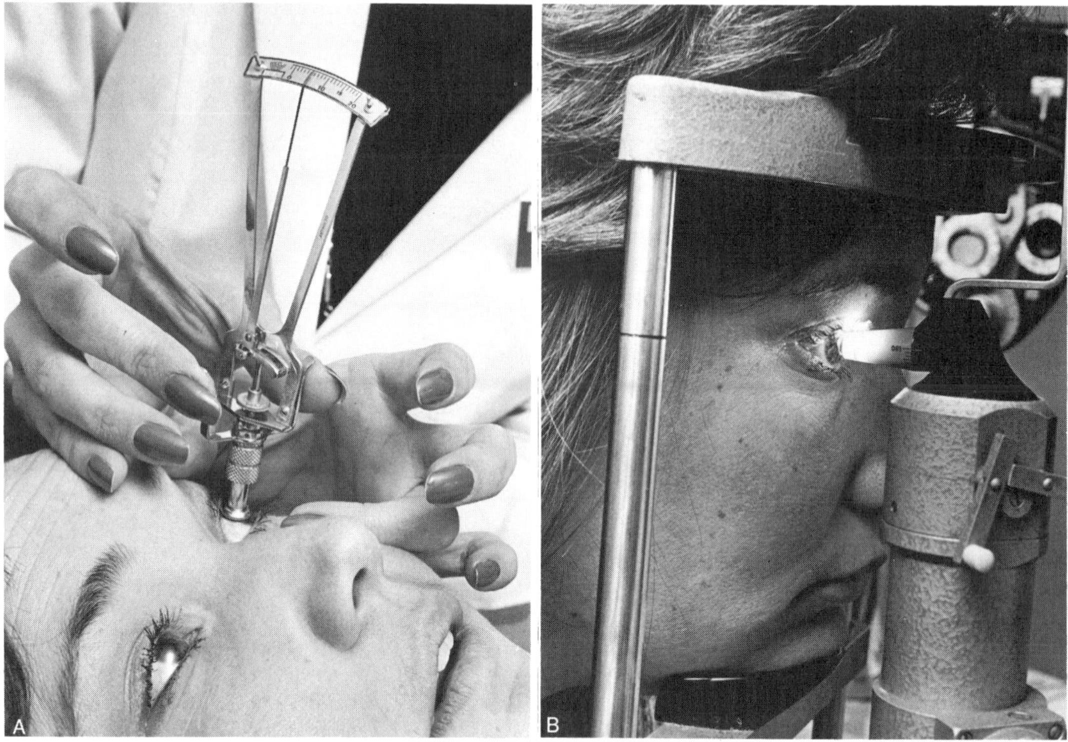

Figure 34-11 *A,* Schiøtz tonometer. *B,* Applanation tonometer. (Photos by Ken Kasper; courtesy of Wills Eye Hospital, Philadelphia, PA.)

reduce intraocular pressure, and a substitute should not be used for the specific drug prescribed.

Whenever glaucoma is being managed by medication, the patient must continue the eyedrops and oral medications on an uninterrupted basis. Patients admitted to the hospital for disorders other than glaucoma often are allowed to keep their glaucoma medication at the bedside if they are able to administer it to themselves.

When drugs do not control glaucoma and increased intraocular pressure persists, surgery is an alternative. The goal is to create openings so that excess fluid can escape. Traditional surgical procedures involve removal of a section of the iris to allow the aqueous to flow into the anterior chamber. The newer laser surgery permits penetration of the iris (iridotomy) for relief of angle-closure glaucoma. The laser beam also can be used to create evenly spaced openings in the collecting meshwork (trabeculoplasty) to facilitate aqueous drainage in open-angle or chronic glaucoma (Fig. 34-12).

The word *laser* stands for *l*ight *a*mplification by *s*timulated *e*mission of *r*adiation. Different types of lasers may be used for trabeculoplasty. Argon or krypton lasers are most commonly employed for this procedure. The basis of laser therapy is that light absorbed by pigment is converted to heat energy. The heat coagulates the protein in the tissue and a thermal burn, known as *photocoagulation,* occurs.

Laser surgery does not require surgical invasion of the eye. Moreover, general anesthesia is not necessary with laser surgery and it can be done much more quickly and with far less trauma to the structures of the eye than invasive techniques.

Care of the patient after laser treatment is relatively simple compared with treatment following more traditional surgical procedures. The patient may experience a mild headache and blurring of vision during the first 24 hours. There is a possibility that IOP may increase because of an inflammatory response. Increasing pain in the eye should be reported to the ophthalmologist immediately. The patient should be instructed to prevent increasing the venous pressure in the head, neck, and eyes by avoiding the Valsalva maneuver, not bending over, keeping the head up, and not making any sudden movements. A stool softener is given to prevent constipation. Strenuous exercise is to be avoided for 3 weeks. The head of the bed should be elevated 15 to 20 degrees to decrease pressure within the eyes during sleep. Elevated intraocular pressure will persist for a week or so in some patients. Glaucoma medications are continued to meet the patient's individual needs. The patient must understand the importance of frequent checkups

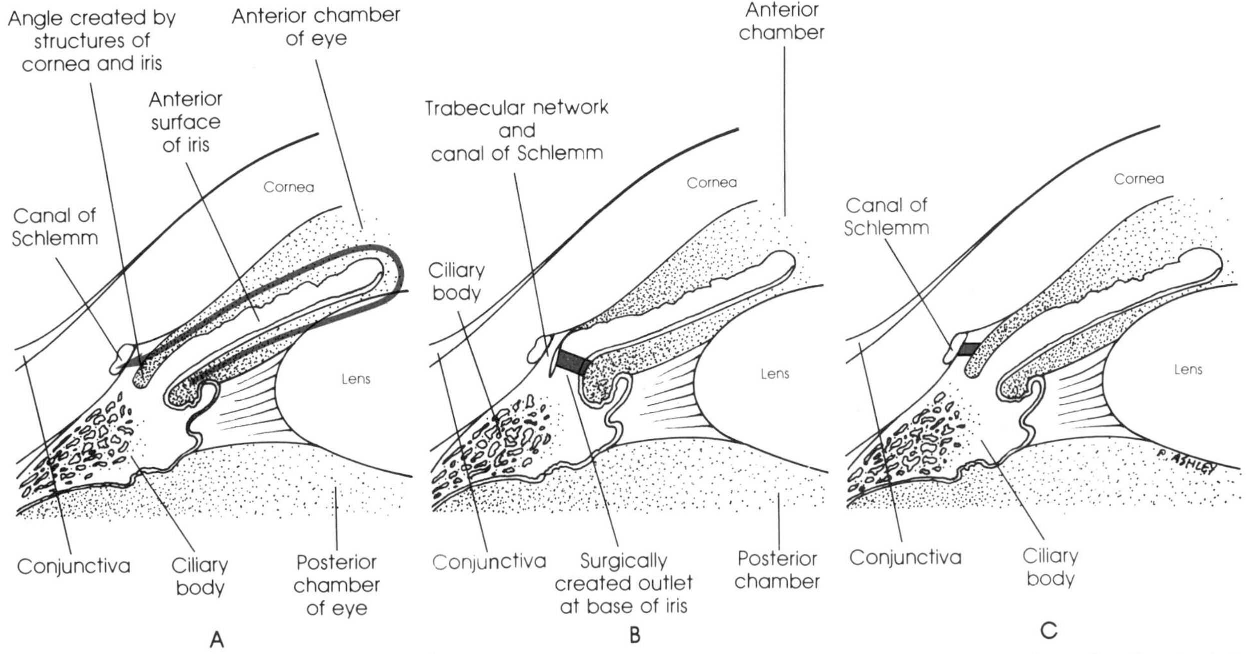

Figure 34-12 Laser surgery for open-angle and angle-closure glaucoma. *A,* Normal flow of aqueous humor from the ciliary body to the posterior chamber, past the surface of the iris, through the trabecular meshwork and canal of Schlemm. *B,* Angle-closure glaucoma. The iris tents up, closing the angle and blocking the flow of aqueous humor through the trabecular meshwork. Laser surgery creates a hole in the base of the iris, thus allowing drainage through the canal. *C,* Open-angle glaucoma. The angle remains normal, but either too much aqueous humor is produced or it cannot get through the trabecular meshwork. Laser surgery creates openings in the meshwork to permit drainage through the canal.

and the necessity of consistently following instructions. In other words, the surgical procedure may relieve the immediate problem of greatly increased intraocular pressure but does not always eliminate the need for medication.

Nursing Intervention

Education of the patient and his family is a major aspect of care, because 90% of all cases of glaucoma are chronic conditions for which there usually is no permanent cure. Failure to follow the prescribed treatment regimen for control of glaucoma and neglecting to maintain regular contact with the physician can result in progressive loss of vision and eventual blindness.

The patient who has glaucoma needs to be fully informed about the nature of this disorder, how it can affect vision, the treatments available, and the expected result of those treatments. Kilroy describes an analogy that is very useful when teaching the patient, his family, and the general public about the normal eye and what happens when there is glaucoma. The eye is compared to a sink with a drain (angle), pipes (trabecular structures), and an open faucet (the ciliary processes). As long as water flows into and out of the sink at the same rate, there is no problem. If, however, something should block the drain or the pipes, the water will fill the sink beyond its capacity.

Carrying the analogy further, medications such as pilocarpine help keep the pipes open so that drainage is possible. Other drugs such as Timoptic eyedrops and diuretic tablets can slow down the rate at which water flows from the tap. If medications do not work or the sink suddenly is blocked by a clogged pipe, it may be necessary for the surgeon to clear the drainage system so that the water can drain from the sink.

In addition to learning about the nature of glaucoma and the expected results of prescribed treatments, the patient also must be made aware of the possibility of vision loss if the condition is not managed. Teaching should emphasize that glaucoma medications prevent further vision loss but cannot restore vision. This must be done with tact and sensitivity for the patient's feelings. The information should never be presented in such a way that the patient feels threatened or becomes so fearful that he is unable to participate in the management of his disorder. He is simply to be made aware of the risks that are inherent in uncontrolled glaucoma. If he cannot or will not use the prescribed eyedrops and oral medications, the help of a family member, neighbor, or visiting nurse must be obtained. Table 34-3 summarizes a teaching plan for patients with glaucoma.

TABLE 34–3 SUGGESTED POINTS FOR TEACHING PLAN FOR A PATIENT WITH GLAUCOMA

- Signs of IOP: pain in eye, redness, tearing, blurred vision, halos around lights, frequent need for change in eyeglasses.
- Measures to prevent increase in IOP: low-sodium diet, little caffeine, prevent constipation and Valsalva maneuver, decrease stress.
- Need to take prescribed medications and refrain from taking over-the-counter or other medications without physician's knowledge. Glaucoma medication must be taken regularly for life.
- Use good aseptic technique when instilling eye medication.
- Wear ID tag or bracelet stating "Glaucoma" and carry card in wallet that states what medications are being taken.
- Keep extra bottle of eye medication on hand. Carry eyedrops.
- Maintain close medical follow-up with physician.
- Practice safety habits; avoid night driving if possible.

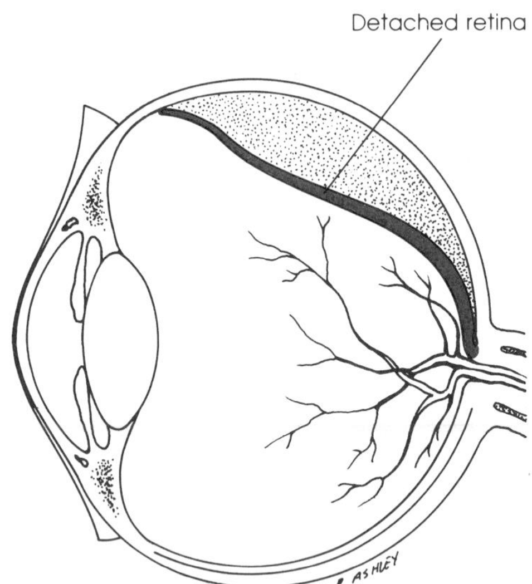

Figure 34–13 Retinal detachment.

RETINAL DETACHMENT

The retina is the innermost layer of the eye. It is composed of (1) a pigmented layer that is in close contact with the choroid (vascular wall) of the eye and that supplies nutrients for both layers and (2) a sensory layer that receives visual stimuli and therefore is essential to normal vision. Retinal detachment is actually not a detachment of the whole retina but a separation of the sensory layers from the pigmented epithelial layer. Retinal detachment can cause vitreous fluid to leak under the retina, separating a portion of it from the vascular wall and thereby depriving it of its blood supply (Fig. 34–13).

Retinal detachments often are classified as either primary or secondary. Primary retinal detachment is the result of spontaneous or degenerative changes in the retina or the vitreous. Secondary retinal detachment is associated with mechanical trauma, inflammation within the eye, or some other ophthalmic disorder. Retinal detachments frequently occur in persons with myopia. The incidence of retinal detachment increases dramatically after 40 years of age and is most common in persons between 50 and 60 years of age.

SYMPTOMS AND MEDICAL DIAGNOSIS

Onset can be either gradual or sudden, depending on the cause and extent of the detachment and location of the area involved. The patient may see flashes of light and then, days or weeks later, notice cloudy vision or loss of central vision. Another common symptom is the sensation of spots or moving particles (drusen) in the field of vision. In severe cases, there may be complete loss of vision.

Diagnosis of detached retina can be made with a direct ophthalmoscope, but it is greatly simplified by a stereoscopic indirect ophthalmoscope. This instrument permits visualization of the entire retina and produces an image of the retina with less magnification and distortion than the direct ophthalmoscope. Ultrasound can be used to detect retinal detachment when the eye is clouded by opacity from cataract or hemorrhage.

SURGICAL TREATMENT

Retinal holes and tears sometimes can be repaired on an outpatient basis with laser therapy that creates an inflammatory reaction, causing the layers to adhere during healing. Those located in the posterior fundus can be coagulated and sealed using a laser beam or photocoagulator. Peripheral retinal holes through which no fluid has leaked can be closed by the application of a freezing probe (cryotherapy). The frozen area scars over in a few days, and the hole is thus sealed.

A third procedure, called *scleral buckling*, requires more extensive surgery. In effect, it places the retinal breaks in contact with the pigmented epithelial layer. Adhesions are formed that bind the sensory, epithelial layers and choroid together.

In some instances when hemorrhage into the vitreous obstructs vision, the surgeon may perform a closed vitrectomy during retinal repair. The purpose of this procedure is to remove the opaque vitreous body and stabilize the retina against the choroid. Inert gas, air, or silicone oil is used to fill the space until aqueous humor eventually refills the area.

NURSING INTERVENTION

Preoperative and postoperative nursing care of the patient having retinal repair and vitrectomy requires a sound knowledge of the kind of detachment affecting the patient and the surgical procedure that is performed to correct the condition. Positioning of the patient and the level of activity allowed after surgery are prescribed by the surgeon.

Before discharge from the hospital, the patient or a family member or both should receive instruction in follow-up care, especially the instillation of eyedrops.

RETINOPATHY

The two major causes of retinopathy are diabetes mellitus and hypertension. Years of elevated blood pressure cause retinal vasospasm, which damages and narrows the retinal arterioles, thereby decreasing the blood supply to the retina.

Diabetic patients experience two different forms of retinopathy: proliferative and nonproliferative retinopathy. In the nonproliferative type of retinopathy, microaneurysms develop on the retinal blood vessels. These eventually swell and rupture, causing hemorrhage into the vitreous, which interferes with vision. The proliferative form of retinopathy occurs later in the course of diabetes. New blood vessels grow from the existing retinal vessels in a process called *neovascularization*. The new vessels are thinner and rupture more easily, causing hemorrhage. The blood from the hemorrhage causes scarring, which also interferes with vision.

Control of blood glucose levels is very important in preventing excessive diabetic retinopathy. There is no other known way to halt the process. The microaneurysms and the neovascularized vessels are treated with laser photocoagulation therapy in an attempt to prevent hemorrhage and the consequent scarring and loss of vision. Vitrectomy can also be done if hemorrhage has caused serious impairment of vision.

CORNEAL TRANSPLANT

Corneal transplants replace corneas that have been damaged by trauma, ulcers, or disease, such as keratitis (inflammation of the cornea), and help restore corneal clarity. Two types of procedures are done: a full-thickness keratoplasty (corneal transplant) or a lamellar keratoplasty, which replaces only a superficial layer of corneal tissue. The full-thickness keratoplasty restores vision in about 95% of patients.

The patient must be "on call" to come for the transplant, as it is unpredictable as to when a matching donor cornea will become available. The patient must realize beforehand that it takes a week or two before improvement in vision will be noticeable, and improvement will continue for several months. Because the cornea does not have an abundant blood supply, healing is very slow and is not complete for about 1 year. Prevention of infection is extremely important. Preoperative care is much the same as for other eye surgeries. Postoperative care may include an overnight hospital stay. A pressure dressing and eye shield are applied in the surgical suite after the procedure and should not be removed by the nurse. Nursing actions focus on caring for a patient with sensory/perceptual alteration (visual). The call bell, telephone, and personal items should be positioned on the side of the patient's uncovered eye. Position the patient on the back and unoperative side only. Should the first transplant fail, the procedure can be redone.

MACULAR DEGENERATION

The macular region of the retina gives us color vision, acute vision, and central vision. Macular degeneration occurs with aging. A fragile vessel network grows into the subretinal space and may bleed into the macular region, causing visual impairment. Laser treatment to destroy the fragile blood vessels can sometimes be done to prevent further bleeding and visual deterioration.

EYE TRAUMA AND EMERGENCIES

A corneal abrasion can cause the patient considerable pain. If he feels he has been "hit in the eye" with a branch, piece of paper, or other object, the nurse should get him in a good light and examine the cornea to see if a scratch can be seen. The eye is then patched to keep contaminants out of the wound and to prevent blinking, which causes more pain, and the patient is referred to his ophthalmologist or an emergency department for treatment. Because infection is always a danger when working with the eyes, the hands should be washed each time before the eye area is approached.

If a foreign body is visible on the cornea, it is best to use irrigation to try to dislodge it. Normal saline is preferred, but tap water can be used if it is the only solution available. Sometimes a speck of foreign matter on the cornea can be removed using a moistened, sterile cotton swab. Have the patient tilt his head back and move his eyes away from the site of the particle. Hold the eyelids open to prevent blinking. If the object appears to be embedded, the eye is patched and the patient sent immediately to the emergency department or to his ophthalmologist.

Chemical burns should be treated by lengthy continuous irrigation. An IV bag of normal saline is the preferred solution; otherwise, tap water will do. Place the patient supine with his head turned to the affected side. With gloves on, direct the stream of fluid to the inner canthus so that the stream flows across the cornea to the outer canthus, holding the lids apart with your thumb and index finger. At intervals, stop and have the patient close his eyes to move secretions and particles from the upper eye to the lower conjunctival sac; then begin again. The patient should be seen by a physician as soon as possible.

REMOVAL OF THE EYE

Surgical removal of the entire eye, including the sclera, is called *enucleation*. If it is possible to preserve the sclera, only the contents of the eyeball are removed *(evisceration)*. This procedure leaves a relatively stable structure for insertion of an artificial eye. Severe trauma to or advanced malignancy of the eye may necessitate a procedure called *exenteration*, in which the eyeball, eyelids, and all contents of the ocular orbit are removed. This type of surgery is so extensive that most patients wear an eyepatch after the surgical wound is healed.

Indications for either enucleation or evisceration include trauma to the eye, malignancy, and severe pain in an eye in which total vision loss occurred from glaucoma or trauma. Also, either type of surgery may be performed as a preventive measure to save an unaffected eye from sympathetic ophthalmia. This condition occurs as a complication of a penetrating injury to one eye. For reasons not fully understood, the ciliary body, iris, and choroid of the uninjured eye become highly inflamed. If the condition cannot be stopped, progressive inflammation can lead to total loss of vision in the eye with sympathetic ophthalmia.

The postoperative care of a patient who has had an eye removed is fairly routine. The chief dangers are hemorrhage and infection, which are relatively uncommon. Most patients are allowed to be up the day of surgery and can go home in a matter of days. However, it is important that the nurse work with the patient on his change in body image and plans for his social adjustment before discharge. A period of grieving over the loss of an eye is common, and the patient and family need to know what to expect. As soon as the eye socket is healed, an artificial eye can be

CARE OF AN ARTIFICIAL EYE

Most patients learn very quickly how to remove and reinsert, clean, and store the artificial eye overnight. However, there will be times when a hospitalized patient will be unable to remove, clean, and reinsert his artificial eye and therefore must depend on members of the nursing staff to care for his prosthesis. The procedure is similar in many ways to care of dentures. Both require basic principles of cleanliness, careful handling, and proper storage.

The prosthesis is removed by depressing the lower lid and allowing the artificial eye to fall into the hands.

The artificial eye is cleansed with gentle soap and water, unless the patient, his family, or the physician directs otherwise. If the eye is not to be reinserted right away, it is stored in a container of water or contact lens solution.

Before the prosthesis is reinserted, it should be cleansed again with soap and water. The patient's upper lid is lifted, and the eye is inserted with the notched end toward the nose. After the prosthesis is placed as far as possible under the upper lid, the lower lid is depressed, allowing the eye to slip into place (Fig. 34–14).

Concerns for the Elderly

Visual acuity decreases to below 20/40 in most people by age 65. Subcutaneous fat decreases with aging, and the eyes appear to be sunken as a result of this loss of fat and decreased elastic tissue and muscle tone. *Arcus senilis*, an opaque ring outlining the cornea, sometimes results from the deposition of fatty globules. Cornea transparency also decreases with age, but more importantly, the cornea flattens and develops an irregular curvature on the surface after age 65. This causes an astigmatism or makes an existing astigmatism worse, and vision becomes blurred.

Fatty deposits give the sclera a yellowish tinge, and thinning of the sclera causes a bluish tinge. With aging the iris has less ability to dilate, which causes difficulty for an older person when he goes from a bright area into a darkened area.

The lens of the eye also changes after age 40, gradually losing water and becoming harder. The ciliary muscle has less ability to allow the eye to accommodate, which is responsible for the gradual extension of distance from the eyes at which an item to be read is held (presbyopia). The farthest point at which an object can be identified also decreases, and the older person has a narrower visual field. Color discrimination also decreases with advancing age.

Moisture secretion diminishes during the senior adult years, placing the eyes at greater risk for irritation and infection. Repeated episodes of keratitis may seriously compromise vision and can lead to loss of independence for an elderly patient.

RESOURCES FOR THE VISUALLY IMPAIRED

Loss of vision need not be devastating for a person if he is given support and encouragement for coping with his handicap. There are resources to help the visually handicapped person learn to care for himself, find employment, and enjoy educational and recreational activities. Many colleges provide special funds to enable blind students to hire readers and tape recorders to help them with their studies.

The Library of Congress in Washington, DC, lends records and recording machines without charge to the blind and maintains a wide selection of recordings. Other resources include:

- American Printing House for the Blind
  1839 Frankfort Ave.
  Louisville, KY 40206

This agency publishes literature for the blind in all media and manufactures tangible aids for the blind. It produces braille books and magazines, music, talking books, large-type books, and educational recorded tapes.

- Helen Keller International
  15 West St.
  New York, NY 10011
  (212)807-5800

This association renders all possible assistance to the promotion of all phases of work for and in the interest of the blind and to the prevention of blindness.

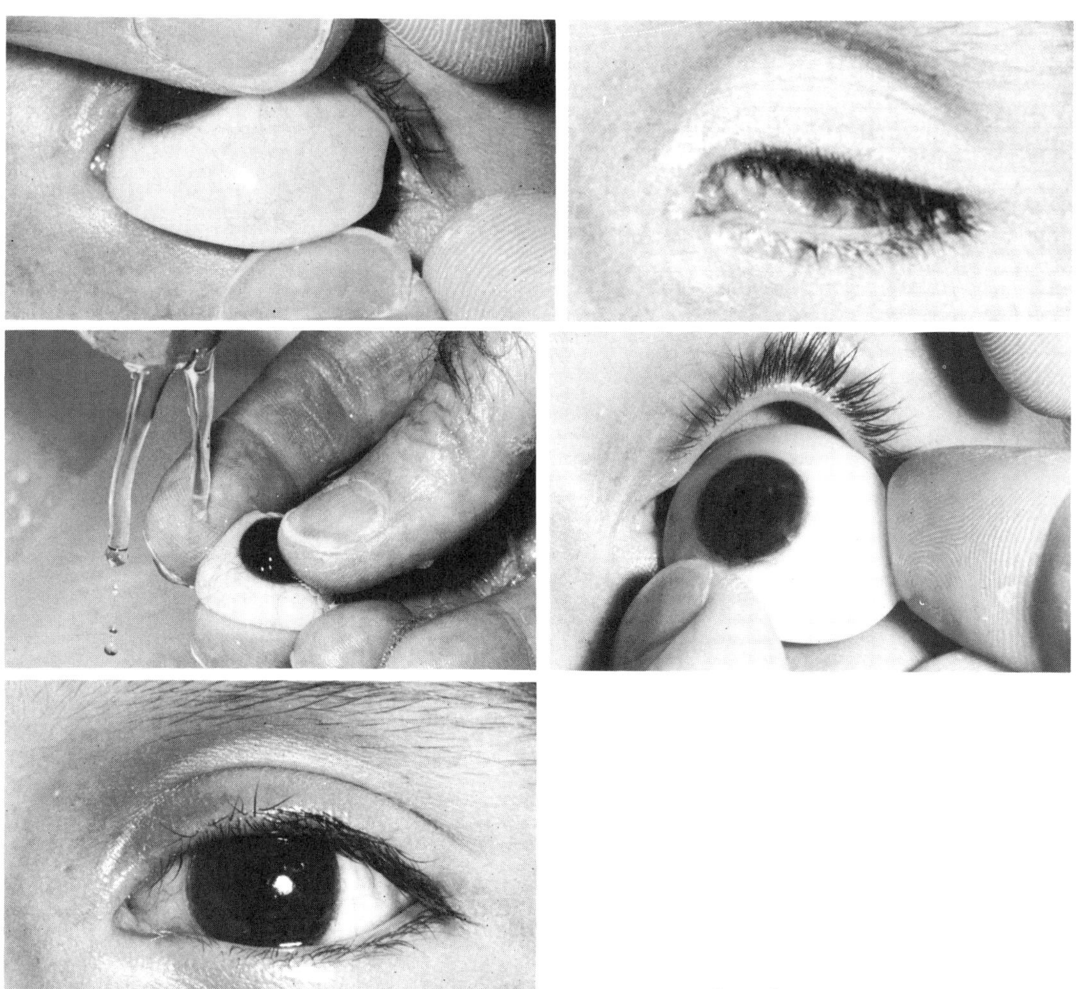

Figure 34-14 Care of an artificial eye.
(From Zucnick, M.: Care of an artificial eye. Am. J. Nurs. May, 1975, p. 835.)

- Guide Dog Foundation for the Blind
  371 E. Jericho Turnpike
  Smithtown, NY 11787
  (516)265-2121

This foundation breeds and trains dogs for the blind and handicapped and trains the blind and handicapped in their use.

- Recording for the Blind
  121 East 58th St.
  New York, NY 10022

This corporation supplies free taped educational textbooks to visually, physically, and perceptually handicapped students and professionals.

BIBLIOGRAPHY

Andreoli, T. E., et al.: Cecil Essentials of Medicine, 2nd ed. Philadelphia, W. B. Saunders, 1990.

Barker-Stotts, K.: Action stat! Hyphema. Nursing 89, Dec., 1989, p. 33.

Beare, P. G., and Myers, J. L.: Principles and Practices of Adult Health Nursing. St. Louis, C. V. Mosby, 1990.

Boyd-Monk, H.: Eye trauma: A close-up on emergency care. RN, Dec., 1989, p. 22.

Boyd-Monk, H., and Steinmetz, C.: Nursing Care of the Eye. Norwalk, CT, Appleton & Lange, 1987.

Bullock, B. L., and Rosendalhl, P. O.: Pathophysiology: Adaptations and Alterations in Function, 2nd ed. Boston, Scott, Foresman, 1988.

Carver, J. A.: Cataract care made plain. Am. J. Nurs., May, 1987, p. 626.

Clark, R. B., et al.: Eye emergencies and urgencies. Patient Care, Jan. 15, 1989, p. 24.

Ignatavicius, D. D., and Bayne, M. J.: Medical-Surgical Nursing. Philadelphia, W. B. Saunders, 1991.

Rakel, R. E., ed.: Conn's Current Therapy 1990. Philadelphia, W. B. Saunders, 1990.

Robertson, C.: Diabetes now: Coping with chronic complications. RN, Sept., 1989, p. 34.

Rosenthal, J. L.: Timely recognition of diabetic retinopathy. Emerg. Med., Jun. 15, 1989, p. 87.

Salisbury, C. S.: Clinical Gerontological Nursing: A Guide to Advanced Practice. Philadelphia, W. B. Saunders, 1991.

Springhouse Corporation: Illustrated Manual of Nursing Practice. Springhouse, PA, 1991.

STUDENT STUDY AIDS

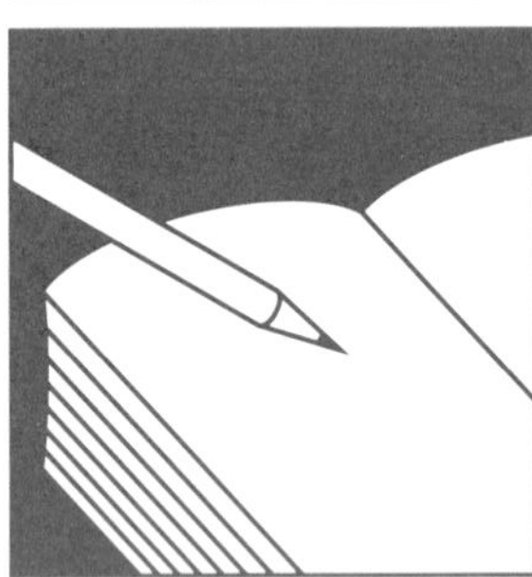

CLINICAL CASE PROBLEMS

Read each clinical situation and discuss the questions with your classmates.

1. Mr. Wilson, age 78, is scheduled for a right cataract extraction and intraocular lens implant. He has bilateral cataracts that have made him legally blind for years. He did not consult a doctor until recently, because he had always heard that cataracts had to be "ripe" before they could be treated, and he felt he could not afford frequent trips to a doctor when nothing could be done for his condition. Mr. Wilson enters the outpatient surgery area, and you are assigned as his nurse.

- How would you approach and orient Mr. Wilson to his surroundings?
- What would you tell Mr. Wilson about the preoperative routine and medications at this time?
- What nursing diagnoses would be appropriate for Mr. Wilson at this time?
- What are the advantages of intraocular lens implants over cataract glasses and/or contact lenses?
- What discharge instructions will need to be given to Mr. Wilson?

---

2. Mr. Lavant, age 52, and his wife, who has diabetes, have heard about a glaucoma screening clinic being held in their community. They are interested in attending the clinic but are very apprehensive about the kind of tests that will be done. They ask you about the tests and whether you think they should go to the screening clinic when they have no symptoms of glaucoma or any other eye disease.

- How would you explain a test with a tonometer?
- How would you explain glaucoma in terms Mr. and Mrs. Lavant could understand?
- Who are among the people at high risk for glaucoma?
- What is the usual treatment for chronic, open-angle glaucoma?

STUDY OUTLINE

I. Introduction

A. Visual loss is one of the most profound and dreaded of disabilities.

B. Nursing care of the visually impaired demands sensitivity to patient's unique needs, gentleness, and creativity in devising ways to help the patient accept and cope with his handicap.
C. Newer surgical techniques and medical treatments have improved the chances for preservation of sight and prevention of blindness.

II. Prevention of eye disorders and impaired vision

A. Nurses share responsibility with other health care providers for preventing eye disease and loss of sight.
B. Two major goals are teaching people how to take care of their eyes and preventing eye injury.
C. Basic eye care and prevention of injury.
   1. It is not possible to strain the eye. Headache, burning, itching, and redness of the eyes are symptomatic of eye disease, not eyestrain.
   2. Adequate nutrition conserves but does not improve eyesight.
   3. Normal eyes do not require irrigation. Persons with "dry eye syndrome" require replacement tears in the form of a solution.
   4. Children do not outgrow crossed eyes. Ambylopia ("lazy eye") requires prompt treatment to avoid permanent loss of vision in the affected eye.
   5. Every person over the age of 40 should have periodic eye examinations.
   6. Teaching children and adults to practice eye safety could prevent many accidental injuries to the eyes.
   7. Cosmetics for the eyelids, eyelashes, and eyebrows can be sources of infection and allergy.
   8. Danger signals of eye disorders:
      a. Persistent redness.
      b. Continued pain about the eye, especially after injury.
      c. Disturbance of vision.
      d. Crossed eyes, especially in children.
      e. Growths on eye or eyelid.
      f. Continuing discharge, crusting, or excessive tearing of the eyes.
      g. Pupil irregularities.

III. Diagnostic tests and examinations

A. Visual acuity: the Snellen chart—made up of rows of progressively smaller type.
   1. Visual acuity is expressed as a fraction, comparing distance at which patient can read a row of type with distance at which a person with normal vision can read the row. Usually tested with patient 20 feet from chart.
   2. 20/20 is normal. A corrected vision of 20/200 in the better eye, or a visual field of less than 20 degrees, is legally defined as blindness.
B. Near vision is tested by reading a card with different sizes of type (Jaeger's Test Types).
C. Refraction: person reads Snellen chart through different shaped lenses.
D. Intraocular pressure: the pressure exerted by fluid within the eyeball.
   1. Normal intraocular pressure is about 15 to 21 mm Hg. However, the pressure varies 3 to 5 mm during the day. In general, a pressure reading that remains in the high 20s suggests glaucoma.
E. Slit lamp or biomicroscopic examination.

1. Examiner can assess exterior and interior of eye through microscopic lens.

F. Topical dyes: used to detect abrasions and tears of the cornea with or without slit lamp examination.

G. Ophthalmoscopy.

1. Direct ophthalmoscope permits inspection of the fundus, retinal blood vessels, macula, and lens.
2. Indirect ophthalmoscope provides stronger light and stereoscopic observation of the interior of the eye. Pupils must be fully dilated for indirect ophthalmoscopy.

H. Fluorescein angiography is used to detect tumors and retinopathy.

IV. Nursing assessment

A. History taking:

1. Note personal history of any systemic disease, notably diabetes mellitus, neurologic disorders, or vascular disease.
2. Some drugs can cause either transient or permanent ocular changes; e.g., digitalis, corticosteroids, indomethacin, and sulfisoxazole.
3. Note family history of eye disease and visual impairment.
4. Patient's recent history of injuries, infections, and changes in activities of daily living (e.g., frequent minor accidents, fatigue, loss of interest in hobbies, work).

B. Subjective data: discomfort, itching, burning or stinging, abnormal tearing, blurred vision, double vision, or other changes in vision.

C. Objective data: redness, swelling of eyelids or periorbital space, excessive tearing, exudate on eyelids, abnormal position of eyelids, exophthalmia.

1. Inflammation or infection (see Table 34–1).
2. Also note patient's posture and general behavior (e.g., tilting the head, squinting, shading the eyes, and matching clothes and colors).
3. Ability to move eyebrows and eyes.

D. Nursing diagnoses associated with eye disorders include those that alter satisfaction of human needs at every level from physiologic to self-actualization needs.

V. Nursing intervention for the visually impaired

A. Give support and encouragement to patient adjusting to loss of eyesight.

B. Guidelines for helping a blind person:

1. Do not shout.
2. Speak to the patient as you enter the room so he will know you are there. Notify him when you are leaving.
3. Remove hazards from environment so patient will not accidentally fall or injure himself.
4. Treat blind person normally; do not express pity.
5. Assess amount of assistance patient will need with self-care activities.
6. Orient patient thoroughly to room at time of admission.
7. Use "clock method" to tell patient about arrangement of food on his plate. Set up tray for him. Feed the patient if necessary.
8. Allow patient to maintain his dignity while his needs are being met.

VI. Common errors of refraction

A. Refraction: light rays are bent so that they are not properly focused on the retina.

1. Myopia (nearsightedness): light rays converge and focus in front of the retina. Person has difficulty seeing distant objects.
2. Hyperopia (farsightedness): light rays converge behind the retina; person has difficulty seeing objects close at hand.
3. Presbyopia: visual defect of old age; improper accommodation of the ciliary muscles and ligaments when switching between distant and near vision.
4. Astigmatism: results from a warped lens or irregular curvature of the cornea.

VII. Foreign bodies in the eye

A. Removed by everting the lid and using cotton swab.

B. Deeply imbedded objects must be removed by ophthalmologist.

VIII. Nursing care of the patient having eye surgery; most eye surgery done on an outpatient basis

A. Preoperative care: nursing care planned according to individual needs.
1. Orient patient to outpatient surgery area and preoperative routine and procedures.
2. Emphasize importance of asepsis in the recovery period.
3. Reinforce teaching of correct manner of instillation of eye medications.
4. Assess for signs of systemic or other infection; surgery may need to be delayed; coughing and sneezing can disrupt suture line.

B. Postoperative care: gentleness very important.
1. No jarring of head when transferring patient.
2. Speak before touching patient who cannot see.
3. Medicate for nausea and vomiting immediately to prevent increased IOP from vomiting.
4. Report sudden pain in eye immediately, as it may indicate hemorrhage.
5. Cold compresses used to reduce swelling.
6. Teach activity restrictions and positioning while in bed (i.e., which side the patient can lie on).
7. Avoid straining, lifting, and other activities that elevate IOP.
8. Follow-up care with physician is essential.
9. Discharge planning is very important.

IX. Cataract: opacity of the lens

A. Symptoms and medical diagnosis: complaint of distortion of vision, floaters, photosensitivity.
1. Diagnosis by examination under slit lamp; lens appears opaque.

B. Surgical treatment: removal of affected lens and prescription of contact lens, intraocular lens, or eyeglasses for aphakic eye.

C. Nursing intervention.
1. Preoperative nursing care: explain expected outcome of surgery. Orient patient to room. Implement safety measures. Administer eyedrops precisely as ordered.
2. Postoperative nursing care.
   a. Observe patient for sudden and severe pain in eye, bleeding, and signs of infection.
   b. Warn patient not to cough, sneeze violently, squeeze eyelids, or make sudden movements of head.
   c. Ambulation and other physical activity usually not restricted unless otherwise ordered by surgeon.
   d. Discharge planning should include instruction of patient about limitations on physical activities, instillation of eye-

drops, and application and removal of eye dressings and shield.

3. Patient warned that adjustment to artificial lens will take time.
   a. Contact lenses provide better vision than cataract glasses but require manual dexterity to remove, care for, and reinsert.
   b. Intraocular lens implanted during surgery. Should not cause discomfort or inconvenience. There is risk of damage to eye.

X. Glaucoma: a complex group of disorders that have in common an increase in intraocular pressure

A. Due to either excessive production or inadequate drainage of aqueous from the chamber of the eye. Increased pressure of accumulating fluid damages optic disc.

B. Two major types: acute or angle-closure glaucoma, and chronic or open-angle glaucoma.

C. Acute, angle-closure glaucoma
   1. Characterized by sudden and severe pain in eye, blurred vision, and regional headache.
   2. Medical and surgical treatment:
      a. Treated as an emergency. Effort is made to reduce pressure immediately by administration of drugs.
      b. As soon as inflammation subsides, surgery is done (peripheral iridectomy) before vision is destroyed.

D. Chronic, open-angle glaucoma more insidious and more common. Can lead to blindness without ever producing an acute attack.
   1. Symptoms and medical diagnosis:
      a. Symptoms relatively mild: blurred vision, trouble adjusting to dark, narrowing of vision, seeing halos around objects and light.
      b. Persons most at risk for glaucoma: diabetics, those with recently controlled hypertension, blacks, those with family history of glaucoma, those with facial hemangioma or nevi, children with large eyes, and victims of eye injury.
      c. Diagnosis confirmed by applanation tonometry.
   2. Medical and surgical treatment:
      a. Chronic glaucoma treated by drugs to enhance outflow of aqueous and decrease its production. Diuretics also may be used.
         (1) Patients with glaucoma being treated in a hospital for unrelated illnesses must continue to receive their eye medication.
      b. Surgical treatment: iridotomy and trabeculoplasty by laser beam to facilitate drainage of aqueous.
   3. Nursing intervention:
      a. Patient education of utmost importance. Failure to follow prescribed treatment can mean loss of vision.
         (1) Nature of disorder and how it affects the eye.
         (2) Treatments available.
         (3) Expected result of currently prescribed treatment.
         (4) Possible outcome of not following prescribed treatment.

XI. Retinopathy: two causes are diabetes mellitus and hypertension

A. Diabetic retinopathy: two types: proliferative and nonproliferative.
   1. Nonproliferative retinopathy: vessels develop microaneurysms, which tend to rupture and hemorrhage into the vitreous.
   2. Proliferative retinopathy: neovascularization with fragile ves-

sels that rupture and hemorrhage into the vitreous or between layers of the retina.

3. Diabetic retinopathy controlled by laser photocoagulation treatments.

XII. Corneal transplant (keratoplasty) done to replace cornea damaged by trauma, ulcers, or disease

A. Two types: full-thickness and lamellar keratoplasty.

B. Keratoplasty performed to restore vision.

C. Cornea is not vascular and heals very slowly; takes up to a year for complete healing.

XIII. Macular degeneration occurs with aging and affects color vision, acute vision, and central vision.

XIV. Eye trauma and emergencies

A. Corneal abrasion very painful; infection is a danger.

B. Removal of foreign body from surface of cornea is best done by irrigation.

C. Foreign body penetrating the cornea should be removed by physician.

D. Chemical burns require extensive irrigation.

XV. Retinal detachment

A. A separation of the sensory layers from the pigmented epithelial layer due to holes or tears in the retina.

B. Incidence increases dramatically after age 40, most common in 50- and 60-year-olds.

C. Symptoms and diagnosis: flashes of light, floaters, cloudy vision, sometimes sudden loss of vision. Diagnosis confirmed by direct ophthalmoscopy.

D. Surgical treatment:

1. Repair of holes and tears by photocoagulation or cryosurgery. More extensive surgery may be required to position retinal breaks in contact with epithelial layer.
2. Vitrectomy: removal of opaque vitreous and stabilization of retina against choroid.

E. Nursing intervention: preoperative and postoperative care require specialized skills and knowledge.

1. Significant nursing interventions and expected outcomes (see Table 25–3).

XVI. Removal of the eye

A. Enucleation is removal of entire eye; evisceration, removal of contents of eyeball, sclera preserved; exenteration, removal of eyeball, eyelids, and all contents of ocular orbit.

B. Indications for eye removal: trauma, malignancy, severe pain in blind eye, and to prevent sympathetic ophthalmia.

C. Postoperative care.

1. Monitor for hemorrhage; prevent infection.
2. Patient allowed out of bed day after surgery; may go home in a few days.
3. After surgical site is healed an artificial eye can be inserted.

D. Care of an artificial eye.

1. Similar to care of dentures; must be handled with great care.
2. Remove carefully, wash with mild soap and water, store in container of water or contact lens solution. Wet prosthesis before reinserting.

XVII. Concerns for the elderly

A. Visual acuity decreases.

B. Arcus senilus may be visible as an opaque ring outlining the cornea.
C. Sclera may become yellowish or bluish.
D. Accommodation ability is decreased, causing difficulty in going from bright to dark areas.
E. Lens of the eye alters; ciliary muscle loses ability to accommodate, and presbyopia occurs.
F. Lack of moisture can cause eye irritation and predispose to infection.

XVIII. Resources for the visually impaired

A. Services, information, and support available to patients and their families.

CHAPTER 35

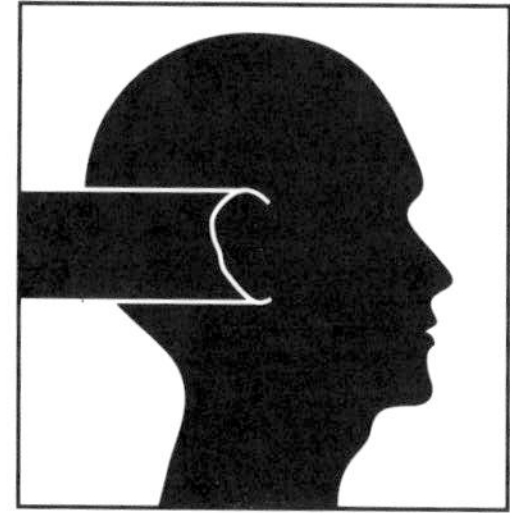

Care of Patients With Disorders of the Ears

VOCABULARY

aural
cerumen
deaf
equilibrium
labyrinthitis
myringotomy
nystagmus
otalgia
otorrhea
presbycusis
tinnitus
vertigo

Upon completion of this part of the chapter the student should be able to:

1. Discuss the impact of hearing loss on an individual and his family.
2. Compare and differentiate conductive and sensorineural hearing loss.
3. Describe nursing responsibilities in the prevention of hearing loss.
4. Discuss common tests used in the diagnosis of impaired hearing.
5. Describe nursing assessment of the sense of hearing and nursing diagnoses commonly associated with impaired hearing.
6. Describe the nursing care plans of patients with selected disorders of the ear (e.g., otitis media, labyrinthitis, Meniere's syndrome, and otosclerosis).
7. Describe specific nursing interventions used for the care of patients who have impaired hearing.
8. Discuss sensory aids and resources for persons with impaired hearing, tinnitus, and dizziness and vertigo.

Approximately 15 million people in the United States have some kind of hearing loss. The National Advisory of Neurologic Diseases and Stroke Council estimates that about 8.5 million Americans have either bilateral or unilateral hearing impairment sufficient to impose a serious handicap. In persons between 30 and 39 years of age, about 1.5% have a problem clearly understanding the spoken word. The figure rises to 4% in persons 50 to 59 years of age.

A loss of hearing, like a loss of sight, burdens its victims with physical, emotional, psychosocial, and financial problems. Hearing allows for communication with others in everyday conversations, in the classroom, and in business transactions. Without the ability to hear, one can be deprived of many of the joys and pleasures of life: music, drama, exchange of ideas, and the thousands of sounds in one's environment. Because hearing warns one of danger, an inability to hear can cause anxiety and fear.

Children who have hearing difficulties can be labeled disobedient, stupid, or even severely retarded. A baby who is deaf at birth must receive intensive speech therapy, because he cannot hear words and repeat them as the normal child does when learning to speak. The adult who has a hearing deficiency might lose his job and alienate friends because of his communication handicap.

TYPES OF HEARING LOSS

CONDUCTIVE LOSS

Normal hearing depends on the ability of the external ear to receive sound waves and transmit them to the eardrum (Fig. 35-1). Sound is described as occurring in waves, because the vibrations of sound are similar to the ripples produced in a pond when a pebble is thrown into the water. The vibrations of sound picked up by the outer ear are conducted through the ear canal to the tiny bones in the middle ear. Their movements produce a pressure wave in the fluid in the inner ear. This fluid surrounds the end organs of hearing and balance. A dysfunction of either the external or the middle ear produces a *conductive* loss of hearing because the external and middle ear are responsible for conducting sound waves. Common causes of conductive hearing loss are listed in Table 35-1.

Treatment of conductive hearing loss includes simple removal of an obstructing foreign body or plug of earwax, reconstructive surgery of the structures of the outer and middle ear, and tympanoplasty (repair of the eardrum).

Sound also is conducted by bones other than those in the middle ear. Vibrations of the temporal bone cause movement of the fluid in the inner ear, but the quality of sound is somewhat

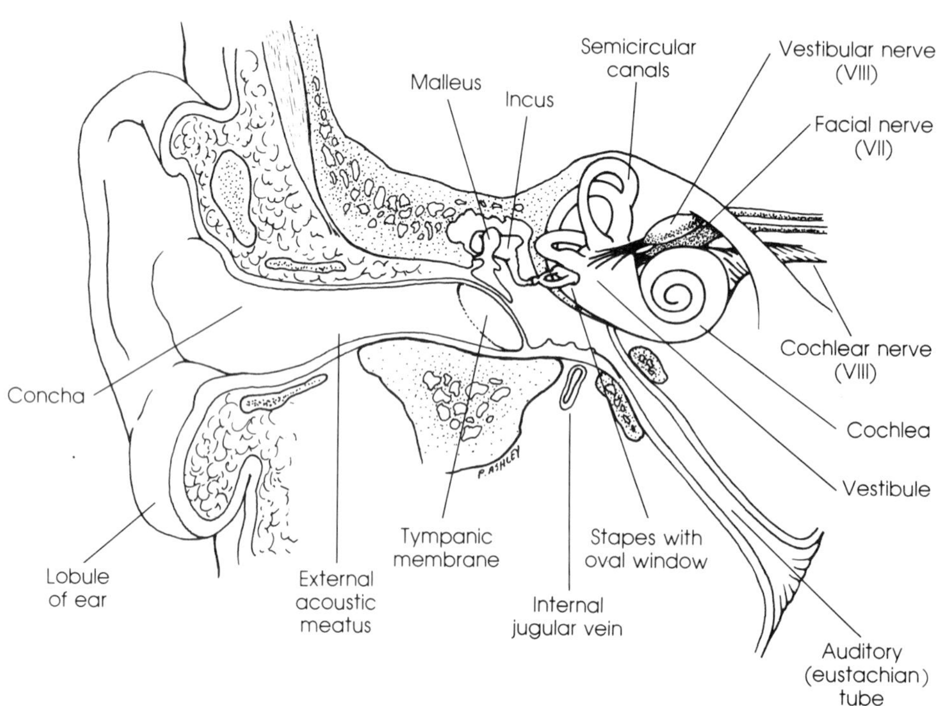

Figure 35-1 Outer, middle, and internal ear.

TABLE 35-1 COMMON CAUSES OF CONDUCTIVE AND SENSORINEURAL HEARING LOSS

Conductive Losses	Sensorineural Losses
Wax plug (cerumen) or foreign object blocking the ear canal	Heredity
Perforated eardrum	Old age (presbycusis)
Middle ear disease (otitis media), recurrent	Noise damage
Otosclerosis	Meningitis
Congenital malformations of outer or middle ear	Childhood diseases (mumps, measles, scarlet fever, viruses, etc.)
	Rubella and Rh incompatibility during fetal life
	Skull fractures and brain damage
	Ototoxic drugs
	Tumors (acoustic neuroma)
	Meniere's syndrome

Adapted from Rosenblum, E. H.: Fundamentals of Hearing for Health Professionals. Boston, Little, Brown, 1980.

distorted when compared with that received through the eardrum.

SENSORINEURAL LOSS

The mechanical energy of sound vibrations received by the external and middle ear is transformed into an electrical energy that stimulates the nerve fibers of the eighth cranial nerve (acoustic nerve). From there the impulses are carried to the brain, where the temporal lobe of the cerebral cortex decodes or interprets the sound. A dysfunction located in the inner ear or in the eighth cranial nerve is called a *sensorineural* loss. The term *sensorineural* simply means that the hearing loss is not due to a malfunction of the outer or middle ear but is a deficit in perception or interpretation of the sound waves. The messages being conducted to the fluid in the inner ear are not perceived normally. Common causes of this type of hearing loss are listed in Table 35-1.

Persons with sensorineural hearing loss typically have more difficulty hearing high-pitched tones than low-pitched ones; thus they frequently can understand the speech of men better than that of women. Another characteristic of sensorineural hearing loss is difficulty hearing softly spoken and poorly enunciated words. Speaking louder to the person with sensorineural hearing loss may help, but it is especially important to speak slowly and clearly and to face the person when communicating with him. Because persons with sensorineural hearing loss do not hear their own voices as well as a person with normal hearing, they tend to speak louder than necessary.

There often is little that can be done to correct sensorineural hearing loss, although a hearing aid helps some patients. Hearing aids can maximize the residual hearing of some persons with this type of hearing loss, especially if the hearing aid is designed to amplify some pitches and block out others that do not need amplification. Hearing aids are not always the answer to a problem of hearing loss, and for some persons the most effective therapy is focused on rehabilitation to facilitate acceptance of the loss and learning of new ways to communicate in spite of some degree of deafness.

CENTRAL HEARING LOSS

This type of hearing loss occurs as a result of some pathologic condition above the junction of the eighth cranial nerve and the brain stem. Central hearing loss can be due to a problem of transmission of stimuli in the brain, an inability to decode and sort signals received from one or both ears, or a failure in the transmission of sounds from one hemisphere of the brain to the other. Underlying causes of these basic pathologic conditions include brain tumors, vascular changes that suddenly deprive the middle ear of its blood supply, cerebrovascular accident, and erythroblastosis fetalis.

SIGNS OF HEARING LOSS

As a member of the health care team, the nurse should be aware of early signs of hearing loss and encourage people with impaired hearing to consult a physician for professional diagnosis and treatment. Not all forms of hearing loss can be corrected, but with professional guidance, many partially deaf people can achieve a more normal level of hearing. Surgical procedures cannot always restore hearing to normal, but measures such as wearing correctly fitted hearing aids, lipreading (also called speech reading), using sign language, and undergoing speech therapy can greatly contribute to one's ability to communicate with others.

Infants and children should be checked frequently for evidence of hearing defects. It is estimated that almost 20% of children in the lower socioeconomic groups, both urban and rural, suffer from some degree of deafness.

Warning signs of impaired hearing in infants and young children:

- Failure to react to loud noises during the first year of life.
- Use of mostly vowel sounds after the first year of life.
- Failure to talk by the age of 2 and scarcely intelligible speech after age 3.
- Speaking in a loud or monotonous tone or using garbled words.
- Habitually saying "what?" and failure to follow instructions.
- Inattentiveness in class and failure to achieve academically.

Some adults do not wish to acknowledge that they are losing their sense of hearing and attempt to conceal the problem rather than seek competent help. Evidence that a person's hearing may be impaired and that consultation with a physician is indicated includes:

- Speaking in either a very loud or a very soft voice.
- Change in awareness of sound (that is, being more aware or less aware than usual).
- Inattentiveness and withdrawal from communication with others.
- Facial expressions indicating difficulty in understanding what is being said.
- Inappropriate response to statements made during a conversation.

PREVENTION OF HEARING LOSS

A glance at the causes of hearing loss listed in Table 35–1 will help identify some of the ways the nurse can participate in prevention of hearing loss. Not all cases of hearing disability can be prevented, of course, but many can with adequate education of the general public and prompt and effective treatment of ear infections and other disorders that can affect hearing.

Children at an early age and adults (who should know better) should be taught not to put objects in their ears. Cleanliness of the outer ear ought to require nothing more than washing with soap and water. Hair pins, the ends of pencils, and other assorted objects are never used to relieve tickling or itching in the ear or to remove cerumen (earwax). Earwax normally moves on its own out of the ear canal to the outer ear, where it can be removed without danger of damaging the delicate lining of the ear canal or the tympanic membrane (eardrum). If there is overproduction of cerumen and blockage of the ear canal, a hearing loss can result. The obstructing collection of cerumen should be removed by a physician or nurse skilled in removal of impacted cerumen. Foreign objects such as beans, peas, and other vegetative substances also should be removed by someone who is experienced and aware of the potential for damage to the ear.

Continued exposure to excessively high levels of sound can produce sensorineural loss called *noise-induced hearing impairment*. This condition is particularly likely to occur in industrial settings where machinery creates a constant din in the working environment. Persons working near airplanes that are landing and taking off also are exposed to high noise levels throughout the day. Since hearing loss can be extremely costly in terms of disability compensation, industries in which there is a potential for damage to the hearing of their employees should and usually do require the wearing of ear protectors at work.

A rather recent phenomenon is the potential damage to the inner ear caused by amplified music. Authorities recommend that continual exposure to music amplified to more than 104 to 111 decibels be avoided.

There are many drugs that can be toxic to the inner ear and cause some hearing impairment. This is especially true if a very high dose of the drug is given or if it is given incorrectly. Among the drugs that can be ototoxic are many of the antibiotics and potent diuretics such as furosemide (Lasix) and ethacrynic acid (Edecrin). Aspirin and other salicylates can produce loss of hearing of high frequencies in both ears and ringing in the ears (tinnitus). Chemotherapeutic agents used for the treatment of malignancies also are likely to be ototoxic.

Nurses should be aware of the potential for damage to the ear by potent drugs. Patients should be monitored carefully while receiving a potentially harmful drug. Any signs of ototoxicity such as ringing in the ears, subtle changes in hearing ability, and difficulty in hearing either high- or low-frequency sounds should be reported immediately and documented on the patient's chart.

DIAGNOSTIC TESTS AND EXAMINATIONS

VISUAL EXAMINATION OF THE EAR

The two instruments most commonly used for examination of the ear canal and tympanic membrane are the otoscope and the aural speculum. The otoscope is fitted with a light and a magnifying lens to facilitate inspection (Fig. 35–2). The aural speculum is used with a special circular, slightly concave head mirror that has a hole in its middle. The head mirror is positioned so that the central hole lies in front of one eye of the examiner. A source of light, such as a lamp, is placed behind the examiner so that it shines on the head mirror and is reflected into the ear.

The simple speculum can be modified by attaching a special tube and inflatable bag (pneumatic otoscope), thereby creating an airtight system. This allows the examiner to determine whether the tympanic membrane responds to positive and negative pressure. The normal eardrum moves in response to pressure. Healed perforations and scars on the eardrum can be seen when the tympanic membrane is moved. Table 35–2 lists the diagnostic tests for the ear.

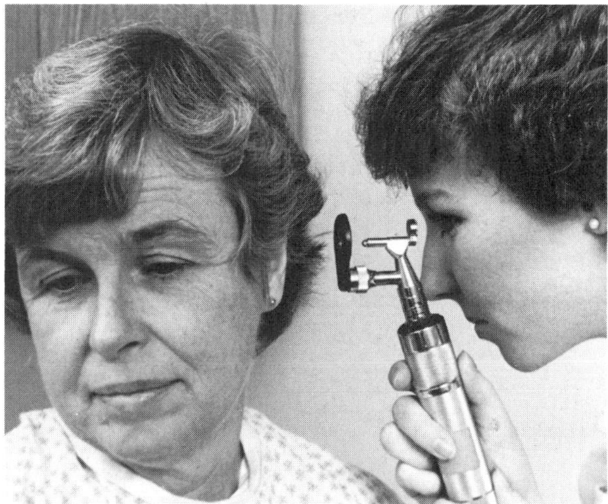

Figure 35–2 Examination of the ear canal with an otoscope. (Photo by Ken Kasper.)

NURSING ASSESSMENT

HISTORY TAKING

Because several local and systemic diseases can produce ear pain (otalgia), ringing in the ears, and dizziness or vertigo, the history taken by the nurse should include questions about any recent episodes of sinusitis, dental problems, and other disorders located in the face or neck. Allergies and recent acute or chronic upper respiratory infections also are noted, as are hypertension and such endocrine disorders as diabetes and hypothyroidism.

Any drugs currently being taken by the patient are significant because of the possibility of toxicity to the ear. Head injuries and exposure to sudden loud noises, as in an explosion, or excessively high levels of noise or amplified music over a period of time are also important to the history of a patient with a hearing disorder. Some patients may not be aware of the possibility that their occupation can contribute to impaired hearing, and so the nurse should ask where the patient works and whether he is routinely exposed to high levels of noise. Recre-

TABLE 35–2 DIAGNOSTIC TESTS FOR EAR PROBLEMS

Test	Purpose	Description	Nursing Implications
Weber test	Determines loss of hearing in one ear or both.	Tuning fork is struck, and then the handle is placed on the patient's forehead. Normal hearing or equal loss in both ears is demonstrated by hearing the sound in the middle of the head.	Explain purpose and procedure to patient.
Rinne test	Determines whether hearing loss is sensorineural or conductive.	Tuning fork is struck, and then the handle is placed on the mastoid bone; the fork is removed and struck again and held beside the ear (Fig. 35–3). The patient is asked in which position he heard the sound better or longer.	Explain procedure to patient.

Table continued on following page

TABLE 35-2 **DIAGNOSTIC TESTS FOR EAR PROBLEMS** *Continued*

Test	Purpose	Description	Nursing Implications
Audiometry	Determines degree of hearing loss in each ear.	Earphones are placed on the patient's ears and with the use of an audiometry machine, the audiologist channels sounds of different decibels and pitch into one ear and then the other of the patient. The patient signals when he hears the tone.	Explain procedure to patient.
Caloric test	Checks for alteration in vestibular function in each ear.	With patient in a seated or supine position, each ear is separately irrigated with a cold and then a warm solution to determine vestibular response. Normal response is nystagmus, vertigo, nausea, vomiting, falling; decreased response indicates abnormality.	Explain procedure to patient; tell him he may experience nystagmus, vertigo, nausea and vomiting, but these will indicate a normal response.
Electronystagmography (ENG)	Assesses for disease of vestibular system.	Electrodes are placed near the patient's eyes. Caloric test is performed; movement of the eyes is recorded on a graph. Decreased response is abnormal.	Explain procedure and equipment to patient. Tell him that nausea, vertigo, etc., indicate a normal response.
Evoked response; auditory and brain stem (ErA and ABR)	Determines abnormality of nerve pathways between eighth cranial nerve and brain stem.	Electrodes are attached to the client's head in a darkened room; similar to EEG. Auditory stimuli are directed to the patient, and a computer is used to track and separate the auditory electrical activity of the brain from other brain waves.	Explain the procedure and the equipment to the patient. Tell him the room will be darkened.
Magnetic resonance imaging	Detects tumor of the eighth cranial nerve, acoustic neuroma.	Huge electromagnet is used to detect radio frequency pulses from the alignment of hydrogen protons in the magnetic field. A computer translates the pulses into cross-sectional images. Provides high-contrast views of soft tissue.	Explain that his head will be placed in a machine that looks like a huge doughnut. He will need to lie very still during the test; all metal must be removed before the test.
FTA-ABS blood test	Blood test for syphilis.	Blood is drawn and sent to the lab for determination of presence of syphilis. Syphilis can cause problems with nerve transmission from the ear.	Explain that a blood sample is needed.

ational activities such as swimming, diving, scuba diving, skeet shooting and hunting, and flying (especially in an unpressurized cabin) can damage the hearing apparatus and produce some hearing loss.

SUBJECTIVE AND OBJECTIVE DATA

Nursing assessment of the ear includes inspection of the ear and observation of the patient for signs of hearing loss. The outer ear is inspected for normal development of the auricles, which should be symmetric. Normally, the top of each auricle is in alignment with the corner of the eye on each side. The surface of the auricle should be free of lesions, nodules, cysts, and tophi, which are hard nodules of varying size located on the margin of the pinna of the ear. Enlarged lymph nodes that can be palpated in front of the ear or over the mastoid process could indicate either infection or malignancy.

There should be no secretions other than cerumen in the ear canal. Otorrhea (drainage or discharge from the ear) is considered abnormal. The color, odor, and approximate amount of any drainage noted are documented on the patient's chart.

The nurse also can notice whether the patient gives any sign of not hearing well. He may report that he cannot hear well, or he may try to mask his disability. If his response to questions and casual remarks do not make sense or are inappropriate, the nurse might suspect that he has a hearing loss.

In addition to subjective reports of inability to hear well, the patient might also complain of pain and discomfort or ringing in the ears or state that he is dizzy or has difficulty maintaining his balance. Ear pain can be referred from other parts of the head and neck. One problem that produces pain in the ear is a disorder of the temporomandibular joint called *temporomandibular joint syndrome* (TMJ).

NURSING DIAGNOSES

Categories of nursing diagnoses associated with ear disorders and varying levels of hearing loss are as follows:

- Activity intolerance related to dizziness, nausea, and vomiting associated with motion. (This condition often occurs when the inner ear is affected, as in Meniere's syndrome and labyrinthitis).
- Anxiety related to inability to hear warnings, perform at work, communicate in social situations.
- Pain related to inflammation.
- Auditory sensory perceptual alteration related to hearing loss.
- Kinesthetic sensory perceptual alteration related to problems with balance.
- Impaired verbal communication related to inability to receive messages or to decode and interpret them.
- Anticipatory and dysfunctional grieving related to refusal to accept hearing loss and participate in rehabilitation efforts.
- Potential for injury related to inability to hear and follow directions or to loss of equilibrium and falls.
- Knowledge deficit related to nature of disability, self-care, availability of community resources for the hearing impaired.
- Disturbance in self-concept related to inability to hear.
- Social isolation related to difficulty in communicating.

COMMON DISORDERS OF THE EAR

In addition to malformations of the outer ear and obstructions to the conduction of sound through the ear canal, such as impacted cerumen and foreign objects, the middle and inner ear are subject to infections and other pathologic conditions. Among the most common are otitis media, labyrinthitis, Meniere's syndrome, and otosclerosis.

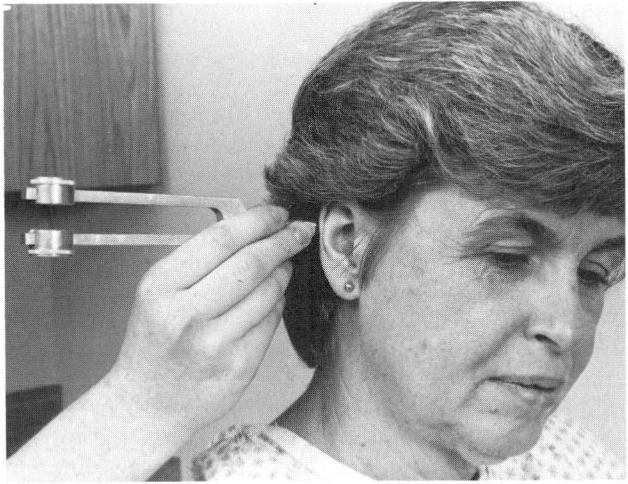

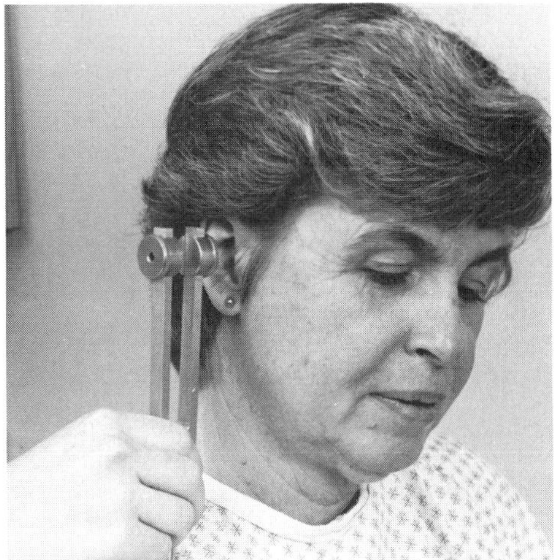

Figure 35-3 The Rinne test.
(Photos by Ken Kasper.)

OTITIS MEDIA

This condition is an inflammation of the middle ear. It occurs most often in infants and young children and is the most common cause of temporary conductive hearing loss. It is classified as serous, secretory, or suppurative. All three types characteristically result in accumulations of fluid behind the eardrum and some impairment of hearing.

Acute serous otitis media usually follows an upper respiratory tract infection or trauma to the ear. It sometimes is accompanied by an allergy or enlarged adenoids or both. Symptoms are mild and may consist only of a feeling of fullness in the ear and evidence of impaired hearing. The eardrum is retracted inward because of negative pressure due to a closed eustachian tube.

Secretory otitis media involves the structures of the middle ear itself. A primary allergic response causes the secretion of large amounts of amber, mucoid, or grayish fluid. The tympanic membrane bulges outward in response to the buildup of pressure from the fluid. The condition is treated conservatively with antihistamines and decongestants. If this approach is not successful, a myringotomy (incision into the eardrum) is done, and ventilating tubes are inserted to permit drainage of the excess fluid in the middle ear.

Suppurative otitis media occurs when pus-producing bacteria infect the middle ear. It usually is associated with an upper respiratory tract infection, most often when organisms from the nasopharynx find their way into the middle ear. Treatment consists of systemic therapy with antibiotics, topical therapy with eardrops, tympanoplasty to repair a ruptured eardrum and damaged ossicles, and, sometimes, mastoidectomy to eliminate all sources of infection and prevent further degeneration of bone.

Infections in the middle ear always have the potential for spreading to the meninges and causing meningitis or to the mastoid bone and causing mastoiditis. With the advent of antibiotics, surgery to scrape and clean infected mastoid bone is performed far less frequently than it was previously. Although otitis media is a fairly common occurrence, it should always be treated immediately.

LABYRINTHITIS

Labyrinthitis is an inflammation involving the labyrinths of the inner ear and occurring as a complication of chronic otitis media or from a viral infection. The symptoms include loss of hearing in the affected ear, severe dizziness with nausea and vomiting, and abnormal jerking movements of the eyes (nystagmus).

Treatment is aimed at removal of the source of infection and control of symptoms. Antibiotics may be given in massive doses to control a bacterial infection. Meclizine (Antivert, Bonine) or another antihistamine that assists in decreasing vertigo and its associated nausea and vomiting is used also. Scopalamine patches behind the ear can be used after the acute phase to control vertigo.

Initially the patient is kept on bed rest to prevent falls and injury. Siderails must be kept up, and the patient is cautioned not to get out of bed without assistance. If the source of the problem is chronic mastoiditis that won't respond to medical treatment, a mastoidectomy may be done.

MENIERE'S SYNDROME

Meniere's syndrome is a group of symptoms in which there is an increase of fluid within the spaces of the labyrinths, with swelling and congestion of the mucous membranes of the cochlea. The symptoms include attacks of dizziness, ringing in the ear (tinnitus), poor coordination that makes walking difficult or impossible, and loss of hearing. Any sudden movement of the head or eyes during an attack usually produces severe nausea and vomiting. The condition occurs most often in people who have had chronic ear disorders and allergic symptoms involving the upper respiratory tract. The exact cause is unknown.

Diagnosis of Meniere's syndrome usually is not difficult, but because these symptoms could indicate a tumor of the auditory mechanism, a *caloric test* is performed, which involves instilling very warm or cold fluid into the auditory canal. A patient with Meniere's syndrome will experience a severe attack; a normal person will complain of only slight dizziness. A person with a tumor of the auditory mechanism will have no reaction at all.

Treatment of Meniere's syndrome is primarily concerned with relief of symptoms; there is no cure for this condition, although it does disappear spontaneously in some cases. For an acute attack with disabling vertigo, atropine may be given subcutaneously. This is followed by diazepam (Valium), dimenhydrinate (Dramamine), meclizine, cyclizine lactate, or other drugs for motion sickness. In order to control edema and reduce pressure in the inner ear, the patient may be placed on a low-sodium diet, his fluid intake may be restricted, and his urinary output may be increased by means of a diuretic drug. The patient is kept quiet and in bed to avoid aggravating his symptoms. He may be very irritable and withdrawn and may refuse to eat or drink because of fear of vomiting. One should be very careful to avoid increasing his irritation by jarring his bed, turning on bright overhead lights, or making loud noises.

These measures help control the severe symptoms during an attack, but the patient's hearing is not improved. If attacks continue and are very severe despite medical treatment, surgical removal of the endolymph sac from the inner ear can be done with microsurgical techniques. When hearing loss is total on the affected side, surgical destruction of the eighth cranial nerve can be done to resolve the symptoms. Although this produces permanent deafness in the affected ear, the severe attacks are eliminated. In most persistent cases of Meniere's syndrome, the patient will eventually suffer a serious or even total loss of hearing regardless of the treatment used.

OTOSCLEROSIS

Otosclerosis is a hereditary degeneration of bone in the inner ear. It occurs principally in white females and is responsible for hearing loss in approximately 10 million persons in the United States. The sense of hearing depends in part on the vibration of very small bones of the inner ear. The *stapes,* or stirrup, is particularly important, because it conducts sound waves to the fluid in the semicircular canals in the inner ear. Otosclerosis is not, as its names implies, a hardening or sclerosis of the bony structures of the inner ear, but rather a degenerative process that makes the bone in the capsule of the labyrinth soft and spongy. During repair of the affected bone, new bone is laid down over the oval window. This causes the footplate of the stapes to be fixed so that it no longer vibrates to transmit sound waves.

Symptoms and Diagnosis

Otosclerosis usually begins when the patient is in the late teens or early 20s. A family history of progressive hearing loss and a personal history of gradual loss of hearing and ringing in the ears (tinnitus) are common.

The patient often complains of difficulty hearing the voices of others, yet his own voice sounds unusually loud. In response to this, he may lower his voice to the point that he can scarcely be heard by others. The patient typically complains that everyone else is mumbling and speaking indistinctly. This reaction can be understood when we realize that because of cranial bone conduction of sound waves, the person with otosclerosis does receive sound waves, but they are of poor quality and are not transmitted along normal pathways in the middle and inner ear. The person can hear fairly well over the telephone or in a noisy environment in which others are speaking loudly above the surrounding noise.

Surgical Treatment

The hearing loss of otosclerosis can sometimes be corrected by the use of a hearing aid. With the advent of microsurgery, surgical intervention can restore air-conductive hearing by providing a new moveable pathway for the sound waves.

During the operation, called a *stapedectomy,* the stapes is removed and is replaced with a prosthetic device. This device may be a steel wire and fat implant, a wire and a segment of vein, or a vein graft with polyethylene tubing. In any case, the prosthesis is attached to one end of the incus (anvil of the middle ear) so that sound can be transmitted to the inner ear (Fig. 35-4).

The surgical procedure is extremely delicate and would not be possible without the dissecting binocular microscope and other modern surgical instruments that allow visualization and manipulation of the very small structures of the middle ear.

Nursing Intervention

Postoperative nursing care is concerned with keeping the patient quiet and flat in bed for 48 hours. The head is turned so that the affected ear is uppermost. When the patient is allowed to move about, he must be warned that dizziness is

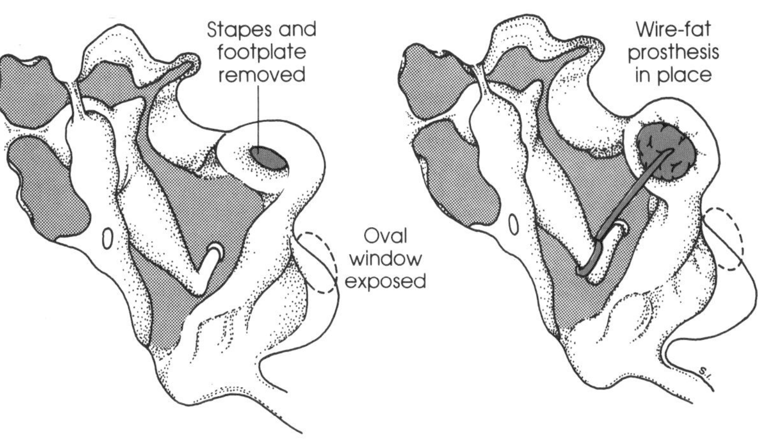

Figure 35-4 Stapedectomy to correct hearing loss caused by otosclerosis. *Left,* Middle ear tissue has been removed. *Right,* Prosthesis is in place.

NURSING CARE PLAN 35–1

Selected nursing diagnoses, goals/outcome criteria, nursing interventions, and evaluations for a patient having a stapedectomy for otosclerosis

Situation: Miss Cook, age 38, is a high school teacher who has had progressive hearing impairment as a result of otosclerosis of the right ear. She is admitted to the hospital for removal of the sclerosed stapes and insertion of a prosthesis.

During her initial assessment, the nurse found Miss Cook to be well-informed about the nature of her disorder but somewhat anxious about the outcome of surgery. Her physical health status is good; her only previous hospitalization was for an appendectomy when she was 19 years old.

Nursing Diagnosis	Goals/Outcome Criteria	Nursing Intervention	Evaluation
Postoperative period Potential for injury related to graft displacement. SUPPORTING DATA Stapedectomy.	Graft will be successful as evidenced by restored hearing in affected ear.	Position patient so that operative ear is uppermost. Reinforce preoperative instructions to remain in bed for 48 hours, avoid sudden movements, blowing nose, sneezing. Check vital signs, especially temperature, for evidence of infection q 4 h. Administer sedative as ordered to promote rest. Provide quiet environment	Temp., 99.2°F.; maintaining bed rest; operative ear up; continue plan.
Potential for activity intolerance related to vertigo and instability. SUPPORTING DATA After stapedectomy, states is very dizzy and nauseous.	Falls and trauma to head will be avoided.	Keep siderails up at all times; repeat explanation for safety precautions. Emphasize importance of having assistance when ambulation is allowed. Caution patient to change positions and turn her head very slowly. Provide well-lighted room when ambulating. Administer medication prescribed for vertigo.	Siderails up; cautioned to turn head slowly; gave dramamine 25 mg IM at 10 and 2 for dizziness and nausea; continue plan.
Knowledge deficit related to self-care after surgery. SUPPORTING DATA Asks about restrictions and self-care.	Patient will verbalize knowledge of home self-care before discharge. Patient will demonstrate dressing change correctly before discharge.	Instruct patient to avoid loud noises and pressure changes for 6 months, especially flying and diving. Stress importance of not blowing her nose for at least 1 week, avoiding an upper respiratory infection if at all possible, protecting her ear against cold, and refraining from any activity that might provoke dizziness or disturb the implant (e.g., straining, bending, and heavy lifting). Teach patient how to change dressing on the external ear and care for surgical incision to avoid infection. Reiterate importance of taking full course of prescribed antibiotic and reporting to surgeon at scheduled times. Reassure patient that due to swelling of tissues and presence of surgical pack it may be several weeks before she can fully evaluate effectiveness of the surgery.	Discharge teaching done; obtain feedback tomorrow and demonstration of changing ear dressing before discharge; continue plan.

likely to occur, especially if he turns his head suddenly. Siderails are applied to the bed, and the patient must have assistance when getting out of bed and walking. Coughing, sneezing, and other violent movements of the head should be avoided, and the patient must be warned not to blow his nose, as this may introduce organisms into the middle ear via the eustachian tube. Before discharge the patient is given instructions about medications to be taken at home and limitations on his physical activities.

Nursing interventions for selected problems in a patient having a stapedectomy for otosclerosis are summarized in Nursing Care Plan 35–1.

DIZZINESS AND VERTIGO

The sense of balance and equilibrium is governed by the vestibular system in the inner ear. Increases in fluid pressure in the inner ear, inflammations, and vascular disorders that interrupt blood supply to the cochlea can produce dizziness, loss of balance, and nausea and vomiting. These symptoms can range from mildly annoying to completely incapacitating and should always be assessed whenever a person has an ear disorder and loss of hearing.

The patient who has dizziness and positional vertigo should be cautioned to avoid sudden turning of the head and other movements that aggravate the vertigo. If he is not on bed rest, he should be told to call for assistance whenever he needs to move from his bed or chair. When helping the patient to his feet, move slowly and give him time to stand for a moment before beginning to walk. Typically, patients with this kind of vertigo feel that the room is spinning around them during an attack, and any motion makes the sensation even worse. While the patient is having an attack of vertigo, he should lie in bed and remain as motionless as possible. Stabilizing his head with a pillow on either side may encourage immobility. Attacks can last from a few minutes to hours.

Medications intended to reduce motion sickness and nausea should be given precisely as ordered. If drugs of this kind are not ordered on a regular schedule of every 3 to 4 hours, they should be given on a preventive basis: that is, *before* the patient's symptoms become severe and as often as necessary to control dizziness.

When increased fluid pressure in the inner ear is suspected as the cause of dizziness, the physician may order a low-salt diet and limitation of fluid intake. Although there is some question about the effectiveness of this form of treatment, it does seem to be helpful in some cases.

Patients with recurrent attacks of vertigo are encouraged to stop smoking if they are habitual tobacco smokers. Emotional upsets and physical stress from overwork also are thought to be associated with the frequency of attacks of vertigo in patients with inner ear disorders. If the patient tends to work extremely long hours without periods of rest and relaxation, he may benefit from a routine of less work. Teaching the patient effective coping mechanisms to handle emotional stress also could be helpful.

TINNITUS

Ringing, buzzing, or other continuous noise in the ear *(tinnitus)* can be mildly annoying or so severe as to interfere with a patient's ability to perform his usual activities of daily living and prevent him from getting sufficient sleep and rest.

Common causes of tinnitus include presbycusis, constant exposure to loud environmental noise, and certain pathologic conditions. Inflammations and infections in the ear, otosclerosis, Meniere's syndrome, and labyrinthitis can produce tinnitus, as can such systemic disorders as hypertension and other cardiovascular disorders, neurologic disease including head injury, and hyper- and hypothyroidism. Tinnitus frequently is one of the first symptoms produced by an ototoxic drug.

Tinnitus is such a universal symptom of so many physiologic and emotional disorders that it is not surprising that most people have experienced the problem at one time or another. Because it is so widespread, and for many persons incapacitating, there is a national association devoted to the study and management of tinnitus. Through the efforts of the American Tinnitus Association (P. O. Box 5, Portland, OR 97207) and similar organizations, measures have been taken to prevent unnecessary environmental noise, for example, in factories and around airports, that may cause tinnitus.

Medical treatment begins with efforts to determine the underlying cause and treat it. When the cause cannot be found or is not amenable to treatment, symptomatic relief is tried. However, some cases of intractable tinnitus resist all modes of conventional therapy. Less traditional measures that have varying degrees of success include biofeedback training and "masking."

Biofeedback training is especially helpful in those cases in which emotional stress and anxiety or hysteria are thought to be the underlying causes of tinnitus. Through visual or auditory signals the person learns to relax and exert some degree of control over his autonomic nervous system. This can lower blood pressure and pulse rate and relax muscles that are very tense.

Masking simply provides a low-level noise to block out, or "mask," the head noise heard by the person complaining of tinnitus. Some examples include playing soft music or a tape of sounds of nature such as a waterfall while the person is resting or sleeping, providing "white sound" in the working environment, using a hearing aid to amplify sound from the outside and overcome head noise, and wearing a special tinnitus instrument that is a combination hearing aid and tinnitus masker for persons who have both hearing loss and tinnitus. The therapeutic effect of masking is highly individualized. Some persons find instant relief, some partial abatement of the head noise, and some do not benefit from any attempts to mask the sounds of tinnitus.

NURSING CARE OF THE PATIENT HAVING EAR SURGERY

PREOPERATIVE CARE

Nursing care of the patient during the preoperative period usually is rather routine except for administration of eardrops or other special medications and treatments. Physical preparation for ear surgery may or may not involve removal of some of the hair from the scalp. Most patients having a mastoidectomy do have some hair removed from the surgical site. Male patients should be clean shaven the morning of surgery. The external ear and surrounding skin should be thoroughly cleansed, preferably with a surgical soap. Female patients with long hair should have it braided or pinned back securely so that it will not become soiled by drainage from the ear or serve as a source of infection at the operative site.

POSTOPERATIVE CARE

Positioning of the patient after ear surgery will depend on specific instructions from the physician. Usually the patient is placed flat in bed, and his head is supported so that he does not turn it from side to side. In addition to noting the vital signs, the nurse should watch for signs of injury to the facial nerve, including inability of the patient to close his eyes, wrinkle his forehead, or pucker his lips. Such symptoms should be reported to the surgeon. If they appear later than 12 hours after surgery, they may be due to edema, and the physician may order a loosening of the dressings.

Precautions such as attaching siderails to the bed should be taken to avoid injury due to dizziness and loss of balance, which can occur temporarily as a result of disturbance to the mechanism that maintains equilibrium. When the patient is allowed to get up and move about, he should have someone in attendance to prevent him from falling.

Because the ear is so near the brain, a special effort must be made to avoid contamination of the surgical site. Dressings may be reinforced to keep them dry, but excessive drainage must be reported to the surgeon. The patient must keep his hands away from the bandages, and if he is unable to do so, he should be restrained.

Sneezing, coughing, and nose blowing are all ways in which the operative site may be disturbed. If sneezing cannot be controlled, the patient should be told to keep his mouth open while sneezing so that the force of the sneeze will exit through the mouth rather than the eustachian tube. Sneezing and blowing the nose also may force bacteria and other infectious material into the operative area.

The nurse should know beforehand exactly what is to be expected from the surgery. If the patient's hearing is slightly impaired immediately after surgery because of edema or bandages but is expected to improve in time, the nurse should know this so that she can reassure the patient. She should be able to give encouragement to her patient but must avoid giving false hopes or telling him that he has nothing to worry about when he will indeed have to make an adjustment to a disability.

NURSING INTERVENTION FOR THE HEARING IMPAIRED

TERMINOLOGY

The terms *deaf* and *hard of hearing* are sometimes taken to mean the same thing, when actually they represent two separate conditions.

Deaf people are those whose sense of hearing is entirely absent; *congenitally deaf* people are born without the sense of hearing, and *adventitiously deaf* people are born with the sense of hearing but, by illness or accident, have lost it. The *hard of hearing* have a hearing deficit, *but they are not deaf.* Persons who are hard of hearing have some functional hearing with or without the help of a hearing aid.

The term *hearing impaired* may be preferred by clinicians and the patients themselves, who could resent being called either deaf or hard of hearing. A hearing-impaired individual is one who has sufficient hearing loss to cause difficulty in communication and in full appreciation of the many sounds in his environment.

Patients who are admitted to an acute or long-term-care facility for unrelated acute or chronic illnesses should be assessed for hearing loss, especially those patients who are over the age of 60. During the initial assessment the nurse should identify each patient's specific type of hearing loss if one is present and find out whether and how the patient has learned to cope with the disability. Hearing aids worn by a patient require special care to avoid damage and ensure maximum benefit.

The "intercom" system used in most hospitals to answer a patient's call light from the nurses' station could be of little or no use to the patient who has a hearing loss. A piece of tape or sign of some kind should be placed over the terminal that designates his room. This will serve to remind the person answering the light to go to the patient's room rather than try to talk with him over the intercom system.

THE PROBLEM OF COMMUNICATION

The patient who is hearing impaired will have unique problems of communication while hospitalized. If he cannot hear well and misunderstands or misinterprets the voices and sounds in the unfamiliar surroundings of the hospital, he is likely to be frustrated, fearful, and anxious. Unless a special effort is made to have frequent contact with the patient, he also can feel socially isolated and out of touch with those caring for him.

When trying to communicate with a person who has a hearing loss, bear in mind that he may try to answer your questions without fully understanding what you are asking. Past experience has taught many hearing-impaired persons that to ask for repetition of questions irritates people and causes them to think the person is stupid. For this reason, many people who cannot hear well frequently smile and say "yes," when such an answer is either incorrect or inappropriate. They do this because they feel that people will tolerate them better if they are pleasant and easy to get along with.

Some guidelines to help the hearing-impaired patient and improve the nurse's ability to communicate with him are given in Table 35–3.

REHABILITATION

Specific measures for rehabilitation of a patient with hearing loss will depend on the age and aptitude of the patient. Children who were born deaf and have never heard the spoken word have no "auditory memory" of the multitude of sounds in language. They require intensive speech therapy to help them learn to communicate verbally. Authorities believe that children with even profound hearing loss benefit from the use of a hearing aid.

Adults who have acquired the skills of speech and language before their loss of hearing occurred are better able to pick up language cues and understand what is being said to them and therefore should have fewer problems with communication of language.

Lipreading

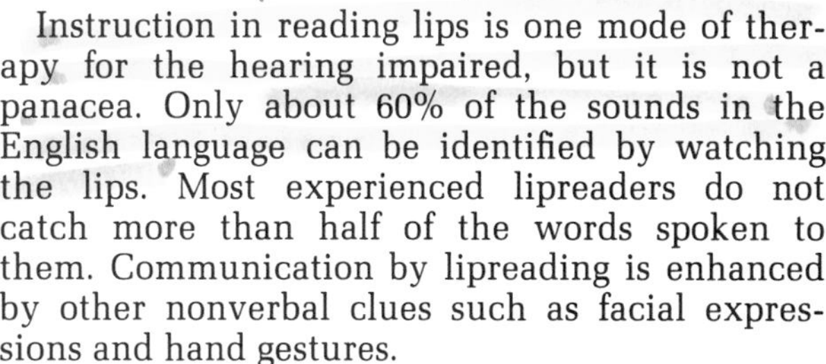

Instruction in reading lips is one mode of therapy for the hearing impaired, but it is not a panacea. Only about 60% of the sounds in the English language can be identified by watching the lips. Most experienced lipreaders do not catch more than half of the words spoken to them. Communication by lipreading is enhanced by other nonverbal clues such as facial expressions and hand gestures.

Learning to lipread is difficult. It requires at least average intelligence, exceptional language skills, excellent eyesight, and much persistence and patience.

Hearing Aids

In 1977 the U. S. Food and Drug Administration ruled that a hearing aid could not be sold in this country without a doctor's prescription. The

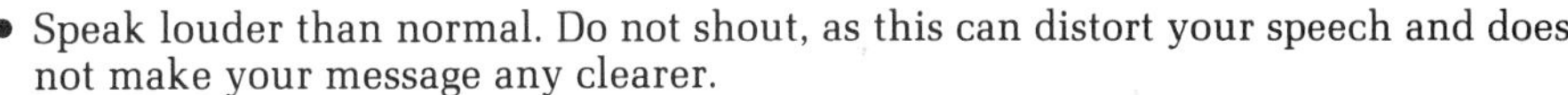

TABLE 35–3 COMMUNICATING WITH THE HEARING-IMPAIRED PERSON

- Speak louder than normal. Do not shout, as this can distort your speech and does not make your message any clearer.
- Speak slowly and distinctly.
- Get the person's attention, making sure he is aware that you are going to speak to him.
- The best distance for speaking to a hearing-impaired person is 3 to 6 feet. Face the person, and place yourself at eye level. If he is seated, seat yourself in front of him or bend down. Never speak directly into the person's ear. This can distort the message and hide all visual cues.
- Be aware of nonverbal communication. Facial expressions, gestures, and lip and body movements all give cues to the meaning of the message.
- Use short, simple sentences. If the person does not appear to understand or responds inappropriately, rephrase your statement. Try to limit each sentence to one subject and one verb. Give the person time to respond to your questions.

purpose of the ruling was to ensure that every person purchasing a hearing aid would have had a medical evaluation of his hearing and some evidence of the need for a hearing aid. Although the impact of the law is somewhat lessened by the fact that a person over the age of 18 can sign a waiver and buy a hearing aid without a prior medical examination, it does protect children. Unscrupulous sellers of hearing aids sometimes talk people into buying such aids when they are either not necessary or potentially dangerous. The person buying the aid may have only a temporary hearing loss due to impacted cerumen or some other easily remedied condition. On the other hand, the person may benefit from a hearing aid but will need a complete evaluation by a reputable audiologist and the prescription of a hearing aid designed to provide the best possible improvement of his hearing.

The hearing aids produced today can improve hearing in a variety of types of hearing loss. For the person who does not have a defect in the middle ear, a hearing aid can transmit amplified sound from the receiver through the eardrum to the inner ear. This is accomplished by amplifying sound waves transmitted by air conduction and bone conduction.

The design of a hearing aid varies. Some are worn in the ear, others behind the ear, and still others are built into the frame of eyeglasses. Persons with binaural hearing loss (both ears are affected) must wear a hearing aid in each ear.

The hearing aid should not be handled roughly or dropped. The ear mold can be cleaned with soap and water, but the other parts of the aid should not get wet. Hair spray can damage the microphone of a hearing aid. Regular servicing by a dealer can keep the aid in good working order.

A hearing aid sometimes is used for only a short while and is then discarded, because the user has not been properly instructed in how to use the appliance or is disappointed in its ability to improve his hearing. It is not reasonable to expect a hearing aid to make sounds clearer or the spoken word more distinct. The aid simply amplifies sound; it does not filter out unwanted sounds such as background noise, nor does it make a garbled sound less garbled. It takes time to become adjusted to a hearing aid and to learn to "troubleshoot" such problems as whistling sounds, scratchy noises, or weak or no amplification of sound.

Concerns for the Elderly

A decrease in hearing acuity occurs with aging for a variety of reasons. Arteriosclerosis can cause decreased blood flow to the otic nerve (cranial nerve VIII), resulting in sensorineural hearing loss. Otosclerosis can become more pronounced, causing a conductive hearing loss. Usually, difficulty perceiving high tones occurs first. Exposure to loud noise over time from machinery, cars, gunfire, etc., can cause sensorineural hearing loss. The majority of people in their senior years (over age 75) state that they have lost some hearing in some frequency ranges.

The loss or decrease of hearing makes it more important for the nurse to pay attention to communication with the senior adult. She should be certain she has his attention, faces him, and speaks distinctly when addressing him. It is essential to validate communication by asking for feedback in order to know that what was said was correctly perceived.

RESOURCES FOR THE HEARING IMPAIRED

There are several possible sources to help for the hearing-impaired person and his family. Universities and medical centers often have departments of speech and hearing that provide lipreading classes, rehabilitation, and hearing aid clinics. Among the societies and organizations devoted to help for the hearing impaired are:

- American Tinnitus Association
  P. O. Box 5
  Portland, OR 97207

This association provides information and support for tinnitus sufferers. It establishes self-help groups in various localities and provides training for health professionals in evaluation and mangement of tinnitus.

- Better Hearing Institute
  Box 1840
  Washington, DC 20013

This institute encourages those with uncorrected hearing problems to seek help. It operates a toll-free "Hearing Helpline": (800) 424-8576.

- National Hearing Aid Society
  20361 Middlebelt
  Livonia, MI 48152

This is a nonprofit association of hearing aid health professionals. It establishes standards, provides consumer information, serves as a data resource center, approves and coordinates educational programs, and provides certification for Certified Hearing Aid Audiologists. It also sponsors a Hearing Aid Helpline to assist the public.

BIBLIOGRAPHY

Andreoli, T. E., et al.: Cecil Essentials of Medicine, 2nd ed. Philadelphia, W. B. Saunders, 1990.

Campbell, S. L.: Some sound advice for managing a hearing impaired patient. Nursing 84, Feb., 1984, p. 46.
Cleveland, P. J., and Morris, J.: Meniere's disease: The inner ear out of balance. RN, Aug., 1990, p. 28.
Deblase, R., and Kucler, M.: Assistive hearing device aids patient-staff communication. Geriatr. Nurs., April, 1985, p. 223.
Guyton, A. C.: Textbook of Medical Physiology, 8th ed. Philadelphia, W. B. Saunders, 1991.
Hanawalt, A., and Troutman, K.: If your patient has a hearing aid. Am. J. Nurs., July, 1984, p. 900.
Ignatavicius, D. D., and Bayne, M. J.: Medical-Surgical Nursing. Philadelphia, W. B. Saunders, 1991.
The Saunders Health Care Directory. Philadelphia, W. B. Saunders, 1984.
Steffee, D., et al.: More than a touch: Communicating with a blind and deaf patient. Nursing 85, Aug., 1985, p. 27.

STUDENT STUDY AIDS

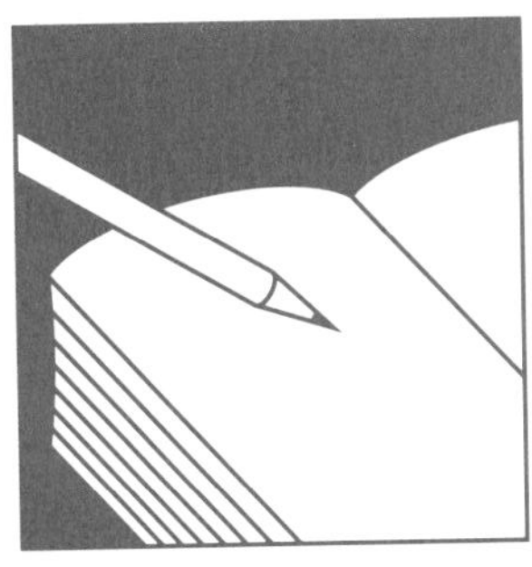

CLINICAL CASE PROBLEMS

Read the following clinical situation and discuss the questions with your classmates.

1. Mrs. Como is admitted to the hospital for management of her hypertension. She has had sensorineural deafness for several years, and it is much worse in her left ear than in her right. Her inability to hear well causes additional stress for Mrs. Como, and she is especially anxious about being in the hospital among strangers. Mrs. Como also suffers from tinnitus, which adds to her stress and inability to relax and rest. This and the stress of not being able to hear adversely affect Mrs. Como's hypertension.

- What evidence would you expect to find that would indicate that Mrs. Como has a hearing impairment?
- What can the nurses do to improve communication with Mrs. Como and help allay her anxiety about being in the hospital?
- What measures might help Mrs. Como cope with her tinnitus?

---

2. Mr. Thompson is suffering from a severe attack of Meniere's syndrome and vertigo. He is severely nauseated and his vertigo prevents him from getting out of bed.

- What nursing actions would be appropriate for him?
- How would you explain this disorder to Mr. Thompson?
- The physician wants to rule out the possibility of tumor as a cause of Mr. Thompson's vertigo, and so he is scheduled for an electronystagmogram (ENG) with a caloric test and a magnetic resonance imaging (MRI) scan. How would you explain these tests to him?

STUDY OUTLINE

I. Introduction

A. About 15 million persons in the United States have some kind of hearing loss. In the 30- to 39-year age group, 1.5% have some degree of hearing loss. In those between 50 and 59 years of age the figure rises to 4%.

B. Loss of hearing can create social, emotional, and financial burdens for the patient and family.

II. Types of hearing loss

A. Conductive: external and middle ear unable to conduct sound waves.

B. Sensorineural: dysfunction located in inner ear of the eighth cranial nerve; not due to malfunction of outer or middle ear.

C. Central hearing loss: pathology above junction of eighth cranial nerve and brain stem.

III. Signs of hearing loss

A. Speech difficulties in young children, inattentiveness, speaking in

loud or monotonous tone, failure in school, tendency to avoid others, habitually saying "what?" and inappropriate responses to questions and statements.
- B. Indicate a need for professional evaluation.

IV. **Prevention of hearing loss**
- A. See Table 35–1 for causes of hearing loss.
- B. Teach children and adults not to put objects in their ears.
- C. Clean ears with soap and water. Impacted earwax should be removed by physician or experienced nurse.
- D. Avoid constant exposure to loud noises.
- E. Monitor patient receiving ototoxic drugs.

V. **Diagnostic tests and examinations** (see Table 35–2)
- A. Visual examination with otoscope.
- B. Tympanocentesis to obtain specimen for study.
- C. Tuning fork tests:
  1. Weber test compares hearing acumen in each ear.
  2. Rinne test determines whether hearing loss is conductive or sensorineural.
- D. Audiometry: measurement of sound perception using audiometer.

VI. **Nursing assessment**
- A. History taking:
  1. Include questions about recent problems of sinusitis, dental problems, and other face or neck disorders.
  2. Note allergies, upper respiratory infections, and such systemic diseases as diabetes mellitus and hypothyroidism.
  3. Record drugs currently being taken because of possible ototoxicity.
  4. Record occupation and recreational activities that could cause hearing loss.
- B. Subjective and objective data:
  1. Outer ear inspected for developmental anomalies, encrustations, and lesions.
  2. Note enlargement of lymph nodes in front of ear and over mastoid process.
  3. Patient reports tinnitus, pain, dizziness, or vertigo.
- C. Common nursing diagnoses:
  1. Activity intolerance.
  2. Anxiety.
  3. Alterations in comfort: pain.
  4. Impaired verbal communication.
  5. Anticipatory and dysfunctional grieving.
  6. Potential for injury.
  7. Knowledge deficit.
  8. Disturbance in self-concept.
  9. Social isolation.

VII. **Common disorders of the ear**
- A. Otitis media: inflammation of the middle ear:
  1. Acute serous otitis media: usually follows upper respiratory infection or trauma.
  2. Secretory otitis media: due to primary allergic response and increased secretions.
     - a. Treatment: antihistamines, decongestants, myringotomy with insertion of ventilating tubes.
  3. Suppurative otitis media: caused by bacterial infection, usually from an upper respiratory tract infection.

a. Treatment: systemic antibiotics, eardrops, tympanoplasty to repair ruptured eardrum, and sometimes mastoidectomy.

B. Labyrinthitis: inflammation of labyrinth of inner ear:
1. Symptoms: loss of hearing, dizziness, nausea and vomiting, nystagmus.
2. Treatment: antibiotics, bed rest, drugs to control motion sickness, possibly mastoidectomy if that bone is involved.

C. Meniere's syndrome: group of symptoms due to an increase of fluid in labyrinthine spaces, with swelling and congestion of cochlear mucosa.
1. Symptoms: tinnitus, headache, poor coordination, hearing loss. Vertigo and nausea and vomiting when head is moved.
2. Treatment: bed rest during attacks of vertigo, drugs to control nausea and motion sickness, restriction of fluid intake, and (rarely) surgical destruction of eighth cranial nerve.

D. Otosclerosis: a hereditary disease of the bone in the labyrinthine capsule. Bone becomes soft and spongy; new bone is laid down, anchoring the stapes in oval window.
1. Symptoms and medical diagnosis:
   a. Progressive hearing loss begins in late teens or early twenties. Patient complains that the voices of others are muffled but can hear his own voice very well.
2. Treatment: some cases respond to a hearing aid; others require stapedectomy and insertion of prosthetic device.
3. Nursing intervention: postoperative care.
   a. Position patient properly for first 48 hours.
   b. Help patient avoid sudden, violent movements.
   c. Instruct in self-care before discharge.

E. Dizziness and vertigo.
1. Caution patient to avoid sudden movements.
2. Assist patient to get up, go to bathroom, ambulate, etc.
3. Administer medication to minimize motion sickness before symptoms become severe.
4. Encourage patient to limit fluid intake if this is recommended.
5. Encourage patient not to smoke.
6. Teach patient coping mechanisms to deal with stress.

F. Tinnitus: noise in the ear, "head noise."
1. Common to many disorders of the ear, cardiovascular disease, neurologic disorders, and thyroid disease.
2. Biofeedback training and masking techniques are sometimes successful when all other treatments fail.

VIII. Nursing care of the patient having ear surgery

A. Preoperative care: physical preparation and administration of eardrops, if ordered.

B. Postoperative care: varies according to surgical procedure:
1. Patient usually kept flat in bed with head kept still for 12 to 24 hours.
2. Watch for signs of injury to facial nerve.
3. Use care to avoid postoperative infection that could spread to brain.
4. Instruct patient to avoid coughing, sneezing, or blowing his nose.

IX. Nursing intervention for the hearing impaired

A. Terminology:
1. Deaf: sense of hearing totally absent.
2. Hard of hearing: hearing deficit.

3. Hearing impaired: have some hearing loss.

B. Guidelines for helping the hearing impaired: (see Table 35–3).

C. Problem of communication: (see Table 35–3).

D. Rehabilitation:

1. Lipreading.
   a. Not a panacea. Experienced lipreaders understand fewer than half the words spoken.
   b. Enhanced by nonverbal cues.
   c. Requires special abilities.
2. Hearing aids.
   a. Require prescription for purchase if under age 18; adult can sign waiver.
   b. Can improve hearing for various kinds of hearing loss.
   c. Must receive special care to avoid damage. Clean ear mold with soap and water. Other parts should not be wet. Avoid hair spray on hearing aid.

X. Concerns for the elderly

A. Some decrease in hearing acuity in all persons over age 75.

B. Arteriosclerotic changes in blood vessels supplying acoustic nerve account for some of the hearing loss.

C. Difficulty in perceiving high tones occurs first.

D. Exposure to loud noise over time is another cause of hearing loss in this age group.

E. Important to validate communication by asking for feedback in order to know that what was said was correctly perceived.

XI. Resources for the hearing impaired

A. Nurse should help patient and family utilize local and national resources.

CHAPTER 36

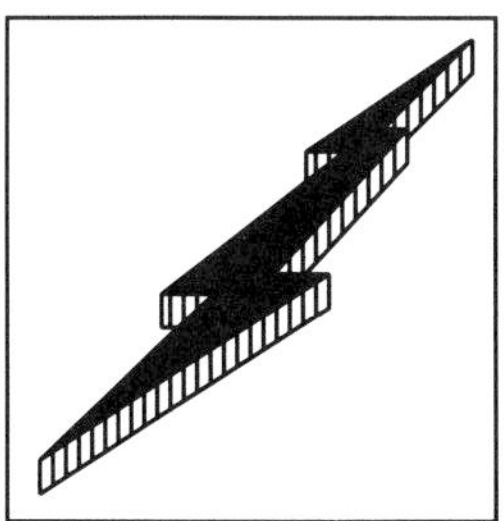

Care of Accident and Emergency Patients

VOCABULARY

bromide
cardiogenic
cardiopulmonary
combative
compression
corrosive
epistaxis
hypovolemic
neurotoxin
paradoxical respirations
prostration
ptomaines
recoil
resuscitation

Upon completion of this chapter the student should be able to:

1. Describe eight specific activities that could be effective in reducing accidental injury and death.
2. List five basic principles of first aid.
3. Describe actions to take in a choking emergency.
4. Describe the appropriate nursing actions and care needed for the patient who has experienced a respiratory or cardiac arrest.
5. Describe proper emergency techniques for control of bleeding, including nosebleed.
6. Describe specific interventions in the emergency care of the more common accidental injuries (e.g., major and minor burns; accidental poisoning by ingestion and inhalation; fractures and sprains; injuries of the eye and ear, head, and neck; abdominal wounds and chest wounds).
7. Describe emergency care of victims of insect stings, tick bites, and snakebites.
8. Discuss prevention of injuries from extremes of heat and cold.
9. Describe first aid treatment of injuries from extremes of heat and cold.
10. State key points in the emergency care of persons suffering from alcohol and drug abuse.
11. Discuss responsibilities and duties of the nurse in the care of disaster victims.

PREVENTION OF ACCIDENTS

HOME SAFETY

According to statistics compiled by the National Safety Council, accidents in the home account for one fourth of all fatal accidents. People under 5 and over 65 years of age are the principal victims of fatal mishaps occurring in the home. Because these individuals spend a large majority of their time inside the house, safety hazards must be identified and removed if accidental deaths are to be avoided.

Nurses, physicians, and others concerned with safety and welfare must take an active part in the education of the public regarding ways in which home accidents can be prevented. The two most dangerous rooms in the house are the kitchen and the bathroom. Table 36–1 shows some of the most common home hazards and how they can be eliminated.

HIGHWAY SAFETY

Motor vehicle accidents are the leading cause of accidental death in the United States (Fig. 36–1). Every year, thousands of Americans are killed in motor vehicle accidents and almost 2 million disabled by some kind of injury sustained in a traffic accident.

The two principal causes of motor vehicle accidents are human failure and mechanical failure. Human failure is by far the greater danger. Improper driving, which causes almost 90% of all accidents, can be caused by the influence of alcohol and/or drugs, fatigue, excessive speed, or emotional instability. Mechanical failure is often not detected as the cause of an accident; however, there has been much interest recently in built-in safety devices and inspection for safety hazards in new automobiles. The use of seat belts, air bags, lowering the speed limit on major highways, and better enforcement of laws against drunk driving have made a significant impact on vehicular deaths. The decrease in the number of

TABLE 36–1 **HOME SAFETY CHART**

Kitchen
For gas, coal, or wood-burning stove, have vents or flues; keep windows open a crack
Never light stove with kerosene or gasoline
Turn off all flames after cooking
Repair any gas leakage
Use potholders, asbestos pads
Keep handles of pots and pans turned away from edge of stove
Keep knives, sharp instruments, and poisons such as bleach out of children's reach
Wipe up spills on floor
Keep electric appliances in good working order

Storage areas
Always keep cellars, attics, garages neat
Throw out newspapers and oily rags at once; they can start fires
Clean and disinfect area where garbage is kept, and dispose of it frequently
Never place poisonous substances in drinking glasses, cold drink bottles, or other containers that have been used for food or drink
Always label poisonous compounds; read labels of poisons you have purchased and store out of reach

Living room
Be sure floors are not slippery
Replace frayed or torn carpets
Use rubber mats under rugs to prevent slipping
Cover electric sockets

Living room (continued)
Replace frayed electric cords
Keep electric cords off floor where people walk
Place heaters a safe distance from walls
Use screens around fireplace
Pad sharp edges on furniture as necessary
Check ashtrays for lit matches or cigarettes when going to bed or leaving house

Furnace
Have it checked every year, especially for leaks in tank of oil-burning furnaces
Never light furnace with gasoline or kerosene

Bathroom
Use rubber mat in tub
Store medicines out of children's reach
Keep all medicines capped and labeled
Throw out old medicines
Dispose of razor blades immediately after use

Bedrooms
Do not smoke in bed
Use rubber mats under scatter rugs

Stairways
Cover with carpeting or rubber safety treads
Replace torn or frayed carpeting
Keep stairs cleared of toys and cleaning equipment
Install handrails, proper lighting
Use gates at top and bottom if there are young children

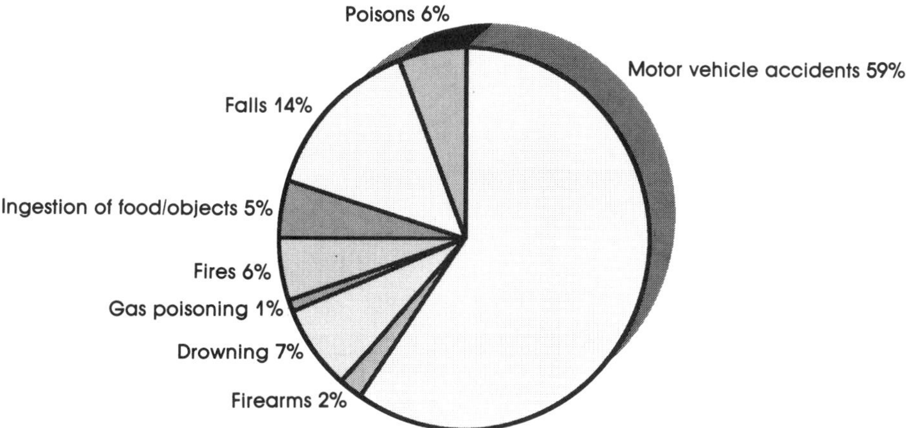

Figure 36-1 Principal types of accidental death, 1988. (Graphic courtesy of Derick Lloyd.)

vehicular deaths also reflects improvements in emergency medical services, which provide prompt and effective first aid and emergency care of accident victims.

WATER SAFETY

The advent of the 40-hour work week and extended vacations has provided more opportunity for Americans to enjoy water sports. With increased participation, there has been a proportionate increase in accidental deaths and injuries in or on the water. Many of these accidents could have been prevented if the simple rules of water safety had been observed. These rules include using good judgment about the choice of swimming area, ensuring proper supervision of children and adults who are not strong swimmers, diving only in areas where the water is sufficiently deep and is free of rocks or other obstacles, never swimming alone, and avoiding overexertion or swimming distances beyond one's ability. Above all, one should know how to handle an emergency should it arise. Panic frequently increases the danger for the victim as well as for the would-be rescuer.

Rescue of a drowning person requires clear thinking and deliberate action. First, the rescuer should call for help. If possible, he should try to reach the victim without going in water over his head. It is often possible to reach him by extending an arm, towel, rope, pole, or any long and sturdy object that is available. When the victim has grasped the object, he can be pulled slowly to safety. If a boat is available, it should be used for rescue of the person who is beyond reach by other methods.

A swimming rescue is very difficult, even for the most experienced swimmer. Because the victim is frightened, he may demonstrate abnormal strength and be quite capable of drowning both himself and his rescuer. After the rescued person is brought out of the water, he must be given cardiopulmonary resuscitation (CPR) if he is not breathing. If he is breathing, he should be placed in a reclining position and covered with a blanket or coat. His head should be turned to one side so that if he vomits, he will not aspirate the vomitus into his lungs.

The ordeal of nearly drowning can place an added burden on the heart. Because near-drowning victims always swallow large amounts of water and because both salt water and fresh water can upset the body's fluid and electrolyte balance, the victim should be transported to a medical facility promptly for evaluation and treatment. There is danger of delayed cardiac irregularities in all persons who have been rescued from drowning, no matter how short a time they might have been struggling in the water.

GENERAL PRINCIPLES OF FIRST AID

The following guidelines explain specific actions to take when called upon to provide first aid.

- *Try to keep calm and think before acting. Concentrate on what should be done first and the manner in which to proceed step by step.* Move slowly and deliberately so that you can gain time to think things through and at the same time instill confidence in those you are trying to help.
- *Identify yourself as a nurse.* This will serve to reassure the victim and the onlookers.
- *Before attending to the victim or victims of an accident, quickly survey the accident scene to determine whether there are further hazards to yourself and the victims.* For example, spillage of gasoline after a motor vehicle accident can cause a fire or explosion,

or there may be danger to the victim, yourself, and onlookers from oncoming traffic and secondary collisions. In both highway and home accidents, live electric wires may be in the vicinity. Whenever there is a high risk of death from hazardous conditions in the immediate environment, the victims should be moved at once, regardless of the nature of their injuries.

One factor that often is overlooked is the heat of the pavement in the summertime. Victims may receive severe burns from lying on a sunbaked street or sidewalk while waiting for the ambulance. Although it may not be safe to move the victim to a shaded area, it is advisable to place clothing, newspaper, or some other protective covering between his skin and the hot pavement.

- *If there are several victims of the accident, make a quick check of each one before beginning treatment.* The most serious and life-threatening injuries must be treated first; those who do not seem to be in immediate danger can be attended to by someone else who is capable of watching the victim and reporting to you any change in his condition.
- *Assess the victim as soon as possible after you are sure that there is no further danger in the immediate environment.*

Look for a MedicAlert bracelet or necklace. If the victim is wearing one or has some other identification showing specific medical needs, bring this to the attention of the ambulance or hospital personnel.

Try to determine the kind of instrument that caused the injury; for example, the column of the steering wheel, a drug or poison, or an electric current. This will give clues as to the type of injury sustained and the treatment required.

When evaluating the victim, begin at the head and work downward to the toes. Refer to the evaluation checklist in Table 36–2.

TABLE 36–2 CHECKLIST FOR EVALUATION OF ACCIDENT AND EMERGENCY PATIENTS

Area of Assessment	Mode of Assessment	Possible Causes
ABCs		
A—Airway	Look and listen for signs of respiratory distress: gasping, wheezing, stridor, choking, restlessness.	Airway obstruction, acute allergic reaction.
	Check mouth and back of throat for obstruction.	Mouth and throat injury.
	Do not tilt head and hyperextend neck if spinal injury is suspected.	
B—Breathing	Put ear close to nose and mouth and listen for breathing.	*Absence of respirations:* cardiac arrest, airway obstruction.
	Watch chest and abdomen for rhythmic rise and fall.	*Rapid, shallow respirations:* hyperventilation, pain.
	Note rate and quality of respirations.	
C—Circulation	Feel for pulse in carotid or femoral artery; note rate and quality.	*Absence of pulse:* cardiac arrest. *Rapid, bounding pulse:* hemorrhage, fright, hypertension. *Rapid, weak pulse:* hemorrhage, shock.
Head-to-toe		
1. General appearance and level of consciousness	Note if alert, oriented to time, place, person. Note response to verbal stimuli. Check for MedicAlert ID.	*Momentarily unconscious:* fainting, mild concussion. *Disoriented, confused, combative:* substance abuse, head injury, cerebral ischemia, insulin reaction, diabetic ketoacidosis. *Comatose:* severe brain damage, poisoning, diabetic ketoacidosis.
2. Pupils	Lift eyelids and check pupils for equality in size and shape, response to light.	*Dilated, fixed:* brain damage, drug overdose, shock, cardiac arrest. *Constricted:* CNS disorder. *Unequal:* intracranial lesion, stroke. *No response to light:* cerebral ischemia, brain damage.
3. Ability to move	If conscious, ask victim to move extremities.	*Paralysis on one side:* stroke, head injury with brain damage, hemorrhage. *Inability to move extremities:* spinal cord injury, severe intoxication, serious metabolic disorder.

TABLE 36–2 **CHECKLIST FOR EVALUATION OF ACCIDENT AND EMERGENCY PATIENTS**
Continued

Area of Assessment	Mode of Assessment	Possible Causes
4. Ears, nose	Look for drainage, note character.	Facial trauma, skull fracture.
5. Skin color and temperature	Note circumoral pallor. In dark-skinned victims evaluate skin changes in conjunctiva, soles of feet, and palms of hands.	*Pallor:* shock, heart attack. *Bright red lips and skin:* carbon monoxide poisoning. *Cyanosis:* asphyxia, electrocution. *Hot, dry skin:* heatstroke. *Cool, dry skin:* hypothermia. *Cold, clammy skin:* shock.
6. Head, mouth, and neck	Check for lacerations, soft depressed area of skull, evulsed tissue. Note breath odor. Check for loose or missing teeth, lacerations inside mouth. Check for pulsating, distended, or collapsed jugular vein.	Skull fracture, hematoma. Alcohol. *Fruity odor:* diabetic ketosis. Facial trauma. Cardiopulmonary pathology, injury.
7. Chest	Check lung sounds, change in position of trachea. Palpate for crepitus. Note skin integrity, open wounds. Check symmetry of chest movement during respirations. Shoulder pain on left side.	Pneumothorax. Pleural effusion. Possible ruptured spleen.
8. Abdomen	Listen for bowel sounds *before* palpation. Check for wounds, drainage. Assess pain.	Abdominal trauma, intestinal irritation, inflammation.
9. Genitalia	Look for lacerations, trauma, discharge, incontinence, bloody urine. Assess pain.	Trauma to genitalia, bladder, or kidney.
10. Extremities	Look for deformities, lacerations, missing fingers and toes. Check for ability to move, abnormal sensations. Assess pain.	Trauma, fractures, nerve damage.

- *Do not move the victim unless, as previously explained, he is in immediate danger or until you have immobilized injured parts.* This is particularly true if spinal injury is suspected.
- *Do not remove an object that has penetrated a part of the body and is still in place.* For example, a knife, piece of metal, or sliver of wood that is protruding from the chest or abdomen should be left as is. Bandages are applied around the object to stabilize it and control bleeding as necessary. The one *exception* to this rule is the presence of an impaled object in the cheek. In this case, the object must be removed to control bleeding.
- *Do not try to give anything by mouth to a person who is unconscious.* It is possible that he may aspirate the material into his air passage.
- *Explain to the victim in a calm and positive tone of voice what you are doing for him and why.* Give honest answers but do not alarm him unduly. You must sound as if you are in control of yourself and the situation.
- *Remember that most states have adopted "good Samaritan" laws that protect medical personnel from malpractice suits in the case of emergency medical care for victims of accidental injury.* These laws prevent litigation for malpractice as long as medically trained individuals act in good faith and to the best of their ability.

Even in states where there are no such protective laws, malpractice suits of this kind very rarely occur. For many people, the advantages derived from knowing that they have used their skills and experience to help someone in need outweigh the risk of a lawsuit.

CARDIOPULMONARY RESUSCITATION (CPR)

The first priority in administering emergency medical care is to check for signs of breathing, as listed in Table 36–2. The second priority is to determine whether the heart is beating. When neither breathing nor circulation is present, cardiopulmonary resuscitation, usually abbreviated CPR, is indicated. The letter C stands for *cardio* (heart), the P for *pulmonary* (lung), and the R for *resuscitation* (revival). Thus CPR means reviving or reestablishing heart and lung action once it has stopped suddenly.

There are many causes of sudden cessation of breathing and circulation, varying from electric shock to drowning to heart attack and cardiac arrest.

The technique for CPR is complex, requiring special knowledge and skills that can be mastered only by diligent study and practice. The following text gives the basic facts about CPR, but anyone intending to administer this procedure in an emergency situation should undergo supervised training to develop the necessary skills.

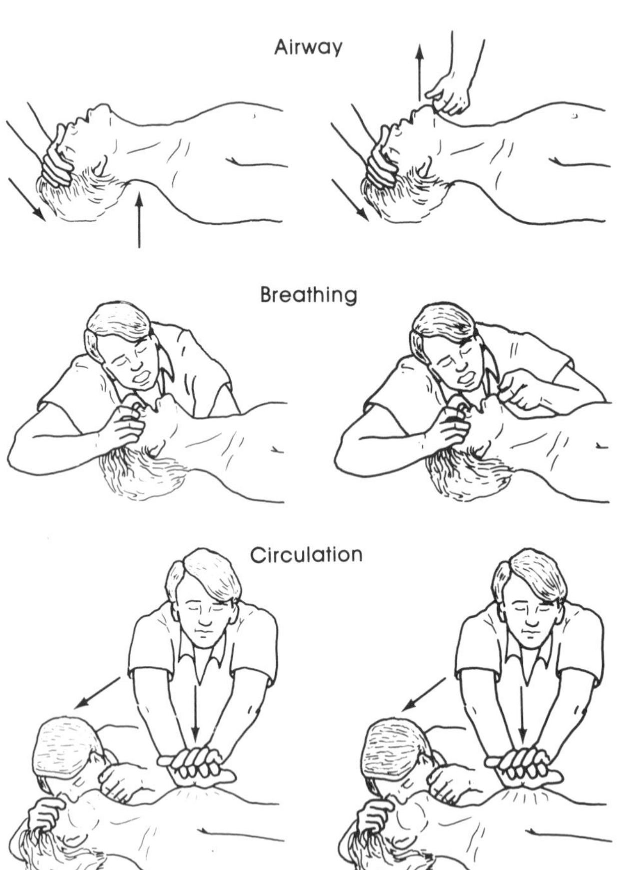

Figure 36–2 Cardiopulmonary resuscitation.

Airway: One hand is placed on the forehead. With the other hand the chin is lifted so that it points upward. Sometimes this maneuver clears the airway and is all that is necessary to reinstate spontaneous breathing.

Breathing: The nostrils are pinched and the chin held in position so that the rescuer's mouth can make a tight seal over the victim's mouth.

Circulation: Compression of the chest with a downward thrust is alternated with breathing. If one person is performing CPR, he or she first blows into the victim's lungs, applies pressure to the sternum 15 times, and then continues a cycle of 2 breaths to 15 compressions.

Prompt action is vitally important to the success of CPR. When a person stops breathing spontaneously and his heart stops beating, "clinical death" has occurred. Within 4 to 6 minutes, the cells of the brain, which are most sensitive to lack of oxygen, begin to deteriorate. If the oxygen supply is not restored immediately, the patient suffers irreversible brain damage and "biologic death" occurs.

Cardiopulmonary resuscitation is indicated when the person shows signs of cardiac arrest. These signs include (1) absence of a carotid pulse, (2) absence of response to stimuli, and (3) absent respirations. Failure of the pupils to react to light eventually will occur as the brain is deprived of its oxygen supply.

The two major components of CPR are artificial respiration and external cardiac compression (heart massage). The mouth-to-mouth technique for artificial respiration is the type recommended and should be used unless it is contraindicated by the patient's condition. In cardiac compression, the heart is squeezed against the spine, and in this way blood is forced out of the heart and into the general circulation.

As an aid to remembering the steps in CPR, the American Heart Association suggests using the *ABC's*. The letter *A* reminds one of "airway," *B* of "breathing," and *C* of "circulation" (Fig. 36–2).

STEPS FOR CARDIOPULMONARY RESUSCITATION (CPR)

- *Establish unresponsiveness.* Gently shake and shout "Are you okay?" Unless he answers immediately, call loudly for help.
- *Check for airflow and establish an airway.* Kneel close to the victim's body, turn him on his back, and place the heel of one hand on the forehead and two fingers of your other hand on the bony prominence of his chin; lift the chin to open the airway. Be careful not to put the fingers on the soft tissue under the chin.
- *Assess for absence of airflow.* Tilt your head down with your ear over the victim's nose and mouth area, and listen and feel for his breath while looking at the chest to see if it rises and falls with respiratory movements. Do this for 3 to 5 seconds.
- *Supply rescue breathing.* If the victim is not breathing, maintain the head tilt/chin lift with the hand on the forehead, and pinch the nose shut. Take a deep breath, and, forming a seal around his mouth, deliver two full breaths lasting about 1½ seconds each of enough volume to make the chest rise; allow exhalation after each breath. If the first

breath will not go into the victim, the airway may have become obstructed; reposition with head tilt/chin lift and try to deliver the breaths again. If the air still cannot be delivered, the Heimlich maneuver will have to be used to open the airway before further intervention can be done. (See description of Heimlich maneuver.) If the two breaths have been delivered successfully, continue with the following steps.

- *Assess for presence of pulse.* Locate the victim's larynx with two fingers and then slide them slightly laterally with gentle pressure to locate the carotid pulse. If the pulse is present but the patient is not breathing, continue rescue breathing at a rate of 12 per minute (one every 5 seconds) and activate the emergency medical system (EMS) for additional help. If there is no pulse, activate the EMS by telling a bystander specifically to call the local emergency number "911" or "0." Begin chest compressions by placing the hand closest to the victim's head on the sternum two fingerbreadths above the xiphoid process. Placing the heel of the other hand over the first hand and keeping the fingers up off the chest, locking your elbows, and keeping your body aligned directly over the hands, depress 1½ to 2 inches on the adult with a smooth downward motion, allowing the sternum to return to a normal position between compressions. Give 15 compressions at a rate of at 80 to 100 per minute. Stop compressions; perform head tilt/chin lift and give two breaths; begin another cycle of compressions. Check the carotid pulse every minute (after four cycles of 15 compressions and two breaths). If the pulse resumes, continue breathing for the patient if he is not breathing on his own. Obtain transport to a medical facility as soon as possible.

In the hospital, initiate CPR and call for help. Have someone alert the full medical emergency team—physician, respiratory therapist, pharmacist, etc.—as soon as possible.

The most common cause of airway obstruction in the unconscious person is the tongue. The head tilt/chin lift maneuver repositions the trachea and tongue so that the airway is open. Because this maneuver also repositions the cervical spine, the jaw thrust method of opening the airway should be used if a spinal injury in the neck area is suspected. For this, kneel at the head of the victim with your elbows on the ground, and place your thumbs on his lower jaw near the corners of the mouth and pointing toward his feet; place your fingertips around the bone of the lower jaw, and lift.

Although transmission of the human immunodeficiency virus (HIV) is highly unlikely via saliva, many health professionals are hesitant to give mouth-to-mouth rescue breathing to strangers. Disposable devices that can be carried in a purse, pocket, or car are available that can be used to provide a barrier while giving rescue breathing.

It is essential to have the victim on a firm surface when giving chest compressions. A board or other firm, flat surface can be placed under the upper back of the victim, or he must be moved to the ground or floor. Otherwise the heart will not be compressed between your hands and the spine.

Hand and body position is very important while giving chest compressions. If the hands slip off the sternum, rib fractures may occur; if the hands are placed too low, the liver may be lacerated, causing internal hemorrhage. The rhythm of compressions should be regular and steady.

TWO-PERSON CPR

This is performed only by trained professionals and is no longer taught to laypersons. As a nurse, you may assist another rescuer by positioning yourself opposite the person performing CPR and offering to help. When CPR is stopped at the end of a cycle and the first rescuer is checking the pulse for 5 seconds, find your hand position for compressions. If the first rescuer says, "No pulse; continue CPR," wait for him to give a breath and then begin compressions. He will then give one breath on the upstroke of your fifth compression. When you tire (after a minimum of 10 cycles), call out, "Switch on five," and count with your compressions, "one—and—two—and—three—and—four—and—switch," as you give the five compressions and then move to the patient's head; check the carotid, indicate the result, and continue CPR by giving a breath.

CHOKING EMERGENCIES

Obstructed airway is the sixth leading cause of accidental death. Adults as well as children can become choking victims and are in need of immediate intervention to prevent death from asphyxiation. Both partial and complete airway obstruction should be treated, especially if there is evidence that there is poor air exchange with the partial obstruction. If the person is conscious and able to cough, he may not need assistance in expelling the object from his throat. In this situation it is best to simply encourage him to cough and breathe as deeply as he can.

A weak and ineffective cough indicates poor air exchange and the need for assistance. The person may make snoring sounds if the airway is obstructed by the tongue. Crowing sounds are

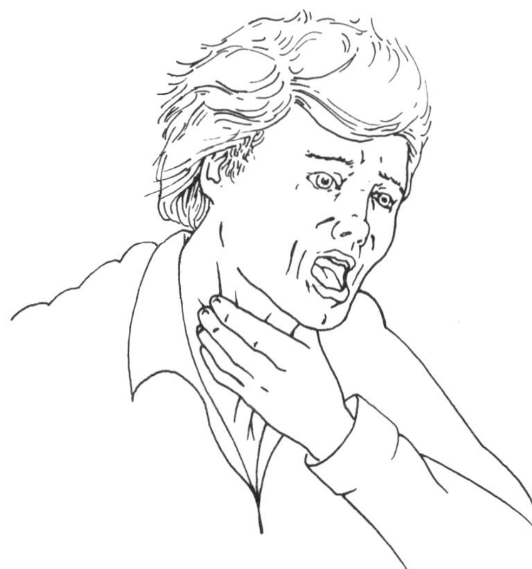

Figure 36-3 Universal distress signal for choking.

indicative of spasm of the larynx, and gurgling sounds indicate foreign matter in the air passages. The victim also may start to become cyanotic, or he may clutch his throat in the universal sign for choking (Fig. 36-3).

When the choking victim cannot speak or cough and is unable to remove the obstructing foreign object in his throat on his own, an attempt must be made to help him expel it.

If the victim is standing, the rescuer positions herself beside or slightly behind him. Tell the victim you can help him, and place your arms around his waist. Make a fist with one hand and place the thumb toward victim just above the umbilicus. Grasp your fist with your other hand and deliver 6 to 10 squeeze-thrusts upward into the abdomen. This is the *Heimlich maneuver* (Fig. 36-4). Each squeeze-thrust should be strong enough to dislodge a stuck foreign body in the airway. These thrusts create an artificial cough, making the diaphragm move and forcing air out of the lungs. Keep a good grip on the victim, as he may lose consciousness and will have to be lowered to the ground.

Heimlich Maneuver for an Unconscious Victim. When you are administering CPR to an unconscious victim and cannot get a breath into the victim because of an obstructed airway, first let go of the head and then reposition with the head tilt/chin lift to clear any tongue obstruction. If you still cannot get a breath in, kneel astride the victim's thighs; place the heel of one hand on top of the other with the hands positioned between the umbilicus and the tip of the xiphoid process at the midline of the body (Fig. 36-5). Push up and in 6 to 10 times forcefully enough to dislodge an obstruction. Then open the

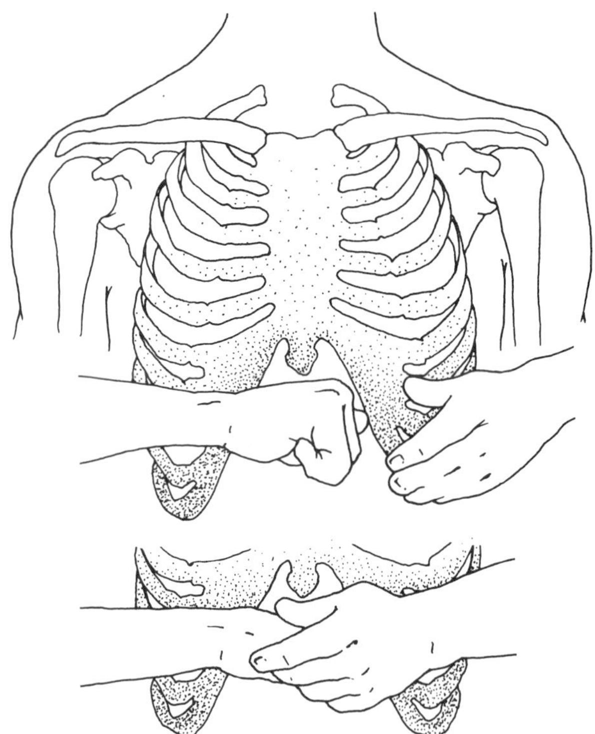

Figure 36-4 Hand placement for abdominal thrust. Rescuer makes a fist with one hand and covers it with the other hand. The flat side of the fist is placed against the upper abdomen. Note its relationship to the sternum and ribs.

airway by grasping the tongue and lower jaw between your thumb and fingers and lifting the jaw. Look into the mouth, and if you see an object, sweep it out with the index finger of your other hand, using a hooking motion to remove the obstruction. Now try to ventilate again. If the airway is still obstructed, give 6 to 10 more abdominal thrusts, open the airway, check the mouth with a sweep, and start the process again.

The initial maneuver alone may dislodge the foreign object so that it can be coughed out by the victim. At this point the rescuer should encourage the victim to persist with coughing until

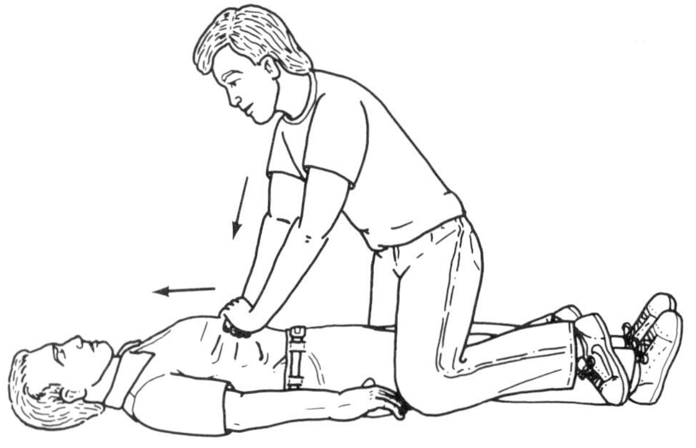

Figure 36-5 Abdominal thrust for an unconscious victim.

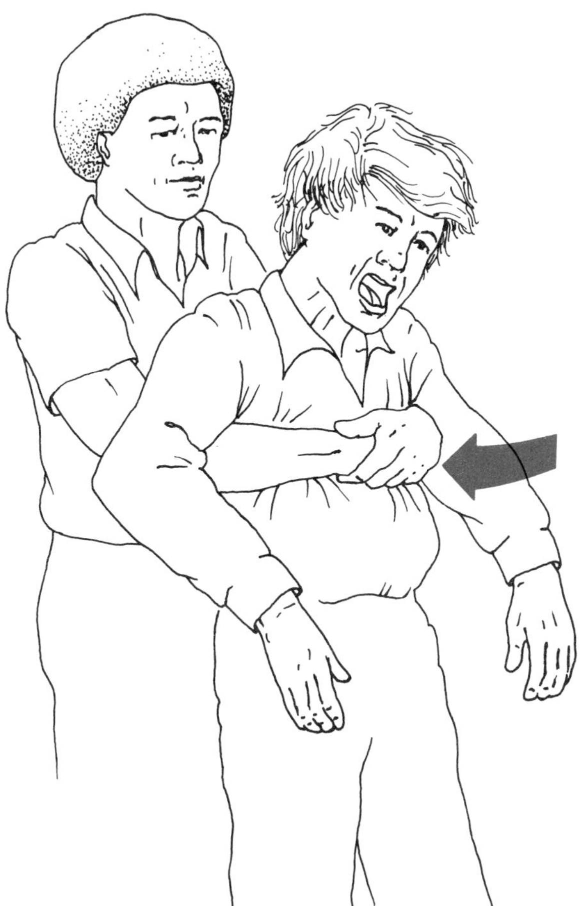

Figure 36-6 Chest thrust, standing. This is an alternative method for removing an obstruction from the airway.

the foreign body is removed. No effort should be made to interfere with the victim's efforts as long as he has good air exchange and his color is good.

An alternative to the abdominal thrust is the chest thrust (Fig. 36-6). This maneuver can be used for pregnant women and others in whom an abdominal thrust is contraindicated.

CONTROL OF BLEEDING

The only emergency conditions that have priority over control of hemorrhage are cessation of breathing and a sucking wound of the chest. Severe bleeding can rapidly lead to irreversible hypovolemic shock from loss of intravascular fluid and to circulatory collapse.

Blood issuing from an artery is bright red and will gush forth in spurts at regular intervals. Blood loss from an artery is more rapid than that from a vein. Blood from a severed or punctured vein leaks slowly and steadily and is dark red.

APPLICATION OF PRESSURE

Even major bleeding can usually be stopped by applying pressure directly over the wound. The palm of the hand is used, preferably after a clean cloth or sterile dressing has been placed over the open wound. However, if no dressing is available and the victim's life is in danger from blood loss, trying to avoid contamination of the wound is not as important as controlling the hemorrhage.

Once the bleeding has stopped, a compression dressing and bandage are gently but snugly tied in place. Do not wrap the body part so tightly as to constrict circulation completely. This would, in effect, be the same as applying a tourniquet, a measure that is used only as a last resort (see the following section).

The amount of blood leaking from a wound can be minimized somewhat by elevating the injured part and immobilizing it so that clots are not disturbed and the pumping action of neighboring vessels is decreased. If ice is available, it could be applied to the wound to aid vasoconstriction and decrease bleeding. The ice should be in a plastic bag or other waterproof container to avoid wetting and contaminating the wound.

Once the bleeding has been controlled, the pressure dressing is left in place so as not to disturb clots and renew the bleeding. If blood soaks through the original dressing, additional dressings are applied over the soaked ones, but none of the dressings should be removed until medical help is available.

If bleeding is copious and cannot be stopped with a pressure bandage and immobilization, the artery leading to the wound can be compressed to decrease or perhaps stop altogether the flow of blood from the wound. Pressure points for control of arterial bleeding are shown in Figure 36-7. If the pressure point has been covered properly, there should be no pulse below the point of pressure, and the victim should notice tingling and numbness in the area. Pressure points in the neck and head must be used with caution, because there is danger of interrupting blood supply to the brain or blocking the intake of air.

USE OF TOURNIQUETS

Application of a tourniquet to prevent hemorrhage is recommended **only as a last resort** when other methods have failed and hemorrhage threatens the life of the victim or when an injured extremity has been amputated, severely crushed, or mangled. In the past, the tourniquet was used more often than it should have been; if you are in doubt, do not apply one. The reason for this is obvious when we realize that a tourniquet can, by obstructing the flow of blood to a part, deprive tissues of vital nutrients and permanently damage them, resulting in loss of the limb.

To apply a tourniquet, one needs several thicknesses of gauze or cloth to make a pad to be placed under the tourniquet, a *wide* strip of fab-

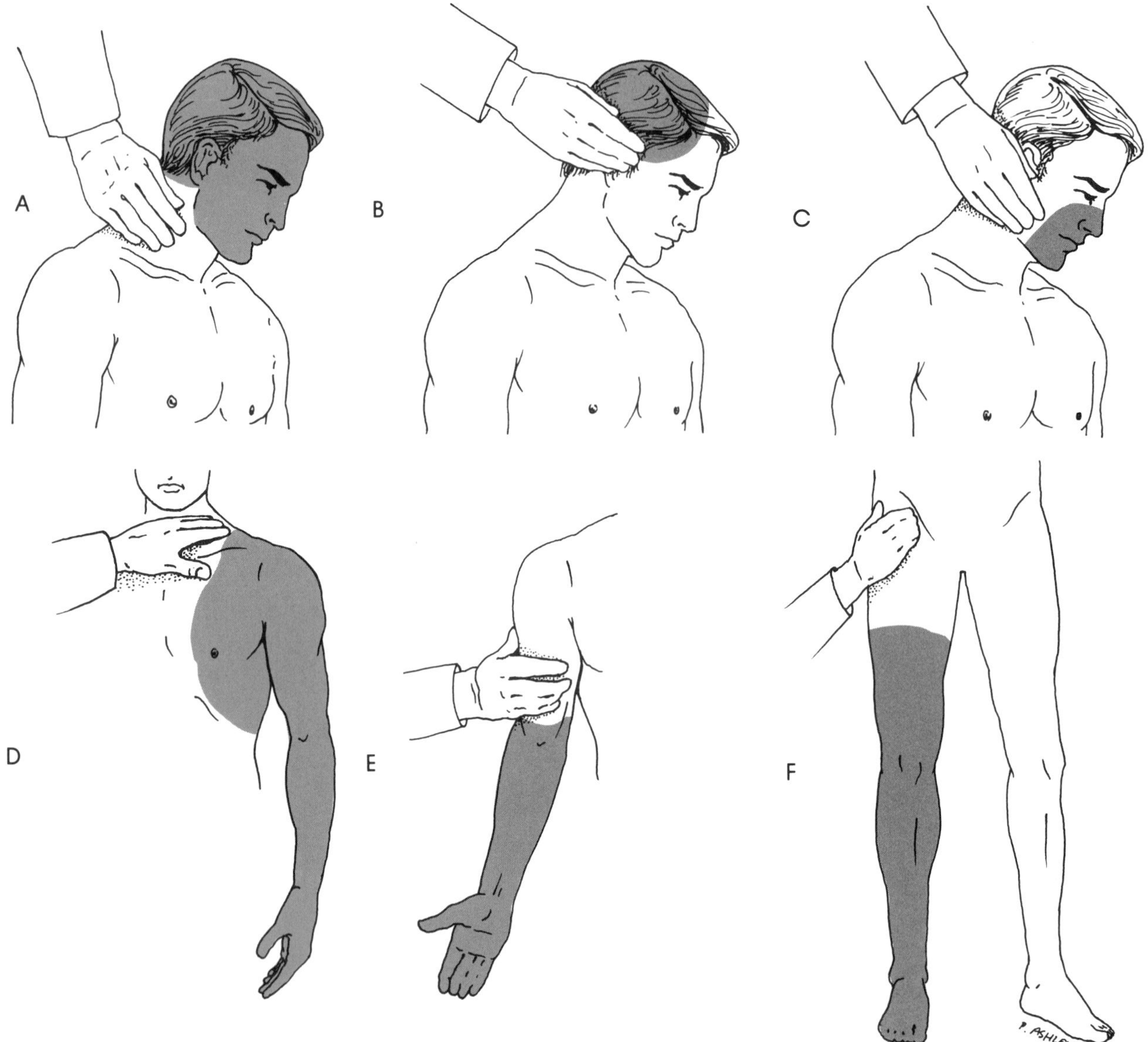

Figure 36-7 Locations of commonly used digital pressure points. The screened areas are those within which hemorrhage may be controlled by pressure on a specific artery. *A*, Carotid artery; *B*, temporal artery; *C*, external maxillary artery; *D*, subclavian artery; *E*, brachial artery; *F*, femoral artery.

ric long enough to go twice around the limb, and a stick or similar heavy, nonbreakable object for tightening the tourniquet. Place the pad on the inside of the limb above the point of bleeding. Wrap the tourniquet around the limb over the pad and then tie the loose end with a half knot (overhand knot). Insert the stick and tie again with a full knot. The tourniquet is then tightened by twisting the stick until bleeding stops. A tourniquet that is too loose may cause an increase in bleeding.

Once the tourniquet has been applied, it should **not** ***be released until the victim has been taken to a medical facility and surgical control of the hemorrhage can be undertaken.***

Although periodic release of a tourniquet was once recommended, it is no longer considered a safe practice.

Always leave the tourniquet uncovered so that it can be seen by others who may not be aware it has been applied. If this is not possible, write the letters *TK* and the location of the tourniquet on the victim's forehead.

CONTROL OF NOSEBLEEDS

Most nosebleeds (*epistaxis*) involve minimal blood loss and are not a cause for alarm. They usually result from crusting, cracking, or irritation of the mucous membrane covering the front

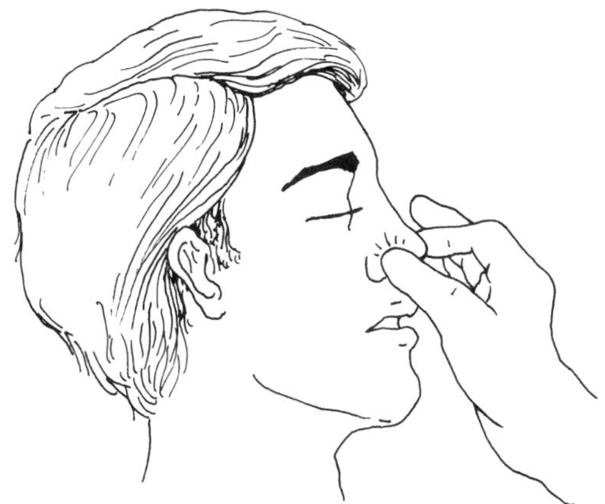

Figure 36-8 Pinching the nose to stop nosebleeding.

of the nasal septum and can easily be stopped by the application of pressure. The person should be seated upright with his head tilted slightly forward. This is done to avoid having blood run down the back of the throat, where it is either swallowed or aspirated into the lungs.

To apply pressure, the nose is gently squeezed closed for 10 to 15 minutes (Fig. 36-8). After the bleeding has stopped, the person should rest quietly for a few hours and avoid blowing the nose or rubbing it and dislodging the clot.

A major nosebleed that does not respond to pressure requires prompt medical attention. Severe epistaxis is a life-threatening condition. The interior of the nose is extremely vascular, and blood loss can be substantial if the point of hemorrhage is in the posterior part of the nose. Blood seeping into the nasopharynx can enter the lacrimal ducts and mouth, giving the impression that the person is bleeding from his eyes and mouth as well as his nose. Emergency medical treatment includes packing the posterior nares, monitoring the vital signs, and reassuring the patient.

SHOCK

The term *shock* is extremely difficult, if not impossible, to define precisely. It has become something of a catchall word that is used to cover a multitude of clinical situations and a variety of symptoms, from simple fainting to total circulatory collapse and death. In emergency nursing, shock is usually *neurogenic* (caused by psychological factors such as pain, fright, or trauma), *hypovolemic* or *hemorrhagic* (caused by decreased blood volume, as in severe bleeding, loss of fluid from nausea and vomiting of gastroenteritis, or loss of plasma, as in burns), *septic* (caused by infection), or *cardiogenic* (caused by decreased cardiac output and collapse of the peripheral vascular system).

SYMPTOMS

Symptoms indicative of shock result from complex pathologic and psychological mechanisms. These involve inadequate blood volume, reduction of the cardiac output, loss of tone in and collapse of the blood vessels near the surface of the body, increased permeability of the capillaries with a shift of the body fluids from one compartment to another, and alterations in the chemical characteristics of the blood.

Not all the signs and symptoms of shock need be present in every patient; they can occur in varying combinations and in different degrees of severity, depending on the cause of shock and the patient's response to it.

The classic symptoms and signs of shock include cold, moist skin, especially in the extremities; pallor, especially of the lips and fingers; and rapid and weak pulse, decreased blood pressure, listlessness, thirst, and oliguria.

MANAGEMENT OF SHOCK

Whenever possible in an emergency situation, the nurse must do what she can to prevent shock or at least to lessen its severity. She can do this by acting quickly to control bleeding, relieving pain through proper splinting or positioning, and treating the wound. The body has several defense mechanisms that are automatically called into action as soon as injury occurs. By supporting these mechanisms through simple nursing measures, the nurse can reduce the severity of shock and mitigate its effects on an accident victim.

Because most emergency cases are accompanied by some degree of psychogenic shock, it is extremely important to reassure and comfort the victim. This will help to keep him calm and reduce physical tension and activity so that his energies can be fully utilized by the natural defense mechanisms of the body. Maintaining normal body heat helps to ensure adequate circulation. To do this, one must protect the patient from cold and dampness, but remember that applications of extreme heat to the surfaces of the body only serve to aggravate circulatory collapse and tend to increase loss of vital body fluids through perspiration. In general, it is best to keep the victim flat, lying on his back. If the victim is bleeding from wounds of the lower face and is unconscious, he should be turned on his side to avoid aspiration of blood and vomitus.

As soon as the patient arrives at a hospital or clinic where equipment is available, other measures are taken to control shock. These may include administration of IV fluids, plasma expanders, or blood products to restore the circulating blood volume; oxygen to relieve respiratory embarrassment; and narcotics for the control of pain.

BURNS

The two hazards to be guarded against in the emergency treatment of burns are infection and shock.

All burns must be considered potentially dangerous because the skin is one of the body's first lines of defense against the invasion of pathogenic organisms. It also plays an important role in the maintenance of fluid balance and body temperature. The destruction of relatively large areas of skin can cause loss of vital body fluids and electrolytes, produce profound changes in the blood vessels, and alter the chemical activities of the cells and tissues of the internal organs.

The severity of complications of a burn will depend on the amount of body surface destroyed by the burn and the depth of the burn. Burn depth and the means by which the extent of a burn is determined are discussed in Chapter 33 of this text.

MINOR BURNS

If the burned area is small and appears to be only superficial (not involving deeper tissues of the skin), the affected area should be immersed in cool water for 2 to 5 minutes. Cold compresses, using cold water and a sterile gauze pad or clean cloth, are continued while the patient is being transported to the hospital or emergency clinic. By applying cold, it is possible to reduce somewhat the pain of the burn and the amount of injury to the tissues.

MAJOR BURNS

If the burn injury is extensive, the burned area should be covered with a clean, dry dressing. This can be a sheet, towel, or other freshly laundered piece of material. It should be made of tightly woven cotton so that air is kept from the wound and the possibility of infection is reduced. The victim should be transported to a hospital as soon as possible.

No attempt should be made to remove clothing from a burned area.* Never *apply absorbent cotton, oily substances, or ointments to a major burn. Blisters should not be disturbed, because they serve as a protective covering over the wound.

Under ordinary circumstances the burned victim is given nothing by mouth until he arrives at a medical facility. However, if there is an unavoidable delay of several hours before getting the patient to a hospital and he is conscious and able to swallow, he should be given fluids to drink. A solution of ½ teaspoon each of salt and baking soda in 1 quart of water is ideal. The patient is encouraged to drink small amounts of the solution at 10- to 15-minute intervals unless nausea develops and vomiting seems likely. Intravenous fluid therapy and more extensive medical treatment of major burns are discussed in Chapter 33 of this text.

CHEMICAL BURNS

Strong chemicals capable of burning the skin and mucous membranes will continue to destroy tissue unless they are diluted and removed immediately. For this reason one must act quickly to irrigate any area burned by chemicals with large amounts of water until all traces of the chemical have been removed. Once this has been done, the burned area is covered with a dressing, and the patient is transported to a hospital.

However, water is not used for burns caused by dry lime or phenol. Dry lime should be brushed from the skin and clothing unless there is enough water to remove *all* traces of the powder. Small amounts of water will only react chemically with the lime to produce a highly corrosive substance. Phenol (carbolic acid) is not water-soluble. The phenol is first removed by alcohol and the burned area is then rinsed with water.

If a corrosive chemical has been ingested, the victim should be given water or milk to drink as soon as possible. Vomiting should **not** be induced or encouraged by overloading the stomach. In general, no more than 6 oz (180 mL) is given if the victim is a child weighing less than 35 pounds and no more than 8 oz (240 mL) if the person weighs more than 35 pounds. No attempt should be made to neutralize a chemical substance, as this can cause further damage to the esophagus and stomach.

POISONING

Poisoning from gases, chemicals, drugs, and other toxic substances accounted for 7% of deaths in the United States in 1988. The death rate for accidental poisoning has not dramatically changed since 1965.

Prevention of accidental poisoning begins with a realization that there are literally hundreds of thousands of poisonous substances in our environment. Every home has a variety of poisons sitting on the shelves of the medicine cabinet, under the kitchen sink, or in the laundry room, utility room, and garage. Children are the most frequent victims of poisoning, and medicines account for half of all accidental poisonings of children under the age of 5. Aspirin has consistently been the leading cause of death in accidental poisoning in children of this age. Other poisons frequently ingested by children include bleaches, soaps and detergents, insecticides, and vitamin and iron preparations. Recently, there has been an increase of poisoning in children who have ingested a parent's prescribed medications.

Since the government began requiring "childproof" caps on all medications and many poisonous substances ordinarily found in households, the incidence of poisoning in children has decreased somewhat, but carelessness on the part of adults continues to be a major factor in the accidental poisoning of children.

Despite this progress in prevention of accidental poisoning in children, acute poisoning is still the most frequently encountered pediatric emergency in this country.

PREVENTION

As a member of the health team, the nurse must do all she can to educate the public in the ways in which accidental poisoning can be prevented. She should remember the following simple rules and use every opportunity to teach them to her friends and neighbors:

- *Destroy all medicines that are no longer being used.* An overdose can be fatal, especially to a child. In some instances, drugs undergo chemical changes with age and become toxic compounds.
- *Store poisons and inedible products separately from edible foods.*
- *Do not transfer poisonous substances from their original container to an unmarked one.* NEVER place a poison in a container (such as a soft drink bottle) that is normally used for edible solids or liquids.
- *Never tell a child that the medicine he is being given is candy.* Tell him it is a drug to make him feel better and that it must be taken only as the doctor has directed.
- *Always read the labels of chemical products before using them.*

SYMPTOMS OF POISONING

The symptoms of poisoning vary according to the substance ingested and the time that has elapsed since it first entered the body. Poisoning should be suspected if the victim becomes ill very suddenly and there is an open container of a poison or a drug nearby. In children, one should be alert to the possibility of poisoning when there is a peculiar odor to the breath or when there is evidence that the child has eaten leaves or wild berries. Always remember that children are naturally very curious and that a substance need not taste good for a child to place it in his mouth and swallow it.

Other symptoms of poisoning include pain or burning sensation in the mouth and throat, nausea, vomiting, disorientation, visual disturbances, loss of consciousness, or a deep, unnatural sleep.

GENERAL PRINCIPLES OF FIRST AID FOR POISONING

All cases of poisoning demand immediate action. The longer the delay before treatment, the greater the chance of the poison being absorbed in the body and permanently damaging body tissues.

Always save the container and any of its contents that may help in identification of the poison. If the container cannot be found and the type of poison is not known, try to save a sample of vomitus for analysis and identification.

Swallowed Poisons

Generally, the first step is *dilution* of the poison, immediately followed by *removal* of the stomach contents. In the absence of a stomach pump, vomiting can be induced, but this is contraindicated for certain kinds of poisons, such as corrosive chemicals and petroleum products. A liquid such as water or milk can usually serve to dilute the poison.

Vomiting is induced by placing a spoon or an index finger down the back of the throat to stimulate the gag reflex. An emetic such as 2 tablespoons of salt in a glass of warm water or 15 mL of syrup of ipecac diluted in a glass of water can be used. Be sure that during the vomiting episode, the victim is positioned so that the vomitus will not be aspirated into the lungs.

Antidotes to specific poisons are often printed on the labels of the containers. A phone call to the nearest hospital emergency department can provide specific instructions on what to do until the patient can reach the emergency department and be treated by a physician. If possible, the specific antidote should be given as soon as the stomach has been emptied of the poison. In the emergency department, activated charcoal is given to absorb any poison remaining in the stomach.

When a patient has swallowed a corrosive poison—for example, a strong acid or alkali—vomiting is contraindicated, because there is the danger of further irritating and damaging the upper intestinal tract. There is

CERTAIN BASIC RULES ARE IMPORTANT IN PREVENTING FOOD POISONING

PERSONAL HYGIENE

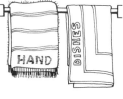

Personal cleanliness and neatness

Nails clean and trimmed

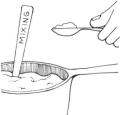

Hands washed before handling food

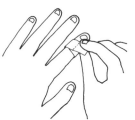

Cover coughs and sneezes

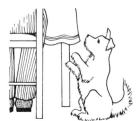

HANDLING OF FOOD

HAND

DISHES

MIXING

Separate towels for wiping dishes and drying hands

Do not put spoon back in mixture after tasting

Cuts and scratches covered with waterproof bandage

Keep pets away from food

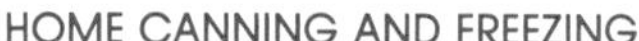

HOME CANNING AND FREEZING

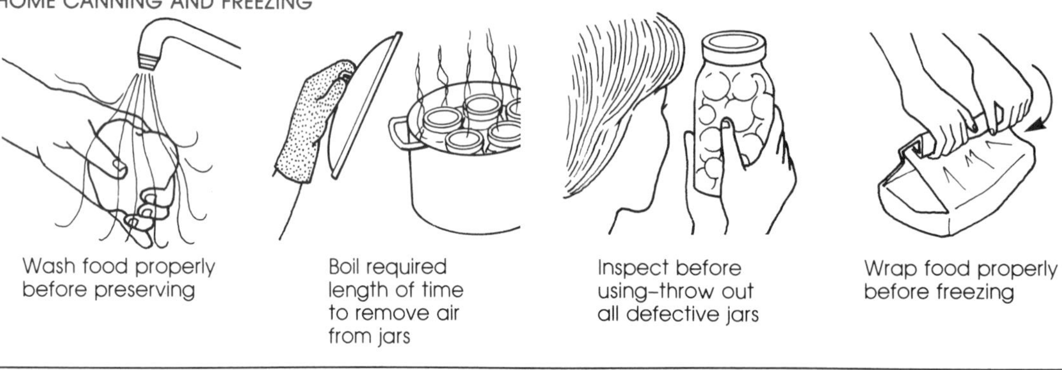

Wash food properly before preserving

Boil required length of time to remove air from jars

Inspect before using–throw out all defective jars

Wrap food properly before freezing

STORAGE AND DISPOSAL OF FOOD

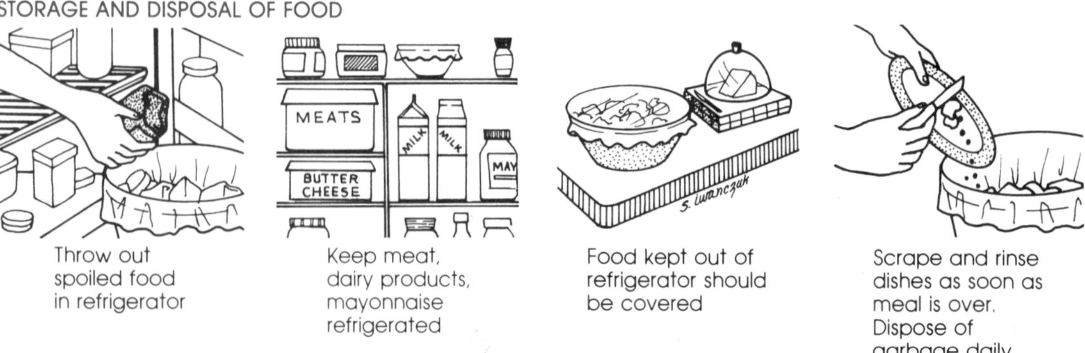

Throw out spoiled food in refrigerator

Keep meat, dairy products, mayonnaise refrigerated

Food kept out of refrigerator should be covered

Scrape and rinse dishes as soon as meal is over. Dispose of garbage daily

Figure 36–9 Basic rules for prevention of food poisoning.
(Redrawn from The Modern Medical Encyclopedia by Benjamin Miller, M.D. © 1965 Western Publishing Company, Inc. Used by permission.)

also a possibility of aspiration of the corrosive substance into the respiratory tract during vomiting.

Corrosive substances should be diluted with milk or water given orally. Never induce vomiting if the victim is unconscious.

Inhaled Poisons

When a patient has inhaled a poisonous substance, he should be transported out into fresh air immediately. Carry him out and loosen any tight clothing. Alert the emergency medical system and obtain transport to a medical facility immediately. Give CPR as needed. If carbon monoxide has been inhaled, the mucous membranes will be cherry red.

Food Poisoning

This type of poisoning is produced by the toxins of bacteria present in contaminated food. The term *ptomaine poisoning*, so frequently associated with food poisoning, is actually misleading. Ptomaines are substances formed by the decomposition, or "spoilage," of protein foods. The digestive system is able to cope with these substances, and they do not necessarily cause illness. Decomposing food is not of itself necessarily harmful, but since foods in the process of decomposition frequently harbor pathogenic organisms and serve as excellent media for their growth, they should be avoided.

Prevention

Cleanliness, good personal hygiene, and proper preparation and handling of foods are essential to the prevention of food poisoning. Figure 36–9 presents the basic rules to follow to avoid this type of poisoning.

Symptoms and Treatment

Food poisoning should be suspected when more than one person in a group, family, or community is affected by an acute febrile gastrointestinal disturbance. The onset is sudden, with nausea, vomiting, diarrhea, and abdominal cramps. Food is withheld, drugs are administered to control diarrhea, and sedation and parenteral fluids are given.

Types

Food poisoning may be bacterial or chemical. The chemical types, however, are not true food poisonings, but toxic conditions caused by poisonous mushrooms, toxic berries, or foods that have not been cleansed of insecticides or other chemicals.

Staphylococcus aureus frequently grows in creamed foods that have not been refrigerated adequately. Custards, cream pies, mayonnaise, and processed foods commonly used for picnics are often the source of this type of food poisoning. The illness is rarely fatal, and symptoms are usually limited to nausea, vomiting, diarrhea, and abdominal cramps. The patient should be kept quiet and given sedation and parenteral fluids as necessary.

TRAUMATIC INJURIES

FRACTURES

A fracture is a break in the continuity of a bone. Types of fractures and their specific treatments are discussed in Chapter 26.

Assessment of a suspected fracture includes noting pain, swelling, and discoloration, as well as a deformity in the contour of the bone. If there is a possibility of a fracture of an extremity, the affected limb is checked for pulse to determine whether circulation has been impaired. Nerve damage in a fractured leg is assessed by having the person flex and extend the foot and by touching a toe and asking the person which toe has been touched. To determine whether the nerve pathways have been damaged by a fracture in the arm, the person is asked to wave his hand, to identify fingers that have been touched by the examiner, and to grip the examiner's hand. Paralysis and total loss of sensation in the extremities may indicate damage to the spinal cord.

Pain is not always present when a fracture has occurred. Numbness and tingling also can accompany a fracture. If there is some question as to whether or not a bone has been broken, it is best to treat the injury as if there were a fracture. Proper first aid will be helpful and will prevent further trauma and pain regardless of the degree of injury to a bone.

Emergency treatment of fractures is aimed at immobilizing the affected part so that soft tissues in the areas adjacent to the bone will not be damaged further.

The term *splint it as it lies* means exactly that. An inexperienced person should never attempt to straighten or set a broken bone. The injured part should be immobilized in the position in which it is found at the time of injury and should be supported firmly so that it will not be jarred when the victim is being moved. If it is available, ice in a plastic bag can be applied to the fracture area to help minimize edema.

If the broken bone has pierced the skin and bleeding is severe, apply direct pressure over the wound or compress the appropriate pressure point (see page 876). Cover the open area with a sterile dressing. Try to avoid introducing infectious agents into the wound, and remember also the need for the prevention and treatment of shock.

HEAD INJURY

The victim of a blow to the head may suffer a skull fracture or concussion. In either case, he should be kept quiet and should not be given any stimulants. Because there can be a delayed reaction in injury to the brain, all head injuries should be considered serious and should receive the attention of a physician. Any person who has received a severe blow to the head should also be evaluated for possible injury to the cervical spine. The symptoms, treatment, and nursing care of head injuries are discussed in Chapter 15.

EYE INJURIES

Although the eye is fairly well protected by the bony structures that make up the eye socket, the eyeball and its coverings are still subject to a variety of injuries. These include foreign matter that becomes lodged under the eyelids or embedded in the outer surface of the eye, sharp objects that penetrate or perforate the ocular globe, lacerations and contusions of the cornea and sclera, and burns from heat, radiation, and chemicals. Facial fractures and other injuries to the bones surrounding the eye also can cause damage to the globe and eventually result in blindness.

Foreign matter, such as small debris and an eyelash, is usually removed by tears that flow when the eye is irritated. If a foreign object cannot be removed by washing the eye or by using a corner of a clean handkerchief or gauze square, a physician should treat the injury.

Perforation of the globe is a very serious injury that can result in blindness. If the penetrating object is still protruding from the globe, it should not be moved or disturbed in any way. A protective guard can be devised using a paper cup, box, or any sturdy device that is large enough to rest against the bony prominences around the eye and long enough so that it does not touch the protruding object. Because the eyes move together, both eyes should be bandaged to prevent motion of the injured eye. With the person thus rendered unable to see, it is necessary to keep him calm and to try to allay his anxiety by explaining why the unaffected eye has been bandaged and to keep him informed of what is being done for him.

Lacerations and contusions of the eyelid or the soft tissues around the eye usually bleed copiously because of their abundant blood supply. Direct pressure is applied to stop the bleeding only if it is obvious that the globe of the eye has not been injured. If the globe has been injured, the eye is covered with a loose dressing to prevent contamination. Repair of contusions and lacerations of the eye and its surrounding structures is done by an ocular plastic surgeon as promptly as possible.

Chemical burns of the eye demand immediate action to avoid permanent damage and loss of vision. The eye is flushed with large amounts of water, preferably sterile, for 15 to 20 minutes from the time of injury. Irrigation continues during the time the person is being transported to a hospital or clinic. If irrigation of the eye with running water is not possible, the patient can submerge his face in a basin of water and blink his eyes continually to help dilute and remove the chemical.

Injuries from radiation and light usually cause severe pain in the eyes. Covering them with bandages or eye patches can minimize the pain, but no other first aid treatment is indicated until the person is in the care of an ophthalmologist. Thermal burns of the eyes are treated by applying loose, moist dressings.

EAR INJURIES

Trauma to the external ear can result in cuts, abrasions, and avulsion (tearing way of part or all of the organ). Injuries to the middle and inner ear may not be so obvious and frequently are associated with explosions and other loud noises or with a skull fracture. Symptoms of inner and middle ear damage include a discharge of either blood or cerebrospinal fluid or a combination of both, severe pain in the ear, and loss of equilibrium.

In general, external lacerations and contusions involving the outer ear are treated as any other open wound. A bulky dressing can be applied if the ear has been severely torn and lacerated. If there is avulsion of the outer ear and the avulsed part can be found, it should be wrapped in plastic and kept cold and dry while being taken to the medical facility with the patient.

NECK AND SPINE INJURIES

In emergency or accident situations, it is not uncommon for severe bleeding, absence of respirations, or other life-threatening conditions to distract the rescuer and cause him to overlook the possibility that the victim might also have a spinal cord injury. If this happens, and the rescuer proceeds to treat the more obvious injuries and moves the victim before properly immobilizing the neck and back, permanent damage and paralysis may result.

Types of accidents in which spinal injury should be suspected are motor vehicle, diving, and sledding mishaps. A person who has been injured by diving into shallow water must be moved by rescuers, because he may be in danger of drowning. Efforts to remove him from the water and to resuscitate him must be gentle and undertaken only after the neck and back have been properly supported in order to avoid further damage to the spinal cord.

The victim of a sledding or skiing accident may not show signs of injury because of bulky clothing, but he should be moved only after careful evaluation and immobilization as indicated.

Evaluation of a victim for a spinal cord injury is described in Table 36-2. If an injury to the neck is suspected, a cervical collar is applied before the person is moved to a stretcher. This should be done only by trained personnel familiar with the techniques of applying and maintaining traction on the head while the collar is being applied. When a cervical collar is not available and the victim must be moved to safety, the neck may be immobilized with any material handy, such as a coat, shirt, or towel, which is rolled in the shape of a collar. The purpose of the collar is to keep the neck as straight as possible, preventing it from flexing or hyperextending.

If injury to the spine below the neck is suspected, the victim should be logrolled onto a flat surface such as a piece of plywood or a door removed from its hinges. He is turned onto his side "in one piece," the backboard is placed beside him, and then he is carefully rolled back onto the board. This should be done slowly and carefully to avoid twisting or bending the spinal column.

CHEST AND ABDOMINAL WOUNDS

Victims of automobile accidents frequently suffer severe chest wounds as a result of violent contact with the steering wheel and column. Fractures of the ribs or sternum are the most common chest injury. Spontaneous pneumothorax may also occur. Victims of stabbings can also have open chest wounds that create serious respiratory difficulties. An open, or "sucking," chest wound is one in which pneumothorax results from penetration of the pleural cavity, which allows air and gas to accumulate there. Symptoms of pneumothorax include labored, shallow respirations and lack of movement on one side of the chest when the person inhales and exhales. A sucking chest wound should be covered at the end of a forceful expiration with an occlusive dressing—that is, one made of plastic wrap, aluminium foil, or any other material that seals the wound and prohibits the flow of air into the pleural cavity. The occlusive dressing is held in place by a pressure dressing, but the bandage must not be so tight that it interferes with normal breathing. Place the patient in the semi-Fowler's position if possible.

A "flail" chest results from the fracture of three or more ribs, each in two places, so that a portion of the rib cage is crushed inward. This type of injury produces "paradoxical respirations," which means that upon inhalation, the affected portion moves inward rather than outward. The condition is temporarily treated by splinting the affected portion of the chest by using a small pillow, folded sheet, or other bulky material and taping it securely in place. The victim is given oxygen to help compensate for respiratory deficiency.

Abdominal injuries resulting from improperly worn seat belts, penetrating objects, blunt instruments, and sharp cutting edges are all potential sources of damage to internal organs and hemorrhage. If internal hemorrhage is suspected, the victim should be observed closely for symptoms of shock and handled very gently when being moved.

Internal abdominal injuries must be treated in an emergency room. External wounds with evisceration are covered with a piece of nonadhering material such as plastic wrap or aluminum foil. This will keep the protruding intestinal contents moist and relatively free of contamination. After the occlusive covering is applied, a clean folded towel or sheet is placed over it to retain body heat in the protruding organs. No attempt should be made to replace the abdominal organs through the wound. The victim is transported to a medical facility as quickly as possible.

ELECTRIC SHOCK

When an electric current passes through the body, it can cause severe shock to the entire body, cessation of breathing, circulatory failure, and serious burns.

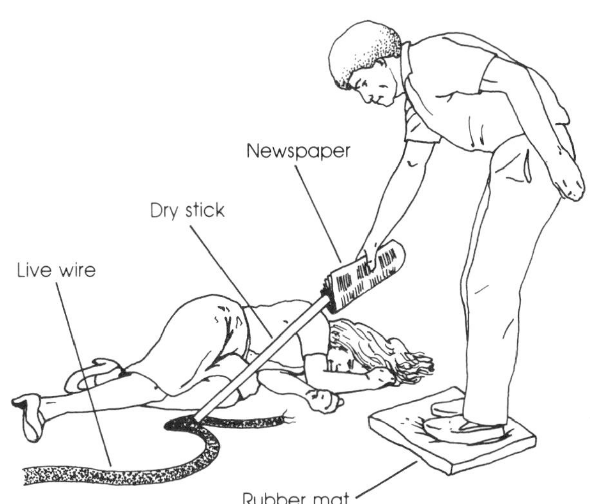

Figure 36-10 Separating a victim from a live electric wire while avoiding similar shock. The rescuer stands on a rubber mat or dry board and wears rubber-soled shoes. The rescuer does not touch the victim until certain that wire contact has been broken.

Emergency treatment of electric shock involves CPR if breathing has ceased or the heart has stopped, general measures to treat shock, and emergency treatment of a major burn if one has been sustained. The proper procedure for separating a victim from a live conductor of electricity is shown in Figure 36–10. Remember that water serves as a conductor of electricity and wet objects can transmit a fatal electric current to a person trying to rescue the victim of electric shock.

A person who is struck by lightning suffers from electric shock.

ANIMAL BITES

Family pets, especially dogs and cats, are the most common source of animal bites. When a wild animal such as a squirrel or fox attacks and bites a human being without provocation, one should always suspect rabies as the cause of the animal's unusual behavior. All animal and human bites should be treated as potentially dangerous because of the presence of pathogenic microorganisms in the mouth that can cause a serious infection.

TREATMENT

Wounds from animal bites should be rinsed immediately with soap and hot running water for 5 to 10 minutes. The affected area is then covered with a clean bandage and immobilized. Medical attention should be given to the wound as soon as possible.

Because the possibility of rabies must always be considered in an animal bite, the animal must be confined and observed for signs of the disease. If it has been killed, its head should be sent to a laboratory for examination. If a diagnosis of rabies in the animal has been confirmed or if there is no proof that the animal has been immunized against rabies, the victim is given a series of injections to build up antibodies against the virus. Newer vaccines require fewer injections and are more effective in stimulating antibody production than the traditional Pasteur treatment.

SNAKEBITE

Although bites from poisonous snakes are rare in the United States, they do occur and can be fatal if not treated promptly and effectively. There are four kinds of poisonous snakes in this country: copperheads, rattlesnakes, and cottonmouths, or water moccasins, which are all called pit vipers because they have pits or depressions behind their nostrils; and coral snakes, which are small snakes with characteristic red, black, and yellow bands. Coral snakes do not have fangs; they inject their venom by a chewing motion.

A venomous snakebite usually can be distinguished by two fang marks (though there may be only one on a small surface, such as the toe or finger), severe pain and swelling in the area, discoloration at the site of injection of venom, nausea and vomiting, respiratory distress, and shock. Nonpoisonous snakebites usually appear as either small scratches or lacerations.

Treatment

Nonpoisonous snakebites are treated as simple wounds, requiring only a cleansing of the wound with soap and water and the application of a mild antiseptic. Venomous snakebites should receive medical attention as quickly as possible.

The victim of a poisonous snakebite should be kept as quiet and calm as possible while being transported, and under no condition should he be given an alcoholic beverage or stimulant.

Current treatment for poisonous snakebite consists of packing the affected area in ice, elevating the extremity or area, and seeking medical attention as quickly as possible. The use of tourniquets, incision, and sucking the area to extract venom is no longer recommended.

Once the snakebite victim reaches a hospital or clinic, the wound is débrided and irrigated to remove the venom and damaged tissues. Skin grafting may be required later. The victim is given antivenin, medications to counteract the specific pharmacologic action of the venom, and other drugs to avoid complications and provide relief of symptoms.

INSECT BITES AND STINGS

Systemic reactions to the bites and stings of insects and bees account for more deaths each year in the United States than do snakebites. A systemic reaction is caused by hypersensitivity to the venom of bees, wasps, hornets, fire ants, or harvester ants.

Symptoms of a systemic reaction include hives, swelling, general weakness, tightness in the chest, abdominal cramps, constriction of the throat, unconsciousness, and possibly death from severe anaphylaxis. Whenever a person suffers from any of these symptoms after a sting or insect bite, treatment must be started immediately. The shorter the interval between the time of the sting or bite and the development of symptoms, the more likely the possibility that death will result. Ice packs may be applied to the area of the bite or sting while medical help is being sought.

Treatment

First aid treatment for a systemic reaction is the injection of aqueous epinephrine—0.001 solution in dosages of 0.3 to 0.4 mL for adults and 0.15 to 0.3 mL for children. An antihistamine such as Benadryl also is given.

The female worker honeybee injects a venom sac that may remain embedded in the victim's skin. This sac may be removed by gently scraping the site with a fingernail or knife blade, being careful not to squeeze the sac and force the venom into the tissues.

An ice pack may be applied to reduce swelling and relieve pain. Patients who appear to be in shock should be kept warm and should remain lying down with the legs elevated and the head flat. If symptoms persist after 20 minutes and the patient has not yet reached a medical facility, a second injection of epinephrine should be given.

An emergency kit that contains the drugs, syringe, constricting band, towelette, and tweezers needed for prompt treatment of a systemic reaction to stings and bites is available by prescription. Individuals known to be hypersensitive to insect and bee venom should keep such a kit with them at all times and be thoroughly familiar with its use *before* the need for it arises. These people also should wear some kind of medical identification that indicates their hypersensitivity.

Any person who has had a systemic reaction or even a severe local reaction with swelling beyond two joints should receive hyposensitization therapy to increase his tolerance to insect and bee stings.

Less serious stings of bees, wasps, yellow jackets, and hornets are treated by the application of a paste of baking soda and water or household ammonia and a cold compress. Meat tenderizer has also been found effective in relieving the symptoms of minor insect sting reactions.

Bites from venomous spiders, scorpions, and other poisonous insects are treated in the same manner as poisonous snakebites.

Ticks, which can carry diseases such as Rocky Mountain spotted fever or Lyme disease, are removed by grasping the tick as close to the skin as possible with tweezers and pulling it straight out without twisting. Some people feel that placing a drop of turpentine, mineral oil, or petroleum jelly on its body makes it let go before pulling it out.

After the tick is removed, wash the area with soap and water and apply a mild disinfectant. If there is some question as to whether or not the tick may be carrying an infectious disease, a physician should be consulted.

INJURIES DUE TO EXTREME HEAT AND COLD

HEATSTROKE

Heatstroke, a rare condition also called *sunstroke*, is the result of a serious disturbance of the heat-regulating center in the brain. Normally, the body responds to higher environmental temperatures by increasing perspiration and by using other internal mechanisms that keep the body temperature within normal limits. In heatstroke, these mechanisms fail to function properly and the patient's temperature rises, the skin becomes dry and hot, and there may be convulsions and collapse. Because the body temperature may go as high as 108°F to 110°F (42°C), the patient is likely to die if his condition is not treated.

A person suffering from heatstroke should be placed in the shade and cooled immediately by being sprinkled with water and fanning. As soon as possible, he should be immersed in cold water or have ice packs applied to his body to lower his temperature. *Care must be taken that his temperature is not lowered too quickly.* The extremities are massaged so that adequate circulation is maintained.

If the body's heat-regulating mechanism is impaired, the person may experience heatstroke any time he is exposed to extremely high temperatures, and he may need to adjust his life so that he can avoid repeated episodes of heatstroke.

HEAT EXHAUSTION (HEAT PROSTRATION)

Heat exhaustion is caused by excessive sweating, which removes large quantities of salt and water from the body. The patient appears to be in shock with cool, damp skin, pallor, increased pulse and heart beat, dizziness, or stupor. He may also have muscle cramps and poor coordination. Treatment is aimed at replacing the essential salts and fluids. A person suffering from heat exhaustion should be placed in a cool area and kept quiet. As much salt and water or tomato juice (1 teaspoon of salt to a glass of liquid) as he can drink is administered. If he is unable to swallow the salt solution, replacement fluids are administered intravenously. Muscular cramps may be relieved by gently massaging the affected muscles.

SUNBURN

Immediate treatment of a minor sunburn involves the application of cool compresses using a solution of magnesium sulfate (Epsom salts) or sodium bicarbonate (baking soda) to relieve the discomfort. If chills, fever, swelling, or gastrointestinal disturbances occur, the patient should receive medical attention.

HYPOTHERMIA

Hypothermia is a serious lowering of the total body temperature caused by prolonged exposure to cold. Persons most at risk for hypothermia are the elderly, very young and thin children, the mentally ill or deficient, alcoholics, the homeless, and drug addicts.

Hypothermia is a chilling of the entire body, but the extremities can withstand lower temperatures (20° to 30° lower) than the torso, where vital organs are located. When the core (central) temperature drops even 2° or 3°, physiologic changes occur that can lead to fatal cardiac arrhythmias and respiratory failure.

Symptoms of hypothermia range from mild shivering and complaints of feeling cold to loss of consciousness and the appearance of death. Indeed, persons in profound hypothermia may be presumed dead, because the body's protective mechanisms have drastically slowed its metabolic processes. The body uses less than half its normal requirement for oxygen in severe hypothermia. Pulse and repiration are barely detected, reflexes are absent, and the person is unconscious.

Prevention

Prevention of hypothermia includes eating high-energy foods, exercising, wearing layers of clothing, and covering the head. From one half to two thirds of the body's heat is lost through the head. Elderly persons are particularly in need of protection from the effects of extreme cold (Table 36–3). Hypothermia in these persons can easily be misdiagnosed because its symptoms resemble those of so many diseases to which the elderly and weak are most susceptible.

Another reason for failing to diagnose profound hypothermia is improper procedure and equipment for measuring body temperature. In profound hypothermia the core temperature can be as low as 86°F (30°C), but clinical thermometers used in hospitals and clinics rarely register temperatures below 94°F (34.5°C), and many times the temperature is taken orally rather than rectally.

Treatment

Once hypothermia is diagnosed, rewarming is begun. The method varies according to the age and physical condition of the patient. Rapid rewarming can create respiratory and cardiac problems. If it is done in an emergency care facility, monitoring equipment must be readily at hand. Rewarming outside a health care facility probably should be more gradual. This must be done properly to avoid sending cold blood that has pooled in the extremities back to the heart, where it can cause deadly arrhythmias. The torso is warmed first by wrapping it in a blanket or submerging it in a tepid bath and leaving the extremities uncovered. Once the "core" temperature has been raised to about 95°F (35°C), the extremities are rewarmed.

FROSTBITE

Frostbite is a localized injury to tissue caused by freezing. Exposure of the tissues to extreme cold brings about constriction of the blood ves-

TABLE 36–3 TIPS FOR HELPING THE ELDERLY PREVENT ACCIDENTAL HYPOTHERMIA

- Room temperature should not be lower than 65°F. An indoor thermometer should be kept in the house and checked daily during the cold season.
- An energy audit by the utility company can identify ways to prevent heat loss from the home. Check with the gas or electric company.
- If heating the entire house presents economic problems, suggest heating one or two rooms adequately and closing off the other rooms of the house.
- Suggest aids such as a quilted snuggle bag (a quilt with snaps or zipper that becomes a bag), extra socks, and warm hats to be worn indoors.
- Recommend several loose layers of clothing to retain body heat.
- Head covering should be worn even while sleeping, as two thirds of the body's heat is lost through the head.
- Advise against using fireplaces in extremely cold weather, unless no other heat source is available; much heat is lost up the flue. If fireplace is used, close damper as soon as fire is completely extinguished.
- Arrange for someone to check in daily with elderly persons who live alone.

sels, damage to vessel walls and tissue cells, and the formation of blood clots. Frostbite occurs most often in the fingers, toes, cheeks, and nose, where exposure usually is greatest and blood supply most easily impeded.

Symptoms of frostbite include numbness and a prickling sensation in the affected area. The skin appears dull and opaque and may have a yellowish cast. Eventually, edema occurs as fluid escapes from the damaged vessel walls.

Prevention

Frostbite, like hypothermia, can be prevented by wearing protective clothing and avoiding exposure to extreme cold. Sometimes this is not possible if a person is caught unaware or unprepared. Those who are intoxicated or under the influence of drugs may not realize they are suffering from frostbite. If the person also is suffering from hypothermia, he cannot think clearly and does not realize that his skin is being exposed to severe cold.

Treatment

The affected area should be warmed by immersion for about 10 minutes in water heated to between 100°F and 110°F (38°C to 43°C). Do not try to hasten the process by using water that is hotter, as this can only add to the damage. Handle the frostbitten part gently. *Never* rub or massage skin that has been frozen. The practice of rubbing snow or ice on the part is dangerous and completely without benefit. Rubbing or rough handling can cause further damage to the fragile tissues.

Wrap the affected area in bulky clean or sterile bandages, being sure to separate skin areas, as between the fingers. Give the person hot tea or coffee to drink. Later on, after emergency treatment has been given, débridement of dead tissue and skin grafting will be necessary if the deeper tissues are destroyed by gangrene resulting from impaired circulation.

THE COMBATIVE PATIENT

The use of tranquilizing drugs has greatly reduced the occurrence of violent behavior in people who are temporarily unable to control their emotions because of a psychological disorder. This does not mean, however, that psychiatric emergencies no longer occur or that the nurse will never need to know how to handle such patients. When a person becomes greatly agitated and experiences an uncontrollable urge to act violently, he may be extremely frightened and usually welcomes help in regaining control if it is offered in the correct way.

Success in dealing with an unruly patient is more easily achieved if help is offered on a one-to-one basis. Several people trying to talk to him or subdue him at once may only add to his fright and disorientation. However, if physical restraint becomes necessary, one should be sure that enough people are on hand to control the patient.

When the nurse is talking to a person who is combative, it is best that she use his name frequently, tell him who she is and what she is trying to do, and express genuine concern about his feelings and the situation he is in.

Patients who are not diagnosed as mentally ill or psychotic also can become "violent" when nurses and other health care personnel fail to respect their rights and needs. Everyone has a right to privacy and to know what is happening to him. Patients should be told what procedures are planned and why they are necessary. When an emergency patient seems to be out of control and combative, it might be that he perceives himself to be in danger from the emergency staff as well as from his injuries.

When a patient gives verbal and nonverbal clues that he is agitated, fearful, and likely to assault a nurse or other staff member, measures should be taken to calm him. This is done by cautiously approaching the patient in a nonthreatening manner, establishing eye contact with him, and in a soft voice explaining what is being done for him and why it is necessary. Taking time to listen as well as talk to the patient can help the nurse understand why a potentially violent or combative patient feels the need to defend himself and regain control over what is happening to him.

It may be necessary to help the patient by exerting some outside controls. These may be verbal or physical, but physical force should be used only after it is apparent that talking with the patient is not going to calm him. One may simply tell him to stop screaming, to sit down, or to put down an object that he apparently intends to use as a weapon. If verbal control does not work, it may be necessary to restrain the patient who is overwrought. If restraints are used, the patient should not be left alone immediately after he has been restrained, as this action will give him the impression that he is being punished for wrongdoing rather than being aided in controlling himself.

It is strongly suggested that any nurse who works regularly in an emergency department, psychiatric unit, or other setting where she will have occasion to deal with violent patients obtain additional information and training in handling such situations. Lack of knowledge and experience in emergency psychiatric situations can be detrimental to the patient as well as to those who are trying to help him.

ALCOHOL AND DRUG ABUSE

Substance abuse is a major health problem in the United States. Chronic abuse of alcohol and prescription, over-the-counter, and illegal, or "street," drugs presents a challenge to every segment of society and costs millions of dollars and thousands of lives each year. In the following paragraphs we will focus on emergencies arising from acute alcoholism and drug overdose, as well as the withdrawal syndromes that occur when chronic users are abruptly deprived of a substance on which they have become physiologically dependent.

ACUTE ALCOHOLISM

Alcohol is a central nervous system (CNS) depressant that affects individuals in different ways. The amount of alcohol consumed is not as relevant to emergency care as is the effect the alcohol has on the brain and its control of coordination, reasoning, and social interaction.

The person who is suffering from acute alcohol intoxication has a decreased level of consciousness that can range from partial to total loss of motor and sensory response to stimuli. In its early stages, acute alcoholism is characterized by deep respirations, bounding pulse, moist skin, and a flushed face. The person who is intoxicated may exhibit inappropriate behavior, as his inhibitions are lowered by the effect of the alcohol. As CNS depression intensifies, respirations become more labored and shallow, the pulse weakens, and the skin becomes pale and dry. The blood pressure begins to drop and the pupils may become dilated.

When a person is extremely intoxicated, he should be treated as one who is semiconscious or totally unconscious. Vomiting, aspiration of vomitus, and asphyxiation are real dangers, and so the first concern is that an open airway and adequate air exchange are maintained.

Because the symptoms of acute alcoholism can be the same as those of a serious illness or injury such as diabetes mellitus or a severe head injury, it is important that those giving emergency care try to get information about the patient's health and medical history and any falls or other accidents he might have suffered. An intoxicated person who cannot be roused or is likely to harm himself or others should be evaluated and treated at a medical facility.

Alcohol Withdrawal Syndrome

Chronic abusers of alcohol may, for one reason or another, suddenly stop drinking alcohol. Perhaps they decide to abruptly quit drinking, are nauseated and unable to keep the alcohol down, or do not have the money to buy the drinks they need. Whatever the reason, sudden withdrawal of alcohol from the body can result in severe CNS agitation.

Symptoms of abrupt withdrawal from alcohol include increased tremors, excitement, anxiety, disorientation, hallucinations, and convulsions. These are typical of the condition called delirium tremens, or DT, which is a very serious complication of withdrawal. Emergency treatment consists of trying to keep the person calm and preventing him from hurting himself. He will need to be admitted to a hospital or clinic where he can be given proper care to alleviate fluid and electrolyte imbalance, nutritional deficits, anxiety and psychomotor agitation, and possibly gastrointestinal irritation and bleeding. The symptoms of delirium tremens can last from 2 to 4 days or longer.

DRUG ABUSE

The list of drugs that might be abused by a chronic substance user is almost endless. In general, there are four groups of drugs that are illicitly obtained and misused: (1) narcotics, which include opium, morphine, heroin, methadone, and other legal prescription drugs such as oxycodone hydrochloride (Percodan) and propoxyphene hydrochloride (Darvon); (2) hallucinogens such as LSD (acid), mescaline and peyote, phencyclidine (PCP or angel dust), and marijuana or hashish; (3) CNS stimulants such as cocaine and the amphetamines; and (4) CNS depressants such as the barbiturates, methaqualone (Quaalude), and tranquilizers such as diazepam (Valium), chlordiazepoxide hydrochloride (Librium), and meprobamate (Equanil, Miltown).

Symptoms of acute narcotic intoxication are those typical of CNS depression; that is, lowered blood pressure and a decrease in other vital signs, pinpoint and fixed pupils, lethargy, and possibly coma. Continued depression of respiration can lead to respiratory arrest.

Hallucinogens are mind-altering agents capable of producing hallucinations and other mental aberrations as well as false sensory perceptions.

Symptoms of acute hallucinogenic intoxication include elevated blood pressure, dilated pupils, increased physical activity, anxiety, and other signs of mental aberration. The person can be very combative because of unexplained fears and possibly paranoia.

CNS stimulants excite the nervous system and produce hyperactivity and increased energy, a feeling of excitement or agitation, chest pain and/or tachycardia, and irritability and talkativeness. The person taking drugs of this kind may become belligerent and dangerously combative. Other symptoms include elevated blood pressure, dilated pupils that react to light, fast pulse, shallow respirations, and high fever.

CNS depressants affect the body in much the same way as narcotics and alcohol. Respiratory depression, diminished gag reflex, and nausea and vomiting jeopardize normal respiration and can lead to either asphyxiation from aspirated vomitus or respiratory arrest from CNS depression.

Emergency care for an acutely ill drug abuser is focused on preventing further injury to the person and those around him. A first concern is adequate air exchange. If possible, the rescuer should try to determine the drug the person has used. Convulsive patients are given support and protection, as is any person having a seizure. Some authorities advocate trying to "talk down" an agitated or panicky drug abuser by sitting calmly with him and assuring him that he will be all right. Restraints are used only as a last resort as they tend to add to the person's panic and make it more difficult for him to regain control of himself.

Evidence of the kind of drug used by the patient should be taken with him to the medical facility. This includes containers of drugs, capsules or pills found near him, and needles and syringes he apparently has used. If the patient vomits while receiving emergency care, the vomitus is taken with the patient in case analysis is necessary to identify the drug or drugs he may have taken. During transport to the medical facility, the patient is monitored closely for signs of shock and respiratory problems.

In general, the emergency care of a person suffering drug withdrawal syndrome is the same as that for alcohol withdrawal syndrome.

DISASTER NURSING

A disaster may be defined as *any catastrophe in which numbers of people are plunged into helplessness and suffering.* Natural disasters include epidemics, earthquakes, explosions, hurricanes, tornadoes, fires, floods, and transportation accidents. War-caused disasters may result from enemy attacks with chemical, biologic, nuclear, psychologic, and conventional weapons.

Whether the disaster is natural or war-caused, it will involve physical injuries, loss of property, and interruption of the normal activities of daily living. Victims often will be in need of food, clothing, shelter, medical and nursing or hospital care, and other basic necessities of life.

The nurse has a definite role in helping to relieve the suffering inflicted by such tragedies, and she should actively participate in community planning and civil defense programs so that, in time of disaster, she will be prepared to function effectively as a member of the health team.

DISASTER PLANNING

The governmental agencies for disaster planning are the Office of Civil Defense and the U.S. Public Health Service. The American Red Cross is a voluntary organization that traditionally provides nursing care and the basic essentials of shelter and food during a natural disaster. In most communities, the local civil defense agency and the Red Cross work together to formulate disaster plans so that their services are coordinated with each other and with other agencies planning for essential services such as transportation, communication, and welfare.

Special courses in civil defense and disaster nursing are usually offered by the Office of Civil Defense, the Red Cross, and professional organizations. These courses help the nurses and volunteer workers in the community to understand the function of each agency in a particular type of disaster and serve to coordinate the planning for each kind of emergency nursing.

PSYCHOLOGICAL RESPONSES TO DISASTER

Since the 1940s there have been many studies conducted to determine the needs and problems of persons trying to cope with a major disaster. Typical responses are not unlike those of any person who is overwhelmed with sudden and profound change, death, or destruction of a former way of life.

One would expect people to panic when they are caught up in a major disaster, but this is not a common reaction except when there is life-threatening danger that occurs in a matter of moments and without warning. More typical of psychological responses to a major disaster are the three states described in the following section.

Stage I is the *impact stage.* Survivors are stunned, apathetic, and disorganized. For several hours after the initial blow they may have difficulty following directions and will need strong support and firm guidance.

Stage II is the *recoil stage.* During this stage individuals are very compliant, want to be helpful, and may minimize or ignore their own injuries. At this stage some persons may need to be protected from themselves if they are indeed injured or exhausted physically and emotionally.

In Stage III, called the *posttrauma stage,* some survivors become elated, grateful that they are still alive. Others might feel guilt when they realize they did not suffer as much as their friends and neighbors. At this stage the attention of the survivors turns toward rebuilding, and they have a strong sense of brotherhood and community spirit.

Later on, victims of a disaster probably will begin to complain about the help provided by

various agencies, governmental and private. If the disaster could have been avoided or at least mitigated by an efficient Civil Defense or similar agency, the psychological effects may be more severe and psychological recovery prolonged.

NURSING INTERVENTION

A booklet published under the direction of the U.S. Department of Health and Human Services includes the following list of nursing responsibilities in regard to planning and implementing health care in the case of disaster.

All nurses should:

- Be prepared for self-survival and for performing emergency nursing measures.
- Know the community disaster plans and organized community health resources.
- Know the meaning of warning signals and the action to be taken.
- Know measures for protection from radioactive fallout.
- Know measures for prevention and control of environmental health hazards.
- Be prepared to interpret health laws and regulations.
- Know and interpret community resources for citizen preparedness, such as first aid and medical self-help courses.

In many types of disaster, the nurse may need to improvise because of lack of equipment. She must always bear in mind the basic principles of nursing that she has been taught and has practiced in the hospital environment. If there is a great disparity between need and availability of medical and nursing personnel, she may be called upon to exercise leadership and judgment in determining the condition of each victim, using supplies and equipment, and detecting changes in the environment that might be hazardous.

The U.S. Department of Health and Human Services recommends that the nurse be competent in the skills described below if she is to be involved in disaster health care.

The nurse participates in planning and providing care for large groups of people under extreme duress in various types of disaster situations. Being a part of the development and revision of nursing procedures aimed at providing comfort and safety during and after a disaster helps the nurse to deal more efficiently with the actual crisis situation.

The emotional and physical comfort and safety of large numbers of disaster victims must be attended to with limited supplies, equipment, utilities, and personnel. The nurse must understand the emotional stress caused by personal fear, problems of displacement and separation of families, increasing anxiety, and continuing danger. She helps people of different cultural backgrounds and religious beliefs to accept and adapt to temporary living conditions in crowded and often adverse situations.

Recognizing and understanding the effect of disrupted social and economic patterns, such as personal and material losses, emotional trauma, and crowded living conditions, helps the nurse to deal with the victims more effectively.

It is helpful to encourage patients to verbalize their concerns and fears and to guide them in performing certain tasks.

Providing basic instruction to disaster victims in the aspects of appropriate self-care and encouraging them to further provide for their own needs and the needs of others are essential responsibilities of the nurse in any disaster situation.

Observing, recording, and reporting information to appropriate people must be carried out in an organized manner. General physical and mental conditions of patients and signs and symptoms that may be indicative of changes in their conditions must be accurately observed. Stresses in relationships between patients, their families, visitors, and personnel must be kept to a minimum.

Performing nursing procedures within the framework of a disaster situation demands skill and judgment in order to provide for the good of the greatest number of people. The nurse must administer medications and treatments as directed and improvise supplies, equipment, and techniques as necessary. She must also carry out precautionary measures, including the maintenance of a safe and sanitary environment and the separation of patients with communicable diseases. Instituting emergency first aid measures is also a duty of the nurse, and usually she is forced to utilize improvised supplies and to observe aseptic techniques such as sterilization under very chaotic conditions.

Working toward restoration of community and family life according to available resources once the disaster has occurred also involves the nurse and other members of the health care team. Individual self-help and work therapy are encouraged, as are activities of family living, with adaptations designed to attain and maintain a sanitary and healthy environment. Deformity prevention must continue to be practiced through the use of improvised equipment and available resources. Existing community facilities and resources must be utilized as much as possible for continued patient care.

The nurse can promote the effectiveness of the health service agency in disaster preparedness by knowing and interpreting the agency's disaster plan. She must understand the relationship between the agency plan, the local government plan, and the local Red Cross plan. Promoting maintenance and restoration of community health by participating in the control of environmental health hazards is also an important responsibility of any nurse.

BIBLIOGRAPHY

American Heart Association and The American Medical Association: Standards and Guidelines for Cardiopulmonary Resuscitation (CPR) and Emergency Cardiac Care (ECC). J.A.M.A., 255, 1988, p. 284.

Anderson, M. R.: The pharmacology of intervention for respiratory emergencies. Emerg. Care Q., May, 1989, p. 23.

Barder-Stotts, K.: Action stat! Hyphema. Nursing 89, Dec., 1989, p. 33.

Budassi, S., and Barber, J.: Emergency Nursing: Principles and Practices, 2nd ed. St. Louis, C. V. Mosby, 1985.

Clark, R. B., et al.: Eye emergencies and urgencies. Patient Care, Jan. 15, 1989, p. 24.

Dubiel, D.: Action stat! Cocaine overdose. Nursing 90, March, 1990, p. 33.

Hoffman, M. S., ed.: The World Almanac and Book of Facts 1990. New York, Pharos Books, 1990.

Huston, C. J.: Action stat! Caustic chemical ingestion. Nursing 90, July, 1990, p. 33.

Huston, C. J.: Action stat! Hypothermia. Nursing 90, Dec., 1990, p. 33.

Jackson D. R.: Action stat! Abdominal stab wound. Nursing 89, Dec., 1989, p. 33.

Jones, S. et al.: Do's and don'ts of a code: Dealing with cardiac arrest. AD Nurse, March/April, 1989, p. 10.

Redheffer, G. M., and Bailey, M.: Assessing and splinting fractures. Nursing 89, June, 1989, p. 51.

Wilson, V.: Action stat! Complications of thrombolytic therapy. Nursing 91, Jan., 1991, p. 41.

STUDENT STUDY AIDS

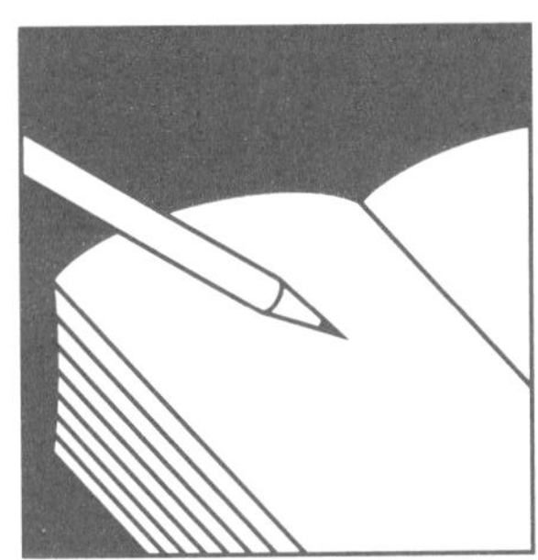

CLINICAL CASE PROBLEMS

Read each clinical situation and discuss the questions with your classmates.

1. While driving home from work one afternoon, you come upon the scene of an accident. There are two victims inside a wrecked automobile and one lying on the side of the road. The two in the car are bleeding moderately from small lacerations. One is unconscious and has a large bruised and swollen area on his forehead. The other person is hysterical and cannot move his leg without great pain. The victim lying on the side of the road has no visible signs of injury, but he is not breathing.

- Which victim is treated first? How is he treated?
- If help is available, what should be done for the apparent fracture?
- If help is not available, what would you say to the victim with the fracture?
- How would you control moderate bleeding?

---

2. While working as a student nurse in the hospital's emergency unit, you notice that patients who have been injured or are very ill sometimes become hostile and combative. Some try to physically assault members of the emergency team and others use abusive and threatening language.

- Discuss with your classmates some reasons why patients may behave in these ways when they are injured or very ill.
- What are some ways in which so-called violent patients who are not mentally ill can be handled so as to calm them and prevent assault on and encourage cooperation with the emergency staff?

---

3. Your community has been hit by a hurricane. There are many people injured, several fatalities, and widespread destruction of property.

- What kinds of psychological responses would you expect to see in the people who have survived the hurricane but have minor injuries, even though many have lost their homes?
- What kinds of nursing intervention would be helpful to people in each of the stages of response to a major disaster?
- What are your responsibilities as a nurse in regard to planning and implementing health care in the case of a disaster?

STUDY OUTLINE

I. Prevention of accidents

A. Home safety.
1. More than one fourth of accidental deaths occur in the home.
2. Principal victims are children and elderly.
3. Education of the public will help prevent accidents.

B. Highway safety.
1. Motor vehicle accidents are leading cause of accidental death in this country.
2. Major causes of such accidents are human and mechanical failure.

C. Water safety.
1. Observing the common-sense rules of water safety helps prevent accidents.
2. Rescue methods vary; attempt a swimming rescue only if you are experienced.
3. Cardiopulmonary resuscitation may be necessary.
4. Have victim lie down, and treat him for shock.
5. Transport near-drowning victim to medical facility for evaluation of fluid and electrolyte status and cardiac irregularities.

II. General principles of first aid

A. Think before acting.
B. Move slowly and deliberately; act with confidence.
C. Evaluate injuries and summon help.
D. Survey scene to determine hazards to victims, onlookers, and rescuers.
E. Check each victim quickly, treat the most serious injuries first.
F. Evaluate condition of victim.
G. Do not move victim unless necessary.
H. Do not remove impaled object unless it is in the cheek and bleeding must be controlled.
I. Do not try to give anything by mouth to an unconscious person.
J. Explain in a calm voice what you are doing for the victim; be honest.
K. "Good Samaritan" law in many states protects medical personnel giving first aid at the scene of an accident.

III. Cardiopulmonary resuscitation (CPR)

A. Reestablishment of heart and lung action.
B. Indicated when there is no breathing and no heart beat in people who have suffered near-drowning, electric shock, or cardiac arrest.
C. Prompt action essential to prevent biologic death.
D. Should be administered only by trained personnel because of possible complications.
E. Indications for CPR:
1. Absence of carotid pulse.
2. Absence of response to stimuli.
3. Absent respiration.

F. Artificial breathing given by mouth-to-mouth technique.
1. Open airway.
2. Breathe into victim's mouth about 12 times per minute.

G. Cardiac compression: applied to lower half of sternum.
1. Press downward to squeeze heart against spinal column.
2. Press without interruption 80 to 100 times per minute.

IV. Choking emergencies

A. Obstructed airway the sixth leading cause of accidental death.

B. Victim may give universal signal for choking, be unable to speak or cough, and begin to turn cyanotic.
C. If victim is able to cough and expel the foreign object on his own, this should be encouraged.
D. Abdominal thrust and chest thrust used.

V. **Control of bleeding**
A. Place clean or sterile dressing over wound.
B. Apply firm, steady pressure with hand.
C. When bleeding has decreased, apply bandage.
1. Do not wrap wound so tightly as to constrict circulation.
D. Elevate and immobilize injured part.
E. If pressure to wound does not decrease blood loss from wound, apply pressure to pressure point above the artery serving the wounded area.
F. Use of tourniquet must be last resort when other methods fail and victim's life is in danger or when limb is amputated, severely mangled, or crushed.
1. Tourniquet should be removed only by physician.
2. Do not cover tourniquet.
3. Write *TK* and location of tourniquet on victim's forehead.
G. Control of nosebleeds (epistaxis).
1. Most respond to gentle pressure for 10 to 15 minutes (by the clock).
2. Major nosebleed a life-threatening condition; requires medical attention.

VI. **Shock**
A. Types are neurogenic, hypovolemic, septic, and cardiogenic.
B. Symptoms due to inadequate blood volume, loss of tone and then collapse of peripheral vessels, and shift of body fluids.
C. Symptoms are pallor, weak pulse, clammy skin, and thirst.
D. Management of shock:
1. Reassure and comfort patient.
2. Maintain body heat.
3. Place patient flat.
4. Restore circulating blood volume, relieve respiratory embarrassment, and control pain.

VII. **Burns**
A. Two dangers are shock and infection.
B. Minor burns should be immersed in cold water or covered with cold compresses.
C. Major burns:
1. Cover with clean, dry dressing and transport victim to hospital or clinic.
2. Give victim fluids to drink only if transport to hospital will be delayed for several hours.
3. Never apply ointments or disturb blisters.
D. Chemical burns:
1. Flush with water; exceptions are burns from dry lime and phenol (carbolic acid).
2. Cover with a dressing and transport victim to hospital.
3. For ingestion of corrosive poison, give victim milk or water to drink. Do not induce or encourage vomiting or try to chemically neutralize the poison.

VIII. **Poisoning**
A. Education can help prevent accidental poisoning.
B. Poisoning should be suspected if victim suddenly becomes ill and

if there is a peculiar odor to the breath and an open container nearby.

1. Save container or vomitus for identification.

C. Swallowed poisons:
   1. Induce vomiting, except for corrosive poisons or petroleum products.
   2. Give specific antidote if it is known; contact Poison Control Center.
   3. Give activated charcoal.

D. Inhaled poisons:
   1. Transport victim to source of fresh air.
   2. Give CPR as necessary.
   3. Keep victim warm and quiet; do not give alcohol or stimulants.

E. Food poisoning due to toxins produced by bacteria in contaminated foods:
   1. Prevented by proper preparation, storage, and handling of food.
   2. Onset is acute with severe gastrointestinal disturbances.
   3. Treatment: begin supportive measures.

IX. Traumatic injuries

A. Fractures:
   1. Immobilize the part before moving victim.
   2. Assess circulation and status of nerve pathways.

B. Head injury:
   1. Keep patient quiet.
   2. Seek medical attention immediately.

C. Eye injuries:
   1. Foreign matter may be removed by irrigation or by touching a corner of a clean handkerchief to the object. No attempt should be made to remove imbedded objects.
   2. Perforation of the globe a serious threat to vision.
      a. Object protruding from the globe should be left in place and stabilized.
      b. Bandage both eyes to minimize eye movement; reassure patient.
   3. Lacerations and contusions of eyelid and soft tissues around the eye will bleed profusely.
      a. Apply pressure only if sure the globe has not been injured.
      b. Cover with loose dressing to prevent contamination if globe has been torn or punctured.
   4. Chemical burns are irrigated immediately and continuously during transport to medical facility.
   5. Injuries from radiation and light: cover with bandage or eye patches.
      a. Cover thermal burns of eye with loose, moist dressing.

D. Ear injuries:
   1. Damage to inner and middle ear indicated by discharge of blood or cerebrospinal fluid or both, severe ear pain, and loss of equilibrium.
   2. External lacerations treated as any open wound.
   3. Apply bulky dressing if ear has been badly torn.
   4. Try to find avulsed part if avulsion occurs. Wrap part in plastic and keep cold while transporting to medical facility with the patient.

E. Neck and spine injuries:
   1. May be accidentally overlooked.
   2. Any person with head injury should be suspected of having spinal injury.

3. Immobilize neck using cervical collar before moving victim.
4. Use backboard for transporting suspected spinal injury victim.

F. Chest and abdominal wounds:
1. Sucking chest wound is treated with occlusive dressing.
2. Impaled objects protruding from a wound are *not* removed; object is stabilized and dressings applied around it.
3. Flail chest is splinted with small pillow or other bulky material.
4. Open wound of abdomen with evisceration is covered with plastic or aluminum foil dressing, which is covered with a folded towel or sheet.

X. Electric shock

A. Give CPR; treat burns as needed.
B. Use caution in separating victim from source of electric current.

XII. Animal bites

A. Treat wound immediately.
B. Vaccinations necessary if examination of the animal reveals the possibility of rabies.
C. Snakebite:
1. Nonpoisonous snakebite is treated as minor wound.
2. Poisonous snakebite is treated by packing affected part in ice and transporting patient to medical facility.

D. Insect bites or stings:
1. Serious stings require immediate attention:
a. Give aqueous epinephrine and Benadryl.
b. Keep victim calm and treat for shock.
2. Apply paste of baking soda and water or meat tenderizer and cold compresses to less serious stings.
3. Apply a drop of turpentine or mineral oil to ticks and remove; wash area with soap and water and apply an antiseptic.

XIII. Injuries due to extreme heat and cold

A. Heatstroke (sunstroke): a disturbance in the heat-regulating mechanism in the brain allows patient's body temperature to become extremely high.
1. Cool with cool water.

B. Heat exhaustion (heat prostration): caused by excessive loss of salt and water through perspiration.
1. Treated by replacement of these substances.

C. Sunburn: treat minor burn with application of solution of baking soda or Epsom salts and water.
1. Major burns require medical attention as soon as possible.

D. Hypothermia: drastic lowering of body temperature.
1. Symptoms: mild shivering and complaints of cold to unconsciousness.
2. Prevention (see Table 36–3).
3. Treatment:
a. Depends on age and physical condition of patient.
b. Rewarm torso before extremities.
c. Submerge in tepid bath or wrap in blanket.
d. Improper warming can cause cardiac arrhythmias and respiratory and cardiac arrest.

E. Frostbite: local condition associated with constriction of blood vessels and damage to tissue and vessel walls.
1. Rewarm quickly by immersion in warm water.
2. Do not rub; handle very gently.

XIV. The combative patient

A. Patient who is violent may be terribly afraid.
B. Identify yourself; speak to the patient, using his name frequently.

C. Try simple commands to help patient gain control of himself.
D. If physical restraint is used, be sure enough people are available to subdue patient.
E. Do not leave him alone immediately after he is restrained.

XV. Alcohol and drug abuse

A. Alcohol is a CNS depressant. Amount consumed not as relevant to emergency treatment of acute alcoholism as is effect alcohol has on brain.
   1. Acute alcohol intoxication characterized by deep respirations, bounding pulse, moist skin, flushed face.
   2. Person may exhibit inappropriate behavior.
   3. As CNS depression intensifies, person becomes semiconscious or totally unconscious.
   4. Major concern is maintaining open airway and adequate air exchange.
   5. Symptoms of acute alcohol intoxication similar to serious diseases and injury (e.g., diabetes and head injury).
   6. Alcohol withdrawal syndrome occurs when intake of alcohol is suddenly stopped.
      a. Symptoms include tremors, excitement, anxiety, disorientation, hallucinations, and convulsions.
      b. Above symptoms typical of delirium tremens or DT.
      c. Emergency treatment consists of monitoring respirations, maintaining adequate air exchange, and protecting person having a seizure from injury. Patient with DT should be evaluated by a physician.

B. Drug abuse.
   1. Major types of drugs frequently abused: narcotics, hallucinogens, CNS stimulants, and CNS depressants.
   2. Symptoms of acute narcotic intoxication or overdose typical of CNS depression. Vital signs decreased, pupils pinpoint and fixed, lethargy, and possible coma. Respiratory arrest a danger as CNS depression becomes more marked.
   3. Symptoms of acute hallucinogenic intoxication include elevated blood pressure, dilated pupils, increased physical activity, anxiety, combativeness.
   4. CNS stimulants excite the nervous system and produce hyperactivity, agitation, irritability, talkativeness. Elevated vital signs, dilated pupils, and high fever also may be present.
   5. CNS depressants produce symptoms similar to those of narcotic intoxication.
   6. Emergency care focused on preventing further injury to patient and those around him.
      a. Adequate air exchange should be assured.
      b. Try to talk patient down; sit calmly with him, reassure him.
      c. Restraints a last resort, as they can make it more difficult for the person to regain control of himself.
      d. Take containers, drugs, needles, and syringes that could contain abused drug to the medical facility with the patient.

XVI. Disaster nursing

A. A disaster involves loss of property, physical injuries, and interruption in activities of daily living on a large scale.
B. Agencies involved in planning disaster nursing are Office of Civil Defense, Red Cross, and other local voluntary organizations.
C. Psychologic responses:
   1. Impact stage: survivors and victims need firm guidance and support.

2. Recoil stage: persons may overextend themselves.
3. Posttrauma stage: survivors compliant, want to be helpful.

D. Nursing intervention:
   1. Know community disaster plans.
   2. Provide leadership and nursing care.
   3. Provide for emotional and physical comfort and safety of victims.
   4. Work to increase effectiveness of local disaster planning agency.

Appendix

TABLE OF MOST COMMON LABORATORY TEST VALUES

INTRODUCTION

The following tables list "normal values," now termed reference values, for the most commonly performed laboratory tests. Clinical laboratories use various forms of tests to derive the needed information, and therefore each laboratory has its own set of reference values.* The International System of Units designated by "S.I. units" has been adopted by clinical laboratories in many countries and represents a modification of the metric system.

The tables are adapted from Conn, R. B.: Laboratory values of clinical importance. *In* Rakel, R. E.: Textbook of Family Practice, 4th ed. Philadelphia, W. B. Saunders Company, 1990.

* The reference values in the Tables of Diagnostic Tests within individual chapters may differ depending on the laboratory used and type of testing procedure.

REFERENCE VALUES IN HEMATOLOGY

	Conventional Units		S.I. Units	
Alkaline phosphatase, leukocyte	Total score 14–100		Total score 14–100	
Cell counts				
Erythrocytes				
Males	4.6–6.2 million/cu mm		$4.6-6.2\times10^{12}$/l	
Females	4.2–5.4 million/cu mm		$4.2-5.4\times10^{12}$/l	
Children (varies with age)	4.5–5.1 million/cu mm		$4.5-5.1\times10^{12}$/l	
Leukocytes				
Total	4500–11,000/cu mm		$4.5-11.0\times10^{9}$/l	
Differential	*Percentage*	*Absolute*		
Myelocytes	0	0/cu mm	0/1	
Band neutrophils	3–5	150–400/cu mm	$150-400\times10^{6}$/l	
Segmented neutrophils	54–62	3000–5800/cu mm	$3000-5800\times10^{6}$/l	
Lymphocytes	25–33	1500–3000/cu mm	$1500-3000\times10^{6}$l	
Monocytes	3–7	300–500/cu mm	$300-500\times10^{6}$/l	
Eosinophils	1–3	50–250/cu mm	$50-250\times10^{6}$/l	
Basophils	0–0.75	15–50/cu mm	$15-50\times10^{6}$/l	
Platelets	150,000–350,000/cu mm		$150-350\times10^{9}$/l	
Reticulocytes	25,000–75,000/cu mm 0.5–1.5% of erythrocytes		$25-75\times10^{6}$/l	
Bone marrow, differential cell count				
	Range	*Average*	*Range*	*Average*
Myeloblasts	0.3–5.0%	2.0%	0.003–0.05	0.02
Promyelocytes	1.0–8.0%	5.0%	0.01–0.08	0.05
Myelocytes: Neutrophilic	5.0–19.0%	12.0%	0.05–0.19	0.12
Eosinophilic	0.5–3.0%	1.5%	0.005–0.03	0.015
Basophilic	0.0–0.5%	0.3%	0.00–0.005	0.003
Metamyelocytes	13.0–32.0%	22.0%	0.13–0.32	0.22
Polymorphonuclear neutrophils	7.0–30.0%	20.0%	0.07–0.30	0.20
Polymorphonuclear eosinophils	0.5–4.0%	2.0%	0.005–0.04	0.02
Polymorphonuclear basophils	0.0–0.7%	0.2%	0.00–0.007	0.002
Lymphocytes	3.0–17.0%	10.0%	0.03–0.17	0.10
Plasma cells	0.0–2.0%	0.4%	0.00–0.02	0.004
Monocytes	0.5–5.0%	2.0%	0.005–0.05	0.02
Reticulum cells	0.1–2.0%	0.2%	0.001–0.02	0.002
Megakaryocytes	0.3–3.0%	0.4%	0.003–0.03	0.004
Pronormoblasts	1.0–8.0%	4.0%	0.01–0.08	0.04
Normoblasts	7.0–32.0%	18.0%	0.07–0.32	0.18
Coagulation tests				
Coagulation time (Lee-White)	5–15 min (glass tubes) 19–60 min (siliconized tubes)		5–15 min (glass tubes) 19–60 min (siliconized tubes)	
Fibrinogen	200–400 mg/dl		5.9–11.7 μmol/l	
Partial thromboplastin time, activated (APTT)	20–35 sec		20–35 sec	
Prothrombin time (one stage)	12.0–14.0 sec		12.0–14.0 sec	
Coombs' test				
Direct	Negative		Negative	
Indirect	Negative		Negative	
Corpuscular values of erythrocytes (values are for adults; in children, values vary with age)				
MCH (mean corpuscular hemoglobin)	27–31 picogm		0.42–0.48 fmol	
MCV (mean corpuscular volume)	80–96 cu micra		80–96 fl	
MCHC (mean corpuscular hemoglobin concentration)	32–36%		0.32–0.36	
Hematocrit				
Males	40–54 ml/dl		0.40–0.54	
Females	37–47 ml/dl		0.37–0.47	
Newborn	49–54 ml/dl		0.49–0.54	
Children (varies with age)	35–49 ml/dl		0.35–0.49	

REFERENCE VALUES IN HEMATOLOGY *Continued*

	Conventional Units	S.I. Units
Hemoglobin		
Males	14.0–18.0 grams/dl	2.17–2.79 mmol/l
Females	12.0–16.0 grams/dl	1.86–2.48 mmol/l
Newborn	16.5–19.5 grams/dl	2.56–3.02 mmol/l
Children (varies with age)	11.2–16.5 grams/dl	1.74–2.56 mmol/l;
Hemoglobin, fetal	Less than 1% of total	Less than 0.01 of total
Sedimentation rate		
Wintrobe: Males	0–5 mm in 1 hr	0–5 mm/h
Females	0–15 mm in 1 hr	0–15 mm/h
Westergren: Males	0–15 mm in 1 hr	0–15 mm/h
Females	0–20 mm in 1 hr	0–20 mm/h
(May be slightly higher in children and during pregnancy)		

REFERENCE VALUES FOR BLOOD, PLASMA, AND SERUM
(For some procedures the reference values may vary depending on the method used)

	Conventional Units	S.I. Units
Adrenocorticotropin (ACTH), plasma		
6 AM	10–80 picogm/ml	10–80 ng/l
6 PM	Less than 50 picogm/ml	Less than 50 ng/l
Ammonia (nitrogen), plasma	15–49 mcg/dl	11–35 μmol/l
Amylase, serum	25–125 milliunits/ml	25–125 units/l
Anion gap	8–16 mEq/liter	8–16 mmol/l
Aspartate aminotransferase, *see* Transaminase		
Base excess, blood	0 ± 2 mEq/liter	0 ± 2 mmol/l
Bicarbonate serum	23–29 mEq/liter	23–29 mmol/l
Bilirubin, serum		
Direct	0.1–0.4 mg/dl	1.7–6.8 μmol/l
Indirect	0.2–0.7 mg/dl (Total minus direct)	3.4–12 μmol/l (Total minus direct)
Total	0.3–1.1 mg/dl	5.1–19 μmol/l
Calcium, serum	4.5–5.5 mEq/liter	2.25–2.75 mmol/l
	9.0–11.0 mg/dl	
	(Slightly higher in children)	(Slightly higher in children)
	(Varies with protein concentration)	(Varies with protein concentration)
Carbon dioxide content, serum		
Adults	24–30 mEq/liter	24–30 mmol/l
Infants	20–28 mEq/liter	20–28 mmol/l
Carbon dioxide tension (Pco_2), blood	35–45 mm Hg	35–45 mm Hg
Chloride, serum	96–106 mEq/liter	96–106 mmol/l
Cholesterol, serum		
Total	150–250 mg/dl	3.9–6.5 mmol/l
Esters	68–76% of total cholesterol	0.68–0.76 of total cholesterol
Cortisol, plasma		
8 AM	6–23 mcg/dl	170–635 nmol/l
4 PM	3–15 mcg/dl	82–413 nmol/l
10 PM	Less than 50% of 8 AM value	Less than 0.5 of 8 AM value
Creatine, serum	0.2–0.8 mg/dl	15–61 μmol/l
Creatine kinase, serum (CK, CPK)		
Males	12–80 milliunits/ml (30°)	12–80 units/l (30 C)
	55–170 milliunits/ml (37°)	55–170 units/l (37 C)
Females	10–55 milliunits/ml (30°)	10–55 units/l (30 C)
	30–135 milliunits/ml (37°)	30–135 units/l (37 C)
Creatine kinase isoenzymes, serum		
CK-MM	Present	Present
CK-MB	Absent	Absent
CK-BB	Absent	Absent
Creatinine, serum	0.6–1.2 mg/dl	53–106 μmol/l

Table continued on following page

REFERENCE VALUES FOR BLOOD, PLASMA, AND SERUM *Continued*
(For some procedures the reference values may vary depending on the method used)

	Conventional Units	S.I. Units
Fatty acids, total, serum	190–420 mg/dl	7–15 mmol/l
nonesterified, serum	8–25 mg/dl	0.30–0.90 mmol/l
Ferritin, serum	20–200 nanogm/ml	20–200 μg/l
Fibrinogen, plasma	200–400 mg/100 ml	5.9–11.7 μmol/l
Glucose (fasting)		
Blood	60–100 mg/dl	3.33–5.55 mmol/l
Plasma or serum	70–115 mg/dl	3.89–6.38 mmol/l
Growth hormone, serum	0–10 nanogm/ml	0–10 μg/l
17-Hydroxycorticosteriods, plasma	8–18 mcg/dl	0.22–0.50 μmol/l
Immunoglobulins, serum		
IgG	550–1900 mg/dl	5.5–19.0 g/l
IgA	60–333 mg/dl	0.60–3.3 g/l
IgM	45–145 mg/dl	0.45–1.5 g/l
IgD	0.5–3.0 mg/dl	5–30 mg/l
IgE	<500 nanogm/ml (Varies with age in children)	<500 μg/l (Varies with age in children)
Insulin, plasma (fasting)	5–25 microunits/ml	36–179 pmol/l
Iodine, protein bound, serum	3.5–8.0 mcg/dl	0.28–0.63 μmol/l
Iron, serum	75–175 mcg/dl	13–31 μmol/l
Iron binding capacity, serum		
Total	250–410 mcg/dl	45–73 μmol/l
Saturation	20–55%	0.20–0.55
Lactate, blood, venous	4.5–19.8 mg/dl	0.5–2.2 mmol/l
arterial	4.5–14.4 mg/dl	0.5–1.6 mmol/l
Lactate dehydrogenase, serum	45–90 milliunits/ml (I.U.) (30°)	45–90 units/l (30 C)
(LD, LDH)	100–190 milliunits/ml (37°)	100–190 units/l (37 C)
LDH_1	22–37% of total	0.22–0.37 of total
LDH_2	30–46% of total	0.30–0.46 of total
LDH_3	14–29% of total	0.14–0.29 of total
LDH_4	5–11% of total	0.05–0.11 of total
LDH_5	2–11% of total	0.02–0.11 of total
Lipids, total, serum	450–850 mg/dl	4.5–8.5 g/l
Lipoprotein cholesterol, serum		
LDL cholesterol	60–180 mg/dl	600–1800 mg/l
HDL cholesterol	30–80 mg/dl	300–800 mg/l
Osmolality, serum	285–295 mOsm/kg serum water	285–295 mmol/kg serum water
Oxygen, blood		
Capacity	16–24 vol % (varies with hemoglobin)	7.14–10.7 mmol/l (varies with hemoglobin)
Content Arterial	15–23 vol %	6.69–10.3 mmol/l
Venous	10–16 vol %	4.46–7.14 mmol/l
Saturation Arterial	94–100% of capacity	0.94–1.00 of capacity
Venous	60–85% of capacity	0.60–0.85 of capacity
Tension, Po_2 Arterial	75–100 mm Hg	75–100 mm Hg
pH, arterial, blood	7.35–7.45	7.35–7.45
Phosphatase, acid serum	0.11–0.60 milliunit/ml (37°) (Roy, Brower, Hayden)	0.11–0.60 units/l
Phosphatase, alkaline, serum (ALP)	20–90 milliunits/ml (30°) (Values are higher in children)	20–90 units/l (30 C) (Values are higher in children)
Phospholipids, serum	6–12 mg/dl (As lipid phosphorus)	1.9–3.9 mmol/l (As lipid phosphorus)
Potassium, serum	3.5–5.0 mEq/liter	3.5–5.0 mmol/l
Protein, serum		
Total	6.0–8.0 grams/dl	60–80 g/l
Albumin	3.5–5.5 grams/dl 52–68% of total	35–55 g/l 0.52–0.68 of total
Globulin		
$Alpha_1$	0.2–0.4 gram/dl 2–5% of total	2–4 g/l 0.02–0.05 of total
$Alpha_2$	0.5–0.9 gram/dl 7–14% of total	5–9 g/l 0.07–0.14 of total
Beta	0.6–1.1 grams/dl 9–15% of total	6–11 g/l 0.09–0.15 of total

REFERENCE VALUES FOR BLOOD, PLASMA, AND SERUM *Continued*
(For some procedures the reference values may vary depending on the method used)

	Conventional Units	S.I. Units
Gamma	0.7–1.7 grams/dl	7–17 g/l
	11–21% of total	0.11–0.21 of total
Sodium, serum	136–145 mEq/liter	136–145 mmol/l
Thyroid-stimulating hormone (TSH), serum	0–7 microunits/ml	0–7 milliunits/l
Thyroxine, free, serum	1.0–2.1 nanogm/dl	13–27 pmol/l
Thyroxine (T_4), serum	4.4–9.9 mcg/dl	57–128 nmol/l
Thyroxine binding globulin (TBG), serum (as thyroxine)	10–26 mcg/dl	129–335 nmol/l
Thyroxine iodine, serum	2.9–6.4 mcg/dl	229–504 nmol/l
Triiodothyronine (T_3), serum	150–250 nanogm/dl	2.3–3.9 nmol/l
Triiodothyronine (T_3) uptake, resin (T_3RU)	25–38% uptake	0.25–0.38 uptake
Transaminase, serum		
SGOT (aspartate aminotransferase, AST)	8–20 milliunits/ml (30°)	8–20 units/l (30 C)
	7–40 milliunits/ml (37°)	7–40 units/l (37 C)
SGPT (alanine aminotransferase, ALT)	8–20 milliunits/ml (30°)	8–20 units/ml (30 C)
	5–35 milliunits/ml (37°)	5–35 units/ml (37 C)
Triglycerides, serum	40–150 mg/dl	0.4–1.5 g/l
		0.45–1.71 mmol/l
Urea nitrogen		
Blood	10–20 mg/dl	7.1–14.3 mmol/l
Plasma or serum	11–23 mg/dl	7.9–16.4 mmol/l

REFERENCE VALUES FOR URINE
(For some procedures the reference values may vary depending on the method used)

	Conventional Units	S.I. Units
Albumin		
Qualitative	Negative	Negative
Quantitative	10–100 mg/24 hrs	10–100 mg/24 h
		0.15–1.5 μmol/24 h
Aldosterone	3–20 mcg/24 hrs	8.3–55 nmol/24 h
Ammonia nitrogen	20–70 mEq/24 hrs	20–70 mmol/24 h
Amylase	1–17 units/hr	1–17 units/h
Amylase/creatinine clearance ratio	1–4%	0.01–0.04
Bilirubin, qualitative	Negative	Negative
Catecholamines		
Epinephrine	Less than 10 mcg/24 hrs	Less than 55 nmol/24 h
Norepinephrine	Less than 100 mcg/24 hrs	Less than 590 nmol/24 h
Total free catecholamines	4–126 mcg/24 hrs	24–745 nmol/24 h
Total metanephrines	0.1–1.6 mg/24 hrs	0.5–8.1 μmol/24 h
Cortisol, free	10–100 mcg/24 hrs	27.6–276 nmol/24 h
Creatinine	15–25 mg/kg body weight/24 hrs	0.13–0.22 mmol·kg^{-1} body weight/24 h
Creatinine clearance		
Males	110–150 ml/min	110–150 ml/min
Females	105–132 ml/min	105–132 ml/min
	(1.73 sq meter surface area)	(1.73 m^2 surface area)
17-Hydroxycorticosteroids		
Males	3–9 mg/24 hrs	8.3–25 μmol/24h
Females	2–8 mg/24 hrs	5.5–22 μmol/24 h
17-Ketosteroids		
Males	6–18 mg/24 hrs	21–62 μmol/24 h
Females	4–13 mg/24 hrs	14–45 μmol/24 h
	(Varies with age)	(Varies with age)
Metanephrines, *see* Catecholamines		
Osmolality	38–1400 mOsm/kg water	38–1400 mmol/kg water
pH	4.6–8.0, average 6.0	4.6–8.0, average 6.0
	(Depends on diet)	(Depends on diet)

Table continued on following page

REFERENCE VALUES FOR URINE *Continued*
(For some procedures the reference values may vary depending on the method used)

	Conventional Units	S.I. Units
Porphyrins		
Coproporphyrin	50–250 mcg/24 hrs	77–380 nmol/24 h
Uroporphyrin	10–30 mcg/24 hrs	12–36 nmol/24 h
Protein		
Qualitative	Negative	Negative
Quantitative	10–150 mg/24 hrs	10–150 mg/24 h
Specific gravity	1.003–1.030	1.003–1.030
Vanillylmandelic acid (VMA) (4-hydroxy-3-methoxymandelic acid)	1–8 mg/24 hrs	5–40 μmol/24 h

REFERENCE VALUES FOR THERAPEUTIC DRUG MONITORING

Drug	Therapeutic Range	Toxic Levels	Proprietary Names
Antibiotics			
Amikacin, serum	15–25 mcg/ml	Peak: >35 mcg/ml Trough: >5–8 mcg/ml	Amikin
Chloramphenicol, serum	10–20 mcg/ml	>25 mcg/ml	Chloromycetin
Gentamicin, serum	5–10 mcg/ml	Peak: >12 mcg/ml Trough: >2 mcg/ml	Garamycin
Tobramycin, serum	5–10 mcg/ml	Peak: >12 mcg/ml Trough: >2 mcg/ml	Nebcin
Anticonvulsants			
Carbamazepine, serum	5–12 mcg/ml	>12 mcg/ml	Tegretol
Ethosuximide, serum	40–100 mcg/ml	>100 mcg/ml	Zarontin
Phenobarbital, serum	10–30 mcg/ml	Vary widely because of developed tolerance	
Phenytoin, serum (diphenylhydantoin)	10–20 mcg/ml	>20 mcg/ml	Dilantin
Primidone, serum	5–12 mcg/ml	>15 mcg/ml	Mysoline
Valproic acid, serum	50–100 mcg/ml	>100 mcg/ml	Depakene
Analgesics			
Acetaminophen, serum	10–20 mcg/ml	>250 mcg/ml	Tylenol Datril
Salicylate, serum	100–250 mcg/ml	>300 mcg/ml	
Bronchodilator			
Theophylline (aminophylline)	10–20 mcg/ml	>20 mcg/ml	
Cardiovascular drugs			
Digitoxin, serum	15–25 nanogm/ml (Specimen obtained 12–24 hrs after last dose)	>25 nanogm/ml	Crystodigin
Digoxin, serum	0.8–2 nanogm/ml (Specimen obtained 12–24 hrs after last dose)	>2.4 nanogm/ml	Lanoxin
Disopyramide, serum	2–5 mcg/ml	>5 mcg/ml	Norpace
Lidocaine, serum	1.5–5 mcg/ml	>5 mcg/ml	Anestacon Xylocaine
Procainamide, serum	4–10 mcg/ml *10–30 mcg/ml (*Procainamide + N-acetyl procainamide)	>16 mcg/ml *>30 mcg/ml	Pronestyl
Propranolol, serum	50–100 nanogm/ml	Variable	Inderal
Quinidine, serum	2–5 mcg/ml	>10 mcg/ml	Cardioquin Quinaglute Quinidex Quinora

REFERENCE VALUES FOR THERAPEUTIC DRUG MONITORING *Continued*

Drug	Therapeutic Range	Toxic Levels	Proprietary Names
Psychopharmacologic drugs			
Amitriptyline, serum	*120–150 nanogm/ml (*Amitriptyline + nortriptyline)	*>500 nanogm/ml	Amitril Elavil Endep Etrafon Limbitrol Triavil
Bupropion	25–100 nanogm/ml	N/A	Wellbutrin
Desipramine, serum	*150–300 nanogm/ml *Desipramine + imipramine)	*>500 nanogm/ml	Norpramin Pertofrane
Fluoxitine	100–800 nanogm/ml (Lower levels may provide adequate clinical response)	N/A	Prozac
Haloperidol	3–20 nanogm/ml	N/A	Haldol
Imipramine, serum	*150–300 nanogm/ml (*Imipramine + desipramine)	*>500 nanogm/ml	Antipress Imavate Janimine Presamine Tofranil
Lithium, serum	0.8–1.2 mEq/liter (Specimen obtained 12 hrs after last dose)	>2.0 mEq/liter	Lithobid Lithotabs
Nortriptyline, serum	50–150 nanogm/ml	>500 nanogm/ml	Aventyl Pamelor
Trazodone	900–2100 nanogm/ml	N/A	Desyrel

REFERENCE VALUES FOR CEREBROSPINAL FLUID

	Conventional Units	S.I. Units
Cells	Fewer than 5/cu mm; all mononuclear	Fewer than 5/μl; all mononuclear
Chloride	120–130 mEq/liter (20 mEq/liter higher than serum)	120–130 mmol/l (20 mmol/l higher than serum)
Electrophoresis	Predominantly albumin	Predominantly albumin
Glucose	50–75 mg/dl (20 mg/dl less than serum)	2.8–4.2 mmol/l (1.1. mmol/less than serum)
IgG		
Children under 14	Less than 8% of total protein	Less than 0.08 of total protein
Adults	Less than 14% of total protein	Less than 0.14 lof total protein
Pressure	70–180 mm water	70–180 mm water
Protein, total	15–45 mg/dl (Higher, up to 0.70 mg/dl, in elderly adults and children)	0.150–0.450 g/l (Higher, up to 0.70 g/l, in elderly adults and children)

REFERENCE VALUES FOR FECES

	Conventional Units	S.I. Units
Bulk	100–200 grams/24 hrs	100–200 g/24 h
Dry matter	23–32 grams/24 hrs	23–32 g/24 h
Fat, total	Less than 6.0 grams/24 hrs	Less than 6.0 g/24 h
Nitrogen, total	Less than 2.0 grams/24 hrs	Less than 2.0 g/24 h
Urobilinogen	40–280 mg/24 hrs	40–280 mg/24 h
Water	Approximately 65%	Approximately 0.65

REFERENCE VALUES FOR IMMUNOLOGIC PROCEDURES

	Conventional Units
Lymphocyte subsets	
T cells	60–85%
B cells	1–20%
T-helper cells	35–60%
T-suppressor cells	15–30%
T-H/S ratio	1.5–2.5
Complement	
C3	85–175 mg/dl
C4	15–45 mg/dl
CH_{50}	25–55 H_{50} units/ml
Tumor markers	
Carcinoembryonic antigen (CEA)	
(Roche)	Less than 5 nanogm/ml
(Abbott)	Less than 4.1 nanogm/ml
Alpha-fetoprotein (AFP)	Less than 10–30 nanogm/ml (depends on method)

ORAL GLUCOSE TOLERANCE TEST

The oral glucose tolerance test (OGTT) may be unnecessary if the fasting plasma glucose concentration is elevated (venous plasma ≥140 mg/dl or 7.8 mmol/l) on two occasions. The OGTT should be carried out only on patients who are ambulatory and otherwise healthy and who are known not to be taking agents that elevate the plasma glucose (Page and Vigourex, 1974). The test should be conducted in the morning after at least 3 days of unrestricted diet (≥150 grams of carbohydrate) and physical activity. The subject should have fasted for at least 10 hours but no more than 16 hours. Water is permitted during the test period; however, the subject should remain seated and should not smoke throughout the test.

The dose of glucose administered should be 75 grams (1.75 grams per kg of ideal body weight, up to a maximum of 75 grams for children). Commercial preparations containing a suitable carbohydrate load are acceptable. If criteria for gestational diabetes are used, a dose of 100 grams of glucose is required.

A fasting blood sample should be collected, after which the glucose dose is taken within 5 minutes. Blood samples should be collected at 30 minute intervals for 2 hours (for gestational diabetes, fasting 1, 2, and 3 hours). The following diagnostic criteria have been recommended by the National Diabetes Data Group:

Normal OGTT in Nonpregnant Adults	Fasting venous plasma glucose <115 mg/dl (6.4 mmol/l); ½ h, 1 h, and 1½ h OGTT venous plasma glucose <200 mg/dl (11.1 mmol/l); 2 h OGTT venous plasma glucose <140 mg/dl (7.8 mmol/l)
Diabetes Mellitus in Nonpregnant Adults	Both the 2 hour sample *and* some other sample taken between administration of the 75 gram glucose dose and 2 hours later must show a venous plasma glucose ≥200 mg/dl (11.1 mmol/l)
Impaired Glucose Tolerance in Nonpregnant Adults	Three criteria must be met: Fasting venous plasma glucose <140 mg/dl (7.8 mmol/l); ½ h, 1 h, or 1½ h OGTT value ≥200 mg/dl (11.1 mmol/l); 2 h OGTT venous plasma glucose between 140 and 200 mg/dl (7.8 and 11.1 mmol/l)
Gestational Diabetes	Two or more of the following values after a 100 gram oral glucose challenge must be met or exceeded: (values are for venous plasma glucose)

Fasting	105 mg/dl	5.8 mmol/l
1h	190 mg/dl	10.6 mmol/l
2h	165 mg/dl	9.2 mmol/l
3h	145 mg/dl	8.1 mmol/l

REFERENCES

AMA Council on Scientific Affairs: J.A.M.A. *253*:2552, 1985.

AMA Drug Evaluations, 6th ed. Chicago, American Medical Association, 1986.

Goodman, A. G., Gilman, L. S., Rall, T. W., and Murad, F.: Goodman and Gilman's The Pharmacological Basis of Therapeutics, 7th ed. New York, Macmillan, 1985.

Henry, J. B.: Clinical Diagnosis and Management by Laboratory Methods, 17th ed. Philadelphia, W. B. Saunders Company, 1984.

Henry, R. J., Cannon, D. C., and Winkleman, J. W.: Clinical Chemistry—Principles and Techniques, 2nd ed. New York, Harper & Row, 1974.

International Committee for Standardization in Hematology, International Federation of Clinical Chemistry and World Association of Pathology Societies: Clin. Chem. *19*:135, 1973.

Lundberg, G. D., Iverson, C., and Radulescu, G.: J.A.M.A. *255*:2247, 1986.

Miale, J. B.: Laboratory Medicine—Hematology, 6th ed. St. Louis, C. V. Mosby, 1982.

National Diabetes Data Group: Diabetes *28*:1039, 1979.

Page, C. H., and Vigourex, P.: The International System of Units (S.I.). U.S. Department of Commerce, National Bureau of Standards, Special Publication 330, 1974.

Physicians' Desk Reference, 43rd ed. Oradell, N. J., Medical Economics Company, 1989.

Scully, R. E., McNeely, B. U., and Mark, E. J.: N. Engl. J. Med. *314*:39, 1986.

Tietz, N. W.: Clinical Guide to Laboratory Tests. Philadelphia, W. B. Saunders Company, 1983.

Tietz, N. W.: Textbook of Clinical Chemistry. Philadelphia, W. B. Saunders Company, 1986.

Williams, W. J., Beutler, E., Erslev, A. J., and Lichtman, M. A.: Hematology, 3rd ed. New York, McGraw-Hill Book Company, 1983.

Some of the values have been established by the Clinical Pathology Laboratories, Emory University Hospital, Atlanta, Georgia, or by the Clinical Laboratories, Thomas Jefferson University Hospital, Philadelphia, Pennsylvania, and have not been published elsewhere.

Glossary

Abduction: Movement away from the midline of the body.
Abrasion: A wound caused by rubbing or scraping the skin or mucous membrane.
Absorption: The passage of liquids or other substances through a body surface and into its tissues and fluids, as in absorption of the end products of digestion into the intestinal villi.
Acceptance: Admission of reality, as in the reality of death; the final stage in the process of dealing with dying and death.
Accommodation: Adjustment, especially of the ocular lens for seeing objects at varying distances.
Acid: A substance that yields hydrogen ions in solution.
Acid-base balance: A normal condition in which the narrow range of normal pH and the normal ratio of carbonic acid to bicarbonate ions are maintained.
Acidosis: A condition in which the pH of body fluids is below normal range because of either a loss of base bicarbonate or an accumulation of acid.
Acquired immunodeficiency syndrome (AIDS): A group of symptoms believed to be caused by a virus (HIV) that infects and destroys T lymphocytes.
Acute myocardial infarction: Ischemic necrosis of an area of the heart muscle resulting from sudden occlusion of blood flow through one or more branches of the coronary arteries.
Adduction: Movement toward the midline of the body.
Adhesion: A fibrous band that binds two parts together that are normally separated; often occurs after surgery in the abdomen.
Adjuvant: That which assists, such as a drug added to a prescription that enhances the principal ingredient.
Adrenergic: Action that mimics that of the sympathetic nervous system.
Adrenocortical: Indicating the cortex of the adrenal gland.
Adulthood: A stage of life at which the individual has reached biologic maturity, usually at age 20.
Aerobe: A microorganism that requires oxygen for survival.
Aerobic: Term for an organism that requires oxygen to live.
Aerosol: A suspension of a drug or other substance that is dispensed in a cloud or mist.
Ageism: Prejudice against aging and aged persons.
Airway: The passage by which air enters and leaves the lungs; also, a device used to secure unobstructed respiration.
Albumin, serum: A plasma protein formed principally in the liver and constituting about 60% of the protein concentration in the plasma.
Alkalosis: A condition in which the pH of body fluids is above normal because of either a loss of acid or an accumulation of base bicarbonate.
Allergen(s): Any substance capable of triggering an exaggerated immune response.
Allergy (allergies): An abnormal and individual hypersensitivity to a particular allergen; acquired by exposure to the allergen and manifested after reexposure.
Alopecia: Baldness or loss of hair.
Amenorrhea: Absence of menstruation.
Anaerobic: Term for an organism that lives in an oxygen-free environment.
Analgesic(s): Pain reliever.
Anaphylaxis: An unusual or exaggerated allergic reaction.
Anastomosis: Communication between two tubular organs; also surgical, traumatic, or pathologic formation of a connection between two normally distinct structures.
Androgen(s): Any steroid hormone that promotes male characteristics.
Anemia(s): Insufficient numbers of functioning red blood cells to meet the oxygen needs of tissues.
Anesthesia: Loss of feeling or sensation.
Aneurysm: Sac formed by localized dilatation of the wall of a blood vessel or the heart.
Anger: A feeling of hostility and bitterness against a situation or person; a second stage in acceptance of death.
Angina pectoris: Exertional chest pain caused by ischemia of heart muscle and increased demand for oxygen.
Angiography: X-ray studies of the arteries, veins, or lymph vessels of the body.
Anion: A negatively charged atomic particle.
Ankylosis: Abnormal immobility and consolidation and obliteration of a joint.
Anorexia: Lack or loss of appetite for food.
Anorexia nervosa: An eating disorder in which there is an aberration of eating patterns, severe weight loss, and malnutrition.
Antiarrhythmic agents: Substances that help return the heart rate and rhythm to more normal values and restore the origin of the heart's electrical activity to its natural pacemaker.
Antibiotic: An agent that is capable of either killing or inhibiting the growth of microorganisms.
Antibody(ies): An immunoglobulin molecule that is capable of adhering to and interacting only with the antigen that induced its synthesis.
Anticoagulants: Substances that suppress, delay, or nullify coagulation of blood.
Antiemetic: An agent that prevents or relieves nausea and vomiting.
Antigen(s): Any substance that can bring about production of an antagonist.
Antifungal(s): Agents destructive to or inhibitive of the growth of fungi.

Antigen-antibody reaction: An immune response that occurs when an antibody comes in contact with the specific antigen for which it was formed. In a transfusion reaction the response is a clumping together, or agglutination, of the red blood cells carrying the antigens.

Antihistamine: An agent that counteracts the effects of histamine; used to relieve the symptoms of an allergic reaction.

Antimicrobial agent: Substance capable of either killing or suppressing the multiplication and growth of microorganisms.

Antineoplastic agent: Substance that inhibits the maturation and proliferation of malignant cells.

Antiseptic(s): Any substance that inhibits the growth of bacteria outside the body; in contrast, a germicide kills the bacteria outright.

Antitoxin: A specific kind of antibody produced in response to the presence of a toxin.

Antitussive: An agent that inhibits the cough reflex in the cough center in the brain.

Antivenin: A substance used to neutralize the venom of a poisonous animal.

Anuria: Diminished or absent production of urine by the kidney.

Aphakic eye: One without a lens, as after a cataract extraction.

Aphasia: A defect in or loss of the power of expression by speech, writing, or signs or in the comprehension of spoken or written language.

Aplastic: Having deficient or arrested development.

Arrhythmia: Variation from the normal rhythm, especially of the heartbeat.

Arteriosclerosis: A group of diseases characterized by thickening and loss of elasticity of the arterial walls.

Arthritis: Inflammation of a joint.

Arthrocentesis: Surgical puncture of a joint cavity for aspiration of synovial fluid.

Arthroplasty: Surgery of a joint to increase mobility or decrease pain.

Arthroscopy: Endoscopic examination of the interior of a joint.

Ascites: Accumulation of edematous fluid within the peritoneal cavity.

Asepsis, medical: Destruction and containment of infectious agents after they leave the body of a patient with an infectious disease.

Assessment, nursing: Data-gathering activities for the purpose of collecting a complete, relevant data base from which a nursing diagnosis can be made.

Astigmatism: Error of refraction in which light rays are not sharply focused on the retina, because of abnormal curvature of the cornea or lens.

Ataxia: Incoordinated motor movements.

Atelectasis: The collapsed or airless state of the lung.

Atherosclerosis: A disease process in which fibrinous plaques are laid down on the inner walls of the arteries, thus narrowing the lumens of the vessels and predisposing them to the development of intravascular clots.

Atrial fibrillation: Rapid, irregular, and ineffective contractions of the atria.

Atrophy: Wasting or a decrease in size from lack of use.

Audiometry: Measurement of sound perception.

Aura: A peculiar sensation preceding the appearance of more definite symptoms, especially a sensation that occurs immediately before an epileptic seizure.

Autoimmune disease: One caused by the body's failure to recognize its own cells, thus rejecting them as it would a foreign substance.

Autonomic dysreflexia: Hyperreflexia, an uninhibited and exaggerated reflex response of the autonomic nervous system to some type of stimulation.

Avulsion: The tearing away of part or all of an organ or structure.

Axon: The process of a neuron that transmits impulses away from the cell body.

Azotemia: Retention in the blood of urea, creatinine, and other nitrogenous protein metabolites that are normally eliminated in the urine.

B lymphocyte: A sensitized lymphocyte that is responsible for antibody formation and the development of humoral immunity.

Babinski reflex: A reflex action elicited by stimulating the sole of the foot and characterized by dorsiflexion of the great toe and flaring of the smaller toes. A positive Babinski indicates an abnormality in the motor control pathways of the nervous sytem.

Bacteria: Microscopically small organisms belonging to the plant kingdom, some of which are capable of producing disease in humans.

Bactericidal: Able to kill bacteria.

Bacteriophage: A virus that destroys bacteria by lysis. The virus is usually of a type specific for the particular kind of bacteria it attacks.

Bacteriostatic: Able to slow duplication of bacteria.

Bargaining: An attempt to make an arrangement whereby one gives something in order to gain something in return; the third stage in acceptance of death.

Base: A substance that combines with acids to form salts.

Behavior: The manner in which one conducts oneself in response to social stimuli, an inner need, or a combination of the two.

Benign: Not very harmful; nonmalignant.

Biliary: Pertaining to bile, the bile ducts, or the gallbladder.

Biliary colic: Acute pain resulting from obstruction of a bile duct, usually caused by cholelithiasis.

Biopsy: Removal of living cells for the purpose of examining them microscopically.

Bladder, cord: Dysfunction of the urinary bladder caused by damage to the spinal cord.

- **neurogenic:** A dysfunction of the urinary bladder caused by a lesion of the central or peripheral nervous system, and characterized by lack of awareness of the need to void.

Blepharitis: Infection of glands and lash follicles along the margin of the eyelid.

Blood gases

- **arterial (ABGs):** The partial pressure exerted by oxygen and carbon dioxide in the arterial blood. ABGs reflect the ability of the lungs to exchange these gases, the effectiveness of the kidneys to retain and eliminate bicarbonate, and the efficiency of the heart as a pump.

Botulism: Food poisoning caused by a neurotoxin produced by *Clostridium botulinum*, sometimes found in improperly canned or preserved foods.

Bradycardia: Slowness of the heart beat, as evidenced by slowing of the pulse rate to less than 60 per minute.

Bronchodilator: A drug that acts directly on the smooth muscles of the bronchi to relax them and relieve bronchospasm.
Bronchogram: An x-ray of the bronchial tree using a radiopaque substance that is introduced into the trachea.
Bronchoscopy: Insertion of an endoscope for diagnosis and treatment of disorders of the bronchi.
Bulla (bullae): A blister; a round, fluid-filled lesion of the skin, usually more than 5 mm in diameter.
Burns
full-thickness: One in which all of the epithelializing elements and those lining the sweat glands, hair follicles, and sebaceous glands are destroyed.
partial-thickness: One in which the epithelializing elements remain intact.

Cachexia: A profound state of general ill health and malnutrition.
Calculus (calculi): An abnormal concretion, usually of mineral salts, occurring mainly in hollow organs or their passages (e.g., renal calculus, or kidney stone).
Callus: A thicknened area of the epidermis caused by pressure or friction.
Carcinoma: A malignant growth made up of epithelial cells.
Cardiac glycosides: A group of compounds containing a carbohydrate molecule (for example, digitalis) that affect the contractile force of the heart muscle.
Cardiac tamponade: Compression of the heart caused by collection of fluid in the pericardial sac.
Cardiogenic shock: Shock state caused by pump failure of the heart.
Cardiopulmonary resuscitation: Reestablishment of heart and lung action after they have suddenly stopped.
Cardiotonic(s): Agent having the effect of strengthening contractions of heart muscle.
Carriers: Persons who harbor infectious organisms within their bodies without manifesting any outward symptoms of the infection.
Catabolism: The phase of metabolism in which larger molecules are broken down and energy is released.
Cataract(s): Opacity of the lens of the eye.
Category-specific precautions: A system of precautionary measures organized according to types of diseases (for example, respiratory or enteric) and employed for the purpose of preventing the spread of disease.
Cations: Positively charged atomic particles.
Cell(s): The basic structural unit of living organisms.
Central hearing loss: Impaired perception of sound caused by pathology above the junction of the eighth cranial nerve and the brain stem.
Chalazion: Infection of the meibomian gland; internal stye.
Chemonucleolysis: Treatment of a herniated intervertebral disk by dissolution of a portion of the nucleus pulposus by injection of a chemolytic agent.
Chemotherapy: Use of chemicals, especially drugs, in the treatment of such diseases as cancer, infection, and some mental illnesses.
Cholecystitis: Inflammation of the gallblader.
Cholelithiasis: Presence of stones within the gallbladder or biliary tract.
Cholinergic: Agent that produces the effect of acetylcholine.
Chorea: Involuntary muscle twitching.
Cirrhosis, of liver: A condition characterized by destruction of normal hepatic structures and their replacement with necrotic tissue and scarring.
Claudication, intermittent: A syndrome characterized by intensification of limb pain as exercise is increased; related to occlusion of arteries in the legs.
Climacteric: Endocrine, somatic, and psychic changes occurring at the end of the female reproductive period (menopause); also normal diminution of testicular activity in the male.
Clonic: Alternating contraction and relaxation of muscles.
Code of ethics: A set of rules governing one's conduct.
Coitus: Sexual intercourse.
Colic: Spasm causing pain; may be biliary, renal, intestinal, or uterine.
Collagen: Fibrous protein found in skin, bone, cartilage, and ligaments.
Colostomy (colostomies): Surgical creation of an opening in the colon to allow for passage of fecal material to the outside.
Colposcopy: Visual examination of the vagina and cervix with a specially designed endoscope that allows for detection of malignant growths in their early stages.
Comedo (comedones): A plug of keratin and sebum within an enlarged pore; a blackhead.
Complement system: A complex series of enzymatic proteins that interact to combine with the antigen-antibody complex, producing lysis of intact antigen cells.
Complete blood count (CBC): The number of each kind of cell in a sample of blood.
Computed tomography (CT) scan: A computer-aided technique in which small sections of tissue within an organ can be visualized by radiograph.
Concept(s): An idea, thought, or notion derived from experiences and information acquired from one's external environment.
Conductive hearing loss: Impaired perception of sound caused by a dysfunction of either the external or the middle ear.
Congestive heart failure: Exhaustion of heart muscle and a resultant engorgement of the heart's chambers and the blood vessels. Eventually, sluggish blood flow leads to retention of fluid and edema in lungs and elsewhere in the body.
Conjunctivitis: Inflammation of the membrane covering the eyeball and lining the eyelids.
Consciousness: Responsiveness of the mind to impressions made by the senses.
Contamination: Presence of a noxious agent such as bacteria or radiation in a place where it is not wanted.
Contracture(s): Adaptive shortening of skeletal muscle tissue that is not subjected to normal stretching and contraction.
Convulsion: State of involuntary muscle contractions and relaxations.
Coronary occlusion: Closing off of a coronary artery and interruption of its blood flow.
Creatinine: A nonprotein substance that is formed in muscle in relatively small and constant amounts, passes into the blood stream, and is eliminated by the kidney. Urine creatinine levels are diminished when glomerular filtration is impaired.

Credé technique: Downward pressure with the open hand over the suprapubic area to facilitate emptying of the urinary bladder.

Crust: An outer layer of solid matter formed by dried exudate or secretion.

Cryoprecipitate: Any precipitate that forms as a result of cooling.

Cryosurgery: Destruction of tissue by application of extreme cold, as in removal of cataracts.

Cryptorchidism (cryptorchism): Failure of one or both of the testes to descend into the scrotum during fetal life.

Culdoscopy: Direct inspection of the female viscera through an endoscope introduced into the pelvic cavity through the posterior vaginal fornix.

Culture: Propagation of microorganisms or living tissue cells in media conducive to their growth.

Curettage: Cleansing of a surface of an organ with a spoon-shaped instrument (curet).

Cyanosis: A bluish tinge to the skin caused by lack of oxygen and accumulation of carbon dioxide in the blood.

Cystogram: Radiograph of the urinary bladder using a contrast medium.

Cystoscopy: Endoscopic examination of the interior of the bladder.

Cytology: The study of cells, their origin, structure, function, and pathology.

Dactylitis: An inflammation of a finger or toe.

Death(s): The cessation of all physical and chemical processes that invariably occurs in all living organisms. See also *Dying*.

Débridement: Removal of all foreign material and dead tissues from or adjacent to a traumatic or infected lesion until healthy tissue is exposed.

Decubitus ulcer(s): A breakdown in the skin and underlying tissues caused by long-standing pressure, ischemia, and damage to the underlying tissue.

Defibrillation: To stop fibrillation of the heart with electrical current.

Dehiscence: Separation of all layers of a surgical wound.

Delirium: An altered state of consciousness that is usually acute and of short duration.

Demyelinization: Destruction of the myelin sheath of nerve tissue.

Dendrite: Any of the threadlike extensions of the cytoplasm of a neuron.

Denial: Defense mechanism in which existence of intolerable conditions are unconsciously rejected; first stage in the acceptance of death.

Depression: A morbid sadness, dejection, or melancholy; a stage in the acceptance of death.

Dermabrasion: Planing of the skin done by mechanical means for the purpose of smoothing the skin and removing scars.

Dermatitis: Inflammation of the skin.

Dermatology: The medical specialty concerned with the diagnosis and treatment of skin disorders.

Developmental task(s): One that should be completed during a specific life period in order to ensure continuing psychosocial growth and maturity.

Diabetic neuropathy: A disorder of the peripheral nerves that is associated with diabetes mellitus and is characterized by sexual impotence in the male, neurogenic bladder, and pain or loss of feeling in the lower extremities.

Diagnosis, nursing: A concise statement of a patient's actual or potential health problems that nurses, by virtue of their education and experience, are capable and licensed to treat.

Dialysis: The diffusion of solute molecules through a semipermeable membrane, the molecules passing from the more concentrated solution to the less concentrated one.

Diaphoresis: Excessive perspiration.

peritoneal: Use of the peritoneum as a dialyzing membrane to remove waste products that have accumulated in the body as a result of renal failure.

Diastole: The phase of the cardiac cycle in which the heart muscle relaxes between contractions; during this phase the two ventricles are dilated by blood flowing through them. Diastolic blood pressure is recorded as the bottom number in the pressure measurement.

Diffusion: The spontaneous mixing of the molecules or ions of two or more substances; the result of random thermal motion.

Digitalization: Initial administration of digitalis to build up a therapeutic blood level of the drug.

Diplopia: Double vision; seeing two images.

Disease-specific precautions: A system of precautionary measures organized according to the specific infectious disease presented by the patient.

Disinfectant(s): An agent that destroys infection-producing organisms.

Dislocation: Stretching or tearing of ligaments around a joint with complete displacement of a bone.

Distal: In a position farthest from the point of reference.

Diuresis: Excretion of excess fluid in the urine.

Diuretic(s): Agents that promote secretion of urine.

Diverticulum (diverticula): Small blind pouches resulting from a protrusion of the mucosa of a hollow organ through weakened areas in the organ's muscle wall.

Documentation: The recording of significant information on a patient's chart.

Down's syndrome: A congenital disorder characterized by physical malformations and some degree of mental retardation; also called trisomy 21 syndrome because there is a defect in chromosome 21.

Dumping syndrome: A group of symptoms caused by too-rapid passage of food through the upper gastrointestinal tract.

Dying: A stage of life; a process that from a medical point of view begins when a person has a disease that is untreatable and inevitably ends in death; or the final stages of a fatal disease. See also *Death(s)*.

Dynamic: Having vital force or inherent power.

Dyscrasia: An imbalance of formed elements, as in blood dyscrasia.

Dyspareunia: Difficult or painful coitus in women.

Dysphagia: Difficulty in swallowing.

Dysphasia: Difficulty speaking; usually caused by a brain lesion.

Dyspnea: Labored or difficult breathing.

Dysuria: Painful urination.

Ecchymosis: Irregularly formed macular areas of hemorrhage in the skin.

ECG: The record produced by amplification of the electrical impulses normally generated by the heart.

Ectopic: Located away from normal position, as in ectopic pregnancy.

Ectropion: Outward turning of the eyelid.

Edema: An accumulation of fluid surrounding the cell.

EEG: A recording of changes in electrical potentials in the brain.

EKG: The record produced by amplification of the electrical impulses normally generated by the heart.

Elastance: The extent to which the lungs are able to return to their original position after being barely distended.

Electrocardiogram: The record produced by amplification of the electrical impulses normally generated by the heart.

Electroencephalogram: A recording of changes in electric potentials in various areas of the brain.

Electrolyte(s): A chemical substance that when dissolved in water dissociates into ions and thus is capable of conducting an electric current.

Electromyography: The recording and study of intrinsic electrical properties of skeletal muscle; useful in diagnosing neuromuscular disorders.

Elimination: Discharge from the body of indigestible materials and waste products of metabolism.

Embolism: Sudden obstruction of arterial blood flow by a blood clot or a mass that has been brought to the site in the blood stream.

Empyema: The presence of infected and purulent exudate within the pleural cavity.

Endarterectomy: Surgical removal of thickened atheromatous areas of the innermost coat of an artery.

Endemic: Present in a community at all times.

Endocarditis: Inflammation of the membrane lining the cavities of the heart and of the connective tissue bed on which it lies.

Endocrine: Secreting internally; refers to glandular function.

Endogenous: Coming from within.

Endometriosis: The presence of endometrial tissue in locations outside the uterus.

Endorphin: One of a group of opiate-like peptides naturally produced by the body.

Endoscopy: Examination by means of an endoscope that allows for direct visual inspection of the interior of hollow organs and body cavities.

Endotoxin(s): Heat-stable toxin that is present in the intact bacterial cell wall, is pyrogenic, and is capable of increasing capillary permeability.

Entropion: Inversion of the eyelid margin.

Enucleation: Removal of an organ or other mass intact, as of the eyeball from the orbit.

Enzyme: Any protein that acts as a catalyst, increasing the rate at which chemical reaction occurs.

Epidemic(s): Disease that simultaneously attacks many people in a geographic area, is widely diffused, and spreads rapidly.

Epidermophytosis: A fungal infection that most often affects the feet, especially between the toes; also called *athlete's foot, dermophytosis.*

Epistaxis: Nosebleed.

Erythema: Redness of the skin.

Erythrasma: A chronic bacterial infection of the major skin folds, marked by red or brownish patches on the skin.

Erythrocyte sedimentation rate: The rate at which red blood cells settle out of unclotted blood in an hour.

Erythropoiesis: Formation of erythrocytes.

Eschar: A cast-out of dead tissue, as from a burn, corrosive application, or gangrene.

Esophageal varices: Varicosities of branches of the azygous vein that connect with the portal vein in the lower esophagus; related to portal hypertension and cirrhosis of the liver.

Estrogens: The female sex hormones, including estradiol, estriol, and estrone.

Etiology: Study of the cause of disease; origin.

Euthanasia: An easy or painless death; active euthanasia, or mercy killing, is the deliberate ending of the life of a person who is incurably and terminally ill; passive euthanasia is the withholding of "heroic" measures and allowing the person to die.

Evaluation:

- **of outcome:** Appraisal of the patient's progress toward achievement of the goals and objectives stated in the nursing care plan.
- **of process:** Appraisal of nursing activities and what has been done to assess, plan, and implement nursing care.
- **of structure:** Appraisal of the physical facilities, equipment, staffing, and other characteristics of an agency that affect the quality of nursing care.

Evisceration: (1) extrusion of internal organs; (2) removal of the contents of the eyeball, leaving the sclera intact.

Excoriation: Any superficial loss of substance, such as that produced by scratching the skin.

Exercise(s)

- **isometric:** Active exercise performed against stable resistance, without change in the length of the muscle.

Exocrine: Secreting externally via a duct.

Exogenous: Coming from outside.

Exotoxin: A potent toxin formed and excreted by the bacterial cell.

Extracellular fluids: Body fluids outside the cell walls that constitute the environment of each cell.

Exudate: Fluid that contains dead cells, serum, phagocytes, bacteria, or pus.

Fecal impaction: Accumulation of puttylike or hardened feces in the rectum or sigmoid colon.

Feedback: The process of providing a system information about its output.

- **negative:** A corrective action in which a system is informed its output is not satisfactory and a change is needed.
- **positive:** Information that tells a system its output is satisfactory.

Fibrocystic breast disease: A condition characterized by single or multiple benign tumors in the breast, sometimes called chronic mastitis.

Fibrosis: Fibrous tissue formation.

Fistula(s): Any abnormal, tubelike passage within the body between two internal organs or leading from an internal organ to the body surface.

Flaccid: Limp, weak, or relaxed.

Fluid(s): The water and substances dissolved in it that form the internal environment.

- **transcellular:** Body fluids that pass through cellular structures and eventually are eliminated from the body.

Fluid balance: Equilibrium between the amount of fluid taken into the body and that lost through urine, feces, the lungs, skin, and possibly vomiting and fistulas.

Fluid deficit(s): Fluid imbalance in which there is not enough fluid in one or more of the body's fluid compartments as a result of either inadequate intake or excessive loss.

Fluid excess: Imbalance in which there is the accumulation of too much fluid in one or more of the body's fluid compartments. See also *Edema.*

Fracture(s): Interruption in the continuity of a bone.

Fungus (fungi): A member of a group of eukaryotic organisms (mushrooms, yeasts, molds, etc.) that thrive in a warm, moist climate and can cause infections difficult to eradicate because they tend to reproduce by means of spores that are resistant to ordinary disinfectants and antiseptics.

Galactosemia: A genetic disorder in which there is a lack of the enzyme necessary for proper metabolism of galactose.

Gastrostomy: Surgical creation of an opening into the stomach to provide for administration of food and liquids.

Gate control theory: The proposal that synapses in the dorsal horn of the spinal cord act as gates, and that pain signals compete with those of other kinds of stimuli for passage through the gate and transmission to the brain.

Gene: One of the self-reproducing biologic units of heredity that make up segments of the DNA molecule, which controls cellular reproduction and function.

Geriatrics: Medical treatment of diseases commonly associated with aging and aged persons.

Gerontology: Study of the problems of aging in all its aspects.

Glaucoma: A group of diseases of the eye, characterized by increased intraocular pressure, that can produce blindness if not managed successfully.

Globulin(s): General term for proteins; separated into five fractions by serum protein electrophoresis and classified in order of decreasing electrophoretic mobility. The fractions are alpha 1-, alpha 2-, beta 1-, and beta 2-globulins, and the gamma globulins.

Glucocorticoid(s): Any hormone released from the adrenal cortex that increases glucogenesis and thus raises the level of liver glycogen and blood glucose.

Glycosuria: Glucose in the urine.

Glycosylated hemoglobin (HGB A-1-C): Hemoglobin with glucose attached to it; periodic measurements of hemoglobin A-1-C can help determine a diabetic patient's average blood glucose level over a period of 3 to 4 months.

Goal(s): A broad statement describing what is to be accomplished over a specified period of time.

Goniometry: Measurement of range of motion in a joint.

Graft(s): Implant or transplant of tissue or an organ.

Granulocyte(s): Leukocyte containing abundant granules in its cytoplasm; granulocytes include neutrophils, eosinophils, and basophils.

Health: The ability to function well physically and mentally and to express the full range of one's potentialities.

Hearing, loss of: Impaired perception of sound.

Heat exhaustion: A disorder resulting from overexposure to heat or to the sun; also called *heat prostration.* It is caused by excessive perspiration and loss of body water and salt.

Heatstroke: A life-threatening condition resulting from prolonged exposure to environmental heat; also called *sunstroke.*

Helping relationship: One in which at least one of the parties intends to promote growth, development, maturity, improved functioning, and improved coping in the life of the other.

Hematemesis: Vomiting of blood.

Hematocrit: The volume percentage of red blood cells in whole blood.

Hematoma(s): A localized collection of blood, usually clotted, that has leaked from adjacent blood vessels into an organ, space, or tissue.

Hematuria: Blood in the urine.

Hemiplegia: Paralysis of one half, or one side, of the body.

Hemodialysis: Removal of nitrogenous wastes from the blood by circulating arterial blood through a dialysate and returning it to venous circulation.

Hemodynamics: Study of the movements of blood and the pressures being exerted in the blood vessels and the chambers of the heart.

Hemoglobin: The protein found in red blood cells that transports molecular oxygen in the blood; oxygenated hemoglobin (oxyhemoglobin) is bright red in color; unoxygenated hemoglobin is darker.

Hemolysis: Rupture of erythrocytes with release of hemoglobin into the plasma.

Hemophilia: An inherited disorder in which there is deficiency of one or more specific clotting factors in the blood.

Hemoptysis: Coughing and spitting of blood that can originate in the lungs, larynx, or trachea.

Hemothorax: Collection of blood in the pleural cavity.

Hepatic encephalopathy: Degenerative changes in the brain associated with liver failure.

Hepatitis: Inflammation of the liver.

Herpesvirus: Any of a large group of DNA viruses found in many animal species. Type 1 herpes simplex virus (HSV) produces lesions that are primarily nongenital. Type 2 HSV lesions are most often genital.

Hiatus hernia: Protrusion of a portion of the stomach through the opening in the diaphragm through which the esophagus passes.

Hierarchy: The arrangement of objects, elements, or values in a graduated series.

Hirsutism: Condition of excessive growth of hair on the body.

Holism: The belief that each person is a unified whole.

Holistic health care: Attention to the mental, social, spiritual, and physical aspects of health and illness.

Homeostasis: A tendency of biological systems to maintain stability in the internal environment while continually adjusting to changes necessary for survival.

Hordoleum: An external stye.

Hormone(s): A chemical produced by the cells of the body and transported by the blood stream to target cells and organs, on which it has a regulatory effect.

Hospice: A program that provides a continuum of home and inpatient care for the terminally ill person and his family.

Human needs: Basic needs for survival and personal growth shared by all humans.

theory: The proposal that basic human needs act as stimuli to human behavior; Maslow postulated five levels of human needs: physiologic, safety and security, love and belonging, esteem, and self-actualization.

Humoral: Pertaining to body fluids or substances contained in them.

Hydronephrosis: Distention of the renal pelvis and calices with urine that cannot flow through obstructed ureters.

Hyperalimentation: Total parenteral nutrition.

Hypercalcemia: An above-normal level of calcium in the blood (i.e., more than 5.5 mEq/L or 11 mg/dL).

Hyperopia: A visual defect in which parallel light rays reaching the eye focus behind the retina; farsightedness.

Hyperplasia: Increase in the number of cells of an organ; extra cell growth.

Hypersensitivity: An exaggerated immune response to an agent perceived by the body to be foreign. See also *Allergy (allergies)*.

Hypertension: Persistently high blood pressure; in adults, a systolic pressure equal to or greater than 140 mm Hg and a diastolic pressure equal to or greater than 90 mm Hg.

Hypertonic solution: One in which the osmotic pressure (concentration) is greater than that of body fluids.

Hypertrophy: Increase in size of a structure or organ.

Hyperventilation: An abnormal breathing pattern in which an above-normal amount of air is inhaled into the lungs.

Hypocalcemia: A below-normal level of calcium in the blood (i.e., less than 4.5 mEq/L or 8.5 mg/dL).

Hypocapnia: A deficit of carbon dioxide in the blood resulting from hyperventilation.

Hypogammaglobulinemia: An immune deficiency characterized by abnormally low levels of generally all classes of serum gammaglobulins with increased susceptibility to infectious diseases.

Hypoglycemic agents: Those that lower the blood glucose level (for example, oral medications that are used to treat some forms of diabetes mellitus).

Hyposensitization: A treatment used in management of hypersensitivity to a known allergen; the program involves regular injections of minute quantities of selected antigens over an extended period of time.

Hypothalamus: That portion of the diencephalon that lies beneath the thalamus at the base of the cerebrum; it activates, controls, and integrates many of the body's vital functions (e.g., regulation of metabolism, volume of body fluids, electrolyte content, and release of hormones).

Hypothermia: A serious loss of body heat caused by prolonged exposure to cold.

Hypotonic solution: One in which the osmotic pressure (concentration) is less than that of body fluids.

Hypoventilation: An abnormal breathing pattern in which insufficient amounts of air are inhaled into the lungs.

Hypoxemia: Insufficient oxygenation of the blood.

Icterus: Bile pigmentation of the tissues, membranes and secretions.

Idiopathic: Of unknown cause.

Ileal conduit: Surgically created passageway that utilizes a portion of the ileum to direct the flow of urine from the ureters to the outside.

Ileostomy(ies): An artificial opening in the ileum, created surgically for the purpose of draining fecal material from the small intestine.

Ileus: Intestinal obstruction, especially failure of peristalsis.

Immune deficiency: A lack of immune bodies and resultant impairment of the immune response to foreign agents.

Immunity: Resistance to a specific disease.

active: That acquired by producing one's own antibody.

passive: That acquired by receiving antibody from a source other than one's own body.

Immunization: The process of rendering an individual immune, as by passive immunity, or becoming immune by active immunity.

Immunocompetence: The capacity to develop an immune response after exposure to antigen.

Immunoglobulin(s): A protein of animal origin with known antibody activity and a major component of humoral immunity. See also *Antibody(ies)*.

Immunosuppression: Deliberate inhibition of the formation of antibody; used in transplantation to prevent rejection of the donor organ.

Immunotherapy: Passive immunity of a person by administration of preformed antibody; also, the administration of immunopotentiators and immunocompetent lymphoid tissue for the treatment of cancer.

Impetigo: An infection of the skin, usually by streptococci or staphylococci.

Impotence: Inability of the male to achieve or maintain an erection.

Incontinence: An alteration in the control of bowel or urinary elimination, or both.

Infarct: Localized area of necrosis produced by ischemia caused by obstructed arterial supply or inadequate venous drainage.

Infection(s): Invasion and multiplication of pathogenic microorganisms in body tissue.

Inflammation: An immediate cellular response to any kind of injury to the cells and tissues.

Ingestion: The taking of any substance—for example, food, drugs, water, chemicals—by mouth or through the digestive system.

Insulin-dependent diabetes mellitus: Type I diabetes; a form of the disease that requires replacement of endogenous insulin with regular injections of exogenous insulin.

Interstitial fluid(s): Body fluids that are located in the tissue spaces around the cells. See also *Edema*.

Intervention: Nursing activities performed by the nurse to meet the specified goals of a nursing care plan.

Intracellular fluids: Body fluids that are within cell walls.

Intraocular: Within the eye.

Intrathecal: Injection into the subarachnoid space of the spinal cord via lumbar puncture.

Intravascular fluids: Body fluids within the blood vessels; they are composed of plasma and the substances it transports.

Intravenous therapy: The administration of fluids through a vein.

Iridectomy: Excision of part of the iris.

Ischemia: Deficiency of blood supply to a part as a result of functional constriction of a blood vessel or to actual obstruction, as by a clot.

Isolation technique: Special precautionary procedures used to set apart patients with communicable diseases; the purpose is to prevent the spread of infectious agents from the patient to others.
Isotonic solution(s): One in which the osmotic pressure is the same as that of intracellular fluid (e.g., normal saline [0.9% concentration]).

Jaundice: A yellowing of the skin and mucous membranes that reflects excessively high blood levels of bilirubin (bile pigment).

Keratitis: Inflammation of the cornea.
Ketoacidosis: Accumulation of ketone bodies in the blood because of incomplete metabolism of fats, resulting in metabolic acidosis.
Kinetic motion: The motion of material bodies and the forces and energy associated with it.
Kupffer's cells: Large, highly phagocytic cells in the liver; they form part of the reticuloendothelial system.
Kyphosis: Abnormally increased curvature of the thoracic spine, which gives a "hunchback" appearance.

Labile: Unsteady, not fixed; easily disarranged.
Labyrinthitis: Inflammation of the internal ear, including the vestibule, cochlea, and semicircular canal.
Laparoscopy: Examination of the peritoneal cavity by means of a fiber-optic instrument that is inserted through a small abdominal incision.
Laryngectomy: Partial or total removal of the larynx by surgical excision; the person who has had a laryngectomy is called a *laryngectomee.*
Laryngography: X-ray examination of the larynx after instillation of a radiopaque medium into the tracheobronchial tree.
Laryngoscopy: Direct or indirect visual examination of the larynx.
Laser: Stands for *l*ight *a*mplification by *s*timulated *e*mission of *r*adiation; converts light wavelengths into one small, intense unified beam of one wavelength radiation; used for diagnosis and surgery.
Latent: Not obvious; hidden.
Leukemia: Malignant disease of the blood-forming organs, marked by abnormal proliferation and development of leukocytes and their precursors in the blood and bone marrow.
Leukocyte(s): A colorless blood cell whose chief function is to protect the body against pathogenic microorganisms.
Leukocytosis: An increase in the number of leukocytes in the blood.
Leukopenia: Reduction in the number of leukocytes in the blood to 5,000 or less.
Leukoplakia: Patches of thickened, white tissue on mucous membrane; considered a precursor to cancer.
Lhermitte's sign: An electric shocklike sensation felt along the spine when the neck is flexed.
Libido: Conscious or unconscious sexual drive.
Lifestyle habits: Entrenched practices related to work, recreation, diet, exercise, and other activities of daily living.
Lipoprotein: Any of the macromolecular complexes that are transported in the blood.
Lithiasis: Formation of stones.
Lordosis: Abnormal forward curvature of the spine.
Lymphadenitis: Inflammation of the lymph nodes.
Lymphangiography: Radiograph of lymphatic vessels after injection of a contrast medium.
Lymphangitis: Inflammation of the lymph vessels.
Lymphatic system: An accessory system by which fluids can flow from tissue spaces into the blood.
Lymphedema: Swelling of tissues drained by the lymphatic system.
Lymph nodes: Small bundles of lymphatic tissue containing lymphocytes, the functions of which are filtration and phagocytosis.
Lymphocyte(s): A mononuclear, nongranulous leukocyte that is chiefly a product of lymphoid tissue and is important in the development of immunity.
  sensitized: A nongranular lymphocyte that has been processed either by the thymus (T lymphocyte) or an unknown processing area (B lymphocyte) and is responsible for either cellular or humoral immunity.
Lymphocyte-transforming factor: A protein-mediator that causes transformation and clonal expansion of nonsensitized lymphocytes that produce a toxin destructive to antigen.
Lymphoma: Any neoplastic disorder of lymphoid tissue.

Macrophage(s): Large, mononuclear phagocytes derived from monocytes; they are components of the reticuloendothelial system.
Macrophage-activating factor: A mediator released by sensitized lymphocytes on contact with an antigen, the function of which is to induce in macrophages an increased content of lysosomal enzymes, more aggressive phagocytosis, and increased mitosis.
Macrophage chemotaxis factor: A protein mediator released by sensitized lymphocytes on contact with antigen, the function of which is to attract macrophages to the antigen site.
Macule (macula): A discolored spot on the skin that is not raised above the surface.
Malignancy: See *Cancer.*
Mammography: X-ray examination of the soft tissues of the breast.
Mammoplasty: Plastic surgery of the breast.
Mean, mathematical: An average (e.g., mean corpuscular hemoglobin concentration, which is the concentration of hemoglobin in the average erythrocyte).
Mediastinum: The mass of tissues and organs separating the sternum in front and the vertebral column behind.
Melena: Black, tarry, stools.
Menarche: Onset of menstruation.
Meniere's syndrome: A group of symptoms produced by an increase in fluid in the labyrinthine spaces with swelling and congestion of the mucosa of the cochlea.
Menopause: The span of time during which the menstrual cycle wanes and gradually stops; the female climacteric.
Menorrhagia: Excessive menstruation.
Metabolic acidosis: A condition in which the pH of body fluids is below 7.4 because of either an excessive production of carbonic acid through the oxidation of fats or because of a loss of bicarbonate.
Metabolic alkalosis: A condition in which the pH of body fluids is above 7.4 owing to excessive loss of acid, above-normal intake or retention of base, or a low level of potassium in the blood.
Metabolism: The sum of the physical and chemical

processes by which living tissue is formed and maintained and by which large molecules are disassembled to provide energy.

Metastasis: The movement of disease from one organ or body part to a distant location; for example, the migration of microorganisms and of malignant cells.

Metrorrhagia: Uterine bleeding occurring at irregular intervals and sometimes for prolonged periods.

Migration-inhibiting factor: A protein mediator released by sensitized lymphocytes on contact with an antigen, the function of which is to inhibit the migration of macrophages, causing them to accumulate at the antigen site.

Mineralocorticoids: A group of hormones elaborated by the adrenal cortex and having an effect on sodium, chloride, and potassium levels in extracellular fluid.

Miotic: Drug that constricts the pupil.

Monocytes: Mononuclear phagocytic leukocytes.

Muscle tone: Readiness of a muscle to contract and relax normally.

Mycosis (mycoses): Any disease caused by a fungus.

Mydriatic: Dilating the pupil.

Myocarditis: Inflammation of the heart muscle.

Myopia: The error of refraction in which parallel light rays focus in front of the retina; nearsightedness.

Myxedema: Condition of low thyroid in the adult.

Nebulizer: An atomizer; a device for delivering drugs or water to the respiratory tract by forcing air or oxygen through a solution.

Necrosis: The changes that occur as a result of death of cells; caused by enzymatic degradation.

Neoplasm: Tumor; any new and abnormal growth.

Nephron: The structural and functional unit of the kidney, which consists of the renal corpuscle, the proximal convoluted tubule, limbs of the loop of Henle, the distal convoluted tubule, and the collecting tubule; each nephron thus is able to form urine independently.

Nephrosclerosis: Atherosclerotic disease of the small renal arteries related to hypertension and eventual destruction of renal cells.

Nephrostomy tubes: Tubes inserted for drainage of the renal pelvis.

Neuron: Any of the conducting cells of the nervous system; consists of a cell body containing the nucleus and cytoplasm and the axon and dendrites.

Neuropathy: Any disease of the nerves.

Neutrophilia: Increase in the number of neutrophils in the blood.

Neutrophils: Granular leukocytes; also called *polymorphonuclear leukocytes.*

Nocturia: Excessive urination during the night.

Nodules: Small masses of tissue that can be detected by touch.

Non–insulin-dependent diabetes mellitus (type II): A form of the disease in which levels of endogenous insulin are adequate and control can be managed by diet and exercise, and perhaps by an oral hypoglycemic agent.

Nosocomial: Pertaining to or originating in a hospital.

Nucchal rigidity: Stiffness and pain in the neck from inflammation of the meninges.

Nursing: The diagnosis and treatment of human responses to actual or potential health problems. See also *Nursing process.*

Nursing care plans: Written plans of care that serve to communicate to the nursing staff and others the specific nursing diagnoses and prescribed nursing orders for directing, and for evaluating the effectiveness of, the care given.

Nursing process: A goal-directed series of activities whereby the practice of nursing accomplishes its goal of alleviating, minimizing, or preventing real or potential problems of health.

Nystagmus: Involuntary, rapid, rhythmic movement of the eyeball.

Objective data: Information obtained through the senses or measured by instruments.

Objectives: Well-defined steps toward the accomplishment of a goal; they should be realistic, be stated in measureable terms, and include the conditions under which they will be accomplished.

Oncology: The study of tumors.

Oophoritis: Inflammation of an ovary; ovaritis.

Ophthalmoscope: An instrument for examining the eye; the direct ophthalmoscope is used to inspect the back portion of the interior of the eyeball; the indirect ophthalmoscope permits stereoscopic inspection of the interior of the eye.

Opportunistic pathogen: Fungi or bacteria, usually harmless, that cause infection in a person with a depressed immune system.

Orchiectomy: Excision of one or both testes.

Orchitis: Inflammation of the testes.

Orthopedic: Referring to the correction of deformities of the musculoskeletal system.

Orthopnea: Ability to breathe easily only in the upright position.

Orthostatic hypotension: A fall in blood pressure that occurs when standing up from a sitting or lying position, or when standing in a fixed position; it is characterized by dizziness, syncope, and blurred vision.

Oscilloscope: An instrument that makes visible on a screen the nature of an electrical current.

Osmosis: The passage of solvent from a solution of lesser concentration to one of greater concentration through a selectively permeable membrane.

Ossification: Formation of or conversion into bone or a bony substance.

Osteoporosis: A porous condition of bone due to demineralization.

Otitis media: Inflammation of the middle ear.

Otoscope: Instrument for examining the ear canal and eardrum.

Pacemaker: Artificial, a mechanical device that provides electrical stimulation when an anatomic pacemaker fails; a cardiac pacemaker provides electrical stimulation when there is heart block.

Pain: A feeling of distress or suffering caused by stimulation of specialized nerve cells; considered to occur whenever a person says it is present.

Palliative: Relief of symptoms when a disease cannot be cured.

Panhysterectomy: Surgical removal of the entire uterus.

Papule: A small, round, solid, elevated lesion of the skin.

Paracentesis: Surgical puncture of a cavity for the aspiration of fluid.

Paradoxical respirations: Those in which, upon inhalation, the traumatized portion of the chest wall moves inward rather than outward.
Paralytic ileus: Absence of peristalsis; paralysis of the intestines.
Paraplegia: Paralysis of the lower extremities.
Parenteral: By a route other than the digestive tract.
Paresthesia: Feeling of tingling or numbness.
Patent: Wide open.
Pathologic: Caused by a disease.
Pediculosis: Infestation with lice.
Pelvic inflammatory disease: Any inflammation in the pelvis that occurs outside the uterus, uterine tubes, and ovaries.
PEMS format: A systematic approach to documentation; the acronym stands for physical problems, emotional needs, mental status, and safety needs.
Peptic ulcer: Loss of tissue lining the esophagus, stomach, or duodenum.
Percutaneous: Through the skin.
Perforation: A hole or break in the retaining walls or membranes of an organ, as in perforated ulcer and perforated eardrum.
Perfusion: Supplying tissues and organs nutrients and oxygen by blood flow through the arteries.
Pericarditis: Inflammation of the fibroserous sac that encloses the heart and the roots of the great vessels.
Peripheral: Pertaining to the area outside the central region or structure.
Peristalsis: Involuntary wavelike contraction of organs with both longitudinal and circular muscle fibers that passes along the organ and propels its contents, as in peristalsis of the digestive tract.
Peritonitis: Inflammation of the serous sac that lines the abdominal cavity and encloses the abdominal organs.
Petechiae: Very small, nonraised, round, purplish spots, caused by intradermal or submucosal bleeding, that later turn blue or yellow.
pH: The concentration of hydrogen (H) in a solution; the higher the concentration of hydrogen ions the lower the pH of the solution.
Phacoemulsification: A technique of cataract extraction in which high-frequency vibrations are used to fragment the lens.
Phagocytosis: The engulfing of microorganisms and other foreign matter by phagocytes.
Phenylketonuria: A genetic disorder in which there is a defect in the metabolism of phenylalanine resulting in the presence of this amino acid in the urine.
Phlebitis: Inflammation of a vein.
Photophobia: Difficulty tolerating light.
Pilonidal sinus: A lesion located at the cleft of the buttocks in the sacrococcygeal region; also called pilonidal cyst.
Placebo(s): A supposedly inactive substance or procedure that can have either positive or negative effects on the relief of symptoms, and that is usually given under the guise of effective treatment, or in clinical trials of new drugs.
Planning: A phase of the nursing process in which a plan is developed with the patient, family, or significant other to provide a blueprint for nursing intervention to achieve specified goals. See also *Nursing care plans.*
Plaque: A patch or flat area.
Plasma: The liquid portion of blood in which formed elements are suspended; it contains plasma proteins, inorganic salts, nutrients, gases, wastes from the cells, and various hormones and enzymes.
Plasma cell: A spherical or ellipsoidal cell involved in the synthesis, storage, and release of antibody.
Plasmapheresis: Separation of the cells and components of the blood.
Platelets: The smallest formed elements in the blood; important in coagulation and clotting of blood.
Plethora: A general term denoting a red florid complexion or an excess of blood.
Pneumocystis carinii: An opportunistic protozoan infection of the lung associated with acquired immunodeficiency syndrome (AIDS).
Pneumothorax: Accumulation of air or gas in the pleural cavity, resulting in collapse of the lung on the affected side.
Polyarteritis: Multiple sites of inflammatory and destructive lesions in the arterial system.
Polycythemia: An elevation in the total number of blood cells.
Polydipsia: Excessive thirst that results in drinking large quantities of water.
Polymorphonuclear leukoctyes: The fully developed cells of the granulocyte series, especially neutrophils of which the nuclei contain three or more lobes.
Polyuria: Production of an excessive amount of urine.
Postictal state: Condition of the person right after a seizure.
Premenstrual syndrome: A group of symptoms experienced by some women for several days before the onset of the menstrual period.
Presbyopia: Farsightedness that occurs normally with aging.
Primary union, of wounds: The joining of two edges of a wound that are close together, resulting in a thin scar after healing; also called healing by first intention.
Problem-oriented medical records (POMR): A system of documentation in which the information is arranged according to specific problems presented by the patient at the time of seeking health care. The four components are database, problem list, initial plan, and follow-up. See also *Progress notes.*
Process: A series of actions that move from one point to another on the way to completion of a goal.
Prodromal stage: Early or very beginning stage of an illness.
Prognosis: Predicted outcome of the course of a disease.
Progress notes: Entries in the medical record describing what has been done in the care of the patient and his response to the intervention.
Prolapse: The falling down or displacement of a part or all of an organ, as in prolapse of a stoma and prolapse of the uterus.
Prophylactic: Something done or used to prevent infection or disease.
Prostaglandins: A group of naturally occurring fatty acids that stimulate contraction of the uterine and other smooth muscle tissue.
Prosthesis: An artificial substitute for a missing part, such as an eye, limb, or tooth, used for functional or cosmetic reasons, or both.
Protective isolation: Special precautionary procedures to minimize exposure to infectious agents in a patient who has an immune deficiency or who is otherwise susceptible to infection.

Proteinuria: An excess of serum proteins in the urine.
Protozoa: A phylum comprising the unicellular eukaryotic organisms; most are free-living, but some lead commensalistic, mutualistic, or parasitic existences.
Proximal: Closest to a point of reference.
Pruritus: Itching.
Ptosis: The dropping of an organ below its usual position, for example, lowering of the eyelid so that it partially or completely covers the cornea.
Pulmonary edema: Diffuse accumulation of fluid in the tissues and air spaces of the lung.
Pulse deficit: The difference between the radial and apical pulse rates.
Purpura: Purplish areas caused by bleeding into the skin or mucous membranes.
Pustule: A small, round, pus-filled lesion of the skin.
Pyelogram: X-ray film of the kidney and ureters after injection of a contrast medium that may be administered intravenously (IV pyelogram) or by way of the ureters (retrograde pyelogram).
Pyelonephritis: Inflammation of the kidney and renal pelvis.
Pyelostomy tube: A tube inserted into the renal pelvis for the purpose of temporarily diverting urine from the ureter.
Pyrogen: Any agent that causes fever.

Quadriplegia: Paralysis of all four extremities.

Rad: Radiation absorbed dose; the unit used for measuring doses of radiation.
Radiation therapy: The use of radiant energy from radioactive materials or high-voltage x-ray for the purpose of treating disease.
Radioimmunoassay: A laboratory method for measurement of minute quantities of specific antibodies or any antigen, such as a hormone or drug, against which antibodies have been produced.
Radiopaque: Not penetrable by x-ray; appears white.
Rales: Abnormal respiratory sounds heard in auscultation with a stethoscope indicating some pathologic condition.
Range of motion: The extent, measured in degrees of a circle, through which a joint can be extended and flexed.
Reflex(es): The sum of any particular autonomic (automatic) response mediated by the nervous system and not requiring conscious movement.
Refraction: Determination of refractive errors (inability to focus light rays on the retina) and their correction with eyeglasses.
Regeneration: The natural renewal of a structure.
Residual urine: Urine that remains in the bladder immediately after urination.
Resorption: Taking in or absorbing again.
Respiratory acidosis: A condition in which the pH of body fluids is below 7.4 because of failure of the lungs to remove sufficient amounts of carbon dioxide.
Respiratory alkalosis: A condition in which the pH of body fluids is above 7.4 due to excessive removal of carbon dioxide by the lungs, as in hyperventilation.
Reticuloendothelial system: A network of cells and tissues found throughout the body, especially in the blood, connective tissue, spleen, liver, lungs, bone marrow, and lymph vessels; these cells play a role in blood cell formation and destruction and in inflammation and immunity.
Retinopathy: A pathologic condition of the retina associated with diabetes mellitus.
Rhonchi: Coarse rattling sounds in the bronchial tubes caused by a partial obstruction.
Rickettsia: A genus of small, rod-shaped-to-round microorganisms found in tissue cells of lice, fleas, ticks, and mites, and transmitted to humans by their bites.

Salpingitis: Inflammation of a uterine tube.
Sarcoma: A tumor, often highly malignant, composed of cells derived from connective tissue.
Scabies: Infestation with the mange mite.
Scintiphotography: A lung scan.
Secondary union: Healing of a wound in which the edges are far apart and cannot be brought together; the wound fills with granulation tissue and heals from the edges inward.
Sedative(s): An agent that calms nervousness, irritability, and excitement.
Seizure(s): An attack of uncontrollable muscular contractions; a convulsion.
Self: The entire person of an individual; the sum of the physiologic, psychological, social, and spiritual dimensions of one's personality.
Self-care: The process whereby one initiates and carries out certain health practices in order to maintain life, health, and personal well-being.
Sensitivity reaction: An exaggerated response to agents perceived by the body as foreign.
Sensorineural hearing loss: Impaired perception of sound caused by a dysfunction in the inner ear or the eighth cranial nerve.
Sensory loss: Impairment of acuity of sight, hearing, taste, touch, and smell.
Septicemia: Invasion of the blood stream by infective microorganisms.
Sequela: Condition resulting from a disease that follows the disease.
Seroma: A collection of serum forming a tumorlike mass.
Serosanguinous: Containing both serum and blood.
Serum (sera): The clear, liquid portion of blood that does not contain fibrinogen or blood cells. Immune serum is blood serum from the bodies of persons or animals that have produced antibody; inoculation with such serum produces passive immunity.
Serum sickness: A hypersensitivity reaction to a foreign serum or other antigen.
Shock: Acute peripheral circulatory failure due to derangement of circulatory control or loss of circulating fluid.
Sickle cell disease(s): All those genetic disorders in which sickle hemoglobin is found in the red cells.
Slit lamp: An instrument for examining the surface of the eye through a biomicroscopic lens.
Smear: A specimen for microscopic and cytologic study; the material is spread thinly and evenly across a slide with a swab or loop.
SOAP: Acronym for subjective and objective data, assessment, and planning.
Somogyi effect: A rebound phenomenon due to overtreatment with insulin.
Source-oriented record keeping: A system of documentation in which information is arranged according to the person, department, or other source of information.
Specific gravity: The weight of a substance compared

with the weight of an equal amount of another substance taken as a standard; for liquids the standard usually is water (specific gravity of 1).

Specificity: The quality of reacting only with certain substances, as antibody with certain antigen (antigen specificity).

Spirometer: Instrument for measuring air taken into and expelled from the lungs.

Sprain: Wrenching or twisting of a joint with partial or complete tearing of the ligaments.

Stapedectomy: Surgical removal of the stirrup of the middle ear and replacement with a prosthetic device.

Stasis: Standing still; stagnation; usually refers to fluid.

Stem cells: Generalized mother cells the descendants of which specialize, often in different functions; an example is an undifferentiated mesenchymal cell that is the progenitor of the blood and fixed-tissue cells of the bone marrow.

Stenosis: Narrowing or contraction of a passageway or opening.

Stereotaxis: Method of precisely locating areas in the brain.

Sterilization, microbe: The process of rendering an article free of microorganisms and their pathogenic products.

Stoma(s): A mouthlike opening, especially one that is created surgically for the elimination of urine or fecal material.

Stomatitis: Generalized inflammation of the oral mucosa.

Strabismus: Deviation of the eye that cannot be controlled voluntarily.

Strain: Pulling or tearing of either muscle or tendon, or both.

Stye: Infected swelling near the margin of the eyelid.

Subluxation: Partial or incomplete disclocation of a bone from its place in a joint.

Subsystem: A system within a larger system.

"Sucking" chest wound: One in which the pleural cavity has been penetrated, allowing air and gas to enter the cavity and produce pneumothorax.

Suprasystem: A highly complex system.

Sympathectomy: Surgical excision or interruption in some portion of the sympathetic nerve pathways.

Syncope: Fainting.

Syndrome: Combination of signs and symptoms associated with a pathologic process or disease.

Synovial fluid: The transparent viscid fluid found in joint cavities, bursae, and tendon sheaths.

System(s): An organized whole composed of interacting parts.

Systole: The phase of the cardiac cycle when the ventricles contract and force blood into the aorta and pulmonary arteries; the systolic pressure is recorded as the top number in a blood pressure reading.

Tachycardia: Abnormally rapid heart rate, usually taken to be over 100 beats per minute.

Tetany: Continuous tonic spasm of a muscle; associated with calcium deficit, vitamin D deficiency, and alkalosis.

Thalamus: Either of two large structures composed of gray matter and situated at the base of the cerebrum and acting as a relay station for impulses traveling from the spinal cord and brain stem to the cerebral cortex.

Thanatology: The medicolegal study of the dying process and death.

Theory(ies): A belief, policy, or principle proposed or followed as the basis of action.

Thoracentesis: Surgical puncture and drainage of the thoracic cavity.

Thrombocytopenia: Condition of decreased number of platelets.

Thrombophlebitis: Inflammation of a vein related to formation of a blood clot within the vessel.

Thrombosis: Formation, development, or presence of a blood clot within a blood vessel.

Thymus: An endocrine gland that lies in the upper chest beneath the sternum and which, during fetal life, sensitizes certain stem cells that eventually become T lymphocytes.

Thyroid crisis: Sudden increase in the output of thyroxine and resultant extreme elevation of all body processes.

Tinea: Ringworm; a name applied to many different kinds of fungal infections of the skin; the specific type usually is designated by a modifying term (e.g., tinea capitis, or ringworm of the scalp).

Tinnitus: Ringing, buzzing, or other continuous noise in the ear.

T lymphocytes: Those white cells destined to provide cellular immunity that have passed through the thymus and migrated to the lymph nodes.

Tonic: State of rigid contraction of the muscles.

Tonometer: An instrument for measuring tension or pressure, especially intraocular pressure.

Topical: Pertaining to a particular area, as in topical medications applied to an area of the skin.

Total parenteral nutrition: Intravenous feeding to provide all nutritional needs over a period of time.

Toxin: Poisonous substance.

Tracheostomy: A surgical incision into the trachea for the purpose of inserting a tube through which the patient can breathe.

Tourniquet: A device for compressing an artery or vein; its use as an emergency measure to relieve hemorrhage is generally recommended only if the victim's life is threatened and other measures fail to stop massive blood loss.

Traction: Exertion of a pulling force, as that applied to a fractured bone or dislocated joint, to maintain proper positioning.

Tranquilizers: A group of agents that provide calm and relief from anxiety.

Transfer factor: A factor occurring in sensitized lymphocytes that recruits additional lymphocytes and transfers to them the ability to confer cell-mediated immunity.

Transfusion(s): The administration of whole blood or blood components directly into the blood stream.

Tuberculin test: An evaluation of sensitivity to the tubercle bacillus; the most common method is intradermal injection of a purified protein derivative of tuberculin (the Mantoux test); a positive reaction indicates the need for further diagnostic procedures.

Tumor node metastasis, staging system for: A system for classifying cancers according to the extent to which the malignancy has spread.

Turgor: Normal tension of a cell; swelling, distention.

Tympanocentesis: Surgical puncture of the tympanic membrane (ear drum).

Ultrasonography: A radiologic technique in which

deep anatomic structures are recorded by depicting the echoes of ultrasonic waves that have been directed into the tissues; the echoes (reflections) returning from the structures are converted into electrical impulses that are displayed on a screen, thus presenting a "picture" of the tissues being examined.

Urea nitrogen: A major protein metabolite that is not recycled by the body but is excreted in the urine; blood urea nitrogen levels indicate the ability of the kidney to filtrate and excrete waste products.

Uremia: Retention in the blood of urea, creatinine, and other nitrogenous wastes normally eliminated in the urine; more correctly called *azotemia*.

Ureterostomy (ureterostomies): Surgical creation of a stoma for purposes of diverting urine to the outside.

Urinalysis: Analysis of a sample of urine, most often done for the purpose of detecting protein, glucose, acetone, blood, pus, and casts.

Urticaria: Hives.

Vaccination: Injection of a vaccine into the body to produce immunity to a specific disease.

Vagotomy: Interruption of impulses carried by the vagus nerve or nerves; may be done to reduce the production of gastric secretions and to inhibit gastric motility, as part of the treatment for peptic ulcer.

Valsalva maneuver: Increase of thoracic pressure by forcible exhalation against the closed glottis, as in straining at stool.

Varicose veins: Enlarged and tortuous veins in which the distorted shape is the result of accumulations of pooled blood.

Vasectomy: Excision of the vas (ductus) deferens, or a portion of it; bilateral vasectomy results in sterility.

Ventilation: The movement of air from the external environment to the gas exchange units of the lung.

Vertigo: A sensation of movement of one's self or of one's surroundings.

Vesicle: A small sac containing a serous liquid; a small blister.

Vesicostomy: Formation of an opening into the urinary bladder.

Virulence: Degree of ability of an organism to cause disease.

Viscera: Internal organs contained within a cavity.

Wart: Epidermal growth of viral origin.

Wheal: Localized area or edema on the body surface.

Xanthoma: Lipid deposit in the skin.

Xerostomia: Lack of saliva; dry mouth.

Yeast: Term for fungi that reproduce by budding.

Zygomatic: Pertaining to zygomatic bone.

Index

Note: Numbers in *italics* refer to illustrations; numbers followed by (t) indicate tables.

C

D

F

J

K

N

O

P

S